Mosby's
Review Questions for the
NCLEX-RN®
EXAMINATION

Mosby's
Review Questions for the
NCLEX-RN® EXAMINATION

Seventh edition

Editors

Patricia M. Nugent, RN, AAS, BS, MS, EdM, EdD

Phyllis K. Pelikan, RN, AAS, BS, MA

Judith S. Green, RN, AAS, BA, MA

Barbara A. Vitale, RN, AAS, BSN, MA

Content Editors

Jane K. Brody, RN, BSN, MSN, PhD
Nassau Community College
Garden City, New York

Catherine R. Coverston, RN, RNC, PhD
Brigham Young University
Provo, Utah

Christina Algiere Kasprisin, RN, MS, EdD
PACE VT, Clinical Director/Home Care
Coordinator
Colchester, Vermont

Barbara A. Vitale, RN, AAS, BSN, MA
Nassau Community College
Garden City, New York

ELSEVIER
MOSBY

ELSEVIER
MOSBY

3251 Riverport Lane
St. Louis, Missouri 63043

Mosby's Review Questions for the NCLEX-RN® Examination, ed 7　　　　ISBN: 978-0-323-07443-8
Copyright © 2011 by Mosby, Inc., an affiliate of Elsevier Inc.

Notice

Knowledge and best practice in this field are constantly changing. As new research and experience broaden our understanding, changes in research methods, professional practices, or medical treatment may become necessary. Practitioners and researchers must always rely on their own experience and knowledge in evaluating and using any information, methods, compounds, or experiments described herein. In using such information or methods they should be mindful of their own safety and the safety of others, including parties for whom they have a professional responsibility.

With respect to any drug or pharmaceutical products identified, readers are advised to check the most current information provided (i) on procedures featured or (ii) by the manufacturer of each product to be administered, to verify the recommended dose or formula, the method and duration of administration, and contraindications. It is the responsibility of practitioners, relying on their own experience and knowledge of their patients, to make diagnoses, to determine dosages and the best treatment for each individual patient, and to take all appropriate safety precautions.

To the fullest extent of the law, neither the Publisher nor the authors, contributors, or editors, assume any liability for the injury and/or damage to persons or property as a matter of products liability, negligence or otherwise, or from any use or operation of any methods, products, instructions, or ideas contained in the material herein.

The Publisher

Previous editions copyrighted 2007, 2004, 2001, 1998, 1995, 1991

Library of Congress Cataloging-in-Publication Data

Mosby's review questions for the NCLEX-RN examination / [edited by] Patricia M. Nugent, Phyllis K. Pelikan, Judith S. Green. — 7th ed.
　p. ; cm.
　Other title: Review questions for the NCLEX-RN examination
　ISBN 978-0-323-07443-8 (pbk. : alk. paper) 1. National Council Licensure Examination for Registered Nurses—Study guides 2. Nursing—Examinations—Study guides. 3. Nursing—Examinations, questions, etc.
I. Nugent, Patricia Mary, 1944- II. Pelikan, Phyllis K. III. Green, Judith S. IV. Title: Review questions for the NCLEX-RN examination.
[DNLM: 1. Nursing—Examination Questions. WY 18.2 M8941 2011]
　RT55.M65 2011
　610.73076--dc22　　　　　　　　　　　　　　　　　　　　　　2010017969

NCLEX® and NCLEX-RN® are registered trademarks and service marks of the National Council of State Boards of Nursing, Inc.

Acquisitions Editor: Kristin Geen
Developmental Editor: Jamie Horn
Publishing Services Manager: Jeff Patterson

Working together to grow
libraries in developing countries

www.elsevier.com | www.bookaid.org | www.sabre.org

ELSEVIER　BOOK AID International　Sabre Foundation

Printed in United States of America　9　8　7　6　5　4　3　2　1

Last digit is the print number:　9　8　7　6　5　4　3　2　1

This book is dedicated to the most important people in our lives
for their love, understanding, and support

To my husband Neil
My children Kelly and Heather, and my grandchildren
Patricia M. Nugent

To my family
The proverbial "Wind Beneath my Wings"
Phyllis K. Pelikan

To my family
Dale and Art, Richard, Eric and Miriam, Cheryl, and Steven
Judith S. Green

To my husband Joe
My grandchildren Joseph, Andie Grace, Andrew, Nathan, and Alexander
Barbara A. Vitale

Linda Carman Copel, PhD, RN, PMH, CNS, BC, CNE, FAPA
Villanova University College of Nursing
Villanova, Pennsylvania

Teresa M. Dobrzykowski, RN, ASN, BSN, MSM, DNS, APRNC
Indiana University at South Bend
South Bend, Indiana

Leann Eaton, RN, BS, MS, ANP
Barnes Jewish Hospital
Saint Louis, Missouri

Jo Elberg, RN, BS, MAE
Iowa Central Community College
Fort Dodge, Iowa

Carol Flaugher, RN, BSN, MSN
State University of New York at Buffalo School of Nursing–Faculty Emeritus
Buffalo, New York

Jane Flickinger, RN, BSN, MSN
Mayo Foundation–Rochester Methodist Hospital, Retired
Rochester, Minnesota

Mary Ann Hellmer Saul, RN, AAS, BS, MS, PhD
Nassau Community College
Garden City, New York

Laurie Gasperi Kaudewitz, RN, RNC-OB, BSN, MSN
Women's Services Director
University Medical Center
Lebanon, Tennessee

Jeanne Millett, RN, BS, MS, EdD, FNP
Capital Care Medical Group
Guilderland, New York

Cynthia C. Small, RN, MSN, APRN-BC
Lake Michigan College
Benton Harbor, Michigan

Judy E. White, RNC, BSN, MA, MSN
Southern Union State Community College
Opelika, Alabama

Deborah Williams, RN, MSN, EdD
Western Kentucky University
Bowling Green, Kentucky

Patricia E. Zander, RN, BSN, MSN, PhD
Viterbo University
La Crosse, Wisconsin

This text was developed to meet the requests of students for "still more questions—with answers and rationales." The seventh edition contains more than 5000 questions and hundreds of new alternate format items (multiple response, fill in the blank, ordered response, hot spot, chart/exhibit, and audio) that reflect the new 2010 NCLEX-RN® Examination Test Plan. The accompanying CD includes all the questions in the book and more than 2000 bonus questions. In addition to the art and science of nursing, questions integrate concepts from the social, biological, and physical sciences. In this edition there is increased emphasis on leadership and management, safety and infection control, and pharmacological and parenteral therapies. Every question has the rationale for the correct and incorrect options and is classified by the categories stipulated in the 2010 NCLEX-RN Examination Test Plan (Client Needs, Cognitive Level, and Integrated Process). These rationales appear with questions in the quizzes and the comprehensive examination in the book and with every question on the CD. Multiple study worksheets are included for students to analyze their testing performance and to help design study strategies. We believe that *Mosby's Review Questions for the NCLEX-RN® Examination* text provides all the necessary tools that students require to prepare for their nursing examinations and the NCLEX-RN examination.

To meet the requirements of students who have different study styles and learning needs, the questions are presented in four distinct formats:

- The questions in Chapters 2 though 5 are grouped according to content categories. These categories reflect specific subject matter, within a broad clinical area, from which the material in the question has been drawn. We have presented these questions in the traditional clinical groupings because we believe that even when preparing for an integrated test similar to the NCLEX-RN examination, most students will need to study each distinct part before attempting to incorporate all the parts into a comprehensive knowledge base.
- One or more 50-item quizzes conclude each clinical nursing chapter in the book and there are 2 or 3 quizzes accompanying each clinical area on the CD. The quizzes combine the subject matter from the various content categories within a specific clinical area. These quizzes provide a bridge for moving from the clinical chapters to the comprehensive examinations.
- Two comprehensive examinations reflect the 2010 NCLEX-RN test plan. One of them is in Chapter 6 of the book and both of them are on the CD. These comprehensive examinations address content included in all the clinical nursing areas (Medical-Surgical, Mental Health, Childbearing and Women's Health, and Child Health). The first part of each test contains 75 questions, the minimum number of questions required to pass or fail the NCLEX-RN examination. The second part of each test contains 190 questions, which when added to the previous 75 questions totals 265 questions. This is the maximum number of questions allowed on the NCLEX-RN examination.
- The CD contains all of the questions in the book plus an additional 2015 bonus questions. These bonus questions include the clinical areas, the 50-item bonus quizzes, and the second 265-item comprehensive examination. The CD allows students to practice their test-taking skills on a computer and build confidence for taking the computerized NCLEX-RN examination.

Finally, the textbook contains two Focus for Study Worksheets. Worksheet 1—Errors in Processing Information—will help the student identify faulty critical thinking patterns. Worksheet 2—Knowledge Gaps—will help the student identify content areas that need further study.

All the questions in this textbook were developed by outstanding, experienced nurse educators and practitioners of nursing. The editorial panel reviewed questions initially submitted, selecting and editing the most pertinent for inclusion. Finally, every question was screened by content reviewers for accuracy of information, relevance of content, and adherence to test construction principles.

We offer our sincere appreciation to our many colleagues for their contributions: Kristin Geen, Senior Acquisitions Editor, for her guidance, patience, and competent supervision of this project from its development to its completion; Jamie Horn, Senior Developmental Editor, for her ability to solve our problems promptly and efficiently and her expert facilitation of the editorial process; Jeanne Genz, Project Manager, for her attention to detail throughout the copyediting and proofing process and her expert advice and support; our content editors for their careful revision of the manuscript; our contributors for their item writing ability; and our manuscript reviewers for their careful reading and thoughtful critique of the manuscript. Finally, we thank our friends and families for their patience, understanding, encouragement, and love.

Patricia M. Nugent
Phyllis K. Pelikan
Judith S. Green
Barbara A. Vitale

Chapter 1: Preparing for the Licensure Examination

(p. 4) Gilbert ES: *Manual of high risk pregnancy and delivery,* ed 4, St. Louis, 2007, Mosby.

Chapter 2: Medical-Surgical Nursing

(pp. 25 and 64) Lewis SM, et al: *Medical-surgical nursing: assessment and management of clinical problems,* ed 7, St. Louis, 2007, Mosby.

(p. 58) Potter PA, Perry AG: *Fundamentals of nursing,* ed 7, St. Louis, 2009, Mosby.

(p. 73) Seidel HM, et al: *Mosby's guide to physical examination,* ed 7, St. Louis, 2011, Mosby.

Chapter 3: Mental Health Nursing

(p. 243) Kaufman DM: *Clinical neurology for psychiatrists,* ed 6, Philadelphia, 2007, Saunders.

Chapter 4: Childbearing and Women's Health Nursing

(p. 313) Dickason EJ, Schultz MO, Silverman BL: *Maternal-infant nursing care,* ed 3, St. Louis, 1998, Mosby.

(p. 315) Tucker SM, Miller LA, Miller D: *Mosby's pocket guide to fetal monitoring and assessment,* ed 6, St. Louis, 2009, Mosby.

Chapter 5: Child Health Nursing

(p 419) Hockenberry M, Wilson D: *Wong's essentials of pediatric nursing,* ed 8, St. Louis, 2009, Mosby.

Chapter 6: Comprehensive Examination

(p. 501) Hockenberry M, Wilson D, Winkelstein ML: *Wong's essentials of pediatric nursing,* ed 8, St. Louis, 2009, Mosby.

CD-ROM Bonus Questions

(Medical-Surgical Questions, Bonus Questions 352 and 353); Lewis SM, et al: *Medical-surgical nursing: assessment and management of clinical problems,* ed 7, St. Louis, 2007, Mosby.

(Exam 1, Question 12): Potter PA, Perry AG: *Fundamentals of nursing,* ed 7, St. Louis, 2009, Mosby.

(Mental Health Questions, Bonus Question 352, Exam 1, Question 26): McKenry LM, Tessier E, Hogan MA: *Mosby's pharmacology in nursing,* ed 22, St. Louis, 2006, Mosby.

(Childbearing and Women's Health Questions, Exam 2, Question 10): Gilbert ES: *Manual of high risk pregnancy and delivery,* ed 4, St. Louis, 2007, Mosby.

(Child Health Questions, Bonus Question 100): Hockenberry M, Wilson D: *Wong's essentials of pediatric nursing,* ed 8, St. Louis, 2009, Mosby.

(Bonus Comprehensive Exam, Bonus Question 10): Lowdermilk DL, Perry SE: *Maternity nursing,* ed 8, St. Louis, 2011, Mosby.

CONTENTS

Preparing for the Licensure Examination

The NCLEX-RN® EXAMINATION

The NCLEX-RN Examination is a computerized test that measures a candidate's level of knowledge, skills, and abilities to determine that the competency level for beginning nursing practice has been achieved. The examination is an individualized testing experience in which the computer chooses the next question based on the ability and competency demonstrated on previous questions. The minimum number of questions is 75 and the maximum number is 265. Each question must be answered before the computer will present the next question, and previously answered questions cannot be revisited. The test length will vary according to each candidate's performance. It is not a timed test, but there is a maximum 5-hour period.

Licensure examinations in the United States and Canada have been integrated and comprehensive for many years. Both contain typical multiple-choice questions that have four options and alternate format items. The alternate format items require the candidate to:

- Fill in the blank
- Identify specific information on a picture or diagram
- Select more than one option as a correct answer
- Place a variety of information in order of priority
- Consider multiple sources of information before answering a question
- Use multimedia such as sound or video before answering a question

The questions on the NCLEX-RN Examination address the domain of nursing care and content from the biological (anatomy, physiology, biology, and microbiology), psychosocial (psychology and sociology), and physical (chemistry and physics) sciences. Questions are classified according to client needs, cognitive levels, and integrated processes (these classifications are discussed in more detail in this chapter). The score on the examination is reported as pass or fail.

The most crucial requisites for doing well on the licensure examination is a sound knowledge of the subject and the ability to comprehend the critical elements within each question. To answer questions appropriately, a candidate must understand and correlate certain aspects of the biological, psychosocial, and physical sciences and the domain of nursing care. The domain of nursing care includes but is not limited to management responsibilities, safety and infection control strategies, the promotion and maintenance of health, maintenance of psychosocial integrity, promotion of basic care and comfort, pharmacological and parenteral therapies, reduction of risk, and identification and interpretation of physiological adaptations. At least three other requirements must be met for test performance to reflect professional competence. First, directions must be followed scrupulously. Second, each question must be analyzed carefully before selecting an answer. Third, answers must be recorded in the manner specified.

Most questions are based on nursing situations similar to those with which candidates have had experiences because both the United States and Canada emphasize the nursing care of clients with representative common national health problems. Some questions, however, require candidates to apply basic principles and techniques to clinical situations with which they have had little, if any, actual experience. Determination to do well and a degree of confidence will further enhance test performance and the ability to pass the NCLEX-RN Examination.

INTRODUCTION TO *MOSBY'S REVIEW QUESTIONS FOR THE NCLEX-RN® EXAMINATION*

To adequately prepare for an integrated comprehensive examination, it is necessary to understand the discrete parts that comprise the universe under consideration. This is one of the major principles on which this text and the accompanying CD have been developed. Using this concept, this book presents questions from each major clinical nursing area (Medical-Surgical, Mental Health, Childbearing and Women's Health, and Child Health) that test your knowledge of principles and theories underlying nursing care in a variety of situations (acute, critical, and long term); in a variety of settings (acute-care hospitals, nursing homes, and the community); and with a variety of nursing approaches to promote health and prevent illness (including primary, secondary, and tertiary care). All of the questions have rationales supporting the correct and incorrect answers. Reviewing the rationales enables you to verify information, reinforce knowledge, correct misinformation, and learn new information.

The format in the book for *Mosby's Review Questions for the NCLEX-RN Examination* is divided into the four basic clinical areas (Chapters 2 through 5). Each chapter concludes with one or more 50-item quizzes reflecting an integration of the chapter's content. Chapter 6 contains a Comprehensive Examination that includes questions that reflect content from all the clinical areas:

Chapter 2: Medical-Surgical Nursing—1000 questions, 2 quizzes

Chapter 3: Mental Health Nursing—500 questions, 1 quiz

Chapter 4: Childbearing and Women's Health Nursing—500 questions, 1 quiz

Chapter 5: Child Health Nursing—500 questions, 1 quiz

Chapter 6: Comprehensive Examination—265 questions

CATEGORIES OF CONTENT IN THE BASIC CLINICAL AREAS

Chapters 2 through 5 are divided into specific content areas within the broad clinical areas from which the material in the question has been drawn. These categories vary somewhat in each clinical area.

Medical-Surgical Nursing and Child Health Nursing

Nursing practice
Growth and development
Emotional needs related to health problems
Blood and immunity
Cardiovascular
Endocrine
Fluids and electrolytes
Gastrointestinal
Integumentary
Neuromuscular
Respiratory
Reproductive and genitourinary
Skeletal
Drug-related responses

Childbearing and Women's Health Nursing

Nursing practice
Emotional needs related to childbearing and women's health
Reproductive choices
Healthy childbearing
High-risk pregnancy
Normal neonate
High-risk neonate
Reproductive problems
Women's health
Drug-related responses

Mental Health Nursing

Nursing practice
Personality development
Therapeutic relationships
Disorders first evident before adulthood
Anxiety, somatoform, factitious, and dissociative disorders
Crisis situations
Dementia, delirium, and other cognitive disorders

Eating and sleep disorders
Disorders of mood
Disorders of personality
Schizophrenic disorders
Substance abuse
Drug-related responses

Comprehensive Examination

Chapter 6 contains a Comprehensive Examination that includes questions that reflect content from all the clinical areas. This 265-question test is similar to the NCLEX-RN Examination because it draws from all the clinical areas and has the same percentages of client needs. Following each set of rationales, the question is categorized by Clinical Area, Client Needs, Cognitive Level, Integrated Process (if relevant to the question), and Nursing Process.

- Management of Care, 16% to 22%
- Safety and Infection Control, 8% to 14%
- Health Promotion and Maintenance, 6% to 12%
- Psychosocial Integrity, 6% to 12%
- Basic Care and Comfort, 6% to 12%
- Pharmacological and Parenteral Therapies, 13% to 19%
- Reduction of Risk Strategies, 10% to 16%
- Physiological Adaptation, 11% to 17%

CLASSIFICATION OF QUESTIONS

Questions are classified according to clinical area, categories of content, and the test plan structure in the NCLEX-RN test plan. The test plan structure consists of client needs, cognitive level, and integrated processes, which includes the nursing process. These classifications appear after the rationales for each question in each quiz and the comprehensive examination in the book and after every question on the CD.

Clinical Areas

Medical-Surgical Nursing
Mental Health Nursing
Childbearing and Women's Health Nursing
Child Health Nursing

Client Needs

Client needs are those health care needs of the client that the nurse must address.

Safe and Effective Care Environment

Management of Care includes but is not limited to coordination among the health team members, the client and the client's significant others, health teaching, and legal, ethical, and managerial responsibilities.

Safety and Infection Control includes but is not limited to accident prevention, errors in care, safety measures, and prevention and control of infection.

Health Promotion and Maintenance includes but is not limited to providing for the achievement of the highest possible level of functioning by promoting and accepting physiological and psychological changes throughout the life cycle, supporting optimum family growth and development including reproduction and childrearing, and facilitating self-care and health maintenance through assessment, education, health programs, and support services.

Psychosocial Integrity includes but is not limited to supporting adaptation to and management of stress; recognizing sociocultural, religious, spiritual, and emotional influences on health; encouraging the use of support systems; using mental health concepts and therapeutic communication; addressing real or imagined threats to self-esteem; using interventions to support the emotional, mental, and social well-being of the client experiencing stress including acute and chronic mental illness; and creating an environment that supports, fosters, and promotes optimum mental health.

Physiological Integrity

Basic Care and Comfort includes but is not limited to activities of daily living consisting of nutrition, hygiene, elimination, rest and sleep, mobility, and nonpharmacological pain control.

Pharmacological and Parenteral Therapies includes but is not limited to purpose, route, range of dosages, interactions, expected side effects, and untoward effects of pharmacological and parenteral interventions.

Reduction of Risk Potential includes but is not limited to prevention of complications and iatrogenic problems, diagnostic testing, evaluation of test results, laboratory values, procedures, treatments, preoperative and postoperative education, and preoperative and intraoperative care.

Physiological Adaptation includes but is not limited to direction and assistance with adaptations to physiological problems based on acute, chronic, or life-threatening conditions consisting of imbalances in fluids and electrolytes, hemodynamics, pathological responses to therapies, and alterations in body systems.

Cognitive Levels

Based on Bloom's taxonomy, the questions reflect the thinking processes required to answer each question.

Knowledge: These questions require the test taker to recall, define, duplicate, and list information from memory. It involves knowledge of facts, principles, terminology, and trends.

Comprehension: These questions require the test taker to comprehend information. It involves classifying, describing, identifying, recognizing, reporting, and paraphrasing data as well as determining the implications and consequences of the information.

Application: These questions require the test taker to use information, principles, or concepts. It involves demonstration, interpretation, and modification and manipulation of data, as well as solving problems involving mathematical calculations, unexpected changes, and scheduling.

Analysis: These questions require the test taker to differentiate among a variety of data. It involves the ability to appraise, compare, contrast, infer, and discriminate among various options. Decisions are based on the recognition of commonalities, differences, and the interrelationships among data, concepts, principles, and situations.

Integrated Processes

The integrated processes are fundamental components critical to the practice of nursing. They include caring, communication and documentation, teaching and learning, and the nursing process.

Caring: These questions reflect the sensitive relationship between the nurse and client or significant others. The nurse offers encouragement, support, and empathy to enhance the development of mutual trust and respect.

Communication and Documentation: These questions involve interactions among clients, families, staff members, and other professionals within and outside the hospital settings. Client status and interactions are reported and/or recorded, to validate clinical findings according to legal and ethical standards.

Teaching/Learning: These questions address the client's need for the knowledge and skills that can change attitudes and lifestyle behaviors that lead to optimum psychosocial and physiological health.

Nursing Process (NP): These questions reflect the use of clinical reasoning. The nursing process consists of the progression of nursing behaviors involved in providing nursing care. Each question is identified by a specific step in the nursing process.

- *Assessment:* This involves gathering subjective and objective data about the client's health status from meaningful sources, grouping the data into categories, and communicating the information to others. The database for making nursing decisions is determined through the assessment phase.
- *Analysis:* This involves interpreting the data obtained during the assessment phase to identify the client's actual or potential health care needs.
- *Planning:* This involves designing strategies to correct, minimize, or prevent problems identified during the assessment and analysis steps, sets priorities for the problems diagnosed, develops both short- and long-term goals with the client and/or client's family, establishes outcome criteria for nursing interventions, and formulates the nursing care plan.
- *Implementation:* This involves initiating and completing the plan of care. The nurse may perform the care or assist, teach, counsel, or supervise the client, the client's significant others, or other health team members to perform specific interventions based on the client's identified needs, diagnoses, priorities, and goals.
- *Evaluation:* This involves determining the effectiveness of nursing intervention. The nurse compares the actual outcomes with the expected outcomes to determine client compliance with and response to the intervention or therapy. The nurse uses the evaluation phase to identify whether the health care needs still exist, whether they require modification of the plan, or whether new health care needs have developed that require new interventions.

QUESTION FORMATS

Most questions on the NCLEX-RN Examination are in the familiar four-option multiple-choice format. The examination also includes alternate format items. These questions include multiple response, fill-in-the blank, drag and drop (ordered response), hot spot, and exhibit items, and items that use multimedia (e.g., sound and/or video).

Multiple-Choice Questions

Multiple-choice items consist of a stem that states the situation in the form of a question or an incomplete sentence. It contains four options, only one of which is correct.

A nurse is caring for a child in the immediate postoperative period after a tonsillectomy. What should the nurse encourage the parents to offer the child?
1. Ginger ale (correct answer)
2. Orange juice
3. Hot chocolate
4. Cherry ice pop

Multiple-Response Questions

Multiple-response items consist of a stem that states the situation in the form of a question. Four to six options are presented and more than one option is correct. The test taker is instructed to select all that apply.

A client who is at risk for seizures secondary to severe preeclampsia is receiving an IV infusion of magnesium sulfate. Which nursing assessments indicate that the client is showing signs of magnesium sulfate toxicity? Select all that apply.
1. _____ Proteinuria
2. _____ Epigastric pain
3. _____ Respirations of 10/min (correct answer)
4. _____ Loss of patellar reflexes (correct answer)
5. _____ Urine output of 40 mL/hr

Fill-in-the-Blank Questions

Fill-in-the-blank items present information that requires the test taker to perform a calculation that relates to pharmacological or parenteral therapies. The test taker must type in numbers that represent the solution to the problem.

A client is to receive 0.25 mg of digoxin IM. The ampule is labeled 0.5 mg = 2 mL. How many mL should the nurse administer?

    Answer: _____mL
    The correct answer is 1 mL.

Hot Spot Questions

Hot spot items pose a question in relation to a picture, diagram, or figure. To answer the question the test taker must place the cursor on the area to be selected and then click the left mouse button.

The partner of a woman experiencing back pain in labor asks what he can do to help. The nurse demonstrates how to apply counterpressure to his partner's back. Mark on the illustration where the counterpressure should be applied.

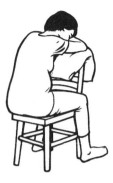

Exhibit Questions

Exhibit items pose a question and then present multiple sources of information. Each exhibit item contains three tabs. The test taker must use the mouse to open each tab to access the attached information. After reviewing and analyzing the information, the test taker then selects an answer to the question.

A client with the diagnoses of schizophrenia and diabetes mellitus has been receiving haloperidol (Haldol) as part of the treatment plan. The nurse identifies a sudden change in the client's health status. The nurse reviews the client's medical history and laboratory results, obtains the client's current vital signs, and performs a physical assessment. What medical emergency does the nurse conclude the client is experiencing?
1. Oculogyric crisis
2. Serotonin syndrome
3. Diabetic ketoacidosis
4. Neuroleptic malignant syndrome (correct answer)

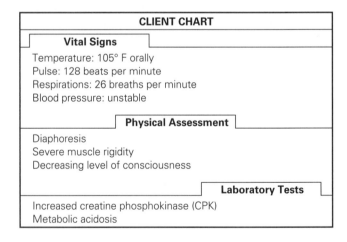

CLIENT CHART
Vital Signs
Temperature: 105° F orally Pulse: 128 beats per minute Respirations: 26 breaths per minute Blood pressure: unstable
Physical Assessment
Diaphoresis Severe muscle rigidity Decreasing level of consciousness
Laboratory Tests
Increased creatine phosphokinase (CPK) Metabolic acidosis

Drag and Drop (Ordered Response) Questions

Drag and drop items present a problem and a list of options. The test taker must place the options in priority order.

An older adult is admitted to the hospital with a tentative diagnosis of pneumonia. The client has a high fever and is short of breath. Bed rest, oxygen via nasal cannula, an IV antibiotic, and blood and sputum specimens for culture and sensitivity (C&S) are ordered. Place these interventions in the order in which they should be implemented.
1. Bed rest
2. Specimens for C&S

3. Oxygen via nasal cannula
4. Administration of an antibiotic
   Answer: _____
   Answer: 1, 3, 2, 4

Multimedia Questions

All question types may include multimedia, such as a chart, table, graph, audio, or video. Three items are included on the CD that use an audio representation of a sound that the nurse may need to interpret in the performance of professional responsibilities. Examples of items that use sound include auscultation of the lungs and heart.

STRATEGIES FOR USING *MOSBY'S REVIEW QUESTIONS FOR THE NCLEX-RN® EXAMINATION*

Guidelines for Using the Textbook

A. Start in one clinical area. Answer all the questions in the area. Do not leave any questions unanswered. Use educated or pure guesses.
B. Circle the option you believe is the correct answer. As you answer each question write a few words about why you think that answer was correct and justify why you selected the answer.
C. Make a special mark if you guess at an answer. This will permit you to identify areas that need further review. Also it will help you to see how correct your guessing can be.
D. Review the answers and rationales for the questions you completed. You may find it easier to tear out the sheets with answers and rationales for the area you are reviewing. If you answered the item correctly, check your reason for selecting the answer with the rationale presented. If you answered the item incorrectly, read the rationale to determine why the answer you selected was incorrect. If you still do not understand your mistake, look up the theory pertaining to the question. In addition, review rationales for all the options. You should carefully review all questions and rationales for items you identified as guesses because you did not have mastery of the material being questioned.
E. Review the area again several days later. If you miss the same question a second time, you need further study of the material.
F. Take the associated quiz or quizzes after you complete each clinical area because they will assist you in applying knowledge and principles from the specific clinical area to any nursing situation.
G. Take the Comprehensive Examination 1 in Chapter 6 after you have completed all the clinical areas, including the quizzes, in Chapters 2 through 5.
H. Analyze your test performance by using the two worksheets at the end of this chapter under Tools for Study.
   Worksheet 1—Errors in Processing Information: This worksheet will help you identify the frequency with which you made particular errors. As you review material in class notes or review books such as *Mosby's Comprehensive Review of Nursing*, pay special attention to correcting those errors that occur repeatedly.
   Worksheet 2—Knowledge Gaps: This worksheet will help you identify the topics you need to review. It is helpful to set priorities. Review the most difficult topics first so that you will have time to review them more than once.
I. Use this opportunity to learn from your mistakes. The mistakes you make on the questions in this text will be as valuable to you as the confident feeling you get from answering questions correctly.
J. Pace yourself when practicing test taking. Because most examinations in schools of nursing have specified time limits, you should pace yourself during the practice testing period accordingly. It is helpful to estimate the time that can be spent on each item and still complete the examination in the allotted time. You can obtain this figure by dividing the testing time by the number of items on the test. For example, a 1-hour (60-minute) testing period with 50 items averages 1.2 minutes per question. The NCLEX-RN is not a timed test. Both the number of questions and the time to complete the test varies according to each candidate's performance. However, if the test taker uses the maximum of 5 hours to answer the maximum of 265 questions, each question equals 1.3 minutes.

Guidelines for Using the CD

Mosby's Review Questions for the NCLEX-RN Examination includes a dual platform (PC and Macintosh) disk. The disk contains seven files. The first five files present all the questions that are included in the book. The sixth file contains the bonus Comprehensive Examination 2. The seventh file is composed of 2015 additional bonus questions that do not appear in the book.

The first four files are divided into Medical-Surgical Nursing, Mental Health Nursing, Childbearing and Women's Health Nursing, and Child Health Nursing. These files contain all the questions that appear in Chapters 2 through 5 in the book. When in each file, questions can be selected by category codes according to specific categories. This allows you to study content within a concentrated area of information selected by you. Also, questions can be selected randomly to cross the spectrum of content within a clinical nursing area. This allows you to prepare for a comprehensive examination at the end of a unit of study. All questions include the rationales for the correct and incorrect answers.

Files 5 and 6 contain Comprehensive Examination 1 and Comprehensive Examination 2, respectively. When in one of these files, you can proceed from questions 1 through 265 at your own pace. These tests reflect computerized examinations that have content that crosses the nursing disciplines. All questions include rationales for correct and incorrect answers. Following each set of rationales the question is categorized by Clinical Area; Client Needs, Cognitive Level, Integrated Process (if relevant to the question), and Nursing Process (NP). At the completion of each comprehensive examination you will receive a personalized review of your performance that identifies your strengths and weaknesses. This information can be used to direct your future study.

When in file 7 you can access questions by category codes according to specific categories selected by you. This allows you to review content guided by your personal study needs. Also, questions can be accessed randomly from all the clinical nursing areas. This simulates the NCLEX-RN Examination. All questions include rationales for correct and incorrect answers. At the completion of a self-constructed, individualized examination in this file, you will receive a personalized review of your performance. This personalized performance review identifies your strengths and weaknesses and should guide your future study. By studying those areas that need improvement, you can use your study time more productively and maximize your ability to pass the NCLEX-RN Examination.

STRATEGIES FOR STUDYING AND TEST TAKING

Develop a Plan of Study

- Develop a realistic plan of study. Do not set rigid, unrealistic goals.
- Do not change your pattern of study. It obviously has contributed to your being here, so it worked. If you have studied alone, continue to study alone. If you have studied in a group, form a study group.
- Identify your problem areas that need attention. Do not waste time on restudying information you know.
- Focus on the common health problems.
- Avoid planning other activities that will add stress to your life between now and the time you take the licensure examination. Enough will happen spontaneously; do not plan to add to it.

Practice Taking Tests

- Become familiar with reading questions on a computer screen. Familiarity reduces anxiety and decreases errors.
- Practice answering questions.

- Pace yourself during the testing period and work as accurately as possible. Do not be pressured into finishing early. Do not rush! Students who achieve higher scores on examinations are typically those who use their time judiciously.
- Do not spend too much time on one question, because it can compromise your overall performance. There is no deduction for incorrect answers, so you are not penalized for guessing. You cannot leave an answer blank; therefore, guess. Go for it! Remember: You do not have to get all the questions correct to pass.
- Monitor questions that you answer with an educated guess or changed your answer from the first option you selected. This will help you to analyze your ability to think critically. Usually your first answer is correct and should not be changed without reason.

Use Test-Taking Skills

- Do not read information into questions, and avoid speculating. Reading into questions creates errors in judgment.
- Make certain that the answer you select is reasonable and obtainable under ordinary circumstances and that the action can be carried out in the given situation.
- Avoid selecting answers that state hospital rules or regulations as a reason or rationale for action.
- Look for answers that focus on the client or that are directed toward the client's feelings.
- If the question asks for an immediate action or response, all the answers may be correct, so base your selection on identified priorities for action.
- Do not select answers that contain exceptions to the general rule, controversial material, or responses that appear to be degrading.

FOCUS FOR STUDY WORKSHEETS

Worksheet 1—Errors in Processing Information

Common errors in processing information are listed in the left column of this worksheet. At the top of the worksheet is a row of blank spaces for inserting the number of the question missed. Directly below each number, check any errors you made in answering that question. You may have made more than one type of error in an answer.

Question number																								
Did not read situation/ question carefully																								
Missed important details																								
Confused major and minor points																								
Defined problem incorrectly																								
Could not remember terms/ facts/concepts/principles																								
Defined terms incorrectly																								
Focused on incomplete/incorrect data in assessing situation																								
Interpreted data incorrectly																								
Applied wrong concepts/ principles in situations																								
Drew incorrect conclusions																								
Identified wrong goals																								
Identified priorities incorrectly																								
Carried out plan incorrectly/ incompletely																								
Was unclear about criteria for evaluating success in achieving goals																								

Worksheet 2—Knowledge Gaps

Types of common knowledge gaps are listed along the top of this worksheet. Write a brief description of topics you want to review in the spaces provided. For example, if you missed a question on administration of a particular drug, write the drug name and problem (e.g., dosage) in the appropriate space under the column labeled *Pharmacology.*

Basic science	Basic skills/ procedures	Basic human needs	Growth and development	Normal nutrition	Psychosocial factors	Clinical area/ topic	Stressors/ coping mechanisms	Patho- physiology	Pharma- cology	Therapeutic nutrition	Legal implications	Other

As you prepare for your course examinations or the NCLEX-RN Examination, consider using a review book such as *Mosby's Comprehensive Review of Nursing.* This book presents information in an abbreviated format that permits you to retrieve and review information quickly. In addition, it contains more than 4000 questions and a CD to practice test taking on a computer.

We wish you success on the NCLEX-RN Examination and as you pursue your career goals.

Medical-Surgical Nursing

Review Questions

NURSING PRACTICE

1. A nurse stops at the scene of an accident and finds a man with a deep laceration on his hand, a fractured arm and leg, and abdominal pain. The nurse wraps the man's hand in a soiled cloth and drives him to the nearest hospital. The nurse is:
   1. Negligent and can be sued for malpractice
   2. Practicing under guidelines of the Nurse Practice Act
   3. Protected for these actions, in most states, by Good Samaritan legislation
   4. Treating a health problem that can and should be addressed by a practitioner

2. When meeting the unique preoperative teaching needs of an older adult, the nurse plans a teaching program based on the principle that learning:
   1. Reduces general anxiety
   2. Is negatively affected by aging
   3. Requires continued reinforcement
   4. Necessitates readiness of the learner

3. A client returns to the surgical unit after a liver biopsy. The nurse identifies a moderately large amount of bile-colored drainage on the dressing. The client also complains of right upper quadrant pain. The nurse should:
   1. Medicate the client for pain as ordered
   2. Ensure the client remains in a supine position
   3. Monitor the client's vital signs every 15 minutes
   4. Notify the practitioner of the client's status immediately

4. A visitor from a room adjacent to a client asks the nurse what disease the client has. The nurse responds, "I will not discuss any client's illness with you. Are you concerned about it?" This response is based on the nurse's knowledge that to discuss a client's condition with someone not directly involved with that client is an example of:
   1. Libel
   2. Negligence
   3. Breach of confidentiality
   4. Defamation of character

5. When approaching homosexual clients with acquired immunodeficiency syndrome (AIDS), it is most important for nurses to:
   1. Establish a meaningful rapport with clients
   2. Have a strong sense of their own sexual identity
   3. Admit their own feelings of discomfort to the clients
   4. Become aware of their own attitudes regarding homosexuality

6. Which statement by the nursing assistant indicates a correct understanding of the nursing assistant role? "I will:
   1. turn off clients' IVs that have infiltrated."
   2. take clients' vital signs after their procedures are over."
   3. use unit written materials to teach clients before surgery."
   4. help by giving medications to clients who are slow in taking pills."

7. A client on hospice care is receiving palliative treatment. A palliative approach involves planning measures to:
   1. Restore the client's health
   2. Promote the client's recovery
   3. Relieve the client's discomfort
   4. Support the client's significant others

8. A nurse observes that a nursing assistant did not use a bag impervious to liquid for contaminated linen from a client who is on contact precautions. The nurse's best way to handle this situation is to:
   1. Place the linen in an appropriate bag
   2. Write an incident report about the situation
   3. Review transmission-based precautions with the nursing assistant
   4. Place an anecdotal summary of the behavior in the nursing assistant's personnel record

9. A client is scheduled for a craniotomy to remove a brain tumor. To prevent the development of cerebral edema after surgery, the nurse anticipates the use of:
   1. Steroids
   2. Diuretics
   3. Anticonvulsants
   4. Antihypertensives

10. During change of shift report the night nurse indicates that a client cannot tolerate the ordered intermittent tube feedings. The nurse receiving report should first:
    1. Suggest that an antiemetic be prescribed
    2. Change the feeding schedule to omit nights
    3. Request that the type of solution be changed
    4. Gather more data from the night nurse about the technique used

11. Before administering preoperative medication to a client, the nurse plans to:
    1. Verify the consent
    2. Have the client void
    3. Check the vital signs
    4. Remove the client's dentures

12. A nurse is caring for a group of clients who are being considered for treatment with a negative pressure wound treatment device. The nurse should discuss this order with the practitioner when the client has which condition?
    1. Neuropathic ulcer
    2. Abdominal dehiscence
    3. Stage IV pressure ulcer with eschar
    4. Treated osteomyelitis within the vicinity of the wound

13. A state's nurse practice act does not allow a registered nurse (RN) to suture wounds. The practitioner offers to teach the RN how to suture and tells the RN that minor wounds may be sutured without supervision. The nurse should:
    1. Refuse to suture wounds
    2. Follow the practitioner's instructions
    3. Report the situation to the state board of nursing
    4. Agree to suture wounds in the practitioner's presence

14. A client refuses to go to the twice-a-day prescribed sessions in physical therapy. The nurse might best approach this problem by:
    1. Having the client observe the progress of a more cooperative client with the same problem
    2. Being the client's advocate and asking the practitioner whether therapy can be decreased to once daily
    3. Ensuring that pain medication is administered to the client before the scheduled physical therapy sessions
    4. Planning a conference with the client, the physical therapist, and the nurse present to discuss the client's feelings

15. During a mass disaster drill simulating a terrorist attack, the nurse must triage numerous severely ill individuals. The client who should receive care first is:
    1. Cyanotic and not breathing
    2. Gasping for breath and conscious
    3. Apneic and has an apical rate of 50
    4. Having a seizure and is incontinent of urine

16. A client is scheduled for surgery. Legally, the client may not sign the operative consent if:
    1. Ambivalent feelings are present and acknowledged
    2. Any sedative type of medication has recently been given
    3. A discussion of alternatives with two physicians has not occurred
    4. A complete history and physical has not been performed and recorded

17. A male client with ascites is to have a paracentesis and has signed the consent. While the nurse is caring for him, he says that he has changed his mind and no longer wants the procedure. The best initial response by the nurse is:
    1. "Why did you sign the consent?"
    2. "Can you tell me why you decided to refuse the procedure?"
    3. "You are obviously afraid about something concerning the procedure."
    4. "Although the procedure is very important, I understand why you changed your mind."

GROWTH AND DEVELOPMENT

18. The nurse considers that a 70-year-old female can best limit further progression of osteoporosis by:
    1. Taking supplemental calcium and vitamin D
    2. Increasing the consumption of eggs and cheese
    3. Taking supplemental magnesium and vitamin E
    4. Increasing the consumption of milk and milk products

19. The nurse recognizes that a common conflict experienced by the older adult is the conflict between:
    1. Youth and old age
    2. Retirement and work
    3. Independence and dependence
    4. Wishing to die and wishing to live

20. A day after an explanation of the effects of surgery to create an ileostomy, a 68-year-old male client remarks to the nurse, "It will be difficult for my wife to care for a helpless old man." This comment by the client regarding himself is an example of Erikson's conflict of:
    1. Initiative vs. guilt
    2. Integrity vs. despair
    3. Industry vs. inferiority
    4. Generativity vs. stagnation

21. An 85-year-old client has just been admitted to a nursing home. When designing a plan of care for this older adult the nurse recalls the expected sensory losses associated with aging. Select all that apply.
    1. _____ Difficulty in swallowing
    2. _____ Diminished sensation of pain
    3. _____ Heightened response to stimuli
    4. _____ Impaired hearing of high-frequency sounds
    5. _____ Increased ability to tolerate environmental heat

22. When teaching about aging, the nurse explains that older adults usually have:
    1. Inflexible attitudes
    2. Periods of confusion
    3. Slower reaction times
    4. Some senile dementia

23. An 80-year-old female is admitted to the hospital because of complications associated with severe dehydration. The client's daughter asks the nurse how her mother could have become dehydrated because she is alert and able to care for herself. The nurse's best response is:
    1. "The body's fluid needs decrease with age because of tissue changes."
    2. "Access to fluid may be insufficient to meet the daily needs of the older adult."

3. "Memory declines with age, and the older adult may forget to ingest adequate amounts of fluid."
4. "The thirst reflex diminishes with age, and therefore the recognition of the need for fluid is decreased."

24. A 75-year-old female client tells the nurse that she read about a vitamin that may be related to aging because of its relationship to the structure of cell walls. The nurse determines that the client is probably referring to:
    1. Vitamin E
    2. Vitamin A
    3. Vitamin C
    4. Vitamin B_1

25. After the removal of a cast from a fractured arm, an 82-year-old client is to receive physical therapy. In an older adult, mild exercise is expected to cause respirations to:
    1. Increase to 24 breaths per minute
    2. Become progressively more difficult
    3. Decrease in rate as their depth increases
    4. Become irregular but stay at 18 breaths per minute

26. Nursing actions for the older adult should include health education and promotion of self-care. Which is most important when working with the older adult client?
    1. Encouraging frequent naps
    2. Strengthening the concept of ageism
    3. Reinforcing the client's strengths and promoting reminiscing
    4. Teaching the client to increase calories and focusing on a high-carbohydrate diet

27. A 90-year-old female resident of a nursing home falls and fractures the proximal end of her right femur. The surgeon plans to reduce the fracture with an internal fixation device. The general fact about the older adult that the nurse should consider when caring for this client is that:
    1. Aging causes a lower pain threshold
    2. Physiological coping defenses are reduced
    3. Most confusional states result from dementia
    4. Older adults psychologically tolerate changes well

28. The nurse recognizes that the mental process most sensitive to deterioration with aging is:
    1. Judgment
    2. Intelligence
    3. Creative thinking
    4. Short-term memory

29. A nurse is preparing a community health program for female senior citizens. The nurse teaches the group that the physical findings that are typical in older people include:
    1. A loss of skin elasticity and a decrease in libido
    2. Impaired fat digestion and increased salivary secretions
    3. Increased blood pressure and decreased hormone production
    4. An increase in body warmth and some swallowing difficulties

30. An 89-year-old client with osteoporosis is admitted to the hospital with a compression fracture of the spine. The nurse identifies that a factor of special concern when caring for this client is the client's:
    1. Irritability in response to deprivation
    2. Decreased ability to recall recent facts
    3. Inability to maintain an optimal level of functioning
    4. Gradual memory loss resulting from change in environment

31. When considering Erikson's psychosocial developmental tasks, a nurse should focus care for middle-aged adults around their need to be:
    1. Productive
    2. Controlling
    3. Independent
    4. Autonomous

32. When nurses are conducting health assessment interviews with older clients, they should:
    1. Leave a written questionnaire for clients to complete at their leisure
    2. Ask family members rather than the clients to supply the necessary information
    3. Spend time in several short sessions to elicit more complete information from the clients
    4. Keep referring to previous questions to ascertain that the information given by clients is correct

33. Considering Erikson's developmental theories, a 21-year-old male client who has sustained a spinal injury below the level of T6 will most likely have difficulty with:
    1. Mastering his environment
    2. Identifying with the male role
    3. Developing meaningful relationships
    4. Differentiating himself from the environment

34. An 82-year-old retired schoolteacher is admitted to a nursing home. During the physical assessment, the nurse identifies an ocular problem common to persons at this client's developmental level, which is:
    1. Tropia
    2. Myopia
    3. Hyperopia
    4. Presbyopia

EMOTIONAL NEEDS RELATED TO HEALTH PROBLEMS

35. When planning discharge teaching for a client who had an ileostomy, the nurse places primary emphasis on:
    1. Informing the client about the ileostomy association
    2. Telling the client whom to contact if assistance is needed
    3. Encouraging the client to return to the workplace as soon as possible
    4. Teaching the client the importance of irrigations to regulate bowel movements

36. The left foot of a client with a history of intermittent claudication becomes increasingly cyanotic and numb. Gangrene of the left foot is diagnosed, and because of the high level of arterial insufficiency, an above-the-knee (AK) amputation is scheduled. The response that demonstrates emotional readiness for the surgery is when the client:
    1. Explains the goals of the procedure
    2. Displays few signs of anticipatory grief
    3. Participates in learning perioperative care
    4. Verbalizes acceptance of future dependency needs

37. When a client who had an above-the-knee amputation (AKA) complains of phantom limb sensations, the nursing staff should:
    1. Reassure the client that these sensations will pass
    2. Explain the psychological component involved to the client
    3. Encourage the client to get involved in diversional activities
    4. Describe the neurological mechanisms in language that the client understands

38. Building confidence in one's worth is important for a client who is scheduled for a below-the-knee amputation (BKA) because an amputation:
    1. Alters a person's sexuality
    2. Implies a lack of wholeness
    3. Increases dependency needs
    4. Affects an idealized self-image

39. A client who recently was diagnosed as having myelocytic leukemia discusses the diagnosis by referring to statistics, facts, and figures. The nurse determines that the client is using the defense mechanism known as:
    1. Projection
    2. Sublimation
    3. Identification
    4. Intellectualization

40. A client with newly diagnosed multiple myeloma asks, "How long do you think I have to live?" The most appropriate response by the nurse is:
    1. "Let me ask your physician for you."
    2. "I can understand why you are worried."
    3. "Tell me about your concerns right now."
    4. "It depends on whether the tumor has spread."

41. A female client who is dying jokes about the situation even though she is becoming sicker and weaker. Which is the most therapeutic response by the nurse?
    1. "Why are you always laughing?"
    2. "Your laughter is a cover for your fear."
    3. "Does it help to joke about your illness?"
    4. "She who laughs on the outside, cries on the inside."

42. A male client is dying. Hesitatingly, his wife says to the nurse, "I'd like to tell him how much I love him, but I don't want to upset him." Which is the best response by the nurse?
    1. "You must keep up a strong appearance for him."
    2. "I think he'd have difficulty dealing with that now."
    3. "Don't you think he knows that without your telling him?"
    4. "Why don't you share your feelings with him while you can?"

43. A nurse identifies that a female client seems to be depressed after a thymectomy for treatment of myasthenia gravis. The nursing action that is most appropriate at this point is:
    1. Recognizing that depression often occurs after surgery
    2. Asking her practitioner to arrange for a psychological consultation
    3. Reassuring the client that she will feel better when her discharge date is set
    4. Talking with the client about her prognosis, emphasizing things that she can do

44. The way individuals cope with an unexpected hospitalization depends on many factors. However, the one that is most significant is:
    1. Cognitive age
    2. Basic personality
    3. Financial resources
    4. General physical health

45. One week after admission to the cardiac care unit a client displays an outburst of anger and tells the nurse to get out of the room. Which is the most appropriate nursing action?
    1. Administer the prescribed sedative
    2. Return when the client has calmed down
    3. Point out that this behavior is inappropriate
    4. Notify the practitioner of the client's behavior

46. A female client has just spent 5 minutes complaining to the nurse about numerous aspects of her hospital stay. Which is the best initial response by the nurse?
    1. Attempt to explain the purpose of different hospital routines to the client
    2. Explain to the client that becoming so upset dangerously blocks her need for rest
    3. Refocus the conversation on the client's fears, frustrations, and anger about her condition
    4. Permit the client to release feelings and then promptly leave to allow her to regain composure

47. A client with hypertension is scheduled for a scan and electrolyte studies. During an interview with the nurse, the client exclaims, "I don't know why the doctor doesn't just give me a prescription for high blood pressure pills; that probably is all it is. I'm missing work by being here." Which is the best response by the nurse?
    1. "It might not be high blood pressure. We have to be sure."
    2. "It's frustrating to miss work and not know for sure what's wrong."
    3. "I know it's frustrating, but you need to have a diagnostic workup."
    4. "Maybe you could ask your physician if the tests could be done on separate days."

48. A client who has recently had an abdominoperineal resection and colostomy accuses the nurse of being uncomfortable during a dressing change because the "wound looks terrible." The nurse identifies that the client is using the defense mechanism known as:
    1. Projection
    2. Sublimation
    3. Compensation
    4. Intellectualization

49. A female client who had abdominal surgery asks if she can return to work after discharge. The most appropriate response by the nurse is:
    1. "No, not for at least two weeks."
    2. "What type of work did you have in mind?"
    3. "Yes, but do you know what it means to take it easy?"
    4. "No, because you must get plenty of rest when you get home."

50. A client who has sustained damage to the bladder is being prepared for diagnostic tests. The client asks, "If I have my bladder removed, how will I ever be able to urinate?" The most therapeutic answer by the nurse is:
    1. "You can still function normally without a bladder."
    2. "I am sure this is very upsetting to you, but it will be over soon."
    3. "The tests will help to determine if your bladder has to be removed."
    4. "I know you're upset, but there are alternatives to removing your bladder."

51. A client is taught how to change the dressing and how to care for a recently inserted nephrostomy tube. On the day of discharge the client states, "I hope I can handle all this at home; it's a lot to remember." The best response by the nurse is:
    1. "I'm sure you can do it."
    2. "Oh, a family member can do it for you."
    3. "You seem to be nervous about going home."
    4. "Perhaps you can stay in the hospital another day."

52. A psychological problem that frequently occurs when a client is on hemodialysis is:
    1. Reactive depression
    2. Postpump psychosis
    3. Superego constriction
    4. Dialysis disequilibrium

53. An 83-year-old client with type 2 diabetes is admitted to the ambulatory surgery unit for elective cataract surgery. Before surgery the client asks the nurse, "How will my diabetes be managed while I am here?" The best response by the nurse is:
    1. "What did your surgeon tell you?"
    2. "Has the anesthesiologist talked to you yet?"
    3. "Your surgeon will write your postoperative orders."
    4. "I'm not quite certain I understand what you are asking."

54. A client's discouragement with the diagnosis of nodular, poorly differentiated lymphocytic lymphoma continues during radiation therapy because of the long time required for treatment and its side effects. What should the nurse emphasize when assisting the client to plan for the future?
    1. Antidepressant medication may be prescribed
    2. Positive beliefs can influence the outcome of therapy
    3. Expected feelings of discouragement will lessen with time
    4. Prognosis for this disease is more favorable than for other cancers

55. A client is newly diagnosed with multiple sclerosis. The client is obviously upset with the diagnosis and asks, "Am I going to die?" The nurse's best response is:
    1. "Most individuals with your disease live a normal life span."
    2. "Is your family here? I would like to explain your disease to all of you."
    3. "The prognosis is variable; most individuals experience remissions and exacerbations."
    4. "Why don't you speak with your physician? You probably can get more details about your disease."

56. A practitioner orders airborne precautions for a client with tuberculosis. After being taught about the details of airborne precautions, the client is seen walking down the hall to get a glass of juice from the kitchen. The most effective nursing intervention is to:
    1. Ensure regular visits by staff members
    2. Explore what the precautions mean to the client
    3. Report the situation to the infection control nurse
    4. Reteach the concepts of airborne precautions to the client

57. A 60-year-old widow living with her daughter, who has seven children, develops heart failure and is referred for home health care. On the first visit by the nurse, the client is feeding a grandchild and preparing dinner for the family. The other children are playing in the area. The best way for the nurse to proceed is to:
    1. Sit down with the client in the living room
    2. Socialize for a few minutes with the client
    3. Make an appointment with the client on a different day
    4. Ask the client if there is a private place to perform the physical assessment

58. The nurse should suspect that a male client who had a recent myocardial infarction is experiencing denial when he:
    1. Attempts to minimize his illness
    2. Lacks an emotional response to his illness
    3. Refuses to discuss his condition with his wife
    4. Expresses displeasure with his activity program

59. The major improvement in body image following early fitting with a prosthesis after amputation usually is related to the:
    1. Acceptance received from others
    2. Client's improved functional abilities
    3. Concept that something is being done to help
    4. Fact that the client appears more complete to others

60. Teaching for clients who have sustained a sudden, traumatic, major loss is often most satisfactorily done during the acceptance or adaptation stage of coping. The rationale for this fact is that clients in this stage are:
    1. Ready for discharge and therefore in need of preparation
    2. At the peak of mental anguish and therefore open to change
    3. Less angry and therefore more compliant and more receptive
    4. Less anxious and more aware of reality and therefore ready to learn

61. On the fourth day after surgery for a fractured hip, a client appears angry and extremely restless and says, "I can't stand this another minute. There's a wrinkle in my sheet, and the water in my pitcher is warm." The client changes position frequently and does not maintain eye contact with the nurse. The best initial interpretation of the client's behavior is that it indicates:
    1. Severe discomfort in hip
    2. Increased levels of anxiety
    3. Anger with perceived poor nursing care
    4. Frustration with the need for leg abduction

62. A nurse who is caring for a male client after head and neck surgery is concerned with the client's anger and depressive episodes about the effects of surgery. The action by the client that indicates that he is reaching acceptance is:
    1. Smiling and becoming more extroverted
    2. Performing self-care of the tracheal stoma
    3. Ambulating in the hall and sitting in the lounge
    4. Allowing a family member to participate in care

63. A young married woman who was hospitalized with partial- and full-thickness burns over 30% of the total body surface area is to be discharged. She asks the nurse, "How will my husband be able to care for me at home?" How should the nurse interpret this statement?
    1. Readiness to discuss her deformities
    2. Indication of a change in family relations
    3. Need for more time to think about the future
    4. Beginning realization of implications for the future

64. A client experiencing thyrotoxic crisis tells the nurse, "I know I'm going to die. I'm very sick." Which is the best response by the nurse?
    1. "You must feel very sick and frightened."
    2. "Tell me why you feel you are going to die."
    3. "I can understand how you feel, but people do not die from this problem."
    4. "If you would like, I will call your family and tell them to come to the hospital."

65. The nurse considers that sensory restriction in a client who is blind can:
    1. Increase the use of daydreaming and fantasy
    2. Heighten the client's ability to make decisions
    3. Decrease the client's restlessness and lethargy
    4. Lead to the use of permanent neurotic behaviors

66. A nurse overhears a nursing assistant talking with a client about the client's marital and family problems. The nurse identifies that the nursing assistant is providing false reassurance when the nursing assistant states:
    1. "I agree; I think you should get a divorce."
    2. "Everything will be fine, just wait and see."
    3. "You should be glad that you have such a loving family."
    4. "In the scheme of things, you do not have a major problem."

67. A female client with chronic renal failure has been on hemodialysis for 2 years. She relates to the nurse in the dialysis unit in an angry, critical manner and is frequently noncompliant with medications and diet. The nurse can best intervene by first considering that the client's behavior is most likely:
    1. An attempt to punish the nursing staff
    2. A constructive method of accepting reality
    3. A defense against underlying depression and fear
    4. An effort to maintain life and to live it as fully as possible

68. Before major abdominal surgery for cancer, a client says to a nurse, "I really don't think this is cancer at all. I'll bet they won't find anything." Which is the most appropriate initial response by the nurse?
    1. "I can understand why you'd like to believe that."
    2. "I hope you're right although tests indicate cancer."
    3. "It must be difficult to be facing such serious surgery."
    4. "You think the physician may have made a wrong diagnosis?"

69. A female client is diagnosed as having cancer of the breast and is admitted to the hospital for a lumpectomy to be followed by radiation. While being admitted to ambulatory surgery by the nurse, the client has tears in her eyes and her chin is quivering. In a shaky voice the client says, "I can't believe this is happening." The nurse's best response is:
    1. "You can't believe this is happening?"
    2. "This must be a very scary time for you."
    3. "Do you have any questions at this time?"
    4. "Cancer of the breast has a high cure rate."

70. After a laryngectomy is scheduled, the most important factor for the nurse to include in the preoperative teaching plan is:
    1. Establishing a means for communicating postoperatively
    2. Explaining that there will be a feeding tube postoperatively
    3. Demonstrating how to care for a permanent laryngeal stoma
    4. Teaching how to cough to expectorate bronchial secretions effectively

71. The nurse identifies that a client who had extensive abdominal surgery appears depressed. The most appropriate nursing action is:
    1. Talking with the client, encouraging exploration of feelings

2. Asking the client's practitioner to prescribe an anti-depressant medication

3. Understanding that the client's depression is an expected response to surgery

4. Reassuring the client that feelings of depression will lift after returning home

72. A nurse is caring for a male client who is hospitalized because of injuries sustained in a major automobile collision. As the client is describing the accident to a friend, he becomes very restless, and his pulse and respirations increase sharply. Which factor is probably related to the client's physical responses?
1. Client's method of seeking sympathy
2. Bleeding from an undiscovered injury
3. Delayed psychological response to trauma
4. Parasympathetic nervous system response to anxiety

73. A male client with a parotid tumor tells the nurse that he is anxious about the surgery to remove the tumor. He states that he is not too sure about delaying surgery until preoperative radiotherapy is completed. The best response by the nurse is:
1. "You are concerned about the delay of surgery?"
2. "You are anxious about the effects of radiotherapy?"
3. "I think you do not have confidence in the physician's decision."
4. "I can understand your anxiety concerning the delay of your surgery."

74. A 54-year-old male police officer who has just had surgery for oral carcinoma indicates to the nurse that he wants only his wife to visit. To support him at this time, the nurse should first:
1. Comply with the client's wishes
2. Ask the client why he does not want others to visit
3. Have the wife explain to the client that everything will be OK
4. Promote communication to find out how the client really feels

75. A male client, who is in a late stage of pancreatic cancer, intellectually understands the terminal nature of the illness. Behaviors that indicate he is emotionally accepting his impending death are:
1. Revising his will and planning a visit to a friend
2. Alternately crying and talking openly about death
3. Getting second, third, and fourth medical opinions
4. Refusing to follow treatments and stating he is going to die anyway

76. A female client with a terminal illness decides to donate her eyes for organ transplantation after she dies. Statutes that address organ transplantation attempt to prevent abuse by:
1. Permitting active euthanasia when necessary
2. Preventing children from giving organs to others
3. Allowing physicians to control donors and recipients
4. Requiring participating institutions to have review boards

77. To be most effective when teaching colostomy care to a client, the nurse must first:
1. Wait until a family member is present
2. Assess barriers to learning colostomy care
3. Begin with simple written instructions concerning the care
4. Wait until the client has accepted the change in body image

78. During the evening after a paracentesis, the nurse identifies that the client, although denying any discomfort, is very anxious. The best nursing approach is to:
1. Offer the client a back rub
2. Administer the prescribed opioid
3. Reinforce the practitioner's explanation of the procedure
4. Explore the client's concerns while administering the ordered anxiolytic

79. A client with recently diagnosed diabetes states, "I feel bad. I don't seem to get along with my husband. He does not care about my diabetes." The nurse's most appropriate response is:
1. "You don't get along with your husband."
2. "I'm sorry. What can I do to make you feel better?"
3. "It may be temporary because he needs more time to adjust."
4. "You are unhappy. I wonder, have you tried to talk to your husband?"

80. A 38-year-old administrative assistant visits a neurologist after experiencing a tonic-clonic seizure. The neurologist suspects a brain tumor, and a CT scan is scheduled. Before the test the nurse should:
1. Withhold routine medications
2. Describe the equipment involved
3. Explain that no radiation is involved
4. Provide the prescribed pre-scan sedative

81. A client with AIDS comments to the nurse, "There are so many rotten people around. Why couldn't one of them get AIDS instead of me?" The nurse's best response is:
1. "It seems unfair that you should be so ill."
2. "It may be helpful to speak with a minister."
3. "I can understand why you're so afraid of death."
4. "I'm sure you really don't wish this on someone else."

82. A client is to be transferred from the coronary care unit to a progressive care unit. The client asks the nurse, "Are you sure I'm ready for this move?" From this statement the nurse determines that the client is most likely experiencing:
1. Fear
2. Depression
3. Dependency
4. Ambivalence

83. On the second day of hospitalization a client is discussing with the nurse concerns about unhealthy family relationships. During the nurse-client interaction the client begins to talk about a job problem. The nurse's

response is: "Let's go back to what we were just talking about." What therapeutic communication technique did the nurse use?

1. Focusing
2. Restating
3. Exploring
4. Accepting

84. A 47-year-old woman with jaundiced skin and abdominal pain is diagnosed with biliary obstruction. She is refusing all visitors. The nurse should first:

1. Listen to her fears
2. Grant her request about visitors
3. Encourage her to visit with relatives
4. Darken the room by pulling the drapes

85. A carpenter with full-thickness burns of the entire right arm confides, "I'll never be able to use my arm again and I'll be scarred forever." The nurse's best initial response is:

1. "The staff is taking steps to minimize scarring."
2. "Think about how lucky you are. You are alive."
3. "Try not to worry for now. Concentrate on your range-of-motion exercises."
4. "I know you're worried, but it is too early to tell how much scarring will occur."

86. A male client with a history of ulcerative colitis is admitted to the hospital because of severe rectal bleeding. He appears to be an angry, demanding person. One day the nursing assistant tells the nurse, "I've had it with that man and all his demands. I'm not going in there again." The nurse's best response to this statement is:

1. "He's frightened. Let's think how we can approach him."
2. "You need to try to be patient with him. He's going through a lot right now."
3. "I'll talk with him. Maybe I can figure out the best way for us to handle this."
4. "Just ignore him and get on with the rest of your work. Let someone else take a turn."

BLOOD AND IMMUNITY

87. Polycythemia is frequently associated with chronic obstructive pulmonary disease (COPD). When assessing for this complication, the nurse should monitor for:

1. Pallor and cyanosis
2. Dyspnea on exertion
3. Elevated hemoglobin
4. Decreased hematocrit

88. The practitioner orders 2 units of packed red blood cells for a client who is bleeding. Before blood administration the nurse's priority is:

1. Obtaining the client's vital signs
2. Letting the blood reach room temperature
3. Monitoring the hemoglobin and hematocrit levels
4. Determining proper typing and crossmatching of blood

89. A client who is scheduled for a modified radical mastectomy decides to have family members donate blood in the event it is needed. The client has type A-negative blood. Blood can be used from relatives whose blood is:

1. Type O positive
2. Type AB positive
3. Type A or O negative
4. Type A or AB negative

90. The practitioner orders a transfusion of 2 units of packed red blood cells for a client. When administering blood, the priority nursing intervention is to:

1. Warm the blood to 98° F to prevent chills
2. Use an infusion pump to increase accuracy of infusion
3. Infuse the blood at a slow rate during the first 10 minutes
4. Draw blood samples from the client after each unit is transfused

91. A client with esophageal varices is admitted with hematemesis, and 2 units of packed red blood cells are ordered. The client complains of flank pain halfway through the first unit of blood. The nurse's first action is to:

1. Stop the transfusion
2. Obtain the vital signs
3. Assess the pain further
4. Monitor the hourly urinary output

92. Halfway through the administration of a unit of blood, a client complains of lumbar pain. After stopping the transfusion and replacing the tubing, the nurse should:

1. Obtain vital signs
2. Notify the blood bank
3. Assess the pain further
4. Increase the flow of normal saline

93. A client demonstrates signs and symptoms of a transfusion reaction. The nurse immediately stops the infusion and next:

1. Obtains blood pressure in both arms
2. Sends a urine specimen to the laboratory
3. Hangs a bag of normal saline with new tubing
4. Monitors the intake and output every fifteen minutes

94. A male client with chronic liver disease reports that his gums bleed spontaneously. In addition, the nurse identifies small hemorrhagic lesions on his face. The nurse concludes that the client needs additional:

1. Bile salts
2. Folic acid
3. Vitamin A
4. Vitamin K

95. During a yearly physical examination a complete blood count (CBC) is performed to determine a client's hematologic status. It is composed of several tests, one of which is the level of:

1. Blood glucose
2. Hemoglobin (Hb)
3. C-reactive protein
4. Blood urea nitrogen (BUN)

96. After years of unprotected sex, a 20-year-old man is diagnosed as having AIDS. The client states, "I'm not worried because they have a cure for AIDS." The best response by the nurse is:
    1. "Repeated phlebotomies may be able to rid you of the virus."
    2. "You may be cured of AIDS after prolonged pharmacologic therapy."
    3. "Perhaps you should have worn condoms to prevent contracting the virus."
    4. "There is no cure for AIDS but there are drugs that can slow down the virus."

97. The nursing staff has a team conference on AIDS and discusses the routes of transmission of the human immunodeficiency virus (HIV). The discussion reveals that there is no risk of exposure to HIV when an individual:
    1. Has intercourse with just the spouse
    2. Makes a donation of a pint of whole blood
    3. Uses a condom each time there is sexual intercourse
    4. Limits sexual contact to those without HIV antibodies

98. The nurse explains to a client that a positive diagnosis for HIV infection is made based on:
    1. Positive ELISA and Western blot tests
    2. Performance of high-risk sexual behaviors
    3. Evidence of extreme weight loss and high fever
    4. Identification of an associated opportunistic infection

99. Blood screening tests of the immune system of a client with AIDS indicates:
    1. A decrease in CD4 T cells
    2. An increase in thymic hormones
    3. An increase in immunoglobulin E
    4. A decrease in the serum level of glucose-6-phosphate dehydrogenase

100. When taking the blood pressure of a client who has AIDS, the nurse must:
    1. Don clean gloves
    2. Use barrier techniques
    3. Put on a mask and gown
    4. Wash the hands thoroughly

101. A client with AIDS and *Cryptococcus* pneumonia frequently is incontinent of feces and urine and produces copious sputum. When providing care for this client, the nurse's priority is to:
    1. Wear goggles when suctioning the client's airway
    2. Use gown, mask, and gloves when bathing the client
    3. Use gloves to administer oral medications to the client
    4. Wear a gown when assisting the client with the bedpan

102. In addition to *Pneumocystis jiroveci*, a client with AIDS also has an ulcer 4 cm in diameter on the leg. Considering the client's total health status, the most critical concern is:
    1. Skin integrity
    2. Gas exchange
    3. Social isolation
    4. Nutritional status

103. When a Schilling test is ordered for a client suspected of having cobalamin deficiency because of pernicious anemia, the nurse plans to:
    1. Give medications on time
    2. Order foods low in vitamin B_{12}
    3. Keep an accurate intake and output
    4. Collect a 24- to 48-hour urine specimen

104. A Schilling test is ordered for a client who is suspected of having pernicious anemia. The nurse considers that the primary purpose of the Schilling test is to determine the client's ability to:
    1. Store vitamin B_{12}
    2. Digest vitamin B_{12}
    3. Absorb vitamin B_{12}
    4. Produce vitamin B_{12}

105. When discussing the therapeutic regimen of vitamin B_{12} for pernicious anemia with a client, the nurse explains that:
    1. Weekly Z-track injections provide needed control
    2. Daily intramuscular injections are required for control
    3. Intramuscular injections once a month will maintain control
    4. Oral tablets of vitamin B_{12} taken daily will provide symptom control

106. The nurse evaluates that the teaching regarding the use of vitamin B_{12} injections to treat pernicious anemia is understood when a client states, "I must take the drug:
    1. when feeling fatigued."
    2. until my symptoms subside."
    3. monthly, for the rest of my life."
    4. during exacerbations of anemia."

107. A client with Hodgkin's disease enters a remission period and remains symptom-free for 6 months when a relapse occurs. The client is diagnosed at stage IV. The therapy option the nurse expects to be implemented at this time is:
    1. Radiation therapy
    2. Combination chemotherapy
    3. Radiation with chemotherapy
    4. Surgical removal of the affected nodes

108. A young woman is admitted to the oncology unit with a diagnosis of Hodgkin's disease. Staging is done and the client's spleen is found to be grossly involved, and it is surgically removed. A complication specifically related to a splenectomy for which the nurse should monitor the client is:
    1. Pulmonary embolism
    2. Inadequate lung aeration
    3. Hypoactive bowel sounds
    4. Postoperative hemorrhage

109. A client receiving chemotherapy and a steroid has a white blood cell count of 12,000/mm³ and a red blood cell count of 4.5 million/mm³. What is the priority instruction that the nurse should teach the client is?
    1. Omit the daily dose of prednisone
    2. Avoid large crowds and persons with infections

3. Shave with an electric rather than a safety razor
4. Increase the intake of high-protein foods and red meats

110. An older adult develops severe bone marrow suppression from chemotherapy for cancer. The nurse should:
1. Monitor for signs of alopecia
2. Encourage an increase in fluids
3. Monitor intake and output of fluids
4. Advise use of a soft toothbrush for oral hygiene

111. The laboratory results of a client following chemotherapy for cancer indicate bone marrow suppression. The nurse should encourage the client to:
1. Use an electric razor when shaving
2. Drink citrus juices frequently for nourishment
3. Increase activity level by ambulating frequently
4. Sleep with the head of the bed slightly elevated

112. A client who is suspected of having leukemia has a bone marrow aspiration. Immediately after the procedure, the nurse should:
1. Apply brief pressure to the site
2. Have the client lie on the affected side
3. Swab the site with an antiseptic solution
4. Monitor vital signs every hour for 4 hours

113. On admission, the bloodwork of a young adult with leukemia indicates elevated blood urea nitrogen (BUN) and uric acid levels. The nurse determines that these laboratory results may be related to:
1. Lymphadenopathy
2. Thrombocytopenia
3. Hypermetabolic status
4. Hepatic encephalopathy

114. When obtaining a health history from a client with probable acute lymphoblastic leukemia (ALL), the clinical manifestation the nurse expects to be present is:
1. Alopecia
2. Insomnia
3. Ecchymosis
4. Splenomegaly

115. A client who was admitted with a diagnosis of acute lymphoblastic leukemia is receiving chemotherapy. Which client manifestations should alert the nurse to the possible development of the life-threatening response of thrombocytopenia? Select all that apply.
1. _____ Fever
2. _____ Diarrhea
3. _____ Headache
4. _____ Hematuria
5. _____ Ecchymosis

116. A client who has bone pain of insidious onset is suspected of having multiple myeloma. The nurse expects that one of the diagnostic findings specific for multiple myeloma is:
1. Occult blood in the stool
2. Low serum calcium levels
3. Bence Jones protein in the urine
4. Positive bacterial culture of sputum

117. The nurse expects that the most definitive test to confirm a diagnosis of multiple myeloma is:
1. Bone marrow biopsy
2. Serum test for hypercalcemia
3. Urine test for Bence-Jones protein
4. X-ray films of the ribs, spine, and skull

118. A client with multiple myeloma is scheduled to have a chest x-ray examination and a bone scan. For this client, the primary responsibility of the nursing and radiology staff is to:
1. Explain the procedure and its purpose
2. Observe the client for the presence of pallor
3. Provide for rest periods during the procedure
4. Handle the client with supportive movements

119. A client diagnosed with multiple myeloma asks the practitioner about what treatment will be administered. The nurse expects the practitioner to reply:
1. "Alpha-interferon therapy."
2. "Radiation therapy on an outpatient basis."
3. "Surgery to remove the lesion and lymph nodes."
4. "Chemotherapy utilizing a combination of drugs."

120. A client with multiple myeloma, who is receiving chemotherapy, has a temperature that has risen 3 degrees during a 6-hour period and is now 102.2° F. The nurse should:
1. Administer the prescribed antipyretic and notify the practitioner
2. Obtain the other vital signs and recheck the temperature in 1 hour
3. Assess the amount and color of urine and obtain a specimen for a urinalysis
4. Note the consistency of respiratory secretions and obtain a specimen for culture

121. A client with multiple myeloma asks how the disease and therapy may progress. When teaching this client, the nurse discusses the possibility that:
1. Blood transfusions may be necessary
2. Frequent urinary tract infections may result
3. IV fluid therapy may be administered in the home
4. The disease is exacerbated by exposure to ultraviolet rays

122. The nurse is caring for a client who is receiving azathioprine (Imuran), cyclosporine, and prednisone before kidney transplant. These medications are administered to:
1. Stimulate leukocytosis
2. Provide passive immunity
3. Prevent iatrogenic infection
4. Reduce antibody production

123. A client has an exacerbation of systemic lupus erythematosus. The dosage of steroid medication is increased, and a home health care nurse is to provide health teaching. To reduce the frequency of exacerbations, the nurse teaches the client:
1. Basic principles of hygiene
2. Techniques to reduce stress
3. Measures to improve nutrition
4. Signs of an impending exacerbation

124. A farmer steps on a rusty nail and the puncture site becomes swollen and painful. Tetanus antitoxin is prescribed. The nurse explains that this is used because it:
    1. Provides antibodies
    2. Stimulates plasma cells
    3. Produces active immunity
    4. Facilitates long-lasting immunity

125. A tuberculin skin test with purified protein derivative (PPD) tuberculin is performed as part of a routine physical examination. The nurse instructs the client to make an appointment so the test can be read in:
    1. 3 days
    2. 5 days
    3. 7 days
    4. 10 days

126. A client is admitted with cellulitis of the left leg and a temperature of 103° F. The practitioner prescribes IV antibiotics. Before instituting this therapy, the nurse should:
    1. Determine whether the client has allergies
    2. Apply a warm, moist dressing over the area
    3. Measure the amount of swelling in the client's leg
    4. Obtain the results of the culture and sensitivity tests

127. After multiple bee stings a client has an anaphylactic reaction. The nurse determines that the symptoms the client is experiencing are caused by:
    1. Respiratory depression and cardiac arrest
    2. Bronchial constriction and decreased peripheral resistance
    3. Decreased cardiac output and dilation of major blood vessels
    4. Constriction of capillaries and decreased peripheral circulation

128. The plan of care for a postoperative client who has developed a pulmonary embolus includes monitoring and bed rest. The client asks why all activity is restricted. The nurse's response is based on the principle that bed rest:
    1. Prevents the further aggregation of platelets
    2. Enhances the peripheral circulation in the deep vessels
    3. Decreases the potential for further dislodgment of emboli
    4. Maximizes the amount of blood available to damaged tissues

129. The nurse teaches a group of clients that nutritional support of natural defense mechanisms indicates the need for a diet high in:
    1. Essential fatty acids
    2. Dietary cellulose and fiber
    3. Tryptophan, an amino acid
    4. Vitamins A, C, E, and selenium

130. After receiving 75 mL of packed red blood cells, the client complains of chills and low back pain. The nurse suspects a hemolytic transfusion reaction and stops the infusion. The blood bag and a urine specimen are sent to the laboratory. The reason for sending a urine specimen to the laboratory is to test for:
    1. Specific gravity
    2. Free hemoglobin
    3. Carboxyhemoglobin
    4. Disseminated intravascular coagulation

131. A client develops internal bleeding after abdominal surgery. Which signs and symptoms of hemorrhage should the nurse expect the client to exhibit? Select all that apply.
    1. _____ Pallor
    2. _____ Polyuria
    3. _____ Bradypnea
    4. _____ Tachycardia
    5. _____ Hypertension

132. When assessing for hemorrhage after a client has a total hip replacement, the most important nursing action is to:
    1. Measure the girth of the thigh
    2. Examine the bedding under the client
    3. Check the vital signs every four hours
    4. Observe for ecchymosis at the operative site

133. A client is brought to the emergency service after an automobile collision. The client's blood pressure is 100/60 mm Hg, and the physical assessment suggests a ruptured spleen. Based on this information, the nurse assesses the client for which early response to decreased arterial pressure?
    1. Warm and flushed skin
    2. Confusion and lethargy
    3. Increased pulse pressure
    4. Reduced peripheral pulses

134. When a client is experiencing hypovolemic shock with decreased tissue perfusion, the nurse expects that the body initially attempts to compensate by:
    1. Producing less ADH
    2. Producing more red blood cells
    3. Maintaining peripheral vasoconstriction
    4. Decreasing mineralocorticoid production

135. After sustaining multiple internal injuries in an automobile collision, the nurse identifies that the client's blood pressure suddenly drops to 80/60 mm Hg. What most likely has caused this drop in blood pressure?
    1. Reduction in the circulating blood volume
    2. Diminished vasomotor stimulation to the arterial wall
    3. Vasodilation resulting from diminished vasoconstrictor tone
    4. Cardiac decompensation resulting from electrolyte imbalance

136. The nurse understands that shock associated with a ruptured abdominal aneurysm is called:
    1. Vasogenic shock
    2. Neurogenic shock
    3. Cardiogenic shock
    4. Hypovolemic shock

137. A client has emergency surgery for a ruptured appendix. After determining that the client is manifesting signs and symptoms of shock, the nurse should:
    1. Prepare for a blood transfusion
    2. Notify the practitioner immediately *Peritonitis + shock P surgery = life-threat!*
    3. Elevate the head of the bed thirty degrees
    4. Increase the liter flow of oxygen being administered

138. During the progressive stage of shock, anaerobic metabolism occurs. The nurse expects that initially this causes:
    1. Metabolic acidosis *d/t accumulated lactic acid*
    2. Metabolic alkalosis
    3. Respiratory acidosis
    4. Respiratory alkalosis

139. A client who is in hypovolemic shock has a hematocrit value of 25%. The nurse anticipates that the practitioner will order:
    1. Ringer's lactate
    2. Serum albumin
    3. Blood replacement *to ↑ O2-carrying capacity of the blood*
    4. High molecular dextran

CARDIOVASCULAR

140. To determine the status of a client's carotid pulse, the nurse should palpate:
    1. Below the mandible
    2. In the lateral neck region
    3. Along the clavicle at the base of the neck
    4. At the anterior neck, lateral to the trachea

141. The practitioner's orders instruct the nurse to monitor the client's apical pulse every 4 hours. Place the following steps in the order that they should be implemented when determining where to place the stethoscope for the point of maximal impulse when taking an apical pulse.
    1. Slide your finger to the edge of the left sternal border to the second intercostal space
    2. Move your finger laterally along the fifth intercostal space to the midclavicular line
    3. Place your index finger in the second intercostal space and continue palpating downward to the fifth intercostal space
    4. Slide your finger down from the sternal notch to the angle of Louis (the bump where the manubrium and sternum meet)
       Answer: _____

142. During auscultation of the heart, the nurse expects the first heart sound (S_1) to be the loudest at the:
    1. Base of the heart
    2. Apex of the heart
    3. Left lateral border
    4. Right lateral border

143. When auscultating a client's heart, the nurse understands that the first heart sound is produced by the closure of the:
    1. Mitral and tricuspid valves
    2. Aortic and tricuspid valves
    3. Mitral and pulmonic valves
    4. Aortic and pulmonic valves

144. A client has a thermodilution pulmonary catheter inserted for monitoring cardiovascular status. With this catheter the most accurate measurement of the client's left ventricular pressure is the:
    1. Right atrial pressure
    2. Cardiac output by thermodilution
    3. Pulmonary artery diastolic pressure
    4. Pulmonary capillary wedge pressure

145. When assessing an 85-year-old client's vital signs, the nurse anticipates a number of changes in cardiac output that result from the aging process. The finding that is consistent with a pathologic condition rather than the aging process is:
    1. A pulse rate irregularity
    2. An equal apical and radial pulse
    3. A pulse rate of sixty beats per minute
    4. An apical rate obtainable at the fifth intercostal space and midclavicular line

146. Thrombus formation is a danger for all postoperative clients. The nurse should act independently to prevent this complication. Check all that apply.
    1. _____ Urging the client to drink more fluids
    2. _____ Massaging the client's extremities with lotion
    3. _____ Placing the client's legs in pneumatic stockings
    4. _____ Encouraging the client to keep the legs uncrossed
    5. _____ Instructing the client to dorsiflex the feet routinely

147. Oxygen by nasal cannula is prescribed for a client in the coronary care unit. The nurse plans to use safety precautions in the room because oxygen:
    1. Is flammable
    2. Supports combustion
    3. Has unstable properties
    4. Converts to an alternate form of matter

148. When interpreting an ECG rhythm strip, the nurse identifies that ventricular contraction is displayed as the:
    1. P wave
    2. T wave
    3. PR interval
    4. QRS interval

149. An electrocardiogram is ordered for a client complaining of chest pain. An early finding in the lead over an infarcted area is:
    1. Flattened T waves
    2. Absence of P waves
    3. Elevated ST segments
    4. Disappearance of Q waves

150. A thallium scan is scheduled for a client who had a myocardial infarction to:
    1. Monitor the mitral and aortic valves
    2. Establish the viability of myocardial muscle
    3. Visualize the ventricular systole and diastole
    4. Determine the adequacy of electrical conductivity

151. After a traumatic accident, a client is admitted to the hospital's emergency department with a blood pressure of 100/60, and the practitioner suspects a ruptured spleen. The nurse should assess the client for an early sign of decreased arterial pressure, such as:
    1. Weak radial pulses
    2. Warm, flushed skin
    3. Lethargy with confusion
    4. Increased pulse pressure

152. A male client has a diskectomy and fusion for a herniated nucleus pulposus (HNP). When getting out of bed for the first time, with assistance from two nurses, the client complains of feeling faint and lightheaded. One nurse instructs the client to:
    1. Sit on edge of the bed so they can hold him upright
    2. Slide to the floor so he will not fall and hurt himself
    3. Lie down immediately, so they can take his blood pressure
    4. Bend forward, because it will increase the blood flow to his brain

153. A client has a right upper lobectomy to remove a cancerous lesion. After this surgery the nurse monitors the client for the most life-threatening complication, which is:
    1. Hemothorax due to decreased thoracic drainage
    2. Dyspnea due to increased intrathoracic pressure
    3. Decreased cardiac output due to mediastinal shift
    4. Pneumothorax due to increased abdominal pressure

154. A man experiences crushing chest pain and is brought to the emergency department. When assessing the ECG tracing, the nurse concludes that the client is experiencing premature ventricular complexes (PVCs). Which abnormalities of the electrocardiogram support this conclusion?
    1. Irregular rhythm; abnormal shaped P wave; normal QRS
    2. Irregular rhythm; absence of a P wave; wide, distorted QRS
    3. Regular rhythm; more than 100 beats per minute; normal P wave; normal QRS
    4. Regular rhythm; 100 to 250 beats per minute; absent P wave; wide, distorted QRS

155. A female client tells the nurse that the physician just told her that her triglycerides and cholesterol are excessively elevated. The client appears discouraged and says, "Well, I guess I'd better cut out all the fat and cholesterol in my diet." Which is the nurse's most appropriate response?
    1. "Well, yes, that will certainly lower the amount of your blood fats."
    2. "That's good, but be sure to compensate by adding more carbohydrates."
    3. "You need some fat to supply the necessary fatty acids, so it's mainly just a need for cutting down the amount."
    4. "You need some cholesterol in your diet because your body cannot manufacture it, so just avoid excessive amounts."

156. The nurse concludes that the gradual occlusion of the internal or common carotid arteries, manifested by transient ischemic attacks, may occur because of:
    1. Acquired valvular heart disease
    2. Atherosclerosis of the vascular system
    3. Emboli associated with atrial fibrillation
    4. Developmental defects of the arterial wall

157. To help reduce a client's risk factors for heart disease, the nurse, when discussing dietary guidelines, teaches the client to:
    1. Avoid eating between meals
    2. Limit unsaturated fats in the diet
    3. Decrease the amount of fat-binding fiber
    4. Increase the quantity of complex carbohydrates

158. A client's diet is modified to eliminate foods that act as cardiac stimulants. What should the nurse teach this client to avoid? Select all that apply.
    1. _____ Iced tea
    2. _____ Red meat
    3. _____ Club soda
    4. _____ Hot cocoa
    5. _____ Chocolate pudding

159. A man is brought to the emergency department by coworkers and is admitted with a possible myocardial infarction. Several hours later the client is experiencing severe chest pain. He is diaphoretic, and his pulse rate is 110 beats per minute. The nurse should immediately:
    1. Increase the oxygen flow
    2. Obtain the blood pressure and an electrocardiogram
    3. Notify the practitioner and administer the ordered morphine
    4. Administer the ordered nitroglycerin tablet until the pain subsides

160. The nurse plans to teach a client receiving a 2g sodium-restricted diet that the foods lowest in sodium are:
    1. Meat and fish
    2. Fruits and juices
    3. Milk and cheese
    4. Dry cereals and grains

161. A 60-year-old client with a long history of cardiovascular problems, including angina and hypertension, is to have a cardiac catheterization. During precardiac catheterization teaching, the nurse explains to this client that the major purpose for this procedure is to:
    1. Obtain the pressures in the heart chambers
    2. Determine the existence of congenital heart disease
    3. Visualize the disease process in the coronary arteries
    4. Measure the oxygen content of various heart chambers

162. A client returns from a cardiac catheterization and is to remain in the supine position for 4 hours with the affected leg straight. These measures prevent:
    1. Orthostatic hypotension
    2. Headache with disorientation
    3. Bleeding at the arterial puncture site
    4. Infiltration of radiopaque dye into tissue

163. After a cardiac catheterization, the client complains of tingling sensations in the affected leg. The nurse should first:
    1. Assess for bleeding at the catheter insertion site
    2. Evaluate the affected leg for signs of inflammation
    3. Compare femoral, popliteal, and pedal pulses in both legs
    4. Obtain the temperature, pulse, respirations, and blood pressure

164. For which expected response should the nurse monitor a client after a cardiac catheterization?
    1. Marked increase in the volume of urine output
    2. Decrease in BP of 25% from precatheterization BP
    3. Complaints of heart pounding with mild chest discomfort
    4. Respiratory distress with an increase in respiratory rate more than 24 breaths per minute

165. For the first several hours after a cardiac catheterization, it is most essential for the nurse to:
    1. Monitor the client's apical pulse and blood pressure
    2. Keep the head of the client's bed elevated 45 degrees
    3. Encourage the client to cough and deep breathe every 2 hours
    4. Check the client's temperature every hour until it returns to normal

166. When developing a plan of care for a client who had a cardiac catheterization via a femoral insertion site, the nurse should include:
    1. Ambulating the client 2 hours after the procedure
    2. Checking the vital signs every 15 minutes for 8 hours
    3. Keeping the client NPO for 4 hours after the procedure
    4. Maintaining the supine position for a minimum of 4 hours

167. A 56-year-old housewife who has a history of angina is scheduled for a cardiac catheterization. Catheter entry will be through the femoral artery. The nurse informs the client that she will:
    1. Remain fully alert during the procedure
    2. Be able to ambulate shortly after the procedure
    3. Experience a feeling of warmth during the procedure
    4. Have to assume the semi-Fowler's position for 12 hours after the procedure

168. A nurse who is caring for a client experiencing anginal pain expects that it will be:
    1. Unchanged by rest
    2. Precipitated by light activity
    3. Described as a knifelike sharpness
    4. Relieved by sublingual nitroglycerin

169. A client with continuous blood loss becomes increasingly diaphoretic, clammy, and pale. The client's blood pressure falls to 90/60. What is the priority nursing intervention?
    1. Place the client in a reclining position
    2. Wait several hours before repositioning the client
    3. Assist the client to assume the semi-Fowler's position
    4. Determine which position is most comfortable for the client

170. An early finding that indicates that a client is hypertensive is:
    1. An extended Korotkoff sound
    2. An irregular pulse of 92 beats per minute
    3. A diastolic blood pressure that remains greater than 90 mm Hg
    4. A throbbing headache over the left eye when arising in the morning

171. A nurse is taking the blood pressure of a client with hypertension. The first sound is heard at 140 mm Hg, the second sound is a swishing sound heard at 130 mm Hg, then a tapping sound is heard at 100 mm Hg, a muffled sound is heard at 90 mm Hg, and the sound disappears at 72 mm Hg. When recording just the systolic and diastolic readings, what is the diastolic pressure?
    1. 72 mm Hg
    2. 90 mm Hg
    3. 100 mm Hg
    4. 130 mm Hg

172. An 82-year-old client, whose baseline blood pressure is 140/90 mm Hg, has the blood pressure taken by the home health nurse. The nurse obtains a sitting blood pressure of 160/100 mm Hg in the left arm. The nurse should initially:
    1. Advise the client to restrict fluid and sodium intake
    2. Call the practitioner and report the blood pressure reading immediately
    3. Understand the result is expected for an older adult and record the information
    4. Take the client's blood pressure in the right arm and then in both arms while standing

173. A businessman makes many long airplane trips. When talking with the occupational nurse he states that he is concerned because his legs swell on these long flights. The nurse should advise him to:
    1. Relax in a reclining position
    2. Sit upright with legs extended
    3. Walk about the cabin at least once every hour
    4. Sit in any position that relieves pressure on the legs

174. A client with a history of hypertension develops pedal edema and demonstrates dyspnea on exertion. The nurse concludes that this probably is:
    1. Caused by cor pulmonale
    2. The result of right atrial failure
    3. The result of left ventricular failure
    4. Associated with obstructive pulmonary disease

175. A client is admitted to the coronary care unit with a tentative diagnosis of myocardial infarction. What type of pain should the nurse expect the client to describe?
    1. Severe, intense chest pain
    2. Burning sensation of short duration
    3. Mild chest pain, radiating to the fingers
    4. Squeezing chest pain, relieved by nitroglycerin

176. A hospitalized client complains of chest pain that feels like a pressure or weight on the chest. The client also states, "I feel nauseated and very weak." The nurse should:
    1. Initiate a rapid response code
    2. Perform a nutritional assessment
    3. Discuss possible sources of stress with the client
    4. Provide reassurance while helping the client to focus on pleasant topics

177. A client, admitted to the cardiac care unit with a myocardial infarction, complains of chest pain. The nursing intervention most effective in relieving the client's pain is to administer the ordered:
    1. Morphine sulfate 2 mg IV
    2. Nitroglycerin sublingually
    3. Oxygen per nasal cannula
    4. Lidocaine hydrochloride 50 mg IV bolus

178. A nurse is teaching a client who has recovered from a myocardial infarction (MI) how to prevent an MI in the future. The nurse evaluates that further teaching is needed when the client states, "I will:
    1. restrict my physical activity."
    2. take one baby aspirin every day."
    3. continue my smoking cessation program."
    4. try to lose the extra weight I'm carrying around."

179. A client is admitted to the coronary care unit complaining of "viselike" chest pain radiating to the neck. Assessment reveals a blood pressure of 124/64, an irregular apical pulse of 64 beats per minute, and diaphoresis. Cardiac monitoring is instituted and morphine sulfate 4 mg IV push stat is ordered. The priority nursing care for this client is directed toward:
    1. Relief of pain
    2. Client teaching
    3. Cardiac monitoring
    4. Maintenance of bed rest

180. A male client who is hospitalized after a myocardial infarction asks the nurse why he is receiving morphine. The nurse replies that morphine:
    1. Dilates coronary blood vessels
    2. Relieves pain and prevents shock
    3. Decreases anxiety and restlessness
    4. Helps prevent fibrillation of the heart

181. A client who is being monitored in the coronary care unit because of a myocardial infarction has to have a bowel movement. The nurse should:
    1. Place the client on a bedpan
    2. Help the client into the bathroom
    3. Roll the client onto a fracture pan
    4. Assist the client to a bedside commode

182. A client who recently had a myocardial infarction is admitted to the cardiac care unit. The nurse can best determine the effectiveness of the client's ventricular contractions by:
    1. Observing anxiety levels
    2. Monitoring urinary output hourly
    3. Evaluating cardiac enzyme results
    4. Assessing breath sounds frequently

183. Isoenzyme laboratory studies are ordered for a client who is suspected of having a myocardial infarction. The most reliable early indicator of myocardial insult is:
    1. AST
    2. Myoglobin
    3. Troponin I and T
    4. CK-MB and CPK totals

184. A client who had a myocardial infarction develops cardiogenic shock despite treatment in the emergency department. Which client response is unrelated to cardiogenic shock?
    1. Tachycardia
    2. Restlessness
    3. Warm, moist skin
    4. Decreased urinary output

185. When a client has a myocardial infarction, one of the major manifestations is a decrease in the conductive energy provided to the heart. When assessing this client, the nurse is aware that the existing action potential is in direct relationship to the:
    1. Heart rate
    2. Refractory period
    3. Pulmonary pressure
    4. Strength of contraction

186. The possibility of death from complications always accompanies an acute myocardial infarction. The most serious complication the nurse monitors the client for during the first 48 hours is:
    1. Pulmonary edema
    2. Pulmonary embolism
    3. Ventricular tachycardia
    4. Failure of the right ventricle

187. A client is admitted to the hospital with the diagnosis of myocardial infarction. The nurse should monitor this client for the signs and symptoms associated with heart failure. Select all that apply.
    1. _____ Weight loss
    2. _____ Unusual fatigue
    3. _____ Dependent edema
    4. _____ Nocturnal dyspnea
    5. _____ Increased urinary output

188. A client who had a myocardial infarction experiences a noticeably decreased pulse pressure. The nurse determines that this is a possible indication of:
    1. Increased blood volume
    2. Hyperactivity of the heart
    3. Increased cardiac efficiency
    4. Decreased force of contraction

189. A client has mitral valve insufficiency (regurgitation). In which area should the stethoscope be placed when auscultating the heart to determine the presence of this problem?
    1. a
    2. b
    3. c
    4. d

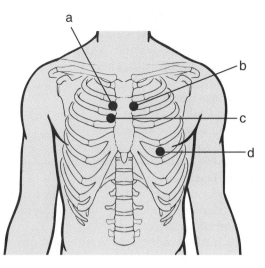

190. A nurse identifies premature ventricular complexes (PVCs) on a client's cardiac monitor and concludes that these complexes are a sign of:
    1. Atrial fibrillation
    2. Cardiac irritability
    3. Impending heart block
    4. Ventricular tachycardia

191. The wife of a client who had emergency coronary artery bypass surgery for the second time asks why her husband has a dressing on his left leg. The nurse explains that:
    1. This is the access site for the heart-lung machine
    2. A filter is inserted in the leg to prevent embolization
    3. A vein in the leg was used to bypass the coronary artery
    4. The arteries in the extremities are examined during surgery

192. A nurse is discussing discharge instructions with a client who had a coronary artery bypass graft (CABG). The client states, "My wife is afraid to have sex with me. When will it be safe to have sex again?" Which is the most appropriate response by the nurse?
    1. "You should wait at least 6 weeks, but check with your physician."
    2. "You will need to talk that over with your physician before you leave."
    3. "When you feel you have recovered enough to resume sexual activity."
    4. "As soon as you can climb one flight of stairs without fatigue or discomfort."

193. It is determined that a client with heart block will require implantation of a permanent pacemaker to assist heart function. The nurse's best response to the client's inquiry as to why a pacemaker is necessary is, "It will:
    1. stimulate a normal heartbeat."
    2. shock the AV node to contract."
    3. slow the heart to a more normal rate."
    4. synchronize action of the heart valves."

194. A client had a ventricular demand pacemaker inserted. The priority nursing intervention immediately after the procedure is to:
    1. Encourage fluids
    2. Assess the implant site
    3. Monitor the heart rate and rhythm
    4. Encourage turning and deep breathing

195. A client's wife arrives at the cardiac care unit and is informed that her husband needs a pacemaker. The wife expresses the concern that her husband could accidentally become electrocuted. The nurse's best response is:
    1. "No one has been electrocuted yet by a pacemaker."
    2. "New technology prevents electrocution from occurring."
    3. "The pacemaker is pretested for safety before it is inserted."
    4. "The voltage emitted is not strong enough to electrocute him."

196. While obtaining a health history, a nurse expects a 78-year-old client admitted to the hospital with chronic heart failure to report a:
    1. Tingling in the upper extremities
    2. Feeling of being bloated after eating
    3. Need to use three pillows at night to sleep
    4. Swelling of the ankles more apparent in the morning

197. A client with a history of hypertension and left ventricular failure arrives for a scheduled clinic appointment and tells the nurse, "My feet are killing me. These shoes got so tight." The nurse's best initial action is to:
    1. Weigh the client
    2. Notify the practitioner
    3. Take the client's pulse rate
    4. Listen to the client's breath sounds

198. A client is admitted with early heart failure. The statement by the client that is uniquely related to heart failure that the nurse can expect is:
    1. "I see spots before my eyes."
    2. "I am tired at the end of the day."
    3. "I feel bloated when I eat a large meal."
    4. "I have trouble breathing when I climb a flight of stairs."

199. Which clinical finding is unexpected when performing a physical assessment of a client with heart failure?
    1. Dependent edema
    2. Progressive fatigue
    3. Moist, clammy skin
    4. Collapsed neck veins

200. The nurse teaches a client that heart failure can best be described as:
    1. A cardiac condition caused by inadequate circulating blood volume
    2. An acute state in which the pulmonary circulation pressure decreases
    3. An inability of the heart to pump blood in proportion to metabolic needs
    4. A chronic state in which the systolic blood pressure drops below 90 mm Hg

201. A 76-year-old client is admitted with the diagnosis of mild chronic heart failure. The sounds indicative of chronic heart failure that the nurse expects to hear when listening to the client's lungs are:
   1. Stridor
   2. Crackles
   3. Wheezes
   4. Friction rubs

202. When assessing a client with the diagnosis of left ventricular failure, the nurse expects to identify:
   1. Crushing chest pain
   2. Dyspnea on exertion
   3. Jugular vein distention
   4. Extensive peripheral edema

203. The teaching plan for a client receiving digoxin for left ventricular failure should include having the client:
   1. Sleep flat in bed
   2. Rest during the day
   3. Follow a low-potassium diet
   4. Take the pulse three times a day

204. A client is admitted to the intensive care unit in pulmonary edema. What should the nurse expect when performing the admission assessment?
   1. Weak rapid pulse
   2. Decreased blood pressure
   3. Radiating anterior chest pain
   4. Crackles at the base of each lung

205. The practitioner prescribes "bathroom privileges only" for a client with pulmonary edema. The client becomes irritable and asks the nurse whether it is really necessary to stay in bed so much. The nurse's best reply is:
   1. "Why do you want to be out of bed?"
   2. "Bed rest plays a role in most therapy."
   3. "Rest helps your body direct energy to healing."
   4. "Would you like me to ask your physician to change the order?"

206. The nurse is assessing a client for signs of right ventricular failure. What should the nurse expect if this occurs?
   1. Slowed pulse rate
   2. Pleural friction rub
   3. Neck vein distention
   4. Increasing hypotension

207. A nurse suggests that a client with right ventricular failure should:
   1. Take a hot bath before bedtime
   2. Avoid emotionally stressful situations
   3. Avoid sleeping in an air-conditioned room
   4. Exercise daily until the pulse rate exceeds 100 beats per minute

208. A client is admitted to the medical unit with a diagnosis of right ventricular heart failure. The nursing assessment that supports this medical diagnosis is:
   1. Nocturnal orthopnea
   2. Distended jugular veins
   3. Shortness of breath on exertion
   4. Decreased arterial blood pressure

209. A home health care nurse is assessing a client with cardiac insufficiency. The nurse identifies that the client's pulse rate increases from 70 to 92 beats per minute while climbing the stairs. The nurse should instruct the client to:
   1. Continue climbing
   2. Stand still and rest
   3. Walk down the stairs
   4. Climb but at a slower rate

210. Which client is considered at the highest risk for a dissecting aneurysm?
   1. 50-year-old white male with moderate hypertension
   2. 55-year-old black male with uncontrolled hypertension
   3. 40-year-old white female with uncontrolled hypertension
   4. 42-year-old black female with peripheral vascular disease

211. During a routine physical examination, an abdominal aortic aneurysm is diagnosed. The client immediately is admitted to the hospital, and surgery is scheduled for the next morning. Which clinical finding should the nurse expect when performing an assessment of this client?
   1. Severe radiating abdominal pain
   2. Pattern of visible peristaltic waves
   3. Palpable pulsating abdominal mass
   4. Cyanosis with other symptoms of shock

212. On the morning of surgery a client is admitted for resection of an abdominal aortic aneurysm. While awaiting surgery, the client suddenly develops symptoms of shock. The nurse should:
   1. Prepare for blood transfusions
   2. Notify the surgeon immediately
   3. Give the client nothing by mouth
   4. Administer the prescribed sedative

213. Postoperatively, a client asks, "Could I have a pillow under my knees? My legs feel stretched." The nurse can best reinforce the preoperative teaching by responding:
   1. "I'll get pillows for you. I want you to be as rested as possible."
   2. "It's not a good idea, but you do look uncomfortable. I'll get one."
   3. "We don't allow pillows under the legs because you will get too warm."
   4. "A pillow under the knees can result in clot formation because it slows blood flow."

214. To prevent thrombus formation after most surgeries, the nurse should plan to:
   1. Keep the client's bed gatched to elevate the knees
   2. Have the client dangle the legs off the side of the bed
   3. Have the client use an incentive spirometer every hour
   4. Encourage the client to ambulate with assistance every few hours

215. The clinical finding the nurse expects when assessing a client with severe varicosities of both legs is:
    1. Increased sensitivity to cold
    2. Pallor of the lower extremities
    3. Increasing ankle edema over the day
    4. Calf pain when the foot is dorsiflexed

216. When collecting data from a client with varicose veins who is to have sclerotherapy, the nurse expects the client to report:
    1. Feelings of heaviness in both legs
    2. Intermittent claudication of the legs
    3. Calf pain on dorsiflexion of the foot
    4. Hematomas of the lower extremities

217. Before having sclerotherapy for varicose veins, a female client who states she is fearful of a chemical injection asks the nurse to explain what is involved if she insisted on a ligation and stripping to correct the problem. The nurse explains that this surgery involves:
    1. Removing the dilated saphenous veins
    2. Cleaning out plaque from within the veins
    3. Anastomosing superficial veins to deep veins
    4. Placing an umbrella filter in the large affected veins

218. A client with a history of thrombophlebitis and varicosities is to have a herniorrhaphy for an incarcerated hernia. What primary nursing action should be implemented postoperatively considering the client's medical history?
    1. Raise the foot of the bed
    2. Help the client to dangle and get out of bed twice daily
    3. Encourage the client to turn often and to exercise the legs regularly
    4. Maintain the body in alignment with firm support of the extremities

219. After a long history of recurrent thrombophlebitis with extensive varicose veins of the lower extremities, surgical intervention is suggested to the client. When asked about the procedure, the nurse explains that this surgery involves:
    1. Removing the dilated superficial veins
    2. Bypassing the varicosities with artificial veins
    3. Stripping the cholesterol deposits from the veins
    4. Creating fistulas between superficial and deep veins

220. Before discharging a client who had an inguinal herniorrhaphy, the nurse teaches the client about exercising to prevent venous stasis. For best results the nurse should:
    1. Demonstrate specific exercises
    2. Suggest frequent moving of the legs
    3. Advise against sitting for prolonged periods
    4. Suggest that the client change position frequently

221. A client with extensive bone and soft tissue injuries to the right leg is on bed rest. When positioning the affected extremity, the nurse should:
    1. Keep the right leg resting straight on the bed, parallel to the left leg
    2. Elevate the entire right leg with pillows, keeping the foot higher than the knee

    3. Maintain both legs on the bed and use an abduction pillow to keep them separated
    4. Attach a padded ankle sling to a Balkan frame to support the right foot and elevate the leg

222. A client reports a history of bilateral blanching and pain in the fingers on exposure to cold. When rewarmed, the fingers become bright red and "tingly" with a slow return to their usual color. The client smokes one to two packs of cigarettes per day. The nurse determines that the client has Raynaud's disease and not Raynaud's phenomenon because of the:
    1. Tingling sensation
    2. Skin color changes
    3. Bilateral involvement
    4. Changes in skin temperature

223. The nurse encourages a client with Raynaud's disease to stop smoking because it causes:
    1. Pain and tingling
    2. Cyanosis and necrosis
    3. Peripheral vasoconstriction
    4. Excessive blood oxygen content

224. A 60-year-old man, who for 40 years drank two alcoholic beverages and smoked two packs of cigarettes daily, comes to the outpatient clinic with an ischemic left foot. It is determined that the cause is arterial insufficiency. The client needs to understand that the pain in his foot is a result of inadequate blood supply, which may be further diminished by:
    1. Drinking alcohol
    2. Lowering the limb
    3. Smoking cigarettes
    4. Consuming excessive fluid

225. A client with arterial insufficiency of both lower extremities is visited by the home health care nurse. An essential nursing intervention is to teach the client to:
    1. Maintain elevation of both legs
    2. Massage the legs when painful
    3. Apply a hot water bottle to the legs
    4. Check arterial pulses in the legs regularly

226. A 55-year-old male bank teller, with a history of occasional pain in the left foot when walking, now has pain at rest. The left foot is cyanotic, numb, and painful. The suspected cause is arteriosclerosis. The nurse teaches the client that the pain in the foot is more likely to decrease if he:
    1. Keeps the left foot cool
    2. Crosses his legs with the left one on top
    3. Complies with the prescribed exercise program
    4. Keeps the foot elevated at a thirty-degree angle

227. When supporting vasodilation by the use of warmth for a client with peripheral arterial insufficiency, the nurse cautions the client to avoid:
    1. Applying a hot water bottle to the abdomen
    2. Using a heating pad to warm the extremities
    3. Drinking a warm cup of tea when feeling chilly
    4. Turning the room thermostat above seventy two degrees

228. A client develops a nonhealing ulcer of the right lower extremity and complains of leg cramps after walking short distances. The client asks the nurse what causes these leg pains. The nurse's best response is:
   1. "Muscle weakness occurs in the legs because of a lack of exercise."
   2. "Edema and cyanosis occur in the legs because they are dependent."
   3. "Pain occurs in the legs while walking because there is a lack of oxygen to the muscles."
   4. "Pressure occurs in the legs because of vasodilation and pooling of blood in the extremity."

229. The practitioner prescribes a progressive exercise program that includes walking for a client with a history of diminished arterial perfusion to the lower extremities. The nurse explains to the client that if leg cramps occur while walking, the client should:
   1. Take one aspirin twice a day
   2. Stop to rest until the pain resolves
   3. Walk more slowly while pain is present
   4. Take one nitroglycerin tablet sublingually

230. A client with peripheral arterial insufficiency is to have surgery. On admission, the client complains of discomfort and aches in the legs and feet. To safely position this client the nurse takes into consideration that the feet and legs should be:
   1. Placed dependent to the torso
   2. Dependent by using a fully extended knee gatch
   3. Raised to a two-pillow height above the buttocks
   4. Elevated by raising the foot of the bed on blocks

231. A client comes to the outpatient clinic with a large leg ulcer. The clinical finding that supports the diagnosis of arterial ulcer is:
   1. Pain at the ulcer site
   2. Bleeding around the ulcer area
   3. Dependent edema of the extremities
   4. Stasis dermatitis on the affected extremity

232. A male client is admitted to the hospital with a large leg ulcer, and a femoral angiogram is performed. After this procedure the nurse should:
   1. Provide passive ROM to all extremities
   2. Elevate the foot of the bed for 36 hours
   3. Assist the client to stand if unable to void
   4. Apply pressure to the catheter insertion site

233. The nurse is caring for a client who has an occlusion of the left femoral artery and is scheduled for an arteriogram. Which sign is most significant when assessing the extremity before the arteriogram?
   1. Mottling of the left leg
   2. Coolness of the left foot
   3. Absence of the left pedal pulse
   4. Thickening of the toenails on the left foot

234. Before a femoral arteriogram is started, the nurse plans to teach the client that:
   1. Radioactive dye will be injected into the femoral vein
   2. Local anesthesia will be used to lessen any pain at the site

3. Contrast media will be injected into a small vessel of the foot
4. Medication will be administered intravenously to induce sleep

235. Six hours after a femoropopliteal bypass graft, the client's blood pressure becomes severely elevated. The nurse notifies the surgeon primarily because the client's:
   1. Blood pressure can cause the graft to occlude
   2. Hypervolemia needs to be corrected immediately
   3. Cardiovascular status can precipitate a brain attack
   4. Intra-arterial pressure may compromise the graft's viability

236. A client with a history of severe intermittent claudication has a femoropopliteal bypass graft. An appropriate postoperative intervention on the day after surgery is to:
   1. Keep the client on bed rest
   2. Have the client sit in a chair
   3. Assist the client with ambulation
   4. Encourage the client to keep the legs elevated

237. A client with peripheral arterial insufficiency tells the nurse that walking sometimes results in severe pain in the calf muscles. The nurse responds that this pain is called:
   1. Rest pain
   2. Intermittent claudication
   3. Phantom limb sensation
   4. Raynaud's phenomenon

238. The nurse provides discharge teaching for a client with a history of hypertension who had a femoropopliteal bypass graft. The nurse evaluates that the teaching is effective when the client says, "I should:
   1. massage my calves and feet every day."
   2. keep my foot elevated when I am in bed."
   3. sit in a hot bath for half an hour twice a day."
   4. assess the color and pulses of my legs every day."

239. The nurse administers oxygen to a client during the early postoperative period after open heart surgery. Why is this necessary?
   1. Clients have closed-chest drainage in place
   2. Hypoxia can precipitate respiratory alkalosis
   3. Reduced oxygen levels can stimulate dysrhythmias
   4. Increased respiratory rates add to postoperative pain

240. The nurse in the ICU is monitoring a client who had an aortic valve replacement. A slow pulse rate during the early postoperative period after open heart surgery can indicate:
   1. Shock
   2. Hypoxia
   3. Heart block
   4. Cardiac failure

ENDOCRINE

241. A 62-year-old client is admitted for hypertension, and serum electrolyte studies have yielded abnormal results. The scheduled workup includes a scan for an

aldosteronoma. The nurse concludes that this scan is ordered to rule out disease of the:

1. Kidney cortex
2. Thyroid gland
3. Pituitary gland
4. Adrenal cortex

242. A client with an aldosterone-secreting adenoma is scheduled for surgery to remove the tumor. The client wonders what will happen if surgery is canceled. The nurse bases a response on the fact that:

1. Heart and kidney damage may occur if the tumor is not removed
2. Surgery will prevent the tumor from metastasizing to other organs
3. Chemotherapy is as reliable as surgery to treat adenomas of this type
4. Radiation therapy or surgery can be just as effective if the tumor is small

243. Late in the postoperative period after resection of an aldosterone-secreting adenoma, the nurse expects the client's blood pressure to:

1. Gradually return to near normal levels
2. Rise quickly above the preoperative level
3. Fluctuate greatly during this entire period
4. Drop very low, then increase rapidly to normal levels

244. The wife of a client who has had a resection of an aldosterone-secreting tumor of an adrenal gland says, "I hope this is the end of the problem and that my husband will be back to work soon." Based on an understanding of the health problem, the nurse should:

1. Caution the wife about high expectations because the outcome for this problem is variable
2. Explain that surgery will effect a cure because the remaining adrenal gland will meet the body's needs
3. Advise the wife to investigate other occupational alternatives for her husband if he plans to return to work
4. Tell her that although her husband will require hormone supplements for the rest of his life, he should be able to work

245. The nurse expects the diagnostic studies of a client with Cushing's syndrome to indicate:

1. Moderately increased serum potassium levels
2. Increased numbers of eosinophils in the blood
3. High levels of 17-ketosteroids in a 24-hour urine test
4. Normal to low levels of adrenocorticotropic hormone (ACTH)

246. A female client has a tentative diagnosis of Cushing's syndrome. The nurse's physical assessment of this client probably will reveal the presence of:

1. Fever and tachycardia
2. Lethargy and constipation
3. Hypertension and moon face
4. Hyperactivity and exophthalmos

247. A 49-year-old female is admitted to the hospital with a possible diagnosis of Addison's disease. What is an important nursing responsibility during a 24-hour urine collection for the client suspected of having Addison's disease?

1. Keep the client quiet and reduce stress
2. Assess the client for signs and symptoms of edema
3. Monitor the client for an elevation in blood pressure
4. Restrict the client's fluid intake during the day of the test

248. A female college freshman visits the health center because she feels nervous, irritable, and extremely tired. She complains that, although she eats large amounts of food, she has frequent bouts of diarrhea and is losing weight. The nurse observes a fine hand tremor, an exaggerated reaction to external stimuli, and a wide-eyed expression. What laboratory tests may be ordered to determine the cause of these signs and symptoms?

1. PTT and PT
2. T_3, T_4, and TSH
3. VDRL and CBC
4. ACTH, ADH and CRF

249. During a home visit to a client, the nurse identifies tremors of the client's hands. When discussing this assessment, the client reports being nervous, having difficulty sleeping, and feeling as if the collars of shirts are getting tight. Which problem should be reported to the practitioner?

1. Increased appetite
2. Recent weight loss
3. Feelings of warmth
4. Fluttering in the chest

250. A client visits the clinic because of concerns about insomnia and recent weight loss. A tentative diagnosis of hyperthyroidism is made. In addition to these changes, the nurse further assesses this client for:

1. Fatigue
2. Dry skin
3. Anorexia
4. Bradycardia

251. Before obtaining blood for protein-bound iodine, T_3, and T_4 tests the nurse should ask a client, suspected of having a hyperactive thyroid, if the client has had:

1. Allergies to seafood
2. More protein intake than usual
3. Anything to drink before the test
4. Recent x-rays using radiopaque dye

252. When assessing a client with Graves' disease, the nurse expects to identify:

1. Constipation, dry skin, and weight gain
2. Lethargy, weight gain, and forgetfulness
3. Weight loss, exophthalmos, and restlessness
4. Weight loss, protruding eyeballs, and lethargy

253. When assessing a female client with Graves' disease (hyperthyroidism) the nurse expects to identify a history of:

1. Diaphoresis
2. Menorrhagia
3. Dry, brittle hair
4. Sensitivity to cold

254. The nurse teaches a client with exophthalmos how to reduce discomfort and prevent corneal ulceration. The nurse evaluates that the teaching is understood when the client states, "I should:
    1. eliminate excessive blinking."
    2. not move my extraocular muscles."
    3. elevate the head of my bed at night."
    4. avoid using a sleeping mask at night."

255. A client is scheduled to have a thyroidectomy for cancer of the thyroid. Preoperative instructions for the postoperative period include teaching the client to:
    1. Cough and deep breathe every two hours
    2. Perform range-of-motion exercises of the head and neck
    3. Support the head with the hands when changing position
    4. Apply gentle pressure against the incision when swallowing

256. A client is diagnosed with hyperthyroidism and surgery is scheduled because the client refuses ablation therapy. While awaiting the surgical date, the nurse plans to instruct the client to:
    1. Consciously attempt to calm down
    2. Eliminate coffee, tea, and cola from the diet
    3. Keep the home warm and use an extra blanket at night
    4. Schedule activities during the day to overcome lethargy

257. A client with cancer of the thyroid is scheduled for a thyroidectomy. Postoperatively the nurse plans to have a:
    1. Quiet, dimly lit room for the client
    2. Tracheostomy set at the client's bedside
    3. Large soft pillow for use under the client's head
    4. Suction machine set on intermittent suction at the client's bedside

258. A client with malignant hot nodules of the thyroid gland has a thyroidectomy. Immediately after the thyroidectomy, the nurse's priority action for this client is to:
    1. Place in low-Fowler's position to limit edema of the neck
    2. Monitor intake and output strictly to assess for fluid overload
    3. Encourage coughing and deep breathing to prevent atelectasis
    4. Assess level of consciousness to determine recovery from anesthesia

259. Immediately after a subtotal thyroidectomy the nurse plans to assess a female client for unilateral injury of the laryngeal nerve every 30 to 60 minutes by:
    1. Checking the throat for edema
    2. Asking her to state her name out loud
    3. Eliciting spasms of her facial muscles
    4. Palpating the neck for seepage of blood

260. When providing care for a client in the first 24 hours after a thyroidectomy, the nurse includes:
    1. Checking the back and sides of the operative site
    2. Supporting the head during mild range-of-motion exercises

    3. Encouraging the client to ventilate feelings about the surgery
    4. Advising the client that regular activities can be resumed immediately

261. During the early postoperative period after a subtotal thyroidectomy, the concern that has the priority is:
    1. Hemorrhage
    2. Thyrotoxic crisis
    3. Airway obstruction
    4. Hypocalcemic tetany

262. On the third postoperative day after a subtotal thyroidectomy for a tumor, a client complains of a "funny, jittery feeling." On the basis of this statement, the nurse's best action is to:
    1. Explain that this reaction is expected and not a concern
    2. Take the vital signs and place the client in a high-Fowler's position
    3. Request stat serum calcium and phosphorus levels and chart the results
    4. Test for Chvostek's and Trousseau's signs and notify the practitioner of the complaints

263. After a thyroidectomy a client should be monitored for thyrotoxic crisis, which is evidenced by:
    1. An increased pulse deficit
    2. A decreased blood pressure
    3. A decreased heart rate and respirations
    4. An increased temperature and pulse rate

264. After treatment with propylthiouracil for hyperthyroidism, a client has the thyroid ablated with ^{131}I. On a visit to the endocrine clinic, the client exhibits signs and symptoms of thyrotoxic crisis (thyroid storm). What is often associated with thyrotoxic crisis?
    1. Deficiency of iodine
    2. Decreased serum calcium
    3. Increased sodium retention
    4. Excessive hormone replacement

265. While assessing a client during a routine examination, a nurse in the clinic identifies signs and symptoms of hyperthyroidism. Which signs are characteristic of hyperthyroidism? Select all that apply.
    1. _____ Diaphoresis
    2. _____ Weight loss
    3. _____ Constipation
    4. _____ Protruding eyes
    5. _____ Cold intolerance

266. When preparing a client for discharge after a thyroidectomy, the nurse teaches the signs of hypothyroidism. The nurse evaluates that the client understands the teaching when the client says, "I should call my physician if I develop:
    1. dry hair and an intolerance to cold."
    2. muscle cramping and sluggishness."
    3. fatigue and an increased pulse rate."
    4. tachycardia and an increase in weight."

267. A client who has had a subtotal thyroidectomy does not understand how hypothyroidism can develop when the

problem was initially hyperthyroidism. The nurse bases a response on the fact that:

1. Hypothyroidism is a gradual slowing of the body's function
2. There will be a decrease in pituitary thyroid-stimulating hormone
3. There may not be enough thyroid tissue to supply adequate thyroid hormone
4. Atrophy of tissue remaining after surgery reduces secretion of thyroid hormones

268. A nurse teaches a client, who has had a thyroidectomy for thyroid cancer, to observe for signs of surgically induced hypothyroidism. What should be included in the teaching plan? Select all that apply.
   1. _____ Dry skin
   2. _____ Lethargy
   3. _____ Insomnia
   4. _____ Tachycardia
   5. _____ Sensitivity to cold

269. When obtaining a health history from a client recently diagnosed with type 1 diabetes, the nurse expects the client to report the classic signs of diabetes, which are:
   1. Irritability, polydipsia, polyuria
   2. Polyuria, polydipsia, polyphagia
   3. Nocturia, weight loss, polydipsia
   4. Polyphagia, polyuria, diaphoresis

270. When obtaining the history of a 24-year-old graduate student recently diagnosed with type 1 diabetes, the nurse expects to identify the presence of:
   1. Edema
   2. Anorexia
   3. Weight loss
   4. Hypoglycemic episodes

271. A client has recently been diagnosed with type 1 diabetes. A glucose tolerance test is ordered. The order reads, "Administer glucose 1g/kg." The client weighs 240 pounds. How much glucose should the nurse administer?
   1. 100 grams
   2. 109 grams
   3. 115 grams
   4. 118 grams

272. The practitioner orders daily fasting blood glucose levels for a client with diabetes mellitus. The goal of treatment is that the client will have glucose levels within the range of:
   1. 40 to 65 mg/dL of blood
   2. 70 to 105 mg/dL of blood
   3. 110 to 145 mg/dL of blood
   4. 150 to 175 mg/dL of blood

273. When assessing the laboratory values of a client with type 2 diabetes, the nurse expects the results to reveal:
   1. Ketones in the blood but not the urine
   2. Glucose in the urine but not in the blood
   3. Urine and blood positive for glucose and ketones
   4. Urine negative for ketones and glucose in the blood

274. A nurse explains to a client with diabetes that self-monitoring of blood glucose is preferred to urine glucose testing because it is:
   1. More accurate
   2. Easier to perform
   3. Done by the client
   4. Not influenced by drugs

275. A client is diagnosed as having type 2 diabetes. A priority teaching goal is, "The client will be able to:
   1. perform foot care daily."
   2. administer insulin as ordered."
   3. test urine for both sugar and acetone."
   4. identify pending hypoglycemia or hyperglycemia."

276. A nurse teaches a client with type 2 diabetes how to provide self-care to prevent infections of the feet. The nurse evaluates that the teaching was effective when the client says, "I should:
   1. massage my feet and legs with oil or lotion."
   2. apply heat intermittently to my feet and legs."
   3. eat foods high in protein and carbohydrate kilocalories."
   4. control my blood glucose with diet, exercise, and medication."

277. A 25-year-old physical fitness instructor is feeling increasingly tired and seeks medical care. Type 1 diabetes is diagnosed. The nurse explains that the increased fatigue is the result of:
   1. Increased metabolism at the cellular level
   2. Increased glucose absorption from the intestine
   3. Decreased production of insulin by the pancreas
   4. Decreased glucose secretion into the renal tubules

278. A client newly diagnosed as having type 1 diabetes is taught to exercise on a regular basis primarily because exercise has been shown to:
   1. Decrease insulin sensitivity
   2. Stimulate glucagon production
   3. Improve the cellular uptake of glucose
   4. Reduce metabolic requirements for glucose

279. A client with type 2 diabetes is taking one oral hypoglycemic tablet daily. The client asks whether an extra pill should be taken before exercise. The best response by the nurse is:
   1. "You will need to decrease your exercise."
   2. "An extra pill will help your body use glucose correctly."
   3. "When taking medicine your diet will not be affected by exercise."
   4. "No, but you should observe for signs of hypoglycemia while exercising."

280. A client who is taking an oral hypoglycemic daily for type 2 diabetes develops the flu and is concerned about the need for special care. The nurse advises the client to:
   1. Skip the oral hypoglycemic pill, drink plenty of fluids, and stay in bed
   2. Avoid food, drink clear liquids, take a daily temperature, and stay in bed

3. Eat as much as possible, increase fluid intake, and call the office again the next day
4. Take the oral hypoglycemic pill, drink warm fluids, and perform a serum glucose test before meals and at hour of sleep

281. An obese client with type 2 diabetes asks about the intake of alcohol or special "dietetic" food in the diet. The nurse teaches the client that:
1. Alcohol can be used, with its calories counted in the diet
2. Unlimited amounts of sugar substitutes can be used as desired
3. Alcohol should not be used in cooking because it adds too many calories
4. Special "dietetic" foods are needed because many regular foods cannot be used

282. A client with type 2 diabetes travels frequently and asks how to plan meals during trips. The nurse's most appropriate response is:
1. "You can order diabetic foods on most airlines and in restaurants."
2. "You should plan your food ahead and carry it with you from home."
3. "You can monitor your blood glucose level frequently and can eat accordingly."
4. "You should make regular food choices and follow your food plan wherever you are."

283. A client with newly diagnosed diabetes indicates a hatred for asparagus, broccoli, and mushrooms. When reviewing the exchange list with the client, the nurse evaluates that the teaching about the exchange list is understood when the client states, "Instead of these foods I can eat:
1. string beans, beets, or carrots."
2. corn, lima beans, or dried peas."
3. baked beans, potatoes, or parsnips."
4. corn muffins, corn chips, or pretzels."

284. While hospitalized, a client with diabetes is observed picking at calluses on the feet. The nurse should immediately:
1. Warn the client of the danger of infection
2. Suggest that the client wear white cotton socks
3. Teach the client the importance of effective foot care
4. Check the client's shoes for their fit in the area of the calluses

285. After a surgical procedure for cancer of the pancreas that included the removal of the stomach, the head of the pancreas, the distal end of the duodenum, and the spleen, the postoperative manifestation by the client that requires immediate attention by the nurse is:
1. Jaundice
2. Indigestion
3. Weight loss
4. Hyperglycemia

286. Four hours after surgery the blood glucose level of a client who has type 1 diabetes is elevated. The nurse can expect to:
1. Administer an oral hypoglycemic
2. Institute urine glucose monitoring

3. Give supplemental doses of regular insulin
4. Decrease the rate of the intravenous infusion

287. A client who has type 1 diabetes is admitted to the hospital for major surgery. Before surgery the client's insulin requirements are elevated but well controlled. Postoperatively, the nurse anticipates that the client's insulin requirements will:
1. Decrease
2. Fluctuate
3. Increase sharply
4. Remain elevated

288. A client is admitted to the hospital with diabetic ketoacidosis. The nurse identifies that the elevated ketone level present with this disorder is caused by the incomplete oxidation of:
1. Fats
2. Protein
3. Potassium
4. Carbohydrates

289. The serum potassium level of a client who has diabetic ketoacidosis is 5.4 mEq/L. When monitoring the ECG tracing, the nurse expects to observe:
1. Abnormal P waves and depressed T waves
2. Peaked T waves and widened QRS complexes
3. Abnormal Q waves and prolonged ST segments
4. Peaked P waves and an increased number of T waves

290. A client with type 1 diabetes is placed on an insulin pump. The most appropriate short-term goal when teaching this client to control the diabetes is: "The client will:
1. adhere to the medical regimen."
2. remain normoglycemic for 3 weeks."
3. demonstrate the correct use of the administration equipment."
4. list 3 self-care activities that are necessary to control the diabetes."

291. When a nurse plans to teach a client with type 1 diabetes about the use of an insulin pump, it is of major importance that the client understand that the:
1. Insulin pump's needle should be changed every day
2. Pump is an attempt to mimic the way a healthy pancreas works
3. Pump will be implanted in a subcutaneous pocket near the abdomen
4. Insulin pump's advantage is that it requires glucose monitoring once a day

292. Which is the best advice regarding foot care to give a client with the diagnosis of diabetes?
1. Remove corns on the feet
2. Wear shoes that are larger than the feet
3. Examine the feet weekly for potential sores
4. Wear synthetic fiber socks when exercising

293. A client with type 1 diabetes of long duration takes Novolin 70/30 (combination of Novolin N 70% and Novolin R 30%) every morning. At noon, before eating lunch, the client is admitted to the emergency department with an acute myocardial infarction. Two hours

later the client's serum glucose level drops to 30 mg/dL, and insulin coma is diagnosed. The nurse concludes that the reason for the development of acute hypoglycemia in this client is that:

1. Glycogenolysis increased when lunch was not eaten after taking Novolin N insulin
2. The stress brought on by the chest pain increases the use of serum glucose available to the client
3. Glucose levels that are controlled by insulin drop more quickly than those controlled by oral antidiabetics
4. The client's body became sensitive to the prescribed dose of insulin after long use causing blood glucose levels to drop erratically

294. When assisting a client with type 1 diabetes, the nurse identifies a 5-cm nodule on the upper arm, where the client states she has been injecting her insulin at home. The nurse concludes that the nodule, which is neither warm nor painful, is a result of:

1. Keratosis
2. An allergy
3. An infection
4. Lipodystrophy

295. The nurse concludes that a client with type 1 diabetes is experiencing hypoglycemia. Which responses support this conclusion? Select all that apply.

1. _____ Vomiting
2. _____ Headache
3. _____ Tachycardia
4. _____ Cool clammy skin
5. _____ Increased respirations

296. A client with diabetic ketoacidosis, who is receiving intravenous fluids and insulin, complains of tingling and numbness of the fingers and toes and shortness of breath. The cardiac monitor shows the appearance of a U wave. The nurse concludes that these symptoms indicate:

1. Hypokalemia
2. Hypoglycemia
3. Hypernatremia
4. Hypercalcemia

297. A nurse evaluates that a client with diabetes understands the teaching about the treatment of hypoglycemia when the client says, "If I become hypoglycemic I should initially eat:

1. fruit juice and a lollipop."
2. sugar and a slice of bread."
3. chocolate candy and a banana."
4. peanut butter crackers and a glass of milk."

FLUIDS AND ELECTROLYTES

298. During an 8-hour shift a client drinks two 6-ounce cups of tea and vomits 125 mL of fluid. Intravenous fluids absorbed equaled the urinary output. What is the client's fluid balance during this 8-hour period?

1. 125 mL
2. 235 mL

3. 360 mL
4. 485 mL

299. At 10 AM the nurse hangs a 1000 mL bag of D_5W with 20 mEq of potassium chloride to be administered at 80 mL/hr. At noon the practitioner orders a stat infusion of an IV antibiotic of 100 mL to be administered via piggyback over 1 hour. How much later than expected will it take the primary bag to empty if the nurse interrupts the primary infusion to use the circulatory access for the secondary infusion of the antibiotic?

1. ¼ hour
2. ½ hour
3. ¾ hour
4. 1 hour

300. A client weighs 210 pounds on admission to the hospital. After 2 days of diuretic therapy the client weighs 205.5 pounds. The nurse estimates that the amount of fluid the client has lost is:

1. 2.0 L
2. 0.5 L
3. 1.0 L
4. 3.5 L

301. A male client with a history of heart failure and atrial fibrillation comes to the clinic for his regular 2-week visit. The client is 9 pounds heavier than his usual weight. The nurse interprets that the most likely cause of this sudden weight gain is:

1. Fluid retention
2. Urinary retention
3. Renal insufficiency
4. Abdominal distention

302. The dietary practice that helps a client to reduce the dietary intake of sodium is:

1. Avoiding carbonated beverages
2. Using steak sauce for flavoring foods
3. Increasing the intake of dairy products
4. Restricting the use of artificial sweeteners

303. An ECG is performed before a client is to have a cardiac catheterization, and hypokalemia is suspected. To confirm the presence of hypokalemia, the nurse expects the practitioner to order:

1. A complete blood count
2. A serum electrolyte level
3. An arterial blood gas panel
4. An x-ray film of long bones

304. A practitioner orders 1000 mL TPN to be infused over 12 hours via a subclavian catheter. When preparing the equipment it is most important for the nurse to obtain:

1. A steady IV pole
2. An infusion pump
3. An infusion set delivering 60 gtt/mL
4. A set of hemostats taped at the bedside

305. An 85-year-old frail woman has had nausea, vomiting, and diarrhea for several days. When she becomes weak and confused she is admitted to the hospital. To

best monitor the client's rehydration status, the nurse should assess the client's:
1. Skin turgor
2. Daily weight
3. Urinary output
4. Mucous membranes

306. When evaluating a client's response to fluid replacement therapy, the clinical finding that indicates adequate tissue perfusion to vital organs is:
1. Urinary output of 30 mL/hr
2. Central venous pressure reading of 2 cm H_2O
3. Pulse rates of 120 and 110 in a 15 minute period
4. Blood pressure readings of 50/30 and 70/40 mm Hg within 30 minutes

307. A practitioner orders total parenteral nutrition for a client with cancer of the pancreas. A right subclavian catheter is inserted. The nurse determines that the most important reason for using a central line is that:
1. It permits free use of the hands
2. It prevents the development of phlebitis
3. The chance of the infusion infiltrating is decreased
4. The amount of blood in a major vein helps to dilute the solution

308. When administering albumin intravenously, the nurse considers that body water will shift from the:
1. Interstitial compartment to the extracellular compartment
2. Intravascular compartment to the interstitial compartment
3. Extracellular compartment to the intracellular compartment
4. Intracellular compartment to the intravascular compartment

309. A nurse identifies that the shift of body fluids associated with the intravenous administration of albumin occurs by the process of:
1. Osmosis
2. Diffusion
3. Active transport
4. Hydrostatic pressure

310. A nurse teaches a client with chronic renal failure that salt substitutes cannot be used in the diet because:
1. A person's body tends to retain fluid when a salt substitute is included in the diet
2. Limiting salt substitutes in the diet prevents a build-up of waste products in the blood
3. Salt substitutes contain potassium, which must be limited to prevent abnormal heartbeats
4. A substance in the salt substitute interferes with the transfer of fluid across capillary membranes, resulting in anasarca

311. A nurse concludes that clients receiving only IV fluids instead of total parenteral nutrition for gastrointestinal problems lose weight because of:
1. Lack of bulk in the diet
2. Deficient carbohydrate intake

3. Insufficient intake of water-soluble vitamins
4. Increasing concentrations of electrolytes in the cells

312. If potassium, an electrolyte, is not added to a basic total parenteral nutrition solution, hypokalemia results. What clinical findings are evidence of hypokalemia? Select all that apply.
1. _____ Muscle weakness
2. _____ Metabolic alkalosis
3. _____ Cardiac dysrhythmias
4. _____ Serum potassium of 5.5 mEq/L
5. _____ Respiratory rate of 24 or higher

313. When a client is receiving total parenteral nutrition, it is important for the nurse to assess the client's:
1. Blood for glucose
2. Stool for occult blood
3. Urine for specific gravity
4. Abdomen for bowel sounds

314. The nurse assesses a client who is receiving total parenteral nutrition for the specific complication of:
1. Infection
2. Hepatitis
3. Anorexia
4. Dysrhythmias

315. A client's clinical signs and symptoms indicate a possible gastric ulcer. Considering the findings of epigastric pain, vomiting, dehydration, weakness, lethargy, and shallow respirations, as well as laboratory results that demonstrate metabolic alkalosis, the primary nursing concern is:
1. Chronic pain
2. Risk for injury
3. Electrolyte imbalance
4. Inadequate gas exchange

316. A client with hypertension is taught to restrict the intake of sodium. The nurse evaluates that the teaching about foods low in sodium is understood when the client states, "I can eat:
1. broiled scallops."
2. bologna on rye bread."
3. shredded wheat cereal."
4. carrot and celery sticks."

317. A 79-year-old male resident of a nursing home has refused to eat or drink for the past few days, and his urinary output has dropped to less than 300 mL/day. He is confused and hypotensive. He is diagnosed as having kidney failure secondary to dehydration. The practitioner orders 50% glucose and regular insulin. The nurse concludes that this is prescribed for a client in kidney failure to:
1. Prevent cardiac arrest
2. Increase urinary output
3. Prevent respiratory acidosis
4. Decrease serum calcium levels

318. A client has a decreased serum sodium level. For which signs of hyponatremia should the nurse assess the client? Select all that apply.
1. _____ Dry skin
2. _____ Confusion

3. _____ Tachycardia

4. _____ Pale coloring

5. _____ Muscle weakness

319. A young male client with a history of ulcerative colitis is admitted to the hospital with severe abdominal pain and loose, bloody stools. Two months after leaving the hospital against medical advice, the client is readmitted for an exacerbation of the illness. At this time he is weak, thin, and irritable and is now willing to consider surgery to create an ileostomy. Which intervention will help meet the client's priority need at this time?
    1. Replace his lost fluids and electrolytes
    2. Help him regain his former body weight
    3. Teach him how to use an ileostomy appliance
    4. Encourage his interaction with other clients with an ileostomy

320. A client with an acute episode of ulcerative colitis is admitted to the hospital. Blood studies reveal that the chloride level is low. How best can this electrolyte deficiency be corrected?
    1. Low-residue diet
    2. Intravenous therapy
    3. Oral electrolyte solution
    4. Total parenteral nutrition

321. When assessing a client with diabetes mellitus, the nurse expects that the primary fluid shift that occurs is:
    1. Intravascular to interstitial because of glycosuria
    2. Interstitial to extracellular because of hypoproteinemia
    3. Intracellular to intravascular because of hyperosmolarity
    4. Intercellular to intravascular because of increased hydrostatic pressure

322. A nurse is reviewing an arterial blood gas report for a client with type 1 diabetes. The nurse expects that the result which reflects diabetic ketoacidosis is:
    1. pH: 7.28; Pco_2: 28; HCO_3: 18
    2. pH: 7.30; Pco_2: 54; HCO_3: 28
    3. pH: 7.50; Pco_2: 49; HCO_3: 32
    4. pH: 7.52; Pco_2: 26; HCO_3: 20

323. A client with a history of atrial fibrillation is admitted to the hospital with the diagnosis of dehydration. The nurse anticipates that the practitioner will order:
    1. A glass of water every hour until hydrated
    2. Small, frequent intake of juices, broth, or milk
    3. Short-term NG replacement of fluids and nutrients
    4. A rapid IV infusion of an electrolyte and glucose solution

324. A client is diagnosed as having kidney failure. During the oliguric phase the nurse should assess the client for:
    1. Hyperkalemia
    2. Hypocalcemia
    3. Hypernatremia
    4. Hypoproteinemia

325. The practitioner prescribes a protein-, sodium-, and potassium-restricted diet for a client with end-stage renal disease who is receiving dialysis. The nurse evaluates that dietary teaching is effective when the client says:
    1. "I should avoid using salt substitutes."
    2. "I should exclude meat from my diet."
    3. "I may not add seasoning to my food."
    4. "I may eat low-sodium canned vegetables."

326. Which assessment by the nurse should be brought to the practitioner's attention before administering a prescribed intravenous solution that contains potassium chloride?
    1. Poor skin turgor with tenting
    2. Behaviors indicating irritability and confusion
    3. Urinary output of 200 mL during the previous 8 hour shift
    4. Oral intake of 300 mL of fluid during the previous 12 hour shift

327. A client with hyperpyrexia who has just been started on IV antibiotics has a diminished urine output. What is the probable cause of the diminished urine output?
    1. Declining blood pressure
    2. Compensatory response to fever
    3. Bacterial invasion of the kidneys
    4. Nephrotoxicity from antimicrobial agents

328. A client is hospitalized with 50% of the body surface area burned. At the beginning of the 48-hour postburn period (acute or diuretic phase) the client's urine specific gravity is 1.015, urine output is 50 mL, hematocrit is 32, albumin is 3.6 g/dL, and the pulmonary arterial wedge pressure is 10 mm Hg. What do these data indicate?
    1. Albumin is critically low
    2. Fluid therapy is successful
    3. Kidney failure is impending
    4. Hemoconcentration is occurring

329. A client with partial- and full-thickness burns over 25% of the total body surface area (TBSA) is hospitalized in the burn unit. A large-bore central venous line is inserted to permit rapid administration of fluids and electrolytes. The large amounts of lactated Ringer's solution and 5% dextrose in saline are administered to:
    1. Prevent fluid shifts
    2. Expand the plasma
    3. Maintain blood volume
    4. Replace electrolytes lost

330. A 34-year-old woman is rescued from a house fire at 2 AM and arrives at the emergency department at 3 AM. The client weighs 132 pounds and is burned over 35% of her body. How much lactated Ringer's solution should be infused within the next 8 hours?
    1. 2100 mL
    2. 4200 mL
    3. 6300 mL
    4. 8400 mL

331. Which sign indicates adequate intravenous fluid replacement for a client with a 30% total body surface area burn?
    1. Increasing hematocrit level
    2. Urinary output of 15 to 20 mL/hr

3. Slowing of a previously rapid pulse rate

4. Central venous pressure progressing from 5 to 1 mm water

332. During the first 48 hours after a client has sustained a thermal injury, the nurse should assess for:

1. Hypokalemia and hyponatremia

2. Hyperkalemia and hyponatremia

3. Hypokalemia and hypernatremia

4. Hyperkalemia and hypernatremia

333. A client's extensive burns are being treated with silver nitrate 0.5% dressings. A week after treatment is begun, the nurse identifies that the client's sodium level is 135 mEq/L and the potassium level is 3.0 mEq/L. The nurse notifies the practitioner and expects to:

1. Add KCl to the current IV of Ringer's lactate

2. Add NaCl to the current IV of Ringer's lactate

3. Change the NaCl with 20 mEq KCl to 5% D_5W

4. Change the 5% D_5W with 40 mEq KCl to 5% D_5W

334. The laboratory findings of a 40-year-old man with burns are BUN 30 mg/dL; creatinine 2.4 mg/dL; serum potassium 6.3 mEq/L; pH 7.1; Po_2 90 mm Hg; and Hgb 7.4 g/dL. The nurse concludes that these findings indicate:

1. Azotemia

2. Hypokalemia

3. Metabolic alkalosis

4. Respiratory alkalosis

335. Thirty-six hours after a young male is admitted with severe burns he is placed on a fluid diet. Considering his potassium level is still 6 mEq/L, the nurse recommends:

1. Milk

2. Jell-O

3. Orange juice

4. Tomato juice

336. A client is receiving a 2-gram sodium diet. The family asks whether they can bring some snacks from home. The nurse suggests that they bring foods low in sodium such as:

1. Ice cream

2. Celery sticks

3. Fresh orange wedges

4. Peanut butter cookies

337. A client with ascites has a paracentesis, and 1500 mL of fluid is removed. What should the nurse monitor the client for immediately after the procedure? Select all that apply.

1. _____ Rapid thready pulse

2. _____ Decreased peristalsis

3. _____ Respiratory congestion

4. _____ Increase in temperature

5. _____ Decreased blood pressure

338. A nurse is monitoring a client who is receiving an IV infusion. What is a serious complication of IV therapy?

1. Bleeding at the infusion site

2. Shortness of breath with wheezing

3. Feeling of warmth throughout the body

4. Infiltration at the catheter insertion site

339. A nurse is assessing an 83-year-old woman who has had diarrhea and vomiting for 48 hours. What should the nurse do when performing a focused assessment for dehydration? Select all that apply.

1. _____ Examine the client's lips for dryness or cracks

2. _____ Observe the client's eyeballs for marked protrusion

3. _____ Ask the client how many glasses of fluid are ingested daily

4. _____ Test the client's skin on the sternum or forehead for tenting

5. _____ Compare the client's current weight with the weight from two days ago

340. A 79-year-old client is admitted for dehydration, and an IV infusion of normal saline at 125 mL/hr is started. One hour later the client begins screaming, "I can't breathe." The nurse should:

1. Discontinue the IV and call the practitioner

2. Elevate the head of the bed and obtain vital signs

3. Call the practitioner and obtain an order for a sedative

4. Assess for allergies and change the IV to an intermittent infusion device

341. A client has received 2500 mL of IV fluid and 300 to 400 mL of oral intake daily for 2 days. The client's urine output progressively has decreased and now is less than 40 mL/hr for the past 3 hours. The nurse should initially:

1. Assess breath sounds and obtain the vital signs

2. Decrease the IV flow rate and increase oral fluids

3. Keep the bladder empty by inserting a retention catheter

4. Check for dependent edema by assessing the lower extremities

342. A hospitalized client receiving a 2-gram sodium diet complains about the bland food and refuses to eat dinner. The nurse should first:

1. Ask the client what foods usually are eaten at home

2. Tell the client about several brands of low-sodium spices

3. Explain to the client that the diet eventually will have to be accepted

4. Urge the client to eat to become accustomed to the diet that must be eaten at home

343. After abdominal surgery a client should be encouraged to turn from side to side and to engage in deep-breathing exercises. These activities are essential to prevent:

1. Metabolic acidosis

2. Metabolic alkalosis

3. Respiratory acidosis

4. Respiratory alkalosis

344. Nasogastric tube irrigations are ordered for a client after abdominal surgery. The nurse instills 30 mL of saline solution and 10 mL is returned. The nurse should:

1. Record 20 mL as intake

2. Increase the amount of suction

3. Reposition the nasogastric tube

4. Irrigate the tube more frequently

345. A client has a nasogastric tube attached to continuous low suction after major abdominal surgery. The nurse is monitoring the client for signs of hypokalemia. Select all that apply.
    1. _____ Irritability
    2. _____ Dysrhythmias
    3. _____ Muscle weakness
    4. _____ Abdominal cramps
    5. _____ Tingling of the fingertips

346. A client's arterial blood gases (ABGs) show the following values: a Po_2 of 89 mm Hg, a Pco_2 of 35 mm Hg, and a pH of 7.37. These findings indicate that the client is experiencing:
    1. Fluid balance
    2. Oxygen depletion
    3. Acid-base balance
    4. Metabolic acidosis

347. A client is diagnosed as having metabolic acidosis. The nurse considers that in metabolic acidosis the:
    1. Blood pH level is increased
    2. Plasma bicarbonates are increased
    3. Excess hydrogen ions are excreted
    4. Respiratory center in the medulla is depressed

348. A client appears anxious, exhibiting 40 shallow respirations per minute. The client complains of feeling dizzy and lightheaded and of having tingling sensations of the fingertips and around the lips. The nurse concludes that the client's complaints are probably related to:
    1. Eupnea
    2. Hyperventilation
    3. Kussmaul's respirations
    4. Carbon dioxide intoxication

349. Nursing intervention for a client who is hyperventilating should focus on providing reassurance and:
    1. Administering oxygen
    2. Using an incentive spirometer
    3. Having the client breathe into a paper bag
    4. Administering an IV containing bicarbonate ions

350. The practitioner orders serum electrolytes. To determine the effect of persistent vomiting, the nurse is most concerned with monitoring the:
    1. Sodium and chloride levels
    2. Bicarbonate and sulfate levels
    3. Magnesium and protein levels
    4. Calcium and phosphate levels

351. A client is hospitalized with epigastric pain, nausea, and vomiting of 4 days' duration. The following laboratory values are obtained: plasma pH of 7.51; Pco_2 of 50 mm Hg; bicarbonate of 58 mEq/L; chloride of 55 mEq/L; sodium of 132 mEq/L; and potassium of 3.8 mEq/L. The nurse determines that the collected data indicate:
    1. Hypernatremia
    2. Hyperchloremia
    3. Metabolic alkalosis
    4. Respiratory acidosis

352. A client with systemic lupus erythematosus is taking prednisone. The nurse anticipates that the steroid may cause hypokalemia. Taking into consideration food preferences, the nurse encourages the client to eat:
    1. Broccoli
    2. Oatmeal
    3. Fried rice
    4. Cooked carrots

353. A 32-year-old woman is brought to the emergency service with complaints of epigastric pain and prolonged vomiting. Her respirations are rapid and shallow, her skin is dry and flushed, and she appears weak and lethargic. As a result of the client's database, the primary nursing concern is:
    1. Acute pain
    2. Risk for injury
    3. Metabolic alkalosis
    4. Ineffective breathing

354. After a gastrectomy, a client has a nasogastric tube to low continuous suction. The client begins to hyperventilate. The nurse anticipates that this pattern will alter the client's arterial blood gases by:
    1. Increasing the Po_2 level
    2. Decreasing the pH level
    3. Increasing the HCO_3 level
    4. Decreasing the Pco_2 level

355. When a client is in profound (late) hypovolemic shock, the nurse assesses the client's laboratory values, especially the arterial blood gases. Which problem will people in late shock develop?
    1. Hypokalemia
    2. Metabolic acidosis
    3. Respiratory alkalosis
    4. Decreased Pco_2 levels

356. A practitioner orders additional diagnostic studies to assess a client's acid-base status. The laboratory value that indicates metabolic acidosis is:
    1. Urine pH of 8.4
    2. Gastric content pH of 6.0
    3. Venous serum pH of 7.28
    4. Arterial plasma pH of 7.40

357. A practitioner determines that a client has metabolic acidosis from severe dehydration. The characteristic respiration that the nurse expects with metabolic acidosis is:
    1. Dyspnea
    2. Hyperpnea
    3. Kussmaul's breathing
    4. Cheyne-Stokes breathing

358. When clients develop respiratory alkalosis, the nurse expects lab values to reflect:
    1. An elevated pH, elevated Pco_2
    2. A decreased pH, elevated Pco_2
    3. An elevated pH, decreased Pco_2
    4. A decreased pH, decreased Pco_2

359. A client with chronic obstructive pulmonary disease (COPD) has a blood pH of 7.25 and Pco_2 of 60. These blood gases require nursing attention because they indicate:
    1. Metabolic acidosis
    2. Metabolic alkalosis

3. Respiratory acidosis
4. Respiratory alkalosis

360. A client has an order for lactated Ringer's solution to run at 150 mL/hr. An IV pump is not available, therefore the nurse uses an administration set that delivers 15 gtt/mL. At how many drops per minute should the nurse set the IV to administer the ordered amount of fluid?
    1. 38
    2. 26
    3. 34
    4. 42

361. Surgery is performed on a client with a parotid tumor. The postoperative arterial blood gas values are pH 7.32; Pco_2 53 mm Hg; HCO_3 25 mEq/L. The nurse should:
    1. Obtain an order for a diuretic
    2. Have the client breathe into a rebreather bag
    3. Encourage the client to take deep, cleansing breaths
    4. Obtain a medical order for the administration of sodium bicarbonate

362. After surgical clipping of a ruptured cerebral aneurysm, a client develops the syndrome of inappropriate secretion of antidiuretic hormone (SIADH). The nurse expects that manifestations of excessive levels of antidiuretic hormone are:
    1. Increased BUN and hypotension
    2. Hyperkalemia and poor skin turgor
    3. Hyponatremia and decreased urine output
    4. Polyuria and increased specific gravity of urine

363. A client with small-cell carcinoma of the lung develops the syndrome of inappropriate secretion of antidiuretic hormone (SIADH). What responses to the secretion of antidiuretic hormone should the nurse expect when preparing care for this client? Select all that apply.
    1. _____ Edema
    2. _____ Polyuria
    3. _____ Bradycardia
    4. _____ Hypotension
    5. _____ Hyponatremia

364. A client with a history of alcoholism and cirrhosis is admitted with severe dyspnea as a result of ascites. The nurse concludes that the ascites is most likely the result of increased:
    1. Secretion of bile salts
    2. Pressure in the portal vein
    3. Interstitial osmotic pressure
    4. Production of serum albumin

365. Because of delayed treatment, a client with hepatitis B (HBV) develops cirrhosis and is admitted to a medical unit. One potential sequela of chronic liver disease is fluid and electrolyte imbalance. The nurse determines that this may be attributed to a decrease in serum albumin level, which leads to:
    1. Hemorrhage with subsequent anemia
    2. Diminished resistance to bacterial insult
    3. Malnutrition of cells, especially hepatic cells
    4. Reduction of colloidal osmotic pressure in the blood

366. A practitioner orders intravenous serum albumin for a client with advanced cirrhosis of the liver. As a result of this treatment, the nurse expects a decrease in:
    1. Urinary output
    2. Abdominal girth
    3. Serum ammonia
    4. Hepatic encephalopathy

367. An agitated, hyperventilating, semicomatose client is brought to the emergency department. The family indicates that they found empty bottles of 100 aspirin tablets and 50 cold tablets and assumes the client took the pills several hours ago. The client's vital signs are BP 160/100, pulse 140, respirations 40, and temperature 101.5° F. An oral airway is in place. Which test is considered the most vital in providing information that will guide the emergency treatment for this client?
    1. Blood glucose
    2. Serum electrolytes
    3. Liver function tests
    4. Twenty-four-hour urine

368. A practitioner orders a client's IV fluids to be delivered at 80 mL/hr. To adjust the drip rate when administering the IV via gravity, the nurse must determine the:
    1. Total volume of fluid in the IV bag
    2. Size of the needle or catheter in the vein
    3. Drops per milliliter delivered by the infusion set
    4. Diameter of the tubing being used to instill the fluid

369. A practitioner orders IV fluids and ciprofloxacin (Cipro) IVPB for a client. The nurse, using gravity to instill the IV, hangs the piggyback ciprofloxacin higher than the primary IV bag. When the piggyback bag is empty, the client observes air in the tubing of the IVPB and becomes frightened. The nurse should explain that:
    1. Air in the tubing, even if it got into the vein, will not be fatal unless it is a large amount
    2. The antibiotic and now the air are flowing into the large IV bag, not into the venous system directly
    3. The solution from the large IV bag begins to flow when the solution from the smaller bag ceases to flow
    4. The clamps on the tubing leading from both bags can be closed for a few minutes to prevent air from entering the vein

370. A client is receiving total parenteral nutrition through a subclavian vein. The nurse should:
    1. Place the client in the supine position before changing the tubing
    2. Monitor the blood pressure frequently to assess for hypovolemia
    3. Decrease the infusion rate if blood glucose levels become elevated
    4. Administer intravenous antibiotics through this central line to prevent infection

371. A client is receiving total parenteral nutrition. Which client response indicates that the client is hyperglycemic?
1. Polyuria
2. Paralytic ileus
3. Respiratory rate below 16
4. Serum glucose of 105 mg/100 mL

GASTROINTESTINAL

372. A 79-year-old client is admitted to the hospital with painful abdominal spasms and severe diarrhea of 2 days' duration. The order of physical skills the nurse should follow when performing an admitting examination of this client should be "inspection" followed by:
1. Percussion, palpation, auscultation
2. Percussion, palpation, auscultation
3. Auscultation, palpation, percussion
4. Auscultation, percussion, palpation

373. When assessing a client's abdomen, the nurse palpates the area directly above the umbilicus. This area is known as the:
1. Iliac area
2. Epigastric area
3. Hypogastric area
4. Suprasternal area

374. A nurse is reviewing preoperative instructions with a client who is scheduled for orthopedic surgery at 8 o'clock the next morning. The nurse advises the client to:
1. Have dinner and then nothing by mouth after 6 PM
2. Drink full liquids tonight and clear liquids in the morning
3. Consume a light evening meal and no food or fluid after midnight
4. Eat lunch the day before surgery and then not drink or eat anything until after surgery

375. What should the nurse do when a client is scheduled for a barium swallow?
1. Give clear fluids on the day of the test
2. Ask the client about allergies to iodine
3. Administer cleansing enemas before the test
4. Ensure a laxative is ordered after the procedure

376. Routine postoperative intravenous fluids are designed to supply hydration and electrolytes and only limited energy. Because 1 L of a 5% dextrose solution contains 50 grams of sugar, 3 L/day will supply approximately:
1. 400 kilocalories
2. 600 kilocalories
3. 800 kilocalories
4. 1000 kilocalories

377. After abdominal surgery a client is to receive a progressive postsurgical diet. This diet is characterized by progressive alterations in the:
1. Caloric content of food
2. Nutritional value of food
3. Texture and digestibility of food
4. Variety of food and fluids included

378. The diet ordered for a client permits 190 grams of carbohydrates, 90 grams of fat, and 100 grams of protein. The nurse calculates that this diet contains approximately how many calories?
1. 920 calories
2. 1970 calories
3. 2470 calories
4. 2970 calories

379. A client's serum albumin value is 2.8 g/dL. The nurse evaluates that teaching is successful when the client says, "For lunch I am going to have:
1. fruit salad."
2. sliced turkey."
3. spinach salad."
4. clear beef broth."

380. The most effective method for the nurse to evaluate a client's response to ongoing serum albumin therapy for biliary cirrhosis is to monitor the client's:
1. Weight daily
2. Vital signs frequently
3. Urine output every half hour
4. Urine albumin level every shift

381. A practitioner orders a high-calorie, high-protein diet for a client who is a heavy smoker. In light of the history of smoking, the nurse encourages the client to eat foods high in:
1. Niacin
2. Thiamine
3. Vitamin C
4. Vitamin B_{12}

382. A client is cautioned to avoid vitamin D toxicity while increasing protein intake. The nurse evaluates that dietary teaching is understood when the client states, "I must increase my intake of:
1. tofu products."   ∅ contain vit. D
2. eggnog with fruit."
3. powdered whole milk."
4. cottage cheese custard."

383. A nurse is assisting a client to plan a therapeutic diet that is high in vitamin C. What excellent sources of vitamin C should be included in the plan? Select all that apply.
1. _____ Lettuce
2. __✓__ Oranges
3. __✓__ Broccoli
4. _____ Apricots
5. __✓__ Strawberries

384. A practitioner tells a client that an increase in vitamin E and beta-carotene is important for healthier skin. The nurse teaches the client that excellent food sources of both of these substances are:
1. Spinach and mangoes
2. Fish and peanut butter
3. Oranges and grapefruits
4. Carrots and sweet potatoes

385. Because of multiple physical injuries and emotional concerns, a hospitalized client is at high risk to develop

a stress ulcer (Curling's). Stress ulcers usually are evidenced by:

1. Unexplained shock
2. Melena for several days
3. Sudden massive hemorrhage
4. Gradual drop in the hematocrit value

386. A client is instructed to avoid straining on defecation postoperatively. The nurse evaluates that the related teaching is understood when the client states, "I must increase my intake of:
   1. ripe bananas."
   2. milk products."
   3. green vegetables."
   4. creamed potatoes."

387. A client with Parkinson's disease complains about a problem with elimination. The nurse should encourage the client to:
   1. Eat a banana daily
   2. Decrease fluid intake
   3. Take cathartics regularly
   4. Increase residue in the diet

388. A practitioner orders three stool specimens for occult blood for a client who complains of blood-streaked stools and a 10-pound weight loss in 1 month. To ensure valid test results, the nurse should instruct the client to:
   1. Avoid eating red meat before testing
   2. Test the specimen while it is still warm
   3. Discard the day's first stool and use the next three stools
   4. Take three specimens from different sections of the fecal sample

389. When a client develops steatorrhea, the nurse documents this stool as:
   1. Dry and rock-hard
   2. Clay colored and pasty
   3. Bulky and foul smelling
   4. Black and blood-streaked

390. Because of chronic crampy pain, diarrhea, and cachexia, a young adult is to receive total parenteral nutrition (TPN) via a central line. Before preparing a client for the insertion of the catheter, the nurse is aware that a:
   1. Parenteral solution may be administered intermittently
   2. Fluoroscopy must be done before the catheter is inserted
   3. Jugular vein is the most commonly used catheter insertion site
   4. Client will experience a moderate amount of pain during the procedure

391. A practitioner orders total parenteral nutrition 1 L every 12 hours. The primary nursing responsibility is to monitor the client's:
   1. Electrolytes
   2. Urinary output
   3. Blood pressure
   4. Serum glucose levels

392. When preparing a client to go home with total parenteral nutrition (TPN), the nurse helps the client plan:
   1. The days to be used for administration
   2. For daily insertion of the circulatory access
   3. For professional help to administer the TPN
   4. A schedule of administration around regular activity

393. After surgical implantation of radon seeds for oral cancer, the nurse observes the client for the side effects of the radiation including:
   1. Nausea and/or vomiting
   2. Hematuria and/or occult blood
   3. Hypotension and/or bradycardia
   4. Abdominal cramping and/or diarrhea

394. A client with cancer of the tongue has radon seeds implanted. The plan of care states that the client is to receive meticulous oral hygiene. This plan can best be implemented by:
   1. Offering a firm-bristled toothbrush
   2. Providing an antiseptic mouthwash
   3. Using a gentle spray of normal saline
   4. Swabbing the mouth with a moistened gauze square

395. When teaching a client how to prevent constipation, the nurse evaluates that the dietary teaching is understood when the client states that the preferred breakfast cereal is:
   1. Froot Loops
   2. Corn Flakes
   3. Cap'n Crunch
   4. Shredded Wheat

396. A client has decided to become a vegan and wishes to plan a diet to ensure adequate protein quality. To provide guidance, the nurse instructs this client to:
   1. Add milk to grains to provide complete proteins
   2. Use eggs and plant foods to provide essential amino acids
   3. Plan a careful mixture of plant proteins to provide a balance of amino acids
   4. Add cheese to grains and beans to increase the quality of the protein consumed

397. To motivate an obese client to eventually include aerobic exercises in a weight-reduction program, the nurse discusses exercise and its relationship to weight loss. The nurse evaluates that this teaching is effective when the client states, "I know that exercise will:
   1. decrease my appetite."
   2. lower my metabolic rate."
   3. raise my resting heart rate."
   4. increase my lean body mass."

398. A client has a body mass index (BMI) of 35 and verbalizes the need to lose weight. The nurse encourages the client to lose weight safely by:
   1. Decreasing portion size and fat intake
   2. Increasing protein and vegetable intake
   3. Decreasing carbohydrate and fat intake
   4. Increasing fruits and limiting fluid intake

399. A client has symptoms associated with salmonellosis. Relevant data to gather from this client include a history of:
1. Any rectal cancer in the family
2. All foods eaten in the past 24 hours
3. Any recent extreme emotional stress
4. An upper respiratory infection in the past 10 days

400. A client is admitted to the hospital with the diagnosis of acute salmonellosis. The nurse expects that the client will receive:
1. Opioids
2. Antacids
3. Electrolytes
4. Antidiarrheals

401. During a health symposium a nurse teaches the group how to prevent food poisoning. The nurse evaluates that the teaching is understood when one of the participants states:
1. "Meats and cream-based foods need to be refrigerated."
2. "Once most food is cooked it does not need to be refrigerated."
3. "Poultry should be stuffed and then refrigerated before cooking."
4. "Cooked food should be cooled before being put into the refrigerator."

402. The nurse teaches the client with gastroesophageal reflux disease that after meals the client should:
1. Drink 8 ounces of water
2. Take a walk for 30 minutes
3. Lie down for at least 20 minutes
4. Rest in a sitting position for 1 hour

403. The laboratory values of a client with cancer of the esophagus show a hemoglobin of 7 g/dL, hematocrit of 25%, and RBC count of 2.5 million/mm³. The outcome that takes priority at this time is, "The client will:
1. be free of injury."
2. remain pain free."
3. demonstrate improved nutrition."
4. maintain an effective airway clearance."

404. Immediately after esophageal surgery the priority nursing assessment concerns the client's:
1. Incision
2. Respirations
3. Level of pain
4. Nasogastric tube

405. A client with achalasia is to have bougienage to dilate the lower esophagus and cardiac sphincter. After the procedure the nurse assesses the client for esophageal perforation, which is indicated by:
1. Tachycardia and abdominal pain
2. Faintness and feelings of fullness
3. Diaphoresis and cardiac palpitations
4. Increased blood pressure and urinary output

406. A 76-year-old obese client arrives at the clinic complaining of epigastric distress and esophageal burning. During the health history the client admits to binge drinking and frequent episodes of bronchitis. After diagnostic studies, a diagnosis of hiatal hernia is made. Which health problems most likely contributed to the development of the hiatal hernia? Select all that apply.
1. _____ Aging
2. _____ Obesity
3. _____ Bronchitis
4. _____ Alcoholism
5. _____ Esophagitis

407. When discussing future meal plans with a client who has a hiatal hernia, the nurse asks what beverages the client usually enjoys. The beverage that should be included in the diet when the client is discharged is:
1. Ginger ale
2. Apple juice
3. Orange juice
4. Cola beverages

408. A client who has a hiatal hernia is 5 feet 3 inches tall and weighs 140 pounds, asks the nurse how to prevent esophageal reflux. The nurse's best response is:
1. "Increase your intake of fat with each meal."
2. "Lie down after eating to help your digestion."
3. "Reduce your caloric intake to foster weight reduction."
4. "Drink several glasses of fluid during each of your meals."

409. A male client is diagnosed with acute gastritis secondary to alcoholism and cirrhosis. When obtaining this client's history, the nurse gives priority to the client's statement that:
1. His pain increases after meals
2. He experiences nausea frequently
3. His stools have a black appearance
4. He recently joined Alcoholics Anonymous

410. When performing the initial history and physical examination of a client with a tentative diagnosis of peptic ulcer, the nurse expects the client to describe the pain as:
1. Gnawing epigastric pain or boring pain in the back
2. Located in the right shoulder and preceded by nausea
3. Sudden, sharp abdominal pain, increasing in intensity
4. Heartburn and substernal discomfort when lying down

411. A client is suspected of having a gastric peptic ulcer. When obtaining a history from this client, the nurse expects the reported pain to:
1. Intensify when the client vomits
2. Occur one to three hours after meals
3. Increase when the client eats fatty foods
4. Begin in the epigastrium, radiating across the abdomen

412. The response after a gastroscopy that indicates a major complication is:
1. Difficulty swallowing
2. Increased GI motility

3. Nausea with vomiting

4. Abdominal distention with pain

413. A traveling salesman develops gastric bleeding and is hospitalized. An important etiologic clue for the nurse to explore while taking this client's history is:

1. Any recent foreign travel

2. The client's usual dietary pattern

3. The medications that the client is taking

4. Any change in the status of family relationships

414. After an acute episode of upper GI bleeding, a client vomits undigested antacids and complains of severe epigastric pain. The nursing assessment reveals an absence of bowel sounds, pulse rate of 134, and shallow respirations of 32 per minute. In addition to calling the practitioner, the nurse should:

1. Start oxygen via nasal cannula

2. Keep the client NPO in preparation for surgery

3. Inquire whether any red or black stools have been noted

4. Place the client in the supine position with the legs elevated

415. A client is diagnosed with cancer of the stomach and is scheduled for a partial gastrectomy. Preoperative preparation for this client should include an explanation about the postoperative:

1. Gastric suction

2. Oxygen therapy

3. Fluid restriction

4. Urinary catheter

416. A client with gastric cancer asks whether this cancer will spread. The nurse identifies that the client is looking for reassurance. When preparing a response to the client's question, the nurse recalls that gastric cancers are most likely to metastasize to the:

1. Liver and lung

2. Bone and brain

3. Pancreas and brain

4. Lymph nodes and blood

417. Twelve hours after a subtotal gastrectomy, a nurse identifies large amounts of bloody drainage from the client's nasogastric tube. The nurse should:

1. Clamp the tube and call the surgeon immediately

2. Report the characteristics of drainage to the surgeon

3. Instill 30 mL of iced normal saline into the nasogastric tube

4. Continue to monitor the drainage and record the observations

418. A nurse assesses for the development of pernicious anemia when a client has a history of:

1. Hemorrhage

2. Diabetes mellitus

3. Unhealthy dietary habits

4. Having had a gastrectomy

419. After a client has a total gastrectomy, the nurse plans to include in the discharge teaching the need for:

1. Monthly injections of vitamin B$_{12}$

2. Regular daily use of a stool softener

3. Weekly injections of iron dextran (Imferon)

4. Daily replacement therapy of pancreatic enzymes

420. After 2 months of self-management for symptoms of gastritis is unsuccessful, a client goes to the practitioner, and extensive carcinoma of the stomach is diagnosed. The client asks the nurse how the disease got so advanced. The nurse's explanation is based on the knowledge that carcinoma of the stomach is:

1. Painful in the early stages of the disease process

2. Difficult to accurately diagnose until late in the disease process

3. Usually diagnosed after the discovery of enlarged lymph nodes in the epigastric area

4. Rarely diagnosed early because the symptoms usually are nonspecific until late in the disease

421. A client with extensive gastric carcinoma is admitted to the hospital for an esophagojejunostomy. What information should the nurse include in the teaching plan when preparing this client for surgery?

1. Chest tube will be in place immediately after surgery

2. Liquids by mouth may be permitted the evening after surgery

3. Complete bed rest may be necessary for two days after surgery

4. Trendelenburg's position will be used on the first day after surgery

422. A client has just undergone a subtotal gastrectomy. Part of discharge teaching includes information about dumping syndrome. What instructions by the nurse will best minimize dumping syndrome? Select all that apply.

1. _____ Drink fluids with meals

2. _____ Eat small frequent meals

3. _____ Lie down for 1 hour after eating

4. _____ Chew food five times before swallowing

5. _____ Increase the carbohydrate component of the diet

423. Immediately after a subtotal gastrectomy a client is brought to the postanesthesia care unit. The nurse identifies small blood clots in the gastric drainage. The nurse should:

1. Clamp the tube

2. Consider this an expected event

3. Instill the tube with iced normal saline

4. Notify the client's surgeon of this finding

424. On the third postoperative day after a subtotal gastrectomy, a client complains of severe abdominal pain. The nurse palpates the client's abdomen and identifies rigidity. The nurse should first:

1. Assist the client to ambulate

2. Obtain the client's vital signs

3. Administer the prescribed analgesic

4. Encourage the use of the spirometer

425. To determine when a client who had a subtotal gastrectomy can begin oral feedings after surgery, the nurse must assess for the:

1. Presence of flatulence

2. Extent of incisional pain

3. Stabilization of hematocrit levels
4. Occurrence of dumping syndrome

426. A client who has a gastric ulcer asks what to do if epigastric pain occurs. The nurse evaluates that teaching is effective when the client states, "I will:
 1. increase my food intake."
 2. take an aspirin with milk."
 3. eliminate fluids with meals."
 4. take an antacid preparation."

427. A client who is diagnosed with a duodenal ulcer asks, "Now that I have an ulcer, what comes next?" The nurse's best response is:
 1. "Most peptic ulcers heal with medical treatment."
 2. "Clients with peptic ulcers have pain while eating."
 3. "Early surgery is advisable, especially after the first attack."
 4. "If ulcers are untreated, cancer of the stomach can develop."

428. A client is diagnosed as having a peptic ulcer. When teaching about peptic ulcers, the nurse instructs the client to report any stools that appear:
 1. Frothy
 2. Ribbon shaped
 3. Pale or clay colored
 4. Dark brown or black

429. After abdominal surgery a client returns to the unit with a nasogastric tube to decompression. The practitioner orders an antiemetic every 6 hours prn for nausea. When the client complains of nausea, the first action by the nurse is to:
 1. Check for placement of the tube
 2. Administer the ordered antiemetic
 3. Irrigate the tube with normal saline
 4. Notify the practitioner of the problem

430. Three hours after a subtotal gastrectomy, a client who has a nasogastric tube to continuous low suction and IV fluids complains of nausea and abdominal pain. The client's abdomen appears distended and there are no bowel sounds. The nurse should first:
 1. Instill air into the tube
 2. Give the prn pain medication
 3. Check bowel movements for blood
 4. Notify the surgeon of absent bowel sounds

431. A client who had a gastric resection for cancer of the stomach is admitted to the postanesthesia care unit with a nasogastric tube. The nurse expects to observe:
 1. Periodic vomiting
 2. Intermittent bouts of diarrhea
 3. Gastric distention after 6 hours
 4. Bloody drainage for the first 12 hours

432. A client progresses to a regular diet after a gastrectomy for gastric cancer. After eating lunch the client becomes diaphoretic and has palpitations. What probably has caused these responses?
 1. Intolerance to fatty foods
 2. Dehiscence of the surgical incision
 3. Extracellular fluid shift into the bowel
 4. Diminished peristalsis in the small intestine

433. After a subtotal gastrectomy a client experiences an episode reflective of dumping syndrome. About 1½ hours after the initial attack, the client experiences a second period of feeling "shaky." The nurse determines that this latter effect is caused by:
 1. A second more extensive rise in glucose
 2. An overwhelmed insulin-adjusting mechanism
 3. A distention of the duodenum from an excessive amount of chyme
 4. An overproduction of insulin that occurs in response to the rise in blood glucose

434. The characteristics that alert the nurse that a client is at increased risk of developing gallbladder disease is a female:
 1. Older than the age of 40, obese
 2. Younger than the age of 40, history of high fat intake
 3. Older than the age of 40, low serum cholesterol level
 4. Younger than the age of 40, family history of gallstones

435. A client with a tentative diagnosis of cholecystitis is discharged from the emergency department with instructions to make an appointment for a definitive diagnostic workup. The recommendation that will produce the most valuable diagnostic information is:
 1. "Keep a journal related to your pain."
 2. "Save all stool and urine for inspection."
 3. "Follow the physician's orders exactly without question."
 4. "Keep a record of the amount and type of fluid you are drinking daily."

436. A nurse asks a client to make a list of the foods that cause dyspepsia. If the client has cholecystitis, the foods that are most likely to be included on this list are:
 1. Nuts and popcorn
 2. Meatloaf and baked potato
 3. Chocolate and boiled shrimp
 4. Fried chicken and buttered corn

437. A client develops a gallstone that becomes lodged in the common bile duct. The practitioner schedules an endoscopic sphincterotomy. Preoperative teaching includes information that for the procedure the client will:
 1. Have a spinal anesthetic
 2. Receive an epidural block
 3. Have a general anesthetic
 4. Receive an intravenous sedative

438. A client has cholelithiasis with possible obstruction of the common bile duct. Before the scheduled cholecystectomy, nutritional deficiencies and excesses should be corrected. A nutritional assessment is conducted to determine whether the client:
 1. Is deficient in vitamins A, D, and K
 2. Eats adequate amounts of dietary fiber
 3. Consumes excessive amounts of protein
 4. Has excessive levels of potassium and folic acid

439. A client undergoes an abdominal cholecystectomy with common duct exploration. In the immediate

postoperative period the nursing action that is the priority for this client is:

1. Irrigating the T-tube frequently
2. Changing the dressing at least twice a day
3. Encouraging coughing and deep breathing
4. Promoting an adequate fluid and food intake

440. A 40-year-old client is admitted with biliary cancer. The associated jaundice gets progressively worse. The nurse is most concerned about the potential complication of:
    1. Pruritus
    2. Bleeding
    3. Flatulence
    4. Hypokalemia

441. After a cholecystectomy to remove a cancerous gallbladder, the client has a T-tube in place that has drained 300 mL of bile-colored fluid during the first 24 hours. The nurse should:
    1. Clamp the tube intermittently to slow drainage
    2. Increase the rate of intravenous fluids to compensate for this loss
    3. Empty the portable drainage system and reestablish negative pressure
    4. Consider this an expected response after surgery and record the results

442. During a laparoscopic cholecystectomy on an obese client, the surgeon encounters difficulty because of the presence of adhesions as a result of the client's having had a previous surgery. An abdominal cholecystectomy is performed. After surgery the nurse plans to alleviate tension on the surgical wound by:
    1. Limiting deep breathing
    2. Maintaining T-tube patency
    3. Maintaining nasogastric tube patency
    4. Encouraging the right side-lying position

443. A client with cholelithiasis has a laser laparoscopic cholecystectomy. Postoperatively it is most appropriate for the nurse to:
    1. Wait about 24 hours to begin clear liquids
    2. Monitor the abdominal incision for bleeding
    3. Offer clear carbonated beverages to the client
    4. Instruct the client to resume moderate activity in 2 to 3 days

444. Because of prolonged bile drainage from a T-tube after a cholecystectomy, the nurse must monitor the client for responses related to a lack of fat-soluble vitamins such as:
    1. Easy bruising
    2. Muscle twitching
    3. Excessive jaundice
    4. Tingling of the fingers

445. A client with cholelithiasis is scheduled for a lithotripsy. Preoperative teaching should include the information that:
    1. Opioids will be available for postoperative pain
    2. Fever is a common response to this intervention
    3. Heart palpitations often occur after the procedure
    4. Anesthetics are not necessary during the procedure

446. A client is to be discharged after a laser laparoscopic cholecystectomy. The nurse evaluates that the discharge instructions are understood when the client states:
    1. "I can change the bandages every day."
    2. "I should stay on a full liquid diet for 3 days."
    3. "I should not clean the surgical sites for a week."
    4. "I may have mild shoulder pain for about a week."

447. After a cholecystectomy a client asks whether there are any dietary restrictions that must be followed. The nurse evaluates that the dietary teaching is understood when the client tells a family member:
    1. "I should avoid fatty foods for the rest of my life."
    2. "I should not eat those foods that upset me before I had surgery."
    3. "I need to eat a high-protein diet for several months after surgery."
    4. "I probably will be able to tolerate a regular diet after this type of surgery."

448. A nurse is caring for a client with acute pancreatitis. Which elevated laboratory test result is most indicative of acute pancreatitis?
    1. Blood glucose
    2. Serum amylase
    3. Serum bilirubin level
    4. White blood cell count

449. A 50-year-old man is admitted to the hospital with severe back and abdominal pain, nausea and occasional vomiting, and an oral temperature of 101°F. He reports drinking six to eight beers a day. A diagnosis of acute pancreatitis is made. Based on the data presented, the primary nursing concern for this client is:
    1. Acute pain
    2. Inadequate nutrition
    3. Electrolyte imbalance
    4. Disturbed self-concept

450. A client is diagnosed with chronic pancreatitis. When providing dietary teaching it is most important that the nurse instruct the client to:
    1. Eat a low-fat, low-protein diet
    2. Avoid foods high in carbohydrates
    3. Avoid ingesting alcoholic beverages
    4. Eat a bland diet of six small meals a day

451. A client who was diagnosed with cancer of the head of the pancreas 2 months ago is admitted to the hospital with weight loss, severe epigastric pain, and jaundice. When performing the admission history and physical assessment, the nurse expects the client's stool to be:
    1. Green
    2. Brown
    3. Red-tinged
    4. Clay-colored

452. When teaching a client about the diet after a pancreaticoduodenectomy (Whipple procedure) performed for cancer of the pancreas, the statement the nurse should include is:
    1. "There are no dietary restrictions; you may eat what you desire."
    2. "Your diet should be low in calories to prevent taxing your pancreas."

3. "Meals should be restricted in protein because of your compromised liver function."

4. "Low-fat meals should be eaten because of interference with your fat digestion mechanism."

453. A long-term complication that a client must be made aware of after a pancreaticoduodenectomy for cancer of the pancreas is hypoinsulinism. The nurse evaluates that the teaching about hypoinsulinism is understood when the client states, "I should seek medical supervision if I experience:
1. oliguria."
2. anorexia."
3. weight gain."
4. increased thirst."

454. After revision of the pancreas because of cancer, total parenteral nutrition is instituted via a central venous infusion route. During the fourth hour of the infusion the client complains of nausea, fatigue, and a headache. The hourly urine output is twice the amount of the previous hour. The nurse should call the practitioner and:
1. Stop the infusion while covering the insertion site
2. Slow the infusion and check the serum glucose level
3. Prepare the client for immediate surgery for possible bowel obstruction
4. Increase fluids via a peripheral intravenous route and give analgesics for the headache

455. After surgery for cancer of the pancreas, the client's nutrition and fluid regimen will be influenced by the remaining amount of functioning pancreatic tissue. Considering both the exocrine and the endocrine functions of the pancreas, the client's postoperative regimen will primarily include managing the intake of:
1. Alcohol and caffeine
2. Fluids and electrolytes
3. Vitamins and minerals
4. Fats and carbohydrates

456. A client with a 20-year history of excessive alcohol use is admitted to the hospital with jaundice and ascites. A priority nursing action during the first 48 hours after the client's admission is to:
1. Monitor the client's vital signs
2. Increase the client's fluid intake
3. Improve the client's nutritional status
4. Determine the client's reasons for drinking

457. A male client with liver dysfunction reports that his gums bleed spontaneously. In addition, the nurse identifies small hemorrhagic lesions on his face. The nurse concludes that the client needs additional vitamin:
1. D
2. E
3. A
4. K

458. A client with ascites is scheduled for a paracentesis. To prepare the client for the abdominal paracentesis the nurse should:
1. Shave the client's abdomen
2. Medicate the client for pain

3. Encourage the client to drink fluids
4. Instruct the client to empty the bladder

459. A client is diagnosed as having hepatitis A. The information from the admitting data that most likely is linked to hepatitis A is the client's history of working:
1. For a local plumber
2. In a hemodialysis unit of a hospital
3. As a dishwasher at a local restaurant
4. With occupational arsenic compounds

460. The nurse instructs a client diagnosed with hepatitis A about untoward signs and symptoms related to hepatitis that may develop. The one that should be reported to the practitioner is:
1. Fatigue
2. Anorexia
3. Yellow urine
4. Clay-colored stools

461. A client with jaundice associated with hepatitis expresses concern over the change in skin color. The nurse explains that this color change is a result of:
1. Stimulation of the liver to produce an excess quantity of bile pigments
2. Inability of the liver to remove normal amounts of bilirubin from the blood
3. Increased destruction of red blood cells during the acute phase of the disease
4. Decreased prothrombin levels, leading to multiple sites of intradermal bleeding

462. A mother whose son has hepatitis A states that there is only one bathroom in their home and she is worried that other members of the family may get hepatitis. The nurse's best reply is:
1. "I suggest that you buy a commode exclusively for your son's use."
2. "There is no problem with your son sharing the same bathroom with everyone."
3. "Your son may use the bathroom, but you need to use disposable toilet covers."
4. "It is important that family members, including your son, wash their hands after using the bathroom."

463. The practitioner orders contact precautions for a client with hepatitis A. What specific interventions are required for contact precautions?
1. Private room and the door must be kept closed
2. Persons entering the room must wear a gown, a mask, and gloves
3. Gown and gloves must be worn when handling articles contaminated by urine or feces
4. Gowns and gloves must be worn only when handling the client's soiled linen, dishes, or utensils

464. A nurse is performing the physical assessment of a client admitted to the hospital with a diagnosis of cirrhosis. What skin conditions should the nurse expect to observe? Select all that apply.
1. _____ Vitiligo
2. _____ Hirsutism
3. _____ Melanosis

4. _____ Ecchymoses

5. _____ Telangiectasis

465. A 64-year-old client is suspected of having carcinoma of the liver, and a liver biopsy is scheduled. A liver biopsy may be contraindicated in certain situations. Therefore, for what should the nurse assess the client?
   1. Confusion and disorientation
   2. Presence of any infectious disease
   3. Prothrombin time of less than 40% of normal
   4. Inclusion of foods high in vitamins E and K in the client's diet

466. When preparing a client for a liver biopsy, the nurse explains that during the test the client will be placed:
   1. In the supine position, with the right arm raised behind the head
   2. On the right side, with the left arm stretched up and over the head
   3. On the left side, with the right arm extended out in front across the bed
   4. In the prone position, with both elbows flexed and the hands resting on the pillow

467. When discussing a scheduled liver biopsy with a client, the nurse explains that for several hours after the biopsy the client will have to remain in:
   1. The left side-lying position with the head of the bed elevated
   2. A high Fowler's position with both arms supported on several pillows
   3. The right side-lying position with pillows placed under the costal margin
   4. Any comfortable recumbent position as long as the client remains immobile

468. A client who has had right upper quadrant pain for several months now experiences clay-colored stools and visits the local clinic. Based on the reported history and elevated liver enzymes, a needle biopsy of the liver is scheduled. The nurse explains that:
   1. The procedure is painless because general anesthesia is used
   2. Disfiguring scars are minimal because a small incision is made
   3. Lying on the right side after the procedure is required because it will decrease the risk of hemorrhage
   4. A light meal should be eaten 2 hours before the procedure because it stimulates gastrointestinal secretions

469. The nurse identifies a small amount of bile-colored drainage on the dressing of a client who has had a liver biopsy. The nurse concludes that:
   1. Fluid is leaking into the intestine
   2. The pancreas has been lacerated
   3. This is a typical, expected response
   4. A biliary vessel has been penetrated

470. The serum ammonia level of a client with hepatic cirrhosis and ascites is elevated. The priority nursing intervention is to:
   1. Weigh the client daily
   2. Restrict the client's oral fluid intake

3. Measure the client's urine specific gravity
4. Observe the client for increasing confusion

471. A client with a long history of alcohol abuse is admitted to the hospital with ascites, jaundice, and confusion. A diagnosis of hepatic cirrhosis is made. A nursing priority is to:
   1. Institute safety measures
   2. Monitor respiratory status
   3. Measure abdominal girth daily
   4. Test stool specimens for blood

472. A client with a history of gastrointestinal varices develops severe hematemesis, and the practitioner inserts a Sengstaken-Blakemore tube. The nurse understands that this tube is a:
   1. Single-lumen tube for gastric lavage
   2. Double-lumen tube for intestinal decompression
   3. Triple-lumen tube used to compress the esophagus
   4. Multi-lumen tube for gastric and intestinal decompression

473. A client with Laënnec's cirrhosis has a Sengstaken-Blakemore tube in place. The client becomes increasingly confused and tries to climb out of bed. The client's breath becomes fetid. What is the nursing priority?
   1. Apply a safety jacket
   2. Give the prn sedative as ordered
   3. Notify the practitioner immediately
   4. Provide oxygen via a nasal catheter

474. A client with cirrhosis of the liver and malnutrition begins to develop slurred speech, confusion, drowsiness, and tremors. With these signs and symptoms, the diet should be limited to:
   1. 20 grams of protein, 2000 calories
   2. 80 grams of protein, 1000 calories
   3. 100 grams of protein, 2500 calories
   4. 150 grams of protein, 1200 calories

475. A client develops peritonitis and sepsis after the surgical repair of a ruptured diverticulum. What signs should the nurse expect when assessing the client? Select all that apply.
   1. _____ Fever
   2. _____ Tachypnea
   3. _____ Hypertension
   4. _____ Abdominal rigidity
   5. _____ Increased bowel sounds

476. When assessing a client who had abdominal surgery, the nurse determines that peristalsis has returned when the client first:
   1. Passes flatus
   2. Has bowel sounds
   3. Tolerates clear liquids
   4. Has a bowel movement

477. One month after abdominal surgery a client is readmitted to the hospital with recurrent abdominal pain and fever. The medical diagnosis is fistula formation with peritonitis. The nurse should maintain the client in the:
   1. Supine position
   2. Right Sims position

3. Semi-Fowler's position
4. Most comfortable position

478. A nurse is performing a physical assessment of a client with ulcerative colitis. The finding most often associated with a serious complication of this disorder is:
1. Decreased bowel sounds
2. Loose, blood-tinged stools
3. Distention of the abdomen
4. Intense abdominal discomfort

479. A client with colitis inquires as to whether surgery will eventually be necessary. When teaching about the disease and its treatment, the nurse should emphasize that:
1. Medical treatment for colitis is curative; surgery is not required
2. Surgery for colitis is considered only as a last resort for most clients
3. Surgery for colitis is done early in the course of the disorder for most clients
4. Medical treatment is all that will be needed if the client can acquire some emotional stability

480. When caring for a client who had abdominal intestinal surgery, it is important for the nurse to consider that:
1. Rectal intubation will relieve vomiting
2. Air swallowing causes gastric distention
3. Preoperative enemas prevent a postoperative ileus
4. Clear liquids a day after surgery stimulate peristalsis

481. When discussing nutrition with a client who has inflammatory bowel disease of the ascending colon, the most appropriate suggestion by the nurse concerning food to include in the diet is:
1. Scrambled eggs and applesauce
2. Barbecued chicken and French fries
3. Fresh fruit salad with cheddar cheese
4. Chunky peanut butter on whole wheat bread

482. A client with colitis has a hemicolectomy performed. After surgery the nurse identifies that, in addition to having vomited 300 mL of dark green viscous fluid, the client has increasing abdominal distention and absent bowel sounds. Immediate care should be directed toward:
1. Replacing fluid losses
2. Decreasing the vomiting
3. Decompressing the bowel
4. Restoring electrolyte balance

483. After surgery for creation of an ileostomy, a client is to be discharged. Before discharge, the primary nursing intervention is to:
1. Coax the client into caring for the ileostomy alone
2. Evaluate the client's ability to care for the ileostomy
3. Ensure the client understands the dietary limitations that must be followed
4. Have the client change the dry sterile dressing on the incision without assistance

484. After the surgical creation of an ileostomy, a client is transferred to a rehabilitation unit. The client asks for help in selecting breakfast. What should the nurse encourage the client to eat or drink?
1. Hot coffee and oranges
2. Shredded wheat and milk
3. Toast and a western omelet
4. Cream of wheat and bananas

485. When teaching a community health class about the signs of colorectal cancer, the nurse stresses that the most common complaint of persons with colorectal cancer is:
1. Rectal bleeding
2. Abdominal pain
3. Change in bowel habits
4. Decrease in diameter of stools

486. A client with the diagnosis of cancer of the transverse colon is transferred from the postanesthesia care unit to a room on a surgical unit after a colon resection with an anastomosis. The nurse on the unit receives the client from the transporting nurse and observes that an IV is in progress and the client has a nasogastric tube and an indwelling urinary catheter. Place the nursing actions in order of priority when receiving this client on the unit.
1. Assess the airway
2. Take the vital signs
3. Check the abdominal dressing
4. Receive the report from the nurse
Answer: _____

487. A 50-year-old executive reports a loss of 20 pounds in 3 months. The stools are black and tarry, and a colonoscopy is scheduled. The nurse prepares the client for this test by:
1. Administering an oil-retention enema just before the test
2. Instructing that a bland diet be eaten the night before the test
3. Explaining that the pretest cathartic will cause diarrhea after the test
4. Telling the client not to eat or drink anything the morning of the test

488. A middle-aged male client has an adenocarcinoma of the colon. The practitioner suspects that this has metastasized and orders a CT scan of the liver. When preparing the client for the CT scan the nurse explains that:
1. After the procedure he must rest in bed for about six hours to prevent complications
2. There will be some discomfort during the procedure but the practitioner will administer an analgesic
3. He will be in twilight sleep during the procedure and may be able to hear people talking in the same room
4. He will be given an IV infusion containing a contrast medium before the procedure and must lie as still as possible for a period of time

489. A client who has cancer of the sigmoid colon is to have an abdominoperineal resection with a permanent colostomy. Before surgery a low-residue diet is ordered. The nurse explains that this is necessary to:
1. Limit production of flatus in the intestine
2. Prevent irritation of the intestinal mucosa

3. Reduce the amount of stool in the large bowel
4. Lower the bacterial count in the gastrointestinal tract

490. A client with carcinoma of the colon is scheduled for an abdominoperineal resection. Preparation of this client several days before surgery should include:
1. Medications to promote diuresis
2. Restriction of fluids to one L daily
3. Antibiotics to reduce intestinal bacteria
4. Abdominal exercises to facilitate recovery

491. An abdominoperineal resection with the creation of a colostomy is scheduled for a client with cancer of the rectum. The nurse anticipates that the client must sign a consent for a:
1. Permanent sigmoid colostomy
2. Permanent ascending colostomy
3. Temporary double-barrel colostomy
4. Temporary transverse loop colostomy

492. On the second day after an abdominoperineal resection, the nurse anticipates that the colostomy stoma will appear:
1. Dry, pale pink, and flush with the skin
2. Moist, red, and raised above the skin surface
3. Dry, purple, and depressed below the skin surface
4. Moist, pink, flush with the skin, and painful when touched

493. The nurse teaches a client to irrigate a new sigmoid colostomy when the:
1. Stool starts to become formed
2. Client can lie on the side comfortably
3. Abdominal incision is closed and contamination is no longer a danger
4. Perineal wound heals and the client can sit comfortably on the commode

494. A client returns from surgery with a permanent colostomy. During the first 24 hours the colostomy does not drain. What does the nurse determine is the probable cause of this response?
1. Intestinal edema after surgery
2. Presurgical decrease in fluid intake
3. Absence of gastrointestinal motility
4. Effective functioning of nasogastric suction

495. A client has a surgical creation of a colostomy for cancer of the rectum. When comparing the procedures of a colostomy irrigation and an enema, the nursing intervention that is unique to a colostomy irrigation is:
1. Positioning the client for evacuation of the bowel
2. Lubricating the catheter tip with a water-soluble jelly
3. Instilling the irrigating solution using a cone-shaped tip catheter
4. Clearing the tubing of air before insertion of the irrigating solution

496. A client has a colostomy after surgery for cancer of the colon. What is the nurse's most therapeutic intervention during the postoperative period?
1. Empty the colostomy bag when it is three fourths full
2. Allow one half inch between the stoma and the appliance
3. Help the client to remove the appliance on the first postoperative day

4. Apply stoma adhesive around the stoma and then attach the appliance

497. The nurse evaluates that dietary teaching for a client with a colostomy is effective when the client states, "It is important that I eat:
1. food low in fiber so that there is less stool."
2. bland foods so that my intestines do not become irritated."
3. everything I ate before the operation and avoid foods that cause gas."
4. soft foods that are more easily digested and absorbed by my large intestine."

498. Part of discharge teaching for a client with a sigmoid colostomy includes how to protect clothing from colostomy leakage. What is the nurse's most appropriate response when the client asks about the use of appliances and dressings?
1. "Appliances are used to avoid soiling your clothing."
2. "Special appliances are expensive but they provide for better bowel control."
3. "I will give you enough appliances to last until your next visit to the physician."
4. "Many people do not need appliances once they regulate their bowels with routine irrigations."

499. A client is admitted for repair of bilateral inguinal hernias. Before surgery the nurse assesses the client for signs that strangulation of the intestine may have occurred. What is an early sign of strangulation?
1. Increased flatus
2. Projectile vomiting
3. Sharp abdominal pain
4. Decreased bowel sounds

500. An 80-year-old male client had surgery for a strangulated hernia. One hour after surgery his blood pressure drops from 134/80 to 114/76. Assessment reveals that he does not have postoperative bleeding. The nurse should:
1. Turn him onto his left side
2. Encourage him to move his legs
3. Call the practitioner immediately
4. Administer his prescribed pain medication

501. After a bilateral herniorrhaphy the nurse should assess a male client for the development of:
1. Hydrocele
2. Paralytic ileus
3. Urinary retention
4. Thrombophlebitis

502. A client receiving a 1500-calorie diet eats these foods for breakfast: 1 cup of milk (12 grams of carbohydrate, 8 grams of protein, 10 grams of fat); ¾ cup corn flakes (15 grams of carbohydrate, 2 grams of protein); and half of an orange (5 grams of carbohydrate). How many calories has this client ingested?
1. 208
2. 258
3. 416
4. 456

INTEGUMENTARY

503. A young male client is admitted to the burn center after incurring electrical burns to both hands while playing golf during a lightning storm. When assessing the entrance and exit wounds, the nurse considers that electrical injury:
1. Causes severe nervous tissue destruction along a path of least resistance
2. Results in severe tissue destruction when the burn is incurred by direct current
3. Causes a line of destruction beginning at the grounding point to the point of contact
4. Results in visible dermal wounds that denote the internal electrical current destruction

504. While starting a barbecue fire a man's shirt ignites. The most effective method for putting out the flames is:
1. Slapping at the flames
2. Log-rolling the man in the grass
3. Pouring cold liquid over the flames
4. Removing the man's burning clothes

505. During a first-aid class, a student asks what should be done when a person rushes out of a house with burning clothes. The nurse explains that after the flames are extinguished it is most important to:
1. Give the person sips of water
2. Assess the person's breathing
3. Cover the person with a warm blanket
4. Calculate the extent of the person's burns

506. A family member suggests that butter be applied to the burns of a relative who experienced extensive burns during a house fire. An appropriate response by a neighbor who is a registered nurse is, "We should just:
1. apply ice."
2. use first-aid cream."
3. wait for the ambulance."
4. cover the area with a bedsheet."

507. A worker is involved in an explosion of a steam pipe and receives a scalding burn to the chest and arms. The burned areas are painful, mottled red, weeping, and edematous. These burns are classified as:
1. Eschar
2. Full-thickness burns
3. Deep partial-thickness burns
4. Superficial partial-thickness burns

508. A client is seen in the emergency department after a barbecue accident. The practitioner diagnoses superficial partial-thickness burns. The family asks what is involved with this type of burn. When considering a response, the nurse remembers that with a superficial partial-thickness burn the:
1. Epidermis is damaged
2. Dermis is partially damaged
3. Epidermis and dermis are destroyed
4. Structures beneath the skin are destroyed

509. A burn victim has waxy white areas interspersed with pink and red areas on the chest and all of both arms.
_18_   _9+9_
     _18_

The nurse calculates that the percentage of total body surface area (TBSA) that has sustained burns is:
1. 20
2. 25
3. 30
4. 36

510. When a female client who has partial-thickness burns on her chest, abdomen, and right leg from a fire at her workplace arrives in the emergency department, the nurse's first responsibility is to:
1. Carefully remove the client's clothing
2. Evaluate whether heat inhalation had occurred
3. Apply sterile saline dressings on burned surfaces
4. Calculate total body surface area that has been burned

511. When a nurse is evaluating the condition of a client with burns of the upper body, a sign that indicates potential respiratory obstruction is:
1. Deep breathing
2. Hoarse quality to the voice
3. Pink-tinged, frothy sputum
4. Rapid abdominal breathing

512. During the first 48 hours after a thermal injury, the nurse should assess the client for:
1. Hypokalemia and hyponatremia
2. Hyperkalemia and hyponatremia ✓
3. Hypokalemia and hypernatremia
4. Hyperkalemia and hypernatremia

513. A client is admitted to the hospital with burns on the trunk and arms. When oral intake is resumed on the fourth day after the injury, the nurse helps the client plan the menu for the next day. Discussion focuses on the need for a diet that includes: ↑ Cal ↑ protein
1. High caloric intake, liberal potassium intake, and 3 grams of protein/kg/day
2. High caloric intake, restricted potassium intake, and 1 gram of protein/kg/day
3. Moderate caloric intake, liberal potassium intake, and 3 grams of protein/kg/day
4. Moderate caloric intake, restricted potassium intake, and 1 gram of protein/kg/day

514. A severely burned client is hospitalized for 2 days. Until now recovery has been uneventful, but the client begins to exhibit extreme restlessness. The nurse determines that this most likely indicates that the client is developing:
1. Renal failure
2. Hypervolemia
3. Cerebral hypoxia
4. Metabolic acidosis

515. A client's partial-thickness burns differ from full-thickness burns in that with partial-thickness burns the burned area will:
1. Require grafting before it can heal
2. Be painful, reddened, and have blisters
3. Have destruction of the epidermis and dermis
4. Take months of extensive treatment before healing

516. A client with burns develops a wound infection. The nurse plans to teach the client that local wound infections are primarily treated with:
    1. Oral antibiotics
    2. Topical antibiotics
    3. Intravenous antibiotics
    4. Intramuscular antibiotics

517. A nurse identifies that a client in the acute phase of burns has eaten only a small portion of each meal. Considering that malnutrition can have a variety of consequences, the nurse should assess the client for:
    1. Dehydration
    2. Dry brittle hair
    3. Prolonged wound healing
    4. Clubbing of the fingertips

518. The method of treatment chosen for a client's burns is the exposure method with application of mafenide (Sulfamylon) twice a day. With this medication the nurse plans to:
    1. Use medical asepsis
    2. Apply a dry sterile dressing
    3. Monitor liver function studies
    4. Give ordered pain medication *b/c burn care is painful*

519. When the exposure method of treatment is used for burns, the nurse explains to the client that:
    1. Bathing will not be permitted
    2. Dressings will be changed daily
    3. Isolation precautions will be required while hospitalized
    4. Room temperature should be kept at a minimum of 72° F

520. When dressing deep partial-thickness burns on a client's hands, the nurse should use:
    1. Cotton-backed gauze and fully extend the fingers with thumb in opposition
    2. Non–cotton-backed gauze and place a hand roll with gauze between each finger *hands in anatomical position of slight flexion w/ each finger separated*
    3. Non–cotton-backed gauze and extend fingers fully with gauze between each finger
    4. Cotton-backed gauze and a hand roll, with fingers completely flexed and thumb in opposition

521. A client with burns tells the nurse that the physician mentioned doing skin grafts and asks when they will be done. The most appropriate response by the nurse is:
    1. "Within seven days."
    2. "Tell me what your physician said."
    3. "As soon as scar formation occurs."
    4. "As soon as signs of infection disappear."

522. A client with burns over 35% of the body complains of chilling. What should the nurse do to promote the client's comfort?
    1. Limit the occurrence of drafts
    2. Keep the room temperature at 80° F *85°*
    3. Place a sterile top sheet over the client
    4. Maintain the room humidity below 40%

523. A nurse understands that a temporary heterograft (pig skin) is used to treat burns because this graft will:
    1. Debride necrotic tissue
    2. Promote rapid epithelialization
    3. Be sutured in place for better adherence
    4. Be used concurrently with a topical antimicrobial

524. A client with a full-thickness burn receives an allograft. Several days later the client points out that the graft is coming off at the edges. What is the nurse's best response?
    1. "It is a temporary graft. I'll notify your physician."
    2. "You must have pulled it loose. I'll notify your physician."
    3. "An infection may be starting. Your physician will be here shortly."
    4. "That was a permanent graft. Your physician probably will replace it."

525. When planning care to prevent deformities and contractures in a client with burns, the nurse expects to begin range-of-motion exercises when the client's:
    1. Pain has lessened
    2. Vital signs are stable
    3. Skin grafts are healed
    4. Emotional status stabilizes

526. When planning a health class about communicable diseases, the nurse includes that under certain circumstances the virus that causes chickenpox also can cause:
    1. Athlete's foot
    2. Herpes zoster
    3. German measles
    4. Infectious hepatitis

527. While obtaining the vital signs of a 30-year-old client, the nurse identifies silvery scales on the client's elbows and knees. To help identify the origin of this rash, the nurse should:
    1. Inquire if the client is using a harsh, irritating soap
    2. Ask the client about any undue stress in recent months
    3. Question the client about recent excursions into uncultivated, weedy areas
    4. Determine if the client has been infected with the human immunodeficiency virus

528. A 40-year-old male client who is receiving combination chemotherapy for stage II Hodgkin's disease is at risk for stomatitis. The nurse's teaching plan should include instructions to:
    1. Rinse his mouth three times a day with lemon juice and water
    2. Brush his teeth once daily and use dental floss after each meal
    3. Vigorously clean his mouth with toothpaste and a firm toothbrush
    4. Frequently cleanse his mouth with a soft toothbrush or a gentle spray

529. What is an expected change that the nurse might identify when assessing the skin of an older adult? Select all that apply.
    1. _____ Scaly skin
    2. _____ Increased wrinkles

3. _____ Signs of ecchymosis
4. _____ Marked flaking of skin
5. _____ Hyperpigmented patches

530. A client who has been in a coma for 2 months is being maintained on bed rest. The nurse concludes that to prevent the effects of shearing force, the head of the bed should be maintained at an angle of:
    1. 30 degrees
    2. 45 degrees
    3. 60 degrees
    4. 90 degrees

531. A practitioner orders bed rest for a client after surgery. The most beneficial method of preventing skin breakdown while the client is confined to bed is for the nurse to:
    1. Massage the skin with cream
    2. Use a sheepskin pad on the bed
    3. Promote passive range of motion
    4. Encourage independent movement

532. A practitioner orders bed rest for a client with cellulitis of the leg. The nurse determines that the primary purpose of bed rest for this client is to:
    1. Decrease catabolism to promote healing at the site of injury
    2. Lower the metabolic rate in an attempt to help reduce the fever
    3. Reduce the energy demands on the body in the presence of infection
    4. Limit muscle contractions that may force causative organisms into the bloodstream

533. A nurse cautions a client with lower extremity arterial disease (LEAD) that minor foot problems easily can become serious. The teaching plan should include the importance of:
    1. Trimming toenails so that they are short and rounded
    2. Checking bathwater temperature by putting the toes in first
    3. Using alcohol to rub hands, feet, legs, and arms at least two times a day
    4. Securing professional treatment for any minor injuries to the extremities

534. A client who has an above-the-knee amputation is fitted for a prosthesis. Two days after using the prosthesis, a small blister develops on the residual limb near the healed incision. The nurse anticipates that the client will be advised to:
    1. Stop using the prosthesis until the blister heals
    2. Increase frequency of limb-toughening exercises
    3. Change the type of covering used to avoid irritation
    4. Bandage the blister before putting the prosthesis back on

535. When planning a teaching session about care of the residual limb after a client had a below-the-elbow amputation, the nurse includes:
    1. Wearing a sling to bed every night
    2. Applying skin lotion and massaging at least twice a day

    3. Washing and drying the residual limb at least once a day
    4. Soaking the residual limb in warm water for half an hour daily

536. A nurse is preparing to change a client's dressing. The statement that best explains the basis of surgical asepsis that the nurse will perform in this procedure is:
    1. Keep the area free of microorganisms
    2. Protect self from microorganisms in the wound
    3. Confine the microorganisms to the surgical incision site
    4. Keep the number of opportunistic microorganisms to a minimum

537. The equipment that is used by the nurse during central venous catheter site care for a client receiving total parenteral nutrition is:
    1. Double sterile gloves
    2. Mask and sterile gloves
    3. Gown and sterile gloves
    4. Mask, gown, and sterile gloves

538. An obese client must self-administer insulin with an insulin syringe. The nurse teaches the client to:
    1. Pinch the tissue and inject at a 45-degree angle
    2. Pinch the tissue and inject at a 60-degree angle
    3. Spread the tissue and inject at a 45-degree angle
    4. Spread the tissue and inject at a 90-degree angle

539. A client develops an infection at a catheter insertion site. The nurse uses the term iatrogenic when describing this infection because it resulted from:
    1. Poor personal hygiene
    2. A therapeutic procedure
    3. Inadequate dietary patterns
    4. The client's developmental level

540. A nurse is caring for a client with a chronic venous stasis ulcer. The practitioner orders a negative-pressure wound treatment device to hasten wound healing. Which nursing action is most appropriate when caring for this client?
    1. Replace the wound sponge every 48 hours
    2. Change the dressing using sterile technique
    3. Overlap the edges of intact skin with the sponge
    4. Set the negative vacuum pressure at 240 mm Hg

541. When reestablishing a portable wound drainage system after emptying its contents, the nurse squeezes the collection container and replaces the stopper to:
    1. Establish positive pressure
    2. Decrease negative pressure
    3. Maintain atmospheric pressure
    4. Increase the difference in pressure

542. A client with the diagnosis of invasive cancer of the head of the pancreas has a permanent biliary drainage tube (T-tube) inserted to provide palliative care. After surgery it is most important for the nurse to:
    1. Cleanse the area around the T-tube to prevent skin breakdown
    2. Maintain intermittent low suction on the T-tube to limit trauma

3. Attach the T-tube to a negative-pressure drainage system to promote drainage

4. Reposition the client frequently to increase the flow of bile through the T-tube

543. A male client is admitted to the hospital for intravenous antibiotic therapy and an incision and drainage of an abscess that developed at the site of a puncture wound. When should the nurse begin to teach the client how to care for the wound?
1. In the preoperative period
2. Several days before discharge
3. On the first postoperative day
4. During the first dressing change

544. The primary nurse tells a client with an infected wound that the nurse epidemiologist will visit daily. The client asks what the nurse epidemiologist does. The nurse correctly explains the role by saying, "The nurse epidemiologist:
1. helps providers of care to control infections."
2. decides what antibiotics should be prescribed for infections."
3. works in the laboratory to identify bacteria causing infection."
4. is responsible for collecting specimens of potentially infectious drainage."

545. A 50-year-old man had a total hip replacement. While the nurse is providing discharge teaching the client states that as soon as he gets home he plans to go swimming at the community pool. The nurse should:
1. Encourage participation in this activity
2. Instruct the client to take a friend along for safety
3. Explain that the wound should not be immersed in water until it has healed
4. Tell the client that if he does this he will not need physical therapy after he is discharged

546. After a choledocholithotomy a client complains that the skin around the T-tube is raw and excoriated. After assessing the skin, the nurse plans to:
1. Reinforce the dressing when it is wet
2. Use a skin barrier around the tube's exit site
3. Cleanse around the site with an antiseptic solution
4. Change the type of adhesive tape used on the dressing

547. A client has a deep soft tissue injury that is open and oozing blood. When managing this wound the nurse should:
1. Replace the dressing when it is completely saturated
2. Reinforce the wound's dressing several times before changing it
3. Change the dressing each time the blood oozes through the outside layer
4. Pack the wound with antimicrobial gauze each time the dressing is changed

548. A client arrives at the emergency department after being bitten by a stray dog. The bite involved tearing of skin and deep soft tissue injury. The first nursing action is to:
1. Inform the owner of the dog about the client's injury
2. Assess the client's injury, vital signs, and past history

3. Notify the appropriate community agency to capture the dog
4. Call the practitioner and obtain an order for human rabies immune globulin

549. A client comes to the clinic after being bitten by a raccoon in an area where rabies is endemic. The nurse understands that rabies is:
1. A bacterial infection characterized by encephalopathy and opisthotonos
2. An acute bacterial septicemia that results in convulsions and a morbid fear of water
3. A nonspecific immunoresponse to organisms deposited under the skin by an animal bite
4. An acute viral infection, characterized by convulsions and difficulty swallowing, that affects the nervous system

550. A client who is to receive radiation for cancer says to the nurse, "My family and friends say that I will get a radiation burn." The best response by the nurse is:
1. "It will be no worse than a sunburn."
2. "A localized skin reaction usually occurs."
3. "Daily application of an emollient will prevent the burn."
4. "They may not have experience with this kind of radiation."

551. A client is scheduled for radiation treatments Monday through Friday. The client asks why the treatments will not be given on Saturday and Sunday. The nurse's best response is:
1. "This schedule gives normal cells time to recover."
2. "The department operates only on Monday through Friday."
3. "Your energy level will be increased greatly by a 5-day schedule."
4. "Side effects are eliminated when treatment is administered for 5 rather than 7 days."

552. A 67-year-old female client with the diagnosis of breast cancer is receiving radiation therapy to the affected area for 6 weeks. The nurse teaches the client about how to care for the area to be irradiated. The nurse determines that further teaching is necessary when the client states that to avoid skin irritation and breakdown, she will:
1. Leave the skin markings intact
2. Protect her skin from sources of heat
3. Wear soft clothing over her upper body
4. Use an oatmeal-based lotion after each treatment

553. Irradiation to the chest wall on an outpatient basis is prescribed for a client after removal of a tumor in the right lung. When teaching skin care to the client, the nurse emphasizes:
1. Keeping the skin dry to protect it from excoriation
2. Massaging four times a day to increase circulation
3. Using skin lotion twice daily to keep the skin supple
4. Washing the area frequently to remove desquamated cells

554. A client with scleroderma complains of difficulty with chewing and swallowing. When providing dietary counseling, the nurse should advise the client to:
1. Puree foods before eating
2. Liquefy the food in a blender
3. Take frequent sips of water with meals
4. Use a local anesthetic mouthwash before eating

555. A female client with scleroderma tells the nurse that she often has numbness and tingling in her hands followed by blanching of her fingers. The nurse concludes that the client has Raynaud's phenomenon, a condition commonly associated with scleroderma. The nurse plans to advise the client to:
1. Bathe her hands frequently in hot water
2. Keep her hands warm by wearing gloves
3. Rub her hands briskly to increase circulation
4. Take her ordered anticoagulants to prevent attacks

556. As part of the teaching plan for a client with scleroderma, the nurse addresses the need for special skin care and advises the client to:
1. Keep the skin well lubricated
2. Use calamine lotion for pruritus
3. Apply warm soaks to the inflamed areas
4. Take frequent baths to remove scaly lesions

557. A practitioner orders a regimen of daily exercises for a client with scleroderma. The nurse teaches the client that these exercises are performed to:
1. Preserve muscle strength
2. Support tissue regeneration
3. Prevent spread of the disease
4. Maintain a sense of well-being

558. A client who has just had a colostomy has an uneventful 24-hour postoperative course. Seventy-two hours after surgery, the primary nursing intervention for this client is:
1. Keeping an accurate record of oral fluid intake
2. Emphasizing the importance of regulating the diet to form stool
3. Teaching care of the incision and how to perform colostomy irrigations
4. Observing and reporting drainage and the condition of the abdominal incision

559. When performing colostomy care, it is important for the nurse to teach the client to care for the skin around the stoma by:
1. Avoiding the use of soap and other irritating agents
2. Rinsing with hydrogen peroxide and applying a gauze pad
3. Pouring saline over the stoma and wiping away the fecal matter
4. Washing the area gently with soap and water before applying an appliance

560. A client returns from surgery with an incisional dressing and a catheter that is attached to a portable wound drainage system exiting from the operative site. The principle underlying the function of a portable drainage system is:
1. Gravity
2. Osmosis
3. Active transport
4. Negative pressure

561. After surgery for cancer, a client is to receive chemotherapy. When teaching the client about the side effects of chemotherapy, the nurse emphasizes that the occurrence of alopecia is:
1. Usually rare
2. Not permanent
3. Frequently prolonged
4. Sometimes preventable

NEUROMUSCULAR

562. A client expresses concern about insomnia. Which activities should the nurse encourage the client to do before bedtime to promote sleep? Select all that apply.
1. _____ Drink a glass of wine
2. _____ Engage in mild exercise
3. _____ Eat foods containing lysine
4. _____ Follow the same bedtime ritual
5. _____ Perform deep-breathing exercises

563. A client with the diagnosis of trigeminal neuralgia comes to the neurological clinic. When assessing the client's trigeminal nerve function, the nurse should evaluate:
1. Corneal sensation
2. Facial expressions
3. Ocular muscle movement
4. Shrugging of the shoulders

564. The nurse in the neurologic clinic assesses for damage to the glossopharyngeal (ninth cranial) and vagus (tenth cranial) nerves by testing the client's ability to:
1. Shrug
2. Smell
3. Smile
4. Swallow

565. A nurse is performing a neurological assessment of a client. Which equipment is required when preparing to assess the vagus nerve (cranial nerve X) of a client?
1. Tuning fork
2. Ophthalmoscope
3. Tongue depressors
4. Cotton and a straight pin

566. A nurse uses a dull object to stroke the lateral side of the underside of a client's left foot and moves upward to the great toe. What reflex is the nurse testing?
1. Moro
2. Babinski
3. Stepping
4. Cremasteric

567. A client recently diagnosed with Bell's palsy has many questions about the course of the disorder. The nurse explains that:
1. Pain occurs with transient ischemic attacks
2. Cool compresses decrease facial involvement
3. Most clients recover from the effects in several weeks
4. Body changes should be expected with residual effects

568. A nurse explains to a client with trigeminal neuralgia that a treatment that is effective on a temporary (6 to 18 months) basis is:
    1. Weekly intravenous injections of cobra venom
    2. A lidocaine injection of the ventral root of the eleventh spinal nerve
    3. Microvascular decompression of the blood vessels at the nerve root
    4. An alcohol injection of the peripheral branch of the fifth cranial nerve

569. A client with pain and paresis of the left leg is scheduled for electromyography. Before the test the nurse explains that:
    1. Your heart rate will be monitored frequently
    2. The involved area will be shaved before testing
    3. The examiner will insert a needle into the muscle being tested
    4. You will be kept flat on your back in bed for a while after the procedure

570. A nurse identifies that a client exhibits the characteristic gait associated with Parkinson's disease. When recording on the client's record, the nurse documents this gait as:
    1. Ataxic
    2. Shuffling
    3. Scissoring
    4. Asymmetric

571. A nurse is performing the history and physical examination of a client with Parkinson's disease. Which assessments identified by the nurse support this diagnosis? Select all that apply.
    1. _____ Nonintention tremors
    2. _____ Frequent bouts of diarrhea
    3. _____ Masklike facial expression
    4. _____ Hyperextension of the neck
    5. _____ Low-pitched monotonous voice

572. A nurse is assessing a client with Parkinson's disease. Which assessment indicates the presence of bradykinesia?
    1. Intention tremor
    2. Muscle flaccidity
    3. Paralysis of the limbs
    4. Lack of spontaneous movement

573. An older adult with a history of parkinsonism has some rigidity and tremors despite medication. At this time the client is admitted to the hospital with pneumonia. In view of the current medical problem and the rigidity, the nursing plan should include:
    1. Gait training in physical therapy department
    2. Isometric exercises every other hour while awake
    3. Active range-of-motion exercises at least every 4 hours
    4. Passive range-of-motion exercises at least once every 8 hours

574. A client with parkinsonism is taking an anticholinergic medication for morning stiffness and tremors in the right arm. During a visit to the clinic the client complains of some numbness in the left hand. What is the nurse's next intervention?
    1. Refer the client to the practitioner if other neurologic deficits are present
    2. Ask the practitioner to increase the client's dosage of the anticholinergic medication
    3. Stress the importance of having the client call the family practitioner as soon as possible
    4. Make arrangements immediately for further medical evaluation by the client's practitioner

575. The nurse evaluates that the teaching about myasthenic and cholinergic crises is understood when a client who is diagnosed with myasthenia gravis states that a characteristic common to both is:
    1. Diarrhea
    2. Salivation
    3. Difficulty breathing
    4. Abdominal cramping

576. When assessing the progress of a client being treated for myasthenia gravis, the nurse expects:
    1. Partial improvement of muscle strength with mild exercise
    2. Fluctuating weakness of muscles innervated by the cranial nerves
    3. Little change in muscle strength regardless of the therapy initiated
    4. Dramatic worsening in muscle strength with anticholinesterase drugs

577. When assisting a client who has myasthenia gravis to bathe, the nurse identifies that the client's arms become weaker with sustained movement. What should the nurse do?
    1. Encourage the client to rest for short periods
    2. Continue the bath while supporting the client's arms
    3. Gradually increase the client's activity level each day
    4. Administer a dose of pyridostigmine bromide (Mestinon)

578. A client with myasthenia gravis comes to the neurology clinic at 4 PM for a routine visit. During an assessment the nurse expects the client to report:
    1. Blurred vision along with episodes of vertigo
    2. Tremors of the hands when attempting to lift objects
    3. Partial improvement of muscle strength with mild exercise
    4. Involvement of the distal muscles rather than the proximal muscles

579. During a routine clinic visit of a client who has myasthenia gravis, the nurse reinforces previous teaching about the disease and self-care. The nurse evaluates that the teaching is effective when the client states that it is important to:
    1. Plan activities for later in the day
    2. Eat meals in a semirecumbent position
    3. Avoid people with respiratory infections
    4. Take muscle relaxants when under stress

580. A nurse is teaching a client with myasthenia gravis how to prevent myasthenic crisis. The nurse evaluates that health teaching is effective when the client says:
    1. "I'll take an antihistamine at the first sign of a cold."
    2. "I can skip a dose of Mestinon if it upsets my stomach."
    3. "We've told our daughter not to let her cold keep her from visiting us."
    4. "The doctor may need to adjust the dosage of my medication if I'm more active."

581. A client is scheduled to have a series of diagnostic studies for myasthenia gravis, including a Tensilon test. The nurse explains to the client that the diagnosis of myasthenia gravis is confirmed if the administration of Tensilon produces a:
    1. Brief exaggeration of symptoms
    2. Prolonged symptomatic improvement
    3. Rapid but brief symptomatic improvement
    4. Symptomatic improvement of just the ptosis

582. A practitioner orders a diagnostic workup for a client who may have myasthenia gravis. The initial nursing goal for the client during the diagnostic phase should be that, "The client will:
    1. adhere to a teaching plan."
    2. achieve psychologic adjustment."
    3. maintain present muscle strength."
    4. prepare for the development of myasthenic crisis."

583. A client is suspected of having myasthenia gravis. What are the most significant initial nursing assessments that should be made?
    1. Ability to chew and speak distinctly
    2. Capacity to smile and close the eyelids
    3. Effectiveness of respiratory exchange and ability to swallow
    4. Degree of anxiety and concern about the suspected diagnosis

584. A client with myasthenia gravis, who is living in a nursing home, experiences inadequate symptomatic control with pyridostigmine bromide (Mestinon) and the practitioner begins long-term steroid therapy. When this type of therapy is being initiated, it is especially important for the nurse to ensure that the client:
    1. Increases sodium intake
    2. Is placed on protective isolation
    3. Decreases total daily fluid intake
    4. Is monitored for an exacerbation of symptoms

585. A client newly diagnosed with myasthenia gravis is concerned about fluctuations in physical condition and generalized weakness. When caring for this client it is most important for the nurse to plan to:
    1. Space activities throughout the day
    2. Restrict activities and encourage bed rest
    3. Teach the limitations imposed by the disorder
    4. Have a member of the family stay and give the client support

586. Which common initial clinical effects should the nurse expect a client with multiple sclerosis to exhibit? Select all that apply.
    1. _____ Headaches
    2. _____ Nystagmus
    3. _____ Skin infections
    4. _____ Scanning speech
    5. _____ Intention tremors

587. A nurse is caring for a client newly diagnosed with Guillain-Barré syndrome. Which procedure should the nurse expect the practitioner to discuss as a potential treatment option?
    1. Hemodialysis
    2. Plasmapheresis
    3. Thrombolytic therapy
    4. Immunosuppression therapy

588. During the neurological assessment of a client with a tentative diagnosis of Guillain-Barré syndrome, the nurse expects that the client will manifest:
    1. Diminished visual acuity
    2. Increased muscular weakness
    3. Pronounced muscular atrophy
    4. Impairment in cognitive reasoning

589. A nurse is caring for a client with Guillain-Barré syndrome. For what essential care related to rehabilitation should the nurse prepare the client?
    1. Physical therapy
    2. Speech exercises
    3. Fitting with a vertebral brace
    4. Follow-up on cataract progression

590. A client with multiple sclerosis is informed that it is a chronic progressive neurological condition. The client asks the nurse, "Will I experience pain?" What is the nurse's best response?
    1. "Tell me about your fears regarding pain."
    2. "Analgesics will be ordered to control the pain."
    3. "Pain is not a characteristic symptom of this condition."
    4. "Let's make a list of the things you need to ask the physician."

591. A 28-year-old woman has known for the past 6 years that she has multiple sclerosis. She has two children, one of whom is an active toddler. The client currently is in remission. At the present time, it is most important for the nurse to encourage the client to:
    1. Schedule periodic quality time with her child
    2. Provide support to other people with multiple sclerosis
    3. Develop a flexible schedule for completion of routine daily activities
    4. Meet with a self-help group for people with the diagnosis of multiple sclerosis

592. When performing a neurological check on a client with a head injury, the nurse identifies a diminished corneal reflex in the left eye. Appropriate nursing care for a client with an absent corneal reflex includes:
    1. Irrigating the eye routinely
    2. Instilling artificial tears frequently

3. Checking the corneal reflex every hour
4. Taping the eyelids open during the day

593. The nurse uses the Glasgow Coma Scale to assess a client with a head injury that resulted from a snowboarding accident. The nurse identifies that the client is in a coma when the Glasgow Coma Scale score is:
   1. 6
   2. 9
   3. 12
   4. 15

594. After an automobile collision a client who is unconscious and exhibiting decerebrate posturing is brought to the emergency department. When assessing this client, the nurse expects to observe:
   1. Hyperextension of both the upper and lower extremities
   2. Spastic paralysis of both the upper and lower extremities
   3. Hyperflexion of the upper extremities and hyperextension of the lower extremities
   4. Flaccid paralysis of the upper extremities and spastic paralysis of the lower extremities

595. A client is admitted to the hospital after sustaining a head injury. The most reliable sign that this client is experiencing an increase in intracranial pressure is a slowly:
   1. Rising respiratory rate
   2. Narrowing pulse pressure
   3. Decreasing level of consciousness
   4. Increasing diastolic blood pressure

596. During the immediate post-trauma period after injury to the frontal lobe of the brain, the nurse places a client in the:
   1. Supine position
   2. Side-lying position
   3. Low Fowler's position
   4. Trendelenburg position

597. A nurse in the emergency department prepares a checklist before transferring an unconscious client with a head injury to the neurological trauma unit. Which nursing action is the priority?
   1. Notifying the receiving unit of the transfer
   2. Having the client's records ready for the transfer
   3. Verifying that the family has been notified of the transfer
   4. Checking that a bag-valve mask is available during the transfer

598. A client who sustained a severe head injury in a diving accident remains unconscious. In addition, the nurse observes bleeding from the left ear and rhinorrhea. The nurse concludes that drainage from the ear and nose indicates a:
   1. Contusion
   2. Concussion
   3. Nose fracture
   4. Basilar fracture

599. A client with a severe head injury is being monitored by the nurse for signs and symptoms of increasing intracranial pressure. Which finding is most indicative of increasing intracranial pressure?
   1. Polyuria
   2. Tachypnea
   3. Increased restlessness
   4. Intermittent tachycardia

600. A young adult who is unconscious after an accident is brought to the emergency department. The client's pupils are equal and responsive to light. As part of the neurological assessment, the nurse applies a painful stimulus to the client's left lower leg. An expected response in a healthy adult is:
   1. Withdrawing the leg
   2. Making no movement
   3. Plantar flexing the left foot
   4. Flexing the upper extremities

601. A client had spinal anesthesia for surgery. On the second day after surgery the client complains of a headache. The nurse should:
   1. Begin an early ambulation program
   2. Supply the client with several containers of juice
   3. Remove any elastic antiembolism stockings being worn
   4. Assist the client to sit at the bedside with the feet dangling

602. A 26-year-old client admitted with the diagnosis of subarachnoid hemorrhage exhibits aphasia and hemiparesis. The nurse concludes that neurological deficits, which may be present immediately after a subarachnoid hemorrhage, primarily are caused by:
   1. Blood loss
   2. Tissue death
   3. Vascular spasms
   4. Electrolyte imbalance

603. In what position should a nurse plan to maintain a client who has experienced a subarachnoid hemorrhage?
   1. In the supine position
   2. On the unaffected side
   3. In bed with the head of the bed elevated
   4. With sandbags on either side of the head

604. After an anterior fossa craniotomy, a client is placed on controlled mechanical ventilation. To ensure adequate cerebral blood flow the nurse should:
   1. Clear the ear of draining fluid
   2. Discontinue anticonvulsant therapy
   3. Elevate the head of the bed thirty degrees
   4. Monitor serum carbon dioxide levels routinely

605. When caring for an unconscious client with increasing intracranial pressure, the nursing intervention that is contraindicated is:
   1. Lubricating the skin with baby oil
   2. Suctioning the oropharynx routinely
   3. Elevating the head of the bed 20 degrees
   4. Cleansing the eyes every 4 hours with normal saline

606. A client who had an infratentorial craniotomy is admitted to the intensive care unit after discharge from the postanesthesia care unit. Frequent assessments reveal that the client's intracranial pressure is increasing. The nurse should first:
1. Notify the surgeon
2. Elevate the head of the bed
3. Reduce the flow rate of IV fluid
4. Administer the next dose of osmotic diuretic early

607. A client has a supratentorial craniotomy for a tumor in the right frontal lobe of the cerebral cortex. Postoperatively, the position that is most appropriate for this client is:
1. Semi-Fowler's with knee gatch elevated
2. Flat on one side with the neck maintained in alignment with a small pillow
3. Head of the bed elevated 30 to 45 degrees with the neck in neutral alignment
4. Head of the bed elevated 20 degrees with the head turned to the operative side

608. A client has surgery for the creation of burr holes after sustaining head trauma from a fall and is at risk for developing an infection. An early clinical manifestation of meningeal irritation for which the nurse assesses the client is:
1. Sunset eyes
2. Kernig's sign
3. Plantar reflex
4. Homans' sign

609. After 3 months of rehabilitation after a craniotomy, a female client is still having motor speech difficulties. To promote the client's use of speech the nurse should:
1. Support her efforts to communicate
2. Correct verbal mistakes immediately
3. Use simple words with short sentences
4. Explain why she is having difficulty speaking

610. A client asks for an explanation about glaucoma. The nurse explains that with glaucoma there is:
1. An increase in the pressure within the eyeball
2. An opacity of the crystalline lens or its capsule
3. A curvature of the cornea that becomes unequal
4. A separation of the neural retina from the pigmented retina

611. When obtaining the nursing history from a client who has open-angle (chronic) glaucoma, a complaint that the nurse should expect is:
1. Flashes of light
2. Intolerance to light
3. Seeing floating specks
4. Loss of peripheral vision

612. A 78-year-old woman who has just been diagnosed with primary open-angle glaucoma (POAG) refuses therapy. The nurse discusses this with the client because if this condition is untreated it may lead to:
1. Cataracts
2. Blindness
3. Retinal detachment
4. Blurred distance vision

613. A client who has open-angle (chronic) glaucoma is scheduled for eye surgery to promote aqueous humor outflow. The nurse evaluates that the client understands the preoperative teaching about the first 24 hours after surgery when the client states, "I should:
1. avoid coughing."
2. lie on my affected side."
3. move around freely in bed."
4. elevate the head of my bed."

614. An older adult has cataracts in both eyes. The left cataract is scheduled to be extracted in several days. The nurse plans to instruct the client that:
1. "Both eyes will be covered for 24 hours after surgery."
2. "You may have to remain on bed rest for 3 to 4 days after your surgery."
3. "You must remember to take deep breaths before coughing several times an hour."
4. "At night you will be wearing a hard patch over your operated eye for about a week."

615. Immediately after cataract surgery a client complains of feeling nauseated. The nurse should:
1. Give the prescribed antiemetic
2. Provide some dry crackers to eat
3. Explain that this is expected after surgery
4. Encourage deep breathing until the nausea subsides

616. After a left cataract extraction, a client complains of severe discomfort in the operated eye. The nurse concludes that this problem may be caused by:
1. Hemorrhage into the eye
2. Expected postoperative discomfort
3. Isolation related to sensory deprivation
4. Pressure on the eye from the protective shield

617. A client is prepared for discharge from an ambulatory surgical unit after cataract removal with an intraocular lens implant. The statement by the client that suggests to the nurse that the discharge teaching was effective is:
1. "I'm driving home because I feel so good."
2. "I can't wait until I get home to wash my hair."
3. "I can expect to see bright flashes of light for a while."
4. "I'll call the surgeon immediately if my eye becomes painful."

618. After cataract surgery a client is taught how to self-administer eye drops before discharge. The nurse approves the technique when the client:
1. Places the drops on the cornea of the eye
2. Raises the upper eyelid with gentle traction
3. Holds the dropper tip above the conjunctival sac
4. Squeezes the eye shut after instilling the medication

619. After an automobile collision a client complains of seeing frequent flashes of light. Which condition should the nurse suspect?
1. Glaucoma
2. Scleroderma
3. Detached retina
4. Cerebral concussion

620. After surgery to repair a retinal detachment, an older adult client is transferred to the postanesthesia care unit

with the affected eye patched. During the first 4 hours after surgery, the nurse should plan to notify the surgeon if the client:
1. Has not voided
2. Cannot open the eye
3. Becomes disoriented
4. Complains of sharp pain in the eye

621. A client who has a detached retina is to have a scleral buckling procedure to attempt to reattach the retina. Before the client is discharged home, the nurse should plan to:
1. Instruct the client to wear dark glasses after the patch is removed
2. Explain to the client that reading will help strengthen the eye muscles
3. Reassure the client that the glasses worn before surgery can still be worn
4. Tell the client that usual activities can be resumed within a couple of weeks

622. A client sustains a vertebral fracture at the T1 level as a result of diving into shallow water. On admission to the emergency department a detailed neurological assessment is performed. Which clinical finding should the nurse expect to identify?
1. Difficulty breathing
2. Inability to move the lower arms
3. Normal biceps reflexes in the arms
4. Loss of pain sensation in the hands

623. A client who sustained a spinal cord injury at the T2 level should be assessed for signs of autonomic hyperreflexia because:
1. The injury results in loss of the reflex arc
2. The injury is above the sixth thoracic vertebra
3. There has been a partial transection of the cord
4. There is a flaccid paralysis of the lower extremities

624. The nurse determines that a client with a spinal cord injury is developing autonomic hyperreflexia when the client has:
1. Flaccid paralysis and numbness
2. Absence of sweating and pyrexia
3. Escalating tachycardia and shock
4. Paroxysmal hypertension and bradycardia

625. During the first week after a spinal cord injury at the T3 level, a male client and the nurse identify a short-term goal. An appropriate short-term goal for this client is, "The client will:
1. understand limitations."
2. consider lifestyle changes."
3. perform independent ambulation."
4. carry out personal hygiene activities."

626. A client who is recuperating from a spinal cord injury at the T4 level wants to use a wheelchair. What should the nurse teach the client to prepare for this activity?
1. Leg lifts to prevent hip contractures
2. Push-ups to strengthen arm muscles
3. Balancing exercises to promote equilibrium
4. Quadriceps-setting exercises to maintain muscle tone

627. A client is admitted to the emergency department after sustaining a spinal cord injury above the T6 level. Which response is most important for the nurse to monitor when concerned about spinal shock?
1. Tachycardia
2. Hypoventilation
3. Bladder distention
4. Elevated blood pressure

628. A client is admitted to the hospital after an automobile collision that caused an injury to the spinal cord. The client is experiencing episodes of autonomic hyperreflexia characterized by a severe headache, paroxysmal hypertension, diaphoresis, nausea, and bradycardia. The client may experience this event if a spinal cord injury occurs at or above a certain level of the spinal cord. Indicate on the illustration by placing an X in the band on the level at which an injury at or above this point can result in episodes of autonomic hyperreflexia.

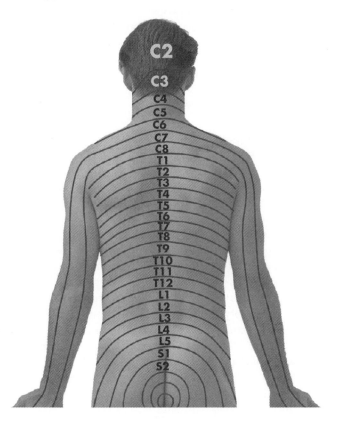

629. A client whose vertebral column at the level of T6 and T7 was completely crushed and whose left leg was traumatically amputated above the knee is admitted to the ICU. When performing an assessment the nurse expects to find that the client is experiencing:
1. Difficulty breathing
2. Discomfort in the residual limb
3. Pain at the level of compression
4. Spastic paralysis of the extremities

630. On the first postoperative evening after a lumbar laminectomy, a male client tells the nurse that his feet are

as numb as they were before the operation. What is the nurse's best response?
1. "Let me elevate your feet so the numbness will decrease more quickly."
2. "That's important to know. I will inform your surgeon about your observation."
3. "Continue to let me know how you feel. It often takes time before this feeling subsides."
4. "There is no cause for concern because the numbness will subside when the anesthesia wears off."

631. A client has a history of progressive carotid and cerebral atherosclerosis and transient ischemic attacks (TIAs). The nurse explains to the client that TIAs are:
1. Temporary episodes of neurological dysfunction
2. Intermittent attacks caused by multiple small clots
3. Ischemic attacks that result in progressive neurological deterioration
4. Exacerbations of neurological dysfunction alternating with remissions

632. A client has carotid atherosclerotic plaques, and a right carotid endarterectomy is performed. Two hours after surgery the client demonstrates progressive hypotension. The nurse should:
1. Notify the surgeon
2. Increase the IV flow rate
3. Raise the head of the bed
4. Put the client in a slight Trendelenburg position

633. After a carotid endarterectomy, the client is monitored for the complication of cranial nerve dysfunction. To monitor for this complication, the nurse assesses the client for:
1. Labored breathing
2. Edema of the neck
3. Difficulty in swallowing
4. Alteration in blood pressure

634. A client is admitted to the hospital with weakness in the right extremities, a slight speech problem, and vital signs that are within expected limits. The practitioner suspects that the client has sustained a brain attack (CVA). During the first 24 hours the nurse gives priority to:
1. Checking the client's temperature
2. Evaluating the client's motor status
3. Monitoring the client's blood pressure
4. Obtaining the client's urine for a urinalysis

635. A client having a brain attack (CVA) is brought to the emergency department. The vital signs are P, 78; R, 16; and BP, 120/80. The change in this client's vital signs that indicates increasing intracranial pressure (ICP) requiring notification of the practitioner is:
1. P, 120; R, 16; BP, 80/60
2. P, 50; R, 22; BP, 140/60
3. P, 60; R, 18; BP, 126/96
4. P, 56; R, 20; BP, 130/110

636. On the evening before discharge from the hospital, a client has a hypertensive crisis and a brain attack (CVA). Initially the nurse should place the client in a:
1. Supine position
2. Contour position
3. Side-lying position
4. Trendelenburg position

637. Initially after a brain attack (CVA), a client's pupils are equal and reactive to light. Later the nurse assesses that the right pupil is reacting more slowly than the left and the systolic blood pressure is beginning to increase. The nurse concludes that these signs are suggestive of:
1. Spinal shock
2. Hypovolemic shock
3. Transtentorial herniation
4. Increasing intracranial pressure

638. What should the nurse do to prevent a client, who had a brain attack (CVA) 2 days ago, from developing plantar flexion?
1. Place a pillow under the thighs
2. Elevate the knee gatch of the bed
3. Encourage active range of motion
4. Maintain the feet at right angles to the legs

639. A female client manifests right-sided hemianopsia as a result of a brain attack (CVA). The nurse should:
1. Correct the client's misuse of equipment
2. Instruct the client to scan her surroundings
3. Teach the client to look at the position of her left extremities
4. Provide the client with tactile stimulation to the affected extremities

640. The husband of a client with expressive aphasia as a result of a brain attack (CVA) asks whether his wife's speech will ever return. What is the best response by the nurse?
1. "It should return in several months."
2. "You will have to ask your physician."
3. "It is hard to say how much improvement will occur."
4. "This probably will be the extent of her speech from now on."

641. When assisting the family to help a member with expressive aphasia regain as much speech function as possible, the nurse instructs them to:
1. Speak louder than usual during visits
2. Tell the client to use the correct words when speaking
3. Give positive reinforcement for correct communication
4. Encourage the client to speak while being patient with each attempt

642. A client, employed as a carpenter, has difficulty holding tools because of carpal tunnel syndrome. Because the client must continue to work, the issue of most concern is:
1. Anxiety
2. Persistent pain
3. Low self-esteem
4. Potential for injury

643. While walking in the hall, a hospitalized client has a tonic-clonic seizure. What should the nurse do during the seizure?
1. Hold extremities firmly
2. Protect the head from injury

3. Insert an airway between the client's teeth
4. Have several staff members move the client to a soft surface

RESPIRATORY

644. A 40-year-old architect with a malignant parotid tumor is treated aggressively with radiation therapy and surgery. Postsurgical laboratory results indicate arterial blood gas values are pH, 7.32; Pco_2, 53 mm Hg; HCO_3, 25 mEq. Which action should be taken by the nurse?
    1. Obtaining an order and administering a diuretic
    2. Having the client breathe into a rebreather bag at a slow rate
    3. Asking the client to cough productively and take deep breaths
    4. Obtaining an order for the administration of sodium bicarbonate

645. The nurse performs preoperative teaching related to a subtotal thyroidectomy. The nurse evaluates that the client understands the teaching about the local effects of the administration of a general anesthetic when the client states, "Immediately after surgery I may experience:
    1. transient headaches."
    2. feelings of chilliness."
    3. paroxysmal hiccoughs."
    4. discomfort swallowing."

646. After a gastroscopy, the nurse assesses the client for the return of the gag reflex by:
    1. Touching the pharynx with a tongue depressor
    2. Giving a small amount of water using a syringe
    3. Observing for when the client gags and spits out airway
    4. Instructing the client to breathe deeply and cough gently

647. When caring for clients in the operating suite, the nurse expects that the last physiological function the client loses during the induction of an anesthetic is:
    1. Gag reflex
    2. Eyelid reflexes
    3. Voluntary control
    4. Respiratory movement

648. When a client returns from a bronchoscopy, the nurse withholds food and fluid for several hours to prevent:
    1. Aspiration
    2. Dysphasia
    3. Projectile vomiting
    4. Abdominal distention

649. An 84-year-old client with a history of hemoptysis and cough for the last 6 months is suspected of having lung cancer. A bronchoscopy is performed. Two hours after the procedure the nurse identifies an increase in the amount of bloody sputum. The nurse's priority is to:
    1. Notify the practitioner of the observation
    2. Continue to monitor the amount of sputum
    3. Monitor vital signs every hour for four hours
    4. Increase the coughing and deep-breathing regimen

650. An older adult confined to bed in a nursing home develops bronchitis and atelectasis of the right lower lobe. When discussing the treatment regimen with the client, the nurse includes the need to:
    1. Lie on the affected side to relieve chest pain
    2. Lie on the unaffected side to promote drainage
    3. Sleep in the position of most comfort to promote rest
    4. Sleep with the head elevated to stimulate deep breathing

651. A client with bronchial pneumonia is having difficulty maintaining airway clearance because of retained secretions. Which intervention will help to decrease retained secretions?
    1. Administering oxygen as ordered
    2. Gargling deeply with warm normal saline
    3. Placing the client in a high Fowler's position
    4. Increasing fluid intake to at least two liters a day

652. After a laryngectomy a client becomes concerned about frequent coughing episodes and copious production of secretions. To what is this increase of coughing and secretions related?
    1. Irritation of the stoma by the tracheostomy tube
    2. Upper respiratory inflammation due to allergies
    3. Inadequate turning, coughing, and deep breathing
    4. The mucous membranes' reaction to air that is dry and unwarmed

653. An important nursing intervention that ensures adequate ventilatory exchange after surgery is:
    1. Maintaining humidified oxygen via nasal cannula
    2. Positioning the client laterally with the neck extended
    3. Assessing for hypoventilation by auscultating the lungs
    4. Removing the airway only when the client is fully conscious

654. Which condition, identified by researchers, is related to the SARS virus?
    1. Malaria
    2. Tularemia
    3. Common cold
    4. Legionnaires' disease

655. The nurse is assessing a client with emphysema. Which sign of COPD does the nurse expect to identify?
    1. Decreased breath sounds
    2. Atrophic accessory muscles
    3. Chest with a decreased AP diameter
    4. Shortened expiratory phase of the respiratory cycle

656. An obese adult, who smokes three packs of cigarettes daily, is admitted for major abdominal surgery. Postoperatively, the most appropriate laboratory value that the nurse should monitor routinely that reflects the client's respiratory status is the:
    1. Po_2
    2. Pco_2
    3. Hemoglobin
    4. Oxygen saturation

657. What should the nurse document after hearing soft swishing sounds of normal breathing when auscultating a client's chest?
   1. Adventitious sounds
   2. Fine crackling sounds
   3. Vesicular breath sounds
   4. Diminished breath sounds

658. A client who had a left-sided pneumonectomy is in the postanesthesia care unit (PACU). The nurse's primary concern at this time is to maintain:
   1. Blood replacement
   2. Ventilatory exchange
   3. Closed chest drainage
   4. Supplemental oxygenation

659. When assessing the breath sounds of a client with chronic obstructive pulmonary disease (COPD), the nurse hears coarse crackles (rhonchi). They are best described as:
   1. Snorting sounds during the inspiratory phase
   2. Moist rumbling sounds that clear after coughing
   3. Musical sounds more pronounced during expiration
   4. Crackling inspiratory sounds unchanged with coughing

660. A client is brought to the emergency department with deep partial-thickness burns on the face and full-thickness burns on the neck, entire anterior chest, and right arm. When assessing for heat inhalation, the nurse should first observe for:
   1. Changes in the chest x-ray findings
   2. Sputum that contains particles of blood
   3. Nasal discharge containing carbon particles
   4. Changes in the arterial blood gases consistent with acidosis

661. The nurse's physical assessment of a client with heart failure reveals tachypnea and bilateral crackles. What should the nurse do next?
   1. Initiate oxygen therapy
   2. Obtain a chest x-ray film immediately
   3. Place client in a high-Fowler's position
   4. Assess the client for a pleural friction rub

662. What is the best method to assess a client for stridor in the immediate postoperative period after a radical neck dissection?
   1. Listen with a stethoscope over the trachea
   2. Determine the client's ability to do neck exercises
   3. Listen with a stethoscope over the base of the lungs
   4. Determine the client's ability to cough and deep breathe

663. A nurse is teaching a preoperative client about postoperative breathing exercises. What information should the nurse include? Select all that apply.
   1. _____ Take short, frequent breaths
   2. _____ Exhale with the mouth open
   3. _____ Plan to do the exercises twice a day
   4. _____ Place a hand on the abdomen while feeling it rise
   5. _____ Hold the breath for several seconds at the height of inspiration

664. A client is admitted to the intensive care unit with a diagnosis of acute respiratory distress syndrome. What should the nurse expect to identify when assessing this client?
   1. Hypertension
   2. Tenacious sputum
   3. Altered mental status
   4. Slow rate of breathing

665. Endotracheal intubation and positive-pressure ventilation are instituted because of a client's deteriorating respiratory status. What is the priority nursing intervention at this time?
   1. Facilitate verbal communication
   2. Prepare the client for emergency surgery
   3. Maintain sterility of the ventilation system
   4. Assess the client's response to the mechanical ventilation

666. A client is admitted to the emergency department with multiple injuries including fractured ribs. Because of the client's fractured ribs, the nurse should assess for signs of:
   1. Pneumonitis
   2. Hematemesis
   3. Pulmonary edema
   4. Respiratory acidosis *d/t Hypovent.*

667. A client is placed on a ventilator. Because hyperventilation can occur when mechanical ventilation is used, the nurse should monitor the client for signs of:
   1. Hypoxia
   2. Hypercapnia
   3. Metabolic acidosis
   4. Respiratory alkalosis

668. A client is on a ventilator. One of the nurses asks what should be done when condensation, resulting from humidity, collects in the ventilator tubing. What should the nurse in charge instruct the other nurse to do?
   1. "Notify the respiratory therapist."
   2. "Empty the fluid from the tubing."
   3. "Decrease the amount of humidity."
   4. "Record the amount of fluid removed from the tubing."

669. After surgery in the inguinal area, the client complains of pain on the right side of the chest, becomes dyspneic, and begins to cough violently. The nurse suspects that a pulmonary embolus has occurred. What is the priority nursing action?
   1. Auscultate the chest
   2. Obtain the vital signs
   3. Elevate the head of the bed
   4. Position the client on the right side

670. A client with a pulmonary embolus is intubated and placed on mechanical ventilation. When suctioning the endotracheal tube, the nurse should:
   1. Apply suction while inserting the catheter
   2. Hyperoxygenate with 100% oxygen before and after suctioning

3. Use short, jabbing movements of the catheter to loosen secretions

4. Suction two or three times in quick succession to remove the secretions

671. The respiratory status of a client with Guillain-Barré syndrome progressively deteriorates and a tracheostomy is performed. Nasogastric tube feedings are ordered. The nurse should:
   1. Deflate the tracheostomy cuff before starting tube feeding
   2. Inflate the tracheostomy cuff for 1 hour before and after each feeding
   3. Deflate the tracheostomy cuff after the tube feeding has been completed
   4. Inflate the tracheostomy cuff before and for 30 minutes after each feeding

672. The nurse considers that when a client has a tracheostomy tube with a high-volume, low-pressure cuff, it is used primarily to prevent:
   1. Leakage of air
   2. Lung infection
   3. Mucosal necrosis
   4. Tracheal secretion

673. A 21-year-old aspiring actress is admitted for a rhinoplasty to improve her appearance and facilitate her breathing. When monitoring for hemorrhage after this surgery, the nurse should assess specifically for the presence of:
   1. Facial edema
   2. Excessive swallowing
   3. Pressure around the eyes
   4. Serosanguineous drainage on the dressing

674. A female college student who had a rhinoplasty is having the nasal packing removed several days after surgery. The nurse should recommend that the client:
   1. Avoid sneezing for two days
   2. Brush her teeth after any intake
   3. Take fluids at a tepid temperature
   4. Sleep on her back with one pillow

675. A client with emphysema is short of breath and is using pursed-lip breathing and accessory muscles of respiration. What does the nurse identify as the cause of the client's dyspnea?
   1. Spasm of the bronchi that traps the air
   2. Increase in the vital capacity of the lungs
   3. Too rapid expulsion of the air from the alveoli
   4. Difficulty in expelling the air trapped in the alveoli

676. A client with an acute emphysemic episode is dyspneic and anxious. To decrease the dyspnea, the nurse's first action is to:
   1. Increase the client's oxygen intake
   2. Have the client breathe into a paper bag
   3. Teach the client to do rhythmic breathing
   4. Check the client's vital signs, including the BP

677. A client with a 10-year history of emphysema is admitted in acute respiratory distress. The nurse's assessment of this client includes monitoring for:
   1. Signs of chest pain

2. Use of accessory muscles of respiration

3. Signs and symptoms of respiratory alkalosis

4. Prolonged inspiration and expenditure of considerable effort

678. A client with chronic obstructive pulmonary disease (COPD) is predisposed to the development of CO_2 intoxication (CO_2 narcosis). Therefore, the nurse should:
   1. Initiate pulmonary hygiene to clear air passages of trapped mucus
   2. Encourage continuous rapid panting to promote respiratory exchange
   3. Administer oxygen at a low concentration to maintain respiratory drive
   4. Encourage slow, deep breathing with inhalation longer than exhalation to increase intake

679. A client with a history of emphysema is in acute respiratory failure with respiratory acidosis. Low level oxygen is administered by nasal cannula. Four hours later the nurse identifies that the client has increased restlessness and confusion followed by a decreased respiratory rate and lethargy. The nurse should:
   1. Question the client about the confusion
   2. Increase the oxygen in small increments
   3. Percuss and vibrate the client's chest wall
   4. Discontinue or decrease the oxygen flow rate

680. If a client undergoing peritoneal dialysis develops symptoms of severe respiratory difficulty during the infusion of the dialysate, the nurse should:
   1. Slow the rate of the client's infusion
   2. Place the client in a low Fowler's position
   3. Auscultate the client's lungs for breath sounds
   4. Drain the fluid from the client's peritoneal cavity

681. A nurse evaluates that a client understands the instructions about an appropriate breathing technique for chronic obstructive pulmonary disease, resulting from emphysema, when the client:
   1. Inhales through the mouth
   2. Increases the respiratory rate
   3. Holds each breath for a second at the end of inspiration
   4. Progressively increases the length of the inspiratory phase

682. A client who is admitted with emphysema has a P_{CO_2} of 60. The nurse determines that this is excessively high and calls the practitioner to obtain an order for:
   1. Mucolytics
   2. Bronchodilators
   3. Mechanical ventilation
   4. Intermittent positive-pressure breathing (IPPB)

683. A nurse is teaching a client how to perform diaphragmatic breathing. The nurse advises the client to:
   1. Take rapid, deep breaths
   2. Breathe with hands on the hips
   3. Expand the abdomen on inhalation
   4. Perform exercises leaning forward while in a sitting position

684. A nurse is teaching a community-based course on smoking cessation. The statement by a male client with chronic obstructive pulmonary disease (COPD) that provides evidence that he is ready to quit smoking is:
    1. "I'll just finish this carton."
    2. "I'll cut back to a half pack a day."
    3. "I am quitting the only relaxation I have."
    4. "I should find this easy because I don't drink when I smoke."

685. A client who has emphysema for many years develops an enlarged liver. The nurse concludes that this results from:
    1. Liver hypoxia
    2. Hepatic acidosis
    3. Esophageal varices
    4. Portal hypertension

686. A nurse is auscultating the chest of a client with chronic obstructive pulmonary disease. What should the nurse expect to hear?
    1. Diminished sounds
    2. Pleural friction rub
    3. Crackles and gurgles
    4. Expiratory wheeze and cough

687. A client with chronic obstructive pulmonary disease complains of a weight gain of 5 pounds in 1 week. The complication that may have precipitated this weight gain is:
    1. Polycythemia
    2. Cor pulmonale
    3. Compensated acidosis
    4 Left ventricular failure

688. A client with chronic obstructive pulmonary disease (COPD) complains of chest congestion especially in the morning. The nurse should suggest that the client:
    1. Use a humidifier in the room
    2. Sleep with two or more pillows
    3. Cough even when it is nonproductive
    4. Deep breathe and cough before retiring

689. A client has chronic obstructive pulmonary disease (COPD) and cor pulmonale. When teaching about nutrition, the nurse instructs this client to:
    1. Eat small meals six times a day to limit oxygen needs
    2. Drink large amounts of fluid to help liquefy secretions
    3. Lie down after eating to conserve energy needed for digestion
    4. Increase the intake of protein to decrease intravascular hydrostatic pressure

690. The nurse is observing a client with chronic obstructive pulmonary disease (COPD) using a nebulizer. What indicates that additional teaching is necessary?
    1. Placing the tip of the nebulizer just beyond the lips
    2. Holding the inspired breath for at least three seconds
    3. Exhaling slowly through the mouth with lips pursed slightly
    4. Inhaling with the lips tightly sealed around the mouthpiece of the nebulizer

691. A 70-year-old client with cancer of the right lung has a lobectomy. After surgery the client has a chest tube attached to suction. What observation should the nurse report to the practitioner?
    1. Clots in the tubing during the first postoperative day
    2. Subcutaneous emphysema on the second postoperative day
    3. Decreased bubbling in the water-seal chamber on the third postoperative day
    4. Bloody fluid in the drainage-collection chamber on the first postoperative day

692. A 21-year-old client comes to the emergency department with the chief complaint of left-sided chest pain after a racquetball game. A chest x-ray examination reveals a left pneumothorax. What should the nurse expect to identify when assessing the client's left chest area?
    1. Dull sound on percussion
    2. Vocal fremitus on palpation
    3. Rales with rhonchi on auscultation
    4. Absence of breath sounds on auscultation

693. A client with a spontaneous pneumothorax asks, "Why did they put this tube into my chest?" The nurse explains that the purpose of the chest tube is to:
    1. Check for bleeding in the lung
    2. Monitor the function of the lung
    3. Drain fluid from the pleural space
    4. Remove air from the pleural space

694. When evaluating the effectiveness of a chest tube inserted in a client with a pneumothorax, the nurse assesses for:
    1. Productive coughing
    2. Return of breath sounds
    3. Increased pleural drainage in the chamber
    4. Constant bubbling in the water-seal chamber

695. When inspecting a dressing after a partial pneumonectomy for cancer of the lung, the nurse observes some puffiness of the tissue around the area. When the area is palpated, the tissue feels spongy, and crackles. When documenting, the nurse describes this assessment as:
    1. Stridor
    2. Crepitus
    3. Pitting edema
    4. Chest distention

696. On the first day after a right pneumonectomy, a male client suddenly sits straight up in bed. His respirations are labored, and he is making a crowing sound. His skin is pale, cool, and moist. The nurse immediately should:
    1. Notify the practitioner
    2. Auscultate the left lung
    3. Inspect the incision for bleeding
    4. Check the chest tube for patency

697. A client in the postanesthesia care unit has just regained consciousness after a right pneumonectomy. The nurse should now:
    1. Assess for pain
    2. Remove the airway
    3. Encourage deep breathing
    4. Place the client on the left side

698. When turning a client after a right pneumonectomy, the nurse plans to place the client in either the:
1. Right or left side-lying position
2. High Fowler's or supine position
3. Supine or right side-lying position
4. Left side-lying or low Fowler's position

699 The nurse should be vigilant for the unique complications associated with a pneumonectomy by observing the client for:
1. Signs of cardiac overload
2. Increased pulse and respirations
3. Cardiac irregularities with premature beats
4. Elevated BP, decreased temperature, and cold, moist skin

700. The most appropriate breathing and coughing routine for a client who has had a pneumonectomy is every:
1. Hour for the first 24 hours and then every 2 hours
2. Two hours for the first 24 hours and then every 3 hours
3. Thirty minutes for the first 24 hours and then every 2 hours
4. Fifteen minutes for the first 24 hours and then every 2 hours

701. A client with oat-cell lung cancer is scheduled for a mediastinoscopy and biopsy. The nurse should:
1. Tell the client chest tubes will be present after the procedure
2. Advise the client that this is an endoscopic examination of lymph nodes
3. Explain to the client that the procedure will visualize the mainstem bronchus
4. Inform the client that some pleural fluid will be removed during the procedure

702. A client arrives in the emergency department and states, "I have a bad cold and chest pain that gets worse when I take a deep breath." In addition to obtaining the vital signs, the nurse auscultates the client's breath sounds. Where should the nurse place the stethoscope to determine the presence of a pleural friction rub?
1. a
2. b
3. c
4. d   lung bases

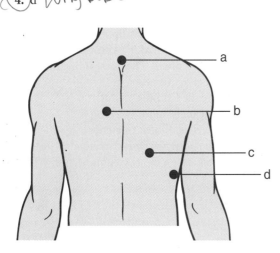

703. When assessing a client with pleural effusion, the nurse expects to identify:
1. Moist crackles at the posterior of the lungs
2. Deviation of the trachea toward the involved side
3. Reduced or absent breath sounds at the base of the lung
4. Increased resonance with percussion of the involved area

704. After a thoracentesis for pleural effusion, a client returns to the outpatient clinic for a follow-up visit. The nurse suspects a recurrence of pleural effusion when the client says:
1. "Lately I can only breathe well if I sit up."
2. "During the night I sometimes get the chills."
3. "I get a sharp, stabbing pain when I take a deep breath."
4. "I'm coughing up larger amounts of thicker mucus for the last several days."

705. A client with an exacerbation of a chronic inflammatory bowel disorder cannot tolerate food. A subclavian catheter is inserted. Immediately after insertion of the catheter, the priority nursing action is to:
1. Obtain a chest x-ray to determine placement
2. Auscultate the client's lungs to evaluate breath sounds
3. Draw a blood sample to assess the client's blood glucose level
4. Assess the upper extremity on the side of insertion for a neurological deficit

706. During the immediate postoperative period after a laryngectomy, a nursing priority for the client is to:
1. Provide emotional support
2. Observe for signs of infection
3. Keep the trachea free of secretions
4. Promote a means of communication

707. After surgery the practitioner orders an incentive spirometer for a client. The nurse evaluates that the spirometer is being used correctly when observing the client:
1. Coughing twice before inhaling deeply through the mouthpiece
2. Using the incentive spirometer for 10 consecutive breaths an hour
3. Inhaling deeply, sealing the lips around the mouthpiece, and exhaling
4. Inhaling deeply through the mouthpiece, holding the breath for 2 seconds, and then exhaling

708. A 60-year-old male is returned to the surgical unit after a laryngoscopy. The primary nurse who is being supervised by the nurse manager, reminds the client not to take anything by mouth until instructed to do so. The nurse manager determines that this nursing intervention is:
1. Inappropriate because the client is not unconscious and may be thirsty after being NPO
2. Appropriate because these clients usually experience painful swallowing for several days

3. Appropriate because early drinking and eating after the client's laryngoscopy may result in aspiration

4. Inappropriate because the client is likely to be anxious and probably will not be aware of feeling thirsty

709. A total laryngectomy and radical neck dissection are scheduled for a client with cancer of the larynx. When reinforcing the surgeon's statements to the client, the nurse should review what the surgery entails and what abilities will be lost. The discussion also should focus on what abilities will be retained, such as the ability to:
1. Blow the nose
2. Sip through a straw
3. Chew and swallow food
4. Smell and differentiate odors

710. After a radical neck resection, a client returns from surgery with two portable wound drainage systems at the operative site. Inspection of the neck incision reveals moderate edema of the tissues. Because of this problem, the nurse should assess the client for:
1. Loss of the gag reflex
2. Cloudy wound drainage
3. Restlessness and dyspnea
4. Edema and dehiscence of the suture line

711. The practitioner orders a progressive diet as tolerated for a client who had head and neck surgery. The nurse should:
1. Keep suction apparatus readily available in case aspiration occurs
2. Administer the diet through a nasogastric tube until the suture line heals
3. Encourage the intake of pureed foods because they promote the swallowing reflex
4. Administer the prescribed pain medication a half hour before meals to limit discomfort that may occur

712. A nurse expects that the initial treatment for a client who has a leak of the thoracic duct after radical neck surgery includes inserting a:
1. Gastrostomy tube to instill feedings, a high-fat diet, and bed rest
2. Chest tube to drain the fluid, total parenteral nutrition, and bed rest
3. Rectal tube to prevent distention, a low-fat diet, and increased activity
4. Nasogastric tube to drain the fluid, a moderate-fat diet, and increased activity

713. A 79-year-old pipe smoker is diagnosed as having cancer of the tongue. A hemiglossectomy and right radical neck dissection are performed. After surgery, the client is transferred to the postanesthesia care unit. When providing for a patent airway, a primary nursing intervention is to:
1. Suction frequently
2. Apply an ice collar
3. Maintain a high Fowler's position
4. Encourage expectoration of secretions

714. A half hour after awakening from anesthesia in the postanesthesia care unit (PACU) a 75-year-old client, who had radical head and neck surgery, becomes agitated, disoriented, and confused. The nurse should:
1. Notify the practitioner
2. Administer the prescribed oxygen
3. Record the observations on the progress notes
4. Medicate the client with the ordered antianxiety medication

715. A client who has a hemiglossectomy and right radical neck dissection arrives in the postanesthesia care unit with two portable drainage catheters in the area of the incision, which are attached to Hemovacs. Six hours later one Hemovac accumulates 180 mL of serosanguineous drainage. The priority nursing intervention is to:
1. Turn the client onto the right side
2. Notify the practitioner immediately
3. Document the output because it is expected
4. Empty the container to reestablish negative pressure

716. A client is scheduled for coronary artery bypass surgery. The nurse explains to the client that chest tubes will be inserted during surgery to:
1. Prevent atelectasis postoperatively
2. Drain fluid from the pericardial sac
3. Reestablish negative intrapleural pressure
4. Monitor the amount of blood loss after surgery

717. When giving a client care on the second day after coronary artery bypass surgery, the nurse observes that the fluid in the water-seal chamber of the chest drainage device stops fluctuating. The nurse should:
1. Look for tube obstructions
2. Increase the amount of suction
3. Add sterile water to the chamber
4. Consider this an expected occurrence

718. A nurse is instructed to measure and document the amount of drainage from a client's chest tube. The nurse should:
1. Mark the time and fluid level on the outside of the drainage collection chamber of the closed chest drainage system
2. Aspirate fluid from the drainage collection chamber of the closed chest drainage system and then measure the drainage
3. Connect a new closed chest drainage system, measure the fluid in the drainage collection chamber of the old system, and discard the old system
4. Clamp the chest tube, empty the fluid from the drainage collection chamber of the closed chest drainage system into a measuring cup, and reconnect the system

719. After thoracic surgery a client has a chest tube connected to a water-seal drainage system attached to suction. When excessive bubbling is observed in the water-seal chamber, the nurse should:
1. Strip the chest tube catheter
2. Check the system for air leaks
3. Decrease the amount of suction pressure
4. Recognize that the system is functioning correctly

720. The nurse evaluates that further teaching is necessary when a client who has had thoracic surgery performs post-thoracotomy exercises by:
    1. Extending the arm up and back, then rotating it to the side
    2. Climbing a wall with fingers of the hand, fully extending the arm
    3. Tying a rope to a doorknob and swinging the arm in wide circles
    4. Extending the arm and bringing it up to touch the nose with a finger

721. A nurse in the emergency department is notified that a person who sustained a gunshot wound to the right side of the chest will arrive soon. What should the nurse plan to do?
    1. Reserve an operating room
    2. Prepare equipment for a tracheotomy
    3. Arrange for a portable x-ray examination
    4. Obtain equipment for chest tube insertion

722. A nurse is caring for a client after a crushing chest injury. A chest tube is inserted. Which observation indicates a desired response to this treatment?
    1. Increased breath sounds
    2. Increased respiratory rate
    3. Crepitus detected on palpation of the chest
    4. Constant bubbling in the drainage collection chamber

723. On the way to an x-ray examination, a client with a chest tube becomes confused and pulls the chest tube out. What is the nurse's immediate action?
    1. Place the client in the supine position
    2. Use a clamp to hold the insertion site open
    3. Obtain sterile Vaseline gauze to cover the opening
    4. Cover the opening with the cleanest material available — quickest

724. A client has a chest tube for a pneumothorax. The nurse identifies that the chest tube is separated from the drainage system and the client is experiencing respiratory difficulty. What should the nurse do?
    1. Obtain a new sterile drainage system
    2. Use two clamps to clamp the drainage tubing
    3. Reconnect the client's tube to the drainage system
    4. Place the client in the high Fowler's position immediately

725. To promote continued improvement in a client's respiratory status after a chest tube is removed, the nurse should:
    1. Continue observing for dyspnea and crepitus
    2. Encourage frequent coughing and deep breathing
    3. Encourage bed rest with range-of-motion exercises
    4. Remind the client to turn from side to side at least every two hours

726. When using personal protective equipment during a physical assessment of a homeless client who is admitted for alcohol withdrawal, the nurse considers that this client also may be at risk for:
    1. Prostatitis
    2. Tuberculosis
    3. Osteoarthritis
    4. Diverticulosis

727. A client has a tentative diagnosis of pulmonary tuberculosis (TB) and the chest x-ray film reveals a lesion in the right upper lobe. Which client complaint supports this diagnosis?
    1. Frothy sputum and fever
    2. Dry cough and pulmonary congestion
    3. Night sweats and blood-tinged sputum
    4. Productive cough and engorged neck veins

728. A nurse administers a Mantoux test for tuberculosis to a client who has chronic obstructive pulmonary disease (COPD) and is HIV negative. The test results indicate a 10-mm area of induration with 5 mm of erythema. The nurse should:
    1. Record a false result and readminister the Mantoux test
    2. Indicate the degree of erythema and record the results as positive
    3. Take the client's history into account and determine that the response to the test is positive
    4. Identify that the extent of induration is significant and the client has been exposed to the pathogen that causes tuberculosis

729. To make a definitive diagnosis of tuberculosis, the nurse expects that the practitioner will order a:
    1. Chest x-ray film
    2. Tuberculin skin test
    3. Pulmonary function test
    4. Sputum for acid-fast testing

730. A client newly diagnosed with tuberculosis has a productive cough. The most appropriate nursing intervention is to teach the client to:
    1. Exercise daily
    2. Use disposable tissues
    3. Avoid foods high in sodium
    4. Monitor blood pressure weekly

731. A client with pulmonary tuberculosis is being treated at home. To help control the spread of the disease, the nurse instructs the client to:
    1. Have visitors sit across the room from the client
    2. Keep personal articles away from the rest of the family
    3. Open the windows slightly to allow air to circulate throughout the house
    4. Avoid putting used dishes in the dishwasher with the rest of the family's dishes

732. A client's purified protein derivative (PPD) test and chest x-ray film results indicate pulmonary tuberculosis. The practitioner orders sputum specimens for acid-fast bacilli. The nurse evaluates that additional teaching is necessary when the client states that the sputum specimens must be:
    1. Coughed up from deep in the lungs
    2. Collected in the early morning hours
    3. Refrigerated until brought to the laboratory
    4. Brought to the clinic as soon as possible after collection

733. When teaching a client with tuberculosis about recovery after discharge from the hospital, the nurse reinforces that the treatment measure with the highest priority is:
    1. Having sufficient rest
    2. Getting plenty of fresh air
    3. Changing the current lifestyle
    4. Consistently taking prescribed medication

734. A client with tuberculosis asks the nurse how long the chemotherapy must be continued. The nurse's most accurate reply is:
    1. "1 to 2 weeks."
    2. "4 to 5 months."
    3. "6 to 12 months."
    4. "3 years or longer."

REPRODUCTIVE AND GENITOURINARY

735. To facilitate micturition in a male client, the nurse should instruct him to:
    1. Use a urinal for voiding
    2. Drink cranberry juice daily
    3. Wash his hands after voiding
    4. Assume the standing position for voiding

736. A nurse is assessing a client who reports frequency and burning when urinating. The nurse performs percussion to determine if there is tenderness that indicates the presence of an ascending urinary tract infection. Which area should be percussed?
    1. Tail of Spence
    2. Suprapubic area
    3. McBurney's point
    4. Costovertebral angle

737. A client is scheduled for an intravenous pyelogram (IVP). The nurse explains that on the day before the IVP the client must:
    1. Avoid fats and proteins
    2. Drink a large amount of fluids
    3. Omit dinner and limit beverages
    4. Take a laxative before going to bed

738 A nurse instructs a client with a history of frequent urinary tract infections to drink cranberry juice to:
    1. Decrease the urinary pH
    2. Exert a bactericidal effect
    3. Improve glomerular filtration
    4. Relieve the symptoms of dysuria

739. To help prevent a cycle of recurring urinary tract infections, the nurse should plan to instruct a female client to:
    1. Increase the daily intake of citrus juice
    2. Douche frequently with alkaline agents
    3. Urinate as soon as possible after intercourse
    4. Cleanse from the vaginal orifice to the urethra

740. A female client who has recurrent urinary tract infections (UTIs) is inquiring about the prevention of future UTIs. What information should the nurse include when teaching the client? Select all that apply.
    1. _____ Avoid fluid intake after 6 PM
    2. _____ Drink 8 to 10 glasses of water each day

3. _____ Urinate immediately after sexual intercourse
    4. _____ Increase the daily intake of carbonated beverages
    5. _____ Clean the perineal area with an astringent soap twice a day

741. A 52-year-old woman 3 hours into a car trip is injured in an automobile collision and is admitted for observation. Damage to her bladder is evident. The history that indicates an increased risk of bladder rupture is:
    1. Multiple bouts of cystitis
    2. Familial history of bladder cancer
    3. Failure to have voided before starting the trip
    4. Drinking two cups of coffee before the accident

742. A client has surgery to repair a bladder laceration. The routine nursing intervention that takes priority in the postoperative care of this client is:
    1. Repositioning frequently
    2. Giving lower back care 3 times daily
    3. Implementing range-of-motion exercises
    4. Placing 3 side rails in the elevated position

743. A male client, age 56, is being assessed for possible cancer of the urinary bladder. Of the client's signs and symptoms, the one most significant for cancer of the urinary tract is:
    1. Dysuria
    2. Retention
    3. Hesitancy
    4. Hematuria

744. A 64-year-old client diagnosed with cancer of the bladder is scheduled for a total cystectomy and the formation of an ileal conduit. When assessing the client 8 hours after surgery, the nurse identifies all of the following findings. Which finding should be promptly reported?
    1. Edematous stoma
    2. Dusky-colored stoma
    3. Absence of bowel sounds
    4. Pink-tinged urinary drainage

745. On the fourth postoperative day after a cystectomy and the formation of a continent diversion, the nurse observes mucous threads in a client's urine. The nurse should:
    1. Expect this response after the diversion
    2. Report this to the practitioner immediately
    3. Obtain a specimen for culture and sensitivity
    4. Increase the client's fluid intake for the next twelve hours

746. A client with an ileal conduit is being prepared for discharge. Before discharge the nurse instructs the client to:
    1. Abstain from beer and alcohol consumption
    2. Maintain fluid intake of at least two liters daily
    3. Notify the practitioner if the stoma size decreases
    4. Avoid getting soap and water on the peristomal skin

747. A client complains of urinary problems. Cholinergic medications are prescribed. Which condition is treated with cholinergic medications?
    1. Kidney stones
    2. Flaccid bladder
    3. Spastic bladder
    4. Urinary tract infections

748. Twenty-four hours after a penile implant the client's scrotum is edematous and painful. The nurse should:
1. Assist the client with a sitz bath
2. Apply warm soaks to the scrotum
3. Elevate the scrotum using a soft support
4. Prepare for an incision and drainage procedure

749. A male client comes to the emergency department because he has a discharge from his penis. The practitioner suspects gonorrhea and asks the nurse to obtain a specimen and to send it for a culture. The nurse should:
1. Instruct the client to provide a semen specimen
2. Swab the discharge when it appears on the prepuce
3. Teach the client how to obtain a clean catch specimen of urine
4. Swab the drainage directly from the urethra to obtain a specimen

750. A client comes to the infectious disease clinic because a sexual partner was recently diagnosed as having gonorrhea. The health history reveals that the client has engaged in receptive anal intercourse. The nurse should assess the client for:
1. Melena
2. Anal itching
3. Constipation
4. Ribbon-shaped stools

751. The nurse should ask the client with secondary syphilis about sexual contacts during the past:
1. 21 days
2. 30 days
3. 3 months
4. 6 months

752. A client is suspected of having late-stage (tertiary) syphilis. When obtaining a health history, the nurse determines that the statement by the client that most supports this diagnosis is:
1. "I noticed a wart on my penis."
2. "I have sores all over my mouth."
3. "I've been losing a lot of hair lately."
4. "I'm having trouble keeping my balance."

753. A 45-year-old client develops acute glomerulonephritis after a recent streptococcal infection. Which sign or symptom should the nurse expect the client to report?
1. Nocturia
2. Mild headache
3. Increased appetite
4. Recent weight loss

754. A client with acute glomerulonephritis complains of thirst. What should the nurse offer the client?
1. Ginger ale
2. Milk shake
3. Hard candy
4. Cup of broth

755. To prevent future attacks of glomerulonephritis, the nurse planning discharge teaching includes instructions for the client to:
1. Take showers instead of bubble baths
2. Avoid situations that involve physical activity

3. Continue the same restrictions on fluid intake
4. Seek early treatment for respiratory infections

756. A nurse is obtaining a health history from a client with the diagnosis of renal calculi. Which factor in the client's history most likely contributed to the development of renal calculi?
1. High-cholesterol diet
2. Excessive exercise program
3. Excess ingestion of antacids
4. Frequent consumption of alcohol

757. A client is admitted to the hospital with a ureteral calculus. What clinical findings should the nurse expect when the client voids?
1. Urgency and pain
2. Foul odor and dark urine
3. Hematuria with sharp pain
4. Frequency with small amounts of urine

758. When planning care for a client with ureteral colic, the goal of preventing future calculi is based on the knowledge that most factors contributing to the development of renal stones can be overcome by:
1. Decreasing serum creatinine
2. Excluding milk products from the diet
3. Drinking 8 to 10 glasses of water daily
4. Excreting 2000 mL of urine per 24 hours

759. A male client is diagnosed as having phosphatic calculi. The nurse teaches the client that his diet may include:
1. Apples
2. Chocolate
3. Rye bread
4. Cheddar cheese

760. A nurse is obtaining the health history of a client with a left ureteral calculus who is scheduled for a transurethral ureterolithotomy. Which description of pain should the nurse expect the client to report?
1. Boring pain in the left flank
2. Pain that intensifies on urination
3. Dull pain that is constant in the costovertebral angle
4. Spasmodic pain on the left side that radiates to the suprapubic area

761. The laboratory values of a client with renal calculi reveal a serum calcium within expected limits and an elevated serum purine. The nurse concludes that the stone is probably composed of:
1. Cystine
2. Uric acid
3. Calcium oxalate
4. Magnesium ammonium phosphate

762. A client is transferred to the postanesthesia care unit after undergoing a pyelolithotomy. The client's urinary output is 50 mL/hr. The nurse should:
1. Record the findings
2. Notify the practitioner
3. Milk the client's nephrostomy tube
4. Encourage the client to drink oral fluids

763. The most essential nursing care for a client with a neph-rostomy tube is:
    1. Ensuring free drainage of urine
    2. Milking the tube every 2 hours
    3. Instilling 2 mL of normal saline every 8 hours
    4. Keeping an accurate record of intake and output

764. A female client is admitted to the hospital with severe renal colic caused by a ureteral calculus. Later that evening the client's urinary output is much less than her intake. When it is confirmed that her bladder is not distended, the nurse should suspect the development of:
    1. Oliguria
    2. Hydroureter
    3. Renal shutdown
    4. Urethral obstruction

765. An obese client with calculi in the calyces of the right kidney is admitted for their removal. The nurse prepares the client for the procedure by explaining that:
    1. The right ureter will be removed
    2. A suprapubic catheter will be in place
    3. The surgery will be performed transurethrally
    4. A small incision will be present in the right flank area

766. A male client who has had recurring renal calculi has a ureterolithotomy. Before discharge the nurse discusses the need to avoid urinary tract infections (UTIs). The nurse evaluates that the signs and symptoms of infection are understood when the client says he will report:
    1. Urgency or frequency of urination
    2. The inability to maintain an erection
    3. Pain radiating to the external genitalia
    4. An increase in alkalinity or acidity of urine

767. A client who had a lithotripsy for a renal calculus is to be discharged from the hospital. The nurse who is providing home care instructions should include:
    1. Drinking at least 3 L of fluid daily for 4 weeks
    2. Removing organ meats from the diet for 6 weeks
    3. Increasing the intake of dairy products for 5 days
    4. Restricting movement for 3 days before resuming usual activities

768. A nurse assesses a newly admitted client with renal colic to determine the signs and symptoms that may be present. The nurse should assess the client for which primary subjective symptom?
    1. Uremia
    2. Nausea
    3. Voiding at night
    4. Flank discomfort

769. When teaching a community health class the nurse informs the group that the person at highest risk of developing prostate cancer is a:
    1. 55-year-old black male
    2. 45-year-old white male
    3. 55-year-old Asian male
    4. 45-year-old Hispanic male

770. A 72-year-old male complaining of dysuria, nocturia, and difficulty starting the urinary stream is scheduled for a cystoscopy and biopsy of the prostate gland. After the procedure the client complains that he is unable to void. The nurse should:
    1. Limit oral fluids until he voids
    2. Assure him that this is expected
    3. Insert a urinary retention catheter
    4. Palpate above the pubic symphysis

771. When admitting a client with benign prostatic hyperplasia, the most relevant assessment made by the nurse is:
    1. Perineal edema
    2. Urethral discharge
    3. Flank pain radiating to the groin
    4. Distention of the lower abdomen

772. A client is scheduled for a transurethral prostatectomy. He is concerned about the operation's effect on his sexual ability. The nurse should reply that he may:
    1. Experience retrograde ejaculations
    2. Have prolonged erections afterward
    3. Be permanently impotent after the operation
    4. Develop a diminishing sex drive after the surgery

773. A client who has had a transurethral prostatectomy (TURP) experiences dribbling after the indwelling catheter is removed. To address this problem, the nurse should state:
    1. "Increase your fluid intake and urinate at regular intervals."
    2. "I know you're worried, but it will go away in a few days."
    3. "Limit your fluid intake and urinate when you first feel the urge."
    4. "The catheter will have to be reinserted until your bladder regains its tone."

774. When planning care for a client with a continuous bladder irrigation after a transurethral vaporization of the prostate, the nurse should:
    1. Measure the output hourly
    2. Monitor the specific gravity of the urine
    3. Irrigate the catheter with saline three times daily
    4. Exclude the amount of irrigant instilled from the output

775. After a transurethral vaporization of the prostate, the client returns to the unit with a urinary retention catheter and a continuous bladder irrigation. What should the nurse do first when the client indicates the need to urinate?
    1. Assess that the tubing attached to the collection bag is patent
    2. Obtain the client's vital signs before notifying the practitioner
    3. Explain that the balloon inflated in the bladder causes this feeling
    4. Review the client's intake and output that was documented in the previous shift

776. The nurse evaluates that a client who had a transurethral vaporization of the prostate understands the discharge teaching when he says, "I should:
    1. sit for several hours daily."
    2. report if my urinary stream decreases."

3. attempt to void every 3 hours when I'm awake."

4. avoid vigorous exercise for 6 months after surgery."

777. In the early postoperative period after a transurethral resection of the prostate, the most common complication the nurse should monitor for is:
1. Sepsis
2. Hemorrhage
3. Leakage around the catheter
4. Urinary retention with overflow

778. A 75-year-old male with a history of cancer of the prostate is admitted for a prostatectomy. The client's prostate specific antigen (PSA) levels have been increasing. This finding should prompt the nurse to plan to:
1. Measure intake and output
2. Institute seizure precautions
3. Monitor his plasma pH for acidosis
4. Handle him gently when turning him

779. A client who had a prostatectomy complains of painful bladder spasms. To limit these spasms the nurse should:
1. Administer the client's ordered opioid every 4 hours
2. Irrigate the indwelling catheter with 60 mL of isotonic solution
3. Encourage the client to avoid contracting his muscles as if he were voiding
4. Advance the urinary catheter to relieve the pressure against the prostatic fossa

780. After prostate surgery a client's indwelling catheter and continuous bladder irrigation (CBI) are to be removed. The nurse discusses the procedure with the client. The nurse evaluates that the teaching is understood when the client states, "After the catheter is removed I probably will:
1. have dilute urine."
2. be unable to urinate."
3. produce dark red urine."
4. experience some burning on urination."

781. A client who had a suprapubic prostatectomy for cancer of the prostate returns to the postanesthesia care unit with a continuous bladder irrigation. The purpose of this irrigation is to:
1. Stimulate continuous formation of urine
2. Facilitate the measurement of urinary output
3. Prevent the development of clots in the bladder
4. Provide continuous pressure on the prostatic fossa

782. After a suprapubic prostatectomy, a client's plan of care must include the prevention of postoperative deep vein thrombosis. This is best achieved by increasing the:
1. Coagulability of the blood
2. Velocity of the venous return
3. Effectiveness of internal respiration
4. Oxygen-carrying capacity of the blood

783. For what common early clinical manifestation should the nurse monitor in clients with renal carcinoma?
1. Flank pain
2. Weight gain
3. Periorbital edema
4. Intermittent hematuria

784. An acute, life-threatening complication for which a nurse should assess a client in the early postoperative period after a radical nephrectomy for cancer of the kidney is:
1. Sepsis
2. Hemorrhage
3. Renal failure
4. Paralytic ileus

785. A nurse's postoperative plan of care for a client who had a nephrectomy should include:
1. Clamping the client's nephrostomy tube when out of bed
2. Giving the client a regular diet on the first postoperative day
3. Replacing the client's original dressing after the first 48 hours
4. Turning the client from the back to the operated side every 2 to 3 hours - prevents resp. complications

786. A client has been receiving hemodialysis for several months. The nurse considers that bleeding into the GI tract is of particular significance to a client with chronic kidney disease because:
1. Hypovolemia can compromise kidney function
2. Blood is digested thereby increasing the kidneys' protein load ↑ is BUN
3. Clotting problems in kidney disease make diagnosis of the bleeding site difficult
4. Usual signs of blood loss will not be manifested in the client with kidney failure

787. A client with chronic kidney disease is on a restricted protein diet and is taught about high-biologic-value protein foods. An understanding of the rationale for this diet is demonstrated when the client states that high-biologic-value protein foods are:
1. Needed to promote weight gain
2. Necessary to prevent muscle wasting
3. Used to increase urea blood products
4. Responsible for controlling hypertension

788. The nurse is caring for a client with acute renal failure. The most serious complication for this client is:
1. Anemia
2. Infection
3. Weight loss
4. Platelet dysfunction

789. A nurse evaluates that a client with chronic kidney disease understands an adequate source of high-biologic-value protein when the food the client selects from the menu is:
1. Apple juice
2. Raw carrots
3. Cottage cheese
4. Whole wheat bread

790. A home health care nurse visits a 40-year-old housewife who is receiving hemodialysis. When reviewing the diet with the client, the nurse encourages her to include:
1. Rice   High carbs, low protein, low Nat, low k+
2. Potatoes

3. Canned salmon

4. Barbecued beef

791. A male client with a history of chronic kidney disease is hospitalized. The nurse assesses the client for signs of related kidney insufficiency, which include:

   1. Facial flushing

   (2.) Edema and pruritus

   3. Dribbling after voiding

   4. Diminished force and caliber of stream

792. A client with uremic syndrome has the potential to develop many complications. Which complication should the nurse anticipate?

   1. Hypotension

   2. Hypokalemia

   (3.) Flapping hand tremors *asterixis*

   4. Elevated hematocrit values

793. A nurse is notified that the latest potassium level for a client in acute renal failure is 6.2 mEq. What is most important for the nurse to do?

   1. Alert the cardiac arrest team

   2. Call the laboratory to repeat the test

   (3.) Take vital signs and notify the practitioner

   4. Obtain an ECG strip and have lidocaine available

794. While the nurse is at the bedside of a client in acute renal failure, the client states, "My doctor said that I will be getting some insulin. Do I also have diabetes?" The response that best demonstrates an understanding of the use of insulin in acute renal failure is:

   (1.) "No, the insulin will help your body handle the increased potassium level."

   2. "Why don't you ask that question when the doctor comes to see you today."

   3. "You probably had an elevated blood glucose level, so your doctor is being cautious."

   4. "No, but insulin will reduce the toxins in your blood by lowering your metabolic rate."

795. The home health care nurse is teaching about peritoneal dialysis to a client who has just started the procedure. The client is informed that if drainage of dialysate from the peritoneal cavity ceases before the required amount has drained out, the client should:

   1. Drink a glass of water

   (2.) Turn from side to side

   3. Deep breathe and cough

   4. Periodically rotate and reposition the catheter

796. The nurse teaches a client receiving peritoneal dialysis that the reason the dialysis solution is warmed to body temperature before it is instilled into the peritoneal cavity is to:

   1. Force potassium back into the cells, thereby decreasing serum levels

   2. Add extra warmth to the body because metabolic processes are disturbed

   3. Help prevent cardiac dysrhythmias by speeding up removal of excess potassium

   (4.) Encourage removal of serum urea by preventing constriction of peritoneal blood vessels

797. A client with acute renal failure moves into the diuretic phase after 1 week of therapy. For which signs during this phase should the nurse assess the client? Select all that apply.

   1. _✓_ Dehydration

   2. _✓_ Hypovolemia

   3. _____ Hyperkalemia

   4. _____ Metabolic acidosis

798. Diet instruction for a client who is being treated with continuous ambulatory peritoneal dialysis (CAPD) for chronic glomerulonephritis includes the need for:

   1. Low-calorie foods

   (2.) High-quality protein

   3. Increased fluid intake

   4. Foods rich in potassium

799. A client with end-stage kidney disease is to begin continuous ambulatory peritoneal dialysis (CAPD). When assessing the client before the institution of CAPD, the nurse should be alert for the presence of:

   (1.) Client motivation

   2. Cardiac problems

   3. Emotional lability

   4. Pulmonary problems

800. When performing a peritoneal dialysis procedure, the nurse should:

   1. Place the client in a side-lying position

   (2.) Warm dialysate solution slightly before instillation

   3. Infuse the dialysate solution slowly over several hours

   4. Withhold the routine medications until after the procedure

801. If a client on peritoneal dialysis develops symptoms of severe respiratory difficulty during the infusion of the dialysate solution, the nurse should:

   1. Increase the rate of infusion

   2. Auscultate the lungs for breath sounds

   3. Place the client in a low Fowler's position

   (4.) Drain the fluid from the peritoneal cavity *to ↓ pressure on diaphragm*

802. A client with end-stage kidney disease is receiving continuous ambulatory peritoneal dialysis. The nurse is monitoring the client for manifestations of complications associated with peritoneal dialysis. Select all that apply.

   1. _____ Pruritus

   2. _____ Oliguria

   3. _✓_ Tachycardia

   4. _✓_ Cloudy outflow

   5. _✓_ Abdominal pain

803. A client has end-stage kidney disease and is receiving hemodialysis. During dialysis the client complains of nausea and a headache and appears confused. Operating on standing protocols, the nurse should:

   1. Give an analgesic

   2. Administer an antiemetic

   (3.) Decrease the rate of exchange *disequilibrium*

   4. Discontinue the procedure immediately

804. A 62-year-old woman who has been on <u>hemodialysis</u> for several weeks asks the nurse what substances are being removed by the dialysis. The nurse informs the client that one of the substances passing through the membrane is:
    1. RBCs
    2. Sodium
    3. Glucose
    4. Bacteria

805. A client has <u>end-stage kidney disease</u> and is admitted for a <u>kidney transplant</u>. The nurse teaches the client that the donor must:
    1. Have the same blood type
    2. Be a member of the same family
    3. Be approximately the same body size
    4. Have matching leukocyte antigen complexes

806. An older adult client is admitted to the hospital with a diagnosis of <u>chronic kidney disease</u>. The nurse reviews the client's medical record and completes a physical assessment. Which clinical finding is a priority to be communicated to the practitioner?
    1. Sodium level
    2. Potassium level
    3. Creatinine results
    4. Elevated blood pressure

CLIENT CHART

Laboratory Results

Sodium 135 mEq/L
Potassium 6 mEq/L
Hemoglobin 8.5 g/dL
Creatinine clearance 20 mL/min

Client Interview

The client complains of lethargy and fatigue

Graphic Sheet

Temperature 99° F
Pulse 84
Respirations 24
Blood pressure 150/100

---

807. When a client returns from the postanesthesia care unit after a <u>kidney transplant</u>, the nurse should plan to measure the client's urinary output every:
    1. 1 hour
    2. 2 hours
    3. 3 hours
    4. 15 minutes

808. After a successful <u>kidney transplant</u> for a client with end-stage kidney disease, the nurse anticipates that laboratory studies will demonstrate:
    1. Increased specific gravity
    2. Correction of hypotension
    3. Elevated serum potassium
    4. Decreasing serum creatinine

809. A nurse teaches the signs of <u>organ rejection</u> to a client who had a <u>kidney transplant</u>. Which sign would the

client have to identify for the nurse to determine that the client understands the teaching?
    1. Weight loss
    2. Subnormal temperature
    3. Elevated blood pressure d/t hypervolemia
    4. Increased urinary output

810. A client who had a <u>kidney transplant</u> develops leukopenia 3 weeks after surgery. The nurse concludes that the leukopenia probably is caused by:
    1. Bacterial infection
    2. High creatinine levels
    3. Rejection of the kidney
    4. Antirejection medications

811. A client who has been receiving <u>hemodialysis</u> for several years is to receive a <u>kidney transplant</u>. The nurse plans to review the essential information that the client should know before surgery. Select all that apply.
    1. ___✓___ Precautions needed to prevent infection
    2. ___✓___ Kidney may not function immediately
    3. ___✓___ Urinary catheter will be present postoperatively
    4. _____ Immunosuppressive medications to be given preoperatively
    5. _____ AV fistula will be used for drawing blood specimens preoperatively

SKELETAL

812. A client with cancer is scheduled for a bone scan to determine the presence of metastasis. The nurse evaluates that the teaching before the scheduled bone scan is effective when the client states that:
    1. "X-rays will be taken to identify where I may have lost calcium from my bones."
    2. "Portions of my bone marrow will be removed and examined for cell composition."
    3. "A radioactive chemical will be injected into my vein that will destroy cancer cells present in my bones."
    4. "A substance of low radioactivity will be injected into my vein and my body inspected by an instrument to detect where it is deposited."

813. A nurse explains to a client that stimulation of calcium deposition in the bone after a distal femoral fracture is best achieved by:
    1. Resting the extremity
    2. Weight-bearing activity
    3. Normal aging processes
    4. Ingesting foods high in calcium

814. A nurse is performing range-of-motion exercises with a client who had a brain attack. The nurse places the client's hand in the position exhibited in the picture. This position is known as:
    1. Flexion
    2. Extension
    3. Adduction
    4. Circumduction

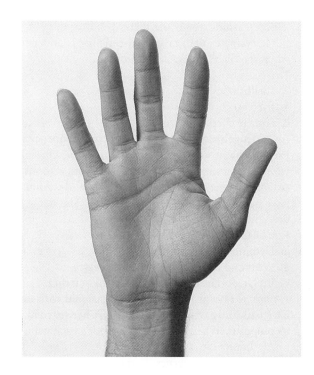

815. A male college basketball player comes to the infirmary complaining of a "click" in his knee when walking. He states that it occasionally gives way when he is running and sometimes locks. He does not recall any specific injury. Which condition should the nurse anticipate that the practitioner primarily will consider when determining the diagnostic tests to order?
1. Cracked patella
2. Ruptured Achilles tendon
3. Injured cartilage in the knee
4. Stress fracture of the tibial plateau

816. A client is scheduled for arthroscopic knee surgery and asks the nurse about the procedure. The statement by the nurse that best describes the procedure is:
1. "It is surgical repair of a joint under direct visualization using an arthroscope."
2. "It is a radiological procedure that will help diagnose the extent of the knee injury."
3. "The procedure will determine the type of treatments the surgeon will prescribe."
4. "You will be anesthetized so that you do not remember anything about the procedure."

817. The practitioner orders non–weight bearing with crutches for a client with a leg injury. Before ambulation is begun, the most important activity the nurse should teach the client to facilitate walking with crutches is:
1. Sitting up in a chair to help strengthen back muscles
2. Keeping the unaffected leg in extension and abduction
3. Exercising the triceps, finger flexors, and elbow extensors
4. Using a trapeze frequently to strengthen the biceps muscles

818. A client with impaired balance is using a walker to provide support when ambulating. While observing the client transferring from a sitting to a standing position and using the walker, the nurse evaluates that further teaching is required when the client:
1. Slides toward the edge of the seat before standing
2. Holds both handles of the walker while rising to the standing position
3. Moves forward into the walker after transferring from sitting to standing
4. Stands in place holding on to the walker for at least 30 seconds before walking

819. A client with multiple injuries from an automobile collision is now permitted out of bed to a chair but is not permitted to bear weight on the lower extremities. When using a mechanical lift to transfer the client, it is essential that the nurse:
1. Fold the client's arms across the chest
2. Place the sling so that the top is below the client's scapulae
3. Call the practitioner to secure an order to use a mechanical lift
4. Raise the lift so that the sling is at least twelve inches above the mattress

820. A nurse performs full range of motion on a client's extremities. When putting an ankle through range of motion, the nurse must perform:
1. Flexion, extension, and rotation
2. Abduction, flexion, adduction, and extension
3. Pronation, supination, rotation, and extension
4. Dorsiflexion, plantar flexion, eversion, and inversion

821. An x-ray film of a client's arm reveals a comminuted fracture of the radial bone. The nurse expects that with a comminuted fracture:
1. Bone protrudes through a break in the skin
2. The bone has broken into several fragments and the skin is intact
3. The bone is broken into two parts and the skin may or may not be broken
4. Splintering has occurred on one side of the bone and bending on the other

822. Clients who have casts applied to an extremity must be monitored for complications. The most significant complication for which the nurse should assess the client's extremity is:
1. Warmth
2. Numbness
3. Skin desquamation
4. Generalized discomfort

823. A nurse is providing teaching about self-care to a client who had a cast applied for a fracture of the right ulna and radius. For which occurrence should the nurse instruct the client to immediately notify the practitioner?
1. Slight stiffness of the fingers
2. Increasing pain at the injury site
3. Small amount of bloody drainage on the cast
4. Bounding radial pulse in the affected extremity

824. A client's right tibia is fractured in an automobile collision, and a cast is applied. For which manifestation related to damage to major blood vessels by the fractured tibia should the nurse assess?
    1. Increased blood pressure
    2. Prolonged edema in the thigh
    3. Increased skin temperature of the foot
    4. Prolonged reperfusion of the toes after blanching

825. Three days after a cast is applied to a client's fractured tibia, the client reports that there is a burning pain over the ankle. The cast over the ankle feels warm to the touch, and the pain is not relieved when the client changes position. The nurse's priority action is to:
    1. Obtain an order for an antibiotic
    2. Report the client's concern to the practitioner
    3. Administer the prescribed medication for pain
    4. Explain that this is typical after a cast is applied

826. After a long leg cast is removed, the client should be instructed to:
    1. Elevate the leg when sitting
    2. Report stiffness of the ankle
    3. Perform full range of motion once a day
    4. Cleanse the leg by scrubbing with a washcloth

827. While a woman with a fractured femur is being prepared for surgery, she exhibits cyanosis, tachycardia, dyspnea, and restlessness. What should the nurse do first?
    1. Call the practitioner
    2. Administer oxygen by mask
    3. Place her in the high Fowler's position
    4. Lower her to the Trendelenburg position

828. A nurse is assisting a client with a full leg cast to use crutches. Which clinical manifestations alert the nurse that the client can no longer tolerate the crutch walking?
    1. Pulse of 100 and deep respirations
    2. Flushed skin and slowed respirations
    3. Profuse diaphoresis and rapid respirations
    4. Blood pressure of 150/88 mm Hg and shallow respirations

829. A client with chronic osteomyelitis in a leg is to have a debridement of the infected bone. When planning for postoperative care the nurse expects that:
    1. Frequent range-of-motion exercises are needed
    2. Septicemia is a common postoperative complication
    3. The client will be allowed out of bed after the first day
    4. The client's leg may be immobilized in a cast or splint

830. A nurse is performing a physical assessment of a client with gout. What parts of the client's body should the nurse assess for the presence of tophi (urate deposits)? Select all that apply.
    1. _____ Feet
    2. _____ Ears
    3. _____ Chin
    4. _____ Buttocks
    5. _____ Abdomen

831. When teaching about the dietary control of gout, the nurse evaluates that the dietary teaching is understood when the client states; "I will avoid eating:
    1. eggs."
    2. shellfish."
    3. fried poultry."
    4. cottage cheese."

832. An older female client is experiencing frequency and uses the bathroom often during the night. One night while attempting to go to the bathroom without assistance, she develops severe back pain and is found to have a vertebral compression fracture. The nurse understands that this is a:
    1. Collapse of vertebral bodies
    2. Demineralization of the spinal cord
    3. Wear and tear of the spinous processes
    4. Bulging of the spinal cord from the vertebra

833. A dock worker is admitted to the hospital with lower back pain and a tentative diagnosis of a herniated nucleus pulposus. When assessing the client's back pain, the nurse should ask:
    1. "Is there any tenderness in the calf of your leg?"
    2. "Have you had any burning sensation on urination?"
    3. "Do you have any increase in pain during bowel movements?"
    4. "Does the pain progress from your flank around to your groin?"

834. A client who is diagnosed as having a herniated nucleus pulposus complains of pain. The nurse concludes that the pain is caused by the:
    1. Inflammation of the lamina of the involved vertebra
    2. Shifting of two adjacent vertebral bodies out of alignment
    3. Compression of the spinal cord by the extruded nucleus pulposus
    4. Increased pressure of cerebrospinal fluid within the vertebral column

835. A client is awaiting surgery for a herniated lumbar nucleus pulposus. The nurse's teaching should include that the pain will most likely increase if the client:
    1. Breathes deeply
    2. Lies on the side
    3. Flexes the knees
    4. Coughs excessively

836. A young adult with a herniated nucleus pulposus is scheduled for a diskectomy with fusion. Preoperatively, the nurse should demonstrate the:
    1. Use of a trapeze
    2. Contour position
    3. Traction apparatus
    4. Log-rolling technique

837. After a client has spinal surgery, it is essential that the nurse:
    1. Encourage the client to drink fluids
    2. Log-roll the client to the prone position
    3. Assess the client's feet for circulation and sensation
    4. Observe the client's bowel movements and voiding patterns

838. The nurse teaches a male client who developed degenerative joint disease of the vertebral column to turn himself from his back to his side, keeping his spine straight. The nurse explains that the least effort will be exerted if he crosses his arm over his chest and:
   1. Uses his overbed table to pull himself to one side
   2. Bends his top knee to the side to which he is turning
   3. Crosses his ankles while turning with both his legs straight
   4. Flexes his bottom knee to the side to which he wishes to turn

839. A male client has a diskectomy and fusion for a herniated nucleus pulposis. When two nurses are assisting the client to get out of bed for the first time he complains of feeling faint and lightheaded. The nurses should have the client:
   1. Sit on the edge of the bed so they can hold him upright
   2. Slide to the floor so he will not hurt himself when falling
   3. Bend forward so that blood flow to his brain is increased
   4. Lie down immediately so they can take his blood pressure

840. When preparing a client for discharge after a laminectomy, the nurse evaluates that further health teaching is necessary when the client says, "I should:
   1. sleep on a firm mattress to support my back."
   2. spend most of day sitting in a straight-back chair."
   3. put a pillow under my legs when sleeping on my back."
   4. avoid lifting heavy objects until the physician tells me I can."

841. A back brace is prescribed for a client who has had a laminectomy. What instruction should the nurse include in the teaching plan?
   1. Apply the brace before getting out of bed
   2. Put the brace on while in the sitting position
   3. Use the brace when the back begins to feel tired
   4. Wear the brace when performing twisting exercises

842. After a cervical neck injury, a male client is placed in a halo fixation device with a body cast. A statement that indicates that the client's concern about body image has been successfully resolved is:
   1. "I hate having everyone else do things for me."
   2. "I've gotten used to the brace. I may even miss it when it's gone."
   3. "I've been keeping my daily calories low in an attempt to lose weight."
   4. "I can't get to sleep. However, I make up for it in the morning by sleeping later."

843. A 30-year-old runner sustains multiple fractures of the left femur when hit by an automobile. At the scene of the accident, an immediate life-threatening systemic complication of injury to the long bones can be minimized by:
   1. Elevating the affected limb
   2. Encouraging deep breathing and coughing

   3. Handling and transporting the client gently
   4. Maintaining anatomic alignment of the client's limb

844. A 67-year-old woman fell while washing windows in her apartment. X-ray films indicate an intertrochanteric fracture of the left femur. She is to be placed in Buck's traction until surgery is performed the next morning. Nursing care is based on the fact that the primary purpose of Buck's traction is to:
   1. Reduce the fracture
   2. Immobilize the fracture
   3. Maintain abduction of the leg
   4. Eliminate rotation of the femur

845. A client sustains a fracture of the femur after jumping from the second story of a building during a fire. The client is placed in Buck's traction until an open reduction and internal fixation is performed. The client keeps slipping down in bed. To alleviate this problem the nurse should:
   1. Elevate the foot of the bed
   2. Shorten the rope on the weights
   3. Release the traction so the client can be repositioned
   4. Move the client toward the head of the bed every couple of hours

846. A 72-year-old male client has a total hip replacement for long-standing degenerative bone disease of the hip. When assessing this client postoperatively, the nurse considers that the most common complication of hip surgery is:
   1. Pneumonia
   2. Hemorrhage
   3. Wound infection
   4. Pulmonary embolism

847. A client has an open reduction and internal fixation for a fractured hip. Postoperatively the nurse should position the client's affected extremity in:
   1. External rotation
   2. Slight hip flexion
   3. Moderate abduction
   4. Anatomical body alignment

848. After surgery for a fractured hip, a client complains of pain. The nurse should:
   1. Notify the surgeon
   2. Use distraction techniques
   3. Medicate the client as ordered
   4. Perform a complete pain assessment

849. A client has an open reduction and internal fixation of a fractured hip. To prevent the most common complication after this type of surgery, the nurse expects the surgeon's order to state:
   1. "Turn from side to side periodically."
   2. "Apply sequential compression stockings."
   3. "Encourage isometric exercises to the extremities."
   4. "Perform passive range of motion to the affected extremity."

850. The most appropriate action by the nurse when assisting a client who has had a hip replacement to get out of bed 4 hours after surgery is to:
1. Tell the client that weight bearing must be on both legs equally
2. Advise the client that the legs must be kept wide apart continually
3. Sit the client in a straight-back chair so that the hips are kept flexed
4. Transfer the client using a mechanical lift because weight bearing on the leg is not allowed

851. A client returns from surgery with a hip prosthesis. An abductor splint is in place. The nurse should remove the splint:
1. When the client gets up in a chair
2. If the client needs a change of position
3. Once the client's edema and pain have ceased
4. During the client's skin care and physical therapy

852. When assisting a client who had a total hip replacement onto the bedpan on the first postoperative day, the nurse should instruct the client to:
1. Turn toward the operative side
2. Flex both knees while slowly lifting the pelvis
3. Extend both legs and pull on the trapeze to lift the pelvis
4. Flex the unaffected knee and pull on the trapeze to raise the pelvis

853. A client has an open reduction and internal fixation (ORIF) of a fractured hip. The nurse monitors this client for signs and symptoms of a fat embolism. Which client assessment reflects this complication?
1. Fever and chest pain
2. Positive Homans' sign
3. Loss of sensation in the operative leg
4. Tachycardia and petechiae over the chest

854. A client with a distal femoral shaft fracture is at risk for developing a fat embolus. The nurse considerss that a distinguishing sign that is unique to a fat embolus is:
1. Oliguria
2. Dyspnea
3. Petechiae
4. Confusion

855. When planning discharge teaching for a client who had a total hip replacement, the nurse should include encouraging the client to avoid:
1. Climbing stairs
2. Stretching exercises
3. Sitting in a low chair
4. Lying prone for half an hour

856. A client sustains a complex comminuted fracture of the tibia with soft tissue injuries after being hit by a car while riding a bicycle. Surgical placement of an external fixator is performed to maintain the bone in alignment. Postoperatively it is most essential for the nurse to:
1. Cleanse the pin sites with alcohol several times a day
2. Perform a neurovascular assessment of both lower extremities

3. Ambulate the client with partial weight bearing on the affected leg
4. Maintain placement of an abduction pillow between the client's legs

857. A client with rheumatoid arthritis asks the nurse about ways to decrease morning stiffness. The nurse should suggest:
1. Wearing loose but warm clothing
2. Planning a short rest break periodically
3. Avoiding excessive physical stress and fatigue
4. Taking a hot tub bath or shower in the morning

858. When assessing a client experiencing an acute episode of rheumatoid arthritis, the nurse observes that the client's finger joints are swollen. The nurse concludes that this swelling most likely is related to:
1. Urate crystals in the synovial tissue
2. Inflammation in the joint's synovial lining
3. Formation of bony spurs on the joint surfaces
4. Escaped fluid from the capillaries that increases interstitial fluids

859. As an acute episode of rheumatoid arthritis subsides, active and passive range-of-motion exercises are taught to the client's spouse. The nurse should teach that direct pressure should not be applied to the client's joints because this may precipitate:
1. Pain
2. Swelling
3. Nodule formation
4. Tophaceous deposits

860. A practitioner orders bed rest for a client with acute arthritis who has bilateral, painful, swollen knee and wrist joints. To prevent flexion deformities during the acute phase, the client's positioning schedule should include placement in the:
1. Sims position
2. Prone position
3. Contour position
4. Trendelenburg position

861. The physiotherapist in a nursing home develops an exercise program for an 82-year-old resident with rheumatoid arthritis. The nurse evaluates that the client understands the purpose of this program when the client states:
1. "I know the exercises are important, so I do them whenever I can."
2. "I do my exercises when I go to physical therapy in the morning and afternoon."
3. "Since I'm stiff in the morning, I do most of my exercises then, so I'm done for the day."
4. "After I eat breakfast, I do one set of exercises slowly, and then I space the rest of them throughout the day."

862. A client with rheumatoid arthritis is in the convalescent stage of an exacerbation. What should the nurse encourage the client to do when the client says, "The only time I am without pain is when I lie perfectly still."
1. Active joint flexion and extension
2. Flexion exercises three times a day

3. Range-of-motion exercises once a day

4. Continued immobility until remission occurs

863. A client who has passed the acute phase of rheumatoid arthritis is now allowed out of bed as tolerated. After assisting the client out of bed, the nurse should place the client in a:
1. Low, soft lounge chair
2. Straight-back armchair
3. Wheelchair with footrests
4. Recliner chair with both legs elevated

864. A nurse is providing health teaching to a client with rheumatoid arthritis. The statement by the nurse that best describes a technique to reduce joint stress is:
1. "Respond to pain in your joints."
2. "Use your smaller muscles most frequently."
3. "Do your heavy tasks at one time to reduce muscle strain."
4. "Increase exercise to reduce swelling when your joints are swollen."

865. After an amputation of a limb, a client begins to experience extreme discomfort in the area where the limb once was. The nurse's greatest concern at this time is:
1. Addressing the pain
2. Reversing feelings of hopelessness
3. Promoting mobility in the residual limb
4. Acknowledging the grieving for the lost limb

866. A client has an above-the-knee amputation because of a gangrenous leg ulcer. To prevent deformities after the second postoperative day the nurse should:
1. Place an abduction pillow between the legs
2. Encourage lying in the supine or prone position
3. Keep the client's residual limb elevated on a pillow
4. Teach the client to press the residual limb against a hard surface several times a day

867. A client who has an above-the-knee amputation is fitted with a prosthesis. The nurse evaluates the client's response to the prosthesis. Which indicates that the prosthesis fits the residual limb correctly?
1. Absence of phantom limb sensation
2. Uneven wearing down of the heels of the shoes
3. Shrinkage of the end portion of the residual limb
4. Darkened skin areas surrounding the end of the residual limb

868. A client with an above-the-knee amputation asks why the residual limb needs to be wrapped with an elastic bandage. The nurse explains that it:
1. Limits the formation of blood clots
2. Decreases the phantom limb sensation
3. Prevents hemorrhage and covers the incision
4. Supports the soft tissue and minimizes swelling

869. A nurse is teaching a client who is to have an above-the-knee amputation about postoperative activities. Which activity is designed to aid in the use of crutches?
1. Lifting weights
2. Changing bed positions
3. Caring for the residual limb
4. Performing phantom limb exercises

870. A client has a below-the-knee amputation. The nurse concludes that a major advantage of a postoperative prosthesis applied immediately is that it:
1. Decreases phantom limb sensations
2. Encourages a normal walking pattern
3. Reduces the incidence of wound infection
4. Allows for the fitting of the prosthesis before discharge

871. A 70-year-old client is scheduled for a below-the-knee amputation because of a 10-year history of impaired arterial circulation to the lower extremities. The skill that the nurse teaches the client preoperatively that can be most helpful during the first several postoperative days is to:
1. Log-roll when turning in bed
2. Toughen the distal residual limb
3. Transfer from the bed to a wheelchair
4. Stand on one leg for five minutes several times a day

872. A 48-year-old farmer is admitted for the repair and revision of a residual limb immediately after the traumatic amputation of the left hand in a corn picker accident. A week after surgery the client complains of constant throbbing in the affected limb. Which is the most appropriate nursing intervention?
1. Applying cool compresses to the limb
2. Securing an order for pain medication
3. Elevating the extremity on two pillows
4. Loosening the bandage around the limb

DRUG-RELATED RESPONSES

873. A female client who is being treated for rheumatoid arthritis arrives in the outpatient clinic stating she has no medical insurance and has not been taking the prescribed drug because it is too expensive. The client reports that a family member has arranged to obtain the drug from Mexico. The nurse should:
1. Discuss alternative solutions with the client
2. Encourage the client to obtain the medication from Mexico
3. Call the practitioner immediately regarding this information
4. Explain that medical regimens must be followed to remain in the clinic

874. In a critical clinical situation, a practitioner tells the nurse to administer a dose of a medication that the nurse identifies as an overdose. Which statement by the nurse is most appropriate?
1. "This is an overdose. I will not feel comfortable administering this dose."
2. "Show me how you arrived at this dose. I think your calculations are incorrect."
3. "You're probably thinking of another drug. This is beyond the safe dosage limits indicated for this drug."
4. "That dose is more than I can legally give. However, if the dose is medically indicated, please administer it yourself."

875. A client has been taking sildenafil (Viagra) 50 mg three times a week for 6 months. He remembers the physician and nurse telling him not to take nitrates while on sildenafil. The client experiences an angina attack and uses a nitroglycerin tablet (Nitrostat) patch that was prescribed for him before his Viagra prescription. The client's physical response to this action will be:
   1. Nausea
   2. Tachypnea
   3. Constipation
   4. Hypotension

876. A client is receiving morphine sulfate (MS Contin) for severe metastatic bone pain. To prevent complications from a common, serious side effect of morphine, the nurse should:
   1. Monitor for diarrhea
   2. Observe for an opioid addiction
   3. Assess for altered breathing patterns
   4. Check for a decreased urinary output

877. A pharmacy technician arrives on the nursing unit to deliver the requested opioids. A primary nurse is entering a client's room and is not available to receive the medications. Which is the most appropriate statement by the nurse to the pharmacy technician?
   1. "I'm sorry. Please wait a few minutes or come back."
   2. "Leave the meds and sign-out sheets by the unit secretary."
   3. "Bring them to me and I'll put them away in a couple of minutes."
   4. "I'll be out in a few minutes. Give them to the nursing assistant in my district."

878. A client is hospitalized with joint pain, loss of hair, yellow pigmentation of the skin, and an enlarged liver. The nurse should suspect and direct further assessment toward an excess intake of:
   1. Thiamine
   2. Vitamin A
   3. Vitamin C
   4. Pyridoxine

879. A client with tuberculosis is to begin Rifater (combination of isoniazid [INH], rifampin [RIF], pyrazinamide [PZA]), and streptomycin sulfate (streptomycin) therapy. The client says, "I've never had to take so much medication for an infection before." The nurse should explain:
   1. "This type of organism is difficult to destroy."
   2. "Streptomycin prevents side effects of Rifater."
   3. "You'll need multiple medications for only a couple of weeks."
   4. "Aggressive therapy is needed when the infection is well advanced."

880. A client with tuberculosis is started on a chemotherapy protocol that includes rifampin (RIF). The nurse evaluates that the teaching about rifampin is effective when the client states:
   1. "I plan to drink a lot of fluid while I take this medication."
   2. "I can expect my urine to turn orange from this medication."

3. "I should have my hearing tested while I take this medication."
4. "I might get a skin rash because it's an expected side effect of this medication."

881. The practitioner prescribes vitamin B$_6$ and isoniazid (INH) as part of the chemotherapy protocol for a client with tuberculosis. The nurse determines that vitamin B$_6$ is used because it:
   1. Improves the nutritional status of the client
   2. Enhances the tuberculostatic effect of isoniazid
   3. Accelerates the destruction of dormant tubercular bacilli
   4. Counteracts the peripheral neuritis that isoniazid may cause

882. A client is diagnosed as having pulmonary tuberculosis, and one of the drugs the practitioner prescribes is pyrazinamide (PZA). The nurse evaluates that the teaching concerning the drug is effective when the client says, "I will:
   1. drink at least 2 quarts of fluid a day."
   2. report changes in vision to my physician."
   3. take the medication 2 hours after each meal."
   4. expect a discoloration of urine, sweat, and tears."

883. A client is diagnosed with tuberculosis associated with HIV infection. The test results that are crucial for the nurse to review before starting antitubercular pharmacotherapy are:
   1. Liver function studies
   2. Pulmonary function studies
   3. Electrocardiogram and echocardiogram
   4. White blood cell counts and sedimentation rate

884. A client with HIV-associated *Pneumocystis jiroveci* pneumonia is to receive pentamidine isethionate (Pentam 300) IV once daily. To ensure client safety, the nurse should monitor the client for the side effect of:
   1. Hypertension
   2. Hypokalemia
   3. Hypoglycemia
   4. Hypercalcemia

885. The practitioner prescribes 50 units of insulin to be added to an IV of glucose and water for a client with diabetes mellitus. The nurse considers that the only insulin that can be used is:
   1. Lispro insulin
   2. Glargine insulin
   3. Novolin N insulin
   4. Novolin R insulin

886. A client newly diagnosed with type 2 diabetes is receiving glyburide (Micronase) and asks the nurse how this drug works. The nurse answers the question about glyburide by telling the client it acts by:
   1. Stimulating the pancreas to produce insulin
   2. Accelerating the liver's release of stored glycogen
   3. Increasing glucose transport across the cell membrane
   4. Lowering blood glucose in the absence of pancreatic function

887. A client with type 1 diabetes self-administers Novolin N insulin every morning at 8 o'clock. The nurse evaluates that the client understands the action of this insulin when the client says, "I should be alert for signs of hypoglycemia between:
   1. 9 AM and 10 AM."
   2. 10 AM and 11 AM."
   3. 2 PM and 8 PM."
   4. 8 PM and 12 AM."

888. A client with newly diagnosed type 1 diabetes is in a self-care teaching group. The nurse evaluates that the client is able to identify signs and symptoms of hypoglycemia when the client states, "I will drink orange juice and eat a slice of bread when I feel:
   1. nervous and weak."
   2. flushed and short of breath."
   3. thirsty and have a headache."
   4. nauseated and have abdominal cramps."

889. A teaching program concerning diabetes and insulin therapy is begun for a client newly diagnosed with type 1 diabetes. The client states, "I hate shots. Why can't I take the insulin in pill form?" What is the nurse's best response?
   1. "Your diabetic condition is too serious for oral insulin."
   2. "Insulin is poorly absorbed and its action is erratic when taken by mouth."
   3. "Insulin by mouth causes a high incidence of allergic and adverse reactions."
   4. "Once your diabetes is controlled, your physician might consider an oral drug."

890. A client with hyperthyroidism is treated first with propylthiouracil (PTU). When teaching the client about this medication, the nurse should include the information that:
   1. This medication will have to be taken for the remainder of the client's life
   2. Symptoms may not subside for up to several weeks after the start of therapy
   3. Milk should be taken with the medication so that gastric irritation does not occur
   4. The medication should be taken between meals so that it is more readily absorbed

891. A client with hyperthyroidism is to receive methimazole (Tapazole). The nurse should instruct the client that:
   1. Initial improvement will take several weeks
   2. There are few side effects associated with this drug
   3. This medication may be taken at any time during the day
   4. Large doses are used to decrease the length of time drug therapy is necessary

892. A client with arthritis is taking ibuprofen (Motrin), a nonsteroidal antiinflammatory drug, and large doses of aspirin (ASA). The nurse teaches the client about the clinical manifestations of aspirin toxicity. Which should the client report to the practitioner?
   1. Feelings of drowsiness
   2. Disturbances in hearing

3. Intermittent constipation
4. Metallic taste in the mouth

893. A client with arthritis states that the prescribed aspirin (ASA) causes stomach irritation even when taken with food. The nurse should instruct the client to take the aspirin:
   1. An hour before a meal
   2. With a full glass of water
   3. With sodium bicarbonate
   4. At the same time as the other drugs

894. A client with arthritis asks the nurse if acetaminophen can be substituted for the aspirin that causes stomach irritation. The nurse explains that acetaminophen (Tylenol):
   1. Lacks anticoagulant action
   2. Has the same action as aspirin
   3. Lacks an antiinflammatory action
   4. Has more severe side effects than aspirin

895. Enoxaparin (Lovenox) 40 mg subcutaneously daily is prescribed for a client who had abdominal surgery. The nurse explains the medication to the client based on the understanding that this drug is given to:
   1. Control expected postoperative fever
   2. Provide a constant source of mild analgesia
   3. Limit the inflammatory response associated with surgery
   4. Provide prophylaxis against postoperative thrombus formation

896. The practitioner prescribes ibuprofen (Motrin) 800 mg PO three times a day for a client with rheumatoid arthritis. The nurse evaluates that the teaching about the side effects of ibuprofen is effective when the client understands that:
   1. Monthly bloodwork is necessary
   2. Exercises must be balanced with rest
   3. Position changes should be made slowly
   4. Administration of the drug should be between meals

897. A client who has a long leg cast for a fractured bone is to be discharged from the emergency department. When discussing pain management, the nurse should advise the client to take the prescribed prn oxycodone and acetaminophen (Percocet):
   1. Just as a last resort
   2. Before going to sleep
   3. As the pain becomes intense
   4. When the discomfort begins

898. A client had a laminectomy and is receiving a skeletal muscle relaxant that will be continued after discharge. After teaching the client about the skeletal muscle relaxant, the nurse evaluates that no further health teaching is necessary when the client says:
   1. "I'm going to take the medication between meals."
   2. "If the medication makes me sleepy, I'll stop taking it."
   3. "If the mediation upsets my stomach, I'll take it with milk."
   4. "I'll take an extra dose of the medication before I do anything active."

899. A practitioner prescribes a low dosage of an opioid to relieve the pain of a client with deep partial-thickness

burns. The nurse determines that the preferred mode of administration for this client is:
1. Oral
2. Rectal
3. Intravenous
4. Intramuscular

900. A hospice client who has severe pain and is receiving analgesics asks for another dose of pain medication. Oxycodone (OxyContin) 40 mg every 4 hours is prescribed. The nurse's primary consideration when responding to the client's request is to:
1. Prevent addiction
2. Determine why the drug is needed
3. Provide alternate comfort measures
4. Help reduce the client's pain immediately

901. A female client is receiving oxandrolone (Oxandrin), an anabolic steroid, for the treatment of the catabolic processes associated with a burn injury. The nurse should monitor the client for signs and symptoms of:
1. Lethargy
2. Virilization
3. Dehydration
4. Hypokalemia

902. The nurse applies mafenide acetate cream (Sulfamylon) to a client's burns as prescribed by the practitioner. Before a dressing change and application of the drug, the nurse should teach the client that this medication will:
1. Inhibit bacterial growth
2. Relieve pain from the burn
3. Prevent scar tissue formation
4. Provide chemical debridement

903. A practitioner decides that a client's burns should be treated by the open exposure method and is contemplating which topical antimicrobial to prescribe. Which medication does the nurse expect the practitioner to order based on the pros and cons of each?
1. Silver sulfadiazine (Silvadene) is easy to apply and has good bactericidal action but it can depress granulocyte formation
2. Mafenide acetate (Sulfamylon) causes no side effects and is effective for both gram-positive and gram-negative organisms
3. Neomycin (Cortisporin) is a strong bactericidal agent effective against most organisms with the fewest number of toxic side effects for the client
4. Silver nitrate paste has strong bacteriostatic properties, and clients respond quickly to these dry dressings because they eliminate odors

904. A nurse attempts to give a male client with chronic arterial insufficiency of the legs the prescribed dose of aspirin (ASA) but the client refuses it stating, "My legs are not painful." The nurse should:
1. Explain the reason for the medication and encourage the client to take it
2. Withhold the medication and tell the client to ask for it if his legs become uncomfortable

3. Withhold the medication at this time and return to check the client again in one-half hour
4. Request that the client take the medication and explain that it prevents him from being uncomfortable in the next few hours

905. The practitioner prescribes isosorbide dinitrate (Isordil) 10 mg prn three times a day and a nitroglycerin transdermal disk once a day for a client with chronic angina pectoris. The client asks the nurse why the isosorbide dinitrate is prescribed. The nurse's best response is, "It:
1. prevents the blood from clotting."
2. suppresses irritability in the ventricles."
3. allows more oxygen to get to heart tissue."
4. increases the force of contraction of the heart."

906. The practitioner prescribes atenolol (Tenormin) for a client with angina. When instructing the client about this medication, the nurse should teach the client about the potential side effect of:
1. Headache
2. Tachycardia
3. Constipation
4. Hypotension

907. The nurse teaches a client about the side effects of furosemide (Lasix), which has just been prescribed. Which client statement about what should be done when taking furosemide alerts the nurse that the teaching is understood? Select all that apply.
1. _____ "I must not eat citrus fruits."
2. _____ "I should wear dark glasses."
3. _____ "I should avoid lying flat in bed."
4. _____ "I should change my position slowly."
5. _____ "I must eat a food that contains potassium every day."

908. At each clinic visit, the nurse should assess a client taking furosemide (Lasix) for:
1. Tinnitus
2. Xanthopsia
3. Hyporeflexia
4. Bronchospasm

909. A client with a history of hypertension comes to the emergency department with double vision and a blood pressure of 260/120 mm Hg. In addition to other drugs, the practitioner prescribes a sodium nitroprusside (Nitropress) infusion. The nurse determines that this drug decreases blood pressure by:
1. Decreasing the heart rate
2. Increasing cardiac output
3. Increasing peripheral resistance
4. Relaxing arterial smooth muscles

910. A client is receiving clonidine (Catapres) for hypertension. The nurse evaluates that the discharge instructions are understood when the client states, "I will call the doctor if I develop:
1. pruritus."
2. diarrhea."
3. euphoria."
4. photosensitivity."

911. A client with hypertensive heart disease, who had an acute episode of heart failure, is to be discharged on a regimen of metoprolol (Toprol-XL) and digoxin (Lanoxin). The nurse expects that Toprol-XL, when administered with Lanoxin, may:
    1. Produce headaches
    2. Precipitate bradycardia
    3. Increase blood pressure
    4. Stimulate nodal conduction

912. An older adult who has been taking digoxin (Lanoxin) for 20 years comes to the emergency department. The client is exhibiting signs of dehydration and laboratory results identify the presence of hypokalemia. For which clinical finding indicating digoxin toxicity should the nurse monitor the client?
    1. Constipation
    2. Blurred vision
    3. Decreased urination
    4. Metalic taste in the mouth

913. When administering warfarin (Coumadin), the nurse understands that the antidote for Coumadin is:
    1. Vitamin K
    2. Fibrinogen
    3. Prothrombin
    4. Protamine sulfate

914. A practitioner prescribes furosemide (Lasix) for a client with hypervolemia. The nurse determines that furosemide exerts its effects in the:
    1. Distal tubule
    2. Collecting duct
    3. Glomerulus of the nephron
    4. Ascending limb of Henle's loop

915. A client is receiving a cardiac glycoside, a diuretic, and a vasodilator and bed rest is ordered by the practitioner. The client's apical pulse rate is 44 beats per minute. The nurse concludes that this pulse rate most likely is a result of the:
    1. Diuretic
    2. Vasodilator
    3. Bed rest regimen
    4. Cardiac glycoside

916. A practitioner prescribes tissue plasminogen activator (t-PA) to be administered intravenously over 1 hour for a client experiencing a myocardial infarction. The nursing priority that is specific to this medication is the assessment of the client's:
    1. Respiratory rate
    2. Peripheral pulses
    3. Level of consciousness
    4. Intravenous insertion site

917. A 42-year-old client is admitted to the cardiac care unit with an anterior lateral myocardial infarction. The practitioner prescribes 500 mL of D_5W with 50 mg of nitroglycerin to be administered intravenously to relieve pain. What is the most common side effect of nitroglycerin for which the nurse should assess the client?
    1. Nausea
    2. Syncope

    3. Bradycardia
    4. Hypotension

918. To hasten the absorption of a nitroglycerin tablet (Nitrostat), the nurse should instruct the client to:
    1. Move the tablet around with the tip of the tongue
    2. Break up the tablet before placing it under the tongue
    3. Swallow saliva before placing the tablet on the tongue
    4. Place the tablet along with warm water under the tongue

919. A client is admitted to the emergency department with crushing chest pain. The nurse expects that the drug most likely to be prescribed to provide analgesia is:
    1. Alprazolam (Xanax)
    2. Midazolam HCI (Versed)
    3. Gabapentin (Neurontin)
    4. Morphine sulfate (Duramorph)

920. A nurse is preparing to teach a client to apply a nitroglycerin patch (Nitro-Dur) as prophylaxis for angina. Which instruction should the nurse include in the teaching plan?
    1. Place the patch on a distal extremity
    2. Remove a previous patch before applying the next one
    3. Massage the area gently after applying the patch to the skin
    4. Apply a warm compress to the site before attaching the patch

921. When administering the prescribed digoxin (Lanoxin) 0.25 mg PO daily to a client with a history of type 1 diabetes who is now in heart failure, the nurse should:
    1. Give the drug with orange juice
    2. Monitor the client for dysrhythmias
    3. Administer it 1 hour after the client's morning insulin
    4. Withhold it if the apical pulse rate is 90 beats per minute

922. A client admitted to the cardiac care unit (CCU) with a myocardial infarction reveals a series of premature ventricular complexes (PVCs) on the monitor. The nurse should anticipate that the client will be receiving:
    1. Atropine
    2. Epinephrine
    3. Sodium bicarbonate
    4. Lidocaine hydrochloride

923. The cardiac monitor indicates that a client's heart rate has increased to 150 beats per minute. Shortly after this increase the nurse identifies that the client is in ventricular tachycardia (VT) and notifies the practitioner. For which intervention should the nurse prepare?
    1. Bolus of lidocaine
    2. Intracardiac epinephrine
    3. Insertion of a pacemaker
    4. Manual cardiopulmonary resuscitation

924. A client is scheduled for an electrophysiology study (EPS) because of persistent ventricular tachycardia. Before the procedure the client is to receive a beta blocker.

The client's response during the procedure that best indicates that the beta blocker is working effectively is:
1. Sinus bradycardia
2. Decreased anxiety
3. Reduced chest pain
4. Ventricular standstill

925. A nurse is administering an intravenous titrated drip of lidocaine HCl (Xylocaine) to a client. What serious side effect must be reported to the practitioner immediately?
1. Tremors
2. Anorexia
3. Tachycardia
4. Hypertension

926. A nurse evaluates that a client understands the side effects of hydrochlorothiazide (HCTZ) therapy when the client states, "I should call the physician if I develop:
1. insomnia."
2. a stuffy nose."
3. an increase in thirst."
4. generalized weakness."

927. A nurse on the arrest team responds to a code for a client experiencing cardiac standstill. In addition to cardiac stimulants, the nurse should expect to prepare:
1. Aminophylline
2. Furosemide (Lasix)
3. Sodium bicarbonate
4. Phenytoin (Dilantin)

928. A client, who has increased intracranial pressure resulting from a traumatic brain injury, is unconscious and has vital signs of P 60, R 16, and BP 142/64. The medication prescription that should be questioned by the nurse is:
1. Mannitol 140 mg IV
2. Dexamethasone 4 mg IV
3. Chlorpromazine 25 mg IM
4. Morphine sulfate 15 mg IM

929. There is a preoperative prescription for midazolam (Versed). For maximum effectiveness, the client's preanesthetic medication should be administered:
1. 2 hours before anesthesia
2. 45 minutes before anesthesia
3. 15 minutes before anesthesia
4. 5 minutes before anesthesia

930. A 32-year-old woman with stage III-B Hodgkin's disease is started on chemotherapy. What response to the chemotherapy should the nurse teach the client to report immediately?
1. Fever of 100° F
2. Sores in the mouth
3. Moderate diarrhea after treatment
4. Nausea for 6 hours after treatment

931. A client with cancer who is receiving a chemotherapeutic regimen that includes vinCRIStine (Oncovin) complains of numbness and loss of feeling in the legs below the knees. The client wants to know if the problem means the cancer is growing or if it is related to the medication. The nurse's answer is based on the fact that:
1. Enlarged lymph nodes in the groin, related to the cancer, may cause these symptoms
2. Most chemotherapeutic regimens do not affect the nervous or peripheral vascular system
3. Vascular occlusion may cause this problem and immediate medical evaluation is indicated
4. Peripheral neuropathies can result from chemotherapy and usually are reversible if addressed early

932. A client who has been taking enteric-coated aspirin (Ecotrin) for rheumatoid arthritis asks if acetaminophen (Tylenol) can be substituted because it is on sale. The nurse's response is based on the fact that:
1. Both are analgesics
2. Both can cause gastritis
3. Aspirin is an antiinflammatory
4. Acetaminophen is an antipyretic

933. Nursing care for a client who is receiving DOXOrubicin (Adriamycin) for acute myelogenous leukemia should include:
1. Serving hot liquids with each meal
2. Providing frequent oral hygiene and increasing oral fluids
3. Emphasizing that the disease will be cured with this treatment
4. Administering medications intramuscularly and encouraging activity

934. A client with small-cell lung cancer is receiving chemotherapy. A complete blood count is ordered before each round of chemotherapy. With this client, the value in a complete blood count that the nurse is most concerned about is:
1. RBCs
2. WBCs
3. Platelets
4. Hematocrit

935. A client with cancer develops pancytopenia during the course of chemotherapy. The client asks the nurse why this has occurred. The nurse explains that:
1. Steroid hormones have a depressant effect on the spleen and bone marrow
2. Noncancerous cells also are susceptible to the effects of chemotherapeutic drugs
3. Lymph node activity is depressed by radiation therapy used prior to chemotherapy
4. Dehydration caused by nausea, vomiting, and diarrhea results in hemoconcentration

936. A male client is receiving imatinib (Gleevec) for chronic myelogenous leukemia (CML). For which complications of this protein-tyrosine kinase inhibitor should the nurse assess the client? Select all that apply.
1. _____ Hair loss
2. _____ Stomatitis
3. _____ Signs of infection
4. _____ Bleeding tendencies
5. _____ Changes indicating feminization

937. A nurse considers that the safe administration of high-dose methotrexate (Rheumatrex) therapy should include:
1. Maintaining an acidic urine
2. Restricting intravenous fluids
3. Providing a diet high in folic acid
4. Monitoring plasma levels of methotrexate

938. A client with the diagnosis of multiple myeloma is being treated with chemotherapy in the oncology clinic. After several months of chemotherapy, the client comes to the emergency department because of confusion, muscle weakness, and diarrhea. A history and physical are obtained, a venous blood specimen is sent to the laboratory, and an ECG is performed. Which complication associated with chemotherapy does the nurse suspect that the client is experiencing after assessing the client and reviewing the medical record?
1. Septic shock
2. Tumor lysis syndrome
3. Superior vena cava syndrome
4. Disseminated intravascular coagulation

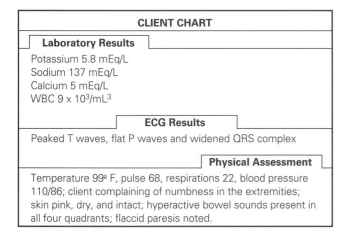

CLIENT CHART

Laboratory Results

Potassium 5.8 mEq/L
Sodium 137 mEq/L
Calcium 5 mEq/L
WBC 9 x 10³/mL³

ECG Results

Peaked T waves, flat P waves and widened QRS complex

Physical Assessment

Temperature 99º F, pulse 68, respirations 22, blood pressure 110/86; client complaining of numbness in the extremities; skin pink, dry, and intact; hyperactive bowel sounds present in all four quadrants; flaccid paresis noted.

939. A client with multiple myeloma who is receiving the alkylating agent melphalan (Alkeran) returns to the oncology clinic for a follow-up visit. For which side effect should the nurse monitor the client?
1. Hirsutism
2. Leukopenia
3. Constipation
4. Photosensitivity

940. The practitioner prescribes finasteride (Proscar) for a 52-year-old client with benign prostatic hyperplasia. The nurse informs the client that:
1. Male pattern baldness can occur
2. Results can be expected in six to twelve weeks
3. Compliance will prevent the development of prostatic cancer
4. Protection should be worn during intercourse with a pregnant female

941. A client with cancer is receiving a multiple chemotherapy protocol. Included in the protocol is leucovorin (Wellcovorin). The nurse concludes that this drug is administered to:
1. Potentiate the effect of alkylating agents
2. Diminish toxicity of folic acid antagonists
3. Limit the occurrence of vomiting associated with chemotherapy
4. Interfere with cell division at a different stage of cell division than the other drugs

942. A client who is receiving chemotherapy for cancer has nausea and vomiting because of the therapy. The client wants to know if it is true that smoking marijuana will help. What is the nurse's best response?
1. "Smoking marijuana is not legal in any state."
2. "Marijuana is more effective for nausea and vomiting if it is injected, but it can cause drowsiness."
3. "Smoking marijuana is not effective in the control of nausea and vomiting caused by chemotherapy."
4. "Tetrahydrocannabinol, the ingredient in marijuana that acts as an antiemetic, can be taken in pill form."

943. A client with metastatic melanoma is being treated with interferon Gamma 1b (Actimmune). The nurse evaluates that the teaching about this drug is understood when the client states, "I:
1. will increase my fluid intake to several quarts every day."
2. need to discard any reconstituted solution at the end of the week."
3. can continue driving my car as before as long as I have the stamina."
4. should be able to continue my usual activity while taking this medication."

944. A client with a parotid tumor that involves the lymph glands in the neck is being treated aggressively with radiation therapy, surgery, and chemotherapy. The practitioner prescribes vinCRIStine (Oncovin), cyclophosphamide (Cytoxan), and prednisone (Meticorten). The nurse should monitor the client routinely for:
1. Peripheral paresthesia
2. Anginal-type chest pain
3. Ophthalmic papilledema
4. Bilateral crackles in the lung

945. A 21-year-old college student with type 1 diabetes requests additional information about the advantages of using penlike insulin delivery devices. The nurse explains that the advantages of these devices over syringes include:
1. Shorter injection time
2. Accurate dose delivery
3. Use of a smaller-gauge needle
4. Lower cost with reusable insulin cartridges

946. A practitioner prescribes oral pancreatic enzymes, pancrelipase (Viokase), for a client. The nurse evaluates that teaching about enzymes is understood when the client states, "I will take them:
1. at bedtime."
2. with meals."
3. 1 hour before meals."
4. on arising each morning."

947. After a course of DOXOrubicin hydrochloride (Adriamycin), the practitioner decides to prescribe cisplatin (Platinol) for a client with metastatic cancer. To prevent toxic effects, the nurse should:

1. Administer the ordered leucovorin
2. Encourage regular vigorous oral care
3. Increase hydration to promote diuresis
4. Provide a high-protein, low-residue diet

948. Which medication should the nurse question when it is prescribed for a client with acute pancreatitis?
1. Ranitidine (Zantac)
2. Cimetidine (Tagamet)
3. Meperidine (Demerol)
4. Promethazine HCl (Phenergan)

949. A client is to receive chemotherapy for cancer of the colon. The practitioner prescribes an intravenous dose of metoclopramide (Reglan) 30 minutes before the chemotherapy infusion. The nurse explains to the client that this medication will:
1. Stimulate production of gastrointestinal secretions
2. Enhance relaxation of the upper gastrointestinal tract
3. Prolong excretion of the chemotherapeutic medication
4. Increase absorption of the chemotherapeutic medication

950. Prednisone (Meticorten), an adrenal steroid, is prescribed for a client with an exacerbation of colitis. What should the nurse tell the client when administering the first dose of prednisone? "This medication:
1. will protect you from getting an infection."
2. may cause weight loss by decreasing your appetite."
3. is not curative but does cause a suppression of the inflammatory process."
4. is relatively slow in precipitating a response but it is effective in reducing symptoms."

951. A client who is scheduled for a bowel resection is to receive antibiotics preoperatively. The nurse teaches the client that the purpose of the antibiotics is to help:
1. Prevent incisional infection
2. Avoid postoperative pneumonia
3. Limit the risk of a urinary tract infection
4. Eliminate bacteria from the gastrointestinal tract

952. Immediately after a bilateral adrenalectomy a client is receiving corticosteroids that are to be continued after discharge from the hospital. The nurse evaluates a need for further teaching when the client states:
1. "I need to have periodic tests of my blood for glucose."
2. "I must take the pills with meals while I have food in my stomach."
3. "Hopefully, the dosage will be regulated so I can take them just once a day."
4. "I should tell the doctor if I am overly restless, depressed, or have trouble sleeping."

953. A client with hepatic cirrhosis develops hepatic encephalopathy. Neomycin sulfate (Mycifradin) is prescribed. The nurse concludes that the purpose of neomycin for a client with cirrhosis is to:
1. Decrease intestinal edema
2. Reduce abdominal distention
3. Diminish the blood ammonia level
4. Limit development of systemic infections

954. The practitioner prescribes propylthiouracil (PTU) for a client with the diagnosis of Graves' disease. What should the nurse include in the teaching plan when discussing the self-administration of this medication?
1. Drink a glass of milk daily
2. Observe for signs of infection
3. Take the drug through a straw
4. Wear sunglasses when exposed to sunlight

955. A nurse suspects that a client who has been taking levothyroxine (Synthroid) for hypothyroidism for 3 weeks needs a decrease in dosage. Which clinical manifestations support this conclusion? Check all that apply.
1. _____ Tremors
2. _____ Bradycardia
3. _____ Somnolence
4. _____ Heat intolerance
5. _____ Decreased blood pressure

956. A practitioner prescribes docusate sodium (Colace) every day for a client. The nurse determines that this drug is prescribed specifically to:
1. Lubricate the feces in the GI tract
2. Create an osmotic effect in the GI tract
3. Stimulate motor activity of the GI tract
4. Lower the surface tension of feces in the GI tract

957. A practitioner prescribes bisacodyl (Dulcolax) for a client with cardiac disease. The nurse explains to the client that this drug acts by:
1. Producing bulk
2. Softening feces
3. Lubricating feces
4. Stimulating peristalsis

958. A practitioner prescribes Maalox by mouth and ranitidine (Zantac) by IVPB for a client with burns and crushing injuries caused by a train accident. The client asks why these medications are being administered. The nurse's best response is:
1. "They decrease irritability of the bowel."
2. "They limit acidity in the gastrointestinal tract."
3. "They're ordered for clients with multiple trauma."
4. "They're what your physician prescribed to calm your stomach."

959. A practitioner prescribes bed rest, loperamide (Maalox), and esomeprazole (Nexium) for a client who just had major surgery. After several days of this regimen, the client complains of diarrhea. Which is the most likely cause of the client's diarrhea?
1. Maalox
2. Nexium
3. Bed rest
4. Diet alteration

960. When caring for a client who has primary open-angle glaucoma, which eye drops should the nurse expect the practitioner to prescribe?
1. Tetracaine (Pontocaine)
2. Cyclopentolate (Cyclogyl)
3. Timolol maleate (Timoptic)
4. Atropine sulfate (Atropisol Ophthalmic)

961. A client has a tonic-clonic seizure that involves all extremities. The nurse anticipates that the practitioner will prescribe the IV administration of:
    1. Naloxone (Narcan)
    2. Diazepam (Valium)
    3. Epinephrine HCl (Adrenalin)
    4. Atropine Sulfate (Atropine)

962. When a client's condition is assessed after a tonic-clonic seizure caused by an overdose of acetylsalicylic acid, the most appropriate nursing action is to:
    1. Check reflexes every 2 hours
    2. Prepare a setup for a CVP line
    3. Insert a urinary retention catheter
    4. Monitor vital signs every 15 minutes

963. The practitioner prescribes phenytoin (Dilantin) for a young mother who had a tonic-clonic seizure of unknown etiology. The nurse should instruct the client to:
    1. Take the medication on an empty stomach
    2. Brush her teeth and gums three times daily
    3. Stop taking the drug if abdominal pain occurs
    4. Note any change in her pulse and respiratory rates

964. A practitioner identifies that a 60-year-old client has Parkinson's disease and prescribes levodopa (L-dopa) therapy. The nurse expects that this medication will relieve and control symptoms by:
    1. Blocking the effects of acetylcholine
    2. Increasing the production of dopamine
    3. Restoring the dopamine levels in the brain
    4. Promoting the production of acetylcholine

965. A client taking levodopa (L-dopa) is taught about the signs of levodopa toxicity. The client and family are instructed to contact the physician if they identify the development of:
    1. Nausea
    2. Dizziness
    3. Twitching
    4. Constipation

966. When teaching a client with severe Parkinson's disease about carbidopa-levodopa (Sinemet), the nurse should state that:
    1. "Multivitamins can be taken daily."
    2. "Alcohol can be used in moderation."
    3. "The drug should be taken with meals."
    4. "A high-protein diet should be followed."

967. Selegiline (Eldepryl) is prescribed for a client with Parkinson's disease who is having an inadequate response to levodopa therapy. When teaching the client and family about the addition of this drug to the regimen, the nurse should explain that the:
    1. Physician should be called immediately if a severe headache occurs
    2. Therapeutic blood level of the drug should be measured every month
    3. Dosage of the drug can be adjusted daily depending on the client's response that day
    4. Side effects of levodopa will decrease when these two drugs are taken concurrently

968. When a client is receiving dexamethasone (Decadron), the nurse should monitor for the development of a negative side effect by:
    1. Auscultating for bowel sounds
    2. Measuring blood glucose levels
    3. Culturing respiratory secretions
    4. Monitoring deep tendon reflexes

969. A client is admitted with head trauma after a fall from a ladder. The client is being prepared for a supratentorial craniotomy with burr holes, and an IV infusion of mannitol (Osmitrol) is instituted. The nurse concludes that this medication primarily is given to:
    1. Lower blood pressure
    2. Prevent hypoglycemia
    3. Increase cardiac output
    4. Decrease fluid in the brain

970. A practitioner prescribes mannitol (Osmitrol) for a client with a head injury. The nurse concludes that the purpose of this medication is to promote cerebral dehydration by:
    1. Decreasing the production of cerebrospinal fluid
    2. Limiting the metabolic requirements of the brain
    3. Drawing fluid from brain cells into the bloodstream
    4. Preventing uncontrolled electrical discharges in the brain

971. A client is receiving IV mannitol (Osmitrol) after sustaining a critical head injury. A nursing assessment specific to the safe administration of mannitol to this client is:
    1. Body weight daily
    2. Urine output hourly
    3. Vital signs every 2 hours
    4. Level of consciousness every 8 hours

972. The wife of a client with a brain attack caused by an intracranial bleed asks why her husband is not receiving anticoagulant therapy. The nurse explains that in her husband's situation anticoagulant therapy:
    1. Is contraindicated because it will increase bleeding
    2. May be necessary to prevent pulmonary thrombosis
    3. Is inadvisable because it may mask signs and symptoms
    4. Will be started if necessary to enhance cerebral circulation

973. To prevent excessive bruising when administering heparin (Hep-Lock) subcutaneously, the nurse should:
    1. Administer the injection via the Z-track technique
    2. Inject the drug into the subcutaneous tissue quickly
    3. Avoid massaging the injection site after the injection
    4. Use 2 mL of sterile normal saline to dilute the heparin

974. A 67-year-old man who had a total hip arthroplasty 4 days ago is being discharged to a rehabilitation facility. He had a pulmonary embolism several months ago and was taking warfarin sodium (Coumadin) 7.5 mg daily as a maintenance dose, which he stopped several days before the arthroplasty. While hospitalized, he received heparin (Hep-Lock) 5000 units subcutaneously

twice a day. His discharge medications do not include an anticoagulant. The nurse should:

1. Call the practitioner for directions about the anticoagulant
2. Arrange for a supply of heparin for the client to take with him
3. Explain that he no longer needs an anticoagulant after discharge
4. Instruct the client to talk about this with his physician when he gets to the new facility

975. A client had a total knee replacement several days ago and has been receiving warfarin sodium (Coumadin) therapy. An international normalized ratio (INR) is performed each afternoon, and the evening warfarin sodium dose is prescribed by the practitioner on a daily basis. The nurse identifies that the afternoon INR is 4.6. The nurse should:

1. Contact the practitioner to request the day's dosage of Coumadin
2. Obtain a blood specimen to have a partial thromboplastin time performed
3. Assist with meal planning to increase the intake of foods high in vitamin K
4. Maintain the client on bed rest until the practitioner reviews the laboratory results

976. One month after an endarterectomy the surgeon instructs the client to take clopidogrel (Plavix) 75 mg once a day. The nurse evaluates that the reason for taking this drug is understood when the client says, "It will:

1. limit inflammation around my incision."
2. help prevent further clogging of my arteries."
3. lower the slight fever I have had since surgery."
4. reduce the discomfort I feel at the surgical incision."

977. A client newly diagnosed with myasthenia gravis is started on pyridostigmine (Mestinon), a cholinesterase inhibitor. Two days later the client develops loose stools and increased salivation. The nurse concludes that these signs are indicative of a:

1. Myasthenic crisis
2. Cholinergic effect
3. Temporary response
4. Toxic effect of the medication

978. A client who has been experiencing double vision, drooping of the eyelids, and fatigue visits the neurological clinic. A diagnosis of myasthenia gravis is made and the practitioner prescribes pyridostigmine (Mestinon). The nurse should teach the client that it is important to take this drug:

1. On an empty stomach
2. One hour before meals
3. According to muscle strength
4. At the exact time intervals prescribed

979. A client with myasthenia gravis who is taking a cholinesterase inhibitor, is admitted to the emergency department in crisis. To distinguish between myasthenic crisis and cholinergic crisis, the nurse expects the practitioner to prescribe:

1. Atropine sulfate
2. Protamine sulfate

3. Naloxone (Narcan)
4. Edrophonium chloride (Tensilon)

980. A client with myasthenia gravis is to receive immunosuppressive therapy. The nurse anticipates that this therapy will be effective because it:

1. Inhibits the breakdown of acetylcholine at the neuromuscular junction
2. Stimulates the production of acetylcholine at the neuromuscular junction
3. Decreases the production of autoantibodies that attack acetylcholine receptors
4. Promotes the removal of autoantibodies that impair the transmission of impulses

981. The practitioner prescribes neostigmine (Prostigmin) for a client with myasthenia gravis. The nurse evaluates that the client understands the teaching about this drug when the client says, "I should:

1. keep the drug in a container in the refrigerator."
2. take the drug at the exact time ordered by my doctor."
3. plan to take the drug between meals to promote absorption."
4. expect that the onset of the action of the drug will occur several hours after I take it."

982. Trimethoprim-sulfamethoxazole (Septra) is prescribed for a client with cystitis. When teaching about the medication, the nurse should recommend that the client:

1. Drink 8 to 10 glasses of water daily
2. Have 2 glasses of orange juice daily
3. Administer the medication with meals
4. Take the medication until symptoms subside

983. A nurse who is preparing a client for discharge after a surgical procedure is teaching about the prescribed ampicillin (Omnipen). The nurse evaluates that the teaching is effective when the client states, "I:

1. can stop taking this medication any time."
2. should take this medication just after eating."
3. must increase my fluid intake while taking this medication."
4. will miss eating grapefruit while I'm taking this medication."

984. A client is informed that he has benign prostatic hyperplasia (BPH) and the practitioner prescribes finasteride (Proscar). The client states that he would like to take saw palmetto instead of the Proscar. The nurse should inform him that this herbal supplement:

1. May be taken after consultation with the practitioner
2. Should be taken on an empty stomach for best results
3. Will relieve symptoms by altering the size of the prostate
4. Can cause a regrowth of hair lost to male pattern baldness

985. The practitioner orders peak and trough levels of an antibiotic for a client who is receiving the medication

IVPB. For peak levels the nurse should have the laboratory obtain a blood sample from the client:
1. Between 30 and 60 minutes after the IVPB
2. Halfway between two IVPB administrations
3. Immediately before administering the IVPB
4. Anytime it is convenient for the client and laboratory

986. A client with hypertension is to take an angiotensin II receptor blocker (ARB). What information related to the need to stop the medication should the nurse plan to include when teaching the client about this medication? Select all that apply.
1. _____ Monitor the BP daily
2. _____ Avoid the use of NSAIDs
3. _____ Stop treatment if a cough develops
4. _____ Stop the medication if swelling of the mouth, lips, or face develops
5. _____ Have blood drawn for potassium levels 2 weeks after starting the medication

987. The medication that the nurse should crush for a client who has difficulty swallowing is:
1. Slow-K
2. Agon SR
3. Toprol-XL
4. Tylenol ES

988. Muromonab-CD3 (Orthoclone [OKT-3]), a murine monoclonal antibody, is administered to a client who is experiencing rejection of a liver transplant. What is the most serious client response to this medication for which the nurse should monitor?
1. Hypothermia
2. Dysrhythmias
3. Anaphylactic shock
4. Subtle neurological changes

989. When preparing discharge teaching for a client who had a kidney transplant, the nurse plans to include the drug regimen that is prescribed to prevent rejection of the kidney. In addition to a corticosteroid, what medications does the nurse include in the plan?
1. Furosemide (Lasix) and sirolimus (Rapamune)
2. Cefazolin (Ancef) and methotrexate (Rheumatrex)
3. Methylprednisolone (Solu-Medrol) and phenytoin (Dilantin)
4. Tacrolimus (Prograf) and mycophenolate mofetil (CellCept)

990. A nurse is administering erythropoietin (Epogen) three times a week to a client receiving chemotherapy for cancer. Which client response is considered most significant?
1. Elevated liver panel
2. Elevated hematocrit level
3. Increase in the WBC count
4. Increase in Kaposi's sarcoma lesions

991. A client who is immunosuppressed is receiving filgrastim (Neupogen). When evaluating the client's response to this medication, the finding that is most significant is an increase in:
1. Platelets
2. Erythrocytes
3. Thrombocytes
4. White blood cells

992. The practitioner orders epoetin (Procrit) for a client who has AIDS. When administering this medication, the nurse should:
1. Obtain the client's pulse rate first
2. Administer the drug via the Z-track technique
3. Shake the vial before withdrawing the solution
4. Use the syringe that has a 1-inch, 25-gauge needle

993. A client is admitted to the hospital with a diagnosis of heart failure and acute pulmonary edema. The client has dependent edema, jugular vein distention, dyspnea, full bounding pulse, and bilateral crackles. The practitioner prescribes furosemide (Lasix) 40 mg IV stat to be repeated in 1 hour. Which nursing action is most important when evaluating the effectiveness of furosemide?
1. Weighing the client daily
2. Auscultating the client's breath sounds
3. Monitoring the client's intake and output
4. Assessing the client for dependent edema

994. A client who has been taking esomeprazole magnesium (Nexium) for several weeks for gastroesophageal reflux disease (GERD), returns to the clinic for a follow-up visit. The nurse's interview of the client reveals that the esomeprazole magnesium has been effective. The practitioner discontinued the drug, a proton pump inhibitor, and prescribed an H_2 receptor antagonist that has fewer long-term side effects. Which medications are within the classification of an H_2 receptor antagonist? Select all that apply.
1. _____ Nizatidine (Axid)
2. _____ Ranitidine (Zantac)
3. _____ Famotidine (Pepcid)
4. _____ Lansoprazole (Prevacid)
5. _____ Metoclopramide (Reglan)

995. A practitioner prescribes 0.2 mg of cyanocobalamin (vitamin B_{12}) IM for a client with pernicious anemia. A vial of the drug labeled 100 mcg = 1 mL is available. How much solution should the nurse administer?
Answer: _____mL

996. A client has a prescription for an antibiotic in an IV piggyback of 50 mL of D_5W to run for 30 minutes. The microdrip has a drop factor of 60 gtt/mL. At what rate should the nurse set the IV infusion?
Answer: _____gtt/mL

997. A practitioner prescribes lidocaine HCl (Xylocaine), 1.5 mg per minute, for a client whose ECG tracing reveals multiple PVCs. The nurse adds 500 mg of lidocaine HCl to 100 mL of D_5W. To administer the correct amount of medication, at what rate should the nurse set the IV infusion pump?
Answer: _____mL

998. A practitioner prescribes cefazolin sodium (Kefzol) 375 mg IVPB every 8 hours. The vial of powder contains 500 mg of the medication. This must be reconstituted with 2 mL of 0.9% sodium chloride. In the resulting solution 1 mL equals 225 mg of Kefzol.

How many mL of Kefzol solution should the nurse administer?

Answer: _____ mL

999. A practitioner prescribes 250 mg of an antibiotic IVPB. A vial containing 1 gram of the powdered form of the medication must be reconstituted with 2.8 mL of diluent to form a withdrawable volume of 3 mL. How many mL of the solution should the nurse administer?

Answer: _____ mL

1000. A client has an IV of D$_5$W 250 mL to which is added 100 mg of morphine. The practitioner prescribes 14 mg of morphine per hour. At how many mL per hour should the nurse set the intravenous pump?

Answer: _____ mL

Additional review questions can be found on the enclosed companion CD.

MEDICAL-SURGICAL NURSING
ANSWERS AND RATIONALES

NURSING PRACTICE

1. 1 **The nurse at the scene of an accident should function in a responsible and prudent manner; the use of a soiled cloth on an open wound is not prudent, nor is the independent transfer of an accident victim from the scene.**

2 Although a nurse practice act defines nursing, it does not provide detailed standards for practice; the nurse's action was not prudent.

3 The nurse's action was not what a reasonably prudent nurse would do, and therefore the nurse is not protected.

4 The nurse's intervention was not prudent and placed the client in jeopardy; the nurse was not practicing medicine but attempting to provide first aid.

2. 3 **Neurologic aging causes forgetfulness and slower response time; repetition increases learning.**

1 This is a general principle applicable to all learning.

2 The older adult has no more difficulty learning than a younger person, although it may take longer.

4 This is a general principle applicable to all learning.

3. 4 **A small amount of bile-colored spotting is expected; a moderately large amount is pathological; this, in conjunction with the presence of pain, needs further assessment.**

1 Although this will be done eventually, it is not the priority.

2 The client should be on the right side, not the supine position; the right side-lying position compresses the liver capsule against the abdominal wall.

3 Although monitoring of vital signs is important, it is not the priority.

4. 3 **The release of information to an unauthorized person or gossiping about a client's activities constitutes a breach of confidentiality and an invasion of privacy.**

1 Libel occurs when a person writes false statements about another that may injure the individual's reputation.

2 Negligence is a careless act of omission or commission that results in injury to another.

4 Defamation of character is the publication of false statements that injure a person's reputation.

5. 4 **Before nurses can help others, they must understand feelings about issues that may affect clients; this is the first step toward providing nonjudgmental care.**

1 Although this is important for all therapeutic relationships, it should follow a self-assessment of attitudes, values, and beliefs.

2 Although it is beneficial for nurses to understand themselves, this does not necessarily mean that the care will be nonjudgmental.

3 Although truthfulness is important in a therapeutic relationship, the nurse should attempt to be nonjudgmental; a nurse who feels uncomfortable should not be caring for the client in the first place.

6. 2 **Monitoring vital signs after procedures is within the scope of a nursing assistant's role.**

1 This intervention should be performed by registered professional nurses or licensed practical nurses, not nursing assistants.

3 This intervention should be performed by registered professional nurses or licensed practical nurses, not nursing assistants.

4 This intervention should be performed by registered professional nurses or licensed practical nurses, not nursing assistants.

7. 3 **Palliative measures are aimed at relieving discomfort without curing the problem.**

1 A cure or recovery is not part of palliative care; with a terminal disease this goal is unrealistic.

2 A cure or recovery is not part of palliative care; with a terminal disease this goal is unrealistic.

4 Although support of significant others is indicated, palliative care is directly related to relieving the client's discomfort.

8. 3 **Standard and contact precautions require specific handling of potentially infectious matter; therefore, the nursing assistant should be reminded that hospital policies concerning these precautions must be followed for personal protection and the protection of others before the mistake is made again.**

1 This can be done by the nursing assistant immediately after relearning appropriate precautions.

2 Because no injury is evident, an incident report in the nursing assistant's personnel record is unnecessary.

4 Because no injury is evident, documentation in the nursing assistant's personnel record is unnecessary.

9. 1 **Glucocorticoids are used for their antiinflammatory action, which decreases the development of cerebral edema.**

2 Diuretics may be used in conjunction with steroids; they reduce edema after it is present.

3 Anticonvulsants prevent seizure activity, not cerebral edema.

4 Antihypertensives control hypertension, not cerebral edema.

10. 4 **Rapid administration, incorrect positioning, and inadequate solution temperature are common causes of intolerance to tube feedings.**

1 Although this may be done eventually, the feeding technique should be assessed first.

2 Feedings generally are better tolerated if given frequently in small amounts over the entire 24 hours.

3   Although this may be done eventually, the feeding technique should be assessed first.

11. 1   **Consent must be acquired when the client is fully oriented and in a clear mental state.**

2   Although important, this can be implemented before surgery even if the client has received medication.

3   Although important, this can be implemented before surgery even if the client has received medication.

4   Although important, this can be implemented before surgery even if the client has received medication.

12. 3   **The nurse should discuss this treatment option with the practitioner because eschar should be removed down to a rich vascular bed before treatment with a negative-pressure wound treatment device.**

1   Research demonstrates that a neuropathic ulcer responds well to negative-pressure wound treatment.

2   Research demonstrates that a wound with dehiscence responds well to negative-pressure wound treatment.

4   A negative-pressure wound treatment device is contraindicated with untreated, not treated, osteomyelitis.

13. 1   **A state's nurse practice act is the ultimate source relative to a nurse's professional practice; a nurse may not function outside of the legal definition of nursing practice.**

2   Performing suturing, with or without supervision, conflicts with the state's nurse practice act, and the nurse would be functioning outside the legal scope of nursing practice.

3   The state board of nursing does not have jurisdiction concerning this procedure.

4   Performing suturing, with or without supervision, conflicts with the state's nurse practice act, and the nurse would be functioning outside the legal scope of nursing practice.

14. 4   **This includes the client in the problem-solving process.**

1   This does not include the client in the problem-solving process; more data should be obtained from the client before deciding on an intervention, which may or may not be appropriate.

2   This does not include the client in the problem-solving process; more data should be obtained from the client before deciding on an intervention, which may or may not be appropriate.

3   This does not include the client in the problem-solving process; more data should be obtained from the client before deciding on an intervention, which may or may not be appropriate.

15. 2   **Disaster triage is based on the principle of the greatest good for the greatest number; those who have a likelihood of survival are treated first.**

People who are gasping for breath and are conscious have priority over those who are cyanotic and not breathing.

1   Clients who are not breathing and cyanotic have low priority because survival requires multiple time-consuming interventions that detract from the care needed by others.

3   Clients who are not breathing and cyanotic have low priority because survival requires multiple time-consuming interventions that detract from the care needed by others.

4   Those having a seizure have low priority because a seizure is not life threatening.

16. 2   **Sedation may interfere with the client's knowledge of the consent form.**

1   Many clients face contradictory feelings regarding their impending surgery, but their consent is legal unless they withdraw the consent.

3   A second opinion is not required for a consent to be legal.

4   A complete history and physical examination are needed before surgery, but they do not affect the legality of consent.

17. 2   **This response attempts to explore why the client is refusing the procedure; it promotes communication.**

1   This response is accusatory; the client has the right to withdraw consent at any time.

3   This is a conclusion without appropriate data; it puts the client on the defensive.

4   This is a conclusion without appropriate data; it may raise the client's anxiety level.

GROWTH AND DEVELOPMENT

18. 1   **Research demonstrates that women past menopause need at least 1500 mg of calcium a day, which is almost impossible to obtain through dietary sources because the average daily consumption of calcium is 300 to 500 mg; vitamin D promotes the deposition of calcium into the bone.**

2   These do not contain adequate calcium to meet requirements to prevent osteoporosis; these do not contain vitamin D unless fortified.

3   If large amounts of magnesium are present, calcium absorption is impeded because magnesium and calcium absorption are competitive; vitamin E is unrelated to osteoporosis.

4   These may not be consumed in quantities adequate to meet requirements to prevent osteoporosis.

19. 3   **A common conflict confronting the older adult is between the desire to be taken care of by others and the desire to be in charge of one's own destiny.**

1   This may occur but is not common.

2   This may occur but is not common.

4   This may occur but is not common.

20. 2 According to Erikson, poor self-concept and feelings of despair are conflicts manifested in those who are older than 65 years of age.
  1 This conflict is manifested in early childhood between 3 and 6 years of age.
  3 This conflict is manifested during the ages from 6 to 11 years.
  4 This conflict is manifested during middle adulthood, 45 to 65 years of age.

21. Answer: 2, 4
  1 An interference with swallowing is a motor, not a sensory, loss, nor is it an expected response to aging.
  2 Due to aging of the nervous system an older adult has a diminished sensation of pain and may be unaware of a serious illness, thermal extremes, or excessive pressure.
  3 There is a decreased, not heightened, response to stimuli in older adults.
  4 As people age they experience atrophy of the organ of Corti and cochlear neurons, loss of the sensory hair cells and degeneration of the stria vascularis, which affects an older person's ability to perceive high-frequency sounds.
  5 There is a decreased, not increased, ability to physiologically adjust to extremes in environmental temperature.

22. 3 A decrease in neuromuscular function slows reaction time.
  1 The ability to be flexible has less to do with age than with character.
  2 Confusion is not necessarily a process of aging, but it occurs for various reasons such as multiple stresses, perceptual changes, or medication side effects.
  4 The majority of older adults do not have organic mental disease.

23. 4 For reasons that are still unclear, the thirst reflex diminishes with age, and this may lead to a concomitant decline in fluid intake.
  1 There are no data to support this statement.
  2 This is not true for an alert person who is able to perform the activities of daily living.
  3 Research does not support progressive memory loss in normal aging as a contributor to decreased fluid intake.

24. 1 Vitamin E hinders oxidative breakdown of structural lipid membranes in body tissues caused by free radicals in the cells.
  2 This assists in the formation of visual purple needed for night vision.
  3 This is used for formation of collagen, which is important for maintaining capillary strength, promoting wound healing, and resisting infection.
  4 This is necessary for protein and fat metabolism and normal function of the nervous system.

25. 1 This increase is a response to the need for oxygen at the cellular level because of the increased metabolic rate associated with exercise.
  2 This should not occur with mild exercise unless the client has cardiac disease.
  3 The rate of respiration will increase with mild exercise; because of inflexibility of the chest in the older adult, the depth will increase only minimally.
  4 Irregular respirations are not an expected response to exercise; this indicates a problem.

26. 3 Reinforcing strengths promotes self-esteem; reminiscing is a therapeutic tool that provides a life review that assists adaptation and helps achieve the task of integrity associated with older adulthood.
  1 Frequent naps may interfere with adequate sleep at night.
  2 Reinforcing ageism may enhance devaluation of the older adult.
  4 A well-balanced diet that includes protein and fiber should be encouraged; increasing calories may cause obesity.

27. 2 Aging causes a lowering of the physiologic coping reserve of various systems of the body.
  1 The pain threshold increases with aging.
  3 There are many etiologies for confusion (e.g., drug intolerance, altered metabolic state, unfamiliar surroundings).
  4 As individuals age they become more entrenched in ideas, environment, and objects that are familiar, and thus do not tolerate change well.

28. 4 During the aging process there is a progressive atrophy of the convolutions of the brain with a decrease in its blood supply, which may produce a tendency to become forgetful, a reduction in short-term memory, and susceptibility to personality changes.
  1 There should be little or no change in judgment.
  2 There is little or no intellectual deterioration; intelligence scores show no decline.
  3 Creativity is not affected by aging; many people remain creative until very late in life.

29. 3 With aging, narrowing of the arteries causes some increase in the systolic and diastolic blood pressures; hormone production decreases after menopause.
  1 There may or may not be changes in libido; there is a loss of skin elasticity.
  2 Salivary secretions decrease, not increase, causing more difficulty with swallowing; there is some impairment of fat digestion.
  4 There may be a decrease in subcutaneous fat, decreasing body warmth; some swallowing difficulties occur because of decreased oral secretions.

30. 3 The onset of disabling illness will divert an older person's energies, making it difficult to maintain an optimum level of functioning.

1 This is an expected response.

2 This can result from the aging process and the change in environment; it is not as important as the loss of function.

4 A gradual memory loss and some confusion are expected; a sudden memory loss is cause for alarm.

31. 1 **A psychosocial task for middle adulthood according to Erikson is generativity; this task is concerned with the sense of productivity and accomplishment.**

2 This is not involved in any task of middle adulthood identified by Erikson.

3 This is not involved in any task of middle adulthood identified by Erikson.

4 This is not involved in any task of middle adulthood identified by Erikson.

32. 3 **Spending time in several short sessions reduces client fatigue and compensates for a shortened attention span, which is common in the older adult.**

1 The questionnaire may never be completed.

2 This is degrading to the client; the client should be asked initially and, if necessary, family can be asked to fill in details later.

4 This may be overwhelming and create feelings of anger and resentment.

33. 3 **This is the young-adult task associated with intimacy vs isolation.**

1 This is a toddler's task associated with autonomy vs. shame and doubt.

2 This is a preschool-age child's task associated with initiative vs. guilt.

4 This is a toddler's task associated with autonomy vs. shame and doubt.

34. 4 **Presbyopia is the decreased accommodative ability of the lens that occurs with aging.**

1 Tropia (eye turn) generally occurs at birth.

2 Myopia (nearsightedness) can occur during any developmental level or be congenital.

3 Hyperopia (farsightedness) can occur during any developmental level or be congenital.

EMOTIONAL NEEDS RELATED TO HEALTH PROBLEMS

35. 2 **The client should know there is help available, even though direct supervision is no longer provided.**

1 This is not the priority at this time.

3 This is not the priority at this time.

4 Ileostomies are not irrigated because stool is liquid.

36. 3 **Active participation in self-care indicates a readiness to learn; it demonstrates that the client is interested in future expectations.**

1 This may indicate intellectual readiness but not necessarily emotional readiness.

2 An expected change in body image precipitates the grieving process; a client may be in denial if no concerns are expressed.

4 The client need not be dependent; this response indicates the need for more teaching and emotional support.

37. 4 **Explanation of the underlying mechanism usually helps calm anxiety about a phantom pain experience.**

1 This is false reassurance because phantom limb sensations may not disappear.

2 This reinforces the idea that there is something psychologically wrong with the client.

3 This may distract the client, but does not foster awareness of the cause.

38. 4 **The loss of a limb affects the idealized self-image because it is difficult to deny the body has not been altered.**

1 Although sexuality is included in self-image, it is concerned with a variety of other factors not affected by amputation.

2 Amputation may signify a lack of wholeness, but feelings about it are influenced by self-image.

3 Amputation may increase dependency needs, but these needs are influenced by self-image.

39. 4 **Intellectualization is the use of reasoning and thought processes to avoid the emotional aspects of a situation; this is a defense against anxiety.**

1 Projection is denying unacceptable traits and regarding them as belonging to another person.

2 Sublimation is a defense wherein the person redirects the energy of unacceptable impulses into socially acceptable behaviors or activities.

3 Identification is the reduction of anxiety by imitating someone respected or feared.

40. 3 **This response encourages the client to review facts and provides an opportunity to talk about feelings.**

1 This suggests the nurse does not want to discuss the subject; it abdicates the nurse's responsibility to explore the issue with the client.

2 Although it is an empathic answer, it does not encourage the client to explore feelings; it may increase anxiety.

4 Although the statement is true, the response does not encourage the client to examine feelings.

41. 3 **This nonjudgmentally points out the client's behavior.**

1 This is too confrontational; the client may not be able to answer the question.

2 This is too confrontational and an assumption by the nurse.

4 This is too judgmental, an assumption, and a stereotypical response.

42. 4 **It is difficult to work through a loss; however, encouraging the sharing of feelings helps both parties to feel better about having to let go.**
   1 This response impedes the work of acceptance of one's finality and the use of the remaining time to the best advantage.
   2 There is no evidence to suggest that the client cannot cope with these emotions; this is a time for closeness and honesty.
   3 This response is demeaning, closes off communication, and does not foster the expression of feelings.

43. 4 **Honest discussion with emphasis on functional and psychological abilities helps promote adjustment.**
   1 Postoperative depression is not a characteristic feature of thymectomy.
   2 This is too soon; it may eventually be necessary if the client has difficulty adjusting to the chronicity of this condition.
   3 This provides false reassurance; there is no guarantee the client will feel better on discharge.

44. 2 **Lifelong coping styles are most important in how a person will deal with stress.**
   1 Age may influence defense mechanisms but lifelong coping styles will most significantly affect a person's behavior.
   3 This is a factor to be considered, but past coping ability is the most significant factor to predict future coping.
   4 This is a factor to be considered, but past coping ability is the most significant factor to predict future coping.

45. 2 **This action indicates recognition that the client's reaction is understandable; it creates a climate of acceptance and eventually promotes expression of feelings.**
   1 This delays the client's use of coping responses.
   3 This creates a situation in which the client will be hesitant to express any feelings.
   4 This suggests that the nurse is unable to deal with the situation; it is not necessary to notify the practitioner.

46. 3 **This provides the opportunity for the client to verbalize the feelings underlying behavior.**
   1 This has no effect on decreasing the client's anxiety or allowing ventilation.
   2 This explanation will not decrease anxiety so that the client can rest.
   4 Although allowing release of feelings is therapeutic, leaving immediately denies the client the opportunity for verbalization and discussion.

47. 2 **This response indicates that the nurse has heard the verbal message and has empathy for the client; it encourages further verbalization.**
   1 This response may increase the client's anxiety.
   3 This response minimizes the client's concerns.

   4 This depersonalizes the client's concerns; it focuses on the tests and the scheduling rather than the client's needs.

48. 1 **Projection is the attribution of unacceptable feelings and emotions to others.**
   2 Sublimation is the substitution of socially acceptable feelings or instincts to replace those that are threatening to the ego.
   3 Compensation is overachievement in a more comfortable area thereby covering up a weakness.
   4 Intellectualization is the use of mental reasoning processes to deny facing emotions and feelings involved in a situation.

49. 2 **The nurse must identify the client's work activities before an appropriate response can be made.**
   1 The client probably can do light work that will not injure the surgical site.
   3 This response is vague and demeaning and gives little direction to the client.
   4 The client probably can do light work as well as rest.

50. 4 **This response offers the best combination of factual information and emotional support.**
   1 This response disregards the client's feelings; it is also inaccurate because if the bladder is removed, urinary function will not be normal.
   2 Although this reflects the client's feelings, further communication is cut off by the second part of the response.
   3 This response is factual but does not answer the question or offer emotional support; it may increase anxiety.

51. 3 **Reflection conveys acceptance and encourages further communication.**
   1 This is false reassurance that does not help to reduce anxiety.
   2 This provides false reassurance and removes the focus from the client's needs.
   4 This is unrealistic, and it is too late to suggest this.

52. 1 **The loss of an established lifestyle and the potential for death may result in depression.**
   2 Paranoia is occasionally seen in the terminal stage of renal failure; this is not known as "postpump psychosis."
   3 The superego is not affected by this illness.
   4 This is neither a concern nor a common reaction.

53. 4 **The nurse needs to know specifically what the client is asking; this response permits clarification.**
   1 Asking what the surgeon has said collects more information, but it will not clarify what the client wants to know.
   2 Asking what the anesthesiologist has said does not relate to what the client wants to know.
   3 The nurse is making an assumption about medical management.

54. 4 **This true statement can be the foundation for developing a positive mental outlook.**
    1 There is no indication that the client needs drugs to combat depression.
    2 Although this is probably true, this response belittles the client's actual concern and physical discomfort.
    3 This is a patronizing response that does not recognize the despair.

55. 3 **This is a truthful answer that provides some realistic hope.**
    1 This provides false reassurance; repeated exacerbations may reduce the life span.
    2 This response avoids the client's question; the family did not ask.
    4 This avoids the client's question and transfers responsibility to the practitioner.

56. 2 **Communication facilitates joint solution of the problem; the nurse must first determine the client's understanding and perceptions before solutions to the problem can be attempted.**
    1 This will not collect data about why the client is leaving the room.
    3 This abdicates the responsibility of the primary nurse.
    4 This may be done but not until further assessment is performed to determine the reason why the client is leaving the room.

57. 4 **Privacy is necessary when the client disrobes; a professional relationship is established more easily if the nurse and client are uninterrupted.**
    1 This does not provide for privacy.
    2 Socializing at this time is an imposition.
    3 This may eventually be necessary, but it is not the initial action.

58. 1 **This is a classic sign of denial; by reducing the importance or extent of the problem, the individual is able to cope; not acknowledging that it is really a problem is a form of denial.**
    2 This indicates repression of affect rather than denial.
    3 Failure to communicate is insufficient evidence to diagnose denial; the husband-wife relationship may be strained, or the husband may be worried about upsetting the wife.
    4 This usually indicates displacement of anger, not denial.

59. 2 **Improved functioning relates most to improved body image, even if the prosthesis is not at all like the original body part.**
    1 Acceptance by others does not guarantee acceptance by self.
    3 Although mood may be improved with aggressive rehabilitation, this in itself does not improve body image.
    4 Acceptance by others does not guarantee acceptance by self.

60. 4 **Anxiety and/or anger associated with other stages of coping interfere with learning.**
    1 This is too late to start preparation for discharge and teaching. Many factors influence readiness for learning; planning for teaching must begin on the day of admission.
    2 The anxiety associated with mental anguish will interfere with the ability to process new information; mental anguish is associated with an earlier stage.
    3 Although clients in the acceptance or adaptation phase are less angry, the reason teaching is most effective is not because of their compliance but because new information can be processed more easily.

61. 2 **When a client is anxious and has a decreased ability to cope, minor environmental irritants are magnified; eye contact is avoided to decrease additional stimuli.**
    1 Pain is indicated by complaints of discomfort, splinting, refusal to move, and alteration in vital signs.
    3 If the client is angry, eye contact will be maintained; prolonged eye contact may be used as a form of intimidation or aggression.
    4 If this is so the client will verbalize about the need to continue the abduction, not about a variety of other annoyances.

62. 2 **The best indicator of acceptance is when the client begins to participate in self-care.**
    1 This does not indicate acceptance and may be an act of pretended courage.
    3 This does not indicate acceptance and may be an attempt to relieve boredom.
    4 This does not indicate acceptance and may indicate dependence.

63. 4 **Once survival needs are met and pain diminishes, there is a realization of lifestyle alterations in the future.**
    1 The client is not talking about deformities; she is beginning to realize the implications of going home.
    2 Information is not adequate to come to this conclusion.
    3 The client is expressing a realistic concern and needs to talk about the future.

64. 1 **This reflects the client's feelings and encourages a further exploration of concerns.**
    2 This response does not reflect the feeling tone of the client's statement; also the client may not be able to answer a "why" question.
    3 This is false reassurance; thyrotoxic crisis is capable of causing death.
    4 This may reinforce the client's anxiety and avoids discussing the client's concerns; it cuts off communication.

65. 1 **Internal self-stimulation increases as external stimuli decrease.**
    2 Blindness is an added stress that can increase anxiety, which impairs decision making; lack of visual stimuli limits data for decision making.

3 Lack of visual stimuli can increase restlessness, lethargy, and apathy.

4 Blindness will not precipitate neurotic behavior unless other emotional factors are present.

66. 2 **Saying that everything will be fine provides false hope.**

1 Agreeing with the client is an example of offering approval.

3 Commenting on how a client should feel is an example of being judgmental.

4 Implying that the problem is minor is an example of minimizing.

67. 3 **Both hostility and noncompliance are forms of anger that are associated with grieving.**

1 The client's behavior is not a conscious attempt to hurt others but a way to relieve and reduce anxiety within the self.

2 The client's behavior is a self-destructive method of coping, which can result in death.

4 The client's behavior is an effort to maintain control over a situation that is really controlling the client; it is an unconscious method of coping, and noncompliance may be a form of denial.

68. 1 **This response indicates recognition of the client's need to use denial and opens the way for a discussion of feelings.**

2 This response forces reality on the client and blocks a discussion of feelings.

3 This reply focuses on the surgery, which is not the concern expressed by the client.

4 This reply focuses on the physician rather than the client's feelings.

69. 2 **This identifies the client's feelings and provides an opportunity for further discussion.**

1 Although this echoes the client's statement, it does not identify a feeling.

3 This denies the client's feelings and focuses on information; the client may be too emotionally distraught to be able to construct or verbalize questions.

4 This provides false reassurance and cuts off communication.

70. 1 **Communication is a priority; it facilitates interaction, limits anxiety, and promotes safety.**

2 A nasogastric tube can cause trauma to the suture lines; total parenteral nutrition may be used.

3 This is done postoperatively as the client begins to accept the laryngectomy.

4 After a laryngectomy the client cannot cough; expectoration occurs through the stoma.

71. 1 **The nurse must first explore the client's feelings; an honest discussion with emphasis on concerns helps promote adjustment.**

2 This may be necessary if the depression continues.

3 Postoperative depression is not an expected response to surgery.

4 This is false reassurance because there is no guarantee that the depression will lift at home.

72. 3 **Reliving the experience brings back the feelings, such as anxiety and fear, associated with it; the alterations described reflect sympathetic nervous system activity.**

1 There are not enough data present to determine the client's usual method of seeking sympathy.

2 The increased pulse and restlessness indicate bleeding; however, the other data presented support anxiety; additional assessment is necessary to confirm bleeding.

4 These changes are indicative of a sympathetic, not a parasympathetic, response.

73. 1 **Reflection of the client's statement will enhance further communication.**

2 The client did not indicate anxiety concerning the effects of radiotherapy; this is an assumption.

3 This is a conclusion that does not reflect the client's stated concern.

4 This may close the opportunity for further exploration and may reinforce the client's concern.

74. 1 **This meets the client's immediate personal needs and demonstrates respect and concern.**

2 This may be explored when planning further support; it is not the priority at this time.

3 This provides false reassurance that may block communication; the nurse, not the wife, should explore this issue with the client.

4 The client's immediate request should be met first; feelings may be explored when the client reflects a readiness to communicate.

75. 1 **These are realistic, productive, and constructive ways of using this time.**

2 These are signs of depression.

3 Going from practitioner to practitioner demonstrates disbelief, denial, or desperation.

4 This indicates anger and hopelessness, not acceptance.

76. 4 **This is a legal requirement of participating institutions to protect the individuals involved.**

1 Active euthanasia is a direct act to shorten a person's life and is illegal.

2 No age restrictions exist; a guardian's signature is required.

3 Legal statutes make certain that this does not occur.

77. 2 **Before a teaching plan can be developed, the factors that interfere with learning must be identified.**

1 Although family members can be helpful, client involvement in care is most important for promoting independence and self-esteem.

3 This is premature. Assessment comes before intervention; written instructions may not be the most appropriate teaching modality.

4 This may be an unrealistic expectation; the client may never accept the change but must learn to manage care.

78. **4 Sharing and discussing concerns often release anxieties; giving the ordered anxiolytic will produce relaxation.**
1 This might relax the client but will do little to reduce the client's level of anxiety.
2 The client is not in pain at this time but needs to share concerns.
3 The procedure is over; this might be appropriate before the paracentesis. Also there are no data to support that this is the client's concern.

79. **4 This response identifies the client's feelings and accepts them but also points out the responsibility of the client to take action.**
1 Although this response identifies one of the client's concerns, the identification of the underlying feeling is more therapeutic.
2 This response makes the nurse responsible for changing the situation, which is not appropriate or therapeutic.
3 This response denies the client's feelings and provides false reassurance.

80. **2 Knowing what to expect should decrease anxiety.**
1 Routine medications are not withheld unless ordered by the practitioner.
3 A small amount of radiation is emitted during the scan; the client should be assured that the procedure is safe.
4 A sedative is not necessary for this test.

81. **1 The client is in the anger or "why me" stage; encouraging the expression of feelings will help the client resolve them and move toward acceptance.**
2 This abdicates the responsibility of talking with the client; a suggestion to speak with a minister ignores the client's need for an immediate supportive response.
3 This does not reflect on what the client said.
4 This judgmental response may precipitate feelings of guilt and block the nurse-client relationship.

82. **1 Fear of a recurrent myocardial infarction or sudden death is common when the client's environment is to be changed to one that appears less vigilant.**
2 Depression is exhibited by withdrawal, crying, anorexia, and apathy, and it usually becomes more evident after discharge from the hospital.
3 Dependency is exhibited by an unwillingness to increase exercise or perform tasks.
4 Ambivalence is exhibited by contrasting emotions; the client's statement does not demonstrate this.

83. **1 Focusing is a technique that directs a client back to the original topic of discussion.**
2 Restating the main idea of what the client has said encourages the client to continue speaking or clarifies what has been said.
3 Exploring permits the nurse to delve deeper into the subject when the client tends to stay on a superficial level.

4 Accepting is a technique used to understand and demonstrate regard for what the client stated.

84. **1 Voicing fears often reduces the associated anxiety.**
2 Although this should be done, it is not the priority.
3 Encouraging socialization when the client has feelings that need exploration is not therapeutic.
4 Avoiding the problem is not therapeutic.

85. **4 This is a truthful answer and validates the client's feelings.**
1 Although true, this response shuts off communication and further ventilation of feelings.
2 This response denies the client's fears.
3 This response denies the client's feelings.

86. **1 This response interprets the client's behavior without belittling the nursing assistant's feelings; it encourages the assistant to get involved with plans for future care.**
2 Although this response recognizes the client's feelings, it does not help the nursing assistant to cope with the client.
3 This assumes the nursing assistant has nothing to contribute and only the nurse can deal with the problem.
4 This does not help the nursing assistant, nor does it demonstrate an understanding of the client's feelings.

BLOOD AND IMMUNITY

87. **3 The body attempts to compensate for decreased oxygen to tissues by increasing the number of blood cells, the oxygen-carrying component of the blood.**
1 With polycythemia, the skin, especially the face, appears flushed, not pale.
2 This is not specific to polycythemia; there is more than one cause of dyspnea on exertion.
4 The hematocrit is increased with polycythemia.

88. **4 This is absolutely necessary to prevent an acute immunological reaction if the donated blood is not compatible with the client's blood.**
1 Although important, this is not the highest priority.
2 Blood must be kept cool until ready to use. If blood is at room temperature for 30 minutes prior to administration it should be returned to the blood bank; after it is started, blood must be administered within 4 hours.
3 This is not the highest priority; these laboratory results were part of the data used to determine the need for the blood.

89. **3 Both A- and O-negative blood are compatible with the client's blood. A-negative is the same as the client's blood type and preferred; in an emergency, type O-negative blood also may be given.**
1 Although type O blood may be used, it will have to be Rh negative; Rh-positive blood is incompatible with the client's blood and will cause hemolysis.

2 Type AB-positive blood is incompatible with the client's blood and will cause hemolysis.

4 Type A-negative blood is compatible with the client's blood but type AB-negative is incompatible and will cause hemolysis.

90. 3 **A slow rate provides time to recognize a reaction that is developing before too much blood is administered.**

1 This is avoided to prevent clotting and hemolysis.

2 Infusion pumps will cause red blood cell damage; blood should flow by gravity through an appropriate filter.

4 This is not necessary.

91. 1 **Flank pain is an adaptation associated with a hemolytic transfusion reaction; it is caused by agglutination of red cells in the kidneys and renal vasoconstriction. The infusion must be stopped to prevent further instillation of blood, which is being viewed as foreign by the body.**

2 Although this will be done eventually, it is not the priority action.

3 Although this will be done eventually, it is not the priority action.

4 Although this will be done eventually, it is not the priority action.

92. 4 **The blood must be stopped first, tubing must be replaced and then normal saline should be infused to keep the line patent and maintain blood volume.**

1 While this assessment is being made, the client's circulating blood volume will decrease.

2 This can be done later.

3 While this assessment is being made, the client's circulating blood volume will decrease.

93. 3 **The tubing must be replaced to avoid infusing the blood left in the original tubing; the normal saline infusion will maintain an open line for any further IV treatment.**

1 All vital signs should be taken eventually; blood pressure may be taken on either arm, not necessarily both.

2 A urine sample is collected after the blood transfusion is stopped, the tubing replaced, and a bag of normal saline hung. The specimen will be analyzed to determine kidney function.

4 Although the intake, and especially the output, should be monitored to assess kidney function, this is not the priority.

94. 4 **Fat-soluble vitamin K is essential for synthesis of prothrombin by the liver; a lack results in hypoprothrombinemia, inadequate coagulation, and hemorrhage.**

1 Although cirrhosis may interfere with production of bile, which contains the bilirubin needed for optimum absorption of vitamin K, the best and quickest manner to counteract the bleeding is to provide vitamin K intramuscularly.

2 Folic acid is a coenzyme with vitamins B_{12} and C in the formation of nucleic acids and heme; thus a deficiency may lead to anemia, not bleeding.

3 Vitamin A deficiency contributes to development of polyneuritis and beriberi, not hemorrhage.

95. 2 **A complete blood count (CBC) includes red blood cell (RBC) count and RBC indices, white blood cell (WBC) count and WBC differential count, hemoglobin (Hb), hematocrit (Hct), and platelet count.**

1 A blood glucose level is not part of a CBC.

3 The C-reactive protein level is not part of a CBC.

4 Blood urea nitrogen (BUN) is not part of a CBC.

96. 4 **This is an honest response that corrects the client's misconception about the effectiveness of the current antiviral medications.**

1 Phlebotomy is not the treatment used to remove the virus from the client's body.

2 Current pharmacological treatment does not eliminate the virus from the body; it can slow its progress and may even effect a remission (although the medications are never discontinued), but there is no known cure.

3 This is a nontherapeutic, judgmental response that can alienate the client and precipitate feelings of guilt.

97. 2 **Equipment used in blood donation is disposable; the donor does not come into contact with anyone else's blood.**

1 The risk depends on the spouse's prior behavior.

3 Although condoms do offer protection, they are subject to failure because of condom rupture or improper use; risks of infection are present with any sexual contact.

4 An individual may be infected before testing positive for the antibodies; the individual can still transmit the virus.

98. 1 **These tests confirm the presence of HIV antibodies that occur in response to the presence of the human immunodeficiency virus.**

2 This places someone at risk but does not constitute a positive diagnosis.

3 These do not confirm the presence of HIV; these adaptations are related to many disorders, not just HIV infection.

4 The diagnosis of just an opportunistic infection is not sufficient to confirm the diagnosis of HIV. An opportunistic infection (included in the CDC surveillance case definition for AIDS) in the presence of HIV antibodies indicates that the individual has AIDS.

99. 1 **The HIV infects helper T-cell lymphocytes; therefore, 300 or fewer CD4 T cells per cubic millimeter of blood or CD4 cells accounting for less than 20% of lymphocytes is suggestive of AIDS.**

2 The thymic hormones necessary for T-cell growth are decreased.

3 This finding is associated with allergies and parasitic infections.

4   This finding is associated with drug induced hemolytic anemia and hemolytic disease of the newborn.

100. 4   **Because this procedure does not involve contact with blood or secretions, additional protection is not indicated.**

1   These are necessary only when there is risk of contact with blood or body fluid.

2   These are necessary only when there is risk of contact with blood or body fluid.

3   A mask and gown are indicated only if there is a danger of secretions or blood splattering on the nurse (for example, during suctioning).

101. 2   These items prevent contact with feces, sputum, or other body fluids during intimate body care.

1   Goggles alone are inadequate because the client is producing copious sputum.

3   Gloves are not necessary because touching body fluids when giving oral medication is not likely.

4   Gloves are necessary when assisting the client with a bedpan because the nurse may be exposed to the client's excreta.

102. 2   *Pneumocystis jiroveci*, now believed to be a fungus, causes pneumonia in immunosuppressed hosts; it can cause death in 60% of the clients. The client's respiratory status is the priority.

1   Although this is a concern, the client's respiratory status is the priority.

3   Although this is a concern, the client's respiratory status is the priority.

4   Although this is a concern, the client's respiratory status is the priority.

103. 4   **This test assesses parietal cell function. After radioactive cobalamin is administered, its excretion is measured; if cobalamin cannot be absorbed as in pernicious anemia, very little is excreted in the urine.**

1   This test is not affected by medications.

2   The results of this test are not affected by food; with pernicious anemia there is a deficiency of intrinsic factor, which is necessary for vitamin B_{12} use.

3   Intake and output records are not necessary with a Schilling test.

104. 3   **Pernicious anemia is caused by the inability to absorb vitamin B_{12} resulting from a lack of intrinsic factor in gastric juices; for the Schilling test, radioactive vitamin B_{12} is administered and its absorption and excretion can be ascertained.**

1   This is not measured by this test.

2   This is not measured by this test.

4   Vitamin B_{12} is not produced in the body.

105. 3   **IM injections bypass the vitamin B_{12} absorption defect (lack of intrinsic factor, the transport carrier component of gastric juices). A monthly dose is usually sufficient because it is stored in active body tissues such as the liver, kidney, heart, muscles, blood, and bone marrow.**

1   The Z-track method need not be used as it is for iron dextran injections.

2   Because it is stored and only slowly depleted, injections once a month usually are sufficient.

4   Vitamin B_{12} cannot be taken by mouth because of the lack of intrinsic factor.

106. 3   **Because the intrinsic factor does not return to gastric secretions even with therapy, B_{12} injections will be required monthly for the remainder of the client's life.**

1   B_{12} injections must be taken for the rest of the client's life.

2   B_{12} injections must be taken for the rest of the client's life.

4   Intramuscular injections of B_{12} must be taken monthly for the rest of the client's life.

107. 2   **A protocol consisting of three or four chemotherapeutic agents that attack the dividing cells at various phases of development is the therapy of choice at this stage; alternating courses of different protocols generally are used.**

1   Radiation, alone or in combination with chemotherapy, is used in stages IA, IB, IIA, IIB, and IIIA.

3   This is recommended for use in stage IIIA.

4   This is not a therapy for Hodgkin's disease at any stage. The nodes may be removed for biopsy or irradiated as part of therapy.

108. 2   **Because of the location of the spleen, postoperative pain will cause splinting and shallow breathing and underaeration of the lung's left lower lobe.**

1   This is true of any abdominal surgery and is not specific to a splenectomy.

3   This is true of any abdominal surgery and is not specific to a splenectomy.

4   This is true of any abdominal surgery and is not specific to a splenectomy.

109. 2   **Moderate leukopenia increases the risk of infection; the client should be taught protective measures.**

1   Leukopenia is a side effect of cyclophosphamide (Cytoxan), not prednisone.

3   The platelet count is not given, so bleeding precautions are not indicated.

4   These are measures to correct anemia; protection from infection takes priority.

110. 4   **Thrombocytopenia occurs with most chemotherapy treatment programs; using a soft toothbrush helps prevent bleeding gums.**

1   Although alopecia does occur, it is not related to bone marrow suppression.

2   Increasing fluids will neither reverse bone marrow suppression nor stimulate hematopoiesis.

3   This is not related to bone marrow suppression.

111. 1   **Suppression of bone marrow increases bleeding susceptibility associated with decreased platelets.**

2   This will not affect the bone marrow. Citrus juices should be avoided by the client receiving chemotherapy because of the side effects of stomatitis.

3   With bone marrow suppression there is a decrease in red blood cells; rest should be encouraged.

4 With bone marrow suppression the red blood cells are decreased in number and there is a decreased oxygen-carrying capacity of the blood. This position will not increase the number of red blood cells.

112. 1 **Brief pressure is generally enough to prevent bleeding at the aspiration site.**
2 Complications are rare; no special positions are required.
3 The site is cleaned prior to aspiration.
4 Complications are rare; frequent monitoring is unnecessary.

113. 3 **The hypermetabolic state associated with leukemia causes more urea and uric acid (end products of metabolism) to be produced and to accumulate in the blood.**
1 Enlarged lymph nodes will not increase blood urea and uric acid.
2 Thrombocytopenia causes a decrease in platelets, which causes bleeding.
4 Hepatic encephalopathy is associated with liver disease, not leukemia.

114. 3 **Bleeding tendencies occur because of bone marrow suppression and rapidly proliferating leukocytes.**
1 There is no change in hair growth in the absence of chemotherapy.
2 The client will more likely be sleeping excessively.
4 Splenomegaly occurs with chronic lymphoblastic leukemia (CLL) and chronic myelogenous leukemia (CML), not acute lymphoblastic leukemia (ALL).

115. Answer: 4, 5
1 Fever is unrelated to thrombocytopenia. Fever is a sign of infection; infection results when the white blood cells are reduced (leukopenia).
2 Diarrhea is unrelated to thrombocytopenia; diarrhea may result from the effects of chemotherapy on the rapidly dividing cells of the gastrointestinal system.
3 Headache is unrelated to thrombocytopenia; headache may be caused by the effects of chemotherapy on central nervous system cells or indicate that the leukemia has invaded the central nervous system.
4 **Hematuria is blood in the urine. Thrombocytes are involved in the clotting mechanism; thrombocytopenia is a reduced number of thrombocytes in the blood.**
5 **Ecchymosis is a superficial bruise caused by bleeding under the skin or mucous membrane. With thrombocytopenia, bleeding occurs because there are insufficient platelets.**

116. 3 **This protein (globulin) results from tumor cell metabolites. It is present in clients with multiple myeloma.**
1 This is not specific for the diagnosis of multiple myeloma; it is a late complication of multiple myeloma related to coagulation defects.
2 Hypercalcemia, not hypocalcemia, occurs with multiple myeloma because of bone erosion.

4 Multiple myeloma is not caused by a bacterial infection.

117. 1 **A definite confirmation of multiple myeloma can only be made through a bone marrow biopsy; this is a plasma cell malignancy with widespread bone destruction.**
2 Although calcium is lost from bone tissue and hypercalcemia results, this is not a confirmation of the disease.
3 Although this protein is found in the urine, it does not confirm the disease.
4 X-ray films will show the characteristic "punched-out" areas caused by the increased number of plasma cells, which contributes to the making of the diagnosis. The definitive diagnosis is made on biopsy.

118. 4 **Because of bone erosion, pathological fractures are a common complication of multiple myeloma.**
1 Although this is done, the priority is to prevent injury.
2 Although this is an adaptation to the associated anemia, it is not life threatening.
3 Although this is important, preventing pathological fractures is the priority.

119. 4 **A variety of drugs affect rapidly dividing cells at different stages of cell division.**
1 Although this is an acceptable therapy, it is not the first treatment used.
2 This is not a primary approach; it may be used to alleviate pain and treat acute vertebral lesions.
3 Multiple myeloma is a disorder of the bone; there are no lesions that can be removed.

120. 1 **Because an elevated temperature increases metabolic demands, the pyrexia must be treated immediately. The practitioner should be notified because this client is immunodeficient from both the disease and the chemotherapy. A search for the cause of the pyrexia can then be initiated.**
2 More vigorous intervention is necessary. This client has a disease in which the immunoglobulins are ineffective and the therapy further suppresses the immune system.
3 This is not the immediate priority, although it is important because the cause of the pyrexia must be determined. Also the increased amount of calcium and urates in the urine can cause renal complications if dehydration occurs.
4 This is not the priority, although important because respiratory tract infections are a common occurrence in clients with multiple myeloma.

121. 1 **Blood products (packed RBCs or platelets) are administered when warranted.**
2 Renal insufficiency, not infections, may occur due to chronic hypercalcemia, proteinemia, and hyperuricemia.
3 Fluid replacement should be provided in carefully supervised clinical settings because if dehydration occurs it may result in renal shutdown.
4 Ultraviolet rays are not related to exacerbations.

122. 4 **These drugs suppress the immune system, decreasing the body's production of antibodies in response to the new organ, which acts as an antigen. These drugs decrease the risk of rejection.**
    1 Leukocytosis is inhibited by these drugs.
    2 These drugs do not provide immunity; they interfere with natural immune responses.
    3 Because these drugs suppress the immune system, they increase the risk of infection.

123. 2 **Systemic lupus erythematosus is an autoimmune disorder and physical and emotional stresses have been identified as contributing factors to the occurrence of exacerbations.**
    1 Although this should be done, inadequate hygiene is not known to produce exacerbations.
    3 Although this should be done, nutritional status is not significantly correlated to exacerbations.
    4 Knowledge of the symptoms will not decrease the occurrence of exacerbations.

124. 1 **Tetanus antitoxin provides antibodies, which confer immediate passive immunity.**
    2 Antitoxin does not stimulate production of plasma cells, the precursors of antibodies.
    3 Passive, not active, immunity occurs.
    4 Passive immunity, by definition, is not long lasting.

125. 1 **It takes this length of time for antibodies to respond to the antigen and form an indurated area.**
    2 This is longer than necessary; the site will reveal induration in 2 to 3 days.
    3 This is longer than necessary; the site will reveal induration in 2 to 3 days.
    4 This is longer than necessary; the site will reveal induration in 2 to 3 days.

126. 1 **Drug hypersensitivity and anaphylaxis are most common with antimicrobial agents.**
    2 This is a dependent function; it is not crucial to starting antibiotic therapy.
    3 This is an important assessment, but it is not crucial to starting antibiotic therapy.
    4 Withholding treatment until culture results are available may extend the infection.

127. 2 **Hypersensitivity to a foreign substance can cause an anaphylactic reaction; histamine is released, causing bronchial constriction, increased capillary permeability, and dilation of arterioles; this decreased peripheral resistance is associated with hypotension and inadequate circulation to major organs.**
    1 These are the problems that result from bronchial constriction and vascular collapse.
    3 Dilation of arterioles occurs.
    4 Arterioles dilate, capillary permeability increases, and eventually vascular collapse occurs.

128. 3 **Activity may encourage the dislodgment of more microemboli.**

    1 Bed rest may enhance platelet aggregation and the formation of thrombi because of venous stasis.
    2 Venous stasis, rather than enhanced circulation, is supported by bed rest.
    4 Bed rest supports venous stasis rather than the circulation of blood to damaged tissues.

129. 4 **These nutrients stimulate the immune system.**
    1 The role of fatty acids in natural defense mechanisms is uncertain.
    2 These have no known effect on natural defense mechanisms.
    3 Tryptophan has no known effect on natural defense mechanisms.

130. 2 **Blood incompatibility causes lysis of red blood cells with the result that hemoglobin is freed into the circulation; if a sufficient (100 mL or more) amount of incompatible blood is transfused, permanent renal damage can occur. Chills and low back pain indicate kidney involvement.**
    1 Specific gravity need not be determined.
    3 Carboxyhemoglobin need not be determined.
    4 Disseminated intravascular coagulation (DIC) is an intravascular clotting disorder that does not occur with a transfusion reaction.

131. Answer: 1, 4
    1 **Pallor occurs with hemorrhage as the peripheral blood vessels constrict in an effort to shunt blood to the vital organs in the center of the body.**
    2 Urinary output decreases with hemorrhage because of a lowered glomerular filtration rate secondary to hypovolemia.
    3 Respirations increase and become shallow with hemorrhage as the body attempts to take in more oxygen.
    4 **Heart rate accelerates in hemorrhage as the body attempts to increase blood flow and oxygen to body tissues.**
    5 Hypotension occurs in response to hemorrhage as the person experiences hypovolemia.

132. 2 **Because of the recumbent position, drainage may flow by gravity under the client and not be noticed unless the bedding is examined.**
    1 This assessment is inaccurate when there is a dressing in place.
    3 In the immediate postoperative period, vital signs should be taken more frequently than every 4 hours; in addition, observation of the site is a more reliable indicator of hemorrhage.
    4 Dressings impede an accurate assessment of the site for ecchymosis.

133. 4 **Hypovolemia results in a decreased cardiac output and a decreased arterial pressure, which are reflected by a feeble, weak peripheral pulse.**
    1 The skin will be cool and pale because of vasoconstriction.

2 These are late signs of shock.

3 The pulse pressure narrows with decreased cardiac pressure associated with hypovolemic shock.

134. 3 With shock, arteriolar vasoconstriction occurs, raising the total peripheral vascular resistance and shifting blood to the major organs.

1 With shock, more antidiuretic hormone (ADH) is produced to promote fluid retention, which will elevate the blood pressure.

2 Although this is a response to hypoxia, peripheral vasoconstriction is a more effective compensatory mechanism.

4 With shock the mineralocorticoids increase to promote fluid retention, which elevates the blood pressure.

135. 1 A decreased intravascular volume results in hypovolemia and hypotension, which is evidenced by a decreased blood pressure and a decreased pulse pressure.

2 Vasomotor stimulation to the arterial walls is increased with shock.

3 This is a description of neurogenic shock, which is unlikely in this situation.

4 Although electrolyte imbalances can precipitate cardiac decompensation, cardiogenic shock is unlikely in this situation.

136. 4 When an abdominal aneurysm ruptures, hypovolemic shock ensues because fluid volume depletion occurs as the heart continues to pump blood out of the ruptured vessel.

1 Vasogenic shock results from humoral or toxic substances acting directly on the blood vessels, causing vasodilation.

2 Neurogenic shock results from decreased neuromuscular tone, causing decreased vasoconstriction.

3 Cardiogenic shock results from a decrease in cardiac output.

137. 2 Peritonitis and shock are potentially life-threatening complications following abdominal surgery; prompt, rigorous treatment is necessary.

1 Fluids, not blood, are needed to expand and maintain the circulating blood volume.

3 The head of the bed should be flat to increase tissue perfusion and oxygenation to the vital organs.

4 The practitioner should be notified; the client is already receiving oxygen and the problem still exists.

138. 1 This occurs during the progressive stage of shock as a result of accumulated lactic acid.

2 Metabolic alkalosis cannot occur with the buildup of lactic acid.

3 Eventually this can result from decreased respiratory function in late shock, further compounding metabolic acidosis.

4 This may occur as a result of hyperventilation during early shock.

139. 3 Blood replacement is needed to increase the oxygen-carrying capacity of the blood; the expected hematocrit for women is 37% to 47% and for men is 42% to 52%.

1 Ringer's lactate does not increase the oxygen-carrying capacity of the blood.

2 Serum albumin helps maintain volume but does not affect the hematocrit level.

4 Although dextran does expand blood volume, it decreases the hematocrit because it does not replace red blood cells.

CARDIOVASCULAR

140. 4 The carotid artery is located along the anterior edge of the sternocleidomastoid muscle at the level of the lower margin of the thyroid cartilage.

1 This is not the anatomical landmark for locating the carotid artery.

2 This is not the anatomical landmark for locating the carotid artery.

3 This is not the anatomical landmark for locating the carotid artery.

141. Answer: 4, 1, 3, 2

This is the order of the procedure that the nurse should follow to identify the point of maximum impulse (PMI). The PMI is located under the fifth intercostal space at the midclavicular line. The apex of the heart lies under the PMI.

142. 2 The first heart sound is produced by closure of the mitral and tricuspid valves; it is heard best at the apex of the heart.

1 This is where the second heart sound (S_2) is best heard; S_2 is produced by closure of the aortic and pulmonic valves.

3 This border covers a large area; the auscultatory areas that lie near it are the pulmonic and mitral areas.

4 This border covers a large area; the only auscultatory area near it is the aortic area.

143. 1 Closure of the atrioventricular valves, the mitral and tricuspid, produces the first heart sound (S_1).

2 These valves do not close simultaneously.

3 These valves do not close simultaneously.

4 These are the semilunar valves; closure of these valves produces the second heart sound (S_2).

144. 4 Pulmonary capillary wedge pressure is an indirect measure of left ventricular end-diastolic pressure, an indication of ventricular contractility.

1 Right atrial pressure measures only the function of the right side of the heart and indirectly its ability to receive blood.

2 Cardiac output by thermodilution does not measure intracardiac pressures.

3 Pulmonary artery diastolic pressure may not be as accurate an indicator of left ventricular pressure if COPD or pulmonary hypertension exists.

145. **1 Dysrhythmias are abnormal and are associated with acute or chronic pathological conditions.**
    2 This is expected; the radial pulse reflects ventricular contractions.
    3 The expected range in adults is 60 to 100 beats per minute.
    4 These are the anatomical landmarks for locating the apex of the heart; they are unaffected by aging.

146. **Answer: 4, 5**
    1 Drinking fluids keeps the client hydrated, preventing dehydration and hypercoagulability; however, this is not an independent function of the nurse because it requires a practitioner's order.
    2 Massaging the client's legs is contraindicated because any developing clot could be dislodged.
    3 This is not an independent function of the nurse. The nurse needs a practitioner's order to apply pneumatic stockings.
    4 Avoiding crossing the ankles and legs relieves pressure against the veins in the legs and facilitates venous return.
    5 Alternating planter flexion and dorsiflexion contracts calf muscles, facilitating venous return.

147. **2 Oxygen is necessary for the production of fire.**
    1 Oxygen does not burn; it supports combustion.
    3 This is irrelevant regarding the need for safety precautions.
    4 This is irrelevant regarding the need for safety precautions.

148. **4 The QRS interval represents time taken for depolarization of both ventricles.**
    1 The P wave represents repolarization of the atria.
    2 The T wave represents repolarization of the ventricles.
    3 The PR interval represents the time taken for the impulse to spread through the atria.

149. **3 This is an early typical finding after a myocardial infarct because of the altered contractility of the heart.**
    1 Flattened or depressed T waves indicate hypokalemia.
    2 This occurs in atrial and ventricular fibrillation.
    4 Q waves may become distorted with conduction or rhythm problems, but they do not disappear unless there is cardiac standstill.

150. **2 This is a radionuclear study that determines viability of myocardial tissue; necrotic or scar tissue does not extract the thallium isotope.**
    1 This information is available from cardiac catheterization with angiography.
    3 This information is available from cardiac catheterization with angiography.
    4 This is determined by a 12-lead ECG.

151. **1 Hypovolemia occurs with decreased cardiac output and the resulting decreased arterial pressure is reflected in weak, thready peripheral pulses.**
    2 The skin will be cool and pale because of vasoconstriction.
    3 This will occur later as a result of hypovolemic shock.
    4 The pulse pressure will be decreased, not increased, with decreased cardiac output associated with hypovolemic shock.

152. **1 Sitting maintains alignment of the back and allows the nurses to support the client until orthostatic hypotension subsides.**
    2 This will induce flexion of the vertebrae, which can traumatize the spinal cord.
    3 Rapid movement can flex the vertebrae, which can traumatize the spinal cord; taking the blood pressure at this time is not necessary.
    4 This will induce flexion of the vertebrae, which can traumatize the spinal cord.

153. **3 If a closed chest drainage tube becomes obstructed there is increased intrathoracic pressure that pushes the heart to the opposite side, thereby reducing venous return and cardiac output.**
    1 Although a hemothorax is serious, it is not as life threatening as a mediastinal shift, which compromises cardiac output.
    2 Dyspnea may develop but is not life threatening.
    4 A pneumothorax is unrelated to abdominal pressure and is not as life threatening as a mediastinal shift, which compromises cardiac output.

154. **2 A premature ventricular complex (PVC) is a contraction originating in an ectopic focus in the ventricles; it is characterized by a premature, wide, distorted QRS complex with the P wave and PR interval buried in the distorted QRS complex resulting in an irregular rhythm.**
    1 These occur with a premature atrial complex.
    3 These occur with sinus tachycardia.
    4 These occur with ventricular tachycardia.

155. **3 The essential fatty acids, linoleic acid and linolenic acid, are necessary for muscle tissue integrity, especially of the myocardium.**
    1 All fats cannot and should not be eliminated from the diet.
    2 Carbohydrates do not contain the essential fatty acids, linoleic acid, and linolenic acid.
    4 The body does manufacture cholesterol.

156. **2 Gradual occlusion of the carotid arteries, manifested by the transient ischemia attacks, is caused almost exclusively by atherosclerotic thrombosis.**
    1 Valvular heart disease, whether acquired or congenital, usually causes cerebral emboli, not gradual occlusion of the carotid arteries.
    3 Emboli resulting from atrial fibrillation cause sudden and complete, not partial, occlusion of the vessels.
    4 Developmental defects of the arterial wall are associated with saccular aneurysms.

157. 4 **The fiber component of complex carbohydrates helps bind and eliminate dietary cholesterol and fosters growth of intestinal microorganisms to break down bile salts and release the cholesterol component for excretion.**
    1 It is what, not when, the client eats that is important.
    2 Saturated fats should be decreased.
    3 Fat-binding fiber should be increased.

158. Answer: 1, 4, 5
    1 **Tea contains caffeine, which stimulates catecholamine release and acts as a cardiac stimulant; tea should be avoided.**
    2 Red meat does not stimulate the myocardium; however, it should be decreased or eliminated if serum cholesterol levels are elevated.
    3 Club soda does not contain caffeine and does not stimulate the myocardium; however, most contain sodium, which promotes fluid retention and should be avoided by a client with a cardiac condition.
    4 **Hot cocoa contains chocolate, which contains caffeine; it stimulates catecholamine release and acts as a cardiac stimulant; cocoa should be avoided.**
    5 **The chocolate in chocolate pudding has a high caffeine content, which may stimulate catecholamine release and act as a cardiac stimulant; chocolate should be avoided.**

159. 3 **The original myocardial infarct may be extending; the client's adaptations require immediate medical intervention and relief of pain.**
    1 This should be done after notification of the practitioner; notification and pain relief are the priorities.
    2 The blood pressure and an ECG will provide additional data but will cause a delay in notification of the practitioner and provision of necessary medical intervention.
    4 Nitroglycerin does not relieve the pain associated with a myocardial infarction.

160. 2 **Of all the basic food groups, fresh fruits and juices are the lowest in sodium.**
    1 Most fresh meat or fish contain approximately 50 to 120 mg of sodium per 100 grams; processed meats contain approximately 1700 to 2000 mg of sodium per 100 grams.
    3 Most aged cheeses contain approximately 300 to 1100 mg of sodium per 100 grams of cheese.
    4 Most dry cereals contain approximately 900 to 1100 mg of sodium per 100 grams of cereal.

161. 3 **Angina usually is caused by narrowing of the coronary arteries; the lumen of the arteries can be assessed by cardiac catheterization.**
    1 Although pressures can be obtained, they are not the priority for this client; this assessment is appropriate for those with valvular disease.
    2 This is appropriate for infants and young adults with cardiac birth defects.
    4 This is appropriate for infants and young children with suspected septal defects.

162. 3 **Bed rest with immobilization of the leg promotes coagulation and healing at the puncture site of the femoral artery.**
    1 In the absence of bleeding and the presence of adequate fluid replacement, a cardiac catheterization does not cause orthostatic hypotension.
    2 These adaptations are not expected after a cardiac catheterization.
    4 A small amount of radiopaque dye is injected (via the catheter) directly into the heart, where it is diluted by the blood; it does not create a problem at the puncture site.

163. 3 **Tingling indicates decreased arterial circulation to the extremity; it may be caused by an embolus distal to the arterial insertion site; checking all pulses will help locate an embolus.**
    1 Tingling sensations of an extremity are not related to bleeding, but rather to lack of circulation.
    2 These signs are associated with thrombophlebitis; tingling is associated with arterial obstruction.
    4 This will be done if there are systemic responses to compromised heart function; tingling in an extremity is a localized response.

164. 1 **There is increased urinary output as a result of the diuretic effect of the contrast medium.**
    2 A decrease of 10% to 20% is expected because of the diuretic effect of the contrast medium; a decrease greater than 20% may be pathologic.
    3 Although this may occur during the procedure because of trauma to the conduction system, it usually does not continue after the procedure.
    4 Respiratory distress may be an indication of a pulmonary embolus from a venous clot and should be reported immediately.

165. 1 **An apical pulse is taken to detect dysrhythmias related to cardiac irritability; blood pressure is monitored to detect hypotension, which may indicate bleeding or shock.**
    2 Flexion of the groin may compromise the clot at the femoral insertion site.
    3 The client did not undergo general anesthesia and will be ambulatory in 4 to 6 hours.
    4 A fever may indicate a bacterial invasion, but this will not be evident during the first few hours after the catheterization.

166. 4 **The supine position prevents hip flexion, limiting injury and promoting healing of the catheter insertion site; if the head of the bed is elevated, it should not exceed 20 degrees.**
    1 Hip flexion when rising to ambulate traumatizes the catheter insertion site and should be avoided for at least 4 hours to promote healing.
    2 This will interfere with rest; the vital signs are measured every 15 minutes until stable, usually for 1 hour.
    3 The gastrointestinal system is not involved and general anesthesia is not used.

167. 3 **A warm flushing sensation that lasts approxi-mately 30 seconds will occur when the contrast medium is injected.**
    1 Medication is given for mild sedation; clients are drowsy but awake enough to follow instructions.
    2 The supine position will be maintained for 4 to 6 hours after the procedure; walking may dislodge clots at the catheter insertion site, resulting in bleeding.
    4 The supine position is maintained 4 to 6 hours after the procedure; the semi-Fowler's position flexes the legs, which may result in bleeding at the femoral insertion site and should be avoided.

168. 4 **This is a classic reaction because it dilates coro-nary arteries, which increases oxygen to the myo-cardium, thus decreasing pain.**
    1 Anginal pain frequently is relieved by immediate rest.
    2 Angina usually is precipitated by exertion, emotion, or a heavy meal.
    3 Angina usually is described as tightness, indigestion, or heaviness.

169. 1 **A reclining position maintains a blood supply to vital centers.**
    2 This is unsafe; maintaining blood flow to vital cen-ters is essential.
    3 While the semi-Fowler's position facilitates breath-ing, it does not assist blood flow to vital centers.
    4 Maintaining blood flow to vital centers, not com-fort, is the priority.

170. 3 **A sustained diastolic pressure exceeding 90 mm Hg reflects pathology and indicates hypertension.**
    1 This is unrelated to hypertension.
    2 This reflects the heart rate and rhythm, not the pressure within the arteries.
    4 Initially hypertension usually is asymptomatic; although headaches can be associated with hyper-tension, there are other causes of headaches.

171. 1 **When the sound disappears at 72 mm Hg it is known as phase five of Korotkoff's sounds; this reflects the diastolic pressure when the artery is no longer compressed and blood flows freely. This number is recorded as the diastolic pressure in adolescents and adults.**
    2 The muffled sound heard at 90 mm Hg is phase four of Korotkoff's sounds; the muffled sound represents the point at which the cuff pressure falls below the pressure within the arterial wall. This number is recorded as the diastolic pressure in infants and children.
    3 The tapping sound heard at 100 mm Hg is known as phase three of Korotkoff's sounds; this reflects blood flow through an increasingly open artery as constriction of the cuff decreases.
    4 The swishing sound heard at 130 mm Hg is phase two of Korotkoff's sounds; this is caused by blood turbulence.

172. 4 **Further assessment is necessary before the nurse can plan a course of action.**
    1 This is not an initial nursing action; further assessment is the priority.
    2 The nurse must gather more data before consulting with the practitioner.
    3 This is not an expected blood pressure for an older adult; both systolic and diastolic pressures are elevated.

173. 3 **Muscle contraction associated with walking prevents pooling of blood in the extremities and dependent edema.**
    1 Movement is required, not inactivity.
    2 Movement is required, not inactivity.
    4 This does not include movement, which is essential to prevent thrombus formation.

174. 3 **The failing left ventricle cannot accept blood returning from the lungs; this results in increased vascular pressure in the lungs.**
    1 This is associated with right ventricular failure.
    2 There is no diagnosis of right atrial failure as a separate entity.
    4 Although dyspnea on exertion is associated with obstructive pulmonary disease, hypertension and pedal edema are related to cardiac, not respiratory, problems.

175. 1 **Blockage of the myocardial blood supply causes accumulation of unoxidized metabolites that affect nerve endings that generally cause pain.**
    2 The pain usually is crushing, severe, and of prolonged duration.
    3 The pain usually is severe.
    4 The pain is unrelieved by nitroglycerin.

176. 1 **These are classic symptoms of a myocardial infarction; further medical evaluation and intervention are needed immediately.**
    2 This response presumes a dietary problem when a more serious situation may exist.
    3 This response considers only an emotional source of the reported symptoms and ignores a potential medical emergency.
    4 This provides false reassurance and ignores a potential medical emergency.

177. 1 **Morphine is an opioid analgesic that acts on the central nervous system by a sympathetic mecha-nism. Morphine decreases systemic vascular resistance, which decreases left ventricular afterload, thus decreasing myocardial oxygen consumption.**
    2 Nitroglycerin sublingually relieves anginal pain, not myocardial infarction pain.
    3 Oxygen administration elevates arterial oxygen tension, potentially improving tissue oxygenation; however, oxygen administration will not relieve the pain.
    4 Lidocaine is an antidysrhythmic, not an analgesic.

178. 1 **Physical activity need not be restricted; clients who have had a myocardial infarction have a cardiovascular rehabilitation exercise program prescribed. Exercises should become a part of the client's lifestyle.**

   2 This is desirable because aspirin decreases platelet aggregation.

   3 This is desirable because cigarette smoking causes arterial constriction.

   4 This is desirable because obesity increases the body's oxygen demands, which increases the workload of the heart.

179. 1 **Unrelieved chest pain increases anxiety, fatigue, and myocardial oxygen consumption with the possibility of extending the infarction.**

   2 The client will not be ready for teaching until the chest pain is relieved.

   3 Cardiac monitoring is important, but it does not take priority over relieving the subjective complaint of chest pain.

   4 Bed rest is necessary to decrease the workload of the heart, but decreasing the cardiac workload will be difficult to achieve unless the chest pain is relieved.

180. 2 **Morphine is a specific central nervous system depressant used to relieve the pain associated with myocardial infarction; it also decreases apprehension and prevents cardiogenic shock.**

   1 This is not the reason for the use of morphine.

   3 This is not the primary reason for the use of morphine.

   4 Lidocaine is given intravenously to accomplish this.

181. 4 **Defecation in the sitting position on a bedside commode uses less energy than walking to the bathroom or getting on and off a bedpan.**

   1 Defecation is difficult on a bedpan and may cause straining and an increase in oxygen demands.

   2 Walking to the bathroom uses more energy than using a bedside commode.

   3 Although the use of a fracture pan takes less energy than using a regular bedpan, it takes more energy than using a commode.

182. 2 **A decreased urinary output reflects a decreased cardiac output; immediate action is indicated if urinary output decreases.**

   1 Although anxiety may occur, the priority is to monitor urinary output, which reflects cardiac effectiveness.

   3 Cardiac enzyme results do not reflect effectiveness of cardiac contractions; they reflect tissue damage.

   4 Although the presence of crackles (rales) will indicate pulmonary edema, it will not determine the effectiveness of ventricular contractions.

183. 3 **Troponin I (cTnI) and troponin T (cTnT) are proteins in the striated cells of cardiac tissue and are therefore unique markers for cardiac damage;** elevations occur within 1 hour of a myocardial infarction (MI) and persist for 7 to 15 days.

   1 Serum aspartate aminotransferase (AST) levels begin to increase in 4 to 6 hours, peak at approximately 24 hours, and remain elevated for 3 to 4 days after an MI.

   2 Myoglobin is the oxygen-binding protein of striated muscle; although it rises within the first few hours after an MI it lacks cardiac specificity.

   4 Creatine kinase (CK) isoenzyme levels, especially the MB subunit, begin to rise within 3 to 6 hours, peak in 12 to 18 hours, and are elevated for 48 hours after the occurrence of an MI.

184. 3 **The skin becomes cool and pale as blood shunts from the peripheral blood vessels to the vital organs.**

   1 The heart rate increases in an attempt to meet the oxygen demands of the body.

   2 Restlessness occurs because of cerebral hypoxia.

   4 The urine output drops to less than 30 mL/hr because of decreased arterial perfusion to the kidneys and the compensatory mechanism of reabsorbing fluid to increase the circulating blood volume.

185. 4 **A direct relationship exists between the strength of cardiac contractions and the electrical conductions through the myocardium.**

   1 The heart rate is related to factors such as SA node function, partial pressures of oxygen and carbon dioxide, and emotions.

   2 This is the period when the heart is at rest, not when it is contracting.

   3 Pulmonary pressure does not influence action potential; it becomes elevated in the presence of left ventricular failure.

186. 3 **At least one half of all deaths occur from the life-threatening dysrhythmia of ventricular tachycardia.**

   1 This can occur, but it can be treated aggressively with expectation of recovery.

   2 This can occur, but it can be treated.

   4 Failure of the left, not right, ventricle is more likely to occur.

187. **Answer: 2, 3, 4**

   1 Weight gain, not loss, occurs because of fluid retention.

   2 **Unusual fatigue is attributed to inadequate profusion of body tissues due to decreased cardiac output in response to cardiac ischemia; unusual fatigue is more commonly reported by women than men.**

   3 **Dependent edema occurs with right ventricular failure because of hypervolemia.**

   4 **Dyspnea at night, which usually requires the assumption of the orthopneic position, is a sign of left ventricular failure. Orthopnea, a compensatory mechanism, limits venous return, which**

decreases pulmonary congestion and promotes ventilation, easing the dyspnea.

    5 Urinary output decreases, not increases, with heart failure because the sympathetic nervous system and the renin-angiotensin-aldosterone system stimulate the retention of sodium and water in the kidneys.

188. 4 **A direct relationship exists between the systolic blood pressure and the force of left ventricular contraction.**
    1 An increased blood volume is indicated by hypertension, not a decreased pulse pressure.
    2 Hyperactivity of the heart is indicated by dysrhythmias and tachycardia.
    3 A decreased pulse pressure indicates decreased cardiac efficiency.

189. 4 **This is the mitral area at the fifth intercostal space at the left midclavicular line (also called apex of the heart); the S₁ heart sound (closure of the mitral and tricuspid valves, the "lub" in the "lub-dub" associated with heart sounds) is heard here. Mitral insufficiency produces a high-pitched blowing sound throughout systole.**
    1 This is the aortic area at the second intercostal space to the right of the sternum. This area best reflects closure of the semilunar valves (pulmonic valve between the right ventricle and pulmonary artery; aortic valve between the left ventricle and the aorta). Ejection clicks associated with aortic stenosis also are heard at this site.
    2 This is the pulmonic area at the second intercostal space to the left of the sternum; this area best reflects problems of the pulmonic valve such as pulmonic stenosis.
    3 This area is not part of the assessment of the heart; this is the area over the right main bronchus, which is used to assess bronchovesicular breath sounds.

190. 2 **This is the cardinal reason for PVCs.**
    1 This is a type of dysrhythmia, not the cause of PVCs; the source of atrial fibrillation is the atrium, not the ventricles.
    3 This type of dysrhythmia is associated with interference with the conduction system.
    4 This is a type of dysrhythmia, not the cause of PVCs.

191. 3 **This response provides information and reduces anxiety; the nurse understands that the greater saphenous vein of the leg is used to bypass the diseased coronary artery because one surgical team obtains the vein while another team performs the chest surgery; this shortens the surgical time and lessens the risks of surgery. The internal mammary arteries are the grafts of choice but the surgery is usually longer because of the necessity of dissecting the arteries from the chest wall. In addition, the internal mammary**

arteries may have been used in the previous bypass surgery.
    1 Cardiopulmonary bypass (extracorporeal circulation) is accomplished by placement of a cannula in the right atrium, vena cava, or femoral vein to withdraw blood from the body; blood is returned to the body via a cannula in the aorta or the femoral artery. Off-pump surgery is used for minimally invasive surgical techniques.
    2 This is not done during a coronary artery bypass graft (CABG).
    4 This is not done during a coronary artery bypass graft (CABG).

192. 4 **This addresses the client's request for information. The energy required for sexual intercourse is equivalent to that of climbing one flight of stairs.**
    1 Each client is different and may require more or less than 6 weeks.
    2 This avoids the client's question and cuts off communication. The nurse has a responsibility to teach.
    3 This answer is too vague and may be dangerous because the client has no basis to make a safe decision.

193. 1 **This type of pacemaker synchronizes impulses to the atria and ventricles to more closely simulate the normal action of the heart; it may be a fixed-rate or, most usually, a demand-mode pacemaker and may stimulate the atria, the ventricles, or both.**
    2 The physiological pacemaker stimulates both the atria and ventricles to contract.
    3 It will increase the heartbeat to a more normal rate.
    4 It affects the electrical conduction system of the heart, not the anatomical structures.

194. 3 **Assessment of the heart's rate and rhythm determines how the newly implanted pacemaker is functioning.**
    1 Unless the client is dehydrated, encouraging fluid will increase the workload of the heart.
    2 Although this is an appropriate action, the priority is to assess the functioning of the pacemaker.
    4 Although this is an appropriate action, the priority is to assess the functioning of the pacemaker.

195. 4 **This information will reduce anxiety. Milliamps are used, not volts of electricity; higher voltages are needed to electrocute.**
    1 This is a patronizing response and minimizes the stated concern.
    2 The voltage used in pacemakers can never cause electrocution; technology is not related.
    3 Although pacemakers are pretested for safety, this does not address the wife's concern about the possibility of electrocution.

196. 3 **Heart failure causes a fluid volume excess that results in pulmonary edema and dyspnea in the supine position.**
    1 This is unrelated to the cardiopulmonary system.
    2 This is unrelated to the cardiopulmonary system.

4 Dependent edema usually occurs after standing or walking; swelling of the ankles is more evident in the evening.

197. 4 **After the assessment protocol of airway, breathing, circulation (ABCs), the nurse should assess the client's breath sounds for crackles that may indicate the development of heart failure.**
1 Although this should be done, it is not the priority. Shoes that become too tight indicate pedal edema, which is a sign of fluid retention; 1 L of fluid weighs 2.2 pounds.
2 Eventually the practitioner will be notified, but the nurse should have more data for the practitioner.
3 With fluid retention the rate is not as significant as a bounding pulse.

198. 4 **Dyspnea on exertion occurs with heart failure because of the heart's inability to meet the oxygen needs of the body.**
1 This is not specific to heart failure.
2 This is not specific to heart failure.
3 This is not specific to heart failure.

199. 4 **With heart failure the veins distend, not collapse, because of congestion of the cardiopulmonary system.**
1 This is an expected adaptation in clients with heart failure.
2 This is an expected adaptation in clients with heart failure.
3 This is associated with clients who are decompensating or exhibiting early signs of cardiogenic shock.

200. 3 **As the heart fails, cardiac output decreases; eventually the decrease will reach a level that prevents tissues from receiving adequate oxygen and nutrients.**
1 Heart failure is related to an increased, not decreased, circulating blood volume.
2 The condition may be acute or chronic; the pulmonary pressure increases and capillary fluid is forced into the alveoli.
4 The blood pressure usually does not drop; the condition may be acute or chronic.

201. 2 **Left-sided heart failure causes fluid accumulation in the capillary network of the lungs; fluid eventually enters alveolar spaces and causes crackling sounds at the end of inspiration.**
1 This is not heard in chronic heart failure, but with tracheal constriction or obstruction.
3 These are not heard with chronic heart failure, but with asthma.
4 These are not heard with chronic heart failure, but with pleurisy.

202. 2 **Pulmonary congestion and edema occur because of fluid extravasation from the pulmonary capillary bed, resulting in difficult breathing.**
1 This is a hallmark of myocardial infarction; it is caused by inadequate oxygen supply to the myocardium.

3 This results from increased pressure in the right atrium associated with right ventricular failure, not left ventricular failure.
4 This is a sign of right, not left, ventricular failure; a weakened right ventricle causes venous congestion in the systemic circulation.

203. 2 **Rest decreases demand on the heart and will prevent fatigue.**
1 Sleeping with the head slightly elevated facilitates respiration.
3 The client needs potassium. A low-potassium diet when the client is taking digoxin predisposes the client to toxicity and dangerous dysrhythmias.
4 To avoid becoming obsessed with the pulse rate, the client should take the pulse less often; once daily is adequate.

204. 4 **Crackles are the sound of air passing through fluid in the alveolar spaces. With pulmonary edema, fluid moves from the intravascular compartment into the alveoli.**
1 With hypervolemia, the pulse is bounding.
2 The blood pressure is increased with hypervolemia.
3 This will occur with angina or a myocardial infarction.

205. 3 **A client's knowledge about the treatment program enhances compliance and reduces stress.**
1 This response does not answer the client's question and might produce frustration.
2 This response does answer the client's question, but does not explain specifically why.
4 This does not support the treatment regimen; the client needs education.

206. 3 **This is caused by hypervolemia and pulmonary hypertension.**
1 The pulse is likely to be rapid and bounding.
2 This is present in pleurisy, not heart failure.
4 Hypertension, not hypotension, will occur because of hypervolemia.

207. 2 **Stressful situations increase the body's oxygen demands.**
1 Clients with low cardiac reserve cannot tolerate extremes of temperature; a hot bath increases the body's oxygen demands.
3 Hot, humid weather is detrimental for those with heart disease; these individuals should use an air conditioner.
4 The heart of a client with low cardiac reserve cannot tolerate a pulse rate this high.

208. 2 **Symptoms of right ventricular heart failure relate to retention of fluid; neck veins become distended because of increased back pressure from the right atrium.**
1 Usually this is associated with left ventricular heart failure because of congestion in the lungs caused by back pressure from the left atrium, which is exaggerated when the client lies down at night.

3 This is associated with both left and right ventricular heart failure.

4 Arterial blood pressure increases because of compensatory mechanisms of the body.

209. 2 **This pulse rate increase indicates that activity tolerance is exceeded. Rest limits muscle contraction and oxygen demands; these allow the heart to return to its preactivity rate.**

1 Activity should be stopped, not continued.

3 Though descending the stairs requires less energy than climbing, rest is essential to permit the heart rate to return to normal.

4 This still constitutes activity, which increases the cardiac workload.

210. 2 **The highest incidence is in people 40 to 70 years of age; it is seen four times more frequently in men than women, with a higher incidence in black men. It occurs most often in older clients with hypertension.**

1 This client is not at as high a risk as a black male.

3 Unless the 40-year-old female is pregnant or in labor, she is not at as great a risk as a black male.

4 This client is not at as high a risk as a black male.

211. 3 **As the heart contracts, an expanding midline mass can be palpated to the left of the umbilicus.**

1 This is not definitive for abdominal aortic aneurysm.

2 There is no problem or pathology in the intestinal tract; this finding is associated with intestinal obstruction.

4 These are not definitive for abdominal aortic aneurysm; pallor occurs with shock.

212. 2 **Immediate surgical intervention to clamp the aorta is necessary for survival; the aneurysm has ruptured.**

1 This may eventually be done, but notifying the surgeon is the priority.

3 The client is already NPO.

4 Sedatives mask important signs and symptoms.

213. 4 **Flexing the hips and pressure against the popliteal space impedes venous return, increasing the risk for clot development.**

1 Although comfort and rest should be encouraged, placing pillows under the knees is contraindicated.

2 Although comfort and rest should be encouraged, placing pillows under the knees is contraindicated.

3 Pillows under the knees produce pressure, not warmth.

214. 4 **Ambulation is essential to promote venous return and prevent thrombus formation.**

1 This causes increased popliteal pressure and impairs venous return.

2 This causes increased popliteal pressure and impairs venous return.

3 This helps prevent atelectasis, not thrombi.

215. 3 **When legs are dependent, gravity and incompetent valves promote increased hydrostatic pressure in leg veins; fluid moves into interstitial spaces.**

1 This reflects inadequate arterial blood supply; arterial circulation is not affected by varicose veins.

2 This reflects inadequate arterial blood supply; arterial circulation is not affected by varicose veins.

4 This pain is referred to as Homans' sign and is associated with thrombophlebitis.

216. 1 **Impaired venous return causes increased pressure, with subjective symptoms of fatigue and heaviness of the legs.**

2 Intermittent claudication, a symptom of cellular hypoxia, is related to impaired arterial, rather than venous, circulation.

3 Homans' sign is indicative of thrombophlebitis.

4 Ecchymosis may occur in some individuals, but there is insufficient bleeding into tissue to cause hematomas.

217. 1 **This is the correct description of this surgery; after ligation, the saphenous vein is removed; however, sclerosing is the treatment of choice.**

2 Plaque is considered an arterial rather than a venous problem.

3 Superficial veins and deep veins are normally attached by communicating veins; surgery involves ligation to isolate the saphenous vein.

4 This prevents emboli from traveling to the lung; it is not a vein ligation and stripping.

218. 3 **Because of the client's history and the site of the surgery, thrombi are likely to develop; activity is a preventive measure.**

1 This alone will not prevent thrombi; activity is necessary.

2 Dangling and getting out of bed will provide little exercise if the client only sits on the bed or in a chair. Also, a practitioner's order is needed.

4 Although body alignment is important for all clients, it will not discourage thrombus formation.

219. 1 **The saphenous vein is ligated at its juncture with the femoral vein; injection sclerotherapy is used as the method of choice, but in chronic venous insufficiency and recurrent thrombophlebitis, surgery may be necessary.**

2 A bypass is unnecessary; the deep veins compensate for the removed saphenous vein.

3 Cholesterol plaques are characteristic of atherosclerosis, an arterial, not venous disease.

4 Communicating veins normally exist between the superficial and deep veins; they are ligated to prevent further engorgement and varicosities.

220. 1 **Seeing the exercises demonstrated will reinforce the verbal explanations.**

2 This statement is too vague; it does not explain how to move them.

3 This statement is too vague and thus may be ineffective; the time period should be stipulated.

4 This response is vague and open to interpretation; nonspecific instructions may be ineffective.

221. 2 **This position supports the leg and promotes venous return by gravity, which reduces edema and pain.**

1 The leg is still in a position that promotes edema.

3 The leg is still in a position that promotes edema.

4 Although this action elevates the foot, it provides no support under the leg and can cause hyperextension of the knee.

222. 3 **Raynaud's phenomenon has unilateral involvement, whereas Raynaud's disease has bilateral involvement.**

1 This indicates return of blood flow and is characteristic of both Raynaud's phenomenon and Raynaud's disease.

2 This indicates blood return and is characteristic of both Raynaud's phenomenon and Raynaud's disease.

4 This indicates lack of blood supply and is characteristic of both Raynaud's phenomenon and Raynaud's disease.

223. 3 **Nicotine causes spasms and constriction of the smooth muscles of the arterial vasculature, compromising blood flow to the distal extremities.**

1 Nicotine does not directly cause pain and tingling, although these may occur as consequences of nicotine-induced vasoconstriction.

2 Vasoconstriction from nicotine will not result in such severe effects.

4 Smoking increases the carboxyhemoglobin level in the blood; carbon monoxide combines with hemoglobin and occupies the sites on the hemoglobin molecule that bind with oxygen, thus decreasing oxygen content.

224. 3 **Nicotine causes vasoconstriction and spasm of the peripheral arteries.**

1 Alcohol may stimulate dilation of blood vessels.

2 Lowering the limb enhances flow of blood into the foot by gravity but does not support the return flow of blood.

4 This will decrease the viscosity of blood, possibly preventing the formation of thrombi.

225. 4 **Altered quantity and quality of pulses are the earliest indications of increasingly limited circulation.**

1 This prevents the use of gravity to carry arterial blood to the legs and feet.

2 This can release an embolus into the circulation and cause tissue trauma.

3 Altered sensation may limit sensitivity to heat, which can result in burns.

226. 4 **An exercise/rest program helps develop collateral circulation, which improves well-being and enables clients to increase their ability to walk longer distances.**

1 A cool environment favors constriction of peripheral blood vessels and further decreases arterial flow.

2 Crossing the legs increases local pressure, which tends to occlude blood vessels.

3 Elevation slows inflow of arterial blood, leading to further oxygen deprivation and pain.

227. 2 **The client's extremities are less sensitive to thermal stress because of peripheral vascular problems, and burns may occur.**

1 Applying heat to the abdomen causes reflex dilation of the arteries in the extremities and increases blood flow without untoward effects.

3 Raising the internal temperature by drinking warm fluid prevents vascular constriction and warms the extremities.

4 Increasing heat of the external environment is an effort to prevent cold, chilling, and further constriction of peripheral vasculature.

228. 3 **Intermittent claudication is the pain that occurs during exercise because of a lack of oxygen to muscles in the involved extremities.**

1 It is exercise, not the lack of exercise, that precipitates muscle weakness.

2 This is related to a venous problem, not an arterial problem.

4 This is related to a venous problem, not an arterial problem.

229. 2 **Decreasing the demand for oxygen by resting will relieve the pain.**

1 Pain will not resolve as long as exercise and, thus muscle hypoxia, is continued, regardless of whether aspirin (ASA) is taken.

3 This is appropriate for venous insufficiency, not arterial insufficiency.

4 Sublingual nitroglycerin is not indicated for leg cramps.

230. 1 **Gravity will assist the flow of blood to the dependent legs and feet.**

2 An extended knee gatch keeps extremities horizontal, not dependent, and does not facilitate blood flow to the feet.

3 Elevation impedes flow of arterial blood to the extremities; it facilitates venous return.

4 Elevation impedes flow of arterial blood to the extremities; it facilitates venous return.

231. 1 **Arterial ulcers are painful because of their depth and interruption of blood supply.**

2 This is characteristic of venous ulcers.

3 This is characteristic of venous ulcers.

4 This is characteristic of venous ulcers.

232. 4 **Pressure promotes coagulation and prevents the complication of bleeding.**

1 Bending the operative leg may cause decreased perfusion to the leg or bleeding at the catheter insertion site.

2 Elevation will resist gravity flow of arterial blood, reducing oxygen to distal tissue.

3 The client should remain in the supine position for 4 to 6 hours to prevent bleeding at the insertion site.

233. 3 **This indicates inadequate circulatory status of the left lower extremity.**
1 This may indicate impaired circulation, but observation of both extremities for comparison is necessary.
2 This is a less significant indication of arterial occlusive disease than the absence of a pulse.
4 This is not as significant as the pulse; this can occur because of inadequate circulation, aging, or fungal infection.

234. 2 **This reassures the client and allays fears of pain.**
1 The contrast medium used is not radioactive.
3 The femoral artery is used.
4 The client will be awake during the procedure.

235. 4 **The client is hypertensive, and the intra-arterial pressure is elevated; this increased pressure can cause the arterial suture line to rupture.**
1 This is unlikely because the blood pressure is elevated and the client is at risk for bleeding.
2 Hypervolemia is an assumption; other causes, such as arterial constriction, can precipitate hypertension.
3 Although this can occur, the priority for this client is protecting the graft.

236. 3 **Mobility will reduce venous stasis and edema as well as promote arterial perfusion and healing.**
1 Bed rest is contraindicated because it promotes the development of thrombophlebitis and pulmonary emboli.
2 This constricts circulation at the hips and knees.
4 This limits arterial perfusion.

237. 2 **Intermittent claudication is pain that results when the arterial system is unable to provide adequate blood flow to the tissues in the presence of increased demands for oxygen and nutrients during exercise; it is relieved by rest.**
1 Rest pain is not a response to exercise; it occurs in the extremities during rest, especially at night.
3 Phantom limb sensation is the presence of unusual sensations or pain in the residual limb after an amputation.
4 This phenomenon is intermittent episodes of constricted arteries and arterioles in response to extreme cold or emotional stress, causing pallor, paresthesias, and pain.

238. 4 **Presence of pulses and a normal skin color indicate adequate arterial perfusion and graft viability.**
1 This is contraindicated in peripheral vascular disease because it may traumatize vessels; it can cause a thrombus to become an embolus.
2 This is appropriate for venous, not arterial, problems.

3 The peripheral dilation produced by a hot bath will increase the workload on the heart, which is undesirable in a client with hypertension.

239. 3 **Inadequate oxygenation can cause premature ventricular complexes.**
1 Although this may be true, it does not explain why adequate oxygenation is important.
2 Hypoxia can precipitate respiratory acidosis; hyperventilation causes respiratory alkalosis.
4 The reverse is true; postoperative pain can increase the respiratory rate.

240. 3 **During open heart surgery the conductive system of the heart can be damaged because of trauma during surgery.**
1 Shock results in a weak, rapid pulse.
2 Hypoxia causes tachycardia.
4 Heart failure causes a rapid pulse rate.

ENDOCRINE

241. 4 **An aldosteronoma is an aldosterone-secreting adenoma of the adrenal cortex.**
1 An aldosteronoma is not a tumor of the kidney cortex.
2 An aldosteronoma is not a tumor of the thyroid gland.
3 An aldosteronoma is not a tumor of the pituitary gland.

242. 1 **Renal and cardiac complications will occur if hypertension is not arrested.**
2 An aldosteronoma is a benign tumor; metastasis is not possible.
3 Drugs are not used; the tumor must be removed.
4 This is not true; the tumor must be removed by surgical means.

243. 1 **Once the excessive secretion of aldosterone is stopped, the blood pressure gradually drops to a near normal level.**
2 The blood pressure drops gradually; it does not rise.
3 Blood pressure will fluctuate if the hypervolemia is overcorrected; this is not expected.
4 The blood pressure drops gradually in response to decreasing serum corticosteroid levels; a rapid drop immediately after surgery may indicate hemorrhage.

244. 2 **The body has two adrenal glands; an aldosteronoma is a unilateral tumor.**
1 The prognosis usually is excellent; this is unnecessarily alarming.
3 This is unnecessary; the prognosis usually is excellent.
4 Hormones are not necessary; there is another adrenal gland that will secrete an adequate amount of hormones.

245. 3 **This is a urinary metabolite of steroid hormones that are excreted in large amounts in hyperaldosteronism.**
1 With aldosterone hypersecretion, sodium is retained and potassium is excreted, resulting in hypernatremia and hypokalemia.

2 With Cushing's syndrome, the eosinophil count is decreased, not increased.

4 ACTH levels usually are high in Cushing's syndrome.

246. 3 Increased glucocorticoids cause sodium and water retention, hypertension, and fat deposition, resulting in a moon face.

1 These characteristics are associated with hyperthyroidism.

2 These characteristics are associated with hypothyroidism.

4 These characteristics are associated with hyperthyroidism.

247. 1 Stress and activity increase the secretion of ACTH and adrenocortical hormones, elevating the urine values for the byproducts of these hormones, thus invalidating the test results.

2 Clients with Addison's disease are chronically dehydrated and do not have edema.

3 Because of fluid deficits, the client will be hypovolemic and the blood pressure will be decreased.

4 Adequate fluid intake is necessary for urine production; Addison's disease involves salt wasting and dehydration, which necessitates an increased fluid intake, not a restriction of fluid intake.

248. 2 These tests provide a measure of thyroid hormone production; an increase is associated with the client's signs and symptoms.

1 Prothrombin time (PT) and partial thromboplastin time (PTT) assess blood coagulation.

3 The VDRL test is for syphilis; the CBC assesses the hematopoietic system.

4 Adrenocorticotropic hormone (ACTH) stimulates the synthesis and secretion of adrenal cortical hormones. Antidiuretic hormone (ADH) increases water reabsorption by the kidney. Corticotropin-releasing factor (CRF) triggers the release of ACTH.

249. 4 Many of these problems are associated with hyperthyroidism; palpitations may indicate cardiovascular changes requiring prompt intervention. The increased metabolism associated with hyperthyroidism can lead to heart failure.

1 Although an increased appetite becomes a compensatory mechanism for the increased metabolism associated with hyperthyroidism, it is not life threatening.

2 Although unexplained weight loss can result from catabolism associated with hyperthyroidism, it is not life threatening.

3 Although a feeling of warmth caused by the increased metabolism associated with hyperthyroidism is uncomfortable, it is not life threatening.

250. 1 Excessive metabolic activity associated with hyperthyroidism causes fatigue.

2 Warm, moist skin is expected because of increased peripheral perfusion associated with increased metabolism.

3 Increased appetite is expected because of the increased metabolism associated with hyperthyroidism.

4 Tachycardia is expected because of the increased metabolism associated with hyperthyroidism.

251. 4 Many radiopaque dyes contain iodine, which will alter the protein-bound iodine test results.

1 The tests ordered do not require this information.

2 This is not specifically related to these studies.

3 This is not specifically related to these studies.

252. 3 Weight loss and restlessness occur because of an increased basal metabolic rate; exophthalmos occurs because of peribulbar edema.

1 These are associated with hypothyroidism because of the decreased metabolic rate.

2 Lethargy and weight gain are associated with hypothyroidism as a result of a decreased metabolic rate; forgetfulness is not related.

4 Although weight loss and exophthalmos occur with hyperthyroidism, the client will be hyperactive, not hypoactive.

253. 1 Increased basal metabolic rate, increased circulation, and vasodilation result in warm, moist skin.

2 This problem is associated with hypothyroidism.

3 This problem is associated with hypothyroidism.

4 This problem is associated with hypothyroidism.

254. 4 The mask may irritate or scratch the eyes if the mask moves during sleep.

1 Blinking of the eyes will bathe the eyes and prevent corneal ulceration.

2 This will not relieve edema or prevent ulceration of the eyes.

3 Although this will help reduce periorbital edema, it will not prevent ulceration of the cornea.

255. 3 This relieves tension on the incision and limits the risk of dehiscence.

1 Coughing should be avoided during the early postoperative period to prevent trauma to the operative site.

2 This should be avoided until advised by the practitioner, usually after initial healing of the incision occurs.

4 Pressure against the operative area is not necessary to promote the integrity of the incision, and it may act to inhibit swallowing.

256. 2 These beverages contain caffeine, which may increase thyroid activity.

1 Hyperactivity is a physiological response; it is not under conscious control.

3 The increased metabolic rate associated with hyperthyroidism will make the client feel warm; a cool environment is needed.

4 Hyperactivity is a problem, and the client should be encouraged to rest.

257. 2 **A tracheostomy set should be available in the event there is excessive edema at the surgical site, which can cause tracheal compression.**
    1 This is not necessary after a thyroidectomy.
    3 The head should be kept in anatomical alignment, the neck not flexed or hyperextended; a small soft pillow can be used to accomplish alignment.
    4 Intermittent suction does not provide the constant suction needed to clear the airway.

258. 1 **The inflammatory response and trauma of surgery may cause edema; elevating the head facilitates drainage preventing compression of the trachea.**
    2 Although this is an important assessment for any postoperative client, it is not the priority for this client.
    3 Although deep breathing should be encouraged, coughing this early in the postoperative period is too traumatic to the operative site.
    4 Although this is an important assessment for any postoperative client, it is not the priority for this client.

259. 2 **If the laryngeal nerve is damaged during surgery, the client will be hoarse and have difficulty speaking.**
    1 This does not indicate injury to the laryngeal nerve; this is part of the assessment for a compromised airway.
    3 Eliciting the Chvostek sign assesses for hypocalcemia resulting from inadvertent removal of the parathyroid glands.
    4 This assesses for bleeding and possible hemorrhage, not laryngeal nerve injury.

260. 1 **Bleeding may occur, and blood will pool in the back of the neck because the blood will flow via gravity.**
    2 ROM exercises will increase pain and put tension on the suture line.
    3 Talking should be avoided in the immediate postoperative period except to assess for a change in pitch or tone, which may indicate laryngeal nerve damage.
    4 Activity should be gradually resumed, and frequent rest periods encouraged.

261. 3 **Maintaining airway patency is always the priority to permit gas exchange necessary to maintain life.**
    1 Although important, it does not exceed patency of the airway in priority.
    2 Although important, it does not exceed patency of the airway in priority.
    4 Although important, it does not exceed patency of the airway in priority.

262. 4 **These symptoms may indicate impending hypocalcemic tetany, a complication after removal of parathyroid tissue during a thyroidectomy.**
    1 These symptoms may be related to postoperative anxiety, but the priority is to assess for impending tetany.

    2 This is not helpful for the complaint made by the client; further assessment for tetany is indicated.
    3 Physical assessment and notification of the practitioner are the priorities.

263. 4 **Thyrotoxic crisis is severe hyperthyroidism; excessive amounts of thyroxine increase the metabolic rate, thereby raising the pulse and temperature.**
    1 During crisis there usually is no increase in the difference between the apical and the peripheral pulse rates (pulse deficit).
    2 The blood pressure will increase to meet the oxygen demand caused by the increased metabolic rate during crisis.
    3 Because of the increased metabolic rate, the pulse and respiratory rates increase to meet the body's oxygen needs.

264. 4 **Thyrotoxic crisis (thyroid storm) is the body's response to excessive circulating thyroid hormones.**
    1 A deficiency of iodine results in a deficiency in thyroid hormone production.
    2 A decreased serum calcium causes tetany.
    3 Sodium retention is unrelated to thyrotoxic crisis; thyrotoxic crisis is caused by excessive circulating thyroid hormones.

265. Answer: 1, 2, 4
    1 **Diaphoresis occurs with hyperthyroidism because of increased metabolism, resulting in hyperthermia.**
    2 **Weight loss occurs with hyperthyroidism because of increased metabolism.**
    3 Diarrhea occurs because of increased body processes, specifically increased gastrointestinal peristalsis.
    4 **Bulging eyes occur with hyperthyroidism and are thought to be related to an autoimmune response of the retro-orbital tissue, which causes the eyeballs to enlarge and push forward.**
    5 Heat intolerance occurs because of the increased metabolism associated with hyperthyroidism.

266. 1 **Dry, sparse hair and cold intolerance are characteristic responses to low serum thyroxine.**
    2 Muscle cramping is associated with hypocalcemia.
    3 Low thyroxine levels reduce the metabolic rate, resulting in fatigue, but do not increase the pulse rate.
    4 Low thyroxine levels reduce the metabolic rate, resulting in weight gain and bradycardia, not tachycardia.

267. 3 **After a subtotal thyroidectomy the thyroxine output may be inadequate to maintain an appropriate metabolic rate.**
    1 Hypothyroidism is a decrease in thyroid functioning, not a slowing of the entire body's functions.
    2 In hypothyroidism the level of thyroid-stimulating hormone (TSH) from the pituitary is usually increased.
    4 Atrophy of the remaining thyroid tissue does not occur.

268. Answer: 1, 2, 5

    1 This is a response to hypothyroidism that is related to the associated decreased metabolic rate.

    2 This is a symptom related to hypothyroidism that is associated with a decreased metabolic rate.

    3 This is related to hyperthyroidism, not hypothyroidism.

    4 This is related to hyperthyroidism, not hypothyroidism.

    5 This is a symptom reflective of hypothyroidism that is associated with a decreased metabolic rate.

269. 2 Excessive thirst (polydipsia), excessive hunger (polyphagia), and frequent urination (polyuria) are caused by the body's inability to metabolize glucose adequately.

    1 Although polydipsia and polyuria occur with type 1 diabetes, lethargy occurs because of a lack of metabolized glucose for energy.

    3 Although polydipsia and weight loss occur with type 1 diabetes, frequent urination occurs throughout a 24-hour period because glucose in the urine pulls fluid with it.

    4 Although polyphagia and polyuria occur with type 1 diabetes, diaphoresis occurs with severe hypoglycemia, not hyperglycemia.

270. 3 Protein and lipid catabolism occur because carbohydrates cannot be used by the cells; this results in weight loss and muscle wasting.

    1 Dehydration, not edema, is more likely to occur because of the polyuria associated with hyperglycemia.

    2 Polyphagia, not anorexia, occurs with diabetes as the client attempts to meet metabolic needs.

    4 Hyperglycemia, not hypoglycemia, is present in both type 1 and type 2 diabetes.

271. 2 The nurse must administer 109 grams of glucose. Solve the problem using ratio and proportion. 2.2 pounds equals 1 kilogram.

$$\frac{240}{2.2} = \frac{x}{1}$$
$$2.2\,x = 240$$
$$x = 109 \text{ grams}$$

    1 This is an incorrect calculation.

    3 This is an incorrect calculation.

    4 This is an incorrect calculation.

272. 2 This is the expected range for blood glucose.

    1 This range is indicative of hypoglycemia.

    3 This range is indicative of hyperglycemia.

    4 This range is indicative of hyperglycemia.

273. 4 The reason for the lack of ketonuria in type 2 diabetes is unknown. One theory is that extremely high hyperglycemia and hyperosmolarity levels block the formation of ketones, stimulating lipogenesis rather than lipolysis.

    1 This does not occur with type 2 diabetes.

    2 This is impossible; if glycosuria is present, there must first be a level of glucose in the blood exceeding the renal threshold of 160 to 180 mg/dL.

    3 This is expected in type 1 diabetes.

274. 1 Blood glucose testing is a more direct and accurate measure; urine testing provides an indirect measure that can be influenced by kidney function and the amount of time the urine is retained in the bladder.

    2 Whereas blood and urine testing is relatively simple, testing the blood involves additional knowledge.

    3 Both procedures can be done by the client.

    4 This is not a factor. Although some urine tests are influenced by drugs, there are methods to test urine to bypass this effect.

275. 4 Knowledge of the signs and treatment for hypoglycemia or hyperglycemia is critical to client health and well-being and essential for survival.

    1 Although this is important, it is not the priority.

    2 The client has type 2 diabetes, which usually is controlled by oral hypoglycemics.

    3 Self-serum glucose monitoring is more accurate than sugar and acetone (S&A) urine measurements to identify serum glucose levels.

276. 4 Controlling the diabetes decreases the risk of infection; this is the best prevention.

    1 If not completely absorbed, these may provide a warm, moist environment for bacterial growth.

    2 Coexisting neuropathy may result in injury from heat application.

    3 Protein, carbohydrates, and fats must be in an appropriate balance; high carbohydrate intake can provide too many calories.

277. 3 Insulin facilitates transport of glucose across the cell membrane to meet metabolic needs and prevent fatigue.

    1 With diabetes there is decreased cellular metabolism because of the decrease in glucose entering the cells.

    2 Glucose is not absorbed from the intestinal tract by the cells; fatigue is caused by decreased, not increased, cellular levels of glucose.

    4 Filtration and excretion of glucose by the kidneys do not regulate energy levels; if insulin production is adequate, glucose does not spill into the urine.

278. 3 Exercise increases the metabolic rate, and glucose is needed for cellular metabolism; therefore, excess glucose is consumed during exercise.

    1 Regular vigorous exercise increases cell sensitivity to insulin.

    2 Glucagon action raises blood glucose but does not affect cell uptake or utilization of glucose.

    4 Cellular requirements for glucose increase with exercise.

279. 4 Exercise improves glucose metabolism; with exercise there is a risk of developing hypoglycemia, not hyperglycemia.

    1 Exercise should not be decreased because it improves glucose metabolism.

2 An extra tablet will probably result in hypoglycemia because exercise alone improves glucose metabolism.

3 Control of glucose metabolism is achieved through a balance of diet, exercise, and pharmacologic therapy.

280. 4 **Physiological stress increases gluconeogenesis, requiring continued pharmacological therapy despite an inability to eat; fluids prevent dehydration; monitoring serum glucose levels permits early intervention if necessary.**

1 Skipping the oral hypoglycemic can precipitate hyperglycemia; serum glucose levels must be monitored.

2 Food intake should be attempted to prevent acidosis; oral hypoglycemics should be taken, and serum glucose levels should be monitored.

3 These are incomplete instructions; oral hypoglycemics should be taken, and serum glucose levels should be monitored; eating as much as possible can precipitate hyperglycemia.

281. 1 **In the overweight individual with type 2 diabetes, occasional alcohol can be ingested with caloric substitution for equivalent fat exchanges in the diet because it is metabolized like fat.**

2 Moderation is vital; these may not be used in unlimited quantities and they must be accounted for in the dietary calculations.

3 Alcohol can be used as long as it is accounted for in the diet.

4 This is untrue; regular foods can be used in the diet of individuals with diabetes.

282. 4 **According to an individual's needs, consistency and regularity in the food plan should be maintained; this is a basic principle of dietary management of diabetes.**

1 This is not necessary; the client can make selections from regular food choices.

2 This cannot always be done; it is unnecessary because choices can be made within the food plan

3 The client should follow the food plan.

283. 1 **These vegetables are in the vegetable exchange, as are asparagus, broccoli, and mushrooms.**

2 These are starchy vegetables and are listed as bread exchanges.

3 These are starchy vegetables and are listed as bread exchanges.

4 These foods are from the bread exchange list.

284. 3 **Inadequate foot care can lead to skin breakdown, poor healing, and subsequent infection.**

1 This can increase anxiety and reduce the client's ability to learn.

2 This is only one aspect of effective foot care; synthetic fibers that wick moisture are preferred.

4 Although important, this is not comprehensive foot care.

285. 4 **When the head of the pancreas is removed, the client has a greatly reduced number of insulin-producing cells and hyperglycemia will occur; immediate treatment is necessary.**

1 This is not immediately life threatening and will take time to develop.

2 This is not immediately life threatening and will take time to develop.

3 This is not immediately life threatening and will take time to develop.

286. 3 **The blood glucose level needs to be reduced; regular insulin begins to act in 30 to 60 minutes.**

1 The client has type 1, not type 2, diabetes, and an oral hypoglycemic will not be effective.

2 Blood glucose levels are far more accurate than urine glucose levels.

4 The rate may be increased because polyuria often accompanies hyperglycemia.

287. 4 **Emotional and physical stress may cause insulin requirements to remain elevated in the postoperative period.**

1 Insulin requirements will remain elevated rather than decrease.

2 Fluctuating insulin requirements are usually associated with noncompliance, not surgery.

3 A sharp increase in the client's insulin requirements may indicate sepsis, but this is not expected.

288. 1 **Incomplete oxidation of fat results in fatty acids that further break down to ketones.**

2 Protein metabolism results in nitrogenous waste production, causing elevated blood urea nitrogen (BUN).

3 Potassium is not oxidized. Ketones do not result when there are alterations in potassium levels.

4 Carbohydrates do not contain fatty acids that are broken down into ketones.

289. 2 **Potassium is the principal intracellular cation, and during ketoacidosis it moves out of cells into the extracellular compartment to replace potassium lost as a result of glucose-induced osmotic diuresis; overstimulation of the cardiac muscle results.**

1 P waves are abnormal because the PR interval may be prolonged and the P wave may be lost; however, the T wave is peaked, not depressed. The T wave is depressed in hypokalemia.

3 Initially, the QT segment is short, and as the potassium level rises, the QRS complex widens. The ST segment becomes depressed.

4 The PR interval is prolonged, and the P wave may be lost. QRS complexes and thus T waves become irregular, and the rate does not necessarily change.

290. 3 **This is a short-term goal, client oriented, necessary for the client to control the diabetes, and measurable when the client performs a return demonstration for the nurse.**

1 This is not a short-term goal.

2 This is measurable, but it is a long-term goal.

4 Although this is measurable and a short-term goal, it is not the one with the greatest priority when a client has an insulin pump that must be mastered before discharge.

291. 2 The basal infusion rate mimics the low rate of insulin secretion during fasting, and the bolus before meals mimics the high output after meals.

1 The subcutaneous needle may be left in place for as long as 3 days.

3 Most insulin pumps are external to the body and access the body via a subcutaneous needle.

4 Blood glucose monitoring is done a minimum of 4 times a day.

292. 4 Research demonstrates that socks with synthetic fibers wick away moisture better than other fabrics when participating in vigorous activities.

1 Self-removal of corns can result in injury to the feet.

2 Shoes that do not fit appropriately will create friction causing sores, blisters, and calluses.

3 The feet should be examined daily, not weekly.

293. 3 The dose of exogenous insulin causes a rapid drop in the blood glucose level, especially if food is not eaten.

1 This leads to hyperglycemia.

2 Stress usually contributes to hyperglycemia because of glycogenolysis and gluconeogenesis.

4 The use of insulin over long periods does not build tolerance to insulin or cause blood glucose levels to fluctuate dramatically.

294. 4 Lipodystrophy is a noninflammatory reaction causing localized atrophy or hypertrophy and a localized increase in collagen deposits.

1 Injections of insulin will not cause a horny growth such as a wart or callus.

2 An allergic response will precipitate a localized or systemic inflammatory response.

3 Hyperthermia and localized heat, erythema, and pain are associated with an infection.

295. Answer: 2, 3, 4

1 Vomiting occurs with hyperglycemia because of the effects of metabolic acidosis.

2 Headache is a neuroglycopenic response directly related to brain glucose deprivation.

3 Tachycardia occurs with hypoglycemia because of a neurogenic adrenergic response; it is a sympathetic nervous system response precipitated by a low blood glucose level.

4 Cool, clammy skin is a neurogenic cholinergic response; it is a sympathetic nervous system response precipitated by a low serum glucose level.

5 Increased respirations are a sign of hyperglycemia and are related to metabolic acidosis; this is a compensatory response in an attempt to blow off carbon dioxide and increase the pH level.

296. 1 These are classic signs of hypokalemia that occur when potassium levels are reduced as potassium reenters cells with glucose.

2 Symptoms of hypoglycemia are weakness, nervousness, tachycardia, diaphoresis, irritability, and pallor.

3 Symptoms of hypernatremia are thirst, orthostatic hypotension, dry mouth and mucous membranes, concentrated urine, tachycardia, irregular heartbeat, irritability, fatigue, lethargy, labored breathing, and muscle twitching and/or seizures.

4 Symptoms of hypercalcemia are lethargy, nausea, vomiting, paresthesias, and personality changes.

297. 2 The suggested treatment of hypoglycemia in a conscious client is a simple sugar (such as two packets of sugar), followed by a complex carbohydrate (such as a slice of bread), and finally a protein (such as milk); the simple sugar elevates the blood glucose level rapidly; the complex carbohydrates and protein produce a more sustained response.

1 These are fast-acting sugars, and neither of them will provide a sustained response.

3 The fat content of chocolate candy decreases the rate of absorption of glucose.

4 Neither of these is a fast-acting sugar; peanut butter crackers and milk can be used to maintain the glucose level after it is raised.

FLUIDS AND ELECTROLYTES

298. 2 235 mL is the correct calculation. The client's intake was 360 mL (6 oz x 30 mL = 360 mL) and the loss was 125 mL of fluid; 360 mL – 125 mL = 235 mL.

1. 125 mL is the amount of fluid output.

3. 360 mL is the amount of fluid intake.

4. 485 mL is the result when the intake is added to the output.

299. 4 An infusion of 1000 mL at 80 mL should take 12.5 hours. Because the primary infusion is interrupted for an hour while the antibiotic is infused, the primary bag will run an hour longer than if it were running uninterrupted.

1 This is an incorrect calculation.

2 This is an incorrect calculation.

3 This is an incorrect calculation.

300. 1 One liter of fluid weighs approximately 2.2 pounds; therefore, a 4.5 pound weight loss equals approximately 2 L.

2 This is approximately a 1 pound weight loss.

3 This is approximately a 2.2 pound weight loss.

4 This is approximately a 7.5 pound weight loss.

301. 1 With the client's history and the large weight gain, this is the most likely cause of the increase in weight.

2 This occurs in the bladder, not the tissues, and does not account for the large weight gain.

3 This can occur with heart failure, but it is not the primary etiological factor of the sudden weight gain.

4 Abdominal distention usually is caused by gas in the intestine and should not contribute to this large a weight gain. If the abdomen is enlarged, assessment by ballottement should be done to determine whether enlargement is caused by fluid in the peritoneal cavity (ascites).

302. 1 **Carbonated beverages generally are high in sodium and should be avoided.**

2 Steak sauce is high in sodium and should be avoided.

3 Many of these products contain sodium and should be avoided.

4 Artificial sweeteners do not contain sodium and do not have to be restricted.

303. 2 **Hypokalemia is suspected when the T wave on an ECG tracing is depressed or flattened; a serum potassium level less than 3.5 mEq/L indicates hypokalemia.**

1 This has no significance in diagnosing a potassium deficit.

3 This has no significance in diagnosing a potassium deficit.

4 This has no significance in diagnosing a potassium deficit.

304. 2 **This hypertonic solution should be administered in a continuous and uniform infusion to prevent hyperosmolar diuresis.**

1 This is true for any intravenous infusion; this is not unique to total parenteral nutrition. Also, infusion pumps can be placed on the bedside table.

3 The tubing set should be specific for the type of infusion pump.

4 Hemostats (clamps) are not necessary when administering total parenteral nutrition; an infusion pump should be used.

305. 2 **A continuous increase in serial weight determinations indicates a movement toward correction in the dehydration; 1 L of fluid weighs 2.2 pounds.**

1 The skin in older adults has less fluid and subcutaneous fat than younger adults, which results in a subjective and inaccurate assessment of rehydration.

3 In older adults there can be a 50% decrease in renal blood flow and tubular function; therefore, urinary output does not provide an accurate assessment of rehydration therapy.

4 The mucous membranes in older adults are drier than in younger adults because of the decrease in salivary secretions and therefore do not provide an accurate assessment of rehydration therapy.

306. 1 **A rate of 30 mL/hr is considered adequate for perfusion of the kidneys, heart, and brain.**

2 A central venous pressure reading of 2 cm H_2O indicates hypovolemia.

3 This indicates improvement but not necessarily adequate tissue perfusion.

4 This indicates improvement but not necessarily adequate tissue perfusion.

307. 4 **Unless diluted, the highly concentrated solution can cause vein irritation or occlusion.**

1 Although this is true, this is not the primary reason for a central line

2 Although this is true, the underlying reason is the large amount of blood in the subclavian vein and the superior vena cava, which dilutes the concentrated solution being administered.

3 This is not the primary reason, although the infusion at this site is more secure than a peripheral site and promotes free use of the arm.

308. 4 **Intravenous albumin increases colloid osmotic pressure, resulting in a pull of fluid from the interstitial and intracellular compartments to the intravascular compartment.**

1 The interstitial compartment is part of the extracellular compartment.

2 This is opposite to the actual shift of fluids when albumin is administered.

3 This is opposite to the actual shift of fluids when albumin is administered.

309. 1 **Osmosis is the movement of fluid from an area of lesser solute concentration to an area of greater solute concentration.**

2 Diffusion is the movement of particles across a semipermeable membrane from an area of greater concentration of particles to an area of lesser concentration of particles.

3 In active transport, molecules move against a concentration gradient; this differs from diffusion and osmosis because metabolic energy is expended.

4 Hydrostatic pressure, the pressure exerted within a closed system, is known as filtration force. Filtration is the passage of fluid through a material that prevents the passage of certain constituents; hydrostatic pressure moves fluid by pressure and concentration gradients.

310. 3 **Salt substitutes usually contain potassium, which can lead to hyperkalemia; dysrhythmias are associated with hyperkalemia.**

1 Sodium, not salt substitutes, in the diet causes retention of fluid.

2 Salt substitutes do not contain substances that influence BUN and creatinine levels; these are the result of protein metabolism.

4 There is no such substance in salt substitutes.

311. 2 **Intravenous fluids supply minimal calories; a client receiving only intravenous fluids will lose weight and become malnourished.**

1 This is not related to weight; lack of bulk in the diet results in constipation.

3 Vitamins are not related to weight loss.

4 Intracellular electrolytes are not related to weight loss.

312. **Answer: 1, 3**
  1 **Potassium is a component of the sodium-potassium pump that is essential for cellular functioning, especially muscle contraction; a deficiency of either potassium or sodium results in weakness.**
  2 Decreased functioning of respiratory muscles may result in respiratory acidosis.
  3 **Potassium is important for muscle contraction; the heart is a muscle and hypokalemia causes dysrhythmias.**
  4 A serum potassium level of 5.5 is within the upper range of normal.
  5 A low respiratory rate, not a rapid one, would be expected because of the weakened respiratory muscles.

313. 1 **Blood glucose that exceeds the renal threshold for glucose reabsorption in the kidney tubules (approximately 160 to 180 mg/dL) will cause cellular osmotic diuresis, resulting in dehydration.**
  2 This determines the presence of digested blood in the stool; it is unrelated to total parenteral nutrition.
  3 An altered specific gravity is nonspecific; increases can result from causes other than glycosuria.
  4 This assesses for increased or decreased peristalsis; it is unrelated to total parenteral nutrition.

314. 1 **The concentration of glucose in the solution (20% to 25%) is a rich culture medium for bacterial and fungal growth.**
  2 This is not associated with total parenteral nutrition.
  3 Anorexia is often present before the medical decision to begin total parenteral nutrition; it is not a complication.
  4 This is not directly related to total parenteral nutrition but rather to concomitant hypokalemia, which can occur if potassium is not added to the solution.

315. 3 **The stomach produces about 3 L of secretions per day. Fluid lost through vomiting can produce inadequate fluid volume and electrolyte imbalance, which can lead to dysrhythmias and death.**
  1 Although pain is associated with gastric ulcers and requires intervention, it is not life threatening as is an electrolyte imbalance.
  2 Although risk for injury is a concern, it is not the priority.
  4 Although respirations may be shallow when the client is experiencing pain, this is not the priority.

316. 3 **This has a low sodium content.**
  1 Shellfish are high in sodium.
  2 Processed meats are high in sodium.
  4 These vegetables are high in sodium.

317. 1 **This treats the hyperkalemia associated with kidney failure; it moves potassium from the intravascular compartment into the intracellular compartment.**
  2 This will not increase urinary output.
  3 This is not a treatment for respiratory acidosis.

4 Insulin and glucose do not decrease serum calcium levels.

318. **Answer: 2, 5**
  1 This is associated with aging and dehydration.
  2 **This is a classic sign of hyponatremia because of its effect on the cerebral cortex; additional symptoms are apprehension and irritability.**
  3 This is associated with hypovolemia.
  4 This is associated with shock and anemia.
  5 **Sodium is a component of the sodium-potassium pump, which is essential for the functioning of cells, especially in relation to muscle contraction. A deficiency in either sodium or potassium will result in weakness.**

319. 1 **Fluid and electrolyte replacement is a life-saving strategy; it must be done before surgery is performed.**
  2 This is not the priority at this time.
  3 The client is neither physically nor cognitively ready to learn the psychomotor skill of how to manage an ileostomy.
  4 The client is not demonstrating a readiness for contact with other persons with ileostomies at this time.

320. 2 **This ensures a well-controlled technique for electrolyte (chloride) replacement.**
  1 There is no assurance that adequate chloride will be ingested and absorbed via a low-residue diet.
  3 This is not a well-controlled method to correct electrolyte deficiencies.
  4 Total parenteral nutrition is not necessary at this point, although it may eventually be used.

321. 3 **The osmotic effect of hyperglycemia pulls fluid from the intracellular and interstitial compartments, resulting in dehydration.**
  1 Hyperglycemia pulls fluid from the interstitial to the intravascular compartment, eventually spilling into the urine.
  2 Interstitial fluid is part of the extracellular compartment; the osmotic pull of glucose exceeds other osmotic forces.
  4 An increase in hydrostatic pressure results in an intravascular to interstitial shift.

322. 1 **A low pH and bicarbonate reflect metabolic acidosis; a low P_{CO_2} indicates compensatory hyperventilation.**
  2 A low pH and elevated P_{CO_2} reflect hypoventilation and respiratory acidosis.
  3 An elevated pH and bicarbonate reflect metabolic alkalosis; an elevated P_{CO_2} indicates compensatory hypoventilation.
  4 An elevated pH and low P_{CO_2} reflect hyperventilation and respiratory alkalosis.

323. 2 **This will provide gradual replacement of both fluid and electrolytes without overloading the intravascular compartment.**
  1 Water does not supply the necessary electrolytes, and hyponatremia may result.

3 No data are present to indicate that the client cannot take fluids orally; an NG tube is not necessary when the client can take fluids by mouth.

4 Rapid correction of a fluid and electrolyte imbalance is dangerous; therapy should promote a gradual correction.

324. 1 **The kidneys retain potassium during the oliguric phase of kidney failure; an elevated potassium level is one of the main indicators of the need for dialysis.**

2 Hypercalcemia occurs.

3 Hyponatremia occurs.

4 Hyperproteinemia occurs.

325. 1 **Commercially prepared salt substitutes are high in potassium.**

2 Some complete protein foods must be included in the diet.

3 Seasoning that contains neither sodium nor potassium, such as lemon juice, pepper, and herbs, can be used to make food more palatable.

4 These contain high potassium concentrations.

326. 3 **A decreased urinary output will result in the retention of potassium, causing hyperkalemia.**

1 This is a sign of dehydration, which can be corrected with appropriate hydration.

2 These indicate dehydration, which is probably the rationale for the fluid ordered.

4 This can precipitate dehydration or aggravate an existing dehydration, which can be prevented by appropriate hydration.

327. 2 **Pyrexia increases fluid loss through the skin; to maintain balance, the body compensates by reducing urinary output.**

1 Blood pressure is not directly affected by antimicrobials.

3 This is unlikely; the client will have to become septic before this can occur.

4 This is a possible, but not probable, side effect of antimicrobial agents; also, nephrotoxicity will not be evident so soon.

328. 2 **All the values provided are within expected limits for an adult.**

1 The albumin is in the expected range for an adult.

3 There is no evidence of kidney failure; all the values provided are within expected limits for an adult.

4 The hematocrit is within the expected limits for an adult; with hemoconcentration the hematocrit is elevated.

329. 3 **Fluids during the first 48 hours are given to replace fluid lost from the intravascular compartment to interstitial spaces.**

1 Administration of fluids treats the fluid shifts, but does not prevent them.

2 Lactated Ringer's solution and 5% dextrose in saline are not plasma expanders, as is albumin.

4 Electrolytes are specifically replaced based on serial assessments of serum electrolytes and arterial blood gases.

330. 2 **In the first 8 hours 4200 mL should be infused. According to the Parkland (Baxter) formula, one half of the total daily amount of fluid should be administered in the first 8 hours. Because the client weighs 60 kg (132 pounds ÷ by 2.2 kg = 60 kg), the calculation is 60 kg x 4 mL/kg x 35% burns = 8400 mL per day; half of this amount should be infused within the first 8 hours.**

1 This is an incorrect calculation.

3 This is an incorrect calculation.

4 This is an incorrect calculation.

331. 3 **The pulse rate is one indicator of optimum vascular fluid volume; the pulse rate decreases as intravascular volume normalizes.**

1 This indicates hemoconcentration resulting from hypovolemia.

2 This indicates inadequate kidney perfusion; if adequate, output should be greater than 30 mL/hr.

4 This indicates hypovolemia.

332. 2 **Massive amounts of potassium are released from the injured cells into the extracellular fluid compartment; large amounts of sodium are lost in edema.**

1 Serum potassium will rise.

3 Serum potassium will rise and a serum sodium deficit will occur.

4 A serum sodium deficit will occur.

333. 1 **Silver nitrate can precipitate electrolyte imbalances; the client's potassium is below the expected range of 3.5 to 5.5 mEq/L and should be supplemented.**

2 The client's sodium level is within the expected range of 135 to 145 mEq/L; additional sodium chloride is not needed.

3 This will cause a further depletion of potassium.

4 This will cause a further depletion of potassium.

334. 1 **The blood urea nitrogen (BUN) is greater than the expected value of 5 to 20 mg/dL. Urea nitrogen is the major nitrogenous end product of protein and amino acid catabolism; azotemia is the accumulation of excessive nitrogenous compounds, such as creatinine, in the blood.**

2 The client has hyperkalemia; the expected value for potassium is 3.5 to 5.5 mEq/L.

3 Although the client does have a metabolic acid-base imbalance, it is acidosis, not alkalosis, because the pH is less than the expected range of 7.35 to 7.45.

4 The pH indicates acidosis, not alkalosis, because it is less than the expected pH of 7.35 to 7.45; the Po_2 is within the expected range of 80 to 100 mm Hg, which indicates that the problem is metabolic, not respiratory.

335. 2 **The client is hyperkalemic, and potassium intake should be limited; potassium is nonexistent in Jell-O.**

1 Milk should be avoided; one cup of milk contains 754 mg of potassium.

3 Orange juice should be avoided; one cup of orange juice contains 496 mg of potassium.

4 Tomato juice should be avoided; one cup of tomato juice contains 550 mg of potassium.

336. 3 **An orange contains only trace amounts of sodium.**

1 One cup of ice cream contains approximately 115 mg of sodium.

2 One cup of celery contains approximately 106 mg of sodium.

4 Four peanut butter cookies contain 142 mg of sodium.

337. Answer: 1, 5

1 **Fluid shifts from the intravascular compartment into the abdominal cavity, causing hypovolemia; a rapid, thready pulse compensates for this shift.**

2 This is not the priority.

3 After a paracentesis, intravascular fluid shifts into the abdominal cavity, not the lungs.

4 Fever is not a concern at this time. If the client were to develop an infection as a result of the procedure, a fever will occur several days after the procedure.

5 **Fluid shifts from the intravascular compartment into the abdominal cavity, causing hypovolemia; the decrease in blood pressure is evidence of hypovolemia.**

338. 2 **Hypervolemia may precipitate pulmonary edema, which produces shortness of breath, wheezing, cough, apprehension, and frothy sputum.**

1 Although this may occur, it is not the most serious complication; an altered respiratory status is the priority.

3 This occurs with the IV administration of dye for diagnostic procedures; it does not occur with IV fluids, such as 0.9% NaCl or D_5W without an additive.

4 Although this may occur, it is not the most serious complication; an altered respiratory status is the priority.

339. Answer: 4, 5

1 There are many factors other than dehydration that can cause dry cracked lips.

2 The eyeballs may be sunken, not protruding, in the presence of dehydration.

3 Although this question may be asked, it does not evaluate the client's physical status in relation to dehydration.

4 **To determine dehydration in the older adult the nurse should test for decreased skin turgor. To assess for dehydration, pinch the skin over a bone with little or no underlying fat, such as the sternum, forehead, or pelvis. If the skin remains tented after it is released, the client is dehydrated.**

5 **One liter of fluid weighs 2.2 pounds; serial weight comparisons will reflect an increase or decrease in body fluid.**

340. 2 **The client's ability to speak indicates that the client is breathing. Elevating the head of the**

bed facilitates breathing by decreasing pressure against the diaphragm. Checking the vital signs after this is the first step in assessing the cause of the distress.

1 Discontinuing the IV access line may cause unnecessary discomfort if it must be restarted; there are too few data to call the practitioner at this time.

3 There is not enough information to support this intervention; further assessment is required.

4 There is no information to support these interventions; assessment for allergies should be done on admission.

341. 1 **The imbalance in intake and output, with a decreasing urinary output, may indicate kidney failure. The retention of excess body fluid can precipitate the development of heart failure. Assessing breath sounds and obtaining the vital signs are necessary when monitoring for these complications.**

2 In the presence of hypervolemia, oral and intravenous fluid intake should be decreased.

3 There are no data to support a problem with excretion of urine; the problem is with insufficient production. The insertion of a urinary retention catheter requires a practitioner's order.

4 This is an appropriate assessment after respirations and vital signs are assessed.

342. 1 **This attempts to collect adequate data to plan the most appealing and appropriate diet.**

2 Low-sodium spices still contain salt and should be avoided when receiving a low-sodium diet.

3 This alone will not guarantee compliance once the client goes home; the client has the right to accept or reject therapy.

4 This alone will not guarantee compliance once the client goes home; the client has the right to accept or reject therapy.

343. 3 **Shallow respirations, bronchial tree obstruction, and atelectasis compromise gas exchange in the lungs; an elevated carbon dioxide level leads to acidosis.**

1 Metabolic acidosis is caused by a loss of bicarbonate from the lower gastrointestinal tract, which is associated with diarrhea.

2 Metabolic alkalosis is caused by excessive loss of hydrogen ions from gastric decompression or excessive vomiting.

4 Respiratory alkalosis is caused by increased expiration of carbon dioxide, a component of carbonic acid.

344. 1 **This 20 mL must be accounted for in the intake and output, either by including it as intake or by subtracting it from the total gastric drainage.**

2 High suction may lead to adherence of mucosa to the tube and potential injury.

3 This is unnecessary.

4 Return of 10 mL indicates patency; more frequent irrigations are not indicated.

345. Answer: 2, 3

1 Irritability, as a result of heightened neuromuscular activity, is a sign of hyperkalemia.

2 **Dysrhythmias are a sign of potassium depletion in cardiac muscle. Other cardiovascular effects include irregular, rapid, weak pulse; decreased blood pressure; flattened and inverted T waves; prominent U waves; depressed ST segments; peaked P waves; and prolonged QT intervals.**

3 **Muscle weakness is a symptom of potassium depletion in skeletal muscles; potassium facilitates the conduction of nerve impulses and muscle activity.**

4 Abdominal cramps, as a result of heightened neuromuscular activity, is a symptom of hyperkalemia.

5 Tingling of the fingertips, as a result of a lowered threshold of excitation of peripheral sensory nerve fibers, is a symptom of hypocalcemia.

346. 3 **All data are within expected limits; Po_2 is 80 to 100 mm Hg, Pco_2 is 35 to 45 mm Hg, and the pH is 7.35 to 7.45.**

1 None of the data are indicators of fluid balance, but of acid-base balance.

2 Oxygen is within expected limits of 80 to 100 mm Hg.

4 With metabolic acidosis the pH is less than 7.35.

347. 3 **The body fights acidosis by hydrogen exchange, which results in excretion of excess hydrogen in the urine, a compensatory mechanism to increase the serum pH level.**

1 With acidosis the pH level of the blood is decreased.

2 Plasma bicarbonates will be decreased with metabolic acidosis.

4 With acidosis the respiratory center in the medulla is stimulated to increase respirations and blow off carbon dioxide, which is carried to the lung as carbonic acid. Lowering carbonic acid increases the serum pH level.

348. 2 **The client is hyperventilating and blowing off excessive carbon dioxide, which leads to these adaptations; if uninterrupted this can result in respiratory alkalosis.**

1 Eupnea is normal, quiet breathing; the client has shallow, rapid breathing.

3 Kussmaul's respirations are deep, gasping respirations associated with diabetic acidosis and coma.

4 These adaptations are related to a decreased carbon dioxide level in the body.

349. 3 **Reassurance decreases anxiety and slows respirations; the bag is used so that exhaled carbon dioxide can be rebreathed to resolve respiratory alkalosis and return the client to acid-base balance.**

1 This is not necessary because there is no evidence of hypoxia.

2 This is used to prevent atelectasis.

4 The client is already alkalotic; bicarbonate ions will increase the problem.

350. 1 **Sodium, which helps regulate the extracellular fluid volume, is lost with vomiting. Chloride, which balances cations in the extracellular compartment, is also lost with vomiting. Because sodium and chloride are parallel electrolytes, hyponatremia will accompany hypochloremia.**

2 These values do not provide significant information in relation to the effects of vomiting.

3 These values do not provide significant information in relation to the effects of vomiting.

4 These values do not provide significant information in relation to the effects of vomiting.

351. 3 **The normal plasma pH value is 7.35 to 7.45; the client is in alkalosis. The normal plasma bicarbonate value is 23 to 25 mEq/L; the client has an excess of base bicarbonate, indicating a metabolic cause for the alkalosis.**

1 The normal plasma sodium value is 135 to 145 mEq/L; the client has hyponatremia.

2 The normal plasma chloride value is 95 to 105 mEq/L; the client has hypochloremia because of vomiting of gastric secretions.

4 With respiratory acidosis the pH is decreased to less than 7.35.

352. 1 **Potassium is plentiful in green leafy vegetables; broccoli provides 207 mg of potassium per half cup.**

2 Oatmeal provides 73 mg of potassium per half cup.

3 Rice provides 29 mg of potassium per half cup.

4 Cooked fresh carrots provide 172 mg of potassium per half cup; canned carrots provide only 93 mg of potassium per half cup.

353. 3 **Prolonged vomiting results in fluid loss; the client's adaptations reflect dehydration and metabolic alkalosis.**

1 Although it is important to address the client's pain, the fluid and electrolyte imbalance must be addressed first because this imbalance is life threatening.

2 Although this is a potential problem, the priority is the fluid and electrolyte problem.

4 The ineffective breathing pattern most likely is caused by the metabolic alkalosis; the fluid and electrolyte imbalance is life threatening and must be addressed first.

354. 4 **Hyperventilation results in the increased elimination of carbon dioxide from the blood.**

1 The Po_2 level is not affected.

2 The pH level will increase.

3 The carbonic acid level will decrease.

355. 2 **Decreased oxygen increases the conversion of pyruvic acid to lactic acid, resulting in metabolic acidosis.**

1 Hyperkalemia will occur because of renal shutdown; hypokalemia can occur in early shock.

3 Respiratory alkalosis can occur in early shock because of rapid, shallow breathing, but in late shock metabolic or respiratory acidosis occurs.

4 The Pco_2 level will increase in profound shock.

356. 3 **The expected range of venous pH is 7.31 to 7.41; any condition that decreases bicarbonate anion concentration in extracellular fluid results in metabolic acidosis.**
  1 This is not an accurate assessment for metabolic acidosis.
  2 This is not an accurate assessment for metabolic acidosis.
  4 This is within the expected range.

357. 3 **Kussmaul's breathing is an abnormally deep, very rapid, sighing type of respiratory pattern that develops as a compensatory response to metabolic acidosis and attempts to raise the pH of the blood by blowing off carbon dioxide.**
  1 Dyspnea is difficult breathing associated with subjective or objective distress in response to oxygen problems.
  2 Hyperpnea is a deep, rapid rate of breathing without a subjective sense of extra effort, usually as a response to strenuous effort.
  4 Cheyne-Stokes respirations are characterized by a waxing and waning of breathing that is usually associated with pathology of the respiratory center in the brain.

358. 3 **In respiratory alkalosis the pH level is elevated because of loss of hydrogen ions; the P_{CO_2} level is low because carbon dioxide is lost through hyperventilation.**
  1 This is partially compensated metabolic alkalosis.
  2 This is respiratory acidosis.
  4 This is metabolic acidosis with some compensation.

359. 3 **The pH of the blood indicates acidosis. CO_2 is the parameter for respiratory function; an acceptable level of arterial P_{CO_2} is 40.**
  1 HCO_3 is the parameter for metabolic functions.
  2 HCO_3 is the parameter for metabolic functions.
  4 A pH of 7.25 is acidic, indicating acidosis, not alkalosis.

360. 1 **Multiply 150 mL (amount to be infused in 1 hour) by 15 (drops per 1 mL delivered by the infusion set) and divide the product by 60 (minutes within 1 hour) = 37.5 mL. Round up to the nearest whole number, which is 38 mL.**
  2 The client will receive an inadequate amount.
  3 The client will receive an inadequate amount.
  4 The client will receive an excessive amount.

361. 3 **The client is in respiratory acidosis, probably caused by the depressant effects of an anesthetic or a compromised airway; deep breaths blow off CO_2 and encourage coughing.**
  1 This will not correct respiratory acidosis and may aggravate hypokalemia if present.
  2 This is the treatment for respiratory alkalosis; the client is in respiratory acidosis.
  4 This is not necessary if clearing of the airway corrects the problem.

362. 3 **Antidiuretic hormone (ADH) causes water retention, resulting in a decreased urine output and dilution of serum electrolytes.**
  1 Blood volume may increase, causing hypertension. Diluting the nitrogenous wastes in the blood decreases rather than increases the BUN.
  2 Water retention dilutes electrolytes. The client is overhydrated rather than underhydrated, so turgor is not poor.
  4 ADH acts on the nephron to cause water to be reabsorbed from the glomerular filtrate, leading to reduced urine volume. The specific gravity of urine is elevated as a result of increased concentration.

363. Answer: 1, 5
  1 **Edema results as fluid is retained because of the increased secretion of antidiuretic hormone.**
  2 A decreased urine output occurs with SIADH because ADH causes resorption of fluid in the kidney glomeruli.
  3 The increased fluid volume associated with SIADH results in tachycardia, tachypnea, and crackles.
  4 The increased fluid volume associated with SIADH results in hypertension, not hypotension.
  5 **Antidiuretic hormone (ADH) causes water retention, which dilutes serum electrolytes such as sodium with a resultant hyponatremia.**

364. 2 **The enlarged cirrhotic liver impinges on the portal system, causing increased hydrostatic pressure and resulting in ascites.**
  1 Bile salts are not responsible for fluid shifts; increased serum bile results from biliary obstruction, not increased secretion of bile.
  3 This pressure is unchanged; decreased intravascular osmotic pressure accounts for fluid movement into interstitial spaces.
  4 The liver's production of serum albumin is decreased with cirrhosis of the liver.

365. 4 **Albumin is an essential component of the bloodstream that helps maintain both osmotic pressure and fluid and electrolyte balance.**
  1 This is not a cause of hemorrhage. Blood components such as platelets, thrombin, and erythrocytes are involved in the prevention of hemorrhage or anemia.
  2 This is not directly involved with immunity and resistance. Blood components such as T and B lymphocytes are involved in this process; the liver synthesizes specific proteins intrinsic to the function of antibodies.
  3 The serum albumin level is not related to nutrition of cells.

366. 2 **An elevated serum albumin level increases the osmotic effect and pulls fluid back into the intravascular compartment, decreasing ascites and edema.**
  1 This therapy will increase blood volume and blood flow to the kidney, thereby increasing urinary output.

3 Albumin therapy has no effect on blood ammonia levels.

4 Albumin will not lower the blood ammonia level; an elevated blood ammonia level causes hepatic encephalopathy.

367. 2 **This is important in determining whether the aspirin has affected the balance of electrolytes.**

1 The blood glucose level is unrelated to an overdose of aspirin or cold tablets. A serum glucose will be done to confirm diabetic ketoacidosis if the client had diabetes mellitus.

3 Toxic hepatic effects of a drug overdose are not apparent so soon after ingestion of the drugs.

4 A test that requires 24 hours is not helpful in an emergency.

368. 3 **Different infusion sets deliver different preset numbers of drops per milliliter. Knowing this is a necessity for calculating the drip rate.**

1 This does not determine the drip rate.

2 This does not determine the drip rate.

4 This determines the size of the drop, not the drip rate.

369. 3 **Air in the secondary line will not enter the vein. Fluid from the primary bottle is under pressure and will flow before air from the secondary line reaches the port in the primary line.**

1 This is possibly true, but this answer may increase anxiety.

2 Cipro bypasses the large IV bag because it is piggybacked into the primary line below the drip chamber and check valve.

4 This is contraindicated because it stops the infusion, which can clog the lumen of the catheter that is inserted into the vein.

370. 1 **This position decreases pressure in the vena cava, which helps prevent an air embolus when the catheter is disconnected.**

2 Infusion of high concentrations of glucose will cause hypervolemia, not hypovolemia.

3 The infusion rate is changed only with a practitioner's order. Although insulin is contained in the parenteral nutrition formula, when blood glucose levels become elevated the practitioner may order insulin coverage.

4 No medications or solutions other than the parenteral nutrition should be administered through this line.

371. 1 **When blood glucose exceeds the renal threshold for glucose reabsorption in the kidney tubules, it acts as an osmotic diuretic resulting in polyuria.**

2 This is not associated with hyperglycemia.

3 With hyperglycemia there is hyperventilation.

4 This level is within the expected range.

GASTROINTESTINAL

372. 3 **Auscultation must be performed before palpation and percussion because they may influence intestinal peristalsis resulting in inaccurate**

results. Palpation is performed before percussion because percussion will have a greater impact on peristalsis.

1 Percussion or palpation performed before auscultation may result in an inaccurate assessment of bowel sounds.

2 Percussion or palpation performed before auscultation may result in an inaccurate assessment of bowel sounds.

4 Although auscultation is performed before percussion or palpation, palpation should precede percussion when assessing the abdomen.

373. 2 **The stomach is located within the sternal angle, known as the epigastric area.**

1 This is in the area of the iliac bones.

3 This is the lowest middle abdominal area.

4 This is the area above the sternum.

374. 3 **Eating a light meal and eliminating food and fluids after midnight limit complications during and after surgery, which include aspiration, nausea, dehydration, and possible ileus.**

1 A large meal the evening before surgery may not clear before peristalsis is slowed by anesthesia, resulting in abdominal distention and discomfort after surgery.

2 Clear liquids in the morning can cause nausea, vomiting, and aspiration.

4 Fluids should not be withheld for more than 8 hours, to prevent dehydration. Not eating or drinking anything after lunch is an excessive amount of time to restrict food and fluids before surgery the next morning.

375. 4 **Barium will harden and may create an impaction; a laxative and increased fluids promote elimination of barium.**

1 The client must be kept NPO.

2 Iodine is not used with barium.

3 This is not part of the preparation; feces in the lower GI tract will not interfere with visualization of the upper GI tract.

376. 2 **Carbohydrates provide 4 kcal/g; therefore, 3 L × 50 g/L × 4 kcal/g = 600 kcal, only about a third of the basal energy need.**

1 This is less than the kilocalories provided by the ordered IV fluid.

3 This is more than the kilocalories provided by the ordered IV fluid.

4 This is more than the kilocalories provided by the ordered IV fluid.

377. 3 **This diet progresses from the one that makes the least metabolic demand on the client (clear liquid) to a regular diet that requires the capability of unimpaired digestion.**

1 The caloric content is not the focus in a progressive postsurgical diet.

2 Initially a progressive diet has little nutritional value; the focus is to rest the gastrointestinal tract immediately after surgery.

4 Initially a limited variety of fluids is presented to rest the gastrointestinal tract; food is not included until later.

378. 2 **This diet contains approximately 1970 calories. There are 9 calories in each gram of fat and 4 calories in each gram of carbohydrate and protein.**
    1 This is an incorrect calculation; this is too few calories.
    3 This is an incorrect calculation; this is too many calories.
    4 This is an incorrect calculation; this is too many calories.

379. 2 **This serum albumin value indicates severe depletion of visceral protein stores; the expected range for serum albumin is 3.5 to 5.5 g/dL; white meat turkey (two slices 4 x 2 x ¼ inch) contains approximately 28 grams of protein.**
    1 A 6-ounce serving of mixed fruit contains approximately 0.5 gram of protein.
    3 A 3-ounce serving of spinach salad contains approximately 9 grams of protein.
    4 A 4-ounce serving of beef broth contains approximately 2.4 grams of protein.

380. 1 **The increased osmotic effect of therapy increases the intravascular volume and urinary output; weight loss reflects fluid loss.**
    2 The vital signs will not change drastically; "frequently" is a nonspecific time frame.
    3 The urinary output is measured hourly; half-hour outputs are insignificant in this instance.
    4 A serum, not urine, albumin level is significant; albumin in the urine indicates kidney dysfunction, not liver dysfunction.

381. 3 **The RDA requirement of vitamin C for an adult male is 90 mg; smoking accelerates oxidation of tissue vitamin C, so smokers need an additional 35 mg/day.**
    1 Niacin is not oxidized more rapidly in the smoker.
    2 Thiamine is not oxidized more rapidly in the smoker.
    4 Vitamin B_{12} is not oxidized more rapidly in the smoker.

382. 1 **Tofu products increase protein without increasing vitamin D because, unlike milk products, tofu does not contain vitamin D.**
    2 Eggnog contains milk, which has vitamin D, and should be avoided.
    3 This contains vitamin D and should be avoided.
    4 This contains milk, which has vitamin D, and should be avoided.

383. Answer: 2, 3, 5
    1 An entire head of lettuce contains 13 mg of vitamin C.
    2 **One cup of fresh orange sections contains 96 mg of vitamin C.**
    3 **Vitamin C (ascorbic acid), an antioxidant, is found in vegetables such as broccoli, tomatoes, and potatoes; 1 cup of broccoli contains 140 mg of vitamin C.**

    4 Apricots contain 11 mg of vitamin C; they are a source of beta-carotene.
    5 **A cup of strawberries contains 106 mg of vitamin C.**

384. 1 **The antioxidants vitamin E and beta-carotene, which help inhibit oxidation and therefore tissue breakdown, are found in these foods.**
    2 These are excellent sources of vitamin E, not beta-carotene.
    3 These are excellent sources of vitamin C, not vitamin E and beta-carotene.
    4 These are excellent sources of beta-carotene, not vitamin E.

385. 3 **Stress ulcers are asymptomatic until they produce massive hematemesis and rectal bleeding.**
    1 Shock is the outcome of massive hemorrhage; it is not unexplained because the sudden gastrointestinal bleeding will be identified.
    2 Sudden massive bleeding occurs, not the slow oozing that causes melena.
    4 A gradual drop in the hematocrit value indicates slow blood loss.

386. 3 **Green vegetables contain fiber, which promotes defecation.**
    1 These have a constipating effect, which results in straining at stool.
    2 These have a constipating effect, which results in straining at stool.
    4 These have a constipating effect, which results in straining at stool.

387. 4 **This produces bulk, which stimulates defecation; the muscles used in defecation are weak in clients with Parkinson's disease.**
    1 Bananas are binding and will intensify the problem of constipation.
    2 This will intensify the problem; fluids need to be increased.
    3 Cathartics are irritating to the intestinal mucosa, and their regular administration promotes dependence.

388. 1 **Red meat can react with reagents used in the test to cause false-positive results.**
    2 This may apply for testing for ova and parasites, not for occult blood.
    3 If the correct procedure is followed, discarding the first specimen is unnecessary.
    4 Random stool testing can be done but must be on three different bowel movements during the screening period.

389. 3 **These characteristics describe steatorrhea, which results from impaired fat digestion.**
    1 This is descriptive of stools resulting from constipation.
    2 This is descriptive of acholic stools occurring with biliary obstruction resulting from an absence of urobilin.
    4 This is descriptive of upper and lower gastrointestinal bleeding.

390. 1 **Although the central venous catheter remains in situ, total parenteral nutrition does not have to infuse continuously. Continuous versus intermittent administration depends on the practitioner's order.**
    2 Placement of the tube after the procedure is verified by x-ray, not fluoroscopy.
    3 The subclavian veins are used most often; the jugular vein is too close to hair-growing areas, which increases the possibility of sepsis, and neck movements may interfere with maintaining placement of the catheter.
    4 Although a feeling of pressure may be experienced, it is not a painful procedure.

391. 4 **This is essential because the solution is hyperosmolar, and a concentrated source of glucose can result in hyperglycemia.**
    1 Although important, it is not the priority.
    2 Although important, it is not the priority.
    3 Although important, it is not the priority.

392. 4 **The less disruptive the procedure, the greater the acceptance by the client.**
    1 Most often, total parenteral nutrition is set up to run daily during sleeping hours.
    2 Depending on the type of circulatory access used, it may not need to be changed for weeks.
    3 The client or a significant other can be taught the principles of administration.

393. 1 **The mucosa of the mouth and the vomiting center in the brainstem may be affected, producing nausea and vomiting.**
    2 These are not side effects of radiation therapy to the oral cavity.
    3 These are not side effects of radiation therapy to the oral cavity.
    4 These are not expected responses because of the distance between the radon seeds and the intestines.

394. 3 **Gentle sprays are effective in cleaning the mouth and teeth without disturbing the sensitive tissues or radon seeds.**
    1 This can dislodge the radon seeds and be traumatic to the compromised oral mucosa.
    2 An antiseptic mouthwash is an astringent that is too harsh for the sensitive oral mucosa.
    4 This can dislodge the radon seeds and be traumatic to the compromised oral mucosa.

395. 4 **Shredded Wheat contains 5.5 grams of fiber per serving, which is more than the other choices.**
    1 Froot Loops contain 0.8 gram of fiber per serving.
    2 Corn Flakes contain 0.7 gram of fiber per serving.
    3 Cap'n Crunch contains 0.7 gram of fiber per serving.

396. 3 **Complementary mixtures of essential amino acids in plant proteins provide complete dietary protein equivalents.**
    1 A vegan does not consume flesh, milk, milk products, or eggs.

2 A vegan does not consume flesh, milk, milk products, or eggs.
    4 A vegan does not consume flesh, milk, milk products, or eggs.

397. 4 **Exercise builds skeletal muscle mass and reduces excess fatty tissue.**
    1 Appetite may increase with exercise.
    2 The metabolic rate will increase with exercise.
    3 During aerobic exercise the heart rate will increase, but between periods of exercise the heart rate will decrease because of the development of collateral circulation.

398. 1 **The most effective and safest method for achieving weight loss is to decrease caloric intake. This is best accomplished by maintaining a balance of nutrients while decreasing portion size and fat intake. A gram of fat is 9 calories, whereas a gram of protein and a gram of carbohydrate are each 4 calories.**
    2 Increasing protein intake can increase fat intake because animal protein also contains fat.
    3 Although decreasing carbohydrate and fat intake will promote weight loss, the diet may result in an imbalance of nutrients, which may jeopardize the client's health.
    4 Fruits are important in any diet, and if a balance of nutrients is to be maintained, fruit intake may need to be increased or decreased depending on the client's eating habits; water intake should not be limited in a weight loss diet; 6 to 8 glasses a day is recommended to enhance weight loss.

399. 2 **The salmonella organism thrives in warm, moist environments; washing, cooking, and refrigeration of food limits the growth of or eliminates the organism.**
    1 Salmonellosis is unrelated to cancer.
    3 Salmonellosis is caused by the salmonella organism, not stress.
    4 The salmonella organism is ingested; it is not an airborne or bloodborne infection.

400. 3 **Fluids of dextrose and normal saline and electrolytes are administered to prevent profound dehydration caused by an excessive loss of water and electrolytes through diarrheal output.**
    1 These are not used when there is a possibility of bacterial infection because slowed peristalsis decreases excretion of the salmonella organism.
    2 Salmonellosis is an infection, not a condition caused by hyperacidity.
    4 These are not used when there is a possibility of bacterial infection because slowed peristalsis decreases excretion of the salmonella organism.

401. 1 **A cold environment limits growth of microorganisms.**
    2 All food should be refrigerated before and after it is cooked to limit the growth of microorganisms.

3 This promotes the growth of microorganisms because the stuffing will still be warm for a period before the refrigerator's cold environment cools the center of the bird. It is advocated that poultry not be stuffed. If it is stuffed, it should be done immediately before cooking.

4 This promotes the growth of microorganisms because microorganisms thrive in warm, moist environments.

402. 4 **Gravity facilitates digestion and prevents reflux of stomach contents into the esophagus.**

1 Water should not be taken with or immediately after meals because it overdistends the stomach.

2 Exercise immediately after eating may prolong the digestive process.

3 Lying down immediately after eating facilitates reflux of the stomach contents into the esophagus.

403. 3 **Based on the presented data, improving nutritional status is the priority at this time. The decreased hemoglobin and hematocrit levels and RBC count may be a result of malnutrition; also cancer of the esophagus can cause dysphagia and anorexia.**

1 Although maintaining the client's safety is a goal, it is not as high a priority as another concern based on the data provided in the question.

2 Data given do not relate to the presence of pain.

4 Data given do not relate to airway obstruction.

404. 2 **Because of the trauma of surgery and the proximity of the esophagus to the trachea, respiratory assessments become the priority.**

1 Although this is important, an adequate airway is the priority.

3 Although this is important, an adequate airway is the priority.

4 Although this is important, an adequate airway is the priority.

405. 1 **An increased heart rate is related to an autonomic nervous system response; pain is related to the trauma of the perforation and possibly gastric reflux.**

2 These are signs of dumping syndrome.

3 These are signs of dumping syndrome.

4 An increased blood pressure may occur, but an increased urinary output has no relationship to esophageal perforation.

406. Answer: 1, 2

1 **Muscle weakness consistent with the aging process is associated with the development of a hiatal hernia.**

2 **Obesity causes stress on the diaphragmatic musculature, which weakens and allows the stomach to protrude into the thoracic cavity.**

3 Inflammation of the bronchi will not weaken the diaphragm.

4 Alcoholism may cause an enlarged liver or pancreatitis but not a hiatal hernia.

5 Esophagitis does not cause a hiatal hernia.

407. 2 **Apple juice is not irritating to the gastric mucosa.**

1 Carbonated beverages distend the stomach and promote regurgitation.

3 The acidity of orange juice aggravates the disorder.

4 Most colas should be avoided because they contain caffeine, which causes increased acidity and aggravates the disorder; also they are carbonated, which distends the stomach and promotes regurgitation.

408. 3 **Weight reduction decreases intra-abdominal pressure, thereby decreasing the tendency to reflux into the esophagus.**

1 Fats decrease emptying of the stomach, extending the period that reflux can occur; fats should be decreased.

2 This increases the pressure against the diaphragmatic hernia, increasing symptoms.

4 This will increase pressure; fluid should be discouraged with meals.

409. 3 **Black (tarry) stools indicate upper GI bleeding; digestive enzymes act on the blood resulting in tarry stools. Hemorrhage can occur if erosion extends to blood vessels.**

1 Investigation of bleeding takes priority; later the nurse should help to identify irritating foods that are to be avoided.

2 Nausea is a common symptom of gastritis, but is not life threatening.

4 Attempts to control alcoholism should be supported but this is a long-term goal; assessment of bleeding takes priority.

410. 1 **Classic symptoms of peptic ulcer include gnawing, boring, or dull pain located in the midepigastrium or back; pain is caused by irritability and erosion of the mucosal lining.**

2 This type of pain is more characteristic of cholecystitis.

3 This type of pain is more characteristic of the complication of a perforated ulcer.

4 This type of pain is more characteristic of a hiatal hernia.

411. 2 **Pain occurs after the stomach empties with a gastric peptic ulcer; ingesting food stimulates gastric secretions, which later act on the gastric mucosa of the empty stomach, causing the gnawing pain.**

1 Vomiting temporarily alleviates pain because acid secretions are eliminated from the body.

3 There is no intolerance of fats; eating generally alleviates gastric peptic pain.

4 Gastric pain is sharply localized in the epigastrium; it can radiate across the abdomen if a gastric peptic ulcer perforates.

412. 4 **Abdominal distention, which may be associated with pain, can indicate perforation, a complication that can lead to peritonitis.**

1 A local inflammatory response to insertion of the fiberoptic tube may result in a sore throat and dysphagia once the anesthesia wears off; this is expected.

2 This, together with cramping, is an expected response.

3 This is not indicative of any particular problem in this situation.

413. 3 **Some medications, such as aspirin, NSAIDs, and prednisone, irritate the stomach lining and may cause bleeding with prolonged use.**

1 Travel to foreign countries may be related to intestinal irritation, causing diarrhea and intestinal bleeding, not gastric bleeding.

2 This is not the cause of gastric bleeding; it is important to ascertain dietary habits when teaching about diet therapy.

4 Although stress may play a part, the use of some medications has a more direct relationship.

414. 2 **These are classic indicators of a perforated ulcer, for which immediate surgery is indicated; this should be anticipated.**

1 Although oxygen may minimize the tachycardia and tachypnea that are related to pain and possible blood loss, keeping the client NPO is the priority.

3 Keeping the client NPO in preparation for surgery is more important than asking about the presence of black, tarry stools or red stools. Although this question should be asked, knowing this information will not change the medical or nursing care of the client at this time.

4 The adaptations are indicative of perforation and the priority is to prepare the client for surgery.

415. 1 **After gastric surgery a nasogastric tube is in place for drainage of blood and gastric secretions.**

2 Oxygen is not required unless the client experiences a complication necessitating its administration.

3 The average client is given about 3500 mL of fluid by IV to meet fluid needs and replace gastric losses.

4 This may or may not be necessary.

416. 1 **Statistics demonstrate that these are the most likely sites for metastasis of this tumor.**

2 It is less likely that the tumor will spread to these areas.

3 It is less likely that the tumor will spread to these areas.

4 These are routes of metastasis.

417. 2 **Large amounts of blood or excessive bloody drainage 12 hours postoperatively must be reported immediately because the client is hemorrhaging.**

1 Clamping the tube is contraindicated; accumulation of secretions causes pressure on the suture line, preventing further observation of drainage.

3 This must be ordered by the practitioner; 50 to 100 mL of normal saline at room temperature instilled every 30 to 50 minutes is the usual therapy to prevent lowering the core body temperature.

4 This is an unsafe intervention at this time; the surgeon should be notified.

418. 4 **Removal of the fundus of the stomach destroys the parietal cells that secrete intrinsic factor (needed**

to combine with vitamin B_{12} preliminary to its absorption in the ileum).

1 Hemorrhaging may cause anemia; however, pernicious anemia occurs when the intrinsic factor is not produced.

2 The beta cells of the pancreas are not involved in secretion of intrinsic factor.

3 Dietary intake does not affect the production of intrinsic factor.

419. 1 **Intrinsic factor is lost with removal of the stomach, and vitamin B_{12} is needed to maintain the hemoglobin level once the client is stabilized; injections are given monthly for life.**

2 Adequate diet, fluid intake, and exercise should prevent constipation.

3 This is not a routine expectation.

4 This surgery does not affect pancreatic enzymes.

420. 4 **This cancer is usually asymptomatic in the early stages; the stomach accommodates the mass.**

1 Gastric cancer is painless in its early stages.

2 It can be accurately diagnosed by gastric washings or biopsy.

3 This is typical of Hodgkin's disease, not gastric carcinoma.

421. 1 **The thoracic cavity usually is entered for a complete resection, necessitating a chest tube.**

2 Fluids are contraindicated until the suture line has healed and nasogastric suction is no longer being used.

3 The client should ambulate early to minimize the hazards of immobility.

4 There is no physiological necessity for this position.

422. Answer: 2, 3

1 Fluids should be taken between meals to decrease the volume within the stomach at one time.

2 **Small, frequent meals keep the volume within the stomach to a minimum at any one time, limiting dumping syndrome. Dumping syndrome occurs after eating because of the rapid movement of food into the jejunum without the usual digestive mixing in the stomach and processing in the duodenum.**

3 **Lying down delays emptying of the stomach contents, which will limit dumping syndrome.**

4 Chewing a set number of times before swallowing is not pertinent to solving this problem.

5 A low-carbohydrate, high-protein, high-fat diet and avoidance of fluids with meals help delay stomach emptying, minimizing this problem.

423. 2 **As a result of the trauma of surgery, some bleeding can be expected for 4 to 5 hours.**

1 Clamping the tube will cause increased pressure on the gastric sutures from a buildup of gas and fluid.

3 Iced saline rarely is used because it causes vasoconstriction, local ischemia, and a reduction in body temperature.

4 This is not necessary; this is an expected occurrence.

424. 2 **Rigidity and pain are hallmarks of bleeding from the suture line and/or of peritonitis; vital signs provide supporting data.**
 1 Ambulation is indicated if the pain is the result of flatulence; however, rigidity is clearly associated with bleeding or peritonitis and more data are needed.
 3 An analgesic may mask the symptoms, delaying diagnosis.
 4 This is unrelated to the adaptations presented.

425. 1 **Bowel sounds and flatulence indicate the return of intestinal peristalsis; peristalsis is necessary for movement of nutrients through the GI tract.**
 2 Incisional pain is unrelated to intestinal peristalsis.
 3 Hematocrit levels indicate blood loss; they are unaffected by GI functioning.
 4 Dumping syndrome occurs after, not before, the ingestion of food and does not indicate readiness to ingest food.

426. 4 **Over-the-counter antacid preparations neutralize gastric acid and relieve pain.**
 1 Although eating food initially prevents gastric acid from irritating the gastric walls, it can precipitate acid production.
 2 Aspirin is contraindicated because it irritates gastric mucosa and promotes bleeding by preventing platelet aggregation.
 3 Reduction of fluids with meals does not affect pain; it helps prevent dumping syndrome.

427. 1 **Treatment with medications, rest, diet, and stress reduction relieves symptoms, heals the ulcer, and prevents complications and recurrence.**
 2 Pain occurs 30 minutes to 1 hour after a meal.
 3 Surgery may be done after multiple recurrences and for treating complications.
 4 Perforation, pyloric obstruction, and hemorrhage, not cancer, are major complications.

428. 4 **Dark brown or black stools (melena) indicate gastrointestinal bleeding.**
 1 Frothy stools are indicative of inadequate fat absorption and are associated with sprue.
 2 Ribbon-shaped stools indicate a bowel mass or obstruction.
 3 Clay-colored stools usually are related to problems that cause a decrease in bile.

429. 1 **With a nasogastric tube for decompression in place, nausea may indicate tube displacement or obstruction. Checking placement can determine whether it is in the stomach; once placement is verified, then fluid can be instilled to ensure patency.**
 2 The antiemetic may relieve the discomfort, but will not determine the cause.
 3 If the tube is displaced it may be in the trachea or bronchi and instillation of fluid will cause respiratory impairment before placement is confirmed.

 4 The nurse should always assess a situation carefully before notifying the practitioner.

430. 1 **Abdominal distention, nausea, and abdominal pain can be signs of nasogastric tube blockage. Instilling 30 mL of air may reestablish patency.**
 2 Although opioids usually are ordered postoperatively, they tend to decrease peristalsis and may increase abdominal distention and nausea.
 3 There will be no stools for several days.
 4 Bowel sounds are not expected for several days after stomach or intestinal surgery.

431. 4 **Drainage is bright red initially and gradually becomes darker red during the first 24 hours.**
 1 If the nasogastric tube is functioning correctly, secretions will be removed and vomiting will not occur.
 2 Because the bowel was emptied before surgery and the client is now NPO, intestinal activity is not expected.
 3 If the nasogastric tube is functioning correctly, gastric distention will not occur.

432. 3 **Hypertonic food increases osmotic pressure and pulls fluid from the intravascular compartment into the intestine (dumping syndrome).**
 1 Increased carbohydrates, not fats, are responsible for the increased osmotic pressure often associated with the dumping syndrome.
 2 This is separation of the wound edges, usually accompanied by a gush of pink-tinged fluid; it is unrelated to dumping syndrome.
 4 Although peristalsis may be decreased because of surgery, it does not account for the adaptations.

433. 4 **The rapid absorption of carbohydrates from the food mass causes an elevation of blood glucose, and the insulin response often causes transient hypoglycemic symptoms. The elevation in insulin usually occurs 90 minutes to 3 hours after eating and is known as late dumping syndrome.**
 1 The physiological adaptations related to late dumping syndrome are caused by an increase in insulin, not glucose.
 2 The insulin-adjusting mechanism is not overwhelmed, but responds vigorously, causing rebound hypoglycemia.
 3 Dumping syndrome is related to the high glucose content of food, not the amount of food, entering the duodenum.

434. 1 **These characteristics are well-established risk factors for gallbladder disease (3 Fs - female, fat, and forty).**
 2 Although these clients usually are older than the age of 40, a high-fat intake does not predispose one to cholecystitis.
 3 The age is correct, but these clients have an increase in serum cholesterol.
 4 Although there is an increased risk with a family history of gallstones, these clients usually are older than the age of 40.

435. 1 **Pain is a cardinal symptom; it is helpful to have as much specific information about it as possible, particularly its description and its relationship to foods ingested.**

2 It is not necessary to save all urine and stool, although changes in color should be reported.

3 The client should be free to question orders that are not understood or agreed with.

4 Although the quality of fluid (e.g., high fat) may be significant, the amount of fluid will not add any valuable information.

436. 4 **Cholecystitis is often accompanied by intolerance to fatty foods, including fried foods and butter.**

1 Because these foods have a high fiber content, they cause flatulence and pain for clients with lower intestinal problems such as diverticulosis.

2 These foods contain less fat than do fried foods or butter.

3 Neither chocolate nor boiled seafood contains as much fat as fried chicken or butter.

437. 4 **During the procedure a sedative is administered intravenously as needed to help the client stay calm.**

1 This is not used during this procedure.

2 This is not used during this procedure.

3 This is not used during this procedure.

438. 1 **Bile promotes the absorption of the fat-soluble vitamins. An obstruction of the common bile duct limits the flow of bile to the duodenum and thus the absorption of these fat-soluable vitamins.**

2 Dietary fiber is not relevant to the situation.

3 Although adequate dietary protein is desirable for wound healing, it is unrelated to cholelithiasis.

4 Elevated potassium and folic acid are not related to cholelithiasis.

439. 3 **Self-splinting results in shallow breathing, which does not aerate the lungs adequately, particularly the lower right lobe.**

1 The T-tube is never irrigated; it drains by gravity until the edema in the operative area subsides; the tube is then removed by the physician.

2 The dressing is not changed by the nurse in the immediate postoperative period; the client's respiratory status takes priority.

4 The client will be NPO immediately after surgery.

440. 2 **Obstruction of bile flow impairs absorption of vitamin K, a fat-soluable vitamin; prothrombin is not produced and the clotting process is prolonged.**

1 Although deposition of bile salts in the skin may lead to pruritus, this is not life threatening.

3 Although there may be an increase in flatulence with biliary disease, it is not life threatening.

4 Obstructive jaundice does not affect potassium levels.

441. 4 **The T-tube provides an outlet for bile produced by the liver and is expected to drain 300 to 500 mL in the first day.**

1 Clamping the tube during the early postoperative period may cause a buildup of pressure and leakage of bile into the peritoneum.

2 The rate of fluid administration is prescribed by the practitioner.

3 Drainage from the T-tube is by gravity; negative pressure is not applied.

442. 3 **Maintaining nasogastric tube patency ensures gastric decompression, thus preventing abdominal distension, which places tension on the incision.**

1 Deep breathing should be encouraged to prevent respiratory complications.

2 Maintaining T-tube patency only ensures a portal of exit for bile drainage; the tube is not irrigated and an obstruction will lead to jaundice rather than tension on the surgical wound.

4 The right-side–lying position after a cholecystectomy can increase, not decrease, tension in the operative area.

443. 4 **Recovery will be rapid because there is no large abdominal incision.**

1 Clear liquids may be started as soon as the client is awake and a gag reflex has returned.

2 With a laparoscopic cholecystectomy there will be one or more puncture wounds, not an incision, on the abdomen.

3 Carbonated beverages will create gas, which will distend the intestines and increase pain.

444. 1 **Vitamin K, a precursor for prothrombin, cannot be absorbed without bile.**

2 This is commonly related to electrolyte imbalances, not fat-soluble vitamin deficiency.

3 Jaundice results from a backup of bile, not a deficiency of fat-soluble vitamins.

4 This may be related to electrolyte imbalances or deficiency of B vitamins, which are water soluble.

445. 1 **Painful biliary colic may occur in the postoperative period as a result of the passage of pulverized fragments of the calculi; this may occur 3 or more days after the lithotripsy.**

2 Fever may indicate pancreatitis, which is a rare occurrence.

3 The delivery of shock waves during the procedure is synchronized with the heartbeat to avoid initiation of dysrhythmias.

4 Light sedation may be used to keep the client comfortable and as still as possible.

446. 4 **Mild shoulder pain is common up to 1 week after surgery because of diaphragmatic irritation secondary to abdominal stretching or residual carbon dioxide that was used to inflate the abdominal cavity during surgery.**

1 The bandages are removed the second day postoperatively.

2 Clients generally tolerate food after 24 to 48 hours.

3 The client may bathe and shower as usual.

447. 4 **The response is individual, but ultimately most people can eat anything they want.**

1 Fats may have to be gradually reintroduced, but most people tolerate them after this surgery.

2 Foods that caused gastric distress before surgery usually are tolerated after surgery.

3 Increased protein is needed only until healing has occurred.

448. 2 **Amylase concentration is increased in the pancreas and is elevated in the serum when the pancreas becomes acutely inflamed; this distinguishes pancreatitis from other acute abdominal problems.**

1 An elevated blood glucose level is not indicative of pancreatitis, but rather diabetes mellitus; however, hyperglycemia and glycosuria may occur in some people with acute pancreatitis if the islets of Langerhans are affected.

3 This occurs in other disease processes, such as cholecystitis.

4 This is not specific to pancreatitis; white blood cells are elevated in other disease processes.

449. 1 **Pain with pancreatitis usually is severe and is the major symptom; it occurs because of the autodigestive process in the pancreas and peritoneal irritation.**

2 Although clients with this medical diagnosis are often malnourished, addressing the client's pain takes priority.

3 There are not enough data for this conclusion; additional data such as skin turgor, serum electrolytes, and I&O are needed to identify whether the client has a fluid and electrolyte imbalance.

4 There are no data to support the presence of a disturbed self-concept.

450. 3 **Alcohol increases pancreatic secretions, which cause pancreatic cell destruction.**

1 Although the diet should be low in fat, it should be high in protein; also it should be high in carbohydrates.

2 The client should be consuming 4,000 to 6,000 calories a day to maintain weight and promote tissue repair.

4 A bland diet is not necessary, but large, heavy meals should be avoided.

451. 4 **Tumors of the head of the pancreas usually obstruct the common bile duct where it passes through the head of the pancreas to join the pancreatic duct and empty at the ampulla of Vater into the duodenum. The feces will be clay-colored when bile is prevented from entering the duodenum.**

1 Green stools may occur with prolonged diarrhea associated with gastrointestinal inflammation.

2 The feces are brown when there is unobstructed bile flow into the duodenum.

3 Inflammation or ulceration of the lower intestinal mucosa results in blood-tinged stools.

452. 4 **A pancreaticoduodenectomy leads to malabsorption because of impaired delivery of bile to the intestine; fat metabolism is interfered with, causing dyspepsia.**

1 These clients are anorexic, require small frequent meals, and should eat a high-calorie, high-protein, low-fat diet.

2 High-calorie meals are needed for energy and to promote use of protein for tissue repair.

3 High protein is required for tissue building; there is no problem with the liver in clients with cancer of the pancreas unless direct extension occurs.

453. 4 **Polydipsia is characteristic of hypoinsulinism (diabetes mellitus) because excessive urine is excreted related to glycosuria.**

1 Polyuria, not oliguria, is characteristic of diabetes mellitus because the kidneys excrete excess fluid with the glucose.

2 Increased appetite is characteristic of diabetes mellitus because of impaired metabolism.

3 Weight loss characterizes diabetes mellitus because of the use of body mass as a source of energy.

454. 2 **Rapid administration can cause glucose overload, leading to osmotic diuresis and dehydration; slowing the infusion decreases the possibility of glucose overload.**

1 Stopping the flow will jeopardize the central line; this site is commonly covered by a transparent dressing to allow for assessment of the site.

3 Signs of bowel obstruction are not present.

4 The client's headache should disappear with oral fluid replacement; analgesics are not indicated.

455. 4 **Formation of lipase necessary for digestion of fats is an exocrine function; the endocrine function is to secrete insulin, which is a hormone essential in carbohydrate metabolism.**

1 Although it is necessary to avoid alcohol, this is not related to pancreatic exocrine functions; caffeine is unrelated to pancreatic function.

2 Fluid and electrolyte problems are not related specifically to exocrine or endocrine pancreatic functioning.

3 Deficiencies of vitamins and minerals may occur because of inadequate intake, but these deficiencies are not specifically related to exocrine or endocrine pancreatic functioning.

456. 1 **A client's vital signs, especially the pulse and temperature, will increase before the client demonstrates any of the more severe symptoms of withdrawal from alcohol.**

2 Increasing intake is contraindicated initially because it may cause cerebral edema.

3 Improving nutritional status becomes a priority after the problems of the withdrawal period have subsided.

4 Determining the client's reasons for drinking is not a priority until after the detoxification process.

457. 4 **Petechiae are evidence of capillary bleeding; the diseased liver is no longer able to metabolize vitamin K, which is necessary to activate blood clotting factors.**

1 Vitamin D is not involved in the clotting process.

2 Vitamin E is not involved in the clotting process.

3 Vitamin A is not involved in the clotting process, even though the transformation of carotene to vitamin A takes place in the liver.

458. 4 **Emptying the bladder of urine keeps the bladder in the pelvic area and prevents puncture when the abdominal cavity is entered.**

1 This is not necessary.

2 This is not necessary.

3 Encouraging fluids is unsafe; the bladder will rise into the abdominal cavity and may be punctured.

459. 1 **Hepatitis A is primarily spread via a fecal-oral route; sewage-polluted water may harbor the virus.**

2 Hepatitis types B, C, and D are more often spread via the bloodborne route; using disposable equipment and proper handling of syringes decreases the risk of spreading the virus.

3 This does not increase the risk of developing the disease, but will increase the risk of an infected individual spreading the disease to others.

4 Exposure to arsenic or carbon tetrachloride can cause toxic hepatitis, which is not communicable.

460. 4 **Clay-colored stools are indicative of hepatic obstruction because bile is prevented from entering the intestines.**

1 It is unnecessary to call the practitioner because this symptom is characteristic of hepatitis from the onset of clinical manifestations.

2 It is unnecessary to call the practitioner because this symptom is characteristic of hepatitis from the onset of clinical manifestations.

3 This is the expected color of urine.

461. 2 **Damage to liver cells affects the ability to facilitate removal of bilirubin from the blood, with resulting deposition in the skin and sclera.**

1 With hepatitis, the liver does not secrete excess bile.

3 Destruction of red blood cells does not increase in hepatitis.

4 Decreased prothrombin levels cause spontaneous bleeding, not jaundice.

462. 4 **Hepatitis A is spread via the fecal-oral route; transmission is prevented by proper handwashing.**

1. This is unnecessary; cleansing the toilet and washing the hands should control the transmission of microorganisms.

2 If the son uses the same bathroom as others, provision must be made for the cleaning of equipment or disposal of contaminated wastes.

3 The use of disposable toilet covers is inadequate to prevent the spread of microorganisms if the bathroom used by the son also is used by others. Handwashing by all family members must be part of the plan to prevent the spread of hepatitis to other family members.

463. 3 **Hepatitis A is transmitted via the fecal-oral route; contact precautions must be used when there are articles that have potential fecal and/or urine contamination.**

1 Neither a private room nor a closed door is required; these are necessary only for respiratory (airborne) precautions.

2 Hepatitis A is not transmitted via the airborne route and therefore a mask is not necessary; a gown and gloves are required only when handling articles that may be contaminated.

4 This is too limited; a gown and gloves also should be worn when handling other fecally contaminated articles, such as a bedpan or rectal thermometer.

464. **Answer: 4, 5**

1 This refers to patches of depigmentation resulting from destruction of melanocytes.

2 This is excessive growth of hair; with cirrhosis, endocrine disturbances result in loss of axillary and pubic hair.

3 Dark pigmentary deposits result from a disorder of pigment metabolism.

4 **Ecchymoses are small areas of bleeding into the skin or mucous membrane forming a blue or purple patch. With cirrhosis there is decreased synthesis of prothombin in the liver.**

5 **Telangiectasis is a vascular lesion formed by dilation of a group of small blood vessels. When cirrhosis causes an increase in pressure in the portal circulation that results in a dilation of cutaneous blood vessels around the umbilicus, it is specifically called *caput medusae*.**

465. 3 **This indicates that the client has a deficiency in clotting, which should be corrected before the biopsy to prevent hemorrhage.**

1 Confusion and disorientation are not a contraindication for a liver biopsy; if present, the client may need support and the examiner may need assistance, but the biopsy can be done.

2 A biopsy is not contraindicated in the presence of an infectious disease.

4 Vitamin K is needed for the production of prothrombin; however, this does not guarantee clotting activity; vitamin E is not involved in clotting.

466. 1 **This position exposes the right intercostal space, making the large right lobe of the liver accessible.**

2 This position will not provide accessibility to the liver; the small left lobe is not anatomically near the left chest wall.

3 In this position the liver will fall away from the chest wall and be less accessible.

4 This will not provide accessibility to the liver.

467. 3 **In this position the liver capsule at the entry site is compressed against the chest wall and escape of blood and/or bile is impeded.**

1 This is unsafe because pressure will not be applied to the puncture site and the client can bleed from the insertion site.

2 This is unsafe because pressure will not be applied to the puncture site and the client can bleed from the insertion site.

4 This is unsafe because pressure will not be applied to the puncture site and the client can bleed from the insertion site.

468. 3 **Because of the vascularity of the liver, compression of the needle insertion site limits the risk of hemorrhage; also it decreases the risk of bile leakage.**

1 The procedure is performed under local anesthesia and some discomfort may be felt during instillation of the anesthetic as well as when the needle enters the liver.

2 There is no scarring because a surgical incision is not necessary for a needle biopsy.

4 The client is kept NPO for at least 6 hours before the procedure to prevent nausea and vomiting.

469. 4 **The flow of bile through the puncture site indicates that a biliary vessel was punctured; this is a common complication after a liver biopsy.**

1 Fluid will leak through the puncture site or into the peritoneum, not the intestine.

2 The pancreas does not contain bile; it is in the upper left, not upper right, quadrant.

3 This is a complication, not an expected outcome.

470. 4 **An increased serum ammonia level impairs the CNS, causing an altered level of consciousness.**

1 Increasing ammonia levels are not related to weight.

2 An alteration in fluid intake will not affect the serum ammonia level.

3 This is not the priority; the priority is to monitor the client's neurological status.

471. 1 **The high ammonia levels contribute to deterioration of mental function and then to hepatic encephalopathy and hepatic coma; safety is the priority.**

2 Although the client may have dyspnea as a result of ascites, it is not life threatening; safety is the priority.

3 Although this is done to monitor ascites, it is not the priority for a confused client; safety is the priority.

4 This is not the priority; providing for client safety is the priority.

472. 3 **One lumen inflates the esophageal balloon, the second inflates the gastric balloon, and the third decompresses the stomach.**

1 It is a triple-, not single-lumen tube.

2 It is a triple-, not double-lumen tube; the stomach, not the intestine, is decompressed.

4 The stomach, but not the intestine, is decompressed.

473. 1 **Measures must be taken immediately to ensure client safety.**

2 Sedatives are contraindicated because they mask the progressive signs of hepatic encephalopathy.

3 Although the practitioner should be notified, the nurse should first take measures to ensure client safety.

4 Hepatic encephalopathy is caused by high serum ammonia levels, not hypoxia.

474. 1 **The signs and symptoms indicate hepatic coma; protein is reduced according to tolerance, and calories are increased to prevent tissue catabolism.**

2 This represents a high-protein diet, which is contraindicated in impending hepatic coma.

3 This represents a high-protein diet, which is contraindicated in impending hepatic coma.

4 This represents a high-protein diet, which is contraindicated in impending hepatic coma.

475. Answer: 1, 2, 4

1 **The metabolic rate will be increased and the temperature-regulating center in the hypothalamus resets to a higher than usual body temperature because of the influence of pyrogenic substances related to the peritonitis.**

2 **Tachypnea results as the metabolic rate increases and the body attempts to meet cellular oxygen needs.**

3 Hypovolemia and therefore hypotension, not hypertension, results because of a loss of fluid, electrolytes, and protein into the peritoneal cavity.

4 **With increased intra-abdominal pressure, the abdominal wall will become rigid and tender.**

5 Peristalsis and associated bowel sounds will decrease or be absent in the presence of increased intra-abdominal pressure.

476. 2 **Bowel sounds are the result of peristaltic movements that propel intestinal contents through the alimentary tract, causing characteristic sounds.**

1 Bowel sounds will be heard before flatus is passed.

3 Liquids should not be given until bowel sounds have returned.

4 Peristalsis will return before the client has a bowel movement.

477. 3 **This position promotes localization of purulent material and inflammation and prevents an ascending infection.**

1 The risk of an ascending infection may be increased in this position because it allows fluid in the abdominal cavity to bathe the entire peritoneum.

2 The risk of an ascending infection may be increased in this position because it allows fluid in the abdominal cavity to bathe the entire peritoneum.

4 The client may choose a position that increases the risk of an ascending infection.

478. 1 **Decreased intestinal motility is associated with serious problems, such as perforation or toxic megacolon.**

2 This is an uncomfortable but less serious manifestation.

3 This is an expected response that is not of primary concern at this time.

4 Intense pain is a symptom of ulcerative colitis, not a complication.

479. **2 Medical treatment is directed toward reducing motility of the inflamed bowel, restoring nutrition, and preventing and treating infection; surgery is used selectively for those who are acutely ill or have excessive exacerbations.**

1 This is untrue; medical treatment is symptomatic, not curative.

3 It is usually performed as a last resort.

4 Although there is an emotional component, the physiological adaptations determine whether surgery is necessary.

480. **2 When anxious, in pain, or performing deep-breathing exercises, it is common for air to be swallowed, which can cause gastric distention.**

1 A rectal tube does not relieve nausea and vomiting; it facilitates expulsion of gas and some secretions trapped in the large intestines because of lack of peristalsis.

3 Preoperative enemas are not given to prevent paralytic ileus postoperatively; they are given to cleanse the lower gastrointestinal tract, decreasing the possibility of peritoneal contamination.

4 Liquids are not given until some peristalsis has returned as evidenced by the presence of bowel sounds.

481. **1 Low-residue foods produce less fecal waste, decreasing bowel contents and irritation; protein promotes healing and calories provide energy.**

2 Barbecued foods are spicy; foods high in fat can increase peristalsis.

3 Fruit and aged, sharp cheese can be irritating to the bowel.

4 Chunky peanut butter and whole wheat bread are high-residue foods.

482. **3 Decompression removes collected secretions behind the nonfunctioning bowel segment (paralytic ileus), thus reducing pressure on the suture line and allowing healing.**

1 Although this is important, the primary concern is decompression of the bowel; the amount of fluid removed will direct fluid and electrolyte replacement therapy.

2 Vomiting will subside as the bowel is decompressed.

4 Although this is important, the primary concern is decompression of the bowel; the amount of fluid removed will direct fluid and electrolyte replacement therapy.

483. **2 The client's feelings, knowledge, and skills concerning the ileostomy must be assessed before discharge.**

1 People should not be pressured into performing self-care before they are physically sand emotionally ready.

3 The diet is not limited; however, the client should be encouraged to eat a high-protein diet or a regular diet with supplemental protein; a high-fluid intake should be maintained.

4 Often the client no longer needs a dressing on the incision at the time of discharge; a collection pouch is used over the stoma.

484. **4 Low-residue foods will not increase motility.**

1 Warmth and the fiber in the orange juice will increase motility and should be avoided.

2 Wheat cereal contains roughage and should be avoided.

3 Toast and the vegetables in a western omelet are high in residue; also the omelet is fried, which should be avoided.

485. **3 Constipation, diarrhea, and/or constipation alternating with diarrhea are the most common signs of colorectal cancer.**

1 This is the second most common complaint that results from destruction of the epithelial lining of the intestine.

2 Pain is reported as a symptom in less than 25% of clients; also it is a late sign after other organs are invaded.

4 This is a later sign that becomes evident when the lumen of the intestine narrows as a result of the enlarging mass.

486. **Answer: 4, 1, 3, 2**
The first step is for the nurse to receive report from the transporting nurse. The receiving nurse should be informed about the type of surgery performed, important events that occurred during surgery, and the client's response and current status. Once the report is completed, the next step is for the receiving nurse to ensure that the client has a patent airway. Vital signs are then taken to assess the client's current cardiopulmonary status and to assess for signs of hemorrhage or other postoperative complications. This assessment follows the ABCs (airway, breathing, circulation) of assessment. After the client's vital signs are determined to be stable, the nurse should assess and monitor the dressing, IV, and the indwelling urinary catheter.

487. **4 The initiation of the gastrocolic reflex can cause intestinal contents to reach the lower GI tract and interfere with visualization of the colon.**

1 An oil-retention enema will interfere with visualization during the colonoscopy and therefore should not be administered.

2 A liquid, not bland, diet should be consumed the night before the test.

3 Diarrhea should not occur after the test.

488. **4 This is an accurate explanation of what the client can expect during the CT scan.**

1 It is not necessary to rest in bed for 6 hours.

2 The procedure causes no physical pain, and an analgesic is not necessary.

3 The client will be awake; neither sedation nor anesthesia is used with a CT scan.

489. 3 **This diet is low in fiber; after digestion and absorption there is only a small amount of residue to be eliminated.**

1 This diet does not promote peristalsis; the products of digestion remain in the intestine longer, and flatus is increased.

2 Although a low-residue diet is less irritating, this is not the primary reason for its use before surgery.

4 Antimicrobials, such as neomycin, are given to do this.

490. 3 **Except in an emergency, the client receives an intestinal antibiotic for several days preoperatively to reduce the amount of intestinal bacteria.**

1 Diuretics are not necessary unless prescribed for a preexisting problem.

2 Fluids usually are restricted after midnight on the day of surgery, not for days before surgery.

4 Abdominal exercises are not part of the surgical preparation.

491. 1 **When intestinal continuity cannot be restored after removal of the anus, rectum, and adjacent colon, a permanent colostomy is formed.**

2 The ascending segment of the colon lies on the right side of the abdomen and has no anatomical proximity to the rectum.

3 This temporary procedure is performed to allow a segment of colon to heal; intestinal continuity is eventually restored.

4 This procedure is commonly performed for inflammation of the colon when intestinal continuity eventually can be restored.

492. 2 **The surface of a stoma is mucous membrane and should be dark pink to red, moist, and shiny; the stoma usually is raised beyond the skin surface.**

1 The stoma should be moist, not dry; pale pink indicates a low hemoglobin level; although some stomas can be flush with the skin, a raised stoma is more common.

3 The stoma should be moist, not dry; purple indicates compromised circulation; a depressed stoma is retracted and unexpected.

4 Although the stoma should be moist and dark pink to red, it should not be painful; although some stomas can be flush with the skin, a raised stoma is more common.

493. 1 **Once stool is formed, peristalsis needs to be stimulated to promote the passage of stool.**

2 The sitting, not side-lying, position is the position of choice for a colostomy irrigation because it facilitates evacuation of the bowel via gravity.

3 Contamination is avoided because fecal elimination flows through the sleeve of the colostomy appliance directly into the commode.

4 The perineal wound may take weeks to heal, and irrigations must be started when the stool is formed.

494. 3 **This is caused by intestinal manipulation and the depressive effects of anesthesia and analgesics.**

1 Edema will not totally interfere with peristalsis; there should be some output.

2 A presurgical decrease in fluid intake will not influence gastric motility 24 hours later.

4 A nasogastric tube decompresses the stomach; it does not directly influence intestinal motility at this time.

495. 3 **A cone-shaped tip controls the depth of insertion of the catheter, which prevents perforation of the bowel and limits leakage of water from the stoma during fluid insertion.**

1 In both procedures the client should be positioned for evacuation of the bowel, which allows gravity to facilitate bowel evacuation.

2 In both procedures the catheter tip should be lubricated with a water-soluble jelly, which limits trauma to the intestinal mucosa.

4 In both procedures the tubing should be clear of air to facilitate the tolerance of a larger volume of irrigating solution.

496. 4 **Stoma adhesive protects the skin and helps to keep the appliance attached to the skin.**

1 The appliance should be emptied when it is one third to one half full.

2 This is too much space between the stoma and the appliance; the enzymes in feces can erode the skin.

3 Initially the nurse should change the appliance; self-care usually is instituted more gradually depending on the client's physical and emotional response to the surgery.

497. 3 **Clients with a colostomy can eat a regular diet; only gas-forming foods that cause distention and discomfort should be avoided.**

1 The amount of stool does not have to be limited; therefore, a low-residue diet is not necessary.

2 The affected tissue has been removed and healthy mucosal tissue lines the intestine and forms the stoma; therefore, bland foods are not necessary.

4 Nutrients are absorbed by the small, not the large, intestine; a regular diet usually is easily digested and absorbed.

498. 4 **Regular irrigation and effective evacuation prevent unexpected bowel movements; generally a drainage pouch is needed only immediately after an irrigation.**

1 Once the colostomy is regulated, an appliance is necessary only immediately after the irrigation (approximately 1 hour).

2 Appliances collect what is evacuated; they do not control the function of the colostomy; a "special" appliance is not needed.

3 This response does not address the client's concern.

499. 3 **Pain is wavelike, colicky, and sharp because of obstruction and localized bowel ischemia.**

1 Flatus is impeded by strangulation.

2 Vomiting is persistent, not projectile.

4 This is not an early sign of obstruction; decreased bowel sounds occur after gas and fluid accumulate.

500. 2 **The lowered blood pressure may be caused by pooling of blood in peripheral vessels; moving the legs will aid venous return.**

1 This will not increase the blood pressure; this intervention is used for pregnant women to move the gravid uterus off the vena cava, which increases placental perfusion.

3 This eventually may be done after performing the initial interventions and evaluating results.

4 Opioid analgesics may decrease the blood pressure further.

501. 3 **Because of pain and the proximity of the operative site to the lower urinary tract, urinary retention is common after this surgery.**

1 Hydrocele is not a complication of a herniorrhaphy.

2 The abdomen was not entered; there should be no interference with peristalsis.

4 Thrombophlebitis should not occur because early ambulation is permitted.

502. 2 **The client has ingested 258 calories. Carbohydrates and proteins each yield 4 calories per gram, and fat yields 9 calories per gram. The total carbohydrate calories are $32 \times 4 = 128$. The total protein calories are $10 \times 4 = 40$. The total fat calories are $10 \times 9 = 90$; $128 + 40 + 90 = 258$ calories.**

1 This is an incorrect calculation.

3 This is an incorrect calculation.

4 This is an incorrect calculation.

INTEGUMENTARY

503. 1 **Nerves are the least resistant tissue, followed by blood vessels, skin, muscle, and bone.**

2 Alternating electrical current, the most prevalent type in the United States, causes the most severe injuries.

3 Electrical current flows from the point of contact to the point of grounding.

4 It is difficult to track the path of electricity by external visualization; it often requires more extensive diagnostic exploration.

504. 2 **This action effectively extinguishes the flames and protects the client from additional injury.**

1 This action will not eliminate the oxygen that supports the fire and will fan the flames.

3 This may extinguish the flames, but not as effectively as rolling in the grass.

4 This may protect the client from further injury, but is dangerous for the rescuer.

505. 2 **A patent airway is most vital; if the person is not breathing, CPR should be instituted.**

1 The person should be kept NPO because large burns decrease intestinal peristalsis and the person may vomit and aspirate.

3 This is not done until assessment for breathing is completed.

4 This is not the priority; this assessment is done after transfer to a medical facility.

506. 4 **A bedsheet is nonfuzzy and nonadhering and will keep the person warm.**

1 Ice can cause additional tissue damage.

2 Cream is difficult to remove and may result in additional damage.

3 Doing nothing does not meet the individual's immediate needs.

507. 3 **In deep partial-thickness burns, destruction of the epidermis and part of the dermis occurs.**

1 Eschar, a dry leathery covering of denatured protein, occurs with full-thickness burns.

2 With full-thickness burns, total destruction of the epidermis, dermis, and some underlying tissue occurs.

4 With superficial partial-thickness burns, the epidermis is destroyed or injured.

508. 1 **This describes a superficial partial-thickness burn.**

2 The dermis is not damaged in superficial partial-thickness burns. The entire epidermis and part of the dermis are affected with deep partial-thickness burns.

3 This describes full-thickness burns.

4 The statement is too vague a description of what is involved.

509. 4 **Using the rule of nines, the percentage of total body surface area burned is 9% for each arm (18% for both arms) and 18% for the chest; thus the total body surface area burned is 36%.**

1 This percentage is too low.

2 This percentage is too low.

3 This percentage is too low.

510. 2 **Heat inhalation can cause edema of the respiratory lumina, interfering with oxygenation; evaluation of respiratory status is a priority.**

1 This is done after the client's respiratory status is evaluated.

3 The practitioner first assesses the client's adaptations to the burn injury and then orders the appropriate therapies. Only then would the nurse apply sterile saline dressings if they were ordered.

4 This is done after the client's respiratory status is evaluated.

511. 2 **Hoarseness is a sign of potential respiratory insufficiency as a result of inhalation burns, which cause edema in the surrounding tissues, including the vocal cords.**

1 This indicates metabolic acidosis, not respiratory insufficiency.

3 Sputum will be sooty, not frothy; pink-tinged, frothy sputum is associated with pulmonary edema.

4 This indicates metabolic acidosis, not respiratory insufficiency.

512. 2 **Massive amounts of potassium are released from the injured cells into the extracellular fluid; large amounts of sodium are lost in edema.**
   1 Although hyponatremia occurs, the serum potassium level increases.
   3 The serum potassium level increases; the serum sodium level decreases.
   4 Although hyperkalemia occurs, the serum sodium level decreases.

513. 1 **A high-calorie diet is needed for the increased metabolic rate associated with burns; the administration of potassium prevents hypokalemia, which can occur after the first 48 hours when potassium moves from the extracellular compartment into the intracellular compartment; protein promotes tissue repair.**
   2 This plan does not meet the body's needs for tissue repair; the calories and potassium are too limited.
   3 This plan does not meet the body's needs for tissue repair; the calories are too limited.
   4 This plan does not meet the body's needs for tissue repair; the calories, potassium, and protein are too limited.

514. 3 **Extreme restlessness in a severely burned client usually indicates cerebral hypoxia.**
   1 With renal failure the client will become progressively confused and lethargic, not restless.
   2 At this stage the client will be hypovolemic rather than hypervolemic.
   4 With metabolic acidosis the client will be lethargic.

515. 2 **Pain is from the loss of the protective covering of the nerve endings; blisters and redness occur because of the injury to the dermis and epidermis.**
   1 Because some epithelial cells remain, grafting is not needed with a partial-thickness burn unless it becomes infected and further tissue damage occurs.
   3 Partial-thickness burns involve only the superficial layers of skin, unless they become infected.
   4 Recovery from partial-thickness burns with no infection occurs in 2 to 3 weeks.

516. 2 **Topical antibiotics are directly applied to the wound and are effective against many gram-positive and gram-negative organisms found on the skin.**
   1 Although these may be administered, they are most effective for systemic rather than local infections; the vasculature in and around a burn is impaired and the medication may not reach the organisms in the wound.
   3 Although these may be administered, they are most effective for systemic rather than local infections; the vasculature in and around a burn is impaired and the medication may not reach the organisms in the wound.
   4 Although these may be administered, they are most effective for systemic rather than local infections; the vasculature in and around a burn is impaired and the medication may not reach the organisms in the wound.

517. 3 **Adequate intake of protein, carbohydrates, vitamin C, and minerals is necessary for tissue building and wound healing.**
   1 There are no data to come to this conclusion; although the client is not eating, the client may be drinking fluids.
   2 This change will take a prolonged period of time; it will not occur during a short period.
   4 This is associated with prolonged hypoxia.

518. 4 **Care of burns is a painful procedure; pain medication should be administered before care to limit discomfort.**
   1 Surgical asepsis should be used.
   2 No dressings are applied when the exposure method is used.
   3 Sulfamylon is not hepatotoxic.

519. 3 **Isolation precautions are essential for the prevention of infection in clients with burns; policies and procedures include specific interventions related to standard and transmission-based precautions, medical asepsis, surgical asepsis, and room assignments.**
   1 Hydrotherapy in a large tank tub may be used to clean burn wounds.
   2 Dressings are not used with the exposure method.
   4 Clients are more comfortable with a room temperature of 85° F.

520. 2 **Non–cotton-backed gauze is less apt to adhere to the wound then does cotton-backed gauze; the hands should be maintained in anatomical position of slight flexion with each finger separated.**
   1 Cotton-filled or cotton-backed gauze should not be used because it may adhere to the wound; the hands should be in anatomical position with fingers slightly flexed.
   3 The hands should not be anatomically positioned in full extension or full flexion; the hands should be slightly flexed in functional alignment.
   4 Cotton-filled or cotton-backed gauze should not be used because it may adhere to the wound. The hands placed in complete flexion can result in contractures; the hands should be in anatomical position with the fingers slightly flexed.

521. 2 **The first step is to determine what the physician has told the client.**
   1 This statement is inappropriate; grafting begins when the granulation bed is formed.
   3 This statement is inappropriate; grafting begins when the granulation bed is formed.
   4 Grafting will not be done until the wound is clean and granulation tissue has formed; there are no data to indicate the presence of an infection.

522. 1 **Limiting drafts minimizes body heat lost by convection; the loss of body heat increases when moistened skin is exposed to slightly moving air.**
   2 The room temperature should be kept at approximately 85° F because heat is lost from burned areas.

3   A sterile sheet is not necessary; some clients may be treated by the open method and have burns exposed.

4   40% to 50% humidity is needed to maximize the warmth of the room.

523. 2   **The graft covers nerve endings, which reduces pain and provides a framework for granulation.**

1   Enzymatic preparations or surgery debride wounds and promote epithelialization.

3   Pig skin grafts are not sutured.

4   Topical antimicrobials will soften the graft and impede healing.

524. 1   **An allograft is a temporary measure; it is expected to come off and the practitioner should be notified that it is happening at this time.**

2   This is an unwarranted accusation that places guilt on the client; allografts are temporary.

3   This is inaccurate information that may frighten the client.

4   An allograft is a temporary, not permanent, measure and is expected to fall off.

525. 2   **Range of motion (ROM) should be instituted as soon as it will not compromise the individual's cardiopulmonary status.**

1   Pain will continue for some time, and if ROM is delayed until it subsides, contractures will develop.

3   If ROM is delayed until skin grafts heal, contractures will develop.

4   Pain and inability to cope may be prolonged; if ROM is delayed, contractures will develop.

526. 2   **Invasion of the posterior (dorsal) root ganglia by the same virus that causes chickenpox can result in herpes zoster or shingles. This may be caused by reactivation of a previous chicken-pox virus that has lain dormant in the body or by recent contact with an individual who has chickenpox.**

1   Athlete's foot is caused by a fungus.

3   German measles is caused by a virus, but not the herpesvirus.

4   Hepatitis type A is caused by a virus, but not the herpesvirus.

527. 2   **The client is exhibiting the clinical manifestations of psoriasis. Psoriasis is characterized by white scaly plaques on the scalp, knees, and/or elbows. The etiology is not known but it is thought to be a multifaceted disease that is related to stress and an immune response.**

1   Harsh soaps may cause dry, itchy, cracked skin, not silvery scales. However, too frequent washing may be irritating; tar-based soaps may be recommended.

3   The client is exhibiting the signs of psoriasis, not Lyme disease.

4   The lesions described are not associated with HIV.

528. 4   **Chemotherapy destroys the rapidly dividing cells of the oral mucosa; frequent gentle oral hygiene limits additional trauma.**

1   Lemon juice is too caustic to the compromised mucosa.

2   Flossing can disrupt and traumatize the gum surfaces; oral hygiene is needed more than once a day.

3   Vigorous cleansing with hard materials can increase mucosal trauma.

529. **Answer: 2, 5**

1   Scaling of the skin is more often associated with psoriasis than aging.

2   **Elastin in the dermis decreases in quality but increases in quantity resulting in wrinkling and sagging of the skin.**

3   Capillary fragility associated with aging contributes to senile purpura; however, ecchymosis indicates ineffective clotting or trauma.

4   Although sweat glands decrease in size, number, and function, contributing to skin dryness, there should not be marked flaking of skin.

5   **Brown pigmented spots (senile lentigines) increase in number, size, and distribution with aging.**

530. 1   **Shearing force occurs when two surfaces move against each other; when the bed is at an angle greater than 30 degrees, the torso tends to slide and causes this phenomenon.**

2   This raises the head of the bed too high, which contributes to the client sliding down in bed.

3   This raises the head of the bed too high, which contributes to the client sliding down in bed.

4   This raises the head of the bed too high, which contributes to the client sliding down in bed.

531. 4   **The client who is confined to bed should be encouraged to move in bed to prevent prolonged pressure on any one skin surface.**

1   Although this will help promote peripheral circulation, prolonged pressure must be avoided.

2   Although it can help decrease skin breakdown by allowing air to circulate under the client, it does not prevent prolonged pressure.

3   Range-of-motion exercises move joints to prevent contractures; they do not relieve prolonged pressure.

532. 4   **Exercise will promote extension of the local infection from the leg into the circulation, causing septicemia.**

1   This is not accomplished by bed rest.

2   Although bed rest does this, it is not the purpose for bed rest in this situation.

3   Although bed rest does this, it is not the purpose for bed rest in this situation.

533. 4   **Because diminished circulation leads to inadequate healing, early treatment of injuries is essential.**

1   Toenails should not be too short and should be trimmed straight across.

2 Bathwater should be checked with a bath thermometer; toes of persons with PAD may be less sensitive to temperature change and a burn may occur.

3 These clients develop trophic skin changes; the drying action of alcohol will potentiate dryness and skin breakdown.

534. 1 **Pressure on the blister will not allow it to heal; use of the prosthesis should be discontinued until healing occurs.**

2 This will neither heal the blister nor alleviate pressure on the blister by the prosthesis.

3 Changing the type of covering will not help heal the blister.

4 The client should not put the prosthesis back on because it causes pressure, which will prevent healing.

535. 3 **Bathing removes microorganisms and promotes circulation, which facilitates wound healing; drying prevents maceration of skin and reduces moisture, which limits bacterial growth.**

1 A sling will interfere with comfort and mobility and can result in elbow or shoulder contractures.

2 Lotion may facilitate adherence of bacteria to wound edges and promote maceration of the skin, which interferes with wound healing.

4 Soaking may cause maceration of the skin and interfere with wound healing.

536. 1 **Surgical asepsis means that the defined area will contain no microorganisms.**

2 This is the purpose of personal protective equipment.

3 This applies to medical, not surgical, asepsis.

4 This applies to medical, not surgical, asepsis.

537. 2 **A mask will protect the catheter insertion site from droplet and airborne microorganisms emanating from the nurse and sterile gloves will protect the insertion site from contact with microorganisms on the nurse's hands.**

1 Although sterile gloves will prevent the introduction of microorganisms into the area of the insertion site, they will not protect the client from droplet or airborne microorganisms.

3 Although sterile gloves will prevent the introduction of microorganisms into the area of the insertion site, they will not protect the client from droplet or airborne microorganisms; a need for a gown depends on institutional protocol.

4 Although a mask and gloves will protect the insertion site from the introduction of microorganisms, the need for a gown depends on institutional protocol.

538. 4 **In the obese individual this helps to inject the medication into subcutaneous tissue, where the absorption of insulin is faster than in adipose tissue.**

1 This will result in the drug being injected into adipose tissue, where it will be inadequately absorbed.

2 This will result in the drug being injected into adipose tissue, where it will be inadequately absorbed.

3 This will result in the drug being injected into adipose tissue, where it will be inadequately absorbed.

539. 2 **An iatrogenic infection is one caused by health care providers or therapy.**

1 This is not the cause of an iatrogenic infection.

3 This is not the cause of an iatrogenic infection.

4 This is not the cause of an iatrogenic infection.

540. 1 **The sponge generally is changed every 48 to 56 hours except when there is a skin graft. The sponge generally is removed on the fourth day when there is a skin graft. Routine changing of the sponge minimizes growth of granulation tissue into the foam sponge and allows for assessment of the wound.**

2 Generally clean technique is considered adequate when changing the dressing.

3 The sponge should be cut to conform to the surface of the wound and should not cover the edges of surrounding intact skin. Moisture associated with fluid pulled from the wound can contribute to maceration of intact skin.

4 Experts agree that vacuum pressure generally should be set at 125 mm Hg. It can be set as low as 50 mm Hg and as high as 200 mm Hg. A negative pressure set less than 50 mm Hg is not enough pressure to effectively draw fluid from the wound. A negative pressure set more than 200 mm Hg contributes to a decrease in blood flow to the wound. Negative pressure is generally set at 75 mm Hg for skin grafts.

541. 4 **This creates negative pressure in the portable wound drainage system; a pressure gradient now promotes the flow of drainage from the client to the collection container.**

1 Positive pressure prevents drainage; it does not promote it.

2 Negative pressure is increased, not decreased.

3 Negative, not atmospheric, pressure promotes drainage via a portable wound drainage system.

542. 1 **Bile is irritating to the skin; this is a priority.**

2 Suction is contraindicated; drainage is via gravity.

3 The T-tube is attached to a bag for straight drainage via gravity, not suction that uses negative pressure.

4 Repositioning the client is vital to avoid venous and pulmonary stasis, not for facilitating the drainage of bile.

543. 1 **Teaching for the postoperative period should begin as soon as the decision for surgery is made; knowledge of what to expect decreases anxiety and may improve adherence to the treatment regimen.**

2 Several days before discharge is too late; the client must have time to ask questions and demonstrate the ability to care for the wound. Teaching begins preoperatively.

3 On the first postoperative day the client may be in too much discomfort to concentrate on learning.

4 During the first dressing change the client may be in too much discomfort to concentrate on learning.

544. 1 **The nurse epidemiologist acts as a consultant to help devise an infection control strategy.**
  2 This is the role of a primary care practitioner.
  3 This is the role of the laboratory technician or technologist.
  4 This usually is done by the nurse.

545. 3 **Because of the risk for infection, the client should avoid tub baths, hot tubs, pools, and bodies of water until after the wound has healed and these activities are approved by the surgeon.**
  1 Immersion in water for a prolonged period interferes with wound healing because water may macerate tissue.
  2 Having a friend along does not change the fact that immersion in water for a prolonged period will interfere with wound healing.
  4 The client needs to continue physical therapy after discharge whether or not the client goes swimming.

546. 2 **Barriers reduce the contact of bile with skin and limit excoriation.**
  1 Dressings should be changed when wet, not reinforced; usually T-tube drainage empties into a collection chamber.
  3 Antiseptics are drying and irritating to excoriated skin, and they sting when applied; this requires a practitioner's order.
  4 This action may help, but the excoriation probably is caused by bile, not adhesive tape.

547. 3 **Moisture promotes the migration of microorganisms through the dressing to the wound, which can result in an infection.**
  1 A warm, moist dressing favors growth of microorganisms; a saturated dressing can be uncomfortable or alarming to the client; it should be changed before saturation occurs.
  2 A warm, moist dressing promotes the proliferation of microorganisms; the dressing should be changed.
  4 This is a dependent function of the nurse and requires a practitioner's order.

548. 2 **To make effective decisions, baseline information about the client's condition, extent of injury, and significant past health history is needed.**
  1 The owner may be unknown because the dog is a stray animal; this is not the priority.
  3 Notification of authorities is done after the injured person has received basic care.
  4 Inoculation for establishment of short-term passive immunity to rabies is done after the initial assessment and treatment of the wound.

549. 4 **This is a viral infection that enters the body through a break in the skin and is characterized by convulsions and choking.**
  1 Rabies is not bacterially caused; its outstanding symptoms are convulsions and choking.
  2 Rabies is not associated with a bacterial septicemia; it is caused by a virus.

  3 The virus specifically attacks nervous tissue and is carried in the saliva of infected animals.

550. 2 **A radiation dermatitis occurs 3 to 6 weeks after the start of treatment.**
  1 The word "burn" may increase the client's anxiety and should be avoided.
  3 Emollients are contraindicated; they may alter the calculated x-ray route and injure healthy tissue.
  4 This response does not answer the client's concern.

551. 1 **Both malignant and healthy cells are affected by radiation; time between courses of treatments allows normal cells to repair.**
  2 Staff are available if necessary for a treatment protocol; many facilities operate 7 days a week.
  3 Fatigue occurs in either a 5- or 7-day schedule.
  4 Some side effects are inevitable, although they vary with each individual.

552. 4 **While undergoing radiation therapy, lotions, powders, and ointments should not be applied to the area because they may redirect the rays, causing unnecessary damage to healthy tissue.**
  1 The skin markings should not be removed because they form the parameters for the delivery of radiation.
  2 To protect the irradiated skin, sunlight and heat should be avoided.
  3 Nonirritating clothing should be worn over the area to prevent trauma to the delicate irradiated skin.

553. 1 **The skin is the first line of defense; keeping it dry and safe from injury promotes skin integrity.**
  2 Massage is traumatic because irradiated skin is fragile and subject to blistering and sloughing.
  3 The skin should be free of emollients because they change the angle or degree of radiation.
  4 Irradiated skin is fragile; if soap is used, a film left after rinsing can change the angle and intensity of radiation.

554. 1 **Scleroderma causes chronic hardening and shrinking of the connective tissues of any organ of the body including the esophagus and face. Pureed foods limit the need to chew, and this facilitates swallowing.**
  2 Although liquids are easier to swallow, they are aspirated easily because of decreased esophageal peristalsis.
  3 Although liquids are easier to swallow, they are aspirated easily because of decreased esophageal peristalsis.
  4 No oral pain is associated with scleroderma.

555. 2 **Raynaud's phenomenon is caused by vasospasm, precipitated by exposure to cold or emotional stress. Keeping the hands warm helps to limit episodes of Raynaud's phenomenon. Raynaud's phenomenon is commonly associated with scleroderma, a connective tissue disorder.**
  1 Frequent exposure to water can lead to skin breakdown; also decreased blood flow interferes with perception of temperature and increases the risk of burns.

3 Trauma to the hands must be avoided; nerve endings are affected by the diminished blood supply.

4 Vasodilators, not anticoagulants, are prescribed to counteract vasospasm and increase blood flow.

556. 1 **With scleroderma the skin becomes dry because of interference with the underlying sweat glands.**

2 Pruritus is not associated with scleroderma.

3 Inflammation is not associated with scleroderma.

4 Scaly skin lesions are not associated with scleroderma.

557. 1 **The changes in connective tissue associated with scleroderma lead to muscle weakness; optimal function must be preserved.**

2 Tissue regeneration will not occur; this is a progressive degenerative disorder.

3 Prevention of extension is not possible in this systemic disease, which involves a number of organs.

4 Exercise of stiff and painful joints causes pain, not a sense of well-being.

558. 4 **Because of the recent trauma of surgery, hemorrhage and infection at the operative site can occur.**

1 The client will have a nasogastric tube to suction and be kept NPO until peristalsis returns; there should be no oral intake.

2 This is inappropriate at this time; observing for bleeding and infection takes priority during the first 48 hours.

3 This is not the appropriate time for this teaching; an abdominal dressing usually is in place.

559. 4 **This removes microorganisms and irritants and maintains skin integrity.**

1 Although irritating agents should not be used, soap is the agent of choice to cleanse the skin around the stoma.

2 Hydrogen peroxide may be irritating and is unnecessary; soap and water are adequate.

3 Wiping the stoma can cause irritation, and a secondary infection caused by bacteria or fungi may develop.

560. 4 **The negative pressure of a portable wound drainage system exerts a sucking force that pulls fluid toward the collection chamber.**

1 Gravity is the environmental force that pulls weight toward the center of the earth. An indwelling urinary catheter uses the principle of gravity to draw fluid from the bladder to the collection bag held below the level of the bladder.

2 Osmosis occurs when a solvent moves from a solution of lesser concentration to one of greater solute concentration when the two solutions are separated by a semipermeable membrane; fluid moving from the interstitial compartment into the intracellular compartment uses osmosis.

3 Active transport occurs when ions move across a cell membrane against a concentration gradient with the assistance of metabolic energy; sodium and potassium ions move into and out of cells via active transport (sodium-potassium pump).

561. 2 **Once the drugs that interfere with cell division are stopped, the hair will grow back; sometimes the hair will be a different color or texture.**

1 Alopecia is a common side effect of chemotherapy.

3 Hair loss persists while the drugs are being received; once the drugs are withdrawn, the hair grows back.

4 Although ice caps on the head and rubber bands around the scalp have been used to try to limit alopecia, they have not been particularly effective.

NEUROMUSCULAR

562. **Answer: 4, 5**

1 People who drink alcohol may fall asleep more quickly but have depressed levels of rapid eye movement, less stage 4 sleep, and interruptions between sleep stages (sleep fragmentation).

2 Physical exercise before bedtime has a stimulating rather than a relaxing effect.

3 Lysine, an amino acid, maintains nitrogen equilibrium and promotes growth and development, but does not influence sleep. L-tryptophan, a precursor of serotonin, one of the neurotransmitters involved in sleep, facilitates a more rapid onset of sleep and reduces the sensitivity to external stimuli.

4 **A bedtime ritual provides a familiar routine that promotes comfort and the self-fulfilling prophesy of sleep.**

5 **Relaxation exercises slow body processes and reduce tension, which facilitate rest and promote sleep.**

563. 1 **The afferent sensory branch of the trigeminal nerve (cranial nerve V) innervates the cornea.**

2 Facial expressions (e.g., smiling, frowning) reflect the functioning of cranial nerve VII.

3 This tests the function of cranial nerves III, IV, and VI.

4 This tests the function of cranial nerve XI.

564. 4 **Having the client swallow or checking the gag reflex is a test of the ninth and tenth cranial nerves.**

1 This tests the accessory nerve (cranial nerve XI).

2 This tests the olfactory nerve (cranial nerve I).

3 This tests the facial nerve (cranial nerve VII).

565. 3 **These are used to depress the tongue to observe the pharynx and larynx, and to assess soft palate symmetry and the presence of the gag reflex; the information obtained provides data about cranial nerve X (vagus).**

1 This is used to assess cranial nerve VIII (auditory).

2 This is used to assess cranial nerve II (optic).

4 These are used to assess sensory function—light touch and pain.

566. 2 **This is the description of how to elicit the Babinski reflex. If it is present in adults it may indicate a lesion of the pyramidal tract. The Babinski reflex is expected in newborns and disappears after 1 year.**

1 The Moro (startle) reflex is expected in newborns. It disappears between the third and fourth months;

if present after 4 months, neurological disease is suspected.

3 The stepping reflex is expected in newborns. It disappears at about 3 to 4 weeks after birth and is replaced by more deliberate action.

4 The cremasteric is a superficial reflex that tests lumbar segments 1 and 2. Stimulation of this reflex is useful in initiating reflex emptying of the spastic bladder after a spinal cord disruption above the second, third, or fourth sacral segment.

567. 3 **The client should be assured that the symptoms are not caused by a stroke; the majority of clients recover in a few weeks.**

1 Bell's palsy is not caused by a transient ischemic attack (TIA). Paresis or paralysis of cranial nerve VII occurs; discomfort may or may not be present.

2 Moist heat, not a cool compress, increases blood circulation to the nerve.

4 The majority of clients recover without residual effects; occasionally some clients are left with evidence of Bell's palsy; exercises may help to maintain muscle tone; also, surgery may be necessary.

568. 4 **A nerve block of the trigeminal (fifth cranial) nerve with alcohol is a conservative approach that lasts 6 to 18 months.**

1 This has been tried but provides little, if any, relief.

2 Lidocaine is not used; cranial nerve XI is the spinal accessory nerve that innervates the sternocleidomastoid and trapezius muscles.

3 This is not a conservative approach; this is the most commonly used surgical procedure for trigeminal neuralgia; neuralgia may recur in 30% of clients within 6 years.

569. 3 **This is done to assess electrical activity and determine whether symptoms primarily are musculoskeletal or neurological.**

1 No special care is required during the procedure.

2 No special preparation for an electromyography is required.

4 No special care is required after the procedure.

570. 2 **With a shuffling gait the steps are short and dragging; this is seen with basal ganglia defects.**

1 Ataxia is a staggering gait often associated with cerebellar damage.

3 Scissoring is associated with bilateral spastic paresis of the legs.

4 An asymmetrical gait is associated with weakness of or pain in one lower extremity.

571. Answer: 1, 3, 5

1 **Tremors associated with Parkinson's disease result from degeneration of the dopaminergic nigrostriatal pathways and excess cholinergic activity in the feedback circuit.**

2 Constipation, not diarrhea, is a common problem because of a weakness of muscles used in defecation.

3 **A masklike facial expression results from nigral and basal ganglial depletion of dopamine, an inhibitory neurotransmitter.**

4 The tendency is for the head and neck to be drawn forward, not hyperextended, because of loss of basal ganglia control.

5 **Amplitude of the voice is reduced because of neuromuscular involvement.**

572. 4 **Bradykinesia is a slowing down in the initiation and execution of movement.**

1 Tremors are more prominent at rest and are known as nonintention, not intention, tremors.

2 Cogwheel rigidity, not flaccidity, occurs because the disorder causes sustained muscle contractions.

3 The limbs are rigid and move with a jerky quality; the limbs are not paralyzed.

573. 4 **This maintains the range of joint movement with a minimum of energy expenditure by the client.**

1 Ambulation may fatigue the client and does not provide sufficient movement of the upper extremities.

2 Isometric exercises do not provide the joint movement necessary to prevent contractures.

3 This increases the client's metabolic rate and need for oxygen; the client's ability to meet increased oxygen demand is decreased in the presence of pneumonia.

574. 4 **Numbness, a sensory deficit, is inconsistent with parkinsonism; further medical evaluation is necessary.**

1 Numbness, even in the absence of other problems, may be indicative of an impending brain attack (CVA).

2 This symptom is not caused by parkinsonism; increasing the dosage of the anticholinergic medication will not be helpful.

3 This can cause a delay in the client's receiving immediate medical attention.

575. 3 **Because of the decrease in tone and strength of the respiratory muscles, this is a prominent feature of both crises.**

1 This occurs in cholinergic crisis; it is an effect of an overdose of the medications (anticholinesterases) used to treat myasthenia gravis.

2 This occurs in cholinergic crisis; it is an effect of an overdose of the medications (anticholinesterases) used to treat myasthenia gravis.

4 This occurs in cholinergic crisis; it is an effect of an overdose of the medications (anticholinesterases) used to treat myasthenia gravis.

576. 2 **Use reduces strength, and rest increases strength; eyelid movement, chewing, swallowing, speech, facial expression, and breathing often are affected and therefore muscle weakness will fluctuate in relation to activity and rest.**

1 Muscle strength decreases, not increases, with activity.

3 Anticholinesterase drugs improve muscle strength.

4 Anticholinesterase drugs improve muscle strength.

577. 1 **Rest will decrease the demands at the synaptic membrane of the neuromuscular junction, reducing fatigue; activity should be paced to prevent fatigue before it begins.**

2 This will aggravate the fatigue; activity and rest should be delicately balanced to prevent fatigue.

3 This will aggravate the fatigue; activity and rest should be delicately balanced to prevent fatigue.

4 This cannot be done without a practitioner's order; rest usually will alleviate the fatigue.

578. 1 **These are symptoms of myasthenia gravis, and they are aggravated by physical activity.**

2 Intentional tremors are associated with multiple sclerosis.

3 Exercise decreases muscle strength.

4 The proximal muscles are more involved than the distal muscles.

579. 3 **Respiratory infections place people with myasthenia gravis at high risk because they do not cough effectively and may develop pneumonia or airway obstruction.**

1 Activity should be conducted earlier in the day before the energy reserve is depleted; periods of activity should be alternated with periods of rest.

2 The client should eat sitting in a chair to prevent aspiration.

4 This is contraindicated; these potentiate weakness because of their effect on the myoneural junction.

580. 4 **Increased activity without an increase in medication can precipitate a myasthenic crisis.**

1 Self-medication may result in drug interactions; a change in medical therapy can have serious consequences.

2 A dose should not be skipped because doing so may result in severe respiratory distress.

3 People with myasthenia gravis should avoid crowds and others with colds; they are more prone to respiratory infections because of an ineffective cough and a potential for aspiration.

581. 3 **Tensilon acts systemically to increase muscle strength with a peak effect in 30 seconds; it lasts several minutes.**

1 Tensilon produces a brief increase in muscle strength; with a negative response the client will demonstrate no change in symptoms.

2 The duration of Tensilon's action is about 3 minutes.

4 Tensilon acts systemically on all muscles, rather than selectively on the eyelids.

582. 3 **Until the diagnosis is confirmed, the primary goal should be to maintain adequate activity and prevent muscle atrophy.**

1 It is too early to develop a teaching plan; the diagnosis is not yet established.

2 This is too early; the client cannot adjust if a diagnosis is not yet confirmed.

4 This is not a goal.

583. 3 **Respiratory failure will require emergency intervention, and inability to swallow may lead to aspiration.**

1 Difficulty with chewing and speaking are signs of myasthenia gravis that may occur but are not life threatening.

2 Ocular palsies and an inability to smile are signs of myasthenia gravis that may occur but are not life threatening.

4 Although the client's level of anxiety and concerns about the diagnosis are important, they are not the most significant assessments.

584. 4 **Exacerbation of myasthenia gravis may occur temporarily at the beginning of steroid therapy, causing respiratory embarrassment and dysphagia.**

1 This is contraindicated because steroids increase sodium retention.

2 Although clients should avoid contact with persons having upper respiratory infections, protective isolation (neutropenic precautions) is not required.

3 This is unnecessary; adequate fluid intake should be maintained.

585. 1 **Spacing activities encourages maximum functioning within the limits of the client's strength and endurance.**

2 Bed rest and limited activity may lead to muscle atrophy and calcium depletion.

3 This is necessary for lifelong psychological adjustment, but does not address the client's concerns at this time.

4 This should be permitted if requested by the client or family, but does not address the concerns voiced by the client.

586. Answer: 2, 4, 5

1 Although this is a neuromuscular disorder, headaches are not a common symptom.

2 **Involuntary, rhythmic movements of the eyes (nystagmus) and other visual disturbances, such as diplopia and blurred vision, are common initial symptoms of optic nerve lesions.**

3 Pressure ulcers may occur late, not early, in the progression of the illness because of immobility, and these pressure ulcers may become infected.

4 **The most common initial signs of multiple sclerosis are scanning speech, intention tremors, and nystagmus; this group of signs is known as Charcot's triad. These adaptations are associated with disseminated demyelination of nerve fibers of the brain and spinal cord.**

5   The most common initial signs of multiple sclerosis are scanning speech, intention tremors, and nystagmus; this group of signs is known as Charcot's triad. These adaptations are associated with disseminated demyelination of nerve fibers of the brain and spinal cord.

587. 2   **A client diagnosed with Guillain-Barré syndrome may have plasmapheresis as part of treatment. Plasmapheresis is the removal of plasma from withdrawn blood followed by the reconstitution of its cellular components in an isotonic solution and the reinfusion of this solution.**

1   A client with Guillain-Barré syndrome, in the absence of kidney disease, does not need hemodialysis.

3   Guillain-Barré syndrome is not a hematological disorder; thrombolytic therapy is not required.

4   Guillain-Barré syndrome is not an autoimmune disorder; immunosuppressive therapy is not required.

588. 2   **Muscular weakness with paralysis results from impaired nerve conduction because the motor nerves become demyelinated.**

1   This usually is not a problem; motor loss is greater than sensory loss, with paresthesia of the extremities being the most frequent sensory loss.

3   Demyelination occurs rapidly early in the disease and the muscles will not have had time to atrophy; this can occur later if rehabilitation is delayed.

4   Only the peripheral nerves are involved; the central nervous system is unaffected.

589. 1   **Rehabilitation needs for a client with Guillain-Barré syndrome focus on physical therapy and exercise for the lower extremities because of muscle weakness and discomfort.**

2   A client with Guillain-Barré syndrome does not need speech or swallowing exercises.

3   A client with Guillain-Barré syndrome does not need vertebral support.

4   Problems with cataracts are not associated with Guillain-Barré syndrome.

590. 3   **This is a truthful answer that provides hope for the client.**

1   This response avoids the client's question and can increase anxiety.

2   Analgesics commonly are not prescribed unless pain results from some other condition.

4   This avoids the client's question; the nurse should respond directly.

591. 3   **The client must be flexible and adjust activities to provide for rest when necessary; activity should cease before the point of fatigue.**

1   Although quality time with children is important, it must be done on a flexible schedule to prevent fatigue.

2   Although laudable, it cannot be done if the client is in need of support or if it overtaxes physical resources.

4   This may not be a need at this time; prevention of fatigue always is important.

592. 2   **Instilling artificial tears frequently lubricates the left eye and prevents drying of the cornea.**

1   Irrigating the left eye is inappropriate; eye irrigations are used to flush foreign matter from the eye.

3   Checking the corneal reflex every hour can lead to corneal abrasion.

4   Taping the left eyelid open can cause corneal ulceration or injury.

593. 1   **The Glasgow Coma Scale is used to assess the extent of neurological damage; it consists of three assessments: eye opening, response to auditory stimuli, and motor response. Consciousness exists on a continuum from full consciousness to coma. A score can be from 3 to 15; the lower the score the more indicative of coma.**

2   To achieve this rating the client must be exhibiting some meaningful responses.

3   To achieve this rating the client must be exhibiting some meaningful responses.

4   A score of 15 represents normal neurological functioning.

594. 1   **Limbs hyperextended and arms hyperpronated (extension posturing, decerebrate posturing) indicate upper brainstem damage; this is a grave sign.**

2   This is associated with an upper motor neuron disease or lesion.

3   This is associated with flexion posturing (decorticate posturing), which indicates damage to the pyramidal motor tract above the brainstem.

4   This is associated with a lower motor neuron disease or lesion.

595. 3   **This occurs because of the brain's acute sensitivity to hypoxia.**

1   The respirations usually are depressed because of brainstem compression.

2   The systolic pressure increases and the diastolic pressure decreases, resulting in a widening, not narrowing, pulse pressure.

4   The peripheral vascular resistance is decreased when hypoxia occurs, thereby decreasing, not increasing, the diastolic blood pressure.

596. 3   **Elevating the head of the bed increases drainage of cerebrospinal fluid and decreases intracranial pressure.**

1   This position will not promote cerebral drainage and may lead to increased intracranial pressure.

2   This position will not promote cerebral drainage and may lead to increased intracranial pressure.

4   This will increase retention of cerebrospinal fluid and increase intracranial pressure.

597. 4   **This is vital in case of respiratory distress; increased intracranial pressure compresses the brainstem, which contains the medulla, the respiratory center.**

1   This is important but not of primary urgency; the respiratory status is the priority.

2 This is important but not of primary urgency; the respiratory status is the priority.

3 This is important but not of primary urgency; the respiratory status is the priority.

598. 4 **A fracture at the base of the cranium can tear meninges, causing nasal leakage of cerebrospinal fluid (rhinorrhea) and bleeding from the ear.**

1 A bruise will not cause these responses.

2 A severe jarring of the brain will not cause these responses.

3 A nose fracture will not produce a clear drainage, and the ears will not be draining.

599. 3 **Increased restlessness indicates a lack of oxygen to the brainstem; cerebral hypoxia impairs the reticular activating system.**

1 Urine output is not related to increased intracranial pressure.

2 The respiratory rate will decrease.

4 The pulse will be slow and bounding.

600. 1 **Withdrawing the leg is an appropriate response, a purposeful withdrawal from pain.**

2 Making no movement may indicate cortical or midbrain compression.

3 Plantar flexion occurs with flexion posturing (decorticate posturing) or extension posturing (decerebrate posturing); these are associated with brain dysfunction.

4 Flexing the upper extremities, with leg extension and plantar flexion, indicates flexion posturing (decorticate posturing); this indicates dysfunction of the cerebral cortex or lesions of the corticospinal tracts above the brainstem.

601. 2 **Encouraging fluids will hydrate the client and contribute to the restoration of cerebrospinal fluid, which cushions the brain; this should ease the pain.**

1 Early ambulation will increase the pain; the client should be maintained in the supine position and kept quiet.

3 This is contraindicated for a postoperative client; the removal of antiembolism stockings will not influence a post–spinal anesthesia headache.

4 This will increase the pain; the client should be maintained in the supine position and kept quiet.

602. 3 **In an attempt to stop the bleeding, adjacent arteries constrict; this in turn contributes to the ischemia responsible for the neurological deficits.**

1 The volume of blood loss is not great enough to significantly alter the oxygen-carrying capability of the remaining blood supply.

2 Although prolonged ischemia may cause necrosis, many of the manifestations of cerebral ischemia are reversed as pressure diminishes, and there may be no permanent damage.

4 Severe electrolyte imbalance may cause generalized weakness; however, hemiparesis and aphasia are not the result of electrolyte loss.

603. 3 **With the head of the bed elevated the force of gravity helps prevent additional intracranial pressure, which will intensify the ischemic manifestations of hemorrhage.**

1 The supine position will not facilitate drainage of cerebral fluid; this position promotes accumulation of fluid, which increases intracranial pressure.

2 Lying on the unaffected side will not facilitate drainage of cerebral fluid; this position promotes accumulation of fluid, which increases intracranial pressure.

4 Vomiting can occur with increased intracranial pressure, and placing sandbags to immobilize the head can result in aspiration.

604. 4 **Controlled ventilation induces hypocapnia; subsequently it causes vasoconstriction and reduced cerebral blood flow.**

1 The fluid may be cerebrospinal fluid; clearing the ear may cause further damage.

2 Because of manipulation during a craniotomy, anticonvulsants are given prophylactically to prevent seizures.

3 Elevating the head of the bed 30 degrees will not increase cerebral blood flow.

605. 2 **Although suctioning is done to maintain an airway, it is not done routinely because it increases intracranial pressure.**

1 Lubricating the skin keeps the skin from drying, which helps prevent skin breakdown.

3 Elevating the head of the bed promotes venous return to the heart and is used to limit increased intracranial pressure.

4 Instilling artificial tears every 2 hours is the appropriate intervention. The corneal reflex may be absent in the unconscious client; a dry cornea is prone to injury.

606. 1 **Immediate corrective therapy based on current assessments must be implemented.**

2 After an infratentorial craniotomy the client is positioned flat on one side with the head on a small firm pillow unless otherwise instructed by the surgeon.

3 Although this is an appropriate action, it is not the priority until the surgeon is notified.

4 Administering a medication is a dependent function of the nurse and the order must be followed exactly.

607. 3 **This position lessens the possibility of hemorrhage, provides for better circulation of cerebrospinal fluid, and promotes venous return.**

1 Gatching the knees is contraindicated because it can increase intracranial pressure.

2 This position is appropriate after infratentorial surgery.

4 This position impedes venous return, thus increasing intracranial pressure.

608. 2 **Kernig's sign, which is an inability to completely extend the legs, is the classic sign of meningeal irritation.**
   1 "Sunset eyes" is associated with hydrocephalus; it occurs when the eyelid falls above the iris, allowing the sclera to show. It occurs only in infants whose cranial bones have not yet fused.
   3 Plantar reflex, a spinal cord reflex, is unrelated to meningeal irritation.
   4 Homans' sign indicates the presence of thrombophlebitis; pain is experienced when the foot is dorsiflexed because of vascular irritability.

609. 1 **Recognition of effort is motivating.**
   2 Correcting mistakes may decrease both self-esteem and motivation.
   3 The problem is a motor, not a sensory (receptive), problem.
   4 Reexplaining the reason for the difficulty may decrease self-esteem and motivation.

610. 1 **An increase in intraocular pressure (IOP) results from a resistance of aqueous humor outflow. Open-angle glaucoma, the most common type of glaucoma, results from increased resistance to aqueous humor outflow through the trabecular meshwork, Schlemm's canal, and the episcleral venous system.**
   2 This is the description of a cataract.
   3 This is the description of astigmatism.
   4 This is the description of a detached retina.

611. 4 **Increased intraocular pressure damages the optic nerve, interfering with peripheral vision.**
   1 Flashes of light may be associated with a detached retina.
   2 There is difficulty in adjusting to darkness, not an intolerance to light.
   3 Seeing floating specks is not specific to glaucoma.

612. 2 **Primary open-angle glaucoma (POAG) progresses gradually without symptoms. Peripheral vision slowly disappears until tunnel vision occurs in which there is only a small center field. Without treatment, eventually all vision is lost.**
   1 POAG is not related to the development of cataracts.
   3 POAG is not related to the development of retinal detachment.
   4 POAG is not related to the development of blurred distance vision.

613. 1 **Coughing is contraindicated; this increases intraocular pressure.**
   2 Lying on the unaffected side or in the supine position will minimize intraocular pressure.
   3 Moving around freely in bed is contraindicated; this increases intraocular pressure.
   4 Elevating the head of the bed is not necessary.

614. 4 **The eye shield will prevent injury to the newly operated eye.**
   1 Only the affected eye will be covered.
   2 This is not necessary.

3 Coughing is contraindicated in clients who have had cataract surgery because it increases intraocular pressure.

615. 1 **An antiemetic will prevent vomiting; vomiting increases intraocular pressure and should be avoided.**
   2 Vomiting increases intraocular pressure, and aggressive intervention is required.
   3 This usually is not expected.
   4 Deep breathing will not minimize nausea and may actually cause respiratory alkalosis; aggressive intervention is required to prevent vomiting.

616. 1 **Acute postoperative pain is a sign of increased intraocular pressure and is caused by hemorrhaging; this is a medical emergency.**
   2 Postoperative discomfort usually is minimal.
   3 Isolation and sensory deprivation will not occur because only one eye is patched.
   4 The shield may be slightly uncomfortable but will not cause severe discomfort.

617. 4 **Postoperatively the client must check daily for signs of rejection, which include redness, irritation, discomfort, or vision loss; the surgeon should be notified if any of these develop; pain after a cataract extraction may indicate infection or hemorrhage and should be reported to the surgeon immediately.**
   1 Driving is contraindicated until the client is given specific permission to do so by the surgeon.
   2 Soap may irritate the eye, and showers or shampooing the hair should be avoided as instructed.
   3 This is a symptom of retinal detachment and is not expected.

618. 3 **To protect against physical injury and infection, the dropper tip should not touch the eye.**
   1 Drops are placed within the lower lid (conjunctival sac).
   2 The lower lid is retracted for placement of eye drops.
   4 Squeezing the eyes shut after administration of the medication should be avoided; this will squeeze medication out of the eye.

619. 3 **This subjective symptom is caused by vitreous traction on the retina.**
   1 Glaucoma causes the individual to see halos around lights.
   2 Scleroderma is a disease of the connective tissue, not the eye.
   4 Cerebral concussions do not result in this ocular symptom.

620. 4 **This indicates that hemorrhage may be occurring in the eye.**
   1 Four hours is too soon to be concerned that the client has not voided.
   2 The eye is patched; in addition, there is edema of the lid, which can interfere with opening the eye.
   3 This may occur in an unfamiliar environment with the eye patched, especially in older adults.

621. 1 The medications usually prescribed for clients with retinal detachment reduce the eye's ability to adjust to light because straining, as well as excess activity, can increase intraocular pressure.

2 The eye movements associated with reading can be uncomfortable and should not be encouraged at this time.

3 Generally, new lenses will be required in 3 months or sooner.

4 Clients should avoid straining and not resume usual activities until given permission.

622. 3 The nerves for arm innervation are at C4, which is above the injury level of T2.

1 Diaphragm innervation is not affected by this injury; the diaphragm is innervated above C4.

2 Innervation of muscles used to move the lower arms is not affected by this injury; these muscles are innervated above C7.

4 Innervation for pain sensation of the hands is not affected by this injury; these nerves are innervated above C7.

623. 2 The T6 level is the sympathetic visceral outflow level. Because the client's injury is above this level (T2), autonomic hyperreflexia is expected.

1 The reflex arc remains intact after spinal cord injury.

3 The important point is not that the cord is transected, but the level at which the injury occurred.

4 This is not related to autonomic hyperreflexia. All cord injuries result in flaccid paralysis during the period of spinal shock; as the inflammation subsides, spasticity gradually increases.

624. 4 These signs occur as a result of exaggerated autonomic responses. If autonomic hyperreflexia is identified, immediate intervention is necessary to prevent serious complications.

1 Paralysis is related to transection, not autonomic hyperreflexia; the client will have no sensation below the injury.

2 Profuse diaphoresis occurs.

3 Bradycardia occurs.

625. 4 If the client has the capability to perform personal hygiene activities, it will help maintain a positive identity. This is necessary for progression to long-term goals.

1 This is a long-term goal.

2 This is a long-term goal.

3 This is a long-term goal.

626. 2 Arm strength is necessary for transfers and activities of daily living and for the use of crutches or a wheelchair.

1 The client does not have neurological control of this activity.

3 Equilibrium is not a problem.

4 The client does not have neurological control of this activity.

627. 2 A cervical spine injury may result in respiratory distress because of impaired muscle function, and respiratory monitoring can guide the decision to use mechanical ventilation. If not treated, atelectasis, pneumonia, and aspiration can occur.

1 The client should be monitored for bradycardia and decreased cardiac output, not tachycardia.

3 Although bladder distention can occur because of loss of autonomic and reflex control, it is not life threatening because an indwelling urinary catheter can ensure emptying of the bladder.

4 Hypotension, not hypertension, will occur.

628. The T6 level is the sympathetic visceral outflow level and any injury at or above this level can result in episodes of autonomic hyperreflexia; the client with an injury below the T6 level is not prone to episodes of autonomic hyperreflexia.

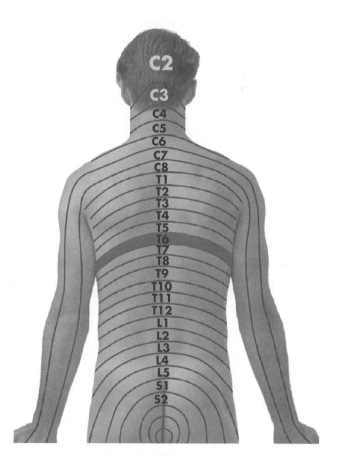

629. 3 Injury and pressure at the nerve roots produce pain.

1 Injury at T6 and T7 is too low to cause paralysis of the respiratory muscles; control of respirations is in the medulla and the cervical plexus (phrenic nerve).

2 With complete crushing at the T6 and T7 level, there is no pain sensation in parts distal to the injury.

4 Initially, paralysis is flaccid; spasticity is a later manifestation.

630. 3 **This response offers the realistic assurance that nothing is wrong and encourages the client to relate information to the nurse.**
   1 This action will not decrease the numbness; nerve root irritation will lessen only with time.
   2 This response tells the client there is a problem when, in reality, there is no reason to call the surgeon.
   4 This provides false reassurance; nerve root numbness lessens only with time.

631. 1 **Narrowing of arteries supplying the brain causes temporary neurological deficits that last for a short period. Between attacks, neurological functioning is normal.**
   2 Emboli result in a brain attack (CVA); with a CVA the damage usually is permanent, not intermittent.
   3 This occurs with multiple small brain attacks; TIAs do not result in permanent damage.
   4 This is not the description of a TIA; remissions and exacerbations occur with progressive degenerative neurological disorders.

632. 1 **The cause of the hypotension must be evaluated by the surgeon.**
   2 Increasing the IV flow rate is a dependent function that requires a practitioner's order.
   3 Raising the head of the bed will further decrease blood flow to the brain.
   4 The Trendelenburg position is contraindicated because it will increase pressure in the carotid arteries.

633. 3 **Muscles used for swallowing are innervated by the ninth (glossopharyngeal) and tenth (vagus) cranial nerves.**
   1 Dyspnea is unrelated to cranial nerves; this is associated with neck edema and potential compromise of the airway.
   2 Edema of the neck will not influence the cranial nerves; some edema is expected because of the inflammatory process at the site of surgery.
   4 Alterations in blood pressure may occur but are not caused by cranial nerve dysfunction.

634. 2 **This assessment will reveal whether there is a progression of symptoms. These data will assist the practitioner in determining a diagnosis.**
   1 An elevation in temperature is not an early sign of an extension of a brain attack (CVA).
   3 The data indicate that the client does not have hypertension. Although vital signs should be monitored, the client's motor status in this instance is most significant.
   4 This is not the priority assessment.

635. 2 **Increasing intracranial pressure is evidenced by an increased pulse pressure and blood pressure and a decreased pulse rate; the practitioner should be notified.**
   1 The pulse rate has increased and the BP has decreased; these are not signs of increased intracranial pressure.

3 Although the pulse rate has decreased, the BP has not increased; these are not signs of increased intracranial pressure.
   4 Although the pulse rate has decreased and the BP has increased slightly, the pulse pressure has narrowed; this is not a sign of increased intracranial pressure.

636. 3 **This position will neither raise intracranial pressure nor interfere with respirations and will permit oral secretions to drain from the mouth by gravity.**
   1 This can compromise the airway by permitting the tongue to fall to the posterior pharynx and obstruct the airway.
   2 Elevating the head of the bed can compromise vital functions by compressing the brainstem.
   4 This is contraindicated because it may increase intracranial pressure.

637. 4 **Increased intracranial pressure is manifested by a sluggish pupillary reaction and elevation of the systolic blood pressure.**
   1 Spinal shock is manifested by a decreased systolic blood pressure with no pupillary changes.
   2 Hypovolemic shock is indicated by a decrease in systolic pressure and tachycardia with no changes in pupillary reaction.
   3 Transtentorial herniation is manifested by dilated pupils and severe posturing.

638. 4 **This position produces dorsiflexion of the feet and prevents the tendons from shortening, preventing footdrop.**
   1 This will not prevent plantar flexion; it can promote hip and knee flexion contractures.
   2 This will not prevent plantar flexion; it can promote hip and knee flexion contractures.
   3 The client will not have the ability or strength to perform range-of-motion exercises unassisted at this time.

639. 2 **The client has lost vision from the right visual field; scanning compensates for this loss.**
   1 This approach is used for clients with apraxia (inability to manipulate objects).
   3 This increases neglect of the affected side.
   4 This approach is used for denial of the right side (unilateral neglect).

640. 3 **Recovery from aphasia is a continuous process; the amount of recovery cannot be predicted.**
   1 This gives false reassurance; it may take a year or longer or may never return.
   2 This response abdicates the nurse's responsibility; the physician cannot predict return of function.
   4 Speech return is a continuous process; it may take a year or longer or may never return.

641. 4 **In addition to the extent of injury, a factor in relearning speech is the client's motivation and effort; the more the client attempts to talk, the**

more likely speech will progress to its optimum level; relearning is a slow process.

1 Clients with aphasia are not deaf.

2 This will create frustration and may infuriate the client.

3 Although the nurse should instruct the family to approve and support the client's efforts to communicate, this support should be for the effort, not for correct communication.

642. 4 **A weak grasp, pain, and uncoordinated movements can result in the dropping of tools, which can be dangerous.**

1 Although this can be a problem, safety is the priority.

2 Although this can be a problem, safety is the priority.

3 Although this may become an issue in the future if the client can no longer work, at this time safety is the priority.

643. 2 **Rhythmic contraction and relaxation associated with a tonic-clonic seizure can cause repeated banging of the head.**

1 This is contraindicated because it can cause broken bones.

3 This is contraindicated because damage to the teeth can occur if force is used to insert an airway.

4 Moving during a seizure can result in physical injuries; the client should be moved after the seizure.

RESPIRATORY

644. 3 **The client is in respiratory acidosis probably caused by the depressant effects of anesthesia or a partially obstructed airway; these activities clear the airway and blow off CO_2.**

1 This will not correct respiratory acidosis and may aggravate it if potassium is depleted.

2 This is the treatment for respiratory alkalosis; the client is in respiratory acidosis.

4 This is not necessary if clearing of the airway rectifies the problem.

645. 4 **A general anesthetic is delivered via an endotracheal tube that irritates the posterior pharynx and larynx and causes discomfort when swallowing.**

1 This is not an effect of general anesthesia.

2 Occasionally this may occur; however, it is a systemic, not a local, effect.

3 Occasionally this may occur; however, it is a systemic, not a local, effect.

646. 1 **Both sides of the posterior pharynx should be touched to elicit the gag reflex; absence of the reflex indicates that the client is at risk for aspiration of secretions or fluid.**

2 If the gag reflex is absent, the client may aspirate.

3 This can happen even in the absence of a gag reflex.

4 The client might be able to breathe deeply and cough without an adequate gag reflex.

647. 4 **There is no respiratory movement in stage 4 of anesthesia; before this stage, respirations are depressed but present.**

1 The gag reflex is lost in stage 3 of anesthesia.

2 Eyelid reflexes are lost in stage 2 of anesthesia.

3 Voluntary control is lost in stage 2 of anesthesia.

648. 1 **To allow for the insertion of the bronchoscope, throat muscles are anesthetized, diminishing the protective gag reflex.**

2 Dysphasia is difficulty in talking and does not occur with a bronchoscopy.

3 This does not occur after a bronchoscopy.

4 A general anesthetic usually is not used; therefore, paralytic ileus is not a complication.

649. 1 **This may be indicative of bleeding and the practitioner should be notified.**

2 Overlooking the first signs of hemorrhage may permit the client to go into shock.

3 Continuing to only monitor the client is unsafe. This is a potentially life-threatening situation; the practitioner should be notified immediately.

4 This can precipitate bleeding because of an increase in intrathoracic pressure.

650. 2 **This facilitates full expansion of the affected area and promotes drainage by gravity.**

1 This position relieves pain but compromises expansion of the affected lung and therefore should be avoided.

3 Lying on the affected side is most comfortable, but it will not promote aeration of the affected lung. Lying on the unaffected side promotes expansion and drainage of the affected lung and should be encouraged.

4 This position does not stimulate deep breathing; gravity keeps secretions lower in the lungs.

651. 4 **Increased fluid intake helps to liquefy respiratory secretions, which promotes expectoration.**

1 Oxygen may dry the mucous membranes, which may thicken secretions; oxygen should be administered only when necessary.

2 Retained secretions are in the bronchi and trachea; gargling lubricates only the oropharynx.

3 This position promotes retention of secretions; supine, prone, and Trendelenburg positions promote removal of secretions via gravity.

652. 4 **Air is moisturized and warmed as it passes through the nasopharynx. With a laryngectomy this area is bypassed and the tracheobronchial tree compensates by producing copious amounts of secretions.**

1 This will produce local irritation and a local response.

2 This is not a response to allergies but to the stress of the air that is entering the tracheobronchial tract. The air is no longer warmed or humidified by passing though the nose.

3 This response occurs regardless of turning, coughing, and deep breathing.

653. 2 **In this position the tongue does not obstruct the airway so that drainage of secretions, and oxygen and carbon dioxide exchange, can occur.**
    1 Oxygen may not be necessary; a patent airway takes priority.
    3 This assesses ventilation but does not support it.
    4 Once the pharyngeal reflex has returned, an in-place airway can cause the client to gag and vomit, and it should be removed; the client may or may not be conscious.

654. 3 **One of the causes of both SARS and the common cold is the coronavirus.**
    1 Malaria is caused by a species of the protozoan *Plasmodium*; it is spread by the bite from an infected female *Anopheles* mosquito (vector).
    2 Tularemia is caused by the bacillus *Francisella (Pasteurella) tularensis*; it can be transmitted by an insect (vector) or by direct contact.
    4 Legionnaires' disease is caused by a bacterium of the genus *Legionella*, a group of gram-negative, aerobic bacilli.

655. 1 **Decreased breath sounds result from reduced airflow, pleural effusion, and destruction of lung tissue.**
    2 There is enlargement of accessory muscles that are used during the expiratory phase to help force air out of the lungs.
    3 There is an increased AP diameter (barrel chest) because of air trapping and enlargement of the lungs with a loss of recoil ability.
    4 There is an increased expiratory phase of the respiratory cycle because of entrapment of air and collapse of airways.

656. 4 **Oxygen saturation is a measure of the relationship between oxygen and hemoglobin; it measures the amount of oxygen available to tissues and provides a pulmonary assessment for clients at risk for hypoxia; pulse oximetry provides a continuous, noninvasive measurement of an individual's oxygen saturation.**
    1 Po_2 is a measure of diffusion across the alveolar membrane. This value may progressively decrease in a heavy smoker, thus it is not the most accurate measure of this client's postoperative respiratory status. Also, it requires an arterial puncture.
    2 Pco_2 is an accurate measure of alveolar ventilation and is elevated with hypoventilation. This may occur in any client after abdominal surgery because deep breathing often is painful. Also an arterial puncture is necessary to acquire a specimen for testing.
    3 Hemoglobin is a measure of the blood's capacity to transport oxygen.

657. 3 **These are normal respiratory sounds heard on auscultation as inspired air enters and leaves the alveoli.**

    1 Adventitious is the general term for all abnormal breath sounds.
    2 Crackles heard at the end of an inspiration are associated with pulmonary edema.
    4 Diminished breath sounds are evidence of a reduction in the amount of air entering the alveoli; this usually is caused by obstruction or consolidation.

658. 2 **Oxygen and carbon dioxide exchange is essential for life and is the priority.**
    1 This is not the priority.
    3 This is unnecessary with a left-sided pneumonectomy because there is no lung to reinflate.
    4 This is not the priority.

659. 2 **Coarse crackles (rhonchi), particularly on expiration, indicate partial airway obstruction because of bronchiolar alterations associated with COPD.**
    1 Snorting sounds are made in the nose.
    3 Wheezes are musical sounds usually heard during expiration; they are caused by rapid vibration of bronchial walls.
    4 Crackling sounds heard on inspiration that are unchanged by coughing are known as fine crackles; they result when air passes through alveoli that are partially filled with fluid.

660. 3 **Singed nasal hair and nasal discharges that contain carbon are warning signs of respiratory inhalation.**
    1 Changes in chest x-ray findings are a late sign of respiratory problems.
    2 This may be a sign of pneumonia or tuberculosis.
    4 Changes in arterial blood gases are late signs of respiratory problems.

661. 3 **This position promotes lung expansion and gas exchange; it also decreases venous return and cardiac workload.**
    1 This may be done, but positioning should be done first because it will have an immediate effect. Time is needed to set up the system for the delivery of oxygen.
    2 Maintaining adequate oxygen exchange is the priority; an x-ray film can be obtained, but after breathing is supported.
    4 A friction rub is related to inflammation of the pleura, not to heart failure.

662. 1 **Stridor is a high-pitched harsh sound caused by an obstruction of the trachea or larynx.**
    2 Neck exercises are important for total rehabilitation; neck exercises do not help identify stridor.
    3 Auscultating the base of the lungs will determine the presence of vesicular breath sounds or crackles.
    4 Although coughing and deep breathing are important, they do not help identify stridor.

663. Answer: 4, 5
    1 Short breaths do not expand the lungs; deep slow breaths at 16 per minute should be encouraged.

2 Exhalation with pursed lips, not with an open mouth, promotes exhalation of air from the lung and minimizes trapping of air in the alveoli.

3 Breathing exercises should be performed at least every 2 hours.

4 Abdominal breathing improves lung expansion because it makes the contraction of the diaphragm more efficient. Placing the hand on the abdomen provides feedback ensuring that abdominal rather than intercostal breathing is accomplished.

5 This action allows several additional seconds for oxygen and carbon dioxide to exchange in the alveoli.

664. **3 This is secondary to cerebral hypoxia, which accompanies acute respiratory distress syndrome (ARDS); cognition and level of consciousness are reduced.**

1 Hypotension occurs because of hypoxia.

2 The sputum is not tenacious, but it may be frothy if pulmonary edema is present.

4 Breathing will be fast and shallow.

665. **4 The effectiveness of therapy is measured by the client's response.**

1 Endotracheal intubation does not permit verbal communication.

2 This is presumptive; the database is inadequate for this conclusion.

3 This is important but not the priority.

666. **4 Fractured ribs cause extreme pain, especially on inhalation; this induces shallow breathing, which results in carbon dioxide retention.**

1 Although decreased respiratory functioning can result in an infection, respiratory acidosis is the immediate concern.

2 Blood in vomitus is unrelated to fractured ribs.

3 Fluid in lung tissue is unrelated to fractured ribs; it is associated with heart failure.

667. **4 Increased rate and depth of breathing result in excessive elimination of CO_2, and respiratory alkalosis can result.**

1 Hypoxia is associated with respiratory acidosis, not respiratory alkalosis, which is related to hyperventilation.

2 With hyperventilation, CO_2 levels will be decreased (hypocapnia), not elevated.

3 Metabolic acidosis results from excess hydrogen ions caused by a metabolic problem, not a respiratory problem.

668. **2 This is necessary to prevent flooding of the trachea with fluid; some systems have receptacles attached to the tubing to collect the fluid and others have to be temporarily disconnected while emptying the fluid.**

1 This circumstance does not require assistance from a respiratory therapist.

3 Humidity is necessary to preserve moistness of the respiratory tract and help liquefy secretions.

4 The amount of condensation is irrelevant when recording total intake and output.

669. **3 This promotes breathing by reducing the pressure of the abdominal organs on the diaphragm and increasing thoracic excursion.**

1 This may confirm diminished breath sounds but will not facilitate breathing.

2 This eventually should be done, but it is not the priority.

4 This will impede aeration of the right lung fields.

670. **2 Suctioning removes not only secretions but also oxygen, which can cause cardiac dysrhythmias; the nurse should try to prevent this by hyperoxygenating the client before and after suctioning.**

1 To prevent trauma to the trachea, suction should be applied only while removing the catheter.

3 Short, jabbing movements can cause tracheal damage.

4 Suction should be performed only as needed to maintain a patent airway; excessive suctioning irritates the mucosa, which increases secretion production.

671. **4 This occludes the tracheal lumen around the tracheostomy tube, preventing aspiration if regurgitation occurs.**

1 This will permit aspiration if regurgitation occurs.

2 Although the cuff must be inflated during the tube feeding as well as after to prevent aspiration, it is done just before feeding, not 1 hour before.

3 This will permit aspiration if regurgitation occurs.

672. **3 These cuffs do not compress the capillary beds and thus do not cause tracheal damage.**

1 A minimal air leak is desirable to ensure the lowest possible pressure in the cuff while still maintaining placement of the tube.

2 Surgical asepsis, not the use of these cuffs, prevents infection.

4 Secretions are increased because the cuff is a foreign body in the trachea.

673. **2 Internal bleeding after nasal surgery may flow by gravity to the posterior oropharynx, where it is swallowed.**

1 Facial edema is expected after the trauma of surgery.

3 The edema that results from the trauma of surgery may be perceived as pressure around the eye; although it is expected, it is not a priority.

4 Pink-tinged drainage on the nasal packing and nasal drip dressing is expected for 24 to 48 hours after surgery.

674. **1 Sneezing involves high pressures in the respiratory passageways during the expulsive phase of a sneeze; this can disrupt sutures or alignment of bone and therefore should be avoided.**

2 This is not a necessity; the client's regular routine may be followed.

3 Fluids that are soothing for the client are given at any temperature; cool or warm temperatures usually are preferred.

4 This position promotes the accumulation of facial edema and possible aspiration of drainage; the semi- to high Fowler's positions are preferred.

675. 4 **Emphysema involves destructive changes in the alveolar walls, leading to dilation of the air sacs; there is subsequent air trapping and difficulty with expiration.**
   1 Bronchospasm is characteristic of asthma, not emphysema.
   2 The vital capacity is decreased because of restriction of the diaphragm and thoracic movement.
   3 Expiration is slowed by pursed-lip breathing to keep the airways open so less air is trapped.

676. 3 **This permits more complete exhalation and emptying of carbon dioxide from the lungs.**
   1 This is contraindicated. It is believed that the client should receive low amounts of oxygen to prevent CO_2 intoxication (CO_2 narcosis). However, the results of one recent study of clients with stable COPD indicate that the hypercarbic drive is preserved. More research is needed before this theory is applied clinically.
   2 This is contraindicated because it increases carbon dioxide retention.
   4 These should be part of assessment, but assessment does not decrease dyspnea.

677. 2 **Accessory muscles are used during respiration because of the increased rigidity of the chest.**
   1 Sudden pleuritic chest pain is associated with pulmonary embolism, not emphysema.
   3 Respiratory acidosis, not alkalosis, is associated with emphysema because of carbon dioxide retention.
   4 Emphysema is accompanied by a prolonged expiratory phase.

678. 3 **With chronically high levels of carbon dioxide it is believed that decreased oxygen levels become the stimulus to breathe; high oxygen administration negates this mechanism. However, the results of one recent study of clients with stable COPD indicate that the hypercarbic drive is preserved. More research is needed before this theory is applied clinically.**
   1 This is an appropriate intervention, but is not directly related to CO_2 intoxication (CO_2 narcosis).
   2 This will not bring oxygen into the alveoli for exchange nor will it adequately remove carbon dioxide because it will increase bronchiolar obstruction.
   4 Inhalation should be of regular depth, and expiration should be prolonged to prevent carbon dioxide trapping (air trapping).

679. 4 **With emphysema it is believed that the respiratory center no longer responds to elevated carbon dioxide as the stimulus to breathe but rather to lowered oxygen levels; therefore, the oxygen being delivered must be lowered to supply enough for oxygenation without being so elevated that it negates the stimulus to breathe. However, the results**
of one recent study of clients with stable COPD indicate that the hypercarbic drive is preserved. More research is needed before this theory is applied clinically.
   1 A confused client cannot answer questions about the confusion.
   2 The client has CO_2 intoxication (CO_2 narcosis); it is believed that increasing oxygen administration will further diminish the respiratory drive. However, the results of one recent study of clients with stable COPD indicate that the hypercarbic drive is preserved. More research is needed before this theory is applied clinically.
   3 There are no indications that respiratory secretions have increased.

680. 4 **Pressure from the dialysate may cause upward displacement of the diaphragm; the dialysate should be drained from the peritoneal cavity.**
   1 Additional fluid will aggravate the respiratory difficulty.
   2 The client should already be in the semi-Fowler's position.
   3 Auscultation is important, but it does not alleviate the respiratory difficulty.

681. 3 **This pause allows added time for gaseous exchange at the alveolar capillary beds.**
   1 Inhalation should be through the nose to moisten, filter, and warm the air.
   2 This decreases the effectiveness of respirations.
   4 The expiratory phase should be lengthened, and exhalation should be through pursed lips.

682. 3 **This indicates progressive respiratory failure; ventilatory support is needed when the P_{CO_2} is more than 40.**
   1 This will liquefy secretions, but will not correct the respiratory failure.
   2 This may dilate bronchi, but will not improve respiratory exchange to decrease CO_2.
   4 This will not correct respiratory failure.

683. 3 **This aids descent of the diaphragm so that more air can enter and fill the lungs.**
   1 Rapid breathing promotes respiratory alkalosis; diaphragmatic breathing includes slow deep breathing.
   2 The hands should be placed lightly on the abdomen to verify abdominal excursion.
   4 Diaphragmatic breathing may be performed in any position other than the prone or Trendelenburg; usually the semi-Fowler's position is used.

684. 2 **This is a positive step in reducing smoking; it is the first step toward stopping.**
   1 The client is postponing the decision to quit.
   3 The client is rationalizing why quitting smoking is too difficult.
   4 This is unrealistic because giving up smoking is difficult regardless of whether the client drinks alcohol.

685. 4 **The enlarged liver is caused by long-term respiratory acidosis with increased pulmonary pressure that eventually causes right ventricular enlargement and failure (cor pulmonale); the elevated pressure causes backup pressure in the hepatic circulation.**

1 Liver hypoxia will cause atrophy and necrosis of cells, not enlargement.

2 Right ventricular failure with increased pressure in the ascending vena cava causes increased pressure in the hepatoportal system, resulting in an enlarged liver, not hepatic acidosis.

3 Esophageal varices, dilated tortuous veins of the esophagus, are caused by hepatic portal hypertension; they are not the cause of an enlarged liver.

686. 1 **Breath sounds will be decreased in clients with COPD because of reduced airflow, pleural effusion, or lung parenchymal destruction.**

2 A pleural friction rub occurs when one layer of the pleural membrane slides over the other during breathing; this is associated with pleurisy.

3 Crackles indicate fluid in the alveoli, which is associated with heart failure or infection; crackles and gurgles (rhonchi) signify airway obstruction, not chronic obstructive lung disease.

4 Expiratory wheezing and coughing are associated with asthma or bronchitis.

687. 2 **A sudden weight gain is an initial sign of right ventricular failure caused by chronic obstructive pulmonary disease.**

1 Polycythemia is associated with polycythemia vera, not chronic obstructive pulmonary disease.

3 A sudden weight gain is not associated with compensated acidosis.

4 Right, not left, ventricular failure occurs with chronic obstructive pulmonary disease.

688. 1 **A humidifier will help liquefy secretions and promote their expectoration.**

2 Sleeping on pillows facilitates breathing; it does not relieve chest congestion.

3 Nonproductive coughing should be avoided because it is irritating and exhausting.

4 Deep breathing and coughing at night will not help relieve early morning congestion.

689. 1 **Eating small meals will decrease the amount of oxygen necessary for ingestion and digestion at any one time; a small volume of food in the stomach will not impede the downward movement of the diaphragm during inhalation.**

2 Although fluids can help liquefy secretions, they should not be encouraged for a client with heart failure.

3 Lying down increases intra-abdominal pressure, pushing a full stomach against the diaphragm and limiting respiratory excursion.

4 Protein maintains or increases hydrostatic pressure; it does not decrease it.

690. 4 **This technique results in nasal breathing, which negates the effects of aerosol medication. The mouthpiece should be gently held in the mouth just past the lips.**

1 The nebulizer tip should be past the lips to deliver the medication.

2 This promotes contact of the medication with the bronchial mucosa.

3 This prolongs and improves delivery of the medication to the respiratory mucosa.

691. 2 **This should not occur; it is evidence of a leak from the chest tube or the lung into the subcutaneous tissue.**

1 Clots are expected initially after surgery.

3 This occurs as the lung is reexpanding; bubbling stops completely when the lung is fully expanded.

4 Bloody drainage is expected immediately after surgery.

692. 4 **The left lung is collapsed; therefore, there are no breath sounds.**

1 A tympanic, not a dull, sound will be heard with a pneumothorax.

2 There is no vocal fremitus because there is no airflow into the left lung as a result of the pneumothorax.

3 These sounds will not be heard because there is no airflow into the left lung as a result of the pneumothorax.

693. 4 **With a pneumothorax, a chest tube attached to a closed chest drainage system removes trapped air and helps to reestablish negative pressure within the pleural space; this results in lung reinflation.**

1 A closed chest drainage system may be inserted to remove blood related to a hemothorax, not to assess for bleeding.

2 This is not the purpose of inserting chest tubes; the function of the lungs is monitored through the assessment of vital signs, breath sounds, arterial blood gases, and chest x-ray.

3 This is the reason for use of a closed chest drainage system when there is fluid in the pleural space.

694. 2 **The return of breath sounds indicates the lung has reinflated.**

1 A cough that raises sputum (productive cough) may indicate a complication such as infection.

3 The drainage should decrease, not increase.

4 Constant bubbling in the water-seal chamber indicates that there is a leak in the closed chest drainage system. Bubbling may occur in this chamber when air exits the pleural space with a cough or forceful expiration; the fluid will rise and fall in this chamber with pleural pressure changes associated with inspiration and expiration (tidaling).

695. 2 **There is air in the tissues, and palpation results in a crackling sound referred to as crepitus.**

1 This is a harsh high-pitched sound usually produced on inspiration because of airway obstruction.

3 This is excessive accumulation of fluid in tissue spaces.

4 The size of the chest is determined by the bony structure; a barrel chest with an increase in the AP diameter is associated with COPD, not cancer of the lung.

696. 2 **A mediastinal shift with airway obstruction may occur because pressure builds up on the operative side, causing the trachea to deviate toward the nonoperative side; assessment of the airway takes priority.**

1 This will eventually be done; further assessment is the priority.

3 This is not the priority; further assessment is the priority.

4 There is no need for a chest tube when a pneumonectomy is performed.

697. 3 **This helps to keep the airway patent and prevents atelectasis of the remaining lung by raising intrapleural pressure.**

1 Although important, it is not the priority.

2 This is done after the gag reflex returns.

4 This will restrict left lung expansion.

698. 3 **These positions permit ventilation of the remaining lung and prevent fluid from draining into the sutured bronchial stump.**

1 Lying on the nonoperative side restricts left lung excursion and may allow fluid to drain into the right bronchial stump.

2 Although the high-Fowler's position promotes ventilation, it is tiring.

4 Lying on the nonoperative side restricts left lung excursion and may allow fluid to drain into the right bronchial stump.

699. 1 **Loss of the large vascular lung and/or the presence of a mediastinal shift can result in cardiac overload.**

2 These signs are associated with hypoxia, which is a common complication of surgery and not unique to a pneumonectomy.

3 These are common complications of thoracic surgeries and are not unique to a pneumonectomy.

4 An elevated BP may be associated with cardiac overload, but the other signs are not unique to a pneumonectomy.

700. 1 **Excessive endotracheal secretions after a pneumonectomy require coughing routines that are effective but not exhausting.**

2 This is not specific for a client who has had a pneumonectomy.

3 This is too exhausting.

4 This is too exhausting.

701. 2 **A mediastinoscopy is an endoscopic examination of mediastinal lymph nodes through a small suprasternal incision; this is generally done to diagnose mediastinal involvement of pulmonary malignancy or other conditions.**

1 Chest tubes are not required unless the lungs are accidentally punctured; the client will have a small incision near the clavicle.

3 A bronchoscopy permits visualization of the mainstem bronchus.

4 Fluid is removed from the pleural space during a thoracentesis.

702. 4 **This is the lower-lateral chest, which is the area of greatest thoracic excursion. With visceral and parietal pleural inflammation (pleurisy), a low-pitched, coarse, grating sound is heard when the client breathes, particularly when approaching the height of inspiration.**

1 Bronchial breath sounds are heard over the trachea and at the nape of the neck on either side of the vertebrae. Bronchial sounds are loud, high pitched and hollow, with a short inspiratory phase and long expiratory phase.

2 Bronchovesicular breath sounds are heard on either side of the sternum or between the scapulae; bronchovesicular sounds have a moderate volume and medium pitch, with equal inspiratory and expiratory phases.

3 This is the area where vesicular breath sounds are heard. Vesicular sounds are soft and low pitched, with a long inspiratory phase and a short expiratory phase; they are heard over most lung fields.

703. 3 **Compression of the lung by fluid that accumulates at the base of the lungs reduces lung expansion and air exchange.**

1 There is no fluid in the alveoli, so no crackles are produced.

2 If there is tracheal deviation, it is away from the involved side.

4 Dullness is produced on percussion of the involved area.

704. 3 **Tension is placed on the pleura at the height of inspiration and causes pain.**

1 This is typical of heart failure.

2 This may indicate a pulmonary infection.

4 This may indicate a pulmonary infection.

705. 2 **The most significant and life-threatening complication of insertion of a subclavian catheter is a pneumothorax because of the proximity of the subclavian vein and the apex of the upper lobe of the lung; a client's respiratory status always is the priority.**

1 Although this may be done before TPN is begun, it is not the priority immediately after insertion of the catheter.

3 A baseline blood glucose level should be obtained before insertion of the catheter. After TPN is started, routine monitoring of blood glucose levels is important.

4 Although this should be done eventually, it is not the priority at this time.

706. 3 **A patent airway is the priority; therefore, removal of secretions is necessary.**

1 This is important, but not the priority immediately after surgery.

2   This is an important postoperative concern, but does not occur immediately.

4   Although important, it is not as important as a patent airway.

707. 4   This is the correct technique; deep inhalation promotes alveolar expansion, holding the breath promotes transfer of gases, and exhalation promotes lung recoil.

1   Coughing is done after deep breathing.

2   The breaths should not be in succession; they should be spaced by several regular breaths to avoid fatigue.

3   Although inhalation should be through the mouthpiece, exhalation should not occur through the mouthpiece.

708. 3   Oral intake should not be attempted after the procedure until the return of the gag reflex.

1   Even an alert person may choke and aspirate if eating or drinking is attempted while the pharyngeal wall is anesthetized.

2   Although some slight irritation may occur after the procedure, there usually is no painful sequela.

4   The client should be informed of the need for being NPO; anxiety is not a reason for withholding this information.

709. 3   There is still a pathway from the mouth to the stomach; eating patterns are not lost when a laryngectomy is performed.

1   There is no passage of air from the lungs to the nose; air is expelled through a tracheal stoma.

2   There is no passage of air from the lungs to the nose; air is expelled through a tracheal stoma.

4   Air passes through a tracheal stoma that bypasses the nose and olfactory organs.

710. 3   The client is at risk for airway obstruction; restlessness and dyspnea indicate hypoxia.

1   This is unimportant. The pharyngeal opening is sutured closed and a tracheal stoma is formed; the trachea is anatomically separate from the esophagus.

2   Cloudy drainage may indicate infection, which is not an immediate postoperative complication.

4   Edema is unlikely to cause dehiscence early in the postoperative period; a patent airway takes priority.

711. 1   Initial attempts at oral feedings may cause a choking feeling, which may produce severe coughing and raise secretions.

2   A nasogastric tube is unnecessary because swallowing does not have an adverse effect on the suture line.

3   Liquids are less obstructive than pureed foods in case aspiration occurs.

4   Pain medication may decrease the respiratory effort and depress the cough reflex.

712. 2   A chest tube drains the leaking chyle from the thoracic area; TPN provides nutrition, boosts immune defenses, and decreases thoracic duct flow.

Bed rest is recommended because lymphatic flow increases with activity.

1   A gastrostomy tube is not used because the client can eat and drink; a high-fat diet is contraindicated, but bed rest is recommended.

3   A rectal tube has no relationship to the drainage of chyle from the thoracic area; a low-fat diet and bed rest are recommended.

4   The nasogastric tube does not drain fluid from the thoracic area; a low-fat diet and bed rest are recommended. A low-fat diet of medium-chain triglycerides will reduce the production and flow of chyle.

713. 1   After a hemiglossectomy a client will have difficulty swallowing and expectorating oral secretions because of the trauma of surgery.

2   Although this may limit edema or pain, it will not maintain patency of an airway that is compromised by secretions.

3   A side-lying position will better facilitate drainage from the mouth.

4   The client may not be reactive or have energy to cough or expectorate; the priority is to prevent secretions from entering the respiratory tract.

714. 2   The cardiovascular and nervous systems of older adults are less flexible than those in a younger age group; postoperative hypoxia responds to oxygen.

1   This is unnecessary because it is a common reaction of older adults to anesthesia, which may be alleviated by oxygen.

3   Although necessary, this will not help the client adapt.

4   An anxiolytic may increase agitation.

715. 2   Serosanguineous drainage of 80 to 120 mL is expected during the first 24 hours; more than this amount of drainage should be reported.

1   Placing the client is this position will have no effect on the portable wound drainage system; it functions via negative pressure, not gravity.

3   Drainage of 180 mL in 6 hours is excessive and should be reported.

4   Although this will be done, it is secondary to notifying the practitioner.

716. 3   During chest surgery the negative pressure around the lung is disrupted and the lungs do not fill adequately during inspiration; chest tubes are inserted to reestablish negative intrapleural pressure.

1   Atelectasis refers to the collapse of alveoli or a lobule caused by a blockage of small airways; chest tubes do not cause or correct atelectasis.

2   Chest tubes are inserted into the intrapleural space, not the pericardial sac.

4   Although the amount of drainage from a chest tube is measured, the reason for a chest tube is to reestablish negative intrapleural pressure.

717. 1 Fluid in the water-seal chamber should rise and fall as the client breathes in and out (tidaling) until the lungs have expanded completely; a lack of tidaling on the second postoperative day indicates that the tube is obstructed.

2 This is contraindicated without an order because it can traumatize pleural tissue.

3 The level of the fluid, as long as it covers the tube in the water-seal chamber, does not affect tidaling.

4 Although full expansion of the lung will eliminate tidaling, an obstruction of the tube should be ruled out.

718. 1 This allows for measuring the output without interrupting the closed drainage system.

2 This is done only to obtain a specimen for diagnostic procedures.

3 This is done only when the drainage collection chamber is full and the closed chest drainage must continue.

4 Clamping the chest tube is contraindicated because it can precipitate a pneumothorax; opening the system destroys the sterility of the closed drainage system.

719. 2 Excessive bubbling indicates an air leak, which must be eliminated to permit lung expansion.

1 This is contraindicated because it can increase the pressure in the pleural space and cause a pneumothorax.

3 Decreased suction pressure results in limiting bubbling in the suction control, not the water-seal chamber.

4 Excessive bubbling in the water-seal chamber is not expected; the system is malfunctioning.

720. 4 This is ineffective because it exercises the elbow rather than the shoulder joint and muscles.

1 This is effective because it exercises the trapezius muscle and shoulder joint.

2 This is effective because it exercises the trapezius muscle and shoulder joint.

3 This is effective because it provides circular range of motion to the shoulder joint.

721. 4 The priority is to stabilize the respiratory status; a chest tube should be inserted.

1 The client must be stabilized before surgery; this may be necessary later.

2 To maintain the airway an endotracheal tube will be inserted.

3 This is secondary to stabilizing respirations.

722. 1 The chest tube normalizes intrathoracic pressure, drains fluid and air from the pleural space, and improves pulmonary function.

2 This may be a sign of pain, respiratory obstruction, or bleeding.

3 This indicates that air has entered the subcutaneous tissue (subcutaneous emphysema).

4 This indicates a probable leak in the drainage system.

723. 4 This is an emergency situation and atmospheric air must be prevented from entering the thoracic cavity; the client's respiratory status takes priority over the potential for infection.

1 This is useless and will further impair the client's breathing.

2 This is unsafe because it allows atmospheric air to enter the thoracic cavity.

3 Although an occlusive dressing is desirable, atmospheric air will enter the thoracic cavity while time is taken to obtain the occlusive dressing.

724. 3 To prevent another pneumothorax, the nurse should reconnect the tube.

1 This is unnecessary.

2 Clamping is appropriate for changing a broken drainage system or to check for an air leak; it should not be done in this situation.

4 This position will not remedy this problem.

725. 2 This prevents atelectasis and collection of secretions and promotes respiratory exchange.

1 Observing for dyspnea is important, but crepitus is unlikely to occur with stabilization of respiratory status.

3 Activity should be promoted within limits of physical ability; bed rest is unnecessary.

4 This is important but not as conducive to improving respiratory status as are coughing and deep breathing.

726. 2 Medically underserved clients such as the homeless, clients who are alcohol and/or drug dependent, and those who have HIV infections are at risk for developing tuberculosis.

1 Being homeless does not increase a person's risk for developing this condition.

3 Being homeless does not increase a person's risk for developing this condition.

4 Being homeless does not increase a person's risk for developing this condition.

727. 3 Blood-tinged sputum, in the absence of pronounced coughing, often is the presenting sign of TB; diaphoresis at night is a later sign.

1 Recurrent fever is present; frothy sputum occurs with pulmonary edema.

2 A productive cough occurs with TB.

4 A productive cough occurs with TB, but engorged neck veins occur with heart failure.

728. 4 The size of the induration determines the clinical significance of the reaction; an induration of 5 mm or more is considered significant, indicating exposure to the tuberculosis bacillus or vaccination with BCG vaccine.

1 An induration of 10 mm is a positive response.

2 The size of the induration, not the amount of erythema, is used to determine the test result.

3 The client history is taken into account with induration of less than 10 mm in high-risk clients, such as those who are HIV positive or who are living with others who have tuberculosis.

729. **4** **When the tubercle bacilli are stained with carbol-fuchsin, an acid, they turn red and are not decolorized by an acid-alcohol wash. The red rods are visible upon microscopic examination.**

    1 This reflects pulmonary status but does not identify the organism if a lesion is found.
    2 This indicates the presence of antibodies but is not diagnostic of the disease.
    3 This reflects pulmonary status but does not identify the organism if a lesion is found.

730. **2** **Sputum can be contained within disposable paper tissues that can then be discarded in fluid-impervious bags.**

    1 Because clients initially diagnosed with TB are typically fatigued and nutritionally compromised, the best approach is to conserve energy and, as the client improves, gradually initiate an exercise program.
    3 Sodium restriction is not necessary.
    4 Weekly blood pressure monitoring is not necessary.

731. **3** **Fresh airflow through the house exchanges the air and lowers the concentration of microorganisms.**

    1 This is not necessary.
    2 Only articles contaminated with infected sputum, such as used tissues, should be contained.
    4 It is permissible to do this because the extreme heat used to clean the dishes will kill the mycobacteria.

732. **3** **The directions need to be clarified because refrigeration is unnecessary.**

    1 The specimen must represent phlegm containing the mycobacterium, which is in the lung, not the oronasopharynx.
    2 For the best results the sputum collection should be made when the client awakens in the morning when mucus secretions are more copious.
    4 Delivery to the laboratory should be made on the same day as close as possible to the time of collection.

733. **4** **Tubercle bacilli are particularly resistant to treatment and can remain dormant for prolonged periods; medication must be taken consistently as prescribed.**

    1 Although this is important, the microorganisms must be eliminated with medication.
    2 Although this is important, the microorganisms must be eliminated with medication.
    3 Although this is important, the microorganisms must be eliminated with medication.

734. **3** **The tubercle bacillus is a drug-resistant organism and takes a long time to be eradicated; usually a combination of three medications is used for a minimum of 6 months and at least 6 months beyond culture conversion.**

    1 This is too short a time for eradication of this organism.

    2 This is too short a time for eradication of this organism.
    4 Usually, the organism can be eradicated in a shorter period of time, unless a resistant strain of the bacillus has developed.

REPRODUCTIVE AND GENITOURINARY

735. **4** **This uses gravity to allow urine to exert pressure on the area of the trigone, initiating relaxation of the urinary sphincter and facilitating micturition.**

    1 Although this may be important when urine is collected to be strained, analyzed, or measured, it will not facilitate micturition.
    2 An acid-ash diet may be used to prevent urinary infection and the formation of calcium stones; it will not facilitate micturition.
    3 This is important after urination but will not help facilitate micturition.

736. **4** **The costovertebral angle (angle formed by the lateral and downward curve of the lowest rib and the vertebral column of the spine itself) is percussed to determine if there is tenderness in the area over the kidney; this can be a sign of glomerulonephritis or severe upper urinary tract infection.**

    1 The tail of Spence extends from the upper outer quadrant of the breast to the axillary area; this is the most common site for tumors associated with cancer of the breast.
    2 The suprapubic area is above the symphysis pubis; it is palpated and percussed to assess for bladder distention.
    3 McBurney's point is 1 to 2 inches above the anterosuperior spine of the ileum on a line between the ileum and umbilicus; external pressure produces tenderness with acute appendicitis, not a kidney infection.

737. **4** **Laxatives remove feces and flatus, providing better visualization.**

    1 An IVP does not require restrictions of fat and proteins.
    2 Large amounts of fluids may dilute the dye, impairing visualization.
    3 A light dinner and beverage are permitted.

738. **1** **Cranberry juice is excreted as hippuric acid, which helps acidify the urine (decrease the pH) and inhibit bacterial growth.**

    2 Although bacterial growth may be inhibited, bacteria are not destroyed.
    3 Glomerular filtration is unaffected by cranberry juice.
    4 Cranberry juice acidifies the urine and may increase the burning sensation associated with urination when an infection is present.

739. 3 **Intercourse may cause urethral inflammation, increasing the risk of infection; voiding clears the urinary meatus and urethra of microorganisms.**
    1 Most fruit juices, with the exception of cranberry juice, cause alkaline urine, which promotes bacterial growth.
    2 Douching is no longer recommended because it alters the vaginal flora.
    4 Perineal care should be accomplished with wipes from the urinary meatus toward the rectum to help prevent microorganisms from the vaginal or rectal areas from reaching the urinary meatus.

740. Answer: 2, 3
    1 Limiting fluid intake contributes to stasis of urine.
    2 **Drinking 8 to 10 glasses of water spaced throughout the day flushes the urinary tract and minimizes urinary stasis.**
    3 **Urination flushes the urethra and urinary meatus limiting the presence of microorganisms.**
    4 Carbonated and caffeinated beverages irritate the bladder and should be avoided.
    5 Cleaning the perineum with harsh soaps is irritating to the skin and mucous membranes, and can contribute to the development of UTIs in susceptible women.

741. 3 **The walls of a full bladder are stretched thinner and are more susceptible to rupture when traumatized.**
    1 A history of cystitis predisposes the client to developing future bladder infections, not to rupturing the bladder.
    2 A family member with bladder cancer might increase the risk of cancer; however, it will not predispose the client to bladder rupture.
    4 This will not result in the production of enough urine to expand the bladder if the client voided before starting the trip.

742. 1 **Frequent position changes are important to ensure efficient urinary drainage; gravity promotes flow, which prevents obstruction.**
    2 Back care is necessary but is not a priority.
    3 ROM is of minimal importance because the client will be able to move without limitation.
    4 Raising three side rails is routine care, particularly if the client is sedated; positioning to promote urinary drainage takes priority.
       Clinical Area: Medical-Surgical Nursing; **Client Needs:** Reduction of Risk Potential; **Cognitive Level:** Application; **Nursing Process:** Planning

743. 4 **Research statistics indicate that hematuria is the most common early sign of cancer of the urinary system, probably because of the urinary system's rich vascular network.**
    1 Dysuria is not specific for bladder cancer; usually it is associated with an enlarged prostate in the male.
    2 Retention is not specific for bladder cancer; usually it is associated with an enlarged prostate in the male.

    3 Hesitancy is not specific for bladder cancer; usually it is associated with an enlarged prostate in the male.

744. 2 **This may denote a compromised blood supply to the stoma and impending necrosis.**
    1 This is expected in the early postoperative period after this surgery.
    3 This is expected in the early postoperative period after this surgery.
    4 Pink-tinged urine may be present in the immediate postoperative period.

745. 1 **This response is expected because mucus continually is secreted by the intestinal mucosa.**
    2 This is not necessary; mucus is expected with an ileal conduit.
    3 This is not necessary; at this point postsurgically the mucus is not an indication of infection; mucus in the urine after ureterostomy may indicate infection.
    4 Although fluids should be encouraged to maintain urine flow, this will not eliminate mucus, which continually is discharged from the intestinal segment.

746. 2 **High-fluid intake flushes the ileal conduit and prevents infection and obstruction caused by mucus or uric acid crystals.**
    1 Alcohol is not contraindicated with an ileal conduit.
    3 This is expected; as edema decreases, the stoma will become smaller.
    4 Soap and water on the peristomal area help prevent irritation from waste products.

747. 2 **Cholinergics intensify and prolong the action of acetylcholine, which increases the tone in the genitourinary tract, preventing urinary retention.**
    1 Cholinergics will not prevent renal calculi.
    3 Anticholinergics are prescribed for the frequency and urgency associated with a spastic bladder.
    4 Preventing urinary tract infections is a secondary gain because cholinergics help prevent urinary retention that can lead to a urinary tract infection, but this is not the primary purpose for administering these drugs.

748. 3 **This increases lymphatic drainage, reducing edema and pain.**
    1 This increases circulation to the area, intensifying edema and pain in this client.
    2 This increases circulation to the area, intensifying edema and pain in this client.
    4 This is not indicated; scrotal swelling is caused by the trauma of surgery, not infection.

749. 4 **This method obtains a specimen uncontaminated by environmental organisms.**
    1 This is not as accurate as obtaining the purulent discharge from the site of origin.
    2 This will contaminate the specimen with organisms external to the body.
    3 This will dilute and possibly contaminate the specimen.

750. 2 Anal itching and irritation are related to erythema and edema of the anal crypts caused by the gonococci.

1 Frank rectal bleeding, not upper GI bleeding, occurs.

3 Diarrhea, not constipation, occurs.

4 The shape of formed stool does not change; however, diarrhea does occur.

751. 4 The client is in the secondary stage, which begins from 6 weeks to 6 months after primary contact; therefore, a 6-month history is needed to ensure that all possible contacts are located.

1 Any time less than 6 months may miss contacts that may have become infected.

2 Any time less than 6 months may miss contacts that may have become infected.

3 Any time less than 6 months may miss contacts that may have become infected.

752. 4 Neurotoxicity, as manifested by ataxia, is evidence of tertiary syphilis, which may involve the CNS; other CNS signs include confusion, paralysis, delusions, impaired judgment, and slurred speech.

1 A sore on the penis occurs in the secondary stage.

2 Sores in the mouth occur in the secondary stage.

3 Alopecia is not a sign of late-stage syphilis.

753. 2 Headaches occur because of the retention of fluid and hypertension.

1 The client will experience oliguria, not nocturia.

3 The client will develop anorexia related to elevated toxic substances in the blood.

4 The client will have a weight gain because of the retention of fluid.

754. 3 Sucking on a hard candy will relieve thirst and increase carbohydrates, but does not supply extra fluid.

1 Carbonated beverages contain sodium and provide additional fluid, which must be restricted.

2 A milkshake contains both fluid and protein, which must be restricted.

4 Broth contains sodium, which increases fluid retention.

755. 4 A common cause of glomerulonephritis is a streptococcal infection. This infection initiates an antibody formation that damages the glomeruli.

1 The alkalinity of bubble baths is linked to urethritis, not glomerulonephritis.

2 Moderate activity is helpful in preventing urinary stasis, which can precipitate urinary infection.

3 Any fluid restriction is moderated as the client improves; fluid is allowed to prevent urinary stasis.

756. 3 An excessive use of antacids may result in hypercalciuria; most calculi contain calcium combined with phosphate or other substances.

1 Cholesterol is unrelated to the formation of renal calculi; cholesterol stones in the gallbladder are the result of increased cholesterol synthesis in the liver.

2 Immobility with the associated demineralization of bone, not exercise, contributes to the formation of renal calculi.

4 Alcohol intake is unrelated to renal calculi formation.

757. 3 Hematuria and pain may result from damage to the ureteral lining as the calculus moves down the urinary tract; the urine may become cloudy or pink tinged.

1 Although severe pain may be present, urgency is not associated with renal calculi; urgency may be associated with an enlarged prostate, cystitis, or other genitourinary problems.

2 The odor of urine is not foul with this condition; the color of urine is not dark with this condition, although it may be cloudy, pink, or red from hematuria.

4 Frequency may occur when the calculus reaches the bladder.

758. 3 Increasing fluid intake dilutes the urine, and crystals are less likely to coalesce and form calculi.

1 An elevated serum creatinine has no relationship to the formation of renal calculi.

2 Calcium restriction is necessary only if calculi have a calcium phosphate or calcium oxalate basis.

4 Producing only 2000 mL of urine per 24 hours is inadequate; urine output should be maintained at 3000 to 4000 mL to limit calculus formation.

759. 1 Apples are low in phosphate.

2 Chocolate contains more phosphate than apples.

3 Rye bread contains more phosphate than apples.

4 Cheese is made with milk, which contains phosphate and should be avoided.

760. 4 Pain with ureteral stones is caused by spasm and is excruciating and intermittent; it follows the path of the ureter to the bladder.

1 Pain is spasmodic and excruciating, not boring.

2 Pain intensifies as the calculus lodges in the ureter and spasms occur in an attempt to dislodge it.

3 Spasmodic pain on the left side that radiates to the suprapubis is typical of pain caused by a stone in the renal pelvis.

761. 2 Purines are precursors of uric acid, which crystallizes.

1 Cystine stones are caused by a rare hereditary defect resulting in inadequate renal tubular reabsorption of cystine (inborn error of cystine metabolism).

3 Serum purine will not be elevated if the stone is composed of calcium oxalate.

4 A struvite stone is sometimes called a magnesium ammonium phosphate stone and is precipitated by recurrent urinary tract infections with coliform bacteria.

762. 1 An output of 50 mL/hr is adequate; when urine output drops below 30 mL/hr, it may indicate renal failure and the practitioner should be notified.

2 This is unnecessary because the output is adequate.

3 This is unnecessary because the output is adequate.

4 This is contraindicated; the client probably will still be under the influence of anesthesia and the gag reflex may be depressed.

763. **1 The tube must be kept patent to prevent urine backup, hydronephrosis, and kidney damage.**
   2 This is unnecessary unless the tube is not functioning.
   3 This is a dependent function and requires a practitioner's order.
   4 Although this is important, it will not ensure free drainage of urine, which is the priority.

764. **2 Calculi may obstruct the flow of urine to the bladder, allowing the urine to distend the ureter, causing hydroureter.**
   1 There is insufficient information to come to this conclusion even though output is less than intake; oliguria is present when the output is between 100 and 500 mL in a 24-hour period.
   3 Calculi do not cause renal shutdown directly; they may obstruct the urinary tract and cause damage indirectly as a result of pressure from urine buildup.
   4 If the urethra is obstructed, the bladder will be distended.

765. **4 If the calculi are in the renal pelvis, a percutaneous pyelolithotomy is performed; the calculi are removed via a small flank incision.**
   1 This is not necessary.
   2 This usually is unnecessary.
   3 This route is used for calculi in the ureters and renal pelvis.

766. **1 These occur with a urinary tract infection because of bladder irritability; burning on urination and fever are additional signs of a UTI.**
   2 This is not related to a UTI.
   3 This is a symptom of a urinary calculus, not infection.
   4 This is not a sign of a UTI; this may be caused by altering the diet to include foods that form acid ash or alkaline ash.

767. **1 Increasing fluid intake aids in the passage of fragments of the calculus that remain after the lithotripsy.**
   2 Organ meats are high in purine, an amino acid, which is a causative factor in the formation of uric acid crystals; they should be avoided by people with gout.
   3 Calcium is the major component of the most common type of calculus; the intake of dairy products, which are high in calcium, should be limited.
   4 Early ambulation is encouraged to aid in the passage of fragments of the calculus that remain after a lithotripsy.

768. **4 A subjective symptom must be experienced and described by the client; flank pain, pain on the side of the body between the ribs and the ileum, accompanies renal colic.**
   1 This is an objective sign that can be verified by observation or measurement.
   2 Although nausea is a subjective symptom and it can occur with the severe pain associated with renal colic, it is not as significant as flank pain.
   3 This is an objective sign that can be verified by observation or measurement.

769. **1 Cancer of the prostate is rare before age 50 but increases with each decade; black men develop cancer of the prostate twice as often and at an earlier age than white men.**
   2 White men develop prostatic cancer half as often as black men, but more commonly than Asian or Hispanic men.
   3 This group of men has a lower incidence of prostatic cancer and lower mortality rate than white and black men.
   4 This group of men has a lower incidence of prostatic cancer and lower mortality rate than white and black men.

770. **4 A full bladder is palpable with urinary retention and distention, which are common problems after a cystoscopy because of urethral edema.**
   1 Fluids dilute the urine and reduce the chance of infection after cystoscopy and should not be limited.
   2 Although urinary retention can occur, it is not expected; the nurse must assess the extent of bladder distention and discomfort.
   3 More conservative nursing methods such as running water or placing a warm cloth over the perineum should be attempted to precipitate voiding; catheterization carries a risk of infection.

771. **4 Distention of the suprapubic area indicates that the bladder is distended with urine and therefore palpable.**
   1 Perineal edema is not related to urinary retention and benign prostatic hyperplasia.
   2 Urethral discharge may be related to sexually transmitted infections.
   3 Radiating flank pain may indicate renal calculi.

772. **1 Ejection of semen into the bladder instead of the urethra is common after a transurethral prostatectomy.**
   2 This surgery will not cause prolonged erections.
   3 Impotence is not usual with this approach; it may occur with the retroperitoneal approach.
   4 This surgery should not interfere with the libido.

773. **1 This will improve bladder tone, which should alleviate dribbling.**
   2 This identifies feelings but does not actively help the client solve the problem.
   3 These interventions do not increase bladder tone; fluids should be increased and the time between voidings should be increased gradually.
   4 Continuous bladder decompression will reduce bladder tone; reduced bladder tone will persist when the indwelling catheter is removed until bladder tone improves.

774. **4 The amount of irrigant instilled into the bladder must be deducted from the total output to determine the amount of urine produced.**
   1 Unless the irrigant is subtracted from the output, the total will be inaccurate.

2 Specific gravity measures the concentration of urine; this measurement will be inaccurate because the urine is diluted with GU irrigant.

3 This is unnecessary; the urinary bladder is constantly being irrigated with GU irrigant.

775. 1 **The drainage tubing may be obstructed. Retained fluid raises intravesicular pressure, causing discomfort similar to the urge to void.**

2 The client's vital signs are not related to the complaint; the practitioner should be called only if a blocked drainage tube is not corrected.

3 Although this is true, the patency of the gravity system should be ascertained before determining the cause of the complaint.

4 Although this might be done, it is not the priority. Whether urine is draining from the tubing at this point in time is significant.

776. 2 **The urethral mucosa in the prostatic area is affected during surgery, and strictures may form with healing.**

1 The client should be ambulating; sitting for several hours is contraindicated because it promotes venous stasis and thrombus formation.

3 The client should void as the need arises; straining can cause pressure in the operative area, precipitating hemorrhage.

4 Although vigorous exercise should be avoided, 6 months is too long for this restriction.

777. 2 **After transurethral surgery, hemorrhage can occur because of venous oozing and bleeding from many small arteries in the area.**

1 Sepsis is unusual and occurs later in the postoperative course.

3 Leaking around the catheter is not a major complication.

4 Urinary retention is unlikely with an indwelling catheter in place.

778. 4 **Increasingly elevated PSA levels may indicate a worsening of the client's condition with possible metastasis to the bone, increasing the risk of pathological fractures; therefore, handling must be gentle.**

1 Although measuring intake and output is necessary for any client with prostatic cancer because of the risk of bladder obstruction, it is not the priority for this client.

2 Seizure precautions are not necessary; a PSA elevation indicates bone, not brain, involvement.

3 Elevated PSA levels do not significantly affect the plasma pH.

779. 3 **This action causes the bladder muscle to contract, initiating painful bladder spasms.**

1 Although opioids may dull the pain, they may not limit muscle spasms.

2 Instillation of fluid may be irritating and can precipitate bladder spasms.

4 Advancing or manipulating the catheter may precipitate bladder spasms.

780. 4 **Because of the trauma to the mucous membranes of the urinary tract, burning on urination is an expected response that should subside gradually.**

1 The urine should no longer be dilute after the continuous bladder irrigation is discontinued and removed. However, the urine may have a slight pink tinge because of the trauma from the surgery and the presence of the catheter.

2 This should not occur unless the indwelling catheter is removed too soon and there is still edema of the urethra.

3 This is a sign of hemorrhage, which should not occur.

781. 3 **A continuous flushing of the bladder dilutes the bloody urine and empties the bladder, preventing clots.**

1 Fluid instilled into the bladder does not affect kidney function.

2 Urinary output can be measured regardless of the amount of fluid instilled.

4 The urinary retention catheter is not designed to exert pressure on the prostatic fossa.

782. 2 **Because venous stasis is the major predisposing factor of pulmonary emboli, venous flow velocity should be increased through activity.**

1 Increasing the coagulability of the blood can lead to the development of deep vein thrombosis.

3 This will not affect the prevention of deep vein thrombosis.

4 This will not affect the prevention of deep vein thrombosis.

783. 4 **This is a classic sign of renal carcinoma; it is due to capillary erosion by the cancerous growth.**

1 Dull flank pain may occur but not as frequently as bleeding.

2 Weight loss, not weight gain, will occur.

3 This will not occur with renal carcinoma; it may occur with glomerulonephritis.

784. 2 **The kidney, an extremely vascular organ, receives a large percentage of the blood flow, and hemorrhage from the operative site can occur.**

1 This may occur later in the postoperative period.

3 This may occur later in the postoperative period.

4 This can occur, but it is not life threatening.

785. 4 **Turning the client prevents respiratory complications.**

1 There is no need for a nephrostomy tube because the kidney has been removed.

2 Because clients are prone to develop paralytic ileus, food and fluid intake are delayed until bowel sounds are auscultated.

3 The first dressing change is performed by the practitioner.

786. 2 **Digested blood is protein which will increase the BUN.**

1 Kidney function already is compromised; dialysis performs the function of the kidneys.

3 Although clients with chronic kidney disease have problems with bleeding, this does not interfere with identifying the site of bleeding.

4 Chronic kidney disease does not affect the signs of GI blood loss, hemorrhage, or shock.

787. 2 **High-biologic-value (HBV) protein contains essential amino acids needed by the body for tissue building and repair; HBV proteins limit the extent of nitrogenous wastes.**

1 A high-calorie diet provides for weight gain.

3 The purpose of a diet for a client with chronic kidney disease is to decrease, not increase, nitrogenous wastes.

4 This is not the purpose of HBV proteins; sodium restriction decreases blood pressure.

788. 2 **Infection is responsible for one third of the traumatic or surgically induced deaths of clients with acute renal failure, as well as for medically induced acute renal failure. Resistance is reduced in clients with kidneys that fail because of decreased phagocytosis, which makes them susceptible to microorganisms.**

1 Anemia occurs often with acute renal failure, but it is not the most serious complication and should be treated in relation to the client's adaptations; erythropoietin and iron supplements usually are prescribed.

3 Weight loss is not life threatening.

4 Platelet dysfunction occurs because of decreased cell surface adhesiveness, but it is not as serious as an infection.

789. 3 **One cup of cottage cheese contains approximately 225 calories, 27 grams of protein, 9 grams of fat, 30 mg of cholesterol, and 6 grams of carbohydrate; proteins of high biologic value (HBV) contain optimal levels of the amino acids essential for life.**

1 Apple juice is a source of vitamins A and C, not protein.

2 Raw carrots are a carbohydrate source and contain beta-carotene.

4 Whole wheat bread is a source of carbohydrates and fiber.

790. 1 **Foods high in carbohydrates and low in protein, sodium, and potassium are encouraged for these clients.**

2 This is high in potassium, which is restricted.

3 This is high in protein and sodium, which usually are restricted.

4 This is high in protein, sodium, and potassium, which usually are restricted.

791. 2 **The accumulation of metabolic wastes in the blood (uremia) can cause pruritus; edema results from fluid overload caused by impaired urine production.**

1 Pallor occurs with chronic kidney disease as a result of anemia.

3 This is a urinary pattern that is not caused by chronic kidney disease; this may occur after prostate surgery.

4 These occur with an enlarged prostate, not kidney disease.

792. 3 **An elevation in uremic waste products causes irritation of the nerves, resulting in flapping hand tremors (asterixis, "liver flap").**

1 Hypertension results from kidney failure because of sodium and water retention.

2 The diseased kidney is unable to excrete potassium ions, resulting in hyperkalemia, not hypokalemia.

4 The hematocrit value will be low because of a decreased production of erythropoietin, a hormone synthesized in the kidney; erythropoietin regulates the production of erythrocytes.

793. 3 **Vital signs monitor the cardiopulmonary status; the practitioner must treat this hyperkalemia to prevent cardiac dysrhythmias.**

1 The cardiac arrest team responds to a cardiac arrest; there is no sign of arrest in this client.

2 A repeat laboratory test will take time and probably reaffirm the original results; the client needs medical attention.

4 These are correct interventions if available, but the priority is medical attention and the practitioner should be notified immediately.

794. 1 **Insulin promotes the transfer of potassium into cells, which reduces the circulating blood level of potassium.**

2 This response halts communication and is not supportive.

3 Blood glucose levels usually are not elevated in acute renal failure.

4 Insulin will not lower the metabolic rate.

795. 2 **Turning from side to side will change the position of the catheter, thereby freeing the drainage holes, which may be obstructed.**

1 Taking fluids into the gastrointestinal tract does not influence drainage of dialysate from the peritoneal cavity.

3 This improves pulmonary ventilation but does not improve flow of dialysate from the catheter.

4 The position of the catheter should be changed by the practitioner.

796. 4 **This promotes vasodilation so that urea, a large-molecular substance, is shifted from the body into the dialyzing solution.**

1 Heat does not affect the shift of potassium into the cells.

2 The removal of metabolic wastes is affected in kidney failure, not the metabolic processes.

3 Excess serum potassium is removed by dialyzing with a potassium-free solution, not by heat.

797. Answer: 1, 2

1 **In the diuretic phase, fluid retained during the oliguric phase is excreted and may reach 3 to 5 L**

daily; dehydration will occur unless fluids are replaced.

2 **In the diuretic phase, fluid retained during the oliguric phase is excreted and may reach 3 to 5 L daily; hypovolemia may occur, and fluids should be replaced.**

3 Hyperkalemia develops in the oliguric phase when glomerular filtration is inadequate.

4 Metabolic acidosis occurs in the oliguric, not diuretic, phase.

798. 2 **Proteins eaten should be high quality to replace those lost during dialysis.**

1 A high-calorie diet is encouraged.

3 Usually there is a modest restriction of fluids when the client is on dialysis.

4 Usually there is a restriction of high-potassium foods when the client is on dialysis.

799. 1 **Lack of motivation is the most serious impediment to successful CAPD.**

2 This is not a contraindication to CAPD.

3 This is not a contraindication to CAPD.

4 This is not a contraindication to CAPD.

800. 2 **The infusion should be warmed to body temperature to lessen abdominal discomfort and promote dilation of peritoneal vessels.**

1 The side-lying position may restrict fluid inflow and prevent maximum urea clearance; the client should be placed in the semi-Fowler position.

3 The infusion of dialysate solution should take approximately 5 to 10 minutes.

4 Routine medications should not interfere with the infusion of dialysate solution.

801. 4 **Pressure from the fluid may cause upward displacement of the diaphragm; draining the solution reduces intra-abdominal pressure, which allows the thoracic cavity to expand on inspiration.**

1 Additional fluid will aggravate the problem.

2 Auscultation is important, but it does not alleviate the problem.

3 The client should be placed in the semi-Fowler's position for peritoneal dialysis; this allows inflow of fluid while not impinging on the thoracic cavity.

802. **Answer: 3, 4, 5**

1 Severe itching (pruritus) is caused by metabolic waste products that are deposited in the skin; dialysis removes metabolic waste products, preventing this adaptation associated with kidney failure.

2 The production of abnormally small amounts of urine (oliguria) is a sign of kidney failure, not a complication of peritoneal dialysis.

3 **Tachycardia can be caused by peritonitis, a complication of peritoneal dialysis; the heart rate increases to meet the metabolic demands associated with infection.**

4 **Cloudy or opaque dialysate outflow (effluent) is the earliest sign of peritonitis; it is caused by the constituents associated with an infectious process.**

5 **Abdominal pain is associated with peritonitis, a complication of peritoneal dialysis; pain results from peritoneal inflammation, abdominal distention, and involuntary muscle spasms.**

803. 3 **These are signs and symptoms of disequilibrium syndrome, which results from rapid changes in composition of the extracellular fluid and cerebral edema; the rate of exchange should be decreased.**

1 Although this may relieve the headache, it will not relieve the other adaptations or the cause of disequilibrium syndrome.

2 Although this may relieve the nausea, it will not relieve the other adaptations or the cause of disequilibrium syndrome.

4 This is unnecessary; reducing the rate of exchange should reduce the adaptations of disequilibrium syndrome.

804. 2 **Sodium is an electrolyte that passes through the semipermeable membrane during hemodialysis.**

1 These do not pass through the semipermeable membrane during hemodialysis.

3 This does not pass through the semipermeable membrane during hemodialysis.

4 These do not pass through the semipermeable membrane during hemodialysis.

805. 4 **Human leukocyte antigen compatibility provides the most specific predictions of the body's tendency to accept or reject foreign tissue.**

1 Although ABO compatibility is necessary, the exact blood type is not.

2 This is unsafe unless the family member has matching leukocyte antigen complexes. This may increase the possibility of a match, but there is no guarantee that a family member will match.

3 Differences in body size do not cause rejection.

806. 2 **The potassium is increased outside the expected range for an adult, which places the client at risk for a cardiac dysrhythmia; the increased potassium level must be treated immediately because elevated levels can be lethal.**

1 A serum sodium of 135 mEq/L is expected because of the electrolyte imbalance and the anemia related to the decreased production of erythropoietin by the kidney in the presence of chronic kidney failure.

3 A creatinine clearance of <20 mL/min is expected with chronic kidney disease; a creatinine clearance level of less than 10 mL/min is reflective of severe kidney impairment.

4 Although these vital signs are increased, they are not as serious a concern as another assessment; fluid overload and hypervolemia associated with chronic kidney disease are reflected in hypertension, tachycardia, and tachypnea and are expected.

807. 1 **Output is critical when assessing kidney function. The urinary output should be monitored every**

30 to 60 minutes; decreasing urinary output is a sign of rejection.

2 This is too infrequent to monitor output immediately after a transplant. It is essential to monitor output more frequently to evaluate whether the new kidney is working or whether it is being rejected.

3 This is too infrequent to monitor output immediately after a transplant. It is essential to monitor output more frequently to evaluate whether the new kidney is working or whether it is being rejected.

4 It is not necessary to monitor urinary output this frequently.

808. 4 **As the transplanted organ functions, nitrogenous wastes are eliminated, lowering the serum creatinine.**

1 As more urine is produced by the transplanted kidney, the specific gravity and concentration of the urine will decrease.

2 With end-stage kidney disease, fluid retention causes hypertension. There should be a correction of hypertension, not hypotension.

3 After the transplant, the serum potassium should correct to within expected limits for an adult.

809. 3 **Hypertension is caused by hypervolemia because of the failure of the new kidney.**

1 Weight gain, not loss, occurs with a rejection of the kidney because of fluid retention.

2 The client will have an elevated temperature exceeding 100° F with kidney rejection.

4 Urine output will be decreased or absent, depending on the degree of kidney rejection.

810. 4 **The WBC count can drop precipitously. If leukocytes are less than 3000/mm³, the drug may have to be stopped to prevent irreversible bone marrow depression.**

1 Leukocytosis, not leukopenia, occurs with an infection.

2 High creatinine levels are related to kidney failure, but do not cause leukopenia.

3 The WBC count is increased, not decreased, with kidney rejection.

811. Answer: 1, 2, 3

1 **Because infection is a major complication of a kidney transplant, prevention begins with the recognition of the earliest signs and symptoms.**

2 **The transplanted kidney does not always function immediately; the client should know that dialysis may have to be continued for several weeks.**

3 **Just prior to surgery a urinary catheter is inserted and an antibiotic is instilled into the bladder to decrease the risk of infection.**

4 Immunosuppressive therapy is started after, not before, surgery.

5 The vascular access is never used for drawing blood, or instilling IV medications.

SKELETAL

812. 4 **A bone scan maps the uptake of a bone-seeking radioactive isotope; an increased uptake is seen in metastatic bone disease, osteosarcoma, osteomyelitis, and certain fractures.**

1 A bone scan measures the uptake of radioactive material, not the absence of calcium, which is seen in an x-ray examination of bone.

2 This is a bone marrow aspiration, when a small amount of marrow is examined to determine the presence of abnormal cells in diseases such as leukemia.

3 A bone scan involves a small diagnostic dosage of a radioactive substance; it is not therapeutic.

813. 2 **Weight bearing and the use of antigravity muscles stimulate bone formation or osteoblastic function.**

1 This will result in bone demineralization, not calcium deposition in the bone.

3 The aging process contributes to a gradual and progressive demineralization of bone.

4 Calcium intake has a relationship to osteoclastic mechanisms in that it inhibits the withdrawal of calcium from bone.

814. 2 **The fingers are flared out in the extended, abducted position.**

1 The fingers are neither bent nor flexed.

3 The fingers are abducted, not adducted, from the midline of the hand.

4 Circumduction is a circular movement of a limb that occurs at a ball and socket joint. The shoulder and hip joints, not the wrist or fingers, can be moved in this way.

815. 3 **These adaptations are consistent with a torn cartilage; this injury is common among basketball players.**

1 A fractured patella will cause pain and usually manifests itself at the time of the injury.

2 A ruptured Achilles tendon is painful and prevents plantar flexion of the foot; adaptations usually are manifested at the time of the injury.

4 A stress fracture is associated with pain, not with a clicking or locking of the knee.

816. 1 **This describes the procedure in which the surgeon uses a scope to visualize and operate on the knee.**

2 Arthroscopic surgery is not a radiological procedure.

3 This is a surgical procedure; the only treatment prescribed is physiotherapy after surgery.

4 Although this is true, it evades the client's concern and does not describe the procedure.

817. 3 **These sets of muscles are used in crutch walking and therefore need strengthening.**

1 Although these muscles keep the person erect, the most important muscles for walking with crutches are the triceps, elbow extensors, finger flexors, and the muscles in the unaffected leg.

2 This will do nothing to promote crutch walking.

4 A pushing, not a pulling, motion is used with crutches; the triceps, not the biceps, are used.

818. 2 **Because of the angle of force applied to a walker when a person uses it to move from a sitting to a standing position, the walker can become unstable and tip over. The arms of the chair should be used for support when rising from a sitting position.**

1 Sliding toward the edge of the seat moves the center of gravity of the body toward the desired direction of movement, which facilitates the transfer.

3 Holding both handles and moving forward into the walker provide the maximum support afforded by a walker.

4 Standing in place after rising allows the body's vasomotor responses to adjust to the vertical position, minimizing orthostatic hypotension.

819. 1 **Folding the arms across the chest maintains both arms in a safe position during the transfer.**

2 During a safe transfer, the sling should extend from above the scapulae to the knees to provide appropriate support.

3 The use of a mechanical lift is an independent function of the nurse.

4 This height is unsafe; during the transfer, the sling should be raised just high enough (3 to 4 inches) to clear the mattress.

820. 4 **These movements include all possible range of motion for the ankle joint.**

1 Although the ankle can be moved in a circular motion, flexion and extension are more specifically called dorsiflexion and plantar flexion in relation to the ankle. Also, eversion and inversion should be done when manipulating the ankle.

2 Flexion and extension are more specifically called dorsiflexion and plantar flexion in relation to the ankle. The ankle cannot be abducted or adducted but can be inverted and everted.

3 These motions refer to the upper extremities.

821. 2 **In a comminuted fracture, the bone is splintered or crushed.**

1 This is a compound fracture.

3 This is a complete fracture.

4 This is a greenstick fracture.

822. 2 **Numbness is a neurological sign because it indicates pressure on the nerves and blood vessels and should be reported immediately.**

1 Warmth is a sign of adequate circulation.

3 Skin desquamation results from inadequate skin care and can be managed with lotion or oil.

4 Some degree of discomfort is expected after cast application.

823. 2 **This may indicate cast pressure on a nerve and should be investigated further.**

1 Some swelling causing stiffness is expected after injury to tissues; it should be noted and monitored further.

3 Some bloody drainage is expected; it should be noted and monitored further.

4 The radial pulse of the affected arm cannot be assessed because of the placement of the cast. Circulation to this extremity is assessed by briefly compressing a fingernail on the affected hand and observing the return of a pink color after releasing the compression.

824. 4 **Damage to the blood vessels may decrease circulatory perfusion of the toes.**

1 Damage to the major blood vessels will more likely cause a decrease in blood pressure.

2 The fracture is between the knee and the ankle, not in the thigh.

3 Decreased circulatory perfusion of the foot causes the skin temperature to decrease.

825. 2 **This indicates tissue hypoxia or breakdown and should be reported to the practitioner.**

1 Other data, such as elevated temperature or increased white blood cells, are not present to support the presence of an infection.

3 Although this will be done to provide relief of pain, the priority is to notify the practitioner.

4 This is not a typical response to a cast and may indicate a complication.

826. 1 **Elevation will help control the edema that usually occurs after an injury or if the injured part is left in a dependent position.**

2 Because the ankle has been at rest, discomfort and stiffness are expected after the cast is removed.

3 The leg should be put through full range of motion more than once daily.

4 Because the skin has not been exposed, it needs gentle washing to prevent injuring the epidermis.

827. 2 **The client probably has a fat embolus; oxygen reduces surface tension of the fat globules and reduces hypoxia.**

1 Oxygen should be administered and the client placed in a semi-Fowler's position before the practitioner is called.

3 This causes hip flexion and stresses the fractured femur; the semi-Fowler's position is preferred.

4 The Trendelenburg position will further compromise the client's respiratory status because the pressure of the abdominal organs against the diaphragm will limit expansion of the thoracic cavity.

828. 3 **Diaphoresis and tachypnea indicate that the client has exceeded tolerance for the activity.**

1 These are expected adaptations to activity.

2 Flushed skin is an expected response to activity; respirations will increase in depth rather than become slow.

4 An increase in blood pressure is an expected response to activity; respirations probably will increase in depth and rate.

829. 4 **The infected bone is placed at rest and may be in a cast or splint to reduce pain and limit motion that promotes spread of the infection.**
  1 This will increase pain and promote spread of the infection.
  2 Osteomyelitis usually is caused by a microorganism traveling through the bloodstream to the bone, not the reverse; the client is already septic.
  3 This is contraindicated; early ambulation may facilitate the spread of the infection.

830. Answer: 1, 2
  1 **Clients with gout may develop deposits of monosodium urate in their tissues (tophi); these consist of a core of monosodium urate with a surrounding inflammatory reaction. Also, urate crystals form in the synovial tissue, typically the metatarsophalangeal joint of the great toe of a foot.**
  2 **Uric acid has a low solubility; it tends to precipitate and form deposits at various sites where blood flow is least active, including cartilaginous tissue such as the ears.**
  3 Urate deposits will not form at this site because the blood flow is ample, and it is not cartilaginous tissue.
  4 Urate deposits will not form at this site because the blood flow is ample, and it is not cartilaginous tissue.
  5 Urate deposits will not form at this site because the blood flow is ample, and it is not cartilaginous tissue.

831. 2 **Shellfish contains more than 100 mg of purine per 100 grams.**
  1 This food is low in purine.
  3 This food is low in purine.
  4 This food is low in purine.

832. 1 **Osteoporotic vertebrae collapse under the weight of the upper body or by improper or rapid turning, reaching, or lifting.**
  2 Bones, not the spinal cord, demineralize in osteoporosis.
  3 This occurs in osteoarthritis.
  4 The spinal cord does not bulge; the nucleus pulposus bulges toward the spinal cord.

833. 3 **The Valsalva maneuver raises cerebrospinal fluid pressure, thereby causing pain.**
  1 Calf tenderness is associated with thrombophlebitis.
  2 Dysuria is associated with urinary problems.
  4 This type of pain is not associated with intervertebral disk problems.

834. 3 **Pain results because herniation of the nucleus pulposus into the spinal column irritates the spinal cord or the roots of spinal nerves.**
  1 This is not involved; the lamina is that portion of the vertebra removed during surgery to gain access to the site.
  2 The vertebral bodies themselves are not shifting.
  4 Circulation of cerebrospinal fluid is not affected.

835. 4 **Coughing raises intervertebral pressure and places strain on the lumbar area, increasing the herniation of the nucleus pulposis.**
  1 This will not increase pressure or pain.
  2 This does not increase intervertebral pressure.
  3 This will not increase pressure or cause pain; lying with the knees flexed usually is a more comfortable position.

836. 4 **Log-rolling to the prone position supports vertebral alignment, decreasing trauma to the operative site.**
  1 Use of a trapeze is contraindicated because it promotes twisting and straining, which are not desirable.
  2 The contour position is contraindicated because it flexes the vertebral column, which may increase intervertebral pressure.
  3 Traction is not used after this surgery.

837. 3 **Alteration in circulation and sensation indicates damage to the spinal cord; if this occurs, the surgeon must be notified immediately.**
  1 After surgery, the surgeon's order should specify if the client is permitted oral fluids.
  2 The prone position is contraindicated because it will hyperextend the vertebral column; log-rolling from side to side is preferred.
  4 Although this will be done, it is not the priority.

838. 2 **Putting the upper arm and leg toward the side to which the client is turning uses body weight to facilitate turning; the spine is kept straight.**
  1 This will result in twisting the spinal column; this is unsafe, an overbed table has wheels and is not a stable object.
  3 This can be done if another person were turning the client; when turning alone in this position, the client will have no leverage and turning will probably result in twisting the spinal column.
  4 This will interfere with turning because the bent leg becomes an obstacle and provides a force opposite to the leverage needed to turn.

839. 1 **Sitting maintains alignment of the back and allows the nurses to support the client until orthostatic hypotension subsides.**
  2 This will induce flexion of the vertebrae, which can traumatize the spinal cord.
  3 This will induce flexion of the vertebrae, which can traumatize the spinal cord.
  4 Rapid movement can flex the vertebrae, which will traumatize the spinal cord; taking the blood pressure at this time is not necessary.

840. 2 **Maintaining the sitting position for a prolonged period places excessive stress on the surgical area.**
  1 This maintains appropriate lordosis of the small of the back and provides support.
  3 This relieves pressure on the back and promotes comfort in bed.

4 This prevents excessive pressure on the musculature and vertebral column.

841. 1 **This is done while in the supine position before the body is subjected to the force of gravity in a vertical position. Anatomical landmarks are easier to locate for correct application of the brace, and intra-abdominal organs have not shifted toward the pelvic floor by gravity.**

2 The brace should be applied while in the supine position, not the sitting position.

3 The brace should be worn as prescribed, not just when the client feels tired.

4 Twisting exercises are contraindicated because they exert excessive pressure on the operative site.

842. 2 **The client is demonstrating acceptance and is looking toward the future.**

1 This relates to low self-esteem, not body image disturbance.

3 This response may indicate that the client is trying to lose weight and may not accept his present body weight.

4 Although this may indicate adaptability, it is not related to body image.

843. 3 **Gentle intervention reduces pain and shock and inhibits the release of bone marrow into the system, which can cause a fat embolism.**

1 Elevation of the affected limb will not prevent a fat embolus; it may limit edema and pain, which are local effects.

2 Deep breathing and coughing will not prevent a fat embolus; they are not a priority at the scene of an accident.

4 Maintaining the client's limb in the position in which it is found is necessary during transport to the hospital.

844. 2 **A continuous pull on the lower extremity keeps bone fragments from moving and causing further trauma, pain, and edema.**

1 The fracture will be reduced by surgery; Buck's traction is a temporary measure before surgery.

3 Moving the leg away from the midline will not keep the leg in alignment; it is not the purpose of Buck's traction.

4 External rotation of the femur may still occur with Buck's traction.

845. 1 **This provides slight countertraction, which will prevent sliding down in bed.**

2 This will have no effect.

3 This is unsafe; an interruption in the traction may result in disruption of bone alignment.

4 This will not alleviate the cause of the problem; it may be necessary more often than every couple of hours.

846. 4 **A pulmonary embolism is the most common complication of hip surgery because of high vascularity and the release of fat cells from the bone marrow.**

1 The occurrence of pneumonia is rare because of early activity after surgery. In addition, the operative area is not in proximity to the diaphragm and lungs; therefore, it does not impede deep breathing.

2 Postoperative hemorrhage with hip surgery is rare because bleeding at the operative site is not covert.

3 The incidence of wound infection is no greater than with other postoperative clients.

847. 3 **Abduction reduces stress on anatomical structures and maintains the head of the femur in the acetabulum.**

1 External rotation places stress on the acetabulum and the head of the femur.

2 Hip flexion may dislodge the head of the femur from the acetabulum.

4 Functional alignment places stress on the bone, soft tissue, and nail plate; it can cause damage and dislocation of the head of the femur.

848. 4 **A complete assessment must be performed to determine the location, characteristics, intensity, and duration of the pain. The pain may be incisional, result from a pulmonary embolus, or be caused by neurovascular trauma to the affected leg, and the intervention for each is different.**

1 This may be done after a complete assessment reveals that this is the appropriate intervention; assessment is the priority.

2 This may be done after a complete assessment reveals that this is the appropriate intervention; assessment is the priority.

3 This may be done after a complete assessment reveals that this is the appropriate intervention; assessment is the priority.

849. 2 **Compressed air inflates the padded plastic stockings systematically from ankle to calf to thigh and then deflates; this promotes venous return and prevents venous stasis and thromboembolism.**

1 Turning on the operative side is contraindicated because it places tension on the hip joint and may traumatize the incision.

3 Isometric exercises may be ordered to promote muscle strength; however, preventing the major complication, thromboembolism, is the priority.

4 Passive ROM is contraindicated immediately after surgery.

850. 2 **Abduction keeps the prosthesis firmly in place; adduction of the extremity may cause the prosthesis to dislocate.**

1 Only partial weight bearing on the affected leg is indicated initially.

3 Sitting flexes the hips to 90 degrees; this is contraindicated initially because it can cause the prosthesis to dislocate.

4 Full weight bearing on the unaffected leg and partial weight bearing on the affected leg generally are permitted on the second or third postoperative day.

851. 4 **Until the order is written to discontinue the abduction splint, it is only removed for mobility such as physical therapy and hygiene; adduction to or beyond the midline is not permitted until allowed by the practitioner.**
1 This splint is needed unless the client can be trusted to maintain abduction; flexing the hip with a prosthesis cannot be beyond 60 degrees for up to 10 days; from then on it cannot be beyond 90 degrees until permitted by the practitioner.
2 This splint helps to maintain position and keep the hip prosthesis in the hip socket.
3 This is inappropriate; there are no criteria for discontinuing abduction of the affected extremity.

852. 4 **The pelvis is elevated by actions involving the unaffected upper extremities and unaffected leg.**
1 This is not permitted because it causes adduction of the leg and can lead to dislocation of the femoral head.
2 This puts pressure on the operative hip, which is contraindicated because it may dislocate the prosthesis.
3 Lifting only with the arms requires strength; the use of both heels puts pressure on the operative hip, which may dislocate the prosthesis.

853. 4 **Tachycardia occurs because of an impaired gas exchange; petechiae are caused by occlusion of small vessels within the skin.**
1 Chest pain is not a common complaint with a fat embolism; fever may occur later.
2 A positive Homans' sign occurs with thrombophlebitis; it is not an indication of a fat embolism.
3 Loss of sensation suggests neurological dysfunction; it is not an indication of a fat embolism.

854. 3 **At the time of a fracture or orthopedic surgery, fat globules may move from the bone marrow into the bloodstream. Also elevated catecholamines cause mobilization of fatty acids and the development of fat globules. In addition to obstructing vessels in the lung, brain, and kidneys with systemic embolization of small vessels from fat globules, petechiae are noted in the buccal membranes, conjunctival sacs, hard palate, chest, and anterior axillary folds; these adaptations only occur with a fat embolism.**
1 This is a sign of an embolus, but it is not specific to a fat embolus.
2 This is a sign of an embolus, but it is not specific to a fat embolus.
4 This is a sign of an embolus, but it is not specific to a fat embolus.

855. 3 **Excessive flexion of the hip can cause dislocation of the femoral head.**
1 This should not cause undue strain on the operative site.

2 These should be encouraged as long as no extremes of positions are implemented.
4 This should be encouraged because it prevents hip flexion contractures.

856. 2 **A neurovascular assessment identifies early signs and symptoms of compartment syndrome. Compartment syndrome is increased pressure within a closed fascial space caused by a fracture and/or soft tissue damage that compresses circulatory vessels, nerves, and tissues compromising viability of the limb. The nurse should monitor for the 6 P's: unrelenting pain, pallor, paresthesia, pressure, pulselessness, and paralysis. In addition, the circumference of the extremity will increase and the leg will feel hard and firm on palpation. Both legs are assessed for symmetry.**
1 There is no established standard of care associated with pin care; some practitioners believe that pin care is contraindicated because it disrupts the skin's natural barrier to infection.
3 Initially the client should use a wheelchair or walk without weight bearing on the affected extremity. As healing occurs the practitioner will order progressive weight bearing.
4 Maintaining abduction of the leg is not necessary with an external fixation of the tibia.

857. 4 **Moist heat increases circulation and decreases muscle tension, which help relieve chronic stiffness.**
1 Although this is advisable for someone with arthritis, it does relieve morning stiffness.
2 Inactivity promotes stiffness.
3 This is related to muscle fatigue, not to stiffness of joints.

858. 2 **The pathological process involved with rheumatoid arthritis is accompanied by vascular congestion, fibrin exudate, and cellular infiltrate, causing inflammation of the synovium.**
1 Urate crystals occur with gouty, not rheumatoid, arthritis.
3 This is unrelated to rheumatoid arthritis.
4 Increased interstitial fluid is only one aspect of the inflammatory response.

859. 1 **Palpation will elicit tenderness because pressure stimulates nerve endings and causes pain.**
2 Pressure will not increase the swelling of already swollen joints.
3 Nodules associated with rheumatoid arthritis are not caused by pressure; they occur spontaneously in about 25% of individuals with rheumatoid arthritis and are composed of collagen fibers, exudate, and cellular debris.
4 These are present in gout, not rheumatoid arthritis; they are composed of sodium urate.

860. 2 **The prone position provides for extension of the hip and knee joints.**
1 The side-lying position promotes flexion of the hip and knee joints.

3 The contour position creates continued flexion of the hip and knee joints.

4 The Trendelenburg position does not prevent flexion contractures.

861. **4 Spacing activity protects joints from overuse, misuse, and stress, limiting inflammation; it provides a balance between rest and activity.**

1 The exercise program should be planned; too much activity can precipitate an exacerbation, and too little may cause contractures.

2 Spaced ROM should be incorporated into daily living activities, not just twice a day.

3 This will cause stress at the joints, which may precipitate an exacerbation.

862. **1 Active exercises (e.g., alternating extension, flexion, abduction, and adduction) mobilize exudate in the joints and relieve stiffness and pain.**

2 Flexion exercises alone will result in contractures.

3 ROM once a day is not enough to prevent contractures.

4 This will increase stiffness, joint pain, and the occurrence of contractures.

863. **2 This chair allows the hips and shoulders to be against the back of the chair while fully supporting the thighs.**

1 This permits the hips and knees to be flexed greater than 90 degrees, which can cause flexion contractures.

3 The thighs are not fully supported in a wheelchair.

4 This permits the hips to be flexed greater than 90 degrees, which promotes flexion contractures.

864. **1 Not neglecting joint pain protects the joints, especially if the pain lasts more than 1 or 2 hours after a particular activity.**

2 The opposite is true; the client should use large muscles, such as pushing doors open with arms rather than fingers.

3 This will increase joint stress; heavy and light tasks should be alternated.

4 When the inflammatory process is active, the joint should be at rest as much as possible.

865. **1 Phantom limb sensation is a real experience with no known cause or cure. The pain must be acknowledged and interventions to relieve the discomfort explored.**

2 There are no data indicating that the client is hopeless.

3 Although this may be effective for some people, it may not be effective for others; all possible interventions should be explored.

4 There are no data indicating that the client is grieving.

866. **2 Lying in the horizontal position stretches the flexor muscle and prevents a flexion contraction of the hip.**

1 This may result in an abduction deformity; the residual limb should be kept in functional alignment.

3 This flexes the hip, which may result in a hip flexion contracture; the residual limb is elevated for only 24 to 48 hours.

4 This type of exercise is started on a soft surface approximately 5 days after surgery; it requires a practitioner's order.

867. **4 The even distribution of hemosiderin (iron-rich pigment) in the tissue in response to pressure of the prosthesis indicates a correct fit.**

1 This is not related to the proper fit of a prosthesis.

2 This indicates that the prosthesis is too long or too short.

3 This will result in an improper fit.

868. **4 Pressure supports tissue, promotes venous return, and limits edema, thus promoting shrinkage of the distal part of the residual limb.**

1 Although it may limit clot formation, its primary purpose is to promote venous return, prevent edema, and shrink the distal part of the residual limb.

2 Bandaging does not decrease the occurrence of phantom limb sensation.

3 Although pressure may prevent hemorrhage, its primary purpose is to prevent edema and shrink the distal part of the residual limb.

869. **1 Preparation for crutch walking includes exercises to strengthen arm and shoulder muscles.**

2 Position changes help prevent hip flexion contractures, but do not prepare the client for crutch walking.

3 Caring for the residual limb promotes healing and helps prepare the limb for the prosthesis; it does not prepare the client for crutch walking.

4 The phantom limb sensation includes a feeling that the absent limb is present; there are no specific exercises for this phenomenon.

870. **2 Without the prosthesis, a walker or crutches will be necessary and require the readjustment of weight bearing on one leg.**

1 Early use of a prosthesis does not affect the development or presence of phantom limb sensation, which can occur in clients with an amputation.

3 Early use of a prosthesis has no effect on wound infection.

4 Although this is true, it is not the major purpose. A prosthesis easily can be fitted after discharge when the residual limb is completely healed and no longer edematous.

871. **3 The ability to transfer ensures mobility and a degree of independence postoperatively.**

1 Log-rolling is necessary for some spinal surgery, but not for amputation.

2 This is not of prime importance while the surgical wound is healing.

4 Standing on one leg in a weakened condition predisposes one to falling.

872. 3 **Elevation of the extremity promotes venous return, which limits edema and the related pressure on nerve endings that causes pain.**

1 Cool compresses limit venous return; vasoconstriction interferes with wound healing.

2 A week after surgery the discomfort probably is due to venous congestion related to the limb's dependent position rather than incisional pain.

4 This is contraindicated because the bandage prevents bleeding and edema and promotes shrinkage of the residual limb.

DRUG-RELATED RESPONSES

873. 1 **The nurse should discuss alternatives in terms of funding such as Medicaid, research projects, and special aid.**

2 Standards outside the United States may be different, and purchasing medications in a foreign country should not be encouraged.

3 Eventually the practitioner may be notified of this situation, but this is not the initial intervention.

4 This is a threatening comment; the nurse should be the client's advocate in this situation.

874. 4 **This response informs the practitioner of the nurse's dilemma and legal position without creating an adversarial professional position.**

1 A confrontational response may make the practitioner look and feel incompetent and jeopardize their collegial relationship.

2 A confrontational response may make the practitioner look and feel incompetent and jeopardize their collegial relationship.

3 A confrontational response may make the practitioner look and feel incompetent and jeopardize their collegial relationship.

875. 4 **Concurrent use of sildenafil (Viagra) and a nitrate, which causes vasodilation, may result in severe, potentially fatal hypotension.**

1 Nausea is not a side effect associated with concurrent use of sildenafil and a nitrate.

2 Tachypnea is not a side effect associated with concurrent use of sildenafil and a nitrate.

3 Viagra may cause diarrhea, not constipation.

876. 3 **Morphine sulfate (MS Contin) is a central nervous system depressant that commonly decreases the respiratory rate, which can lead to respiratory arrest.**

1 Morphine, an opioid, will cause constipation, not diarrhea.

2 Addiction is not a concern for a terminally ill client.

4 Although morphine sulfate may cause urinary retention, it is not a common side effect and is not life threatening.

877. 1 **The transfer of controlled substances from one authorized person to another must occur**

according to protocol. In this situation the controlled substance must be returned to the pharmacy and delivered at a later time.

2 The unit secretary does not have the authority to receive controlled substances.

3 The nurse cannot delay the securing of controlled substances; if time is not available when the medications are delivered, they must be returned to the pharmacy.

4 The nursing assistant does not have the authority to receive controlled substances.

878. 2 **These adaptations as well as anemia, irritability, pruritus, and an enlarged spleen occur with vitamin A toxicity.**

1 Excess thiamine is excreted in the urine and rarely, if ever, causes toxicity; an excessive dose may elicit an allergic reaction in some individuals.

3 Excess vitamin C (ascorbic acid) does not cause these adaptations or toxicity; however, vitamin C may cause diarrhea or renal calculi.

4 Pyridoxine (vitamin B_6) is relatively nontoxic, and excess amounts are excreted in the urine.

879. 1 **Multiple drugs are administered because of the concern regarding drug resistance.**

2 Streptomycin sulfate (Streptomycin) is an antibiotic; it does not prevent the side effects of Rifater therapy.

3 Multiple antitubercular drugs are necessary for an extended period, approximately 6 to 8 months depending on the individual.

4 This may increase anxiety and may not be true.

880. 2 **Rifampin (RIF) causes the body fluids, such as sweat, tears, and urine, to turn orange.**

1 It is not necessary to drink large amounts of fluid with this drug; it is not nephrotoxic.

3 Damage to the eighth cranial nerve is not a side effect of rifampin; it is a side effect of streptomycin sulfate, sometimes used to treat tuberculosis.

4 This is not a side effect of rifampin.

881. 4 **One of the most common side effects of isoniazid (INH) is peripheral neuritis, and vitamin B_6 will counteract this problem.**

1 It does help nutrition, but that is not the specific reason it is given.

2 It counters the side effects of isoniazid; it does not act to enhance its action.

3 It does not speed the destruction of the causative organism.

882. 1 **This medication causes hyperuricemia, leading to joint swelling and pain; fluids dilute the urine and help remove the uric acid.**

2 This is not a side effect of this medication.

3 This medication causes GI irritation and should be taken with food.

4 This is a side effect of rifampin (RIF), not pyrazinamide (PZA).

883. 1 **Antitubercular drugs such as isoniazid (INH) and rifampin (RIF) are hepatotoxic; liver function**

should be assessed before initiation of pharmacological therapy.

2 Although these studies might be done, the results
of these tests are not crucial for the nurse to review
before administering antitubercular drugs.

3 Although these studies might be done, the results
of these tests are not crucial for the nurse to review
before administering antitubercular drugs.

4 These tests will not provide information relative to
starting antitubercular therapy or to its side effects.

884. 3 **Pentamidine isethionate (Pentam 300) can cause
either hypoglycemia or hyperglycemia even after
therapy is discontinued, and therefore blood
glucose levels should be monitored.**

1 Hypotension, not hypertension, occurs with pentamidine isethionate.

2 Hyperkalemia, not hypokalemia, occurs with
pentamidine isethionate.

4 Hypocalcemia, not hypercalcemia, occurs
with pentamidine isethionate.

885. 4 **Novolin R insulin acts rapidly and is compatible
with intravenous solutions.**

1 Lispro (Humalog) insulin is not compatible with
intravenous solutions; it is a rapid-acting insulin.

2 Glargine (Lantus) insulin is not compatible with
intravenous solutions; it is a long-acting insulin.

3 Novolin N insulin is not compatible with intravenous solutions; it is an intermediate-acting insulin.

886. 1 **Glyburide (Micronase), an antidiabetic sulfonyl-
urea, stimulates insulin production by the beta
cells of the pancreas.**

2 This occurs when serum glucose drops below normal levels.

3 This occurs in the presence of insulin and potassium. Antidiabetic medications of the chemical
class of biguanide improve sensitivity of peripheral
tissue to insulin, which ultimately increases glucose
transport into cells.

4 Beta cells must have some function to enable this
drug to be effective.

887. 3 **The action of intermediate-acting insulins peak in
6 to 12 hours.**

1 This is too soon for Novolin N to produce a hypoglycemic response. A hypoglycemic response that
occurs in 45 to 60 minutes after administration is
associated with rapid-acting insulins.

2 This is too soon for Novolin N to produce a hypoglycemic response. A hypoglycemic response that
occurs in 2 to 3 hours after administration is associated with short-acting insulins.

4 Novolin N will have produced a hypoglycemic
response before this time frame.

888. 1 **These are the most commonly reported symptoms
of hypoglycemia and are related to increased sympathetic nervous system activity.**

2 These are adaptations of hyperglycemia.

3 These are symptoms of hyperglycemia.

4 These are symptoms of hyperglycemia.

889. 2 **The chemical structure of insulin is altered by
gastric secretions, rendering it ineffective.**

1 There is no such thing as oral insulin; this comment
about the seriousness of the diabetic condition may
increase anxiety.

3 There are no data to support this statement, and
insulin is given parenterally, not orally.

4 Insulin is not absorbed but is destroyed by gastric
secretions; there is no insulin that is effective if
taken by mouth.

890. 2 **This drug does not interfere with thyroxine already stored in the gland; symptoms remain until
the hormone is depleted.**

1 Duration of therapy varies depending on the severity
of the disease and the client's response to therapy.

3 This drug is not irritating to mucosal tissue, and no
special precautions are necessary.

4 Absorption is not affected by the presence of food
in the stomach.

891. 1 **Methimazole (Tapazole) blocks thyroid hormone
synthesis; it takes several weeks of medication
therapy before the hormones stored in the thyroid
gland are released and the excessive level of thyroid hormone in the circulation is metabolized.**

2 There are many common side effects that include
nausea, vomiting, diarrhea, rash, urticaria, pruritus,
alopecia, hyperpigmentation, drowsiness, headache,
vertigo, and fever.

3 Methimazole (Tapazole) should be spaced at
regular intervals because blood levels are reduced in
approximately 8 hours.

4 Large doses cause toxic side effects that can be
life threatening, including nephritis, hepatitis,
agranulocytosis, leukopenia, thrombocytopenia,
hypothrombinemia, and lymphadenopathy.

892. 2 **Ringing in the ears occurs because of its effect on
the eighth cranial nerve and is a classic symptom
of aspirin toxicity.**

1 This is not a side effect of aspirin; ASA promotes
comfort, which may permit rest.

3 Aspirin may cause diarrhea, nausea, and vomiting.

4 This is not a side effect of salicylates such as aspirin.

893. 2 **This helps to decrease gastric irritation by diluting
the acidic substances in the stomach.**

1 If aspirin (ASA) is taken on an empty stomach,
gastric irritation is increased.

3 Although this will limit gastric irritation, it will decrease
the effect of aspirin by increasing its renal excretion.

4 Aspirin has a gastric-irritating and ulcerogenic
effect, which may be potentiated by other drugs.

894. 3 **Although acetaminophen (Tylenol) reduces pain,
it lacks the antiinflammatory action needed to
limit joint inflammation associated with arthritis.**

1 People with arthritis do not need anticoagulants
unless prescribed for a concomitant cardiovascular
problem or cardiovascular prophylaxis.

2 Although they are both analgesics, acetaminophen is not an antiinflammatory agent.

4 There are fewer side effects with acetaminophen than with aspirin.

895. 4 **Enoxaparin (Lovenox), a low-molecular-weight heparin, prevents the conversion of fibrinogen to fibrin and prothrombin to thrombin by enhancing the inhibitory effects of antithrombin III.**

1 Enoxaparin is not an antipyretic.

2 Enoxaparin is not an analgesic.

3 Enoxaparin is not an antiinflammatory drug.

896. 1 **Diagnostic tests are necessary because ibuprofen (Motrin) is nephrotoxic, hepatotoxic, and prolongs the bleeding time.**

2 This is important for all clients with arthritis; it is not related to ibuprofen.

3 Ibuprofen does not cause postural hypotension.

4 Ibuprofen causes epigastric distress and occult bleeding; it should be taken with meals or milk to reduce these adverse reactions.

897. 4 **Pain is most effectively relieved when an analgesic is administered at the onset of pain, before it becomes intense; this prevents a pain cycle from occurring.**

1 Analgesics are less effective if administered when pain is at its peak.

2 This may or may not be necessary; the medication should be taken when the client begins to feel uncomfortable within the parameters specified by the practitioner's prescription.

3 Analgesics are less effective if administered when pain is at its peak.

898. 3 **These drugs tend to irritate the gastric mucosa and should be taken with milk or food.**

1 These drugs should be taken with food or milk to limit GI irritation.

2 This is an expected side effect; safety precautions are indicated, but the drug should not be discontinued.

4 This can result in toxicity if the extra dose in addition to the prescribed dose exceeds the therapeutic range; the dosage prescribed by the practitioner should be followed.

899. 3 **The intravenous route provides for the quickest onset of action of the opioid; pain relief occurs almost immediately.**

1 Nausea, vomiting, and paralytic ileus may occur postburn, making oral medications impractical.

2 The rectal route does not provide uniform absorption; also relief of pain will be delayed.

4 The medication may be sequestered in the tissues, and with fluid shifts it takes time for the medication to take effect.

900. 4 **Hospice clients with severe pain need increasing levels of analgesics and should be maintained at a pain-free level, even if addiction occurs.**

1 Pain management, not the prevention of addiction, is the priority.

2 The client has severe pain and the priority is to relieve the pain.

3 Comfort measures should augment, not be substitutes for, pharmacological interventions when clients are experiencing severe pain.

901. 2 **Anabolic agents are synthetic androgenic steroids that may produce masculinizing effects in women.**

1 With an increase in muscle mass and stimulation of erythropoiesis, the client should have an increase in energy.

3 Oxandrolone will cause sodium retention that will result in edema, not dehydration.

4 The client may become hyperkalemic, not hypokalemic, because potassium is retained with this drug.

902. 1 **Mafenide acetate (Sulfamylon) is effective against a wide variety of gram-positive and gram-negative organisms including anaerobes.**

2 This is an antimicrobial, not an analgesic; topical application may cause pain.

3 This is an antimicrobial that inhibits bacterial growth. Preventing scar tissue formation is not its action; however, by facilitating healing it may minimize the need for skin grafting.

4 This medication is an antimicrobial; it does not provide chemical debridement.

903. 1 **Silver sulfadiazine (Silvadene) is effective against gram-positive, gram-negative, and fungal organisms; however, it causes agranulocytosis, a serious side effect.**

2 Mafenide acetate (Sulfamylon) is effective against gram-negative and gram-positive organisms, but not fungi; it has serious side effects such as acidosis.

3 Neomycin (Cortisporin) has serious side effects; it is ototoxic, which can cause hearing loss, and it is nephrotoxic, which can cause kidney failure.

4 Silver nitrate is a component of silver sulfadiazine (Silvadene). It is not as effective if used alone. Drugs with silver nitrate must be kept moist.

904. 1 **Aspirin (ASA) is given to this client to prevent platelet aggregation and possible deep vein thrombosis. The client needs information to make an educated decision.**

2 The ASA is not prescribed to relieve pain. The client should receive information and support before making the decision to refuse the medication.

3 The ASA is not prescribed to relieve pain. The client should receive information and support before making the decision to refuse the medication.

4 The ASA is not prescribed to relieve pain. Clients should never be pressured to take medication, especially when they do not have an understanding of the risks and benefits of the medication.

905. 3 **Isosorbide dinitrate (Isordil) dilates the coronary vasculature, improving the supply of oxygen to the hypoxic myocardium.**

1 This is the action of anticoagulants.

2 This is the action of antidysrhythmics.

4 This is the action of cardiac glycosides.

906. 4 **Atenolol (Tenormin) competitively blocks stimulation of beta-adrenergic receptors within vascular smooth muscles, which lowers the blood pressure.**
   1 This drug does not cause headaches; this drug may be used to relieve vascular headaches.
   2 This drug may cause bradycardia, not tachycardia.
   3 This drug may cause diarrhea, not constipation.

907. Answer: 4, 5
   1 Citrus fruits, particularly oranges, are high in potassium and should be encouraged when the client is taking furosemide (Lasix) because this medication can cause hypokalemia.
   2 Furosemide does not cause photophobia.
   3 Lying horizontally has no relationship to furosemide.
   4 **Furosemide may cause hypovolemia, which can result in orthostatic hypotension with sudden changes in position.**
   5 **With loop diuretics, such as furosemide, an increased sodium load is presented to the distal tubule; this prompts an increase in sodium secretion as well as a corresponding increase in potassium secretion.**

908. 3 **Furosemide (Lasix) enhances the excretion of potassium, producing signs and symptoms of hypokalemia, such as hyporeflexia.**
   1 This is not a side effect of furosemide.
   2 This is not a side effect of furosemide.
   4 This is not a side effect of furosemide.

909. 4 **This drug decreases blood pressure by relaxing venous and arteriolar smooth muscle and is used for immediate reduction of blood pressure.**
   1 This drug may increase the heart rate as a response to vasodilation.
   2 It decreases cardiac workload by decreasing preload and afterload.
   3 It decreases peripheral resistance by dilating peripheral blood vessels.

910. 1 **Pruritus is a common side effect of clonidine (Catapres). Additional integumentary side effects include rash, hives, edema, alopecia, and facial pallor.**
   2 This drug causes constipation, not diarrhea.
   3 This drug may cause depression, anxiety, fatigue, and drowsiness, not euphoria.
   4 This is not a side effect of this medication.

911. 2 **Metoprolol (Toprol XL) and Lanoxin both exert a negative chronotropic effect, resulting in a decreased heart rate.**
   1 Metoprolol reduces, not produces, headaches.
   3 These drugs may cause hypotension.
   4 These drugs may depress nodal conduction.

912. 2 **Blurred vision, as well as yellow/green vision, is a sign of toxicity.**
   1 Constipation is not a sign of toxicity; gastrointestinal signs and symptoms of toxicity include anorexia, nausea, vomiting, and diarrhea.
   3 This is not a sign of toxicity. The client will have a decrease in urination because of dehydration.

   4 Digoxin (Lanoxin) does not cause a metal taste in the mouth.

913. 1 **Warfarin sodium (Coumadin) inhibits vitamin K; therefore, vitamin K is the antidote for warfarin sodium.**
   2 This is a blood-clotting factor, not the antidote for warfarin sodium.
   3 This is a blood-clotting factor, not the antidote for warfarin sodium.
   4 This is the antidote for heparin, not warfarin sodium.

914. 4 **Furosemide (Lasix) acts in the ascending limb of Henle's loop in the kidney.**
   1 Thiazides act in the distal tubule in the kidney.
   2 Potassium-sparing diuretics act in the collecting duct in the kidney.
   3 Plasma expanders and xanthines act in the glomerulus of the nephron in the kidney.

915. 4 **A cardiac glycoside such as digoxin (Lanoxin) decreases the conduction speed within the myocardium and slows the heart rate.**
   1 The primary effect of a diuretic is on the kidneys, not the heart; it may reduce the blood pressure, not the heart rate.
   2 A vasodilator can cause tachycardia, not bradycardia, which is an adverse effect.
   3 This does not drastically reduce the heart rate.

916. 4 **The most common adverse effect of a tissue plasminogen activator is bleeding because of the thrombolytic action of the drug.**
   1 Although this is important for any client with a decreased cardiac output, it is not specific to the administration of a tissue plasminogen activator.
   2 Although this is important for any client with a decreased cardiac output, it is not specific to the administration of a tissue plasminogen activator.
   3 Although this is important for any client with a decreased cardiac output, it is not specific to the administration of a tissue plasminogen activator.

917. 4 **The major action of intravenous nitroglycerin (Nitrostat IV) is venous and then arterial dilation, leading to a decrease in blood pressure.**
   1 This is not a common side effect of intravenous nitroglycerin.
   2 This is an infrequent effect when nitroglycerin is given intravenously.
   3 Reflex tachycardia may occur with the decrease in blood pressure.

918. 2 **Breaking the tablet increases the surface area of the tablet, which permits it to dissolve faster.**
   1 This may slow absorption because the tablet may move away from the absorption site.
   3 This will slow absorption because saliva helps to dissolve the tablet. Also the tablet should be placed under the tongue, where it is more readily absorbed.
   4 If taken with water, the tablet is washed away from the site of absorption or may even be swallowed.

919. 3 **Gabapentin (Neurontin) is an anticonvulsant and is not the drug of choice to relieve the pain associated with an MI.**
1 Alprazolam (Xanax) is an anxiolytic that is used for its calming effect, but it will not relieve the pain of an MI.
2 Midazolam HCl (Versed) is a sedative-hypnotic that is used for its calming effect, but it will not relieve the pain of an MI.
4 For severe MI, morphine sulfate (Duramorph) is a potent narcotic that relieves pain quickly and reduces anxiety.

920. 2 **Removing the previous patch before applying the next patch ensures that the client receives just the prescribed dose. Ideally, a patch should be removed after 12 to 14 hours to avoid the development of tolerance.**
1 The patch should be rotated among hair-free and scar-free sites; acceptable sites include chest, upper abdomen, proximal anterior thigh, or upper arm.
3 The patch should be gently pressed against the skin to ensure adherence; it should not be massaged.
4 This is unnecessary and can result in an excessive absorption of the medication.

921. 2 **The speed of conduction is decreased when digoxin is given, and this can result in premature beats, atrial fibrillation, and first-degree heart block.**
1 Digoxin (Lanoxin) does not deplete potassium and therefore orange juice does not need to be given; orange juice is high in calories and needs to be calculated in the diet.
3 Insulin and digoxin can be given at the same time.
4 The purpose of the drug is to reduce a rapid heart rate and therefore be administered; it should be withheld when the client's heart rate decreases below a parameter set by the practitioner (e.g., 60 beats per minute).

922. 4 **Lidocaine hydrochloride (Xylocaine) suppresses ventricular activity; therefore, it is used for treatment of PVCs.**
1 Atropine sulfate (Atropine) blocks vagal stimulation; it increases the heart rate and is used for bradycardia, not PVCs.
2 Epinephrine HCl (Adrenalin) increases myocardial contractility and heart rate; therefore, it is contraindicated in the treatment of PVCs.
3 Sodium bicarbonate increases the serum pH level; therefore, it combats metabolic acidosis.

923. 1 **Lidocaine HCl (Xylocaine) will interrupt the VT before it progresses to ventricular fibrillation.**
2 Epinephrine HCl (Adrenalin) is not used for VT; it is used for cardiac arrest and may even precipitate ventricular fibrillation.
3 A pacemaker is used for supraventricular tachycardia and bradycardia.
4 CPR is used for cardiac arrest, not VT.

924. 1 **A decreased heart rate or sinus bradycardia is the expected response to a beta-blocker. Beta-blockers inhibit the activity of the sympathetic nervous system and of adrenergic hormones, decreasing the heart rate, conduction velocity, and workload of the heart.**
2 A beta-blocker is not an anxiolytic and does not reduce anxiety.
3 A beta-blocker is not an analgesic and does not reduce chest pain.
4 Ventricular standstill indicates that the client is in cardiac arrest.

925. 1 **Tremors are a precursor to the major adverse effect of seizures.**
2 Although anorexia can occur, it is not a serious side effect.
3 Bradycardia occurs, which can lead to heart block.
4 Hypotension, not hypertension, occurs.

926. 4 **Generalized weakness is a symptom of significant hypokalemia, which may be a sequela of diuretic therapy.**
1 Insomnia is not known to be related to hypokalemia or hydrochlorothiazide (HCTZ) therapy.
2 Although a stuffy nose is unrelated to hydrochlorothiazide therapy, it can occur with other antihypertensive drugs.
3 Increased thirst is associated with hypernatremia. Because this drug increases excretion of water and sodium in addition to potassium and chloride, hyponatremia, not hypernatremia, may occur.

927. 3 **Sodium bicarbonate counteracts the acidosis that occurs secondary to tissue anoxia that accompanies cardiac standstill.**
1 Aminophylline (DBL) relaxes smooth muscle of the bronchial airways and pulmonary blood vessels, which is not indicated in this instance.
2 Furosemide (Lasix) is a diuretic commonly used for heart failure.
4 Phenytoin (Dilantin) is used after resuscitation to counteract seizures if they occur.

928. 4 **Morphine sulfate (Duramorph) is contraindicated for an unconscious, neurologically impaired client because it depresses respirations.**
1 Mannitol (Osmitrol), an osmotic diuretic, is used to reduce increased intracranial pressure.
2 Dexamethasone (Decadrone), a corticosteroid antiinflammatory agent, is used to help reduce increased intracranial pressure.
3 Chlorpromazine (Thorazine), an antipsychotic/neuroleptic/antiemetic, can be given safely to a neurologically impaired client for restlessness.

929. 2 **Administration of midazolam (Versed) 45 minutes before anesthesia allows for maximum effectiveness of its action.**
1 Administration of midazolam 2 hours before anesthesia is too long a time for maximum effectiveness of its action.

3 Administration of midazolam 15 minutes before anesthesia does not permit sufficient time for maximum effectiveness of the medication.

4 Administration of midazolam 5 minutes before anesthesia does not permit sufficient time for maximum effectiveness of the medication.

930. **2 Stomatitis is a common response to chemotherapy and should be brought to the practitioner's attention because a swish-and-swallow anesthetic solution can be prescribed to make the client more comfortable.**

1 Although a low-grade fever may occur, it does not require immediate medical attention.

3 Moderate diarrhea is expected and is not a cause for concern unless dehydration results.

4 Nausea is expected but should be reported if it lasts more than 24 hours.

931. **4 Muscle weakness, tingling, and numbness are related to drugs like vinCRIStine (Oncovin); neuropathies usually are transient if the drug is stopped or reduced.**

1 Nodal enlargement produces vascular rather than neural side effects.

2 This is untrue; neuropathies and peripheral vascular adaptations are potential side effects of chemotherapy.

3 Tingling and numbness are characteristic of neuropathy, not vascular occlusion.

932. **3 Aspirin (ASA) has an antiinflammatory action that relieves the inflammation and pain associated with arthritis. Acetaminophen (Tylenol) does not have antiinflammatory properties.**

1 Although both drugs are analgesics, acetaminophen does not have an antiinflammatory action.

2 Acetaminophen does not cause gastritis; this is an effect of aspirin.

4 Although true, this drug does not have the antiinflammatory properties of aspirin.

933. **2 Stomatitis and hyperuricemia are possible complications of therapy; therefore, oral care and hydration are important.**

1 Food and fluids with extremes in temperature should be avoided because of the common occurrence of stomatitis.

3 This may provide false reassurance.

4 Abnormal bleeding is a common problem and thus injections are contraindicated; rest is important for increased fatigability.

934. **2 Antineoplastic drugs depress bone marrow, which causes leukopenia; the client must be protected from infection, which can be life threatening.**

1 RBCs diminish slowly and can be replaced with a transfusion of packed red blood cells.

3 Platelets decrease as rapidly as WBCs, but complications can be limited with infusions of platelets.

4 RBCs diminish slowly and can be replaced with a transfusion of packed red blood cells.

935. **2 Chemotherapy destroys erythrocytes, white blood cells, and platelets indiscriminately along with the neoplastic cells because these are all rapidly dividing cells that are vulnerable to the effects of chemotherapy.**

1 This is not a true description of the side effects of steroids.

3 This is not the cause for fewer erythrocytes, white blood cells, and platelets.

4 Although true, this does not explain pancytopenia.

936. **Answer: 3, 4**

1 Hair loss is a complication associated with antimetabolites.

2 Stomatitis is a complication associated with antimetabolites and antitumor antibiotics.

3 **Imatinib (Gleevec) affects the bone marrow, causing thrombocytopenia; an adequate number of thrombocytes are necessary to prevent bleeding.**

4 **Imatinib affects the bone marrow, causing neutropenia; an adequate number of neutrophils are necessary to fight bacterial infections.**

5 Feminization is a complication when estrogens are administered to men.

937. **4 Plasma levels indicate whether therapeutic or toxic levels are present.**

1 Methotrexate (Rheumatrex) crystallizes in the kidneys if urine becomes acidic.

2 The regimen should include hydration with a minimum of intravenous fluids of 125 mL/hr 6 to 12 hours before and during therapy.

3 The effectiveness of methotrexate, a folic acid antagonist, is minimized by a diet high in folic acid.

938. **2 Hyperkalemia occurs when large quantities of tumor cells are destroyed, rapidly releasing potassium and purines quicker than the body can manage them (tumor lysis syndrome). A serum potassium of 5.8 mEq/L is more than the expected range of 3.5 to 5.3 mEq/L, resulting in the abnormal ECG results. Hyperkalemia can cause a pulse in the lower range of that expected for an adult, numbness in the extremities, flaccid paresis, hyperactive bowel sounds, and diarrhea.**

1 There are no adaptations indicating septic shock. The WBC count and vital signs are all within the expected range. A rapid, weak pulse, rapid respirations, increased temperature, hypotension, and cold, clammy skin are associated with septic shock.

3 Superior vena cava syndrome occurs when a tumor obstructs or compresses the superior vena cava resulting in blockage of blood flow to the venous system of the head, neck, and upper trunk. Edema of the face (especially periorbital edema) and eventually edema of the arms and hands, dyspnea, epistaxis, and erythema occur. Lastly hemorrhage, cyanosis, hypotension, and heart failure can result in death.

4 With disseminated intravascular coagulation (DIC) there is abnormal coagulation resulting in bleeding

from many sites and clot formation decreasing blood flow to major organs. Decreased circulation to organs causes pain, strokelike adaptations, dyspnea, tachycardia, oliguria, bowel necrosis, and multiple organ failure.

939. 2 **Melphalan (Alkeran) depresses the bone marrow, causing a reduction in white blood cells (leukopenia), red blood cells (anemia), and thrombocytes (thrombocytopenia); leukopenia increases the risk of infection.**

1 Hirsutism occurs with the administration of androgens to women.

3 Diarrhea, not constipation, occurs with melphalan.

4 Photosensitivity occurs with 5-fluorouracil, floxuridine, and methotrexate, not with melphalan.

940. 4 **A pregnant woman having contact with the semen of a client taking finasteride (Proscar) can adversely affect a developing male fetus.**

1 Finasteride helps prevent male pattern baldness.

2 Results may take 6 to 12 months.

3 Finasteride medication can mask the occurrence of prostatic cancer because it decreases prostatic specific antigen (PSA).

941. 2 **Leucovorin (Wellcovorin) limits toxicity of folic acid antagonists, such as methotrexate sodium, by competing for transport into cells.**

1 Leucovorin does not potentiate the effect of alkylating agents; however, leucovorin promotes binding of fluorouracil (5-FU) to target tumor cells.

3 Antiemetics such as prochlorperazine maleate (Compazine) and ondansetron (Zofran) minimize nausea and vomiting associated with chemotherapeutic agents.

4 Leucovorin does not interfere with cell division; this is the purpose of a multiple drug protocol.

942. 4 **Tetrahydrocannabinol, an ingredient in marijuana, acts as an antiemetic in some persons and can be absorbed through the gastrointestinal tract or inhaled.**

1 This does not answer the client's question.

2 Marijuana is not injected.

3 Tetrahydrocannabinol, an ingredient in marijuana, is an effective antiemetic for some clients.

943. 1 **This helps flush the kidneys and prevent nephrotoxicity, especially during the early phase of treatment.**

2 Reconstituted solution can be stored in the refrigerator for 1 month.

3 Confusion, dizziness, and hallucinations are side effects of this drug; the client should avoid hazardous tasks, such as driving or using machinery.

4 Activity may have to be altered because fatigue and other flulike symptoms are common with this drug.

944. 1 **Peripheral paresthesia is an indication of toxicity from a plant alkaloid such as vinCRIStine (Oncovin).**

2 This is not a side effect of any of the drugs listed.

3 This is not a side effect of any of the drugs listed.

4 This is not a side effect of any of the drugs listed.

945. 2 **Penlike insulin delivery devices are more accurate because they are easy to use; also they promote adherence to insulin regimens because the medication can be administered discreetly.**

1 One disadvantage of the penlike insulin delivery device is that the injection time will be longer; the device must remain in place for several seconds after the insulin is injected to ensure that no insulin leaks out.

3 Pain and discomfort are decreased with the penlike insulin delivery device because it has a larger-gauge needle that has a smaller diameter.

4 The insulin cartridges of a penlike insulin delivery device are single use and disposable.

946. 2 **The pancreatic enzymes (amylase, trypsin, and lipase) must be present when food is ingested for digestion to take place.**

1 At bedtime the food eaten for dinner has passed beyond the duodenum; at bedtime the enzyme is given too late to aid digestion.

3 The client will have no chyme in the duodenum on which the enzyme can act.

4 The client will have no chyme in the duodenum on which the enzyme can act.

947. 3 **Cisplatin (Platinol) is nephrotoxic and can cause kidney damage unless the client is adequately hydrated to flush the kidneys.**

1 Leucovorin, a form of folic acid, is used to combat toxic effects of methotrexate; cisplatin does not interfere with folic acid metabolism.

2 Gentle, not vigorous, oral care is needed to cleanse the mouth without further aggravating the expected stomatitis.

4 A low-residue diet is unnecessary. Prolonged gastrointestinal irritation is not the major concern; nausea and vomiting last about 24 hours, and although diarrhea may occur and last longer, it is not the primary concern.

948. 3 **Meperidine (Demerol) should be avoided because accumulation of its metabolites can cause CNS irritability and even tonic-clonic seizures (grand mal seizures).**

1 Ranitidine (Zantac) is useful in reducing gastric acid stimulation of pancreatic enzymes.

2 Cimetidine (Tagamet) is useful in reducing gastric acid stimulation of pancreatic enzymes.

4 Promethazine HCl (Phenergan) is useful as an antiemetic for clients with pancreatitis.

949. 2 **The relaxation effect increases the passage of food through the gastrointestinal tract limiting reverse peristalsis, gastroesophageal reflux, and vomiting, all of which are precipitated by chemotherapeutic agents.**

1 Metoclopramide does not stimulate the production of gastrointestinal secretions.

3 Metoclopramide has no effect on the excretion of chemotherapeutic medications.

4 Metoclopramide has no effect on the absorption of chemotherapeutic medications.

950. 3 **Prednisone (Meticorten) inhibits phagocytosis and suppresses other clinical phenomena of inflammation; this is a symptomatic treatment that is not curative.**

1 Prednisone suppresses the immune response, which increases the potential for infection.

2 The appetite is increased with prednisone; weight gain may result from the increased appetite or from fluid retention.

4 Generally the response to prednisone is rapid.

951. 4 **The GI tract contains numerous bacteria; antibiotics are given to decrease the number of microorganisms in the bowel before surgery.**

1 This is a potential complication prevented by the use of sterile technique when changing the dressing.

2 This is a potential complication prevented by coughing, deep breathing, and early ambulation postoperatively.

3 This is a potential complication prevented by hygiene, meatal care, and increased hydration postoperatively.

952. 3 **Usually a larger dose is given at 8 AM and the second dose is given before 4 pm to mimic expected hormonal secretion and prevent insomnia.**

1 This is necessary because long-term administration of steroids leads to elevated blood glucose levels and possible steroid-induced diabetes.

2 Oral corticosteroids should be taken with food or antacids to prevent gastric irritation and gastric hemorrhage.

4 Neurological and emotional side effects such as euphoria, mood swings, and sleeplessness are expected.

953. 3 **Neomycin sulfate (Mycifradin) reduces bacterial activity on blood and wastes in the GI tract, thereby reducing the level of blood ammonia, a byproduct of protein metabolism; hepatic encephalopathy is a result of elevated ammonia levels in the blood.**

1 Neomycin sulfate interferes with bacterial protein synthesis but has little or no effect on intestinal edema.

2 Neomycin sulfate reduces bacterial action in the GI tract but does not reduce abdominal distention.

4 Neomycin sulfate does not limit the development of a systemic infection when it is ingested because it is not absorbed systemically.

954. 2 **Propylthiouracil (PTU) may lower the white blood cell count, making the client prone to infection.**

1 Propylthiouracil does not cause hypocalcemia; milk does not facilitate absorption of the drug.

3 Taking the drug through a straw is necessary with iodine preparations to prevent staining of the teeth; propylthiouracil does not contain iodine.

4 Propylthiouracil does not cause photosensitivity.

955. Answer: 1, 4

1 **Excessive levothyroxine (Synthroid) produces adaptations similar to hyperthyroidism including tremors, tachycardia, hypertension, heat intolerance, and insomnia. These adaptations are related to the increase in the metabolic rate associated with hyperthyroidism.**

2 Bradycardia is a sign of hypothyroidism and a need to increase the dose of levothyroxine.

3 Somnolence is a sign of hypothyroidism and a need to increase the dose of levothyroxine.

4 **Heat intolerance is a sign of hyperthyroidism and a need to decrease the dose of levothyroxine.**

5 Hypotension is a sign of hypothyroidism and a need to increase the dose of levothyroxine.

956. 4 **The detergent action of docusate sodium (Colace) promotes the drawing of fluid into the stool which softens the feces.**

1 This is the action of lubricant laxatives such as mineral oil.

2 This is the action of saline laxatives such as magnesium hydroxide (Milk of Magnesia).

3 This is the action of peristaltic stimulants such as cascara.

957. 4 **Bisacodyl (Dulcolax) stimulates nerve endings in the intestinal mucosa, precipitating a bowel movement.**

1 Dulcolax is not a bulk cathartic. Bulk-forming laxatives, such as psyllium hydrophilic mucilloid (Metamucil), form soft, pliant bulk that promotes physiologic peristalsis.

2 Bisacodyl is not a stool softener. Stool softeners, such as docusate sodium, permit fat and water to penetrate feces, which softens and delays the drying of the feces.

3 Bisacodyl is not an emollient. Emollient laxatives, such as mineral oil (Kondremul), lubricate the feces and decrease absorption of water from the intestinal tract.

958. 2 **Increased acidity caused by the stress occurring with burns and crushing injuries contributes to the formation of Curling's ulcer; ranitidine (Zantac), an H_2 antagonist, decreases the formation of gastric acid, and Maalox, an antacid, neutralizes gastric acid once it is formed.**

1 These drugs do not decrease irritability of the bowel; their purpose is to decrease gastrointestinal acidity.

3 This does not explain how these drugs work.

4 This does not explain how these drugs work.

959. 1 **Loperadine (Maalox), a combination antacid, contains magnesium hydroxide, which may cause diarrhea; it also contains aluminum hydroxide, which may cause constipation.**

2 Esomeprazole (Nexium), a proton pump inhibitor, may cause constipation, not diarrhea.

3 Immobility causes constipation, not diarrhea.

4 Although diet can affect elimination, no data are presented to support this conclusion.

960. 3 **Timolol maleate (Timoptic) is a beta-adrenergic antagonist that decreases aqueous humor production and increases outflow, thereby reducing intraocular pressure.**
    1 Tetracaine (Pontocaine) is a topical anesthetic; it will not reduce the increased intraocular pressure associated with glaucoma.
    2 Cyclopentolate (Cyclogyl) is contraindicated because it dilates the pupil and paralyzes ciliary muscles.
    4 Atropine sulfate (Atropisol Ophthalmic), a mydriatic, is contraindicated because it dilates the pupil, obstructing drainage, which increases intraocular pressure.

961. 4 **Parenterally administered diazepam (Valium) is a benzodiazepine that has muscle relaxant and anticonvulsant effects that help limit massive muscular spasms.**
    1 Atropine sulfate (Atropine) is not used for seizures. It is used for bradycardia resulting from vagal overstimulation, but does not reverse bradycardia caused by metabolic changes such as acid-base imbalances or electrolyte imbalances.
    2 Epinephrine HCl (Adrenalin) does not limit seizures; it increases contractility of the heart.
    3 Naloxone (Narcan) does not limit seizures; it is an opioid antagonist and is used for morphine, meperidine, and methadone overdose.

962. 4 **Because of the lethal toxicity of aspirin (ASA) overdose, hypotensive crisis and cardiac irregularities can occur.**
    1 The central nervous system is not involved at the reflex level at this time.
    2 Central venous pressure readings are not indicated in this situation.
    3 This is not the priority at this time.

963. 2 **Adequate dental hygiene is essential to control or prevent the common side effect of hypertrophy of gums.**
    1 This medication should be taken with food or milk to decrease GI side effects.
    3 The practitioner should be consulted before the drug is discontinued or the dosage is adjusted; usually in this situation, a gradual dosage reduction is prescribed.
    4 These are unrelated to phenytoin (Dilantin) therapy.

964. 3 **Levodopa (L-dopa) is a precursor of dopamine, a catecholamine neurotransmitter; it increases dopamine levels in the brain that are depleted in Parkinson's disease.**
    1 Blocking the effects of acetylcholine is accomplished by anticholinergic drugs.
    2 Increasing the production of dopamine is ineffective because it is believed that the cells that produce dopamine have degenerated in Parkinson's disease.
    4 Levodopa does not affect acetylcholine production.

965. 3 **Abnormal involuntary movements (dyskinesias), such as muscle twitching, rapid eye blinking, facial grimacing, head bobbing, and an exaggerated protrusion of the tongue, are signs of toxicity; these probably result from the body's failure to readjust properly to the reduction of dopamine.**
    1 Nausea is a side effect of therapy, not toxicity.
    2 Dizziness is a side effect of therapy, not toxicity.
    4 Constipation is unrelated to levodopa toxicity.

966. 3 **Carbidopa-levodopa (Sinemet) should be taken with meals to reduce the nausea and vomiting that commonly are caused by this drug.**
    1 Multivitamins are contraindicated; vitamins may contain pyridoxine (vitamin B_6) that diminishes the effects of levodopa.
    2 Moderate amounts of alcohol will antagonize the drug's effects; a rare, occasional drink is not harmful.
    4 A high-protein diet is contraindicated. Sinemet contains levodopa, an amino acid that may increase blood urea nitrogen (BUN) levels. Also some proteins contain pyridoxine, which increases peripheral metabolism of levodopa, decreasing the amount of levodopa crossing the blood-brain barrier.

967. 1 **A severe headache is a sign of an MAOI-induced hypertensive crisis and should be reported to the physician immediately.**
    2 Monthly blood tests are unnecessary, but routine medical evaluations of the client should be scheduled.
    3 Adjusting the dose of the drug daily is unsafe; the recommended daily dose of the drug should be taken as prescribed.
    4 The opposite is true; the side effects of levodopa will increase when these two drugs are taken concurrently.

968. 2 **Corticosteroids, such as dexamethasone (Decadron), have a hyperglycemic effect, and blood glucose levels should be routinely monitored.**
    1 Assessing bowel sounds is unnecessary; corticosteroids are not known to precipitate cessation of gastrointestinal activity.
    3 Although corticosteroids may increase the risk of developing an infection, routine culturing of respiratory secretions is unnecessary. Culturing respiratory secretions becomes necessary when the client exhibits adaptations of a respiratory infection.
    4 Monitoring deep tendon reflexes is required when administering magnesium sulfate, not dexamethasone.

969. 4 **Osmotic diuretics remove excessive cerebrospinal fluid (CSF), reducing intracranial pressure.**
    1 Osmotic diuretics increase, not decrease, the blood pressure by increasing the fluid in the intravascular compartment.
    2 Osmotic diuretics do not directly influence blood glucose levels.
    3 Although there is an increase in cardiac output when the vascular bed expands as CSF is removed,

it is not the primary purpose for administering the medication.

970. **3 Mannitol (Osmitrol), an osmotic diuretic, pulls fluid from the white cells of the brain to relieve cerebral edema.**

  1 Mannitol's diuretic action does not decrease the production of cerebrospinal fluid.
  2 Mannitol does not affect brain metabolism; rest and lowered body temperature reduce brain metabolism.
  4 Preventing uncontrolled electrical discharges in the brain is the action of phenytoin sodium (Dilantin), not mannitol.

971. **2 Mannitol (Osmitrol), an osmotic diuretic, increases the intravascular volume that must be excreted by the kidneys. The client's urine output should be monitored hourly to determine the client's response to therapy.**

  1 Although with mannitol there is an increase in urinary excretion that is reflected in a decrease in body weight (1 L of fluid is equal to 2.2 pounds), a daily assessment of the client's weight is too infrequent to assess the client's response to therapy. Urine output can be monitored hourly and is a more frequent, accurate, and efficient assessment than is a daily weight.
  3 Vital signs should be monitored every hour considering the severity of the client's injury and the administration of mannitol.
  4 Although the level of consciousness should be monitored with a head injury, assessments every 8 hours are too infrequent to monitor the client's response to therapy.

972. **1 Administration of an anticoagulant to a client who is bleeding will interfere with clotting and increase bleeding.**

  2 Anticoagulants are not used in this situation because they will increase bleeding; they may be used for a client with a cerebral, not pulmonary, thrombosis.
  3 Although contraindicated, if given it will increase bleeding and its associated signs and symptoms.
  4 Anticoagulants are not used in this situation because they will increase bleeding; anticoagulants may be used with cerebral thrombosis.

973. **3 The site of the injection should not be massaged to avoid dispersion of the heparin (Hep-Lock) around the site and subsequent bleeding into the area.**

  1 The Z-track technique and the intramuscular route are not used with heparin; subcutaneous injection and intravenous administration are the routes appropriate for heparin administration.
  2 The drug should be injected into the subcutaneous tissue slowly, not quickly.
  4 Diluting heparin with normal saline is unnecessary. Generally heparin is provided by the pharmacy department in single dose syringes.

974. **1 Failure to clarify this omission can be life threatening because of the potential for an embolus.**

  2 It is the practitioner's role, not the nurse's, to decide if the client needs or does not need an anticoagulant.
  3 It is the practitioner's role, not the nurse's, to decide if the client needs or does not need an anticoagulant.
  4 Waiting until the client is in the new facility to discuss the administration of an anticoagulant may jeopardize the client's status. It is the nurse's, not the client's, responsibility to discuss this situation with the practitioner.

975. **4 An INR of 4.6 is higher than the desired therapeutic level of 2 to 3.5. It is prudent to maintain bed rest to prevent injury until the practitioner evaluates the client's INR result.**

  1 Another dose of warfarin sodium (Coumadin) may be contraindicated in light of the client's increased INR result.
  2 A partial thromboplastin time is performed to evaluate a client's response to the administration of heparin.
  3 Increasing the intake of food high in vitamin K is contraindicated; vitamin K is the antidote for warfarin sodium. The client should have a consistent, limited intake of food high in vitamin K.

976. **2 Clopidogrel (Plavix) interferes with platelet aggregation, which impedes the formation of thrombi.**

  1 Clopidogrel is a platelet aggregation inhibitor, not an antiinflammatory.
  3 Clopidogrel is a platelet aggregation inhibitor, not an antipyretic.
  4 Clopidogrel is a platelet aggregation inhibitor, not an analgesic.

977. **2 Because this drug inhibits the destruction of acetylcholine, parasympathetic activity may be increased.**

  1 Myasthenic crisis, like cholinergic crisis, is characterized by increasing muscle weakness.
  3 Side effects continue as long as the drug is continued; the dosage may be adjusted or an anticholinergic given to limit side effects.
  4 Toxicity or cholinergic crisis is manifested by increased muscle weakness, including muscles of respiration.

978. **4 Taking the medication as prescribed promotes an even therapeutic blood level, which maintains muscle strength.**

  1 Because of drug-related nausea and gastric irritation, the drug should be taken with crackers or milk.
  2 Thirty, not 60 minutes before meals is recommended for maximum chewing and swallowing function.
  3 This is unsafe because it will not maintain constant therapeutic drug levels.

979. 4 **A decrease in symptoms in response to the administration of edrophonium chloride (Tensilon) indicates myasthenic crisis; an increase in the severity of symptoms indicates cholinergic crisis.**
   1 Atropine sulfate (Atropine) is the treatment for cholinergic crisis.
   2 Protamine sulfate is the antidote for heparin.
   3 Naloxone (Narcan) is an opioid antagonist.

980. 3 **Steroids decrease the body's immune response, limiting the production of antibodies that attack acetylcholine receptors at the neuromuscular junction.**
   1 This is the action of anticholinergic medications.
   2 This is not the action of immunosuppressives.
   4 This is the rationale for plasmapheresis.

981. 2 **Neostigmine (Prostigmin) should be taken as prescribed, usually before meals, to limit dysphagia and possible aspiration.**
   1 Keeping neostigmine refrigerated is not necessary; it may be kept at room temperature.
   3 Neostigmine should be taken with milk to prevent GI irritation; usually it is taken about 30 minutes before meals.
   4 The onset of the action of neostigmine occurs 45 to 75 minutes after administration; the duration of its action is 2½ to 4 hours.

982. 1 **A urinary output of at least 1500 mL daily should be maintained to prevent crystalluria (crystals in the urine).**
   2 Orange juice produces an alkaline ash, which results in an alkaline urine that supports the growth of bacteria.
   3 Trimethoprim-sulfamethoxazole (Septra) should be taken 1 hour before meals for maximum absorption.
   4 A prescribed course of antibiotics must be completed to eliminate the infection, which can exist on a subclinical level after symptoms subside.

983. 3 **The client should increase fluid intake when taking ampicillin (Omnipen) to prevent nephrotoxicity; side effects include oliguria, hematuria, proteinuria, and glomerulonephritis.**
   1 An antibiotic should be continued until the entire prescription is completed; discontinuing before completion lowers its serum level, thereby decreasing its effectiveness.
   2 Ampicillin should be taken when the stomach is empty, either 1 to 2 hours before eating or 3 to 4 hours after eating.
   4 There are no restrictions on eating grapefruit when taking an antibiotic; this is contraindicated when taking some calcium channel blockers because grapefruit juice increases their serum level.

984. 1 **Finasteride (Proscar) and saw palmetto both have antiandrogenic and antiproliferative properties in prostate tissue. Saw palmetto has comparable efficacy to Proscar. The practitioner must be** consulted regarding the client's desire to change the prescribed therapy.
   2 Saw palmetto should be taken with food to limit gastrointestinal side effects.
   3 Saw palmetto does not alter the size of the prostate gland.
   4 Finasteride (Proscar), an androgen inhibitor, not saw palmetto, promotes the regrowth of hair that is lost.

985. 1 **Because the drug was just administered, the blood level of the drug will be at its highest level.**
   2 The result will reveal a drug blood level halfway between the peak and trough levels.
   3 This is done for a trough level when the drug level is at its lowest.
   4 This will produce inaccurate results; peak and trough levels are measured in relation to the time a drug is administered.

986. Answer: 4, 5
   1 Daily monitoring is not indicated. The blood pressure should be monitored at routine office visits.
   2 There is no need to avoid the use of NSAIDs while taking an angiotensin II receptor blocker (ARB).
   3 A dry cough may occur during treatment with ARBs; however, it is not necessary to discontinue the medication because the cough usually resolves.
   4 **The medication should be stopped if angioedema occurs, and the practitioner notified.**
   5 **Electrolyte levels of potassium, sodium, and chloride should be obtained 2 weeks after the start of therapy and then periodically thereafter.**

987. 4 **Tylenol ES (extra strength) is not coated or intended to be released slowly; crushing this medication will not cause a bolus of the medication to be administered to the client.**
   1 Crushing of potassium chloride (Slow K) will cause a bolus of medication to be given at once rather than slowly; if crushing is necessary, another form of the medication or another medication should be requested from the practitioner.
   2 Crushing an SR (sustained release) medication will cause a bolus of medication to be administered at once rather than slowly as intended; if crushing is necessary, another form of the medication or another medication should be requested of the practitioner.
   3 Crushing of an XL (extended release) medication will cause a bolus to be given; if crushing is necessary, another form of the medication or another medication should be requested of the practitioner.

988. 3 **Anaphylaxis is an acute, adverse, life-threatening reaction to this immunosuppressant; it is manifested by dyspnea, seizures, and shock.**
   1 Hypothermia is a common side effect of this medication.
   2 Dysrhythmias are not a side effect of this medication, although chest pain can occur.

4 The neurological side effects of this medication are not subtle. Pyrexia, chills, tremors, and aseptic meningitis can occur, but they are not immediately life threatening as is anaphylactic shock.

989. 4 **Standard triple therapy includes a corticosteroid (prednisone [Meticorten], methylprednisolone [Solu-Medrol]), an antimetabolite, mycophenolate [CellCept], and a calcineurin inhibitor (tacrolimus [Prograf], cyclosporine [Sandimmune]).**
1 Although sirolimus (Rapamune) is used for immunosuppression, furosemide (Lasix) is a diuretic.
2 Neither of these medications are immunosupressives. Cefazolin (Ancef) is an antibiotic and methotrexate (Rheumatrex) is a folic acid antagonist used in cancer chemotherapy.
3 Although methylprednisolone (Solu-Medrol) is used for immunosuppression, phenytoin (Dilantin) is an antiseizure medication.

990. 2 **Epogen stimulates red blood cell production, thereby increasing the hematocrit level.**
1 An elevated liver panel is not related to Epogen because Epogen is not hepatotoxic.
3 Epogen increases RBCs, not WBCs.
4 Increased Kaposi's sarcoma lesions are a sign of AIDS progression and are not affected by Epogen.

991. 4 **Filgastrin (Neupogen), a granulocyte colony-stimulating factor, increases the production of neutrophils with little effect on the production of hematopoietic cells.**
1 The production of platelets is not stimulated by filgastrin.
2 The production of erythrocytes is not stimulated by filgastrin.
3 The production of thrombocytes is not stimulated by filgastrin.

992. 4 **Epoetin (Procrit) is administered via the subcutaneous or intravenous route; a 1-inch, 25-gauge needle is appropriate for either method of administration.**
1 The client's vital signs, particularly the blood pressure, need to be monitored only routinely to determine the effectiveness of the medication.
2 Epoetin is not administered via the intramuscular route.
3 Shaking the vial denatures the glycoprotein, making the medication biologically inactive and therefore ineffective.

993. 2 **Maintaining adequate gas exchange and minimizing hypoxia with pulmonary edema are critical; therefore, assessing the effectiveness of furosemide (Lasix) therapy as it relates to the respiratory system is most important. Furosemide inhibits the reabsorption of sodium and chloride from the loop of Henle and distal renal tubule causing diuresis; as diuresis occurs fluid moves out of the vascular compartment thereby reducing pulmonary edema and the bilateral crackles.**
1 Another nursing action will more quickly reflect the effectiveness of furosemide therapy. Although a liter of fluid weighs approximately 2.2 pounds and weight loss will reflect the amount of fluid lost, it will take time before a change in weight can be measured.
3. Although identifying a greater output versus intake indicates the effectiveness of furosemide, it is the client's pulmonary status that is most important with acute pulmonary edema.
4. Although the lessening of a client's dependent edema reflects effectiveness of furosemide therapy, it is the client's improving pulmonary status that is most important.

994. Answer: 1, 2, 3
1 **Nizatidine (Axid) is an H₂ receptor antagonist that reduces gastric acid secretion and provides for symptomatic improvement in GERD.**
2 **Rinitidine (Zantac) is an H₂ receptor antagonist that reduces gastric acid secretion and provides for symptomatic improvement in GERD.**
3 **Famotidine (Pepcid) is an H₂ receptor antagonist that reduces gastric acid secretion and provides for symptomatic improvement in GERD.**
4 Metoclopramide (Prevacid) is a proton pump inhibitor that inhibits gastric secretion up to 90% with one dose daily and provides for symptomatic improvement in GERD.
5 Metoclopramide (Reglan) is a prokinetic agent that increases the rate of gastric emptying; it has multiple side effects and is not appropriate for long-term treatment of GERD.

995. Answer: 2 mL. First convert milligrams (mg) to micrograms (mcg) and then use ratio and proportion (0.2 mg = 200 mcg).

$$\frac{200 \text{ mcg}}{100 \text{ mcg}} = \frac{x \text{ mL}}{1 \text{ mL}}$$

$$100 \text{ x} = 200$$

$$x = 2 \text{ mL}$$

996. Answer: 100 gtt/minute. The total drops per minute should be divided by the total time in minutes:

$$\frac{50 \text{ ml} \times 60 \text{ gtt/mL}}{30 \text{ minutes}} = \frac{3000}{30} = 100 \text{ gtt/minute}$$

997. Answer: 18 mL/hr. The practitioner prescribed 1.5 mg of lidocaine HCl (Xylocaine) to be administered per minute. Multiply the 1.5 mg times 60 minutes to determine the hourly dosage to be administered. Then solve the problem using ratio and proportion.

$$\frac{90 \text{ mg}}{500 \text{ mg}} = \frac{x \text{ mL}}{100 \text{ mL}}$$

$$500 \text{ x} = 9000$$

$$x = \frac{9000}{500}$$

$$x = 18 \text{ mL/hr}$$

998. Answer: 1.7 mL. Use ratio and proportion to calculate the desired amount of solution.

$$\frac{375 \text{ mg}}{225 \text{ mg}} = \frac{x \text{ mL}}{1 \text{ mL}}$$

$$225 \text{ x} = 375$$

$$x = 1.67 \text{ (this result should}$$
$$\text{be rounded up to 1.7 mL)}$$

999. Answer: 0.8 mL. Use ratio and proportion to answer the question.

$$250 \text{ mg} = 0.25 \text{g}$$

$$\frac{0.25 \text{ mg}}{1 \text{ g}} = \frac{x \text{ mL}}{3 \text{ mL}}$$

$$x = 0.75 \text{ mL or } 0.8 \text{ mL}$$

1000. Answer: 35 mL/hr. 1 mg = 2.5 mL; therefore, 14 mg = 35 mL.

$$\frac{14 \text{ mg}}{100 \text{ mg}} = \frac{x \text{ mL}}{250 \text{ mL}}$$

$$100 \text{ x} = 3500$$

$$x = 35 \text{ mL}$$

MEDICAL-SURGICAL NURSING
QUIZ 1

1. A client with rheumatoid arthritis calls the outpatient clinic to report that the pain lasts for 2 to 3 hours after exercise. What is the nurse's most appropriate initial response?
   1. "Stop exercising for a day."
   2. "Increase the number of repetitions of each exercise."
   3. "Decrease the number of repetitions of your exercises."
   4. "Limit progressive resistive exercises to three times a day."

2. When preparing a client for a liver biopsy, the nurse should instruct the client to:
   1. Turn onto the left side after the procedure
   2. Breathe normally throughout the procedure
   3. Hold the breath at the moment of the actual biopsy
   4. Bear down during the insertion of the biopsy needle

3. A 40-year-old client visits a neurologist with complaints of blurred, double vision and muscular weakness. After multiple sclerosis is diagnosed, the client, visibly upset, reports this diagnosis to a friend, who is a nurse. Which is the best response by the nurse?
   1. "Don't worry; early treatment often alleviates symptoms of the disease."
   2. "See another physician. I've heard of several treatments that aid recovery."
   3. "That must have really shocked you. Tell me what the physician told you about it."
   4. "You should see a psychiatrist, who will help you cope with this overwhelming news."

4. The major nursing concern when caring for a client with the diagnosis of hyperthyroidism is:
   1. Providing an adequate diet
   2. Keeping the bed linen neat
   3. Modifying hospital routines
   4. Arranging for sufficient rest periods

5. The practitioner prescribes propylthiouracil (PTU) for a client with hyperthyroidism. The nurse explains that this drug:
   1. Increases the uptake of iodine
   2. Causes the thyroid gland to atrophy
   3. Interferes with the synthesis of thyroid hormone
   4. Decreases the secretion of thyroid-stimulating hormone

6. A male client with the diagnosis of multiple myeloma is told by the practitioner that he has a poor prognosis. He and his wife decide to travel, attend the theater, and go to sporting events. When preparing a teaching plan for this client, the nurse should take into consideration that:
   1. Travel will cause depletion of his already exhausted energy stores
   2. A positive mental attitude will decrease the effects of stress and improve his prognosis
   3. He is prone to develop infections when exposed to large crowds, which may shorten his life
   4. As long as he does not have an accident that causes a hemorrhage, his travel will not affect his prognosis

7. A client who is suspected of having Cushing's syndrome is admitted to the hospital. The nurse plans to monitor this client for:
   1. Hypokalemia
   2. Hypovolemia
   3. Hypocalcemia
   4. Hyponatremia

8. A person sustains burns of the arms from a barbecue accident in the park. A bystander emerges from the crowd and suggests to a nurse, who has come to the person's assistance, that butter be applied to the burns. An appropriate response by the nurse is, "Thanks, but:
   1. we'll just wait for the ambulance."
   2. it is better to use some first-aid cream."
   3. a tablecloth should be used. It will act as a blanket."
   4. we should apply ice to the burns. Please get me some."

9. The nurse is assigned to a client who has had surgery. Nalbuphine (Nubain) is prescribed for pain. For which side effects/adverse reactions should the nurse assess this client after administering this medication? Select all that apply.
   1. _____ Oliguria
   2 _____ Dry mouth
   3. _____ Palpitations
   4. _____ Constipation
   5. _____ Urinary retention
   6. _____ Orthostatic hypotension

10. A client who is complaining of severe midsternal pain is brought to the emergency department. The practitioner makes the diagnosis of myocardial infarction. Which drug can the nurse expect to be prescribed because it is the drug of choice to control the pain associated with myocardial infarction?
    1. Xanax
    2. Demerol
    3. Morphine
    4. Lidocaine

11. The nurse identifies that 2 weeks after full-thickness burns, a client is losing 1 pound of weight daily. The nurse's best action is to discuss the needs of the client with the practitioner and request that the diet be adjusted to include:
    1. Low-sodium milk
    2. High-protein drinks
    3. Fruit juices low in potassium
    4. Ten percent more calories in the form of fats

12. A client is diagnosed with cancer of the larynx. Before a total laryngectomy, an important aspect of preoperative nursing care includes:
    1. Answering questions
    2. Having a speech therapist visit
    3. Teaching postoperative breathing exercises
    4. Explaining the nature of the surgery to be performed

13. A client has a tracheostomy tube attached to a tracheostomy collar for the delivery of humidified oxygen. The nurse identifies that the client will need suctioning primarily because the:
    1. Humidified oxygen is saturated with fluid
    2. Tracheostomy tube interferes with effective coughing
    3. Inner cannula of the tracheostomy tube irritates the mucosa
    4. Weaning process increases the amount of respiratory secretions

14. A nurse is caring for a client with ascites who is to receive IV albumin to replace each liter of fluid removed via paracentesis. The nurse expects that albumin replacement will decrease:
    1. Ascites and blood ammonia level
    2. Capillary perfusion and blood pressure
    3. Venous stasis and blood urea nitrogen level
    4. Tissue fluid accumulation and hematocrit level

15. A client arrives in the emergency department with multiple crushing wounds of the chest, abdomen, and legs. The nursing assessments that assume the greatest priority are:
    1. Level of consciousness and pupil size
    2. Characteristics of pain and blood pressure
    3. Quality of respirations and presence of pulses
    4. Presence of abdominal contusions and other wounds

16. A nurse is caring for a client who has just had kidney surgery. One of the functions of the nurse is evaluating the adequacy of the client's kidney function after surgery. Essential to this nursing assessment is the understanding that the healthy kidney filters a number of blood components. Which component identified as being abnormally present in the client's urine should the nurse report to the practitioner?
    1. Sodium
    2. Potassium
    3. Urea nitrogen
    4. Large proteins

17. A client with the tentative diagnosis of Hodgkin's disease asks how the practitioner will know that it is definitely this disease. The nurse explains that the diagnosis is confirmed by a:
    1. Bone scan
    2. Lymph node biopsy
    3. Computed tomography (CT) scan
    4. Radioactive iodine (^{131}I) uptake study

18. A nurse who is working in a neighborhood health clinic is caring for a client who was just diagnosed with a gastric ulcer. The nurse determines that a teaching plan is needed to address diet therapy for this client. Which diet should the nurse expect the practitioner to order?
    1. Soft diet
    2. Low-fat, high-protein liquid diet
    3. Hourly feedings of dairy products
    4. Regular diet with foods that are tolerated

19. A client with diabetes, who has been diagnosed as having lower extremity arterial disease (LEAD), tells the nurse that before hospitalization, exercise resulted in severe cramplike pain in both legs. The nurse includes in the teaching plan specific measures the client can use to increase arterial blood flow to the extremities. These measures should include:
    1. Exercises that promote muscular activity
    2. Meticulous care of minor skin breakdown
    3. Elevation of the legs above the level of the heart
    4. Daily cleansing of the feet by soaking in hot water

20. A nurse is assigned to care for a client who has just returned from Hong Kong with pneumonia and a cough. To reduce the risk of acquiring an infection, what protective clothing should the nurse wear when caring for this client?
    1. Gown and gloves
    2. Gown, mask, cap, and gloves
    3. Gloves, barrier mask, and gown
    4. Gloves, gown, barrier mask, eye shield, and cap

21. A nurse is caring for a client who is scheduled to have a paracentesis. Immediately before the procedure, the nurse asks the client to void because a full bladder:
    1. Decreases the intra-abdominal pressure
    2. Decreases the amount of fluid in the abdominal cavity
    3. Increases the danger of puncture during the procedure
    4. Increases the presence of urea in the intra-abdominal fluid

22. A nurse anticipates occasional but serious problems with hypoxia among postoperative clients. When caring for a client after surgery, the client reports shortness of breath and chest pain. Which is the most appropriate initial response by the nurse?
    1. Initiate oxygen via a nasal cannula
    2. Administer the prescribed morphine
    3. Prepare the client for endotracheal intubation
    4. Place a nitroglycerin tablet under the client's tongue

23. A nurse is caring for a client who was diagnosed with a myocardial infarction. While caring for the client 2 days after the event, the nurse identifies that the client's temperature is elevated. The nurse concludes that this increase in temperature is most likely the result of:
    1. Tissue necrosis
    2. Venous thrombosis
    3. Pulmonary infarction
    4. Respiratory infection

24. The primary responsibility of a nurse when caring for a client with a chest tube attached to a three-chamber underwater seal drainage system is to:
    1. Ensure maintenance of the closed system
    2. Maintain mechanical suction to the system
    3. Encourage the client to deep breathe and cough
    4. Keep the client in the dorsal recumbent position

25. The nurse is caring for a male client who recently was diagnosed with urinary phosphate calculi. What should the nurse plan to teach this client to include in his diet?
    1. Pears
    2. Hamburgers
    3. Split pea soup
    4. Cheddar cheese

26. The practitioner discusses with a male client the need for an abdominoperineal resection and a colostomy. Later, the client tells the nurse that he is pleased only minor surgery is necessary. The nurse concludes that the client's reaction is an example of:
   1. Reflection
   2. Regression
   3. Repudiation
   4. Reconciliation

27. One week after an above-the-knee amputation, a client refuses to go to physical therapy and tells the nurse, "I'll never be a whole person again!" What is the nurse's best response?
   1. "You're still the same person you've always been. Just relax."
   2. "You've lost a part of yourself. That must be very difficult for you."
   3. "You may feel that way, but I'm sure your family considers you a whole person."
   4. "You must go to physical therapy every day or you will develop muscle contractures."

28. A 67-year-old client is diagnosed as having a right-sided brain attack (cerebrovascular accident) and is admitted to the hospital. When preparing to care for this client, the nurse should:
   1. Apply elastic stockings to prevent flaccid leg muscles
   2. Utilize a bed cradle to prevent dorsiflexion of the feet
   3. Implement passive range-of-motion exercises to prevent muscle atrophy
   4. Use a hand roll while supporting the left upper extremity on a pillow to prevent contractures

29. The nursing assistant assigned to the 7 AM shift has not been coming to work until 8 AM. Nursing care is delayed and assignments are started late. What is the most appropriate action by the nurse in charge?
   1. Discuss the issue with a friend from another unit
   2. Remind the nursing assistant of the expected start time
   3. Report the problem to the Human Resources department
   4. Document the information before discussing it with the nursing assistant

30. A client is diagnosed as having type 2 diabetes, and the practitioner prescribes an oral hypoglycemic. The nurse should include in the teaching plan that people taking oral hypoglycemics:
   1. Should not work where food is readily available
   2. May tend to relax dietary rules on an unconscious level
   3. Do not need to be concerned about serious complications
   4. Have less fear of their condition than those who take insulin

31. A client is to receive an IV antibiotic in 50 mL of 0.9% sodium chloride to be administered over 20 minutes. At what rate should the nurse set the infusion pump?
   Answer: _____ mL/hr

32. A male client, who has been living in a foreign country for 10 years, is undergoing diagnostic testing to identify the causative organisms of the infection that he has acquired. When discussing the concept of immunity, the client asks, "When does active immunity occur?" The nurse responds, "Active immunity occurs when:
   1. protein antigens are formed in the blood to fight invading antibodies."
   2. protein substances are formed within the body to neutralize antigens."
   3. blood antigens are aided by phagocytes in defending the body against pathogens."
   4. sensitized lymphocytes from an immune donor act as antibodies against invading pathogens."

33. A client with the diagnosis of inhalation anthrax is admitted to the intensive care unit. Which category of adaptations is most important for the nurse to make a focused assessment?
   1. Mental
   2. Hydration
   3. Neurologic
   4. Respiratory

34. A nurse is caring for a client who just had surgery for a parotid tumor. Which nursing intervention is the priority in the immediate postoperative period?
   1. Offering psychological support
   2. Monitoring the client's fluid balance
   3. Keeping the client's respiratory passages patent
   4. Providing a pad and pencil for writing messages

35. A client is admitted to the hospital with a history of cancer of the liver and jaundice. In relation to the jaundice, the nurse expects the client to report the presence of:
   1. Pruritus
   2. Diarrhea
   3. Blurred vision
   4. Bleeding gums

36. During a teaching session about insulin injections, a client asks the nurse, "Why can't I take the insulin in pills instead of taking shots?" What is the nurse's best response?
   1. "Insulin cannot be manufactured in pill form."
   2. "The physician will prescribe pills when you are ready."
   3. "The route of administration is decided on by the physician."
   4. "Insulin is destroyed by gastric juices, rendering it ineffective."

37. A 50-year-old client is admitted to the hospital with a suspected brain tumor. Based on the history of loss of equilibrium and coordination, the nurse suspects the tumor is located in the:
   1. Cerebellum
   2. Parietal lobe
   3. Basal ganglia
   4. Occipital lobe

38. The nurse checks for hypocalcemia by placing a blood pressure cuff on a client's arm and inflating it. After

about 3 minutes the client develops carpopedal spasms. The nurse records this finding as a positive:

1. Homans' sign
2. Romberg's sign
3. Chvostek's sign
4. Trousseau's sign

39. A client is admitted for a coronary artery bypass graft. The client states that the physician said that pacemaker wires will be inserted during surgery as a precautionary measure and asks, "What is the purpose of the pacemaker?" The best response by the nurse is, "The pacemaker:

1. prevents a rapid heart rate."
2. provides access for defibrillation."
3. maintains a constant cardiac rhythm."
4. manages an abnormally slow heart rate."

40. A male client with a brain attack (cerebrovascular accident) has regained control of bowel movements but is still incontinent of urine. To help reestablish bladder control, the nurse should encourage the client to:

1. Assume a standing position for voiding
2. Void every 4 hours and attempt to hold urine between set times
3. Attempt to void more frequently in the afternoon than in the morning
4. Drink a minimum of 4 L of fluid daily and divide it equally among the hours while awake

41. A client is admitted to the emergency department with a stab wound of the left thorax. The nurse should position the client:

1. On the left side with the head of the bed elevated
2. In the Trendelenburg position with knees gatched
3. In the high-Fowler's position with the left side supported
4. On the right side flat in bed with a pillow supporting the left arm

42. A client is admitted to the emergency department with a stab wound of the chest. What is the priority when the nurse performs a focused assessment of the client's response to this injury?

1. Level of pain
2. Quality and depth of respirations
3. Amount of serosanguineous drainage
4. Blood pressure and pupillary response

43. A 35-year-old male who sustained a closed head injury is being monitored for increased intracranial pressure. Arterial blood gases are obtained and the results include a Pco_2 of 33 mm Hg. It is most important for the nurse to:

1. Encourage the client to slow his breathing rate
2. Auscultate the client's lungs and suction if indicated
3. Advise the practitioner that the client needs supplemental oxygen
4. Inform the practitioner of the results and continue to monitor for signs of increasing intracranial pressure

44. A 42-year-old mentally challenged individual with the intellectual capacity of a 5-year-old child is brought to the emergency department after an accident. The nurse can best assess the client's pain level by:

1. Asking the client's mother
2. Using Wong's "Pain Faces"
3. Observing the client's body language
4. Explaining the use of a 0 to 10 pain scale

45. A debilitated, older male client with glaucoma who places great value on independence is being prepared for discharge from the hospital. What should the nurse encourage the client to do to promote independence?

1. Perform his own household chores and shopping
2. Learn to administer his eye medications correctly
3. Prevent stressful events that can increase his symptoms
4. Conserve his eyesight by not reading or watching television

46. A client undergoes removal of a pituitary tumor through a transsphenoidal approach. Postoperatively the nurse should:

1. Provide oral hygiene and include brushing the teeth
2. Encourage the client to deep breathe and cough frequently
3. Maintain the head of the bed at a thirty-degree angle continuously
4. Continue giving nothing by mouth until the nasal packing is removed

47. A nurse is providing preoperative teaching for a client who is scheduled for a transurethral resection of the prostate. What should the nurse tell the client that he can expect after the surgery?

1. Urine that is bright red for 24 to 48 hours
2. Spasms of the bladder during the first 24 to 48 hours
3. Need to perform the Valsalva maneuver to decrease bladder contractions
4. Decrease in oral fluids because of the need for continuous urinary irrigation

48. A 52-year-old engineer is admitted to the hospital with Laënnec's cirrhosis and chronic pancreatitis. Bile salts (Bile Acid factor) are prescribed, and the client asks why they are needed. The nurse replies, "They:

1. stimulate prothrombin production."
2. aid absorption of fat-soluble vitamins."
3. promote bilirubin secretion in the urine."
4. stimulate contraction of the common bile duct."

49. Clients are encouraged to perform deep-breathing exercises after most types of surgery. The nurse teaches clients that the reason for these exercises is to help:

1. Stimulate red blood cell production
2. Expand the residual volume in the lungs
3. Decrease partial pressure of oxygen in the blood
4. Prevent the buildup of carbon dioxide in the body

50. An older client is hard of hearing and has severe, painful rheumatoid arthritis. The client is admitted to a nursing home after becoming incontinent of urine. The primary consideration in the care of this client is the need for:

1. Control of pain
2. Immobilization of joints
3. Motivation and teaching
4. Bladder training and control

MEDICAL-SURGICAL NURSING QUIZ 1
ANSWERS AND RATIONALES

1. **3 Exercise should be to tolerance only; limiting the amount of exercise should decrease pain.**
   1 This will increase stiffness.
   2 Exercises should be decreased, not increased.
   4 Resistive exercises usually are not part of the regimen for clients with rheumatoid arthritis.
   Client Needs: Health Promotion and Maintenance; **Cognitive Level:** Application; **Integrated Process:** Teaching/Learning; **NP:** Implementation

2. **3 Holding the breath at the moment of the actual biopsy ensures that the liver does not move as it normally does with regular respiratory excursions; minimizing movement reduces potential injury to the liver.**
   1 Lying on the right side after the procedure applies pressure at the insertion site, preventing hemorrhage.
   2 Movement or breathing increases the danger of damage to the liver.
   4 Bearing down (Valsalva maneuver) during the insertion of the biopsy needle is unnecessary; holding the breath at the moment of the actual biopsy is all that is necessary to help minimize injury to the liver.
   Client Needs: Reduction of Risk Potential; **Cognitive Level:** Application; **Integrated Process:** Teaching/Learning; **NP:** Implementation

3. **3 This acknowledges the effect of the diagnosis on the client and explores what is known.**
   1 This statement provides false reassurance.
   2 This statement provides false reassurance.
   4 There is no evidence of ineffective coping.
   Client Needs: Psychosocial Integrity; **Cognitive Level:** Application; **Integrated Process:** Communication and Documentation; **NP:** Implementation

4. **4 Promotion of rest to reduce metabolic demands is a challenging but essential task for a client who has hyperthyroidism.**
   1 The diet can be increased to meet metabolic demands; the client usually has an excellent appetite.
   2 The neatness of linen is not an important aspect of care; the client usually is hyperactive, and it is more important to promote rest.
   3 Hospital routines are not considered a nursing problem; routines should be flexible to meet client needs.
   Client Needs: Basic Care and Comfort; **Cognitive Level:** Application; **NP:** Planning

5. **3 Propylthiouracil (PTU), used in the treatment of hyperthyroidism, blocks the synthesis of thyroid hormones by preventing iodination of tyrosine.**
   1 Propylthiouracil does not increase the uptake of iodine.
   2 Iodine solutions reduce the size and vascularity of the thyroid gland.
   4 Thyroid-stimulating hormone (TSH), secreted by the anterior pituitary, is not affected by propylthiouracil.
   Client Needs: Pharmacological and Parenteral Therapies; **Cognitive Level:** Comprehension; **Integrated Process:** Teaching/Learning; **NP:** Implementation

6. **3 The bone marrow is impaired with multiple myeloma; the effectiveness of white blood cells and immunoglobulins is reduced, which increases susceptibility to bacterial infections.**
   1 Travel can be accomplished with careful planning and adequate rest periods.
   2 Although a positive mental attitude can contribute to quality of life and may even extend life, generally it does not change the prognosis.
   4 Although coagulation is impaired, it is not as life threatening as exposure to infection.
   Client Needs: Physiological Adaptation; **Cognitive Level:** Application; **Integrated Process:** Teaching/Learning; **NP:** Planning

7. **1 With glucocorticoid excess, aldosterone hypersecretion occurs and sodium is retained; therefore, potassium is excreted, leading to hypokalemia.**
   2 Hypervolemia occurs because of sodium and water retention precipitated by aldosterone.
   3 Hypocalcemia is not associated with aldosteronism.
   4 Aldosterone hypersecretion causes sodium retention and hypernatremia, not hyponatremia.
   Client Needs: Physiological Adaptation; **Cognitive Level:** Application; **NP:** Planning

8. **3 A tablecloth is nonfuzzy and nonadhering and will keep the burned person warm.**
   1 Doing nothing is inappropriate; body heat should be conserved with a nonadhering covering.
   2 Cream is difficult to remove and may result in additional damage.
   4 This is contraindicated because ice can result in additional tissue damage.
   Client Needs: Physiological Adaptation; **Cognitive Level:** Application; **Integrated Process:** Communication and Documentation; **NP:** Implementation

9. **Answer: 2, 3, 4, 6**
   1 _____ The ability to form urine is not affected; an increased urinary output or frequency may occur.
   2 _____ **Dry mouth is a side effect of Nalbuphine HCl (Nubain).**
   3 _____ **Palpitations are a side effect of Nalbuphine HCl.**
   4 _____ **Constipation is a common side effect of Nalbuphine HCl.**
   5 _____ Urinary urgency, not retention, is a reaction to Nalbuphine HCl.
   6 _____ **Orthostatic hypotension may occur with Nalbuphine HCl.**

NP: Nursing process.

Client Needs: Pharmacological and Parenteral Therapies; **Cognitive Level:** Analysis; **NP:** Evaluation

10. **3** **Morphine sulfate is the drug of choice because it reduces severe pain, lowers systemic vascular resistance, and decreases venous return.**
    1 Alprazolam (Xanax), a benzodiazepine, lowers anxiety, which may reduce some pain, but it is not an effective analgesic.
    2 Although meperidine (Demerol) is an analgesic, morphine sulfate is the preferred drug in this situation.
    4 Lidocaine hydrochloride is used to control ventricular ectopic activity, not pain.
    Client Needs: Pharmacological and Parenteral Therapies; **Cognitive Level:** Analysis; **NP:** Planning

11. **2** **High-protein drinks have twice the calories per volume of other fluids and provide protein for wound healing.**
    1 Low-sodium milk does not contain adequate calories to help meet the high metabolic rate associated with burns.
    3 Potassium is restricted during the first 48 to 72 hours after a burn injury, not 2 weeks after the injury.
    4 Increased calories in the form of protein and carbohydrates, not fats, are needed.
    Client Needs: Management of Care; **Cognitive Level:** Analysis; **Integrated Process:** Communication and Documentation; **NP:** Planning

12. **1** **Before teaching, the nurse must determine the client's areas of concern; knowledge generally reduces anxiety and learning increases when anxiety decreases.**
    2 Having a speech therapist visit is not beneficial for all preoperative clients scheduled for a laryngectomy.
    3 The client will be dependent on a respirator postoperatively; breathing exercises are not necessary immediately after surgery.
    4 Although this may be part of the information included in preoperative teaching, the teaching should begin at the client's level.
    Client Needs: Reduction of Risk Potential; **Cognitive Level:** Application; **Integrated Process:** Teaching/Learning; **NP:** Implementation

13. **2** **Because the tracheostomy tube enters the trachea below the glottis, the client is unable to close the glottis to retain air in the lungs; this prevents an increase in the intrathoracic pressure and the ability to open the glottis to expel an explosive cough.**
    1 Humidified oxygen decreases the need for suctioning because it liquefies secretions, which are then easier to expel.
    3 The outer, not inner, cannula of a tracheostomy tube irritates the mucosa.
    4 Weaning begins when the respiratory status improves and the amount of respiratory secretions subsides.
    Client Needs: Physiological Adaptation; **Cognitive Level:** Application; **NP:** Planning

14. **4** **Serum albumin is administered to maintain serum levels and normal oncotic (osmotic) pressure; it**

does this by pulling fluid from the interstitial spaces into the intravascular compartment.
    1 Serum albumin does affect blood ammonia levels; fluid accumulated in the abdominal cavity is removed via a paracentesis.
    2 The administration of albumin results in a shift of fluid from the interstitial to the intravascular compartment, which probably will increase the blood pressure.
    3 Albumin administration does not affect venous stasis or the blood urea nitrogen level.
    Client Needs: Pharmacological and Parenteral Therapies; **Cognitive Level:** Application; **NP:** Planning

15. **3** **Assessing breathing and circulation are the priorities in trauma management; basic life functions must be maintained or reestablished (ABCs: Airway, Breathing, Circulation).**
    1 Level of consciousness and pupil size are assessments associated with head injury; in this situation these follow determination of respiratory and circulatory status, which are the priorities.
    2 Although blood pressure is an important assessment associated with adequacy of circulation, it is obtained after assessments associated with patency of airway and breathing; a client's pain is addressed after airway, breathing, and circulation needs are assessed and interventions implemented to support life.
    4 Assessment for abdominal injury and other wounds follows determination of respiratory and circulatory status, which are the priorities.
    Client Needs: Physiological Adaptation; **Cognitive Level:** Analysis; **NP:** Assessment

16. **4** **The glomeruli are not permeable to large proteins such as albumin or red blood cells (RBCs) and it is abnormal if albumin or RBCs are identified in the urine; their presence should be reported.**
    1 The proximal tubules are responsible for regulating water, electrolytes (including sodium and potassium), urea nitrogen, and pH; the byproducts of this regulation appear in normal urine.
    2 The proximal tubules are responsible for regulating water, electrolytes (including sodium and potassium), urea nitrogen, and pH; the byproducts of this regulation appear in normal urine.
    3 The proximal tubules are responsible for regulating water, electrolytes (including sodium and potassium), urea nitrogen, and pH; the byproducts of this regulation appear in normal urine.
    Client Needs: Reduction of Risk Potential; **Cognitive Level:** Comprehension; **Integrated Process:** Communication and Documentation; **NP:** Evaluation

17. **2** **The diagnosis depends on the identification of characteristic histologic features of an excised lymph node.**
    1 A bone scan is a diagnostic device to assess bony metastasis of cancers.
    3 CT scans identify the extent of the disease in the abdominal and thoracic cavities.

4 These are not indicated for Hodgkin's disease; they are used for radiotherapy or diagnosis of thyroid diseases.
Client Needs: Reduction of Risk Potential; **Cognitive Level:** Comprehension; **Integrated Process:** Teaching/Learning; **NP:** Implementation

18. **4 No specific diet is recommended; the client is encouraged to avoid meals that overdistend the stomach and foods that cause GI distress.**
    1 There is no need for a soft diet; a soft diet is appropriate for those who have difficulty with chewing and swallowing.
    2 The client does not require a liquid diet.
    3 High-fat dairy products increase GI secretions and should be avoided.
    Client Needs: Basic Care and Comfort; **Cognitive Level:** Application; **Integrated Process:** Teaching/Learning; **NP:** Planning

19. **1 Arterial blood flow is improved with exercise by fostering the development of collateral circulation.**
    2 Meticulous care of minor skin breakdown is important for the person with diabetes, but it does not improve arterial blood flow.
    3 Elevating the legs above the heart reduces arterial blood flow; the legs should be kept dependent to facilitate tissue perfusion.
    4 Soaking the feet in hot water is contraindicated because it can burn the skin and/or cause drying; also, individuals with diabetes may have neuropathies, which alter the perception of temperature.
    Client Needs: Physiological Adaptation; **Cognitive Level:** Application; **Integrated Process:** Teaching/Learning; **NP:** Planning

20. **4 Gloves, gown, barrier mask, eye shield, and cap protect the nurse from respiratory droplets. The client's recent travel and clinical adaptations suggest that the client may have severe acute respiratory syndrome (SARS), which is spread by respiratory droplets and has been known to infect health care workers through exposure of the eyes.**
    1 Because of the nature of this droplet-transmitted infection, these precautions are inadequate. A barrier mask, eye shield, and cap should be worn in addition to the gown and gloves for adequate protection from infection.
    2 Because of the nature of this droplet-transmitted infection, these precautions are inadequate. A barrier mask, not just a mask, and eye shield in addition to the gown, gloves, and cap are necessary for adequate protection from infection
    3 Because of the nature of this droplet-transmitted infection, these precautions are inadequate. An eye shield and cap are necessary in addition to the gloves, barrier mask, and gown for adequate protection from infection.
    Client Needs: Safety and Infection Control; **Cognitive Level:** Analysis; **NP:** Planning

21. **3 When the bladder contains large amounts of urine, it becomes distended and may push upward into the abdominal cavity, where it can be punctured accidentally.**
    1 This is not the rationale for emptying the bladder.
    2 The amount of fluid in the bladder has no relationship to ascites.
    4 Urea is present in blood and urine, not ascitic fluid.
    Client Needs: Reduction of Risk Potential; **Cognitive Level:** Application; **Integrated Process:** Teaching/Learning; **NP:** Implementation

22. **2 Supplemental oxygen supports the body while the cause of the problem is identified; supplemental oxygen can be instituted without an order in an emergency.**
    1 Morphine is used in the treatment of chest pain, but it is not the priority intervention.
    3 Endotracheal intubation is not the priority intervention. If the client's condition deteriorates and the client becomes unconscious or experiences respiratory failure or obstruction, endotracheal intubation is warranted.
    4 Nitroglycerin is available in most client acute care areas and does lessen chest pain if the pain is cardiac in origin, but it is not the priority intervention and requires a prescription.
    Client Needs: Physiological Adaptation; **Cognitive Level:** Application; **NP:** Implementation

23. **1 The body's inflammatory response to myocardial necrosis causes an elevation of temperature as well as leukocytosis within 24 to 48 hours after the event.**
    2 Venous thrombosis is not an expected finding after a myocardial infarction.
    3 Pulmonary infarction is not an expected finding after a myocardial infarction.
    4 Respiratory infection is not common after myocardial infarction.
    Client Needs: Physiological Adaptation; **Cognitive Level:** Analysis; **NP:** Evaluation

24. **1 An airtight system is needed to reestablish negative pressure and reinflate the lung.**
    2 Drainage can be maintained without mechanical suction.
    3 Encouraging coughing and deep breathing is important, but not the priority.
    4 Any position is acceptable as long as the tube is not compressed or pulled.
    Client Needs: Reduction of Risk Potential; **Cognitive Level:** Application; **NP:** Planning

25. **1 All fresh fruits are low in phosphate.**
    2 Beef contains phosphate.
    3 Split pea soup contains a significant amount of phosphate.
    4 Cheddar cheese is made with milk, which contains phosphate.
    Client Needs: Basic Care and Comfort; **Cognitive Level:** Analysis **Integrated Process:** Teaching/Leaning; **NP:** Planning

26. **3 A refusal to recognize anticipated loss in an attempt to protect oneself against the overpowering stress of illness is called repudiation.**
    1 The data do not suggest that the client has contemplated consequences related to the illness.
    2 There are no data to support that the client is demonstrating behavior characteristic of an earlier stage of development.
    4 The data do not suggest that the client has made a realistic adjustment to the illness.
    Client Needs: Psychosocial Integrity; **Cognitive Level:** Analysis; **NP:** Analysis

27. **2 This response acknowledges and reflects the client's feelings and encourages further communication.**
    1 This response negates the client's feelings.
    3 The nurse does not know how the client's family members feel; this response takes the focus off the client.
    4 This is true, but telling the client this serves no therapeutic purpose at this time.
    Client Needs: Psychosocial Integrity; **Cognitive Level:** Analysis; **Integrated Process:** Communication and Documentation; **NP:** Implementation

28. **4 These interventions maintain the affected left arm in functional alignment; the left side of the body will be affected with a right-sided brain attack.**
    1 Elastic stockings promote venous return rather than prevent flaccid muscles; also, this requires a prescription.
    2 Plantar flexion (foot drop), not dorsiflexion, may occur with a brain attack; high-top sneakers or splints, not a bed cradle, more appropriately prevent plantar flexion contractures.
    3 Passive range-of-motion (ROM) exercises prevent contractures rather than muscle atrophy; the institution of ROM exercises should be discussed with the practitioner because activity during the acute phase can increase intracranial pressure and should be avoided.
    Client Needs: Basic Care and Comfort; **Cognitive Level:** Application; **NP:** Implementation

29. **4 Documentation is the best initial response; documentation should include both the missed time and the effect on client care.**
    1 Discussing the issue with a friend from another unit is not a professional or appropriate response to the problem.
    2 Reminding the nursing assistant of the expected start time may be helpful but will not address the issue if the problem continues.
    3 Reporting the event to the Human Resources department may be a later response to the problem.
    Client Needs: Management of Care; **Cognitive Level:** Application; **Integrated Process:** Communication and Documentation; **NP:** Implementation

30. **2 Taking a pill may give the client a false sense that the disease is under control, and this can lead to dietary indiscretions.**
    1 A person's ability to follow dietary restrictions is highly individual; the employment setting is not a universal factor in such behaviors.
    3 Diabetes is a chronic disease, and its complications can affect all individuals with the disease, particularly those who do not follow the prescribed regimen.
    4 Having to take any medication for a chronic illness every day can be threatening to some people whether the medication is taken orally or by injection.
    Client Needs: Pharmacological and Parenteral Therapies; **Cognitive Level:** Application; **Integrated Process:** Teaching/Leaning; **NP:** Planning

31. **Answer: 150 mL per hour. An infusion device delivers a specific volume of fluid to be infused over the period of 1 hour; calculate the answer by using ratio and proportion:**

$$\frac{50 \text{ mL}}{20 \text{ min}} = \frac{x \text{ mL}}{60 \text{ min}}$$
$$20x = 50 \times 60$$
$$x = 3000 \div 20$$
$$x = 150 \text{ mL/hr}$$

    Client Needs: Pharmacological and Parenteral Therapies; **Cognitive Level:** Application; **NP:** Planning

32. **2 Active immunity occurs when the individual's cells produce antibodies in response to an agent or its products; these antibodies will destroy the agent (antigen) should it enter the body again.**
    1 Antigens do not fight antibodies; they trigger antibody formation that in turn attacks the antigen.
    3 Antigens are foreign substances that enter the body and trigger antibody formation.
    4 Sensitized lymphocytes do not act as antibodies.
    Client Needs: Physiological Adaptation; **Cognitive Level:** Comprehension; **Integrated Process:** Teaching/Learning; **NP:** Implementation

33. **4 Because respiratory collapse is an early sign of inhalation anthrax, a client's respiratory status requires immediate assessment and continued monitoring.**
    1 Development of a CNS problem such as anthrax-related meningitis is a late sign of inhalation anthrax.
    2 Although assessing hydration status is important for any client who is acutely ill, it is not a nursing assessment that is specific to anthrax.
    3 Neurologic adaptations are late signs of inhalation anthrax.
    Client Needs: Physiological Adaptation; **Cognitive Level:** Application; **NP:** Assessment

34. **3 A patent airway is always the priority; therefore, removal of secretions is imperative.**
    1 Offering psychological support is an important postoperative intervention, but it is not the priority immediately after removal of a parotid tumor.
    2 Monitoring the client's fluid balance is an important postoperative intervention, but it is not the priority immediately after removal of a parotid tumor.
    4 Providing for a means of communication is an important postoperative intervention, but it is not the priority immediately after removal of a parotid tumor.

Client Needs: Physiological Adaptation; **Cognitive Level:** Application; **NP:** Planning

35. 1 **Itching associated with jaundice is believed to be caused by accumulating bile salts in the skin.**
    2 This is not related to jaundice.
    3 This is not related to jaundice.
    4 This is not related to jaundice.
    Client Needs: Physiological Adaptation; **Cognitive Level:** Application; **Integrated Process:** Communication and Documentation; **NP:** Assessment

36. 4 **Insulin in tablet form is inactivated by gastric juices; insulin given by injection avoids exposure to digestive enzymes.**
    1 Insulin is not given orally at this time because it is inactivated by digestive enzymes.
    2 This is incorrect information and provides false reassurance; the client currently is insulin dependent.
    3 This response does not answer the client's question; insulin is administered IV or subcutaneously, and the route depends on the client's needs.
    Client Needs: Pharmacological and Parenteral Therapies; **Cognitive Level:** Application; **Integrated Process:** Teaching/Learning; **NP:** Implementation

37. 1 **The cerebellum is involved in synergistic control of the skeletal muscles and the coordination of voluntary movement.**
    2 The parietal lobe is concerned with localization and two-point discrimination; tumors here cause motor seizures and sensory function loss.
    3 Basal ganglia are concerned with large subconscious movements and muscle tone; damage here may cause paralysis, as in a brain attack or involuntary movements and uncontrollable shaking, as in Parkinson's disease.
    4 The occipital lobe is concerned with special sensory perception; tumors here cause visual disturbances, visual agnosia, or hallucinations.
    Client Needs: Physiological Adaptation; **Cognitive Level:** Analysis; **NP:** Analysis

38. 4 **Peripheral muscular hypoxia precipitates carpopedal spasms in the presence of hypocalcemia.**
    1 This indicates thrombophlebitis when pain results from dorsiflexing the foot.
    2 This indicates the loss of position sense; swaying results when the client stands still with the feet close together and the eyes closed.
    3 Although this sign indicates hypocalcemia, it is elicited by tapping over the facial nerve.
    Client Needs: Reduction of Risk Potential; **Cognitive Level:** Analysis; **NP:** Analysis

39. 4 **Vagal stimulation during surgery may cause a severe bradycardia; in anticipation, pacemaker wires are inserted into the right atrium to be used to initiate impulses if the natural rate decreases below the preset rate of the pacemaker; this will ensure that the heart beats at the rate set for the pacemaker.**
    1 This pacemaker initiates an impulse if the heart rate drops below a certain rate; the concept underlying this pacemaker is to speed up the heart, not to slow it down.

2 There are no data to support the fact that this is a defibrillator pacemaker. The pacemaker wires are not used for defibrillation; defibrillator paddles are placed so that electricity affects the entire heart muscle.
3 The rhythm can be irregular; however, if the pause between two beats is too long, the pacemaker will initiate an impulse.
Client Needs: Reduction of Risk Potential; **Cognitive Level:** Application; **Integrated Process:** Teaching/Learning; **NP:** Implementation

40. 1 **Assuming a standing position for voiding reduces tension (physical and psychological), facilitates the movement of urine into the lower portion of the bladder, and relaxes the external sphincter (increasing pressure and initiating the micturition reflex).**
    2 Bladder training should be instituted by encouraging voiding every 1 to 2 hours and progressively increasing the time between attempts.
    3 Voiding should be encouraged at regular and frequent intervals during waking hours, not just in the afternoon.
    4 Four liters is a large fluid intake and is unnecessary; it will result in a large volume of urine, probably increasing the frequency of incontinence.
    Client Needs: Basic Care and Comfort; **Cognitive Level:** Application; **Integrated Process:** Teaching/Learning; **NP:** Implementation

41. 1 **When the client lies on the affected side, the unaffected lung can expand to its fullest potential; elevation of the head facilitates respirations by reducing the pressure of the abdominal organs on the diaphragm, allowing the diaphragm to descend with gravity on inspiration.**
    2 Maximum lung expansion is inhibited when the head is not elevated.
    3 Although the high-Fowler's position facilitates diaphragmatic movement, it is unclear as to what "left side supported" means.
    4 Pressure against the right thorax limits right intercostal expansion and gaseous exchange in the right lung. The abdominal organs restrict contraction of the diaphragm when lying flat in bed; also, lying flat in bed does not permit the diaphragm to drop by gravity as it does when in the high-Fowler's position.
    Client Needs: Safety and Infection Control; **Cognitive Level:** Application; **NP:** Implementation

42. 2 **The rate and characteristics of respirations, in addition to the presence or absence of breath sounds, oxygen saturation and unilateral chest movements, should be assessed so that the client's respiratory status can be determined. The concern is to identify a pneumothorax caused by the injury, which can be life threatening.**
    1 Although important, pain is not a life-threatening symptom.
    3 Bleeding may accumulate in the pleural space, but it is inaccessible to direct observation.

4 Excessive blood loss will cause a decreased blood pressure, but bleeding is indicated first by respiratory changes because the blood will accumulate in the pleural space; pupillary response is unaffected.
Client Needs: Physiological Adaptation; **Cognitive Level:** Application; **NP:** Assessment

43. **4 A lower than expected Pco_2 actually will benefit the client because it reduces intracranial pressure by preventing cerebral vasodilation; the results should be reported, and monitoring for signs and symptoms of increased intracranial pressure should continue (restlessness, confusion and lethargy, pupillary and oculomotor dysfunction, hemiparesis or hemiplegia of the contralateral side, projectile vomiting without nausea, increased systolic pressure, widening pulse pressure and bradycardia, and altered breathing pattern).**
   1 Instructing the client to slow the breathing rate is inappropriate because it will elevate the Pco_2, which will increase intracranial pressure.
   2 There is no evidence that suctioning is indicated; suctioning increases intracranial pressure and therefore should be avoided unless absolutely necessary to maintain a patent airway.
   3 There is no evidence that supplemental oxygen is needed; an abnormal Pco_2 does not indicate the need for supplemental oxygen.
   Client Needs: Management of Care; **Cognitive Level:** Application; **Integrated Process:** Communication and Documentation; **NP:** Planning

44. **2 An adult client with the mental capacity of a 5-year-old child may not understand the concept of numbers as an indicator of levels of pain; Wong's "Pain Faces" uses pictures to which the individual can relate.**
   1 The client, irrespective of mental capacity, is the primary source from whom to obtain information about pain because it is a personal experience.
   3 Body language provides some information, but may not accurately reflect the client's level of pain.
   4 A client functioning at the level of a 5-year-old child may not understand the concept of numbers.
   Client Needs: Basic Care and Comfort; **Cognitive Level:** Application; **Integrated Process:** Communication and Documentation; **NP:** Assessment

45. **2 The responsibility for correctly doing this task will foster independence.**
   1 This goal is too ambitious for a debilitated, older client.
   3 This is a laudable goal but it does not relate to independence.
   4 Moderate use of the eyes is not contraindicated in clients with glaucoma.
   Client Needs: Psychosocial Integrity; **Cognitive Level:** Application; **Integrated Process:** Teaching/Learning; **NP:** Planning

46. **3 This decreases pressure on the sella turcica and promotes venous return, thus limiting cerebral edema.**
   1 Gentle oral hygiene is performed, excluding brushing of teeth, to prevent trauma to the surgical site.

2 Although deep breathing is encouraged, initially coughing is discouraged to prevent increasing intracranial pressure.
   4 There is no need to limit oral fluids because of the presence of nasal packing.
   Client Needs: Reduction of Risk Potential; **Cognitive Level:** Application; **NP:** Implementation

47. **2 Spasms result from irritation of the bladder during surgery; they decrease in intensity and frequency as healing occurs.**
   1 This is too long; this indicates hemorrhage; drainage should be dark red and after the first few hours gradually turn pink.
   3 The Valsalva maneuver should be avoided because it may initiate prostatic bleeding, not bladder contractions.
   4 The presence of a continuous bladder irrigation (CBI) is unrelated to the amount of oral fluids that should be consumed; once the continuous bladder irrigation is discontinued, oral fluids should be encouraged.
   Client Needs: Reduction of Risk Potential; **Cognitive Level:** Application; **Integrated Process:** Teaching/Learning; **NP:** Implementation

48. **2 Bile salts (Bile Acid Factor) are used to aid digestion of fats and absorption of the fat-soluble vitamins A, D, E, and K.**
   1 Bile salts are not involved in stimulating prothrombin production.
   3 Bile salts are not involved in promoting bilirubin secretion in the urine.
   4 Bile salts are not involved in stimulating contraction of the common bile duct.
   Client Needs: Physiological Adaptation; **Cognitive Level:** Comprehension; **Integrated Process:** Teaching/Learning; **NP:** Implementation

49. **4 Retention of carbon dioxide in the blood lowers the pH, causing respiratory acidosis; deep breathing maximizes gaseous exchange, ridding the body of excess carbon dioxide.**
   1 Deep breathing improves oxygenation of the blood, but it does not stimulate red blood cell production.
   2 Although regular deep breathing improves the vital capacity of the lungs, residual volume is unaffected.
   3 Deep breathing increases, not decreases, the partial pressure of oxygen.
   Client Needs: Physiological Adaptation; **Cognitive Level:** Application; **Integrated Process:** Teaching/Learning; **NP:** Implementation

50. **1 After the need to survive (air, food, water), the need for comfort and freedom from pain closely follow; care should be given in order of the client's basic needs.**
   2 Joints must be exercised, not immobilized, to prevent stiffness, contractures, and muscle atrophy.
   3 Motivation and learning will not occur unless basic needs, such as freedom from pain, are met.
   4 Although bladder training should be included in care, it is not the priority when the client is in pain.
   Client Needs: Basic Care and Comfort; **Cognitive Level:** Application; **NP:** Planning

MEDICAL-SURGICAL NURSING
QUIZ 2

1. A client is admitted with 50% of the body surface area burned after an industrial explosion and fire. The client's serum albumin is 1.5 g/dL, the hematocrit is 30%, the urine specific gravity is 1.025, and the serum globulin is 3 g/dL. When evaluating the client's response to fluid replacement, the nurse should prepare to administer a colloid when the:
   1. Globulin is 3 g/dL
   2. Albumin is below 2 g/dL
   3. Hematocrit is below 32%
   4. Urine specific gravity is 1.018

2. A client is admitted to the hospital with a diagnosis of laryngeal cancer. What is a common early sign of laryngeal cancer for which the nurse should assess this client?
   1. Aphasia
   2. Dyspnea
   3. Dysphagia
   4. Hoarseness

3. The nurse stops at an accident scene to administer emergency care for a person who has sustained partial- and full-thickness burns to the chest, right arm, and upper legs as the result of a car fire. What should the nurse do first when caring for this person?
   1. Cover the person with a blanket
   2. Wrap the person in a clean, dry sheet
   3. Apply sterile dressings to burned areas
   4. Remove clothing from the areas that are burned

4. A male client with thrombophlebitis is apprehensive about the possibility of a clot reaching his lungs and causing sudden death. The nurse's initial intervention should be to:
   1. Discuss his concerns
   2. Clarify his misconception
   3. Explain preventive measures
   4. Teach recognition of early symptoms

5. On entering a hospital room to administer a capsule of hydroxyzine (Vistaril) to a client, the nurse observes the client vomiting. The nurse decides that the injectable form of the medication should be administered rather than the oral form, and calls the practitioner to secure an order to change the route. Proper and safe disposal of the oral capsule of hydroxyzine requires the nurse to:
   1. Drop the tablet into a sharps container
   2. Crush the tablet and flush it into the sewer system
   3. Drop the tablet into a red biohazard bag and tie it shut
   4. Return the tablet to the pharmacy, where it can be discarded safely

6. A client with a history of excessive alcohol use develops hepatic portal hypertension and an elevated serum aldosterone level. For which complications should the nurse assess this client?
   1. Chloride depletion and hypovolemia
   2. Potassium retention and dysrhythmias
   3. Sodium retention and fluid accumulation
   4. Calcium depletion and pathological fractures

7. A female client who is scheduled for a thyroidectomy is concerned that the surgery will interfere with her ability to become pregnant. The nurse should base a response on the understanding that:
   1. As long as medication is continued, ovulation will occur
   2. Hyperthyroidism can cause abortions and fetal anomalies
   3. Pregnancy is not advisable for the client with a thyroidectomy
   4. Pregnancy affects metabolism and will require decreased thyroid hormone

8. A nurse is providing postoperative care for a client who just had a thyroidectomy. For what response should the nurse assess the client when concerned about the potential risk of thyrotoxic crisis?
   1. Elevated serum calcium
   2. Sudden drop in pulse rate
   3. Hypothermia and dry skin
   4. Rapid heartbeat and tremors

9. A nurse is caring for a client who has sustained full-thickness and deep partial-thickness burns. While the nurse is caring for the client the client asks, "What is the difference between my full-thickness and deep partial-thickness burns?" Which is the best response by the nurse?
   1. "Full-thickness burns extend into the subcutaneous tissue and deep partial-thickness burns affect only the epidermis."
   2. "Deep partial-thickness burns extend through the epidermis and full-thickness burns involve superficial layers of the epidermis."
   3. "Deep partial-thickness burns extend into the subcutaneous tissue and full-thickness burns extend through the epidermis and only part of the dermis."
   4. "Full-thickness burns extend into the subcutaneous tissue and deep partial-thickness burns extend through the epidermis and involve only part of the dermis."

10. A client with chronic obstructive pulmonary disease is admitted to the hospital with a tentative diagnosis of pleuritis. When caring for this client the nurse should:
    1. Administer opioids frequently
    2. Assess for signs of pneumonia
    3. Give medication to suppress coughing
    4. Limit fluid intake to prevent pulmonary edema

11. The nurse identifies that a client who was admitted to the hospital after experiencing an anterior septal myocardial infarction does not have a prn prescription for a stool softener. The nurse decides to obtain a prescription for docusate sodium (Colace) primarily because the client:
    1. Is receiving digoxin
    2. Has poor peripheral perfusion
    3. May be kept NPO for several days
    4. Will probably become constipated

12. A client has had a right pneumonectomy. For which postoperative complication that is specific to this type of surgery should the nurse assess this client?
    1. Brain attack
    2. Renal failure
    3. Internal bleeding
    4. Cardiac overload

13. The nurse is caring for a client who had a wedge resection of a lobe of the lung and now has a chest tube with a three-chamber underwater drainage system in place. The nurse considers that the main purpose of the third chamber of the underwater drainage system is to:
    1. Act as a drainage container
    2. Provide an airtight water seal
    3. Control the amount of suction
    4. Allow for escape of air bubbles

14. The nurse is caring for a client with a diagnosis of acute kidney failure associated with drug toxicity. What should the nurse offer the client when the client complains of thirst?
    1. Ice chips
    2. Warm milk
    3. Hard candy
    4. Carbonated soda

15. When a client with severe chronic rheumatoid arthritis reports that pain lasts for 2 to 3 hours after exercising, the nurse should teach the client to:
    1. Substitute isometric exercises for isotonic exercises
    2. Stop the exercises for one day and then resume them
    3. Delay doing aerobic exercises until the pain subsides
    4. Decrease the total time and number of repetitions of the exercise

16. Acetylsalicylic acid (aspirin) is prescribed for a client with rheumatoid arthritis. The nurse understands that the major rationale for this treatment is:
    1. Reduction of fever
    2. Preservation of bone integrity
    3. Reduction of joint inflammation
    4. Prevention of flexion contractures

17. When assessing a client for respiratory involvement during the first 2 days after a burn injury, the nurse observes for sputum that is:
    1. Sooty
    2. Frothy
    3. Yellow
    4. Tenacious

18. A client who is receiving multiple medications for a myocardial infarction complains of severe nausea, and the heartbeat is irregular and slow. The nurse determines that these signs and symptoms are toxic effects of:
    1. Digoxin
    2. Lidocaine
    3. Morphine
    4. Furosemide

19. A female client with type 2 diabetes tells the nurse that she takes Robitussin (guaifenesin) cough syrup when she has a cold. The nurse should teach her that she:
    1. Can substitute an elixir for the syrup
    2. Must calculate the glucose in her daily carbohydrate allowance
    3. Can increase her fluid intake and humidify her bedroom to control a cough
    4. Monitor her serum glucose level; if it remains within an acceptable range, she may take the cough syrup

20. A client has laparoscopic surgery to remove a calculus from the common bile duct. What postoperative client response indicates to the nurse that bile flow into the duodenum is reestablished?
    1. Stools become brown
    2. Liver tenderness is relieved
    3. Colic is absent after ingestion of fats
    4. Serum bilirubin level returns to the expected range

21. A 59-year-old client with type 1 diabetes is admitted to the hospital in ketoacidosis. With medical supervision the client has been adjusting insulin dosage at home based on blood glucose levels. Based on the statements made by the client during the health history, the nurse concludes that the best explanation of the etiology of the ketoacidosis is that the client has:
    1. Become a vegan
    2. Chronic sinusitis
    3. Planned to retire next year
    4. Been taking steroids for a rash

22. When receiving chemotherapy for non-Hodgkin's lymphoma a client states, "I get so sick to my stomach. The medication is useless." The best response by the nurse that uses the technique of paraphrasing is:
    1. "You get sick to your stomach."
    2. "Tell me more about how you feel."
    3. "I'll get a prescription for an antiemetic."
    4. "You don't think the medication is helping you."

23. A nurse is administering vaccines at the local influenza prevention clinic. A client arrives for a vaccination, and a nursing assessment identifies a current febrile illness with a cough. The nurse should:
    1. Give the vaccine
    2. Administer aspirin with the vaccine
    3. Hold the vaccine and notify the practitioner
    4. Reschedule administration of the vaccine for the next month

24. A client has a fracture of the right tibia and a cast is applied. What nursing intervention should the nurse implement when caring for this client?
    1. Cover the cast with plastic wrap until dry
    2. Assist with weight bearing when the client ambulates
    3. Elevate the client's right leg above the level of the heart
    4. Insert a finger inside the edges of the cast to check for skin abrasions

25. A client, admitted to the hospital with a fractured hip, is scheduled for surgery for a total hip replacement.

In which position should the nurse place the client's affected limb after surgery?
1. Adduction and flexion
2. Abduction and extension
3. Adduction and internal rotation
4. Abduction and external rotation

26. A male client who had a brain attack (cerebrovascular accident) had varying moods. These moods ranged from anger to depression and concern about his aphasia, hemiparesis, and need for gavage feedings. Which behavior observed by the nurse indicates the client's acceptance of his physical limitations?
1. Performing his own tube feedings
2. Smiling and becoming more extroverted
3. Allowing his wife to participate in his care
4. Walking in the hall and sitting in the lounge

27. A client with type 2 diabetes, who is taking an oral hypoglycemic agent, is to have a serum glucose test early in the morning. The client asks the nurse, "What do I have to do to prepare for this test?" Which statement by the nurse reflects accurate information?
1. "Eat your usual breakfast."
2. "Have clear liquids for breakfast."
3. "Take your medication before the test."
4. "Do not ingest anything before the test."

28. After surgery a client's fever does not respond to antipyretics. The practitioner orders that the client be placed on a hypothermia blanket. The nurse expects that one reaction to hypothermia therapy that should be prevented is:
1. Shivering
2. Vomiting
3. Dehydration
4. Hypotension

29. A client has an excision of a thrombosed external hemorrhoid. What should the nurse teach the client to use when cleaning the anus after a bowel movement?
1. Betadine pads
2. Soft facial tissue
3. Medicated pads (Tucks)
4. Sterile 4×4-inch gauze pads

30. A client with a rigid and painful abdomen is diagnosed with a perforated peptic ulcer. A nasogastric tube is inserted and surgery is scheduled. Before surgery, the nurse should place the client in the:
1. Sims position
2. Flat-lying position
3. Semi-Fowler's position
4. Dorsal recumbent position

31. A client is admitted to the cardiac care unit with a diagnosis of myocardial infarction. When caring for the client, the client asks the nurse, "What is causing the pain I am experiencing?" The most appropriate response by the nurse is, "The pain is the result of:
1. compression of the heart muscle."
2. release of myocardial isoenzymes."
3. rapid vasodilation of the coronary arteries."
4. inadequate oxygenation of the myocardium."

32. A client with Crohn's disease is admitted to the hospital with a history of chronic, bloody diarrhea, weight loss, and signs of general malnutrition. The client has anemia, a low serum albumin level, and signs of negative nitrogen balance. The nurse concludes that the client's health status is related to a major deficiency of:
1. Iron
2. Protein
3. Vitamin C
4. Linoleic acid

33. A client is admitted to the ambulatory surgery unit for a laparoscopic cholecystectomy. While in the postanesthesia care unit the client experiences nausea and vomiting and is admitted overnight for hydration and observation. The nurse arriving at 7 AM receives report, reviews the medical record, and assesses the client. The nurse concludes that the nausea and vomiting are probably precipitated by:
1. Pain
2. Dilaudid
3. Hemorrhage
4. Dehydration

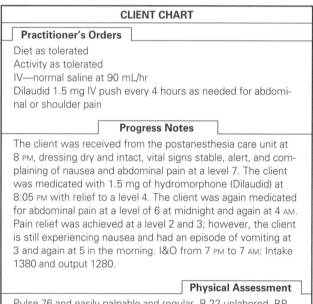

CLIENT CHART

Practitioner's Orders

Diet as tolerated
Activity as tolerated
IV—normal saline at 90 mL/hr
Dilaudid 1.5 mg IV push every 4 hours as needed for abdominal or shoulder pain

Progress Notes

The client was received from the postanesthesia care unit at 8 PM, dressing dry and intact, vital signs stable, alert, and complaining of nausea and abdominal pain at a level 7. The client was medicated with 1.5 mg of hydromorphone (Dilaudid) at 8:05 PM with relief to a level 4. The client was again medicated for abdominal pain at a level of 6 at midnight and again at 4 AM. Pain relief was achieved at a level 2 and 3; however, the client is still experiencing nausea and had an episode of vomiting at 3 and again at 5 in the morning. I&O from 7 PM to 7 AM: Intake 1380 and output 1280.

Physical Assessment

Pulse 76 and easily palpable and regular, R 22 unlabored, BP 120/76. Client states that pain is tolerable with medication but is still experiencing nausea. Dressing is dry and intact. Client is ambulating to the bathroom and voiding sufficient quantities. Hypoactive bowel sounds noted in all four quadrants.

34. An older adult, who is complaining of fatigue, is admitted to the hospital with a diagnosis of chronic obstructive pulmonary disease (COPD). What should the nurse plan to do to address the client's fatigue?
1. Provide small, frequent meals
2. Encourage pursed-lip breathing
3. Schedule nursing activities to allow for rest
4. Encourage bed rest until energy level improves

35. A client is admitted to the hospital with a possible diagnosis of myocardial infarction. What description of the character of pain should the nurse expect when assessing this client's pain?
    1. Severe, intense chest pain
    2. Burning chest pain of short duration
    3. Mild chest pain, radiating toward the abdomen
    4. Squeezing chest pain, relieved by nitroglycerin

36. A client who is receiving a 2 g sodium diet asks for a glass of juice. Pear nectar and apple and tomato juice are available in the unit pantry. Which intervention by the nurse is most appropriate?
    1. Offer the client apple juice or pear nectar
    2. Suggest that the client drink the tomato juice
    3. Tell the client that juice is not permitted on a low-sodium diet
    4. Explain that juice between meals is not calculated into the client's diet, and offer water

37. A nurse is caring for a client who was admitted to the hospital with a diagnosis of incarcerated hernia. The client asks the nurse, "What does incarcerated hernia mean?" The nurse's best response is, "Incarcerated hernia means that the:
    1. bowel has twisted on itself."
    2. protruding hernia cannot be reduced."
    3. intestinal blood supply has been cut off."
    4. involved intestine has developed an erosion."

38. A nurse is caring for a client who just had surgery to repair an inguinal hernia. What should the nurse do to limit a common complication after the repair of an inguinal hernia?
    1. Apply an abdominal binder
    2. Place a support under the scrotum
    3. Teach the client to cough several times an hour
    4. Encourage the client to eat a high-carbohydrate diet

39. A male client, recovering from hepatitis A, asks the nurse when he can return to work. Which is the best response by the nurse?
    1. "As soon as you're feeling less tired, you may go back to work."
    2. "Unfortunately, few people fully recover from hepatitis in less than 6 months."
    3. "Gradually increase your activities because relapses may occur in those who return to full activity too soon."
    4. "You cannot return to work for 6 months because the virus will still be in your stools and you are still communicable."

40. A client newly diagnosed with cancer of the pancreas is scheduled for surgery. When arranging for the next appointment, the client says to the nurse, "Wouldn't I be better off with some other treatment instead of surgery?" The nurse's best response is:
    1. "Why don't you explore the other acceptable treatments for your cancer with the physician?"
    2. "Surgery is the recommended approach. Why don't you discuss this further with the physician?"

3. "Maybe you will be more confident with a second opinion. I think you need a referral to another physician."
4. "With your disease your prognosis will improve if you follow the physician's suggestion to have the recommended surgery."

41. A client is admitted to the hospital with a diagnosis of COPD, and medication that is delivered via a nebulizer is prescribed by the practitioner. What should the nurse teach the client to do when using a nebulizer?
    1. Hold the breath while spraying the medication into the mouth
    2. Position the lips loosely around the mouthpiece and take rapid, shallow breaths
    3. Seal the lips around the mouthpiece and breathe in and out taking slow, deep breaths
    4. Inhale the medication from the nebulizer, remove the mouthpiece from the mouth, and then exhale

42. A 60-year-old client is admitted to the hospital for a needle biopsy of the liver. The practitioner suspects cancer of the liver. What should the nurse teach the client about a needle biopsy in preparation for this procedure?
    1. Midline abdominal incision will be used
    2. Bed rest must be maintained after the procedure
    3. General anesthesia will be used during the biopsy
    4. Supine position will be maintained after the procedure

43. A client is taught the signs and symptoms of a hypoglycemic reaction. Which signs and symptoms identified by the client indicate to the nurse that the teaching is effective? Select all that apply.
    1. _____ Fatigue
    2. _____ Nausea
    3. _____ Weakness
    4. _____ Nervousness
    5. _____ Increased thirst
    6. _____ Increased perspiration

44. A client with Hodgkin's disease, stage III, is started on ABVD therapy, a multiple drug regimen. The client wonders why so many drugs have to be used at once. Which is the best response by the nurse?
    1. Using groups of drugs reduces the likelihood of serious side effects
    2. Each drug destroys the cancer cell at a different time in the cell cycle
    3. Several drugs are used to destroy cells that are not susceptible to radiation therapy
    4. Because there are stages of Hodgkin's disease, if one drug is ineffective, another will work

45. A client develops thrombophlebitis in the right calf. Bed rest is prescribed, and an IV of heparin is initiated. When describing the purpose of this drug to the client, the nurse explains that it:
    1. Prevents extension of the clot
    2. Reduces the size of the thrombus
    3. Dissolves the blood clot in the vein
    4. Facilitates absorption of red blood cells

46. A nurse is preparing to discharge a client who had a transurethral prostatectomy for benign prostatic hyperplasia. The nurse evaluates that the client understands the discharge teaching when he states:
1. "I will drink 8 cups of fluid daily and none after 9 PM."
2. "I am so glad this is over so I don't have to keep going to the doctor."
3. "I will use stool softeners regularly for 1 to 2 months after I get home."
4. "I was so worried and now I can hardly wait to get home to have sex with my wife."

47. A nurse is caring for a client who has just had surgery on the ear. For what early response associated with potential damage to the motor branch of the facial nerve should the nurse assess the client?
1. Pain behind the ear
2. Bitter metallic taste
3. Dryness of the mouth
4. Inability to wrinkle the forehead

48. During the first 36 hours after surgery for cancer of the pancreas, a client complains of severe pain and is medicated with 10 mg of morphine sulfate via IV infusion every 4 hours. What conclusion should the nurse make when the client rests or sleeps between infusions?
1. Pain management is effective
2. Dosage of the drug is excessive
3. Another opioid should be prescribed
4. Oral analgesics probably can be substituted for the opioid

49. A client is admitted to the hospital with a diagnosis of atrial fibrillation, and the practitioner suspects mitral valve stenosis. When obtaining a health history, the nurse determines that it is most significant if the client presents a history of:
1. Cystitis at age 28
2. Pleurisy at age 20
3. Strep throat at age 12
4. German measles at age 6

50. A client is admitted to the hospital for replacement of the mitral valve. Postoperatively the pulses in the client's legs are assessed frequently by the nurse. The primary purpose of this intervention is to detect:
1. Atrial fibrillation
2. Postsurgical bleeding
3. Arteriovenous shunting
4. Peripheral thrombophlebitis

MEDICAL-SURGICAL NURSING QUIZ 2
ANSWERS AND RATIONALES

1. **2 Administration of a colloid is indicated when the serum albumin decreases below 2 g/dL; then, albumin must be administered to increase the level to the expected range of 3.5 to 5.5 g/dL; this increases the oncotic pressure and prevents the shift of fluid out of the intravascular compartment.**
   1 A globulin of 3 g/dL is within the expected parameters of 2.3 to 3.4 g/dL.
   3 A hematocrit level of 32% is low and indicates overhydration; administration of a colloid will increase this problem.
   4 The urine specific gravity is within the expected limits of 1.010 to 1.030.
   Client Needs: Pharmacological and Parenteral Therapies; **Cognitive Level:** Analysis; **NP:** Planning

2. **4 Hoarseness is caused by the inability of the vocal cords to move adequately during speech when a tumor exists.**
   1 Aphasia refers to an expressive or receptive communication deficit as a result of cerebral disease; it is not related to laryngeal cancer.
   2 Dyspnea is a late, not early, adaptation that occurs with laryngeal cancer when a tumor is large enough to obstruct air flow.
   3 Dysphagia is a late, not early, adaptation that occurs when the tumor is large enough to compress the esophagus.
   Client Needs: Physiological Adaptation; **Cognitive Level:** Application; **NP:** Assessment

3. **2 Covering exposed burned surfaces limits contamination by microorganisms and prevents exposure to air, which increases pain.**
   1 A blanket is not smooth in texture and is more apt to adhere to the burned areas and traumatize wounds when removed.
   3 The decision about open or closed treatment of burns will be made by the practitioner after the individual is transferred to a burn unit.
   4 Removing clothing from the areas that are burned is unsafe; it will further traumatize the wounds.
   Client Needs: Physiological Adaptation; **Cognitive Level:** Application; **NP:** Implementation

4. **1 Addressing the client's feelings and then exploring preventive measures should reduce anxiety.**
   2 The risk of a pulmonary embolus is a real concern, not a misconception, associated with thrombophlebitis.
   3 Explaining measures to prevent a pulmonary embolus is not the client's concern; this response does not address the client's feelings concerning the risk of sudden death.
   4 Teaching recognition of early signs and symptoms of pulmonary emboli disregards the client's expressed fears and may increase anxiety.

Client Needs: Psychosocial Integrity; **Cognitive Level:** Application; **Integrated Process:** Teaching/Learning; **NP:** Implementation

5. **4 Medication taken from a stock supply cannot be returned; it should be returned to the pharmacy for safe disposal.**
   1 The purpose of a sharps container is for safe disposal of sharp objects; a tablet dropped into a sharps container can be retrieved.
   2 Wasted medications should not be disposed of through the sewer system because this can contaminate underground water sources.
   3 Placing the tablet into a biohazard bag does not render it unusable.
   Client Needs: Pharmacological and Parenteral Therapies; **Cognitive Level:** Application; **NP:** Implementation

6. **3 Aldosterone, a corticosteroid, causes sodium and water retention and potassium excretion by the kidneys.**
   1 Hypovolemia will not occur with increased aldosterone levels because sodium and water are retained.
   2 Potassium is excreted in the presence of aldosterone and therefore will not accumulate and cause dysrhythmias.
   4 Calcium is unaffected by aldosterone.
   Client Needs: Physiological Adaptation; **Cognitive Level:** Analysis; **NP:** Assessment

7. **1 Medication is regulated to maintain the usual blood levels of thyroxine; therefore, ovulation is not affected, and future pregnancy is possible.**
   2 The client will no longer be hyperthyroid after surgery because the overactive tissue is excised; therefore, pregnancy is not contraindicated.
   3 Pregnancy is not contraindicated after a thyroidectomy because the overactive tissue is excised.
   4 Pregnancy is not contraindicated; however, thyroid hormone therapy may have to be increased during pregnancy.
   Client Needs: Physiological Adaptation; **Cognitive Level:** Application; **Integrated Process:** Teaching/Learning; **NP:** Implementation

8. **4 Thyrotoxic crisis (thyroid storm) refers to a sudden and excessive release of thyroid hormones, which causes pyrexia, tachycardia, and exaggerated symptoms of thyrotoxicosis; surgery, infection, and ablation therapy can precipitate this life-threatening condition.**
   1 Hypercalcemia is not related to thyrotoxic crisis; hypocalcemia results from accidental removal of the parathyroid glands.
   2 Tachycardia is an increased, not decreased, heart rate, which occurs with thyrotoxic crisis because of the sudden release of thyroid hormones; thyroid hormones increase the basal metabolic rate.

NP: Nursing process.

3 Fever, not hypothermia, and diaphoresis, not dry skin, occur with thyrotoxic crisis because of the sudden release of thyroid hormones, which increase the basal metabolic rate.
Client Needs: Reduction of Risk Potential; Cognitive Level: Application; NP: Evaluation

9. **1 Whereas full-thickness burns extend into the subcutaneous tissue, deep partial-thickness burns affect both the epidermis and dermis.**
2 Deep partial-thickness burns not only extend through the epidermis but also involve part of the dermis; superficial partial-thickness, not full-thickness, burns affect the superficial layers of the epidermis.
3 The reverse is true of both these types of burns.
4 This correctly describes the difference between full-thickness and deep partial-thickness burns.
Client Needs: Physiological Adaptation; Cognitive Level: Comprehension; Integrated Process: Teaching/Learning; NP: Implementation

10. **2 Clients with pleuritic disease are prone to develop pneumonia because of impaired lung expansion, air exchange, and drainage.**
1 Opioids are contraindicated because opioids depress respirations.
3 Coughing should not be suppressed; it enhances lung expansion, air exchange, and lung drainage.
4 Oral fluids should be encouraged; pulmonary edema does not develop unless the client has severe cardiovascular disease.
Client Needs: Physiological Adaptation; Cognitive Level: Application; NP: Implementation

11. **4 Inactivity and opioids decrease peristalsis, which may precipitate constipation; straining at stool should be avoided to prevent the Valsalva maneuver, which increases demands on the heart.**
1 Digoxin is unrelated to intestinal peristalsis and the potential for constipation.
2 This is unrelated to constipation; in addition, there is no indication the client has poor peripheral circulation.
3 Being NPO is only one factor that can contribute to constipation; opioid analgesics and bed rest are the primary causes of constipation in this situation.
Client Needs: Pharmacological and Parenteral Therapies; Cognitive Level: Analysis; Integrated Process: Communication and Documentation; NP: Planning

12. **4 Cardiac overload can be caused by the loss of the large vascular lung or a mediastinal shift.**
1 A brain attack is not unique to a pneumonectomy.
2 Renal failure is not unique to a pneumonectomy.
3 Internal bleeding is not unique to a pneumonectomy.
Client Needs: Reduction of Risk Potential; Cognitive Level: Analysis; NP: Evaluation

13. **3 The first chamber collects drainage; the second chamber provides for the underwater seal; the third chamber controls the amount of suction.**
1 The first chamber, not the third chamber, collects drainage.

2 The second chamber, not the third chamber, provides an underwater seal.
4 Although this occurs in a three-chamber system, the purpose of the third chamber is to control suction.
Client Needs: Physiological Adaptation; Cognitive Level: Application; NP: Planning

14. **3 Sucking on candy will relieve thirst and provide calories without supplying extra fluid.**
1 Ice chips add to the restricted fluid intake.
2 Milk contains both fluids and proteins, which should be restricted with acute kidney failure.
4 Carbonated beverages may be high in sodium and provide additional fluid; both should be restricted.
Client Needs: Physiological Adaptation; Cognitive Level: Analysis; NP: Implementation

15. **4 Exercise should be decreased to a level of tolerance.**
1 Isometric exercises promote muscle contraction, not joint movement.
2 The exercise should not be stopped.
3 The purpose of aerobic exercises is to improve cardiovascular functioning, not joint movement; there is no reason to interrupt aerobic exercises if they are tolerated.
Client Needs: Basic Care and Comfort; Cognitive Level: Application; Integrated Process: Teaching/Learning; NP: Implementation

16. **3 The antiinflammatory action of aspirin reduces joint inflammation.**
1 Aspirin reduces fever but this is not the rationale for prescribing it for clients with rheumatoid arthritis.
2 Aspirin does not preserve bone integrity.
4 Flexion contractures are prevented by exercise, not aspirin.
Client Needs: Pharmacological and Parenteral Therapies; Cognitive Level: Application; Integrated Process: Communication and Documentation; NP: Implementation

17. **1 The mucous membranes of the respiratory tract may be charred after inhalation burns; this is evidenced by the production of sooty sputum.**
2 Frothy sputum usually is indicative of pulmonary edema.
3 Yellow sputum usually is indicative of a respiratory infection.
4 Tenacious sputum usually is indicative of respiratory infection.
Client Needs: Physiological Adaptation; Cognitive Level: Application; NP: Assessment

18. **1 Signs of digoxin toxicity include cardiac dysrhythmias, anorexia, nausea, vomiting, and visual disturbances.**
2 Although nausea and heart block may occur with lidocaine, these symptoms rarely are seen; drowsiness and CNS disturbances are more common.
3 Toxic effects of morphine are slow, deep respirations; stupor; and constricted pupils; nausea is a side effect, not a toxic effect.
4 Toxic effects of furosemide are renal failure, blood dyscrasias, and loss of hearing.

Client Needs: Pharmacological and Parenteral Therapies; **Cognitive Level:** Analysis; **NP:** Evaluation

19. **2 Cough syrup contains a glucose base; the client should use a glucose-free product or account for the glucose.**

    1 Elixirs contain natural sweeteners.

    3 Although increasing fluid intake and using a room humidifier will loosen secretions, it will not suppress a cough.

    4 Additional glucose may increase serum glucose levels beyond the desired range; once control is achieved, it is unwise to alter dietary intake or medications without supervision.

    Client Needs: Pharmacological and Parenteral Therapies; **Cognitive Level:** Application; **Integrated Process:** Teaching/Learning; **NP:** Implementation

20. **1 The return of brown color to the stool indicates that bile is entering the duodenum and being converted to urobilinogen by bacteria.**

    2 Liver tenderness is unrelated to bile flow.

    3 The absence of biliary colic is related to the removal of the calculus, not the flow of bile.

    4 The serum bilirubin level is not affected.

    Client Needs: Physiological Adaptation; **Cognitive Level:** Application; **NP:** Evaluation

21. **4 Steroids cause gluconeogenesis and glycogenolysis, both of which increase blood glucose levels.**

    1 A vegan diet will not increase blood glucose levels.

    2 Chronic sinusitis is a chronic condition that probably has been incorporated into the client's coping patterns; it will not cause sufficient stress to increase the serum glucose to the level of ketoacidosis.

    3 Planning retirement is an event that is in the future and will not cause sufficient stress to increase the serum glucose level enough to cause ketoacidosis; retirement may be welcomed and may not cause undue stress.

    Client Needs: Pharmacological and Parenteral Therapies; **Cognitive Level:** Analysis; **Integrated Process:** Teaching/Learning; **NP:** Analysis

22. **4 Rewording of the client's statement is paraphrasing that promotes further verbalization.**

    1 This response is not paraphrasing; this repeats the client's exact words.

    2 This response is clarifying, a therapeutic technique; it is not paraphrasing.

    3 This response is not an interviewing technique; it does not address the theme in the client's statement and it cuts off communication.

    Client Needs: Psychosocial Integrity; **Cognitive Level:** Analysis; **Integrated Process:** Communication and Documentation; **NP:** Implementation

23. **4 The appropriate response is to delay the administration of the vaccine until the client is healthy.**

    1 Vaccines should not be administered during a febrile illness.

    2 Vaccines should not be administered during a febrile illness; administering an aspirin is a dependent function of the nurse and requires a practitioner's prescription.

    3 Although holding the vaccine and administering it after the fever and cough are resolved is appropriate, notifying the practitioner is not necessary.

    Client Needs: Pharmacological and Parenteral Therapies; **Cognitive Level:** Application; **NP:** Analysis

24. **3 Elevating the affected leg will help reduce the formation of edema via the principle of gravity.**

    1 Plastic wrap holds moisture and will interfere with drying of the cast.

    2 Full weight bearing should not start until ordered by the practitioner.

    4 Nothing should be inserted under the cast; this can cause tissue injury.

    Client Needs: Reduction of Risk Potential; **Cognitive Level:** Application; **NP:** Implementation

25. **2 Abduction and extension reduce stress on the joint capsule, preventing the hip prosthesis from becoming dislocated.**

    1 Adduction and flexion strain the joint capsule, promoting dislocation of the hip prosthesis.

    3 Adduction and internal rotation strain the joint capsule, promoting dislocation of the hip prosthesis.

    4 Although abduction helps prevent dislocation of the prosthesis, external rotation puts strain on the joint capsule, promoting dislocation of the hip prosthesis.

    Client Needs: Reduction of Risk Potential; **Cognitive Level:** Application; **NP:** Implementation

26. **1 The best indicator of acceptance is when the client begins to participate in self-care.**

    2 The nurse cannot assume that physical limitations have been accepted just because a client smiles.

    3 Allowing others to provide care does not indicate acceptance.

    4 Walking in the hall and sitting in the lounge do not indicate acceptance; they may be an attempt to relieve boredom.

    Client Needs: Psychosocial Integrity; **Cognitive Level:** Application; **NP:** Evaluation

27. **4 Fasting before the test is indicated for accurate and reliable results; food before the test will increase serum glucose levels through metabolism of the nutrients.**

    1 Food should not be ingested before the test; food will increase the serum glucose level, negating accuracy of the test.

    2 Instructing the client to have clear liquids for breakfast is inappropriate; some clear fluids contain simple carbohydrates, which will increase the serum glucose level.

    3 Medications are withheld before the test because of their influence on the serum glucose level.

    Client Needs: Reduction of Risk Potential; **Cognitive Level:** Application; **Integrated Process:** Teaching/Learning; **NP:** Implementation

28. 1 **Shivering should be prevented; peripheral vasoconstriction increases the temperature, the circulatory rate, and oxygen consumption.**
    2 Vomiting is not a response to hypothermia therapy.
    3 Dehydration is not a response to hypothermia therapy; presence of a fever can cause dehydration if oral or parenteral fluid intake is inadequate to maintain fluid balance.
    4 Hypotension is not a response to hypothermia therapy; hypotension can occur with dehydration if oral or parenteral fluid intake is inadequate to maintain fluid balance.
    Client Needs: Reduction of Risk Potential; **Cognitive Level:** Application; **NP:** Planning

29. 3 **Witch hazel–moistened pads (Tucks) are not irritating and are soothing to the anal mucosa.**
    1 Betadine may cause excessive drying and irritation; the rectum always is contaminated; external cleansing with Betadine will not appreciably affect the bacteria present.
    2 Dry facial tissue is irritating and can cause trauma.
    4 Sterile gauze pads are unnecessary; the rectal area is considered contaminated.
    Client Needs: Pharmacological and Parenteral Therapies; **Cognitive Level:** Analysis; **Integrated Process:** Teaching/Learning; **NP:** Implementation

30. 3 **The semi-Fowler's position will localize the spilled stomach contents in the lower part of the abdominal cavity.**
    1 The Sims position will exert pressure on the abdomen, which may be uncomfortable for the client.
    2 Lying flat in bed exerts pressure against the diaphragm from abdominal organs; this will inhibit breathing and intensify discomfort. Also, it allows spilled stomach contents to spread throughout the abdominal cavity.
    4 The dorsal recumbent position exerts pressure against the diaphragm from abdominal organs; this will inhibit breathing and intensify discomfort. Also, it allows spilled stomach contents to spread throughout the abdominal cavity.
    Client Needs: Reduction of Risk Potential; **Cognitive Level:** Application; **NP:** Implementation

31. 4 **Cessation of blood flow, which normally carries oxygen to the myocardium, results in pain because of ischemia of myocardial tissue.**
    1 Myocardial infarction does not involve compression of the heart.
    2 The release of myocardial isoenzymes is indication of myocardial damage; this does not cause myocardial pain.
    3 Vasodilation will increase perfusion and contribute to pain relief, not cause myocardial pain.
    Client Needs: Physiological Adaptation; **Cognitive Level:** Application; **Integrated Process:** Teaching/Learning; **NP:** Implementation

32. 2 **Protein deficiency causes a low serum albumin level, which permits fluid shifts from the intravascular to the interstitial compartment, resulting in edema. Decreased protein also causes anemia; protein intake must be increased.**
    1 Although a deficiency of iron will result in anemia, it will not cause the other adaptations.
    3 Vitamin C is unrelated to these adaptations.
    4 Linoleic acid is unrelated to these adaptations.
    Client Needs: Physiological Adaptation; **Cognitive Level:** Analysis; **NP:** Analysis

33. 2 **Nausea and vomiting are common side effects of hydromorphone (Dilaudid); the nurse should notify the practitioner and obtain a prescription for an antiemetic and a different drug for pain relief.**
    1 The client reports that pain is tolerable on a level of 3 or 4 with medication.
    3 With hemorrhage the pulse is weak and rapid with a decrease in BP; this client's vital signs are in the expected range and the dressing is dry and intact.
    4 With dehydration there is a weak, rapid pulse and a decrease in blood pressure; the client's intake is more than the output and the client is receiving 90 mL of IV solution hourly along with some oral intake, which is adequate to prevent dehydration.
    Client Needs: Pharmacological and Parenteral Therapies; **Cognitive Level:** Analysis; **NP:** Evaluation

34. 3 **Rest limits muscle contractions, which diminishes oxygen needs and decreases fatigue.**
    1 Although small frequent meals may decrease pressure on the diaphragm and facilitate breathing, it does not address the client's fatigue.
    2 Although encouraging pursed-lip breathing facilitates gas exchange, it does not reduce the metabolic demand for oxygen.
    4 Bed rest promotes pooling of pulmonary secretions, which may aggravate the client's respiratory status.
    Client Needs: Basic Care and Comfort; **Cognitive Level:** Application; **NP:** Planning

35. 1 **Blockage of myocardial blood supply causes accumulation of unoxidized metabolites in the muscle; this affects nerve endings and causes severe, intense chest pain.**
    2 Burning chest pain is not the type of pain associated with a myocardial infarction.
    3 Mild chest pain, radiating toward the abdomen is not the type of pain associated with a myocardial infarction.
    4 Nitroglycerin relieves pain associated with angina, not pain associated with myocardial infarction.
    Client Needs: Physiological Adaptation; **Cognitive Level:** Application; **NP:** Analysis

36. 1 **Apple juice and pear nectar are low in sodium and therefore are better choices for this client.**
    2 Tomato juice has a high sodium content; it should be avoided to prevent fluid retention.
    3 Low-sodium juices are permitted.

4 The client is permitted low-sodium juice between meals.

Client Needs: Basic Care and Comfort; **Cognitive Level:** Analysis; **NP:** Implementation

37. 2 **When the intestine cannot be manually returned to the body cavity, the hernia is considered incarcerated.**

 1 A twisted bowel is called a volvulus.

 3 When blood supply is cut off to the intestine, it is called a strangulated hernia.

 4 Erosion of intestinal tissue may be caused by a variety of conditions; one condition that can cause erosion of the bowel is a strangulated hernia, not an incarcerated hernia.

 Client Needs: Physiological Adaptation; **Cognitive Level:** Comprehension; **Integrated Process:** Teaching/Learning; **NP:** Implementation

38. 2 **After inguinal hernia repair, the scrotum commonly becomes edematous and painful; drainage is facilitated by elevating the scrotum on rolled linen or using a scrotal support.**

 1 An abdominal binder will not support the operative site; the incision is too low.

 3 Coughing increases intra-abdominal pressure and should be avoided because it strains the operative site.

 4 Obesity is a factor in the development of hernias; high-carbohydrate diets should be discouraged.

 Client Needs: Reduction of Risk Potential; **Cognitive Level:** Application; **NP:** Implementation

39. 3 **Relapses are common; they occur after too early ambulation and too much physical activity.**

 1 Fatigue is a cardinal symptom; if the client tires at rest, a return to work must be delayed.

 2 The majority of clients recover in 3 to 16 weeks with no further problems.

 4 The majority of clients recover in 3 to 16 weeks; hepatitis A is most communicable before the onset of symptoms and during the first few days of fever.

 Client Needs: Physiological Adaptation; **Cognitive Level:** Application; **Integrated Process:** Teaching/Learning; **NP:** Implementation

40. 2 **This response provides needed information and establishes an opportunity for further discussion of surgery.**

 1 This implies the other approaches are as effective as surgery; this places doubt in the client's mind that surgery is the most effective option.

 3 This is an inappropriate response; the competence of the physician was not questioned, but there exists a need for further discussion of the treatment; making this type of referral is not the nurse's role.

 4 This is false reassurance; it cuts off communication and does not address the need for further discussion.

 Client Needs: Psychosocial Integrity; **Cognitive Level:** Analysis; **Integrated Process:** Communication and Documentation; **NP:** Implementation

41. 3 **Sealing the lips around the mouthpiece ensures that medication is delivered on inspiration; slow, deep breaths promote better deposition and efficacy of medication deep into the lungs.**

 1 The breath should not be held; a nebulizer treatment delivers medication by inhaling it into the mouth through a mouthpiece.

 2 Positioning the lips loosely around the mouthpiece may allow room air to be inhaled, which will dilute the aerosolized medication; rapid, shallow breaths mainly will deposit medication in the oral cavity and will not effectively deliver medication deep into the lung.

 4 This technique allows valuable aerosolized medication to be deposited into the air when the client removes the mouthpiece from the mouth to exhale; the client will not receive the full dose of aerosolized medication.

 Client Needs: Pharmacological and Parenteral Therapies; **Cognitive Level:** Application; **Integrated Process:** Teaching/Learning; **NP:** Implementation

42. 2 **Bed rest in the right side-lying position for 2 hours after the procedure applies pressure to the insertion site and reduces the risk of bleeding.**

 1 A needle biopsy requires a stab wound over the liver, not an abdominal incision.

 3 A liver biopsy is done with local anesthesia.

 4 The supine position is contraindicated. The client should be positioned in the right side-lying position for 2 hours after the procedure because this applies pressure to the insertion site and reduces the risk of bleeding.

 Client Needs: Reduction of Risk Potential; **Cognitive Level:** Application; **Integrated Process:** Teaching/Learning; **NP:** Implementation

43. **Answer: 3, 4, 6**

 1 Fatigue is related to hyperglycemia, not hypoglycemia.

 2 Nausea is related to hyperglycemia, not hypoglycemia.

 3 **Weakness is related to a decrease in glucose within the central nervous system.**

 4 **Nervousness is caused by increased adrenergic activity and increased secretion of catecholamines.**

 5 Increased thirst with an excessive oral fluid intake (polydipsia) is associated with hyperglycemia and is one of the cardinal signs of diabetes mellitus.

 6 **Increased perspiration is related to increased adrenergic activity and increased secretion of catecholamines.**

 Client Needs: Physiological Adaptation; **Cognitive Level:** Analysis; **Integrated Process:** Teaching/Learning; **NP:** Evaluation

44. 2 **Cells are vulnerable to specific drugs through the stages of mitosis, and a combination bombards the malignant cells at various stages.**

 1 The side effects of a drug are not ameliorated by a combination with others.

3 Although this is true, it is not the reason for using a combination of drugs.

4 Although there is more than one stage of Hodgkin's, this is not the reason for using a combination of drugs.

Client Needs: Pharmacological and Parenteral Therapies; **Cognitive Level:** Application; **Integrated Process:** Teaching/Learning; **NP:** Implementation

45. 1 **Heparin interferes with activation of prothrombin to thrombin and inhibits aggregation of platelets.**

2 Heparin does not reduce the size of a thrombus.

3 Heparin does not dissolve blood clots in the veins.

4 Heparin does not facilitate the absorption of red blood cells.

Client Needs: Pharmacological and Parenteral Therapies; **Cognitive Level:** Application; **Integrated Process:** Teaching/Learning; **NP:** Planning

46. 3 **Straining at stool should be avoided for 4 to 6 weeks after surgery, or until permitted by the practitioner; avoiding straining supports healing and limits precipitation of bleeding.**

1 Eight glasses of fluid a day is insufficient fluid; between 2500 and 3000 mL/day should be consumed to ensure adequate flushing of the bladder and urethra.

2 The client should have continued medical supervision.

4 Sexual intercourse should be avoided until permitted by the practitioner.

Client Needs: Reduction of Risk Potential; **Cognitive Level:** Application; **Integrated Process:** Teaching/Learning; **NP:** Evaluation

47. 4 **The motor fibers of the facial nerve innervate the superficial muscles of the face and scalp.**

1 This is a sensory response that may be manifested when the injury is to the sensory, not motor, branch of the facial nerve.

2 This is a sensory response that may be manifested when the injury is to the sensory, not motor, branch of the facial nerve.

3 This is a sensory response that may be manifested when the injury is to the sensory, not motor, branch of the facial nerve.

Client Needs: Physiological Adaptation; **Cognitive Level:** Application; **NP:** Evaluation

48. 1 **Sleeping between doses of the pain medication indicates that the client is comfortable; therefore, the medication regimen is effective.**

2 Ten milligrams of morphine sulfate via IV infusion every 4 hours is a recommended dose; no data exist to indicate that it is excessive for this client.

3 Changing the medication is not necessary; the medication regimen is effective.

4 Earlier than 36 hours after this major surgery is too soon to change the pain medication from an opioid to a less effective oral analgesic.

Client Needs: Pharmacological and Parenteral Therapies; **Cognitive Level:** Application; **NP:** Evaluation

49. 3 **Streptococcal infections occurring in childhood may result in damage to heart valves, particularly the mitral valve. Group A streptococcal antigens bind to receptors on heart cells, where an autoimmune response is triggered, damaging the heart.**

1 Cystitis usually is caused by *Escherichia coli*, which does not affect heart valves.

2 Pleurisy usually follows pulmonary problems unrelated to streptococcal infection; it does not result in damage to heart valves.

4 The rubella virus does affect the valves of the heart.

Client Needs: Physiological Adaptation; **Cognitive Level:** Analysis; **NP:** Analysis

50. 4 **Because blood pools in the extremities, there is an increased hazard of peripheral emboli in clients who have received a mitral valve replacement.**

1 A peripheral pulse alone will not reveal atrial fibrillation; to detect the presence of a pulse deficit, one must compare a peripheral pulse with the apical pulse.

2 Bleeding is detected by checking the wound dressing and observing for signs of shock (e.g., lowered BP, tachycardia, restlessness).

3 Arteriovenous shunting is not a danger after mitral valve replacement.

Client Needs: Reduction of Risk Potential; **Cognitive Level:** Analysis; **NP:** Evaluation

CHAPTER

3

Mental Health Nursing

Review Questions

NURSING PRACTICE

1. A housekeeping staff member in a mental health unit reports to the nurse that food was found hidden in a client's room. Knowing that the client was admitted with a fluid and electrolyte imbalance because of anorexia nervosa, the nurse should ask housekeeping personnel to:
   1. Point this out to the client and remove the food
   2. Keep the nursing staff informed if this happens again
   3. Disregard this because it is common behavior of clients with anorexia
   4. Keep a record of when this happens and report to the nursing staff weekly

2. A client is admitted to a psychiatric hospital because of a recurrent mental health problem. During admission the nurse determines expected client outcomes. The nurse concludes that expected outcomes are:
   1. Long-term goals
   2. Variances of care
   3. Clinical pathways
   4. Measurable objectives

3. The nurse is explaining the Client Bill of Rights for Psychiatric Patients to a female client whose psychiatrist has admitted her to an inpatient facility. Her admission is voluntary. The statement that is not a client right is the "Right to:
   1. personal mail"
   2. refuse treatment"
   3. written treatment plans"
   4. select health team members"

4. A client is presented with the treatment option of electroconvulsive therapy (ECT). After discussion with staff members, the client requests that a family member be called to help with the decision for undergoing this treatment. What ethical principle does the nurse consider when supporting the client's request?
   1. Justice
   2. Veracity
   3. Autonomy
   4. Beneficence

5. A 13-year-old boy, who recently was suspended from school for consistently bullying other children, is brought to the pediatric mental health clinic by his mother. The child is assessed by the psychiatrist and referred to a psychologist for psychological testing. The day after the tests are completed the mother returns to the clinic and asks the nurse for results of the tests. The nurse should:
   1. Refer the mother to the psychiatrist
   2. Explain to the mother the results of the tests
   3. Suggest that the mother call the psychologist
   4. Teach the mother about the variety of tests administered

6. After caring for a terminally ill client for several weeks, a nurse becomes increasingly aware of a need for a respite from this assignment. What is the nurse's best initial action?
   1. Request vacation time for a few days
   2. Seek support from colleagues on the unit
   3. Withdraw emotional involvement with the client
   4. Stay with the client while trying to work through feelings

7. A 34-year-old woman who was sexually assaulted is examined in the emergency department within 2 hours of the assault. During assessment she freely discusses the incident, her past psychiatric history, and her past sexual history with the sexual assault nurse examiner (SANE). What data are inappropriate for the nurse to document in the client's medical record?
   1. Details of the client's previous sexual history
   2. Verbatim statements made by the client regarding the assault
   3. Observation of the client's physical trauma using a body map and/or photographs
   4. Signs of emotional trauma, including the client's present condition and cooperative behavior

8. A nurse has been working double shifts to pay for a new car. These extra shifts are stopped when frequent headaches and fatigue ensue. The nurse manager identifies that the care the nurse is providing is barely adequate, even when staying an extra hour every day. The nurse manager handles this situation by stating:
   1. "Don't you think you are trying to do too much?"
   2. "What can I do to help you finish your work on time?"
   3. "I'll help you get organized so you can leave on time."
   4. "I've noticed that you have been staying late every night."

9. A client with moderate dementia often assaults the nursing staff, and the staff decides to develop a plan to minimize this behavior. What should the plan include?
   1. Limiting the time staff and client spend together
   2. An outline of the consequences for uncooperative behavior
   3. The client's preferences for use as a reward or a punishment
   4. Identification of nursing staff members whom the client prefers

10. The nurse should first discuss terminating the nurse-client relationship with a client during the:
    1. Working phase when the client initiates this
    2. Orientation phase when a contract is established
    3. Working phase when the client shows some progress
    4. Termination phase when discharge plans are being made

11. On a home visit to an older adult who has chronic heart failure, the nurse observes that a 6-month-old grandchild lies quietly in a crib, rarely smiles or babbles, and barely has basic needs attended. The client is the primary caregiver for the infant. The nurse should:
    1. Advise purchasing appropriate toys designed for this age level
    2. Inform the client that the child will be retarded if not stimulated
    3. Explain the need for the family to hire a mother's helper for the home
    4. Initiate a referral to an appropriate agency to assess the need for a home health aide

12. When planning nursing care for a client with severe agoraphobia, the nurse should first:
    1. Determine the client's degree of impairment
    2. Support the client's self-esteem through verbal interactions
    3. Expose the client gradually to anxiety-provoking situations
    4. Teach the client biofeedback techniques for reducing anxiety

13. A nurse revises the care plan based on the client's responses that show evidence that goals were not attained. What phase of the nursing process is being applied?
    1. Planning
    2. Evaluation
    3. Assessment
    4. Implementation

14. After speaking with the parents of a child dying from leukemia, the practitioner gives a verbal DNR order but refuses to put it in writing. What should the nurse do?
    1. Follow the order as given by the practitioner
    2. Refuse to follow the practitioner's order, unless the nursing supervisor approves it
    3. Ask the practitioner to write the order in pencil on the child's chart before leaving the room
    4. Determine whether the family is in accord with the practitioner while following hospital policy

15. A young client who is a mother for the first time is anxious about her new parenting role. With the nurse's encouragement, she joins the new mothers' support group at the local "Y." What kind of prevention does this activity reflect?
    1. Primary prevention
    2. Tertiary prevention
    3. Secondary prevention
    4. Therapeutic prevention

16. The nurse manager of an emergency department who is helping a nurse with "burnout" should facilitate confrontation of the problem by urging the nurse to:
    1. Work on a primary nursing care unit
    2. Choose a nursing position on a low-stress unit
    3. Attend educational programs as often as possible
    4. Identify personal responses to daily work stresses

PERSONALITY DEVELOPMENT

17. One afternoon the nurse on the unit overhears a young female client having an argument with her boyfriend. A while later the client complains to the nurse that dinner is always late and the meals are terrible. The nurse identifies that the defense mechanism the client is using is:
    1. Projection
    2. Dissociation
    3. Displacement
    4. Intellectualization

18. Although upset by a young client's continual complaints about all aspects of care, the nurse ignores them and attempts to divert the conversation. Immediately following this exchange with the client, the nurse discusses with a friend the various stages of development of young adults. What defense mechanism is the nurse using?
    1. Substitution
    2. Sublimation
    3. Identification
    4. Intellectualization

19. According to Erikson, a child's increased vulnerability to anxiety in response to separations or pending separations from significant others results from failure to complete a developmental stage. What does the nurse call this stage?
    1. Trust
    2. Identity
    3. Initiative
    4. Autonomy

20. The nurse explains to the mother of a preschool child that Erikson identified the developmental conflict of children from 3 to 5 years as:
    1. Initiative vs. guilt
    2. Industry vs. inferiority
    3. Breaking away vs. staying at home
    4. Sexual impulses vs. psychosexual development

21. According to Erikson, a young adult must accomplish the tasks associated with the stage known as:
    1. Trust vs. mistrust
    2. Intimacy vs. isolation
    3. Industry vs. inferiority
    4. Generativity vs. stagnation

22. A 23-year-old female client is admitted to a psychiatric unit after several episodes of uncontrolled rage at her parents' home. She is diagnosed as having borderline personality disorder. While watching a television newscast describing an incident of violence in the home, the client states, "People like that need to be put away before they kill someone." The nurse identifies that the client is using:
    1. Denial
    2. Projection
    3. Introjection
    4. Sublimation

23. A 65-year-old individual is admitted to the hospital with a history of depression. The client, who speaks little English and has few outside interests since retiring, states, "I feel useless and unneeded." The nurse identifies that the client is in Erikson's developmental stage of:
    1. Initiative vs. guilt
    2. Integrity vs. despair
    3. Intimacy vs. isolation
    4. Identity vs. role confusion

24. A 7-year-old hospitalized boy wakes up crying because he has wet his bed. It is most appropriate for the nurse to:
    1. Allow the child to change his bed and pajamas
    2. Change the child's bed while he changes his pajamas
    3. Take the child to the bathroom and change his pajamas
    4. Remind the child to call the nurse next time to avoid changing his pajamas

25. The mother of an 18-year-old male comes to the local mental health center. She is extremely upset because of her son's behavior since returning from his freshman year at college. He takes his brother's clothing, comes in at all hours, and refuses to get a job. However, sometimes he is happy and outgoing, and other times he is withdrawn. The mother asks why her son is like this. While contemplating this situation, the nurse considers that adolescents usually are:
    1. Anxious and unhappy
    2. Angry and irresponsible
    3. Impulsive and self-centered
    4. Hyperactive and self-destructive

26. According to Erikson, an individual who fails to master the maturational crisis of adolescence will most often:
    1. Rebel at parental orders
    2. Experience role confusion
    3. Be interpersonally isolated
    4. Become a substance abuser

27. A constructive and lengthy method of confronting the stress of adolescence and preventing a negative and unhealthy developmental outcome is:
    1. Role experimentation
    2. Adherence to peer standards
    3. Sublimation through schoolwork
    4. Development of dependency on parents

28. The parents of an overweight adolescent female tell the nurse that they are concerned that their daughter feels inferior to her sister who is an attractive, successful college senior. They ask the nurse what they can do about this problem. The nurse should:
    1. Suggest that they appear to be creating a problem where none exists
    2. Tell them to avoid talking about their older child's accomplishments
    3. Encourage the parents to give the adolescent recognition for her strong points
    4. Advise the parents to tell the adolescent to view her sister's success as a challenge

29. A nurse, along with an adolescent girl and her parents, set bolstering the adolescent's self-esteem as a high-priority goal. The girl expresses an interest in earning money. What nursing action will contribute to the achievement of this goal?
    1. Telling the adolescent how much her parents love her
    2. Urging the adolescent to join a neighborhood volunteer group
    3. Supporting the adolescent's interest in enrolling in a babysitting course
    4. Encouraging the adolescent to talk about feelings of pride in her successful siblings

30. When a person who is unathletic and uncoordinated is successful in a musical career, it may be related to the defense mechanism of:
    1. Sublimation
    2. Transference
    3. Compensation
    4. Rationalization

31. The nurse evaluates that the plan for bolstering an overweight adolescent's self-esteem was effective when, 3 months later, the adolescent's mother reports that the adolescent:
    1. Seems to be doing average work in school
    2. Has asked her how to bake bread and cookies
    3. Imitates a sibling's manner of speech and dress
    4. Joined a dirt bike group that meets at the school

32. According to Erikson, a person's adjustment to the period of senescence will depend largely on the adjustment the individual made to the developmental stage of:
    1. Trust vs. mistrust
    2. Industry vs. inferiority
    3. Generativity vs. stagnation
    4. Identity vs. identity diffusion

33. When helping an older adult (ages 65 to 75 years) successfully complete Erikson's task of this stage, the nurse should assist the client to:
   1. Invest creative energies in promoting social welfare
   2. Redefine a role in society that offers something of value
   3. Look to recapture those opportunities that were not experienced
   4. Feel a sense of satisfaction when reflecting on past achievements

34. The nurse's role in maintaining or promoting the health of the older adult should be based on the principle that:
   1. Some physiological changes that occur as a result of aging are reversible
   2. Thoughts of impending death are frequent and depressing to most older adults
   3. Older adults can better accept the dependent state that chronic illness often causes
   4. There is a strong correlation between successful retirement and maintaining health

35. When planning care for an older client, the nurse considers that aging has little effect on a client's:
   1. Sense of taste or smell
   2. Muscle or motor strength
   3. Capacity to handle life's stresses
   4. Ability to remember recent events

36. Survivors of a major earthquake are being interviewed on admission to the hospital. The nurse identifies that they exhibit a flattened affect, make minimal eye contact, and speak in a monotone. These behaviors are indicative of the defense mechanism known as:
   1. Isolation
   2. Splitting
   3. Introjection
   4. Compensation

THERAPEUTIC RELATIONSHIPS

37. A nurse plans to use family therapy as a means of assisting a family to cope with their child's terminal illness. The nurse's basis for this choice is that:
   1. It is more efficient to interact with the whole family together
   2. The entire family is involved because what happens to one member affects all
   3. The nurse can control manipulation and alliances better by using this mode of intervention
   4. It will prevent the parents from deceiving each other about the true nature of their child's condition

38. A client who has recently been diagnosed with HIV infection comments to the nurse, "There are so many terrible people around. Why couldn't one of them get HIV instead of me?" What is the best nurse's response?
   1. "It seems unfair that you should have this disease."
   2. "I'm sure you really don't wish this on someone else."

   3. "It might be good if you speak with your religious leader."
   4. "I'm sure you know that HIV infection is now considered a chronic illness."

39. The parents of an autistic child begin family therapy with a nurse therapist. The father states that the family members wish to share their religious beliefs with the therapist. The nurse should:
   1. Limit the father's discussion of religion
   2. Include the mutual discussion of religious beliefs
   3. Keep the sessions focused on the family's concerns
   4. Invite the family's religious leader to a therapy session

40. A 17-year-old is diagnosed as having anorexia nervosa. The psychiatrist, in conjunction with the client and the parents, decides to institute a behavior modification program. The nurse identifies that a major component of behavior modification is that it:
   1. Rewards positive behavior
   2. Decreases necessary restrictions
   3. Deconditions fear of weight gain
   4. Reduces anxiety-producing situations

41. When caring for a client with a major depressive disorder, the nurse's priority intervention should be to help the client to:
   1. Feel comfortable with the nurse
   2. Investigate new leisure activities
   3. Participate in small-group activities
   4. Initiate conversations about feelings

42. The nurse manager is evaluating a primary nurse's ability to develop a therapeutic relationship. A client with a bipolar mood disorder, manic phase, has been hyperactive and sarcastic. This behavior has been decreasing and the client states, "My husband and I have problems because we see things differently." What response indicates to the nurse manager that the primary nurse is not being therapeutic?
   1. "Do you know why you are feeling calmer today?"
   2. "Not getting along with one's spouse is upsetting."
   3. "Can you explain what you mean by seeing things differently?"
   4. "Tell me about a specific time when you have had problems with your husband."

43. A nurse on the psychiatric unit is planning a discharge conference with a client and the client's family. The priority nursing action that should be included in the discharge plan is:
   1. Obtaining a more complete family history
   2. Teaching the client about the medication to be taken
   3. Discussing new issues that could be worked on at home
   4. Exploring what has been learned from this hospitalization

44. In an attempt to remain objective and support a client during a crisis, the nurse uses imagination and determination to project the self into the client's emotions.

The nurse accomplishes this by using the technique known as:

1. Empathy
2. Sympathy
3. Projection
4. Acceptance

45. After a traumatic event, a client is extremely upset and exhibits pressured and rambling speech. What therapeutic technique can the nurse use when a client's communication rambles?
    1. Touch
    2. Silence
    3. Focusing
    4. Summarizing

46. When a newly admitted client with paranoid ideation tells the nurse about people coming through the doors to commit murder, the nurse should:
    1. Ignore the client's stories
    2. Listen to what the client is saying
    3. Explain that no one can get through the door
    4. Ask for an explanation of where the information was obtained

47. When communicating with a client with a psychiatric diagnosis, the nurse uses silence. When silence is used in therapeutic communication, clients should feel:
    1. Unhurried to answer
    2. It is their turn to talk
    3. The nurse is thinking about the interaction
    4. The nurse expects that further communication is unnecessary

48. When speaking with a client diagnosed with schizophrenia, the nurse identifies that the client keeps interjecting sentences that have nothing to do with the main thoughts being expressed. The client asks whether the nurse understands. What is the nurse's best response?
    1. "You aren't making any sense; let's talk about something else."
    2. "You are so confused; I cannot understand what you are saying to me."
    3. "Why don't you take a rest, then we can talk about your concerns again later this afternoon."
    4. "I'd like to understand what you are saying, but I'm having difficulty following what you are saying."

49. A mother visiting her hospitalized teenage daughter gets into an argument with her. Leaving her daughter's room in tears, the mother meets the nurse and relates the argument, stating, "I can't believe I got so angry I could have hit her." The nurse's most therapeutic response is:
    1. "Teenagers can really drive you to distraction."
    2. "You can't compare yourself to an abusing parent."
    3. "You should bring a surprise for your daughter to make her feel better."
    4. "Sometimes we find it difficult to live up to our own expectations of ourselves."

50. A husband is upset that his wife's alcohol withdrawal delirium has persisted for the second day. What is the most appropriate initial response by the nurse?
    1. "I see that you are very worried. Medications are being used to lessen your wife's discomfort."
    2. "This is expected. I suggest that you go home because there is nothing you can do to help at this time."
    3. "Are you afraid that your wife may die? I assure you that very few alcoholics die during the detoxification process."
    4. "Do you think that your wife is uncomfortable while she is undergoing the withdrawal process? I am sure that your wife is not in pain."

51. A newly admitted client looks at but does not respond to the nurse. Which is the most appropriate statement by the nurse?
    1. "You may prefer to be alone for now. I will return later so we can talk."
    2. "I am talking to you. You must be having trouble understanding what I am saying."
    3. "This is the mental health unit of the hospital. Let me tell you about the many services we have to offer."
    4. "I am here to offer you my help. I am now going to tell you about the services available to you on the mental health unit."

52. A newly admitted client quietly listens to a nurse's explanation of the services and activities available on the mental health unit. When the nurse is finished, the client looks around and states, "So this is where they keep the crazies." What is the nurse's most appropriate initial response?
    1. "These people are emotionally ill. They are not crazy."
    2. "Some people feel that way. Let's talk about mental health."
    3. "Do you want me to explain the purpose of a mental health unit?"
    4. "Are you feeling that a person has to be crazy to need mental health services?"

53. The nurse tells a client that talking with the staff members is part of the therapy program. The client responds, "I don't see how talking to you can possibly help." What is the nurse's most appropriate response?
    1. "I can see how you feel that way now, but hopefully you'll change your mind."
    2. "You will never know whether or not it is helpful unless you are willing to give it a try."
    3. "The one-to-one relationship has proven to be helpful for others and you should give it a try."
    4. "Hopefully, I can help you sort out your thoughts and feelings so you can better understand them."

54. The nurse can best handle the answering of personal questions asked by the client in any phase of the nurse-client relationship by:
    1. Reviewing the positive and negative aspects of the subject

2. Providing brief, truthful answers and redirecting the focus of conversation

3. Offering an honest, brief expression of personal views on the subject raised

4. Reminding the client gently that the nurse's feelings are not the client's concern

55. After admitting a confused 80-year-old client to the mental health unit, the nurse considers that a factor associated with the aging process is:
1. Slowing of responses
2. Changing of personality
3. Lowering of intelligence
4. Diminishing of long-term memory

56. A male client with dementia due to Parkinson's disease has been placed in a nursing home. His wife appears tired and angry on her first visit with her husband. As she is leaving she says to the unit nurse in a sarcastic tone, "Let's see what you can do with him." Which is the nurse's most therapeutic response?
1. "It sounds like it has been difficult for you."
2. "I don't understand what you mean by that comment."
3. "I have experience in caring for clients such as your husband."
4. "It's too bad you didn't realize you needed help to care for him."

57. An overweight 12-year-old boy is brought to the clinic by his parents. The child tells the nurse that he dislikes school because his classmates tease him about his weight. He states rather sadly, "I'm always last when they choose up sides in gym." The nurse's most therapeutic response is:
1. "That hurts a lot when you want to be liked."
2. "Have you tried letting them know how that makes you feel?"
3. "Not everybody's a great athlete and you have other strengths."
4. "Won't it be great when you lose weight and can do better in gym?"

58. Occasionally silence will occur during a group therapy session. To manage this situation in a growth-promoting way, the leader should:
1. Be willing to sit indefinitely to wait out the silence
2. Call on specific members to talk when silence occurs
3. Go around the group and require each member to talk in turn
4. Comment on the silence or nonverbal behavior related to the silence

59. When working with clients during group therapy, the working phase usually begins when the group displays:
1. Cohesiveness
2. Confrontation
3. Imitative behavior
4. Corrective recapitulation

60. At a therapy group session a group member, using a teasing manner, makes several negative remarks about the nurse's appearance. The nurse can best respond by saying to:
1. The group, "What do you think this client is trying to tell me?"
2. The group, "Do you think this client's behavior is appropriate today?"
3. The client, "You should not talk to me this way. Why are you so angry at me?"
4. The client, "You seem very interested in my appearance. What's this all about?"

61. A registered nurse who is a beginning group leader in a community mental health center has been assigned to start a new group with regressive long-term clients. The nurse manager explains that in the beginning new group leaders are expected to:
1. Talk extensively about their own experiences
2. Confront group members about a variety of issues
3. Feel uncomfortable handling conflicts between members of the group
4. Have little difficulty with long-term clients who do not have acute emotional problems

62. A nurse-group leader in a mental health center uses a variety of techniques in an effort to promote group cohesion. The nurse identifies the presence of group cohesion when the group members:
1. Withdraw from disliked members
2. Accept new members by saying "welcome"
3. Socialize more when productivity decreases
4. Use the phrase "our group" during discussions

63. During a therapy group session, after several members relate traumatic incidents that happened during the week, a client with a smile states, "Things haven't gone well in my life this week either." It is most appropriate for the nurse to:
1. Ask the client to share what has been happening during this week
2. Make a note of the incongruity of the client's message but remain silent
3. Comment, "This seems to have been a bad week for several group members."
4. Say to the client, "You say things have been bad this week, yet you are smiling."

64. As a young male client is receiving a dialysis treatment, the nurse observes he is not talking with the other clients and his eyes are lowered and his jaw is clenched. The nurse states, "You look discouraged." The client replies, "I'm a bother. My wife will at least get some insurance money if I die." Which is the nurse's most therapeutic response?
1. "I can understand how you feel."
2. "You feel so bad you wish you were dead."
3. "We all have days we feel like that. Let's talk about your diet."
4. "I know it's hard. Don't let it get you down because you need time to adjust."

65. When the behavior of a visiting family member creates anxiety in a depressed client, the nurse should:
    1. Take the client to the coffee shop for a treat
    2. Distract the client by providing another activity
    3. Limit the family member's contact with the client
    4. Discuss the family member's behavior with the client

66. A client in a psychiatric hospital requests an unaccompanied pass and it is denied. The client vocalizes anger toward the staff for this response. The nurse concludes that this anger results from feelings of:
    1. Hopelessness
    2. Indecisiveness
    3. Powerlessness
    4. Worthlessness

67. A nurse at the crisis intervention center asks a new female client, who has come because her husband is planning a divorce, her reasons for seeking help. The client responds by describing her first meeting with her husband when they were both teenagers. What is the nurse's most therapeutic response?
    1. "You're avoiding talking about the divorce."
    2. "And now your husband is asking for a divorce."
    3. "What does this have to do with your situation now?"
    4. "Would you like to tell me more about the early years?"

68. A nurse enters the room of an agitated, angry client to administer the prescribed antipsychotic medication. The client shouts, "Get out of here!" The nurse's best approach is to:
    1. Say, "I'll be back in 15 minutes and we can talk."
    2. Get assistance and give the medication by injection
    3. Explain why it is necessary to comply with the practitioner's order
    4. State, "You must take the medicine that has been prescribed for you."

69. An older female who has been a widow for 20 years comes to the community health center with a vague list of complaints. Her only child, a son, died at birth. She has lived alone since her husband's death and performs all of her own daily tasks of living. She had a very active social life in the past but has outlived many of her friends and family members. When taking this client's health history, it is important for the nurse to ask:
    1. "Do you feel alone?"
    2. "Do you still miss your husband?"
    3. "What unfulfilled hopes do you have?"
    4. "How did you feel when your son died?"

70. Alprazolam (Xanax) is prescribed for a client with the diagnosis of panic disorder. The client refuses to take the medication because of fear of addiction. Initially the nurse should:
    1. Provide the client information about alprazolam
    2. Assess the client's feelings about alprazolam further
    3. Ask the practitioner about changing the client's medication

    4. Have the practitioner speak with the client about the safety of this medication

71. In addition to hallucinating, a client yells and curses throughout the day. The nurse should:
    1. Ignore the client's behavior
    2. Isolate the client until the behavior stops
    3. Explain the meaning of the behavior to the client
    4. Seek to understand what the behavior means to the client

72. At times a client's anxiety level is so high it blocks attempts at communication and the nurse is unsure of what is being said. To clarify understanding, the nurse states, "Let's see whether we both mean the same thing." This is an example of the technique of:
    1. Reflecting feelings
    2. Making observations
    3. Seeking consensual validation
    4. Attempting to place events in sequence

73. Which psychotherapeutic theory uses hypnosis, dream interpretation, and free association as methods to release repressed feelings?
    1. Behaviorist model
    2. Psychoanalytic model
    3. Psychobiologic model
    4. Social-interpersonal model

74. A nurse considers that the focus of environmental (milieu) therapy is to:
    1. Role-play life events to meet individual needs
    2. Use natural remedies rather than medications to control behavior
    3. Allow freedom to determine the extent of involvement in activities
    4. Manipulate the environment to bring about positive changes in behavior

75. A widow of 6 months is brought to a psychiatric hospital. During the assessment interview the client avoids eye contact, responds in a low voice, and is tearful. What is the nurse's best initial approach?
    1. "You'll find that you'll get better faster if you try to help us to help you."
    2. "I am your nurse. I'll take you to the dayroom as soon as I get some information."
    3. "Hold my hand. I know you are frightened, but I will not allow anyone to harm you."
    4. "I know that this is difficult, but as soon as we are finished I'll take you to your room."

76. The nurse and client have entered the working phase of a therapeutic relationship. What can the nurse expect the client to do during this phase? Select all that apply.
    1. _____ Initiate topics for discussion
    2. _____ Focus the conversation on the nurse
    3. _____ Repress emotionally charged material
    4. _____ Accept limits on unacceptable behavior
    5. _____ Express emotions related to transference

77. A client who is being treated in a mental health clinic is to be discharged after several months of therapy. The client anxiously tells the nurse, "I don't know what

I will do when I can't see you anymore." The nurse determines that the client is:
1. Expressing thanks to the nurse
2. Reacting to the planned discharge
3. Attempting to manipulate the nurse
4. Indicating a need for further treatment

78. A male client is preparing to leave the hospital and return to college. When saying good-bye, he hugs and kisses the nurse on the cheek. What is the nurse's most appropriate response?
1. Hug the client in return
2. Smile at the client but say nothing
3. Encourage him to visit periodically
4. Wish him well with his future studies

79. Three days after a stressful incident a client can no longer remember why it was stressful. The nurse, in relating to this client, can be most therapeutic by identifying that the inability to recall the situation is an example of the defense mechanism of:
1. Denial
2. Regression
3. Repression
4. Dissociation

80. The parents of a female client in a psychiatric hospital send an unwrapped birthday gift to the unit for their daughter but do not stay to visit with her. The client responds to this situation by crying. The best response by the nurse is to:
1. Limit her contact with the parents
2. Discuss her parents' behavior with her
3. Distract her by engaging her in an activity
4. Take her to the coffee shop for a birthday treat

81. A goal for a client who has difficulty with verbal communication precipitated by psychological barriers is that the client will:
1. Be free of injury
2. Demonstrate decreased acting-out behavior
3. Identify consequences of acting-out behavior
4. Interact with other people in the environment

82. A 15-year-old male is being assessed in the adolescent clinic. He is known for drug abuse, stealing, refusal to comply with rules, and an inability to get along with others in any setting. When obtaining the health history, the nurse may be prevented from accurately listening to what the client is saying. This may be caused by the:
1. Client's disease process
2. Nurse's personal cultural beliefs
3. Pressure of time to complete care
4. Personal need to secure information

83. Before effectively responding to a sexually abused victim on the phone, it is essential that the nurse in the rape crisis center:
1. Get the client's full name and address
2. Call for assistance from the psychiatrist
3. Know some myths and facts about sexual assault
4. Be aware of any personal bias about sexual assault

84. A nurse anticipates that value clarification is a technique useful in therapeutic communication because initially it helps clients to:
1. Become aware of their personal values
2. Gain information related to their needs
3. Make correct decisions related to their health
4. Alter their value systems to make them more socially acceptable

85. A reasonable short-term goal for clients who are functioning below the optimum level of mental health is to help them become better able to:
1. Understand the dynamics behind their inadequate interpersonal relations
2. Confront their inadequacies in interpersonal relations and be more sociable
3. Discuss feelings regarding their life experiences and their significant others
4. Take actions that will increase their satisfaction with their relationships with others

86. A terminally ill client is moving gradually toward resolution of feelings about impending death. Basing the plan of care on Elisabeth Kübler-Ross's research, the nurse should use nonverbal interventions after having assessed that the client is in the:
1. Anger stage
2. Denial stage
3. Bargaining stage
4. Acceptance stage

87. A terminally ill client tells the nurse, "I would love to learn to speak German before I die." The nurse's response to the client's desire to learn a foreign language should be based on an understanding that:
1. Interests should focus on pursuits that are easily attainable
2. Activities that support the client's denial should not be encouraged
3. Clients should be encouraged to set meaningful goals for themselves
4. Energies expended on such an activity would not justify the outcome

88. It is most helpful to the nurse who is attempting to apply the principles of mental health to consider that:
1. People with emotional illnesses can empathize easily with others
2. Emotionally ill people will initially reject psychological support
3. Mental illness is characterized by signs and symptoms of socially inappropriate behavior
4. Emotional health is promoted when there is a sense of mastery of self and the environment

89. With the client's permission, the nurse should inform the family about what is happening. The main reason for this action is that informed families:
1. Decrease the client's anxiety
2. Are better equipped to assist the client
3. Appear more relaxed with the situation
4. Commonly cause fewer nursing problems

90. A nurse anticipates that when a client is a member of a different ethnic community it is important to:
    1. Ensure that the nurse's biases are understood by the family
    2. Make plans to counteract the client's misconceptions about therapies
    3. Offer a therapeutic regimen compatible with the lifestyle of the family
    4. Recognize that the client's responses will be similar to other clients' responses

91. The nurse is scheduled to be the co-leader of a therapy group being formed in the mental health clinic. When planning for the first meeting, it is of primary importance that the nurse consider the:
    1. Number of clients in the group
    2. Needs of the clients being included
    3. Diagnoses of the clients being included
    4. Socioeconomic status of the clients in the group

92. A newly admitted client with schizophrenia has a treatment plan that includes participation in a physical activity group for several days before being assigned to an analytic group. The basis for this decision is that the client will:
    1. Develop skills in managing leisure time
    2. Have time to develop insight into personal problems
    3. Be too disruptive to benefit from group therapy at this time
    4. Cultivate trust before moving into a potentially anxiety-producing group

93. The nurse is planning therapeutic group sessions for regressed long-term clients. The nurse considers that these clients need to:
    1. Experience a structured setting
    2. Learn how to confront interpersonal conflict
    3. Develop the sense that they can control the group
    4. Have opportunities for an expression of deep feelings

94. When leading the first session of a newly formed group of clients in a mental health clinic, the nurse identifies that group members frequently assume self-serving roles. The nurse anticipates that:
    1. Early group development consists of these behaviors
    2. Some group members will need to be placed in another group
    3. Certain group members may be emerging to control attention seekers
    4. The group is attempting to reconcile conflicting viewpoints among its members

95. During the first session of a therapy group one of the clients asks, "What is supposed to happen in this group?" What is the most appropriate response by the nurse leader?
    1. "Before I answer that, I'd like for you to tell me what you want to happen."
    2. "This is your group and your participation will determine what will happen."
    3. "The purpose of this group is to examine the way each of you interacts with the others."
    4. "You and the others are supposed to discuss any reality-based concerns you have about your illness."

96. The best initial approach to take with a self-accusatory, guilt-ridden client is to:
    1. Contradict the client's persecutory delusions
    2. Accept the client's statements as the client's beliefs
    3. Medicate the client when these thoughts are expressed
    4. Redirect the client whenever a negative topic is mentioned

97. An older female client desires to remain independent but is concerned about maintaining her independent living status. What initial intervention strategy is of primary importance?
    1. Reinforcing routines and supporting her usual habits
    2. Helping her secure assistance with cleaning and shopping
    3. Writing down and repeating important information for her use
    4. Setting clear goals and time limitations for her visits with the nurse

DISORDERS FIRST EVIDENT BEFORE ADULTHOOD

98. A school nurse knows that school-age children often use defense mechanisms to cope with situations that might negatively affect their self-esteem. The nurse hears a child who is not invited to a sleepover say, "I don't have time to go to that sleepover. I have better things to do." The nurse concludes that the student is using the defense mechanism of:
    1. Denial
    2. Projection
    3. Regression
    4. Rationalization

99. A nurse expects a child with a diagnosis of reactive attachment disorder to:
    1. Have been physically abused
    2. Try to cling to the mother on separation
    3. Be able to develop just superficial relationships with others
    4. Have a more positive relationship with the father than with the mother

100. The nurse manager is evaluating a primary nurse who is working with a hospitalized adolescent client with the diagnosis of conduct disorder. Which intervention by the primary nurse should the nurse manger question?
    1. Discussing rules of the unit
    2. Allowing opportunities for choices
    3. Explaining the consequences for not following unit regulations
    4. Encouraging the verbalization of negative feelings toward others

101. When assessing disturbed children, the clue that the nurse finds most indicative of severe emotional problems is the child's:
    1. Physical complaints
    2. Behavioral outbursts
    3. Inadequate school performance
    4. Lack of response to the environment

102. A school-age child is brought to the clinic by the mother, who states, "Something is very wrong. My child never seems happy and refuses to play." When assessing this child for depressed behavior, the nurse initially begins with the statement:
    1. "Tell me about yourself."
    2. "Let's talk about what you do after school."
    3. "Can you tell me what is making you so unhappy?"
    4. "Why does your mother think that you are unhappy?"

103. When teaching parents about childhood depression the nurse should say, "It:
    1. may appear as acting-out behavior."
    2. looks almost identical to adult depression."
    3. is short in duration with an early resolution."
    4. does not respond to conventional treatment."

104. When implementing a tertiary preventive program for mentally retarded individuals the nurse should:
    1. Teach mentally retarded children how to feed themselves
    2. Refer children for evaluation if they fail to meet developmental milestones
    3. Encourage the use of birth control methods by women who are mentally retarded
    4. Use the Denver Developmental Screening Test to evaluate children attending well-child clinics

105. A toddler has a history of frequent temper tantrums. The mother asks how to limit this acting-out behavior. The nurse's most therapeutic response should focus on:
    1. Restraining the child whenever a tantrum begins
    2. Telling the mother to ignore the tantrum whenever possible
    3. Moving the child to a quiet area before the tantrum escalates
    4. Asking the practitioner to prescribe medication for behavioral control

106. A 3-year-old child has a possible diagnosis of pervasive developmental autistic disorder. Which characteristic would the nurse find most unusual when assessing this toddler?
    1. Interest in music
    2. Ritualistic behavior
    3. Attachment to odd objects
    4. Responsiveness to the parents

107. A mother of a 6-year-old boy with the diagnosis of attention deficit hyperactivity disorder (ADHD) tells the nurse that when reading storybooks to her son, about halfway through the story he becomes distracted, fidgets, and does not pay attention. The nurse suggests that the mother:
    1. Talk with a louder voice
    2. Shorten the rest of the story

    3. Encourage her son to pay attention
    4. Use therapeutic holding for the rest of the story

108. A nurse considers that language development in the autistic child resembles:
    1. Echolalia
    2. Stuttering
    3. Scanning speech
    4. Pressured speech

109. A 7-year-old girl is brought to the clinic by her mother, who tells the nurse that her child has been having trouble in school, has difficulty concentrating, and is falling behind in her schoolwork since she and her husband separated 6 months ago. The mother reports that lately her daughter has not been eating her dinner and she often hears her crying in her room. The nurse concludes that the child:
    1. Feels different from her classmates
    2. Would be happier living with her father
    3. Is working through her feelings of anger
    4. May blame herself for her parents' breakup

110. When assessing the mental status of a 7- or 8-year-old child, it is most important for the nurse to:
    1. Listen to the parents' description of the child's behavior
    2. Compare the child's functioning from one time to another
    3. Engage the parents in a discussion about the child's feelings
    4. Determine the child's mental status by using direct questions

111. An only child who lives with the mother (the custodial parent) begins demonstrating school and emotional problems after the parents' marital breakup. It is decided that the child may benefit from family therapy. The nurse informs the mother that the first session will include the:
    1. Parents
    2. Mother and the child
    3. Parents and the child
    4. Mother, the child, and the child's teacher

112. A 12-year-old child who has a history of school failure and destructive acting out is admitted to a child psychiatric unit with the diagnosis of conduct disorder. The youngest of three children, the child is identified by both the parents and the siblings as the family problem. The nurse identifies the family's pattern of relating to the child as:
    1. Controlling
    2. Patronizing
    3. Scapegoating
    4. Overburdening

113. To help a disturbed, acting-out child develop a trusting relationship, the nurse should:
    1. Inquire as to the child's feelings about the parents
    2. Implement a half hour one-to-one interaction daily
    3. Initiate limit-setting and explain the rules to be followed
    4. Offer periodic support and emphasize safety in play activities

114. A 6-year-old child recently started school but has been refusing to go for the past 3 weeks. The nurse determines that an appropriate intervention for this child is to:
    1. Explain that school is a place to have fun
    2. Delay return to school for several months
    3. Enroll the child in a special education program
    4. Develop a behavior modification program with the child

115. A school nurse is requested to present an educational program on attention deficit hyperactivity disorder (ADHD) to the teaching staff of an elementary school. The nurse should emphasize that this disorder:
    1. Becomes evident before 4 years of age
    2. Affects around 3% to 7% of the school-age population
    3. Occurs more frequently in lower socioeconomic groups
    4. Causes affected children to sleep more than unaffected children

116. An acting-out hyperactive 9-year-old boy is started on a behavior modification program that uses tokens for acceptable behavior. When playing a game that he is losing, he begins to kick the other children under the table and call them names. Which is the most appropriate behavior modification technique the nurse should use?
    1. Ignore the child's behavior
    2. Place the child in a short time-out
    3. Take the child's daily allotment of tokens away
    4. Engage the child in a conversation about good sportsmanship

117. A hyperactive self-destructive child is to be discharged from an inpatient setting in a few days. In preparation for the child's discharge, it is most important for the nurse to plan to:
    1. Establish, maintain, and enforce limits on behavior
    2. Meet with the child's teacher to review the child's needs
    3. Schedule a team conference with the child and the parents
    4. Help the child begin to terminate relationships with the nursing team

ANXIETY, SOMATOFORM, FACTITIOUS, AND DISSOCIATIVE DISORDERS

118. In an outpatient mental health clinic, a nurse is working with a client who is beginning to address more effective ways to handle stressful situations. The best nursing action to include in the plan of care is to have the client:
    1. Identify unhealthy habits that need to be altered
    2. Determine the benefits of a rehabilitation program
    3. Learn about the benefits of antianxiety medications
    4. Develop a consistent method for performing self-care

119. The nurse considers that a primary gain is distinguished from a secondary gain because a primary gain's main function is to:
    1. Reduce anxiety
    2. Gain benefits from others
    3. Fulfill unconscious desires
    4. Control unacceptable impulses

120. When the nurse considers a client's placement on the continuum of anxiety, a key in determining the degree of anxiety being experienced is the client's:
    1. Memory state
    2. Creativity level
    3. Perceptual field
    4. Delusional system

121. An older adult who lives alone tells a nurse at the community health center, "I really don't need anyone to talk to. The TV is my best friend." The nurse identifies that the client is using the defense mechanism known as:
    1. Denial
    2. Projection
    3. Sublimation
    4. Displacement

122. Some clients repeatedly perform ritualistic behaviors throughout the day to limit anxious feelings. The nurse determines that these behaviors are:
    1. Obsessions
    2. Compulsions
    3. Under personal control
    4. Related to rebelliousness

123. A nurse evaluates that a client has successfully achieved the long-term goal of mobilizing effective coping responses when the client states, "When I feel myself getting anxious I will:
    1. perform a relaxation exercise."
    2. get involved in some type of quiet activity."
    3. avoid the situation that precipitated the anxiety."
    4. examine carefully what precipitated my anxiety."

124. When working with a client who has a phobia about black cats, the nurse anticipates that a problem for this client is:
    1. Denying that the phobia exists
    2. Anger toward the feared object
    3. Anxiety when discussing the phobia
    4. Distortion of reality when completing daily routines

125. The nurse identifies that the major defense mechanism used by an individual with a phobic disorder is:
    1. Splitting
    2. Regression
    3. Avoidance
    4. Conversion

126. The nurse determines that the therapy that has the highest success rate for people with phobias is:
    1. Desensitization using relaxation techniques
    2. Insight therapy to determine the origin of the fear
    3. Psychotherapy aimed at rearranging maladaptive thought processes

4. Psychoanalytic exploration of repressed conflicts of an earlier developmental phase

127. Many clients who call a crisis hotline are extremely anxious. The nurse answering the hotline phone considers that the characteristics distinguishing posttraumatic stress disorders from other anxiety disorders are:
   1. Lack of interest in family and others
   2. Reexperiencing the trauma in dreams and flashbacks
   3. Avoidance of situations and activities that resemble the stress
   4. Depression and a blunted affect when discussing the traumatic situation

128. A female accountant comes to the health clinic for a preemployment physical. During the health history the new employee frequently states, "I feel so nervous about starting this job." She is able to connect with her feelings, thoughts, and actions but constantly focuses her attention on starting the new job. The nurse determines that the client is exhibiting:
   1. A moderate level of job-related anxiety
   2. A severe level of anxiety related to new situations
   3. An inappropriate response to handling new situations
   4. An ineffective coping mechanism in handling job-related stress

129. A client with a generalized anxiety disorder is hospitalized. The nurse determines that an environment conducive to reducing emotional stress and providing psychological safety is one in which:
   1. Needs are met
   2. Realistic limits and controls are set
   3. The client's requests are met promptly
   4. The client's environment is kept neat and orderly

130. A client comes to the hospital because of intense feelings of unrest, inability to sleep, and frequent episodes of panic. The client tells the nurse, "I admitted myself because I think I'm going crazy." The nurse identifies the client's remark as a:
   1. Plea for support
   2. Reflection of insight
   3. Symptom of depression
   4. Test of the nurse's trustworthiness

131. A client who is to begin a physical therapy regimen after orthopedic surgery verbally expresses anxiety about starting this new therapy. The nurse responds that some of this apprehension can be an asset because it will:
   1. Increase alertness to the environment
   2. Slow down physiological functioning
   3. Mobilize automatic behavioral responses
   4. Promote the use of ego defense mechanisms

132. A nurse is accompanying a client with a diagnosis of substance-induced anxiety disorder who is pacing the halls and crying. When the client's pacing and crying increase, the nurse suddenly feels uncomfortable and experiences a strong desire to leave. The probable reason for this feeling is:
   1. A desire to go off duty after a busy day
   2. A fear of the client becoming assaultive

3. An empathic communication of anxiety
4. An inability to tolerate more bizarre behavior

133. A client is admitted to the hospital with the diagnosis of severe anxiety. The nurse's plan of care for a client with an anxiety disorder should include:
   1. Promoting the suppression of anger by the client
   2. Supporting the verbalization of feelings by the client
   3. Encouraging the client to limit anxiety-related behaviors
   4. Restricting the involvement of the client's family during the acute phase

134. The husband of a young mother who has attempted suicide asks if he may bring their 26-month-old daughter to visit his wife. Which is the nurse's best response?
   1. "Probably so, but you better check with her physician first."
   2. "Of course, children of all ages are welcome to visit relatives."
   3. "It may be very upsetting for your child to see her mother so depressed."
   4. "Tell me what your wife said when you offered to bring your child for a visit."

135. A client is pacing the floor and appears extremely anxious. The nurse approaches in an attempt to alleviate the client's anxiety. The most therapeutic initial question by the nurse is:
   1. "What has made you so upset?"
   2. "Where would you like to walk with me?"
   3. "Shall we sit down to talk about your feelings?"
   4. "How would you like to go to the gym to work out?"

136. A client with the diagnosis of panic disorder jumps when spoken to, complains of feeling uneasy, and states, "It's as though something bad is going to happen." It is most therapeutic at this time for the nurse to:
   1. Stay with the client to be a calming presence
   2. Encourage the client to communicate with the staff
   3. Allow the client to set the parameters for the interaction
   4. Help the client to understand the cause of the feelings described

137. A client, who had a panic attack on the previous day, says to the nurse, "That was a terrible feeling I had yesterday. I'm so afraid to talk about it." The nurse's most therapeutic response is:
   1. "It's best that you try to talk about it."
   2. "Why don't you want to talk about it now?"
   3. "What were you doing yesterday when you first noticed the feeling?"
   4. "I understand you are upset, but don't be concerned because that feeling probably won't come back."

138. A female client is admitted to the acute care psychiatric unit with a diagnosis of panic disorder with agoraphobia. During the initial assessment phase the nurse should focus on:
   1. Reducing the client's anxiety so that further interviewing can occur
   2. Learning about the client's home life to facilitate planning future care

3. Suggesting to the client that she rest for a while before taking her health history
4. Helping the client identify the source of her anxiety so the source can be avoided

139. When talking with a female client who displays many of the emotional and physiological symptoms associated with a panic disorder, the nurse should:
   1. Use short sentences with an authoritative voice
   2. Describe for her the possible reasons for her anxiety
   3. Keep asking questions because she probably is not going to volunteer much information
   4. Suggest that she refrain from crying, because most of the time crying makes matters worse

140. A client is admitted to the hospital because of incapacitating obsessive-compulsive behavior. The statement that best describes how clients with obsessive-compulsive behavior view this disorder is:
   1. "I know there's no reason to do these things, but I can't help myself."
   2. "I don't know why everyone is upset with me. I'm doing nothing wrong."
   3. "The things I do take a little time, but they make me a productive person."
   4. "The devil makes me do it. It's not my fault that I constantly act this way."

141. A client, recently admitted to the psychiatric unit with the diagnosis of an obsessive-compulsive disorder, engages in a handwashing ritual. When the nurse interrupts the ritual, the client becomes angry and acts out. The most probable cause for the behavior is that the:
   1. Client's personality is clashing with the nurse
   2. Client is feeling overwhelmed in this situation
   3. Client resents the nurse's authoritarian manner
   4. Client's response reflects an aggressive personality

142. The nurse plans to teach a client to use healthier coping behaviors that consciously can be used to reduce anxiety. These include:
   1. Eating, dissociation, fantasy
   2. Sublimation, fantasy, rationalization
   3. Exercise, talking to friends, suppression
   4. Repression, intellectualization, smoking

143. A nurse on the psychiatric unit evaluates that the staff's approach to setting limits for a demanding, angry client is effective when the client:
   1. No longer calls the nursing staff for assistance
   2. Understands the reasons why frequent calls to the staff were made
   3. Apologizes for disrupting the unit's routine when something is needed
   4. Discusses concerns regarding the emotional condition that required hospitalization

144. A nurse should reassess an older adult client's needs and current plan of care when the client's behavior indicates the development of:
   1. Confusion
   2. Hypochondriasis

3. Additional complaints
4. Increased socialization

145. During the first meeting of a therapy group, the members become quite uncomfortable. The nurse identifies frequent periods of silence, tense laughter, and nervous movement in the group. The nurse assesses that these responses:
   1. Require active leader intervention to relieve signs of obvious stress
   2. Indicate unhealthy group processes with an unwillingness to relate openly
   3. Are expected group behaviors because relationships are not yet established
   4. Should be addressed immediately so members will not become too uncomfortable

CRISIS SITUATIONS

146. A nurse working in a crisis center identifies that a crisis can best be defined as:
   1. A threat to equilibrium
   2. An imbalance of emotions
   3. The perception of the problem by the client
   4. The circumstance that requires help other than personal resources

147. When working with families encountering problems, it is most important that the nurse have a:
   1. Precise memory for details
   2. Common social background
   3. Warm nature and loving personality
   4. Sense of self and empathy for others

148. An adolescent client seeks help at a crisis intervention clinic. The client relates, "I dropped out of college because the instructors were dumb. I tried waiting on tables but got fired. The boss said I was nasty to the customers. They were the nasty ones. If people were nicer, I wouldn't be in this mess." In relation to crisis theory, this client's stressful events can be seen as:
   1. Experiential
   2. Age-related and frequent
   3. Usually noncrisis producing
   4. Situational and maturational

149. A nurse is assessing a client who enters a walk-in mental health clinic. Which statement supports the assessment that the client may be experiencing a crisis?
   1. "I have these feelings of uneasiness. They come and go."
   2. "Everything I try does not work. It just keeps getting worse."
   3. "Things have been building up slowly. I don't know what is causing it."
   4. "I feel tense and irritable. When I concentrate on my work I feel better."

150. A psychiatric nurse anticipates that a situational crisis usually will resolve within:
   1. 1 to 4 days
   2. 2 to 3 weeks
   3. 1 to 2 months
   4. 2 to 6 months

151. A single mother of two children, who recently lost her job because her company is downsizing, comes to the emergency department. The woman does not know what to do and is in crisis. The most critical factor for the nurse to determine during crisis intervention is the client's:
    1. Developmental history
    2. Available situational supports
    3. Underlying unconscious conflict
    4. Willingness to restructure the personality

152. A young mother of three children, each born 1 year apart, has been hospitalized after attempting to hang herself. The client is being treated with milieu therapy. The nurse identifies that this therapeutic modality consists of:
    1. Providing individual and family therapy
    2. Using positive reinforcement to reduce guilt
    3. Uncovering unconscious conflicts and fantasies
    4. Manipulating the environment to benefit the client

153. A nurse suggests a crisis intervention group to a client experiencing a developmental crisis. The nurse determines that these groups are successful because the:
    1. Client is encouraged to talk about personal problems
    2. Crisis group supplies a workable solution to the client's problems
    3. Client is assisted to investigate alternative approaches to solving the identified problem
    4. Crisis intervention worker is a psychologist who understands common behavior patterns

154. A nurse is taking calls at a local crisis center hotline and receives a telephone call from a suicidal adolescent. The nurse can safely terminate the call when the client:
    1. Wishes to terminate the conversation
    2. Has responded to the nurse's initial assessment of suicidal risk
    3. Begins repeating the same information that has already been discussed
    4. Can state a preventive plan of action for dealing with self-destructive behaviors

155. A young college student tells the nurse in the school's health service that his girlfriend's period is late and they both think she is pregnant. The client, with a broad smile on his face, states loudly and angrily, "If she is pregnant I will drop out of school, marry her, and get a full-time job." The nurse's best initial assessment of the client's verbal and nonverbal behaviors is that they are:
    1. Uniform
    2. Consistent
    3. Incongruent
    4. Inappropriate

156. When talking to a nurse about his decision to drop out of school and marry his girlfriend who is pregnant, a young college student says, "It's really the best decision. It is important for a child to have two parents." The nurse identifies that the client is using the defense mechanism known as:
    1. Projection
    2. Introspection
    3. Displacement
    4. Intellectualization

157. A 24-year-old secretary, pregnant for the first time, receives a letter from her boyfriend with a check for $500 and the news that he has left town. The client, who is very upset and feels overwhelmed, calls the crisis intervention center for help. The nurse concludes that the client is experiencing a crisis because the:
    1. Client is under a great deal of stress
    2. Client is going to have to raise her child alone
    3. Client's past methods of coping are ineffective for this situation
    4. Client's boyfriend left her when he found out that she was pregnant

158. An unmarried pregnant adolescent who is attending a crisis intervention group has decided to continue the pregnancy and keep the baby. Now the crisis intervention nurse's primary responsibility is to:
    1. Support the client for making a wise decision
    2. Explore other problems the client may be experiencing
    3. Make an appointment for the client to visit a prenatal clinic
    4. Provide information about where the client may receive assistance

159. An unmarried, pregnant client, who has been attending a crisis intervention clinic, has decided to keep the baby and is looking forward to motherhood. The nurse identifies that the decision to attend prenatal childcare classes is an example of:
    1. Intrinsic motivation
    2. Extrinsic motivation
    3. Operant conditioning
    4. Behavior modification

160. A client who has been pregnant for 5 months spontaneously aborts after an accident. The client tells the nurse she feels depressed over the loss of her son. She describes how he would have looked and how bright he would have been. What is the client demonstrating?
    1. Panic level of anxiety
    2. Typical grief syndrome
    3. Pathological grief reaction
    4. Diminished ability to test reality

161. A client who has just experienced her second spontaneous abortion expresses anger toward the practitioner, the hospital, and the "rotten nursing care." When assessing the situation, the nurse concludes that the client may be using the coping mechanism of:
    1. Denial
    2. Projection
    3. Displacement
    4. Reaction formation

162. A nurse is with the parents of a 3-year-old child who has just died. The nurse is most therapeutic when asking the parents:
    1. "Do you feel ready to consent to an autopsy?"
    2. "Has a decision been made about organ donation?"

3. "Would you like to talk about how you will tell your other children?"

4. "Can I be of some help with any traditional practices that are important to you?"

163. The parents of an 11-month-old infant diagnosed with failure to thrive are referred to the crisis intervention clinic. What is the primary crisis intervention the nurse should use?
    1. Problem solving
    2. Analytic therapy
    3. Prescriptive work
    4. Exploratory therapy

164. A nurse who suspects that a newly admitted infant is the victim of child abuse, assesses the parents' interaction with their baby. What typical parental behavior might support the diagnosis of child abuse? Select all that apply.
    1. _____ Displaying sensitivity about their child care ability
    2. _____ Taking the initiative in meeting their child's needs
    3. _____ Having difficulty in showing concern for their child
    4. _____ Demonstrating heightened interest in their child's welfare
    5. _____ Procrastinating about getting help for their child's injuries

165. Child physical maltreatment is suspected in a 3-year-old girl admitted to the hospital with many poorly explained injuries. Which statement by the mother further supports this suspicion?
    1. "When I get angry, I take her for a walk."
    2. "I have no problems with any of my other children."
    3. "When she misbehaves, I send her to her room alone."
    4. "I make her stand in the corner when she doesn't eat her dinner."

166. The nurse is assessing a client who enters a walk-in mental health clinic. Which statements support an existent crisis situation? Select all that apply.
    1. _____ "I feel so overwhelmed. I don't know what to do."
    2. _____ "I feel very tense and irritable. I can't concentrate."
    3. _____ "I have vague feelings of uneasiness. They seem to come and go."
    4. _____ "This has been building up slowly. I don't know what's causing it."
    5. _____ "Nothing I have tried has helped the situation. It keeps getting worse."

167. An emergency department nurse assesses a male client brought in by a law enforcement officer. The client was in jail and attempted to hang himself with his shirt. Physically the client is stable but emotionally he continues to state he wants to die. The nurse assesses high-risk suicidal factors. The risk factor that is considered to be most "lethal" is:
    1. History of alcohol and drug abuse
    2. Previous high-risk suicide attempts

3. History of withdrawal from friends and co-workers
4. Recent family disorganization due to his incarceration

168. When counseling the 20-year-old parents of a 13-month-old child, the nurse considers that the defense mechanism most often used by physically abusive parents is:
    1. Idealization
    2. Transference
    3. Manipulation
    4. Displacement

169. A nurse is interviewing a mother accused of physical child abuse. When speaking with this mother, the nurse expects her to:
    1. Attempt to rationally explain her behavior
    2. Reveal the belief that her child needed to be disciplined
    3. Offer a detailed explanation of how her child was injured
    4. Ask how she can arrange to visit her child on the pediatric unit

170. When a diagnosis of child abuse is established, a nursing care priority should be:
    1. Promoting bonding with the child
    2. Staying with the parents while they visit
    3. Protecting the total well-being of the child
    4. Teaching methods of discipline to the parents

171. A nurse may best assist abusing parents to alter behavior toward an abused 2-year-old child by helping the parents to:
    1. Recognize what behavior is appropriate for a toddler
    2. Learn appropriate ways of punishing a toddler's inappropriate behavior
    3. Identify the specific ways in which the toddler's behavior provokes frustration
    4. Ignore the toddler's negative, nondestructive behavior while supporting acceptable behavior

172. A nurse on the pediatric unit is assigned to care for a 2-year-old child with a history of being physically abused. The nurse expects the child to:
    1. Smile readily at anyone who enters the room
    2. Be wary of physical contact initiated by anyone
    3. Begin to scream when the nurse nears the bedside
    4. Pay little attention to the nurse standing at the bedside

173. A nurse is working with children who have been sexually abused by a family member. What overwhelming feelings do these children usually express? Select all that apply.
    1. _____ Guilt
    2. _____ Anger
    3. _____ Revenge
    4. _____ Disbelief
    5. _____ Self-blame

174. A 15-year-old adolescent tearfully states that her father has been sexually abusing her for the past 8 years. Initially the nurse should respond:
    1. "Which type of incidents preceded the abuse?"
    2. "What actions are involved in the sexual abuse?"

3. "Sharing this information is a positive step in getting help."
4. "This must be reported immediately to Child Protective Services."

175. When the pediatric nurse practitioner examines the genital area of a 5-year-old child suspected of being sexually abused, the primary nurse is most therapeutic by:
    1. Explaining the procedure and remaining with the child during the examination
    2. Asking if the child prefers the nurse or the mother to be present during the examination
    3. Telling the child that the nurse practitioner wants to see if there is "anything wrong down there"
    4. Requesting that the mother explain the examination and the findings in terms the child will understand

176. A young child suspected of being sexually abused says to the nurse, "Did I do something bad?" What is the nurse's most therapeutic reply?
    1. "Who said you did something bad?"
    2. "What do you mean something bad?"
    3. "Do you think that you did something bad?"
    4. "Do you think that I think you did something bad?"

177. A 13-year-old female student tearfully reveals to the school nurse that her brother has been forcing her to have intercourse. The nurse should:
    1. Suspect that this revelation is a cry for help related to some other crisis
    2. Recognize that this revelation is an attention-getting method to meet unmet needs
    3. Assume that this revelation is true and follow the school's protocol for investigation
    4. Accept that this revelation may be a way to explain a suspected pregnancy and refer her for a pregnancy test

178. A woman is admitted to the emergency department with trauma that indicates possible abuse. List in priority order the appropriate nursing interventions.
    1. Gather a more in-depth history
    2. Provide information about safe houses
    3. Encourage the client to ventilate feelings
    4. Assist in the treatment of physical injuries
    Answer: _____

179. During a nurse's interview with a client who has been sexually assaulted, the woman states that she should have fought back. What is the nurse's most therapeutic response?
    1. "You are feeling guilty about submitting."
    2. "You may have submitted, but you had few options."
    3. "It's over so let's not explore what you could have done."
    4. "It is hard to know, but what is important is that you are alive."

180. A recently married 22-year-old woman is brought to the trauma center by the police. She had been robbed, beaten, and sexually assaulted. The client, although very anxious and tearful, appears in control. The practitioner orders an anxiolytic for agitation. The nurse should administer this medication when the:
    1. Client requests something to calm her
    2. Client's crying and trembling seem to increase
    3. Practitioner is ready to perform a vaginal examination on the client
    4. Nurse determines the anxiety and fearfulness the client is experiencing are increasing

181. The husband of a woman who has been sexually assaulted arrives at the hospital after being called by the police. After reassuring him about his wife's condition, the nurse should give priority to:
    1. Arranging for the rape counselor to meet with the wife
    2. Discussing with him his own feelings about the situation
    3. Helping him to understand how his wife feels about the situation
    4. Making him comfortable until the practitioner has completed examining his wife

182. A 15-year-old girl is brought to the high school health office by two of her friends, who state, "We think she just took a handful of pills." The adolescent appears alert and refuses to speak. The school nurse's initial response should be to:
    1. Ask the friends where she got the pills
    2. Ask the adolescent if she took any pills
    3. Call the rescue squad to stand by for an emergency
    4. Call the adolescent's parents to tell them they must come immediately

183. The biggest problem for an older female client, immediately after the sudden death of her husband, probably will be her inability to cope with:
    1. Anger
    2. Finances
    3. Loneliness
    4. Estrangement

184. A male client is brought to the psychiatric emergency department after attempting to jump off a bridge. The client's wife states that he lost his job several months ago and has been unable to find another job. The primary nursing intervention at this time is to assess for:
    1. Feelings of failure
    2. Marital difficulties
    3. Past episodes of depression
    4. Plans of committing suicide

185. Which is the nurse's most appropriate response to a parent's question about childhood suicide?
    1. "Suicide threats in children should be taken seriously."
    2. "Children do not have readily available means to kill themselves."
    3. "Children younger than age six may threaten but do not attempt suicide."
    4. "Suicide attempts in young children are manipulative behaviors to control their parents."

186. A child has been diagnosed as having acute myelogenous leukemia. The practitioner has discussed the diagnosis and prognosis with the parents. Later, after visiting their child, they have a severe argument. The nurse identifies that they are using the defense mechanism of:
1. Denial
2. Projection
3. Displacement
4. Compensation

187. An 8-year-old child with a terminal illness is demanding of the staff. The child asks for many privileges that other children on the unit do not have. The staff members know the child does not have long to live. The nurse can best help the staff members cope with the child's demands by encouraging them to:
1. Provide as many extra treats as possible because the child is dying
2. Set reasonable limits to help the child feel more secure and content
3. Give the child some extra treats so they will feel less anxiety after the child dies
4. Understand that the dying child has unique needs and special privileges can provide the necessary security

188. A child dies after an explosion at school. The parents arrive at the hospital a few minutes later and are told what happened. The parents ask the nurse whether they can see their child. What is the best response by the nurse?
1. "It's best to wait awhile."
2. "You can see your child now if you want."
3. "You'll have to wait until the physician can be with you."
4. "It will be less traumatic if you see your child at the funeral home."

189. A mother whose daughter is killed in a school bus accident tells the nurse that her daughter was just getting over the chickenpox and did not want to go to school, but she insisted that she go. The mother cries bitterly and says her child's death is her fault. The nurse considers that perceiving a death as preventable most often will influence the grieving process in that it may:
1. Grow in intensity and duration
2. Progress to a psychiatric illness
3. Be easier to understand and to accept
4. Cause the mourner to experience a pathological grief reaction

190. A hospice nurse is caring for a dying client while several family members are in the room. When the client dies, the initial nursing intervention during the shock phase of a grief reaction is focused on:
1. Staying with the individuals involved
2. Directing the individuals' activities at this time
3. Mobilizing the support systems of the individuals
4. Presenting the full reality of the loss to the individuals

191. Shortly after the death of her husband after a long illness, the wife visits the mental health clinic complaining of malaise, lethargy, and insomnia. The nurse, knowing that it is most important to help the wife cope with her husband's death, should attempt to determine the:
1. Age of the wife
2. Timing of the husband's death
3. Socioeconomic status of the couple
4. Adequacy of the wife's support system

192. A female client's stream of consciousness is occupied exclusively with thoughts of her mother's death. The nurse plans to help the client through this stage of grieving, which is known as:
1. Resolving the loss
2. Shock and disbelief
3. Developing awareness
4. Restitution and recovery

193. A nurse expects that when an individual successfully completes the grieving process after the death of a significant other, the individual will be able to:
1. Accept the inevitability of death
2. Go on with life while forgetting the past
3. Remember the significant other realistically
4. Focus mainly on the good qualities of the person who died

194. A nurse discusses the plan of care with a depressed client whose husband has recently died. The nurse determines it is most helpful to:
1. Involve the client in group exercises and games
2. Encourage the client to talk about and plan for the future
3. Talk with the client about her husband and the details of his death
4. Motivate the client to interact with male clients and the nursing staff

195. A nurse completes the assessment of a female client who cannot function because of an impending divorce. What is the most effective nursing intervention for this client at this time?
1. Help her to identify precipitating factors
2. Assist her to explore new coping abilities
3. Limit her support systems to promote independence
4. Develop her plan of care to fit her perception of the events

196. A depressed client, whose spouse recently died, attends an inpatient group therapy session in which the nurse is a co-leader. When another client talks about being divorced and the resulting feelings of abandonment, the nurse notices that tears are running down the depressed client's face. What should the nurse do to support this client?
1. Ask group members to return to discuss this client's feelings
2. Have another client stay and spend time talking with the client
3. Observe the client's behavior carefully during the next several hours
4. Accompany the client to her room and encourage a discussion of her feelings

197. An older female comes to the mental health clinic. The client states, "I've not been feeling right and haven't been able to sleep or eat since my husband died 8 months ago." The nurse determines that the client is experiencing grieving associated with the loss of the husband. What supports this conclusion?
    1. Inability to talk about her loss
    2. Difficulty in expressing her loss
    3. Lack of sleep and the presence of symptoms of depression
    4. Prolonged period of grief and mourning after her husband's death

198. A client with an inoperable temporal lobe tumor is experiencing frightening audio hallucinations, especially when alone. How can the nurse best help the client to cope with these hallucinations?
    1. Move the client to a four-bed room closer to the nurses' station
    2. Suggest that the client turn on the radio or television when alone
    3. Work out a schedule for visitors so that the client will not be alone
    4. Have family or friends remain with the client until hallucinations stop

199. An older widow with lung cancer is now in the terminal stage of her illness. Her family is puzzled by her mood changes and apparent anger at them. The nurse explains to the family that the client is:
    1. Trying to avoid her situation
    2. Coping with her impending death
    3. Attempting to reduce family dependence on her
    4. Hurting because the family will not take her home to die

200. A 76-year-old widower is terminally ill. He is very quiet and is unwilling to have visitors. During the initial contact with this client, the nurse should:
    1. Assess what the client knows about death and the dying process
    2. Avoid talking about his condition unless he initiates the discussion
    3. Encourage him to accept phone calls from those who wish to visit with him
    4. Explore the extent to which he knows of his condition and what it means to him

201. A client who has been sexually abused tearfully states, "I'm no good now; there is nothing to live for." What is the nurse's most therapeutic response?
    1. "Tell me more about your feelings."
    2. "I can understand why you feel worthless."
    3. "Why do you feel there is nothing to live for?"
    4. "Do you feel this way because of what has happened?"

202. The nurse determines that to help a couple work through their feelings about the husband's terminal illness, it is important to:
    1. Refer the husband to the psychotherapist for assistance in coping with his anger
    2. Assist the couple to express their feelings about his terminal illness to each other

    3. Encourage the wife to verbalize her feelings to a therapist during a therapy session
    4. Place the couple in a couples' therapy group that addresses the terminal illness of one partner

203. The grieving wife of a client who has just died says to the nurse, "We should have spent more time together. I always felt the children's needs came first." The nurse identifies that the wife is experiencing:
    1. Displaced anger
    2. Shame for past behaviors
    3. Expected feelings of guilt
    4. Ambivalent feelings about her husband

204. Why should the nurse question a prescription for a benzodiazepine for an individual undergoing acute grief?
    1. The depression is magnified and the risk of suicide increases
    2. Brain activity is suppressed and the risk of depression increases
    3. Lethargy results and it prevents the return to interpersonal activity
    4. The period of denial is extended and the grieving process is suppressed

205. A 68-year-old client who has metastatic carcinoma is told by the practitioner that death will occur within a month or two. Later, the nurse enters the client's room and finds the client crying. The nurse's action should take into consideration that:
    1. Crying relieves depression and helps the client face reality
    2. Crying releases tension and frees psychic energy for coping
    3. Nurses should not interfere with a client's behavior and defenses
    4. Accepting a client's crying maintains and strengthens the nurse-client bond

206. A terminally ill 76-year-old client is very quiet and unwilling to have visitors. During the initial contact with the client, the nurse should:
    1. Attempt to understand what death means to the client
    2. Avoid talking about the client's condition unless the client initiates the discussion
    3. Determine how much pain the client is experiencing and what medications have been prescribed
    4. Explore the extent to which the client is aware of the prognosis and the client's feelings about the situation

207. A female client terminally ill with cancer says to the nurse, "My husband is avoiding me. He doesn't love me anymore because of this awful tumor!" What is the nurse's most appropriate response?
    1. "What makes you think he doesn't love you?"
    2. "Avoidance is a defense. He needs your help to cope."
    3. "Do you think he is having difficulty dealing with your illness?"
    4. "You seem very upset. Tell me how your husband is avoiding you."

DEMENTIA, DELIRIUM, AND OTHER COGNITIVE DISORDERS

208. A client with a history of atrial fibrillation has a brain attack and vascular dementia (multi-infarct dementia) is diagnosed. When comparing assessments of clients with vascular dementia and dementia of the Alzheimer's type, which factor is unique to vascular dementia?
1. Memory impairment
2. Abrupt onset of symptoms
3. Difficulty making decisions
4. Inability to use words to communicate

209. A 70-year-old retired man has difficulty remembering his daily schedule and finding the right words to express himself. He is diagnosed as having dementia of the Alzheimer's type. The nurse expects that symptoms of this disorder:
1. Occur fairly rapidly
2. Have periods of remission
3. Begin after a loss of self-esteem
4. Demonstrate a progression of disintegration

210. When assessing a client with a cognitive disorder, the nurse identifies a behavior related to an alteration in mood when the client:
1. Loses interest in eating
2. Tells sexually explicit jokes
3. Has delusions and hallucinations
4. Reverses day and night activities

211. An 84-year-old widow with dementia, who had been living with her daughter before hospitalization, is being discharged with a referral to the visiting nurse. When the nurse visits, the client is in bed sleeping at 10 AM. Her daughter states that she gives her mother sleeping pills to stop her wandering at night. The nurse should:
1. Explore hiring a home health aide to stay with the client at night
2. Discuss the possibility of having the client placed in a nursing home
3. Suggest moving the client among family members on a monthly basis
4. Empathize with the daughter but suggest that wrist restraints would be preferable

212. When the nurse is communicating with a client with substance-induced persisting dementia, the client cannot remember facts and fills in the gaps with imaginary information. The nurse identifies that this is typical of:
1. Concretism
2. Confabulation
3. Flight of ideas
4. Associative looseness

213. When taking a health history from a client who has a moderate level of cognitive impairment due to dementia, the nurse expects the presence of:
1. Hypervigilance
2. Increased inhibition
3. Enhanced intelligence
4. Accentuated premorbid traits

214. An 84-year-old woman is admitted to the hospital with a diagnosis of dementia of the Alzheimer's type. The nurse determines that this disorder is a:
1. Problem that first emerges in the third decade of life
2. Nonorganic disorder that occurs in the later years of life
3. Cognitive problem that is a slow and relentless deterioration of the mind
4. Disorder that is easily diagnosed through laboratory and psychologic tests

215. An older client is admitted to the hospital with the diagnosis of dementia of the Alzheimer's type and depression. Which signs of depression does the nurse identify? Select all that apply.
1. _____ Loss of memory
2. _____ Increased appetite
3. _____ Neglect of personal hygiene
4. _____ "I don't know" answers to questions
5. _____ "I can't remember" answers to questions

216. When planning activities for a nursing home resident with a diagnosis of vascular dementia, the nurse should:
1. Plan varied activities that will keep the resident occupied
2. Provide familiar activities that the resident can successfully complete
3. Ensure that the resident actively participates in the unit's daily activities
4. Offer challenging activities to maintain the resident's contact with reality

217. A client with the diagnosis of dementia of the Alzheimer's type, stage 1, is living at home with a grown daughter. To best address the functional and behavioral changes associated with this stage, the nurse should encourage the daughter to:
1. Place the mother in a long-term care facility
2. Provide for the mother's basic physical needs
3. Post a schedule of the mother's daily activities
4. Perform care so that the mother does not need to make decisions

218. An older client's family tells the nurse that the client has suffered some memory loss in the past few years. They say that the client is sensitive about not being able to remember and tries to cover up this loss to avoid embarrassment. When attempting to increase the client's self-esteem, the nurse should try to avoid discussing events that require memory of the client's:
1. Married life
2. Work years
3. Recent days
4. Young adulthood

219. During the first month in a nursing home, a client demonstrates numerous disorganized behaviors related to disorientation and cognitive impairment. The nurse's plan of care should continue to take into consideration the client's:
1. Level of interest in unit activities
2. Orientation to time, place, and person
3. Ability to perform tasks while not becoming frustrated

4. Cognitive impairment, which will increase until adjustment to the home is accomplished

220. An older female client who is confused and often does not recognize her children is admitted to a nursing home. The client appears slovenly in attire, often soiling her clothing with feces and urine. How can the nurse best manage this problem?
1. Toilet the client every two hours
2. Place the client in orientation therapy
3. Supervise the client's bathroom activities closely
4. Explain to the client how offensive her behavior is to others

221. A 65-year-old retired baker is admitted to the hospital with the diagnosis of dementia. The nurse's question that best tests the client's ability for abstract thinking is:
1. "How are a television and a radio alike?"
2. "Can you give me today's complete date?"
3. "What would you do if you fell and hurt yourself?"
4. "Can you repeat the following numbers: 8, 3, 7, 1, 5?"

222. What should the nurse assess first when evaluating memory impairment in a client with dementia?
1. Disorientation of self
2. Recollection of past events
3. Remembrance of recent events
4. Impaired ability to name objects

223. An older nursing home resident with the diagnosis of early onset dementia likes to talk about olden days and at times has a tendency to confabulate. The nurse determines that confabulation serves to:
1. Prevent regression
2. Increase self-esteem
3. Attract the attention of others
4. Reminisce about achievements

224. What should be a priority of nursing care for a client with a dementia resulting from AIDS?
1. Assessing for pain frequently
2. Planning for re-motivational therapy
3. Arranging for long-term custodial care
4. Providing for basic intellectual stimulation

225. When planning care for a 72-year-old client who has been admitted to the hospital because of bizarre behavior, forgetfulness, and confusion, the nurse should give priority to:
1. Preserving the dignity of the client
2. Promoting a structured environment
3. Determining or ruling out organic etiology
4. Limiting the acceleration of symptomatology

226. A 54-year-old man has demonstrated increasing forgetfulness, irritability, and antisocial behavior. After being found disoriented and semi-naked walking down a street, the diagnosis of dementia of the Alzheimer's type is made. He expresses fear and anxiety when he is admitted to a long-term care facility. What is the best nursing intervention considering the client's diagnosis?
1. Explore with him the reasons for his concerns
2. Reassure him by the frequent presence of staff members

3. Provide him with a written schedule of planned interactions
4. Explain to him why the admission to the facility is necessary

227. Nursing management of a forgetful, disoriented client with inappropriate behaviors signifying dementia should be directed toward:
1. Restricting gross motor activity to prevent injury
2. Preventing further deterioration in the client's condition
3. Maintaining scheduled activities through behavior modification
4. Rechanneling the client's energies into more appropriate behaviors

228. A 79-year-old widow with dementia living in a nursing home is to join a group in recreational therapy. The nurse identifies that the client has laid out several dresses on her bed but has not changed from her nightgown. What is the nurse's best approach by the nurse?
1. Helping her select appropriate attire and assisting her with dressing
2. Reminding her to dress more quickly to avoid delaying the other clients
3. Allowing her as much time as she needs and explaining that she will be late
4. Telling her which dress to wear while reminding her that she is expected in the activity room soon

229. The nurse is caring for a client with dementia who has an alteration in the expression of emotions. Which behavior is unexpected with this client?
1. Lability
2. Passivity
3. Curiosity
4. Withdrawal

EATING AND SLEEP DISORDERS

230. A mental health nurse is admitting a client with anorexia nervosa. When obtaining the history and physical assessment, the nurse expects the client's condition to reveal:
1. Edema
2. Diarrhea
3. Hypotension
4. Amenorrhea

231. When caring for clients with the diagnosis of anorexia nervosa or bulimia nervosa, it is important that nurses understand the sociocultural influences related to eating disorders in the United States. What are these influences? Select all that apply.
1. _____ Diet industry
2. _____ Fashion trends
3. _____ Fast-food industry
4. _____ Over-the-counter medications
5. _____ Competitive women's athletics

232. A nurse who works in a mental health facility determines that the priority nursing intervention for a newly admitted client with bulimia nervosa is to:
    1. Monitor the client continually
    2. Observe the client during meals
    3. Teach the client to measure intake and output
    4. Involve the client in developing a daily meal plan

233. The nurse is interviewing a female adolescent with anorexia nervosa, who is malnourished and severely underweight. The nurse identifies that the client is experiencing secondary gains from her behavior when she says:
    1. "I am fat as a house."
    2. "I get straight A's in school."
    3. "My mother keeps trying to get me to eat."
    4. "My hair is beginning to fall out in clumps."

234. A major recognizable difference between anorexia nervosa and bulimia nervosa is that clients with anorexia nervosa usually:
    1. Tend to be more extroverted than clients with bulimia
    2. Seek intimate relationships, whereas clients with bulimia avoid them
    3. Are at greater risk for fluid and electrolyte imbalances than are clients with bulimia
    4. Deny the problem, whereas clients with bulimia generally recognize that their eating pattern is abnormal

235. An adolescent, who is extremely underweight and disappears into the bathroom after meals, angrily says to the nurse, "I don't need to be here. I don't have any problems. Stop watching me." To reduce the client's feeling of being threatened, the nurse is most therapeutic when responding:
    1. "I hear how frustrated you are to be here."
    2. "If you do not follow the rules, you will lose your privileges."
    3. "Your feelings are part of your illness; later you will feel better."
    4. "I'll get you the medication your physician prescribed for anxiety."

236. A client is admitted to the mental health unit with the diagnosis of anorexia nervosa. What typical signs and symptoms of anorexia nervosa does the nurse expect the client to exhibit?
    1. Slow pulse, mild weight loss, and alopecia
    2. Compulsive behaviors, excessive fears, and nausea
    3. Amenorrhea, excessive weight loss, and abdominal distention
    4. Excessive activity, memory lapses, and an increase in the pulse rate

237. A 5-foot, 5-inch-tall 15-year-old female who weighs 80 pounds is admitted to a mental health facility with a diagnosis of anorexia nervosa. The nurse identifies that her problem most likely is caused by:
    1. A desire to control her life
    2. The wish to be accepted by her peers
    3. The media's emphasis on the beauty of thinness
    4. A delusion in which she believes she must be thin

238. What characteristic of an adolescent girl suggests to the nurse that she may have bulimia?
    1. History of gastritis
    2. Positive self-concept
    3. Excessively stained teeth
    4. Frequently reswallowing food

239. Clients with eating disorders often exhibit similar symptoms. What should the nurse expect an adolescent with anorexia nervosa to exhibit?
    1. Affective instability
    2. Repetitive motor mechanisms
    3. Depersonalization and derealization
    4. Disheveled and unkempt physical appearance

240. What nursing intervention is the priority in the period immediately after an emaciated 13-year-old child's admission to the hospital for starvation secondary to anorexia nervosa?
    1. Ensuring the child's rest and nutrition needs are met
    2. Correcting the child's fluid and electrolyte imbalances
    3. Obtaining more data about the child's diet and exercise program
    4. Completing an assessment of the child's physical and mental status

241. A nurse in the mental health unit is working with a group of adolescent girls with the diagnosis of anorexia nervosa. The nurse considers that the major health complication associated with intractable anorexia nervosa is:
    1. Endocrine imbalance, causing amenorrhea
    2. Decreased metabolism, causing cold intolerance
    3. Cardiac dysrhythmias, resulting in cardiac arrest
    4. Glucose intolerance, resulting in protracted hypoglycemia

242. While admitting a young client with anorexia nervosa to the unit, the nurse finds a bottle of assorted pills in the client's luggage. The client tells the nurse they are antacids for stomach pains. What is the best initial response by the nurse?
    1. "Let's talk about your drug use."
    2. "These pills don't look like antacids."
    3. "Some people take pills to lose weight."
    4. "Tell me more about these stomach pains."

243. A nurse is assessing a client with bulimia nervosa. What should the nurse ask to obtain information about the client's intake habits and patterns?
    1. "Are you trying to control other people through the use of food?"
    2. "When you socialize, do you find that you eat more than when you eat by yourself?"
    3. "Do you find yourself eating more right before the beginning of your menstrual cycle?"
    4. "How frequently are you eating in response to your feelings rather than because you are hungry?"

244. What is the priority nursing intervention when planning care for an adolescent client with anorexia nervosa?
    1. Rewarding weight gain by increasing privileges
    2. Discussing the importance of eating a balanced diet

3. Encouraging the client to include high-caloric foods in the diet
4. Family therapy focusing on the influence of the client's behavior on the family

245. The parents of an adolescent female are upset about their daughter's diagnosis of anorexia nervosa and the treatment plan proposed. What should the nurse respond when the client's parents ask, "May we bring our daughter some food from home?"
   1. "Your concerns about food contribute to her problem."
   2. "While in the hospital, she should eat the hospital food."
   3. "For now, allow the hospital staff to handle her food needs."
   4. "It is important that you bring in whatever you think she'll eat."

246. When distinguishing whether a client may have anorexia nervosa or bulimia nervosa, the nurse should identify those characteristics that relate only to anorexia nervosa. Select all that apply.
   1. _____ Cachexia
   2. _____ Binge eating
   3. _____ Constipation
   4. _____ Decreased blood pressure
   5. _____ Delayed psychosexual development

247. When interacting with an adolescent client with the diagnosis of anorexia nervosa, it is most important that the nurse:
   1. Show empathy
   2. Maintain control
   3. Set and maintain limits
   4. Focus on food and nutrition

248. The multidisciplinary team decides to use a behavior modification approach for a young woman with anorexia nervosa. Which planned nursing intervention is an appropriate behavior modification approach to use with this client?
   1. Have the client role-play interactions with her parents
   2. Provide the client with a high-calorie, high-protein diet
   3. Restrict the client to her room until she gains 2 pounds
   4. Force the client to talk about her favorite foods for 1 hour a day

249. What should the nurse do when an adolescent female client with the diagnosis of anorexia nervosa starts to discuss food and eating?
   1. Listen to the client's list of favorite foods and secure these foods for her
   2. Tell the client gently but firmly to direct her discussion of food to the nutritionist
   3. Use the client's current interest in food to encourage her to increase her food intake
   4. Let the client talk about food as long as she wants and limit discussion about her eating

250. The nurse notes that a young female with anorexia nervosa telephones home just before each mealtime. She ignores reminders to eat and continues talking until the other clients are finished eating. She then refuses to eat "cold food." The nurse should initially:
   1. Insist that the client eat the food
   2. Remove the client's telephone privileges
   3. Hang the telephone up when meals are served
   4. Schedule a family meeting to discuss the problem

251. A young male client with anorexia nervosa telephones home just before mealtime. The client uses the phone calls to avoid eating. The nurse evaluates that the nursing plan to set limits on this avoidance behavior is effective when the client:
   1. Begins clipping recipes from magazines
   2. Organizes an aerobic group for the clients
   3. Arrives on time for meals without being called
   4. Contacts his family frequently by telephone between meals

252. The parents of a male adolescent diagnosed with anorexia nervosa ask the nurse, "How long will our son's treatment take?" What is the most therapeutic response by the nurse?
   1. "Progress depends on determining what triggered his desire to lose weight."
   2. "Treatment of anorexia nervosa takes a long time, including frequent setbacks."
   3. "Most anorectic adolescents respond favorably to treatment within a few weeks."
   4. "Length of the treatment depends on your willingness to become involved in therapy."

253. A nurse at the mental health center has been counseling the family of an adolescent client with anorexia about nutrition. The statement made by a family member that demonstrates an adequate understanding of the needs of the client is, "We:
   1. do not have to worry about this passing fad for long."
   2. will monitor the exercise habits of both our teenagers."
   3. need to watch more closely when we are eating together."
   4. should allow our daughter to have input into food planning."

DISORDERS OF MOOD

254. A nurse has been caring for a female client with the diagnosis of major depressive disorder. The nurse evaluates that a trusting relationship is beginning to develop when the client:
   1. Establishes eye contact with the nurse
   2. Accompanies the nurse to the dining room
   3. Responds to the nurse when asked a question
   4. Permits the nurse to get her dressed in the morning

255. How can a nurse minimize agitation in a disturbed client?
   1. Ensure constant staff contact
   2. Discuss the reasons for suspicious beliefs

3. Increase environmental sensory stimulation

4. Limit unnecessary interactions with the client

256. A client is experiencing feelings of sadness and is having difficulty concentrating and sleeping. What are additional common signs and symptoms of depression that the nurse should expect when performing an assessment of this client?
    1. Rigidity and a narrowing of perception
    2. Alternating episodes of fatigue and high energy
    3. Diminished pleasure in activities and alteration in appetite
    4. Excessive socialization and interest in activities of daily living

257. A nurse is caring for several extremely depressed clients. The nurse determines that these clients seem to do best in settings where they have:
    1. Multiple stimuli
    2. Varied activities
    3. Simple daily routines
    4. Opportunities for decision making

258. When caring for a client with major depression, nurses usually have the most difficulty dealing with the:
    1. Client's lack of energy
    2. Negative nonverbal responses
    3. Client's psychomotor retardation
    4. Pervasive quality of the depression

259. When working with a client who is depressed, the nurse should initially:
    1. Accept what the client says
    2. Attempt to keep the client occupied
    3. Keep the client's surroundings cheery
    4. Try to prevent the client from talking too much

260. When planning continuing care for a moderately depressed client, the nurse should include:
    1. Encouraging the client to determine leisure time activities
    2. Offering the client an opportunity to make some decisions
    3. Relieving the client of the responsibility of making any decisions
    4. Allowing the client time to be alone to decide in which activities to engage

261. The nurse identifies establishing trust as a major nursing goal for a depressed client. How can this goal be best accomplished?
    1. Spending the day with the client
    2. Asking the client at least one question daily
    3. Waiting for the client to initiate conversation
    4. Spending short periods of time with the client every day

262. One day the nurse sits by a depressed client's bed and states, "I will be spending some time with you today." The client responds angrily, "Go talk to someone else. They need you more." What is the nurse's most therapeutic response?
    1. "Why are you angry with me?"
    2. "I'll go but I will be back tomorrow."
    3. "I will be spending the next ten minutes with you."

4. "Don't you think you are just as important as the others?"

263. One morning a client with the diagnosis of acute depression states, "God is punishing me for my past sins." What is the nurse's best response?
    1. "Why do you think that?"
    2. "You sound very upset about this."
    3. "Do you believe God is punishing you for your sins?"
    4. "If you feel this way then you should talk to your clergyman."

264. An older widower in a nursing home, who is sitting by himself in a lounge, states, "I am all alone; no one has any use for me." Which response by the nurse is most therapeutic?
    1. "You seem upset. Let's talk about what is bothering you."
    2. "We need to be alone sometimes. It helps to get to know ourselves better."
    3. "Try doing something to avoid feeling lonely. I think you should socialize more."
    4. "You should focus on ways to change this. Let's play some games to improve your morale."

265. A depressed client has feelings of failure and a low self-esteem. What is an initial activity in which the client should be encouraged to become involved?
    1. Joining other clients in playing a board game
    2. Singing in the karaoke contest to be held at the end of the week
    3. Assisting a staff member working on the monthly bulletin board
    4. Selecting the movie to be played during the evening recreation period

266. Two weeks after a client has been admitted to the mental health hospital, the client's depression begins to lift. The nurse encourages involvement with unit activities, primarily because this type of activity:
    1. Supports self-confidence
    2. Provides for group interaction
    3. Limits opportunities for suicide
    4. Allows verbalization of repressed feelings of hostility

267. On the fifth hospital day, the nurse observes that a depressed client remains lying on the bed when the other clients are called to the dining room for lunch. What can the nurse do to encourage the client to eat?
    1. Simply state, "I will accompany you to the dining room."
    2. Bring a tray to the client's room, then leave it without comment
    3. Provide information about the importance of eating to maintain health
    4. Firmly state, "All clients are expected to go to the dining room for meals."

268. A client is admitted to the mental health hospital with the diagnosis of major depression. What is a common problem that clients experience with this diagnosis?
    1. Loss of faith in God
    2. Visual hallucinations

3. Decreased social interaction

4. Ambivalent feelings about the future

269. A depressed, withdrawn female client exhibits sadness through nonverbal behavior. The nurse should plan to help the client to:
    1. Increase her structured physical activity
    2. Cope with painful feelings by sharing them
    3. Decide which unit activities she can perform
    4. Improve her ability to communicate with significant others

270. A depressed client is very resistive and complains about inabilities and worthlessness. The nurse's best approach is to:
    1. Involve the client in activities in which success can be ensured
    2. Listen to the client while postponing a planned activity for later
    3. Encourage the client to select an activity in which there is some interest
    4. Schedule the client's activities so that they can be implemented independently

271. The nurse working on the mental health unit finds a depressed client crying. What is the most therapeutic approach to help the client explore feelings?
    1. "Does crying help?"
    2. "I know you are upset."
    3. "Tell me what you are feeling now."
    4. "Do you want to tell me why you are crying?"

272. A woman who has severe rheumatoid arthritis becomes depressed and is admitted to the psychiatric unit. The nurse begins to work with her in one-to-one sessions to help her cope with her depressive episode. The best long-term goal for this client is that she will:
    1. Eat at least two meals per day with other clients
    2. Maintain self-care and attend structured activities
    3. Make a positive verbal comment to another client daily
    4. Decrease negative thinking about herself, others, and life

273. A client remains depressed even after an 8-week trial on several antidepressant medications. A decision to initiate electroconvulsive therapy (ECT) is being considered by the treatment team. Which condition is a contraindication for administering ECT?
    1. Brain tumor
    2. Type 1 diabetes
    3. Hypothyroid disorder
    4. Urinary tract infection

274. To further assess a client's suicidal potential, the nurse should be especially alert to the client's expression of:
    1. Anger and resentment
    2. Loneliness and anxiety
    3. Frustration and fear of death
    4. Helplessness and hopelessness

275. A client whose wife recently died appears extremely depressed. The client states, "What's the use in talking? I'd rather be dead. I can't go on without my wife." What is the nurse's best response?
    1. "Would you rather be dead?"
    2. "What does death mean to you?"
    3. "Are you thinking about killing yourself?"
    4. "Do you understand why you feel that way?"

276. A hospitalized, depressed, suicidal client has been taking a mood-elevating medication for several weeks. The client's energy is returning and the client no longer talks about suicide. What should the nurse do in response to this client's behavior?
    1. Keep the client under closer observation
    2. Arrange for the client to have more visitors
    3. Engage the client in preliminary discharge planning
    4. Observe the client for side effects of the medication

277. A nurse becomes aware of an older client's feeling of loneliness when the client states, "I only have a few friends. My daughter lives in another state and couldn't care whether I live or die. She doesn't even know I'm hospitalized." The nurse identifies that the client's communication is probably a:
    1. Call for help to prevent acting on suicidal thoughts
    2. Manipulative attempt to persuade the nurse to call the daughter
    3. Reflection of depression that is causing feelings of hopelessness
    4. Request for information about community social support groups

278. When caring for a newly admitted depressed client, a nurse arranges for a staff member to remain with the client continuously. What information supports the nurse's decision to institute this precaution? Select all that apply.
    1. _____ Refusal to eat any food
    2. _____ Inability to concentrate
    3. _____ Agitated pacing in the hall
    4. _____ History of suicide attempts
    5. _____ Statements that life is not worth living

279. A female client who is clinically depressed reports that she has not experienced sexual orgasm in the past 3 years. The nurse describes this condition as:
    1. Diminished libido
    2. Dysfunctional hypo-orgasmia
    3. Primary orgasmic dysfunction
    4. Situational orgasmic dysfunction

280. A female client is admitted to the hospital because she attempted suicide. She reveals that her desire for sex has diminished since her child's birth 3 years ago. What is most directly related to the client's disinterest in sex?
    1. Depression
    2. Dependency
    3. Marital stress
    4. Identity confusion

281. A clinically depressed female client on a psychiatric unit of a local hospital uses embroidery scissors to cut her wrists. After treatment, when the nurse approaches, the

client is tearful and silent. What is the best initial intervention by the nurse?
1. Note client's behavior, record it, and notify the practitioner
2. Sit quietly next to the client and wait until she begins to speak
3. Say, "You are crying. I guess that means you feel badly about attempting suicide and really want to live."
4. Comment, "I notice you seem sad. Tell me what it's like for you and perhaps we can begin to work it out together."

282. A male client with the diagnosis of a bipolar disorder, depressed episode, is found lying on the floor in his room in the psychiatric unit. He states, "I don't deserve a comfortable bed; give it to someone else." The nurse's best response is:
1. "Everyone has a bed. This one is yours."
2. "You are not allowed to sleep on the floor."
3. "I don't understand why you are on the floor."
4. "You're a valuable person. You don't need to lie on the floor."

283. A nurse on a psychiatric unit has been working with a suicidal college student for 2 days. The student's comment that indicates relief from suicidal thinking is, "I:
1. can be a burden to others."
2. feel very alone sometimes."
3. plan to go to school next semester."
4. don't know if I can talk about my feelings."

284. A client is admitted with a bipolar disorder, depressed episode. The nursing history indicates a progressive increase in depression over the past month. What should the nurse expect the client to display?
1. Elated affect related to reaction formation
2. Loose associations related to a thought disorder
3. Physical exhaustion related to decreased physical activity
4. Paucity of verbal expression related to slowed thought processes

285. A client with a bipolar mood disorder, manic episode, says to the nurse, "I don't know what I'm doing here. I never felt better in my life; I've got the world on a string around my finger." What is the nurse's most therapeutic response to this comment?
1. "Have you ever felt this way before?"
2. "You are feeling pretty elated right now."
3. "You've got the whole world on a string."
4. "Why do you think you're feeling so good?"

286. A woman with a bipolar disorder, manic episode, has been spending thousands of dollars on clothing and makeup. She has been partying in bars every night and rarely sleeps or eats. The nurse in the outpatient clinic, identifying that this client rarely eats, recognizes that her eating problems most likely result from her:
1. Feelings of guilt
2. Need to control others
3. Desire for punishment
4. Excessive physical activity

287. When selecting a room for a client with the diagnosis of bipolar I disorder who is hyperactive and talking non-stop in a loud demanding voice, the nurse determines that the most important factor is that the:
1. Room have a pleasant view
2. Atmosphere be quiet and restful
3. Location be close to the nurses' desk
4. Roommates have similar diagnoses and behaviors

288. A female client with bipolar I disorder, manic episode, is admitted to the mental health unit of a community hospital. When developing an initial plan of care for this client, the nurse should plan to:
1. Increase her gym time
2. Isolate her from her peers
3. Encourage increased nutritional intake
4. Reinforce her participation in unit programs

289. A male client diagnosed with a bipolar disorder is aggressive and disruptive in group and social settings. Initially, the nurse works with him to develop social skills by:
1. Facilitating one-to-one interactions
2. Encouraging self-care with support
3. Developing guidelines for his behavior
4. Helping him to decrease his activity level

290. When a client who has a bipolar mood disorder is hyperactive, it is difficult to entice the client to sit still long enough to eat a complete meal. The plan of care states, "Provide finger foods such as carrots, celery, and cheese sticks at 10 AM, 2 PM, and 7 PM." Recent assessment of this client indicates that all of the food at mealtime is eaten but snacks have been refused. The nursing staff should:
1. Change the plan based on the evaluation
2. Ask the client if the finger foods should still be provided
3. Continue the present plan so that the client's nutritional status will improve
4. Reassess the client's nutritional status in one week so that changes can be made

291. A nurse is caring for a client with bipolar I disorder. What should the plan of care for this client include? Select all that apply.
1. _____ Touching the client to provide reassurance
2. _____ Providing a structured environment for the client
3. _____ Ensuring that the client's nutritional needs are met
4. _____ Engaging the client in conversation about current affairs
5. _____ Designing activities that require the client to maintain contact with reality

292. A female client is hospitalized for a bipolar mood disorder, manic episode. She is hyperactive and obnoxious, calls the nurse names, is sarcastic to the staff, and taps the nurse playfully on the buttocks. When caring for this client, it is most important for the nurse to:
1. Spend extra time with the client
2. Place the client alone in a quiet room

3. Disregard the client's acting-out behavior
4. Be aware of own feelings toward the client

293. A man with a bipolar disorder, manic episode, has been traveling around the country, dating multiple women and buying his dates expensive gifts. He is admitted to the hospital when he becomes exhausted and is out of money. The nurse anticipates that during a manic episode the client is most likely experiencing feelings of:
   1. Guilt
   2. Grandeur
   3. Worthlessness
   4. Self-deprecation

294. A 32-year-old woman is hospitalized with a diagnosis of a bipolar disorder, manic episode. She becomes loud and vulgar and disturbs the other clients. What is the nurse's best reaction to this situation?
   1. State, "You are bothering the other clients."
   2. Ignore the vulgar talk because it is part of the illness
   3. Segregate the client until this phase of her illness passes
   4. Comment, "We don't like that kind of talk around here."

295. A client who has been diagnosed with bipolar disorder, manic episode, has been sleeping very little and has not eaten for 2 weeks prior to hospitalization. The nurse concludes that in the overactive client, feeding problems frequently result from the client's:
   1. Feeling of unworthiness
   2. Inability to take the time to eat
   3. Unconscious desire for punishment
   4. Preoccupation with ritualistic behavior

296. A nurse identifies that the environment is important when caring for a client with the diagnosis of bipolar II disorder with hypomanic episodes. What should the nurse do when caring for clients with this disorder?
   1. Provide a quiet atmosphere by placing the client in a private room
   2. Ensure a cheerful environment by having bright drapes in the client's room
   3. Promote access to activities by assigning the client to a room near the dayroom
   4. Encourage interaction with others by having the client share a room with other clients

297. A client demonstrating manic behavior is elated and sarcastic. The client is constantly cursing and using foul language and has the other clients on the unit terrified. Initially the nurse should:
   1. Demand that the client stop the behavior immediately
   2. Tell the client firmly that the behavior is unacceptable
   3. Ask the client to identify what is precipitating the behavior
   4. Increase the client's medication or get a prescription for another drug

298. Nursing care for a client with a bipolar mood disorder, manic episode, is sometimes difficult. An important fact for the nurse to consider when planning care is that these clients are:
   1. Aware of reality
   2. Embarrassed by their behavior
   3. Out of contact with the environment
   4. Able to control the acting-out behavior

299. Encouragement and praise should be given to hyperactive clients to help them increase their feelings of self-esteem. When a client has behaved well within a group, the nurse should acknowledge the improvement by saying:
   1. "I knew you could behave."
   2. "Everyone likes you better when you behave like this."
   3. "Your behavior today was much better than it was yesterday."
   4. "You behaved well today when you sat through the community meeting."

300. A male client with the diagnosis of bipolar I disorder, manic episode, is hospitalized because he has been stopped by the police several times for reckless driving. He rarely eats or sleeps, and talks constantly. The second day of hospitalization he is attempting to organize the other clients in the lounge to form a softball team. What is the most therapeutic nursing intervention?
   1. Take him for a walk
   2. Suggest a time-out in his room
   3. Have him play cards with another client
   4. Explain that there is no place for him to play softball

301. A male client with cyclothymic disorder with hypomanic symptoms is admitted to the psychiatric unit. He progressively has lost weight and does not take the time to eat his food. How can the nurse best respond to this situation?
   1. Provide a tray for him in his room
   2. Assure him that he is deserving of food
   3. Order food that he can hold in his hand to eat while moving around
   4. Point out that the energy he is burning up must be replaced by eating food

302. A client with a diagnosis of bipolar I disorder with rapid cycling is readmitted 4 months after discharge. On the first day on the unit the client consistently interrupts the nurse and is increasingly talkative and loud. What is the most therapeutic response by the nurse?
   1. "You seem to have a need to interrupt me."
   2. "How is your relationship with your spouse?"
   3. "Do you realize your speech is loud and rapid?"
   4. "Tell me about the medicine you have been taking."

303. Nurses on a psychiatric unit have secluded a client who has the diagnosis of bipolar I disorder, manic episode, and who has been losing control and throwing objects while in the dayroom. The most important intervention for the client who is given a prn medication and confined to involuntary seclusion is to:
   1. Continue intensive nursing interactions
   2. Ascertain if any staff member has been injured
   3. Evaluate the client's progress toward self-control
   4. Observe for side effects of the prn medication given to the client

DISORDERS OF PERSONALITY

304. A client has a diagnosis of schizoid personality disorder. During the assessment the nurse should expect that the client's behavior is:
   1. Rigid and controlling
   2. Dependent and submissive
   3. Detached and socially distant
   4. Superstitious and socially anxious

305. A hospitalized psychiatric client with the diagnosis of histrionic personality disorder demands a sleeping pill before going to bed. After being refused the sleeping pill, the client throws a book at the nurse. The nurse identifies this behavior as:
   1. Exploitive
   2. Acting out
   3. Manipulative
   4. Reaction formation

306. A client comes to the mental health clinic with the complaint of a progressing inability to be in enclosed spaces. The practitioner makes the diagnosis of claustrophobia and prescribes desensitization therapy. The nurse considers that desensitization therapy is used successfully with clients experiencing phobias because it focuses on:
   1. Imagery
   2. Modeling
   3. Role playing
   4. Assertiveness training

307. A client comes to the mental health clinic for treatment of a phobia about large dogs. The nurse should anticipate that this client will demonstrate:
   1. Fear of discussing the phobia
   2. Resentment toward the feared object
   3. Inadequate impulse control when threatened
   4. Distortion of reality when discussing the phobia

308. A 30-year-old female client asks the nurse to change her room, stating that she hates her roommate and can't stand to be in the same room with her. Just as she finishes speaking, her roommate enters and the client tells her she missed her and has been all over the unit looking for her. The nurse identifies that the client is using:
   1. Projection
   2. Sublimation
   3. Passive aggression
   4. Reaction formation

309. The mother of a hospitalized female adolescent leaves a bag at the desk saying, "This is for my daughter's birthday. I'm too busy to visit today." The gift is an unwrapped expensive purse with the price tag attached. The daughter becomes upset after being given the message and seeing the gift. The mother's action is an example of:
   1. Maternal rejection
   2. Projective behavior
   3. Double-bind message
   4. Passive-aggressive behavior

310. A nurse on a mental health unit has developed a therapeutic relationship with an acting-out, manipulative client. One day as the nurse is leaving, the client says, "Please stay. I'm afraid the evening staff doesn't like me. They often punish me." What is the nurse's most therapeutic response?
   1. "I'll ask the staff not to punish you."
   2. "Tell me more about what you're feeling now."
   3. "Don't worry. I told you everything will be all right."
   4. "You know I leave at this time. We'll talk about this in the morning."

311. A client with the diagnosis of borderline personality disorder has been exhibiting manipulative, inappropriate behavior and consistently attempting to take advantage of the other clients. What should the nurse consider first before confronting the client?
   1. Last time medication was given
   2. Depth of their working relationship
   3. Client's ability to be empathic toward others
   4. Amount of self-awareness exhibited by the client

312. After a conference with the psychiatrist, a client with a borderline personality disorder cries bitterly, pounds the bed in frustration, and threatens suicide. What is the most helpful response by the nurse?
   1. Leave the client for a short period and wait until the client regains control
   2. Pat the client reassuringly on the back and say, "I know it is hard to bear."
   3. Ask about the client's troubles and answer, "Other people also have problems."
   4. Stay with the client and listen attentively if the client wishes to talk about the problem

313. A client is exhibiting withdrawn patterns of behavior. The nurse anticipates that this type of behavior eventually produces feelings of:
   1. Anger
   2. Paranoia
   3. Loneliness
   4. Repression

314. A nurse concludes that a client's withdrawn behavior may temporarily provide a:
   1. Defense against anxiety
   2. Basis for emotional growth
   3. Time for internal problem solving
   4. Delay to organize personal resources

315. A nursing team has a conference to develop goals for the care of a withdrawn, shy male client with low self-esteem who is afraid to talk to members of the opposite sex. Which objective should be given priority and documented in the client's plan of care? "The client will:
   1. increase his self-esteem."
   2. understand his sexual disorder."
   3. examine his feelings toward women."
   4. increase his knowledge of sexual functioning."

316. A female client with severe incapacitation because of obsessive-compulsive behavior has been admitted to the mental health hospital. The client's compulsive

ritual involves changing her clothing 8 to 12 times a day. She continually asks the nurse for advice regarding her problems but then ignores it. This is an example of the conflict of:

1. Apathy vs. anger
2. Trust vs. mistrust
3. Intimacy vs. isolation
4. Dependence vs. independence

317. A client misses breakfast because of an elaborate handwashing ritual. During the early stage of the client's hospitalization, it is most therapeutic for the nurse to:

1. Prevent the client from beginning the ritual until after breakfast
2. Wake the client early so the ritual can be completed before breakfast
3. Encourage the client to interrupt the ritual for meals at the scheduled times
4. Allow the client to choose between eating breakfast or completing the ritual

318. A female client with obsessive-compulsive disorder has become immobilized by her elaborate handwashing and walking rituals. The nurse considers that the basis of obsessive-compulsive disorder often is feelings of:

1. Anxiety and guilt
2. Anger and hostility
3. Embarrassment and shame
4. Hopelessness and powerlessness

319. An executive secretary experiences an overwhelming impulse to count and arrange the rubber bands and paper clips in the desk. The client feels something dreadful will occur if the ritual is not carried out. Considering the client's symptoms, the nurse concludes that rituals:

1. Are useful in our society as long as they can be controlled
2. Serve to control anxiety resulting from unconscious impulses
3. Are a displacement of general anxiety onto an unrelated specific fear
4. Serve to consciously limit the associated behavior that otherwise is overwhelming

320. A client who uses a ritual of counting paper in the printer tells the nurse, "I am spending 30 minutes counting each time I photocopy and my boss is getting very upset. What should I do?" What is the nurse's best response?

1. "Limit photocopying by clustering it to 2 or 3 times a day."
2. "Arrive at work 30 minutes early for counting the paper in the printer."
3. "Substitute another activity at home such as counting shoes or other objects."
4. "Talk with the boss to ask for tolerance until the mental health treatments help."

321. A client who uses a complex ritual says to the nurse, "I feel so guilty. None of this makes any sense. Everyone must really think I'm crazy." What is the most therapeutic response by the nurse?

1. "Your behavior is bizarre. However, it serves a useful purpose."
2. "You are concerned about what other people are thinking about you."
3. "I am sure people understand that you cannot help this behavior right now."
4. "Guilt serves no useful purpose. It just helps you stay stuck where you are."

322. A female client with a diagnosis of obsessive-compulsive personality disorder goes to the mental health center. She is restless, irritable, and angry at her adolescent children because they do not do the household chores correctly and she has to do all the work again. What is the nurse's most therapeutic response?

1. "You look exhausted. Can you take some time off from work to rest?"
2. "Don't get so excited. Why do you feel you have to do everything yourself?"
3. "It must be frustrating. How can you help them learn to do the chores correctly?"
4. "I know that you are upset. Do you really think your children are not typical teenagers?"

323. When planning care for a client who uses ritualistic behavior, the nurse recalls that the ritual:

1. Helps the client control anxiety
2. Is under the client's conscious control
3. Is used by the client primarily for secondary gains
4. Helps the client focus on the inability to deal with reality

324. It is observed that at times a client with a personality disorder clings to the nurse and at other times maintains a noticeable distance. The nurse concludes that this pattern of behavior illustrates that the client has conflicting fears of:

1. Shame vs. rejection
2. Lost self-esteem vs. hostility
3. Abandonment vs. identity loss
4. Engulfment vs. interdependence

325. At 10 PM a client with a personality disorder is in the lounge playing cards. When the nurse enters, the client requests a sleeping pill. The nurse responds, "First go to bed and attempt to sleep." The nurse's response is directed toward:

1. Setting limits
2. Reality testing
3. Routinizing care
4. Conditioning behavior

326. A client with a personality disorder is playing cards with another person in the lounge. When the other person cheats at cards, the client responds by aggressively scattering the deck of cards around the room. The nurse assesses that the client has:

1. Poor reality testing
2. A violent personality
3. An antisocial personality
4. Inadequate impulse control

327. An adolescent with a long history of drug abuse, stealing, refusal to comply with rules, and an inability to get

along with peers is admitted to an adolescent unit for evaluation. The most appropriate plan of care at this time is for the nurse to:

1. Act as a role model for mature behavior while providing a structured setting
2. Allow as much freedom as possible, setting few rules and minimum structure
3. Provide activities that ensure immediate gratification as well as social stimulation
4. Behave in a moralistic, punitive manner toward the adolescent when rules are not followed

328. Personality disorders are identified in the DSM-IV-TR in clusters. How should the nurse describe the behaviors of an individual with a cluster A personality disorder?
1. Odd and eccentric
2. Anxious and fearful
3. Dramatic and erratic
4. Hostile and impulsive

329. A male adolescent with the diagnosis of antisocial personality disorder spends a great deal of time with a female adolescent client on the unit. One day the nursing assistant enters the female client's room and finds them in bed together. The nursing assistant reports the incident to the nurse. The nurse should:
1. Lock the bedroom doors
2. Arrange a discussion with both adolescents
3. Assign the same staff member to observe both clients several times an hour
4. Call a unit meeting to talk about sexual activity among the clients on the unit

330. An adolescent female with an antisocial personality disorder plans to live with her parents after discharge. The parents request advice on how to respond to their daughter's unruly behavior. What is the most therapeutic response by the nurse?
1. "Discuss her behavior with her and encourage her to develop self-control."
2. "Avoid setting expectations for her behavior and react to each situation as it arises."
3. "Help her find new friends, encourage her to get a job and assume responsibility for herself."
4. "Set clear limits, explain to her the consequences of disregarding them, and firmly and consistently apply them."

331. For the past week a young male client has been threatening vulnerable clients on the unit and trying to manipulate the female staff members to obtain special privileges. What is the best nursing approach?
1. Assign a nursing assistant to watch him when he is awake
2. Ignore the client's behavior while protecting the vulnerable clients
3. Set firm limits on the client's behavior and consistently confront him
4. Assign a male staff member to the client and limit his contact with other clients

332. One afternoon a male client on the inpatient psychiatric service complains to the nurse that he has been waiting for more than an hour for someone to accompany him to activities. The nurse replies, "We're doing the best we can. There are a lot of other people on the unit who need attention, too." This response demonstrates the nurse's use of:
1. Impulse control
2. Defensive behavior
3. Reality reinforcement
4. Limit-setting behavior

333. The personality characteristics of a client with an antisocial personality disorder make it difficult for family members to interact and maintain a healthy relationship. What are common characteristics of an antisocial personality? Select all that apply.
1. _____ Aloof
2. _____ Suspicious
3. _____ Perfectionist
4. _____ Irresponsible
5. _____ Manipulative

334. An adolescent client with an antisocial personality disorder is admitted to the hospital because of drug abuse and repeated sexual acting-out behavior. The nurse evaluates that interventions directed toward modifying the behavior of this client have been successful when the client:
1. Promises never to take drugs again
2. Discusses the need to seduce other adolescents
3. Recognizes the need to conform to society's norms
4. Identifies underlying feelings of the acting-out behavior

335. A nurse in an outpatient mental health setting has been assigned to care for a new client who is diagnosed with an antisocial personality disorder. During assessment the nurse expects to observe that the client:
1. Pays great attention to detail and demonstrates high levels of anxiety
2. Has scars from self-mutilation and a history of many negative relationships
3. Is charming, has an above-average intelligence, and tends to manipulate others
4. Demonstrates suspiciousness, avoids eye contact, and engages in limited conversation

336. A male client with a diagnosis of antisocial personality disorder is admitted to the mental health hospital. What is the priority nursing intervention?
1. Encouraging interactions with others
2. Having a united, consistent staff approach
3. Assuming a nurturing, forgiving tone in disputes
4. Using seclusion when manipulative behaviors are exhibited

337. A client with a dissociative identity disorder is to be discharged after a 2-week hospitalization. The nurse, evaluating the effectiveness of the short-term therapy, expects the client to verbalize:
1. The ability to deal openly with feelings
2. That many of the personalities can be ignored
3. The need for long-term outpatient psychotherapy
4. That the personalities serve no protective purpose

SCHIZOPHRENIC DISORDERS

338. Despite repeated nursing interventions to improve reality orientation, a client insists that he is the commander of an alien spaceship. What is the client experiencing?
    1. Illusion
    2. Delusion
    3. Confabulation
    4. Hallucination

339. A newly admitted client is apathetic and exhibits an inappropriate affect. A diagnosis of acute schizophrenic reaction is made. Considering the diagnosis, a symptom the nurse expects to identify in the client's communication or behavior is:
    1. Logical deductions
    2. Suicidal preoccupation
    3. Absence of self-criticism
    4. Autistic magical thinking

340. A female graduate student who has become increasingly withdrawn and neglectful of her studies and personal hygiene is brought to the psychiatric hospital by her roommate. After a detailed assessment, a diagnosis of schizophrenia is made. Which characteristic is unlikely to be demonstrated by this client?
    1. Weak ego
    2. Low self-esteem
    3. Concrete thinking
    4. Effective self-boundaries

341. A client who has been admitted with a diagnosis of schizophrenia says to the nurse, "Yes, it's March. March is Little Women. That's literal you know." These statements illustrate:
    1. Echolalia
    2. Neologisms
    3. Flight of ideas
    4. Loosening of associations

342. The nurse is caring for a client newly diagnosed with an acute schizophrenic reaction. What factor in the client's history indicates a greater potential for recovery?
    1. A precipitating event
    2. Insidious onset of the illness
    3. A relative with schizophrenia
    4. Vague prepsychotic symptoms

343. The nurse is interviewing the family about the onset of problems in a young client with the diagnosis of schizophrenia. In what stage of development does the nurse expect that the client's difficulties began?
    1. Puberty
    2. Adolescence
    3. Late childhood
    4. Early childhood

344. A client with schizophrenia sees a group of visitors sitting together talking. The client tells the nurse, "I know they are talking about me." Which altered thought process should the nurse identify?
    1. Flight of ideas
    2. Ideas of reference

3. Grandiose delusion
    4. Thought broadcasting

345. A client with schizophrenia repeatedly says to the nurse, "No moley, jandu!" The nurse determines that this is called:
    1. Echolalia
    2. Neologism
    3. Concretism
    4. Perseveration

346. After 2 days on the unit, a female client with the diagnosis of schizophrenic reaction refuses to take a shower. What is the most appropriate intervention by the nurse?
    1. Simply state she must shower now
    2. Have the staff give the client a shower
    3. Tell her she can shower when she feels more comfortable
    4. Gently point out that her appearance is upsetting the other clients

347. A client is admitted to a psychiatric unit with the diagnosis of schizophrenia, undifferentiated type. When assessing the client, the nurse identifies the presence of the characteristics related to this disorder. Select all that apply.
    1. _____ Bizarre behavior
    2. _____ Extreme negativism
    3. _____ Disorganized speech
    4. _____ Persecutory delusions
    5. _____ Auditory hallucinations

348. A client who has been hospitalized with schizophrenia tells the nurse, "My heart has stopped and my veins have turned to glass!" What should the nurse conclude that the client is experiencing?
    1. Echolalia
    2. Hypochondriasis
    3. Somatic delusion
    4. Depersonalization

349. A female client with acute schizophrenia tells the nurse, "Everyone hates me." What is the best response by the nurse?
    1. "Tell me more about this."
    2. "Everyone does not hate you."
    3. "That feeling is part of your illness."
    4. "You may be promoting this feeling yourself."

350. Breaks with reality, such as those experienced by clients with schizophrenia, necessitate that the nurse first realize that:
    1. Extended institutional care is necessary
    2. Clients believe what they feel they are experiencing is real
    3. Electroconvulsive therapy produces remission in most clients with schizophrenia
    4. The clients' families must cooperate in the maintenance of the psychotherapeutic plan

351. A man is admitted to the psychiatric unit after attempting suicide. The client's history reveals that his first child died of SIDS 2 years ago, he has been unable to work since the death of the child, and he has attempted suicide

before. When talking with the nurse he states, "I hear my son telling me to come over to the other side." What should the nurse conclude the client is experiencing?

1. Fixed delusion
2. Magical thought
3. Pathological regression
4. Command hallucination

352. By identifying common behaviors exhibited by the client who has a diagnosis of schizophrenia, the nurse can anticipate:

1. Disorientation, forgetfulness, and anxiety
2. Grandiosity, arrogance, and distractibility
3. Withdrawal, regressed behavior, and lack of social skills
4. Slumped posture, pessimistic outlook, and flight of ideas

353. A client in the psychiatric hospital is attempting to communicate by stating, "Sky, flower, angry, green, opposite, blanket." The nurse concludes that this type of communication is:

1. Echolalia
2. Word salad
3. Confabulation
4. Flight of ideas

354. A nurse is caring for a client with the diagnosis of schizophrenia. What is a common problem for clients with this diagnosis?

1. Chronic confusion
2. Inability to trust others
3. Rigid personal boundaries
4. Violence directed toward others

355. On admission a disturbed, unkempt female client refuses to remove her clothing. What should the nurse do to best meet the client's needs?

1. Get assistance and remove her clothing to meet her basic hygiene needs
2. Provide her with two outfits to encourage the client to reach a simple decision
3. Tell her she will look more attractive in clean clothing to increase her self-esteem
4. Wait and allow her to undress whenever she is ready to help the client maintain her identity

356. The nurse documents that a client has been experiencing a somatic delusion. Which statement led to this conclusion?

1. "I am Jesus Christ."
2. "I know I am dead."
3. "This food has been poisoned."
4. "My stomach has disintegrated."

357. A nurse is writing a plan of care on the medical record of a paranoid male client who has unjustifiably accused his wife of having many extramarital affairs. An intermediate goal for this client is, "The client will develop:

1. faith in his wife."
2. better self-control."
3. feelings of self-worth."
4. insight into his behavior."

358. A 25-year-old male client is being treated for an anxiety disorder and issues related to impaired social interaction. The client accuses the health care providers of being homosexuals. This behavior indicates that the client most likely is:

1. Attempting to keep the focus off his problems
2. Having difficulty handling unacceptable feelings about himself
3. Exploring emotionally charged reactions to threatening situations
4. Trying to embarrass those people he perceives as authority figures

359. The nurse finds an acting-out, disturbed male client in the fetal position. What is the most appropriate intervention for the nurse?

1. Tap him gently on the shoulder to get his attention and then stay with him
2. Sit down beside him on the floor saying, "I'm here to spend time with you."
3. Go to him saying, "I'll be waiting for you by the chairs, so please get up and join me."
4. Leave him alone because the behavior demonstrates he is too regressed to benefit from verbal communication

360. Schizophrenia type II is associated with negative symptoms. When assessing a client with schizophrenia, which symptoms are classified as negative symptoms? Select all that apply.

1. _____ Lack of energy
2. _____ Poor grooming
3. _____ Illogical speech
4. _____ Ideas of reference
5. _____ Agitated behavior

361. During an assessment, the nurse identifies that the client is experiencing a hallucination when the client says:

1. "I am going to save the world because I am God."
2. "My insides smell like they are going to rot away."
3. "Unless I gamble at least once a week I feel extremely anxious."
4. "It's crazy, but I keep thinking something terrible will happen to my baby."

362. The nurse believes an emotionally disturbed client is ready to begin participating in therapeutic activities. What should the nurse initially suggest?

1. Drawing pictures with the nurse
2. Attending a class on medications
3. Participating on the softball team
4. Watching television in the dayroom

363. A client with schizophrenia says to the nurse, "I've been here 5 days. There are five players on a basketball team. I like to play the piano." How should the nurse document this cognitive disorder?

1. Word salad
2. Loose association
3. Thought blocking
4. Delusional thinking

364. A female client with schizophrenia is going to occupational therapy for the first time. She tells the nurse she doesn't want to go. What is the most therapeutic response by the nurse?
   1. "I will go with you to occupational therapy."
   2. "It is only for an hour, then you will be back."
   3. "Try it once. If you don't like it, you do not have to go back."
   4. "The physician ordered it as part of your treatment. You should go."

365. A client is experiencing hallucinations. What therapeutic intervention should the nurse plan to help the client cope with the hallucinations?
   1. Reinforce the perceptual distortions until the client develops new defenses
   2. Provide an unstructured environment and assign the client to a private room
   3. Avoid helping the client make connections between anxiety-producing situations and hallucinations
   4. Distract the client's attention by providing a competing stimulus that is stronger than the hallucinations

366. What should a nurse do first when managing interpersonal relationships with a client who has schizophrenia?
   1. Allow the client to be alone when desired, but provide quiet activities
   2. Insist that the client join group meetings and activities with other clients
   3. Establish a one-to-one relationship and then bring the client into group activities
   4. Encourage dependency by the client initially, but set limits on the extent of this behavior

367. A newly admitted male client diagnosed with schizophrenia appears to be responding to internal stimuli when laughing and talking to himself. What is the best initial response by the nurse?
   1. Ask the client if he is hearing voices
   2. Encourage the client to engage in unit activities
   3. Tell the client the voices he is hearing are not real
   4. Give the client his prescribed prn antipsychotic medication

368. A delusional client is actively hallucinating and worried about being stalked by a terrorist group. What defense mechanism does the nurse identify is the most prominent in this situation?
   1. Splitting
   2. Undoing
   3. Projection
   4. Sublimation

369. A male client claims the voices he hears are clearly telling him what actions and decisions to make. What is the nurse's most therapeutic response?
   1. Play soft music when the client starts hearing voices
   2. Begin talking to the client when he is hearing the voices
   3. Explain to the client that his perception of voices is wrong
   4. Indicate acceptance that the client may be frightened by the voices

370. What should a nurse do when a client with the diagnosis of schizophrenia talks about being controlled by others?
   1. Express disbelief about the delusion
   2. Acknowledge the feeling tone of the delusion
   3. Respond to the verbal content of the client's delusion
   4. Institute an activity that will compete with the delusion

371. A nurse is obtaining a health history from a woman who is known to be verbally abusive. The client tells the nurse, "You're ugly and you're probably stupid too. Why am I stuck with you for my nurse?" What is the nurse's best response?
   1. "It does not matter what you think, because I know I am a capable nurse."
   2. "Tell me more about why my caring for you today is so upsetting to you."
   3. "You are talking inappropriately, which makes it harder for us to work together."
   4. "If you like I will arrange to switch assignments so you can have another nurse."

372. A 22-year-old male client with the diagnosis of schizophrenia has been in a mental health facility for approximately 2 weeks. After his parents visit he is observed pacing in the hall talking loudly to himself. What should be the nurse's initial intervention?
   1. Obtain an order for a tranquilizer
   2. Ask the client about the events of his day
   3. Call the parents to find out what happened
   4. Assign a nursing assistant to remain with the client

373. At mealtime a client with schizophrenia moves to the counter to choose food but is unable to decide what to do next. The nurse, identifying the client's ambivalence, assists by using:
   1. Nonverbal communication
   2. Simple declarative statements
   3. Basic questions requiring simple choices
   4. Rewards for each of the food items chosen

374. A client with the diagnosis of schizophrenia watches the nurse pour juice for the morning medication from an almost empty pitcher and screams, "That juice is no good! It's poisoned." What is the most therapeutic response by the nurse?
   1. Remark, "You sound frightened."
   2. Assure the client, "The juice is not poisoned."
   3. Pour the client a glass of juice from a full pitcher
   4. Take a drink of the juice to show the client that it is alright

375. When a disturbed acting-out female client's condition improves, the practitioner suggests discharge to a halfway house. The client's family is worried that she will continue to act out at the halfway house. What is the nurse's best intervention at this time?
   1. Have the social worker talk with the family
   2. Cancel the discharge plans until the family is reassured

3. Have the client promise the nurse and family that acting out will not occur
4. Discuss the concern at a meeting with both the client and the family present

376. One morning a nurse finds a disturbed client curled up in the fetal position in the corner of the dayroom. The most accurate initial evaluation of the behavior is that the client is:
1. Feeling more anxious today
2. Attempting to hide from the nurse
3. Tired and probably did not sleep well last night
4. Physically ill and experiencing abdominal discomfort

377. An extremely agitated male client hospitalized in a mental health unit begins to pace around the dayroom. What should the nurse do?
1. Lock the client in his room to limit external stimuli
2. Let the client pace in the hall away from other clients
3. Get the client involved in a card game to distract his thoughts
4. Encourage the client to work with another client on a unit task

378. A nurse identifies that a male client sitting alone in the corner is smiling and talking to himself. Concluding that the client is hallucinating, the nurse should:
1. Ask the client why he is smiling
2. Leave the client alone until he stops talking
3. Invite the client to help decorate the dayroom
4. Tell the client it is not good for him to talk to himself

379. The nurse is planning a group session for three chronically ill clients who have the diagnosis of schizophrenia. Considering the symptoms and general characteristics of schizophrenia and long-term mental illness, one of the most helpful topics for this group is:
1. Relaxation techniques
2. Rational behavior therapy
3. Assertiveness in relationships
4. Social skills in the group setting

380. A nurse is caring for a client with the diagnosis of schizophrenia. What should the nurse plan to do to increase the self-esteem of this client?
1. Reward healthy behaviors
2. Explain the treatment plan
3. Identify various means of coping
4. Encourage participation in community meetings

381. A young client with schizophrenia states, "I am starting to hear voices." What is the nurse's most therapeutic response?
1. "How do you feel about the voices, and what do they mean to you?"
2. "You are the only one hearing the voices. Are you sure you hear them?"
3. "I understand you are hearing voices talking to you, and that they are very real to you."
4. "The health team members will observe your behavior. We will not leave you alone."

382. When being admitted to a mental health facility, a young male adult tells the nurse that the voices he hears

frighten him. The nurse identifies that clients tend to hallucinate more vividly:
1. Before meals
2. After going to bed
3. During group activities
4. While watching television

383. One morning a client tells the nurse, "My legs are turning to rubber because I have an incurable disease called schizophrenia." The nurse identifies that this is an example of:
1. Hallucinations
2. Paranoid thinking
3. Depersonalization
4. Autistic verbalization

384. A client with schizophrenia who has auditory hallucinations is withdrawn and apathetic. What should the nurse say to involve this client in an activity?
1. "I need a partner when I go for my walk today."
2. "You will receive a reward if you go to the gym."
3. "Those voices you hear would like it if you did a little exercise."
4. "There is a positive relationship between exercise and mental health."

385. The nurse is caring for a female client who is confused and delirious. What is the most therapeutic intervention when interacting with this client?
1. Reassure the client that she will get better
2. Direct the client's daily activities on the unit
3. Help the client to clarify her experience and gain insight into her behavior
4. Provide the client with solutions to past and current problems experienced

386. A male client in a mental health facility is tugging on his ear during a unit meeting. When the nurse comments about it, the client replies, "You know, it's that microcomputer those foreign agents implanted in my ear." Based on this statement, the nurse determines that the client is experiencing:
1. Illusions
2. Hallucinations
3. Delusional thoughts
4. Neologistic thinking

387. The nurse identifies that paranoid delusions usually are related to the defense mechanism of:
1. Projection
2. Regression
3. Repression
4. Identification

388. A client with schizophrenia tells the nurse, "There are foreign agents conspiring against me; they're out to get me at every turn." How should the nurse respond?
1. "It must be scary to believe that people are out to trick you at every opportunity."
2. "Those people you call foreign agents are out to do you in. What else is happening?"
3. "What's happened to make you believe these people you call foreign agents are after you?"

4. "I can understand how frightening your thoughts are to you. However, your thoughts do not seem factual to me."

389. When establishing a plan of care, the nurse should identify that a male client's delusion that he is an important government adviser is most likely related to:
1. A psychotic loss of touch with his real identity
2. An attempt at wish fulfillment created to manipulate others
3. A need to feel a sense of importance within his environment
4. An effort to compensate for feelings of depression about his problems

390. During the admission procedure a client who has paranoid ideation refuses to answer the nurse's questions, stating, "You are in a conspiracy to kill me." The nurse concludes these feelings are related to the client's:
1. Low self-esteem
2. Need to be alone
3. Lack of acceptance
4. Necessity for attention

391. The nurse is caring for a client who is using paranoid ideation. When planning care, the nurse determines the importance of:
1. Not placing demands on the client
2. Removing stress so that the client can relax
3. Giving the client difficult tasks to provide stimulation
4. Providing the client with activities in which success can be achieved

392. During a one-to-one interaction with a client with schizophrenia, paranoid type, the client says to the nurse, "I figured out how foreign agents have infiltrated the news media. They want to shut me up before I spill the beans." How should the nurse describe this statement?
1. Nihilistic delusion
2. Delusion of grandeur
3. Auditory hallucination
4. Overvaluation of the self

393. A disturbed male client is admitted to the hospital for evaluation. When obtaining the history, the nurse asks why he was brought to the hospital by his parents. The client states, "They lied about me. They said I murdered my mother. You killed her. She died before I was born." What does the nurse identify that the client is experiencing?
1. Ideas of grandeur
2. Confusing illusions
3. Persecutory delusions
4. Auditory hallucinations

394. A nurse is caring for a client with the diagnosis of schizophrenia of the paranoid type. How should the nurse plan for the client's initial care?
1. Discuss prominent life events
2. Provide a nonthreatening environment
3. Concentrate on the content of delusions
4. Limit topics for discussion to recent situations

395. A nurse is caring for a client who is using paranoid ideation. To establish a trusting relationship, the nurse should begin by:
1. Seeking the client out frequently to spend long blocks of time together
2. Sitting in the unit and observing the client's behavior throughout the day
3. Being available on the unit continually and waiting for the client to approach
4. Calling the client into the office to establish a contract for regular therapy sessions

396. A client with schizophrenia, paranoid type, is delusional, withdrawn, and negativistic. The nurse should plan to:
1. Invite the client to play a game of ping-pong
2. Explain to the client the benefits of a group activity
3. Encourage the client to become involved in group activities
4. Mention to the client that the psychiatrist has ordered increased activity

397. A client refuses to eat and states, "The food is poisoned." The nurse should:
1. Ask the client what foods are desired so they can be ordered
2. Encourage the client's family to bring favorite foods from home
3. Suggest going to the cafeteria and selecting foods the client feels safe eating
4. Go with the client to the cafeteria and taste the food to show that it is not poisoned

398. Lunch is being served, and the clients must walk to the dining room. The nurse finds one client sitting alone with the head slightly tilted as if listening to something. The nurse should state:
1. "I know you're busy. However, it's lunchtime."
2. "Get going. You don't want to miss lunchtime."
3. "It's lunchtime. I'll walk with you to the dining room for lunch."
4. "Those voices are bothering you again. I'll help you get ready for lunch."

399. The nurse is talking with a delusional client who has been hospitalized for 2 weeks. In the middle of the conversation the client stops talking and suddenly seems preoccupied and then states, "I hear voices." What is the nurse's most therapeutic response?
1. Ask the client, "What are the voices saying?"
2. Tell the client, "I did not hear any voices," and focus back to the conversation
3. Say nothing, remain observant, and later document the incident in the client's record
4. Challenge the client by emphasizing that there's nobody there, reminding her that there are just the two of them

SUBSTANCE ABUSE

400. A 20-year-old carpenter falls from a roof and incurs fractures of the right femur and left tibia. The client reveals a history of substance abuse. What is the

primary consideration for the nurse who is caring for this client?

1. Confronting the client about substance abuse
2. Avoiding calling attention to the client's drug abuse
3. Communicating in the same speech pattern that the client uses
4. Realizing that this client will need more pain medication than a nonabuser

401. A mental health nurse is working on a unit where many clients have the diagnosis of alcoholism. The nurse identifies that the defense mechanism most commonly used by clients who are alcoholics is:
    1. Denial
    2. Projection
    3. Displacement
    4. Compensation

402. A client with the diagnosis of alcoholism explains to the nurse that alcohol has a calming effect and states, "I function better when I'm drinking than when I'm sober." What defense mechanism does the nurse identify that the client is using?
    1. Sublimation
    2. Suppression
    3. Compensation
    4. Rationalization

403. Within a few hours of alcohol withdrawal the nurse should assess the client for the presence of:
    1. Irritability and tremors
    2. Yawning and convulsions
    3. Disorientation and paranoia
    4. Fever and profuse diaphoresis

404. A client is admitted to an alcohol rehabilitation center. On the fourth day after admission, the nurse detects a strong odor of alcohol on the client's breath. What is the nurse's first action?
    1. Ask where the client got the alcohol
    2. Locate and remove the alcoholic substance
    3. Convey the staff's disappointment in this behavior
    4. Document and notify the practitioner about the client's drinking

405. A 42-year-old adult with a long history of alcohol abuse seeks help in one of the local hospitals. The nurse considers that the major underlying factor for success in an alcohol treatment program will be the client's:
    1. Family
    2. Motivation
    3. Practitioner
    4. Self-esteem

406. A 65-year-old male is admitted to a mental health facility with a diagnosis of substance-induced persisting dementia resulting from chronic alcoholism. When conducting the admitting interview, the nurse determines that the client is using confabulation. The nurse takes into consideration that the use of confabulation is precipitated by the client's:
    1. Ideas of grandeur
    2. Need for attention

3. Marked memory loss
4. Difficulty in accepting the diagnosis

407. A nurse is planning care for a client with substance-induced persisting dementia resulting from chronic alcohol ingestion. Which nutritional problem, in addition to the effect of alcohol on brain tissue, has contributed to substance-induced persisting dementia?
    1. Increase in serotonin
    2. Deficiency of thiamine
    3. Reduction in iron intake
    4. Malabsorption of riboflavin

408. A nurse identifies that for individuals who are alcoholics, alcohol is a substance that is used to:
    1. Blunt reality
    2. Precipitate euphoria
    3. Promote social interaction
    4. Stimulate the central nervous system

409. A nurse, planning care for a client who is an alcoholic, considers that the most serious life-threatening symptoms from alcohol withdrawal usually begin after a specific time interval. How many hours after the last drink do they occur?
    1. 8 to 12
    2. 12 to 24
    3. 24 to 72
    4. 72 to 96

410. A salesman with a history of heavy drinking is on a detoxification unit. He asks the nurse's permission to skip the Alcoholics Anonymous (AA) meeting held daily. What is the nurse's initial response?
    1. "What are your feelings about going to AA meetings?"
    2. "What is it that you dislike about going to AA meetings?"
    3. "It's all right to wait until you feel like going to AA meetings."
    4. "An important part of your treatment is attending AA meetings."

411. A client with a history of heavy drinking is brought to a psychiatric facility in a stupor. On the day after admission the client is confused, disoriented, and delusional. The nurse concludes that the client may be developing alcoholic:
    1. Amnesia
    2. Hallucinations
    3. Withdrawal delirium
    4. Uncomplicated dementia

412. The nurse is caring for a client who is now hospitalized in a rehabilitation unit for the third time for alcoholism. The nurse identifies that the reason some alcoholics relapse even though they attend AA meetings is that they:
    1. Need attention from family members
    2. Are trying drastically to alter a long-standing habit
    3. Physiologically require the substance in their body
    4. Often have a character defect that defeats their willpower

413. When working with a client who is in an alcohol detoxification program, it is most important for the nurse to:
    1. Support the client's need for nurturing
    2. Accept the client as a worthwhile person

3. Discuss with the client the negative effects of alcohol
4. Promote the client's compliance with the program through gentle prodding

414. What should the nurse initially plan to do to give clients with histories of long term alcohol abuse greater responsibility for maintaining sobriety?
1. Confront them about their substance abuse
2. Administer medications exactly as prescribed
3. Explain what to expect in detoxification programs
4. Assist them to adopt more healthful coping patterns

415. Two days after admission to the detoxification program, a client with a long history of alcohol abuse tells the nurse, "I don't know why I came here." What is the nurse's most therapeutic response?
1. "You feel you don't need this program?"
2. "You realize you are trying to avoid your problem."
3. "I thought you admitted yourself into the program."
4. "Don't you remember why you decided to come here?"

416. After an automobile accident, a male client is arrested for driving while intoxicated and is admitted to the hospital. When the client becomes angry and blames his family for his problems, the nurse can be most therapeutic by stating:
1. "You know you are to blame for your alcohol abuse."
2. "You need help now or you are going to get even sicker."
3. "I can see that you are upset and I want to help you feel better."
4. "I will talk to your family about their behavior if you want me to."

417. A client who is on the third day of detoxification therapy becomes agitated and restless. What are the signs and symptoms that indicate impending alcohol withdrawal delirium? Select all that apply.
1. _____ Polydipsia
2. _____ Drowsiness
3. _____ Diaphoresis
4. _____ Tachycardia
5. _____ Hypertension

418. A man has completed an alcohol detoxification program and is setting goals for rehabilitation. When setting goals it is important for this client to understand the need to:
1. Plan to avoid people who drink
2. Accept that he is a fragile person
3. Develop new social drinking skills
4. Restructure his life without alcohol

419. A 19-year-old adolescent is admitted to the emergency department with multiple fractures and potential internal injuries. The client's history reveals multiple drug abuse for the past 8 months. When caring for this client, the nurse determines that the most serious life-threatening responses during withdrawal usually result from:
1. Heroin
2. Methadone
3. Barbiturates

4. Amphetamines

420. When planning care for a client who has just completed withdrawal from multiple-drug abuse, the nurse should take into consideration that this client probably is:
1. Unable to give up drugs
2. Unconcerned with reality
3. Unable to delay gratification
4. Unaware of the danger of drug addiction

421. A 37-year-old man has been remanded by the court to the drug rehabilitation unit of a psychiatric facility for treatment of cocaine addiction. When taking his health history, what characteristics should the nurse expect the client to report? Select all that apply.
1. _____ Anxiety
2. _____ Weight loss
3. _____ Palpitations
4. _____ Sedentary habits
5. _____ Difficulties with speech

422. As a client addicted to cocaine withdraws from the drug, the nurse should expect to observe behavior related to:
1. Insomnia
2. Depression
3. Disinhibition
4. Hyperactivity

423. A school nurse is teaching a high school health class about drug abuse. What serious effect of inhaling cocaine should the nurse include?
1. Esophageal varices
2. Acute electrolyte imbalances
3. Extrapyramidal tract symptoms
4. Deterioration of the nasal passages

424. When a recently hospitalized client has a tentative diagnosis of opioid addiction, the nurse should assess the client for signs and symptoms related to opioid withdrawal. List them in the order that they will occur as the client progresses through withdrawal.
1. Runny nose
2. Muscle twitching
3. Return of appetite
4. Flulike syndromes
Answer: _____

425. After a binge with cocaine, an individual is found unconscious and is admitted to the hospital with acute cocaine toxicity. What should the initial nursing action be directed toward?
1. Being understanding
2. Maintaining a drug-free environment
3. Providing the necessary physical care
4. Establishing a therapeutic relationship

426. After a visit from several friends a nurse on the mental health unit finds a client with a known history of opioid addiction in a deep sleep and unresponsive to attempts at arousal. The nurse assesses the client's vital signs and determines that an overdose of an opioid occurred. Which findings support this conclusion?
1. Blood pressure of 70/40 mm Hg, a pulse of 120, and respirations of 10

2. Blood pressure of 120/80 mm Hg, a pulse of 84, and respirations of 20

3. Blood pressure of 140/90 mm Hg, a pulse of 76, and respirations of 28

4. Blood pressure of 180/100 mm Hg, a pulse of 72, and respirations of 18

427. A nurse working on a substance abuse unit identifies that opioids most commonly are used because the individual:

1. Desires independence

2. Attempts to reduce stress

3. Wants to fit in with the peer group

4. Enjoys the social interrelationships that occur

428. A client who is a regular user of cocaine is admitted to a rehabilitation facility. Which common side effects of regular cocaine use should the nurse expect when assessing this client?

1. Nausea, fatigue, and extreme hunger

2. Anxiety, dysphoria, and suspiciousness

3. Seizures, hoarseness, and electrolyte imbalance

4. Lethargy, sexual arousal, and hormone imbalance

429. A client with a known history of opioid addiction is treated for multiple stab wounds to the abdomen. After surgical repair the nurse notes that the client's pain is not relieved by the prescribed morphine injections. The nurse identifies that the failure to achieve pain relief indicates that the client is probably experiencing the phenomenon of:

1. Tolerance

2. Habituation

3. Physical addiction

4. Psychological dependence

430. At a staff meeting the question of a staff nurse returning to work after a drug rehabilitation program is discussed. The nurse manager helps the staff to decide that the most therapeutic way to handle the nurse's return is to:

1. Offer the nurse support in a direct, straightforward manner

2. Avoid mentioning the problem unless the nurse brings up the topic

3. Assign another staff member to keep the nurse under close observation

4. Make certain the nurse is assigned to administer only non-narcotic medications

431. It is determined that a staff nurse has a drug abuse problem. As an initial intervention the staff nurse should be:

1. Counseled by the staff psychiatrist

2. Dismissed from the job immediately

3. Referred to the employee assistance program

4. Forced to promise to abstain from drugs in the future

432. A male client with the dual diagnosis of major depression and polysubstance abuse has been attending group therapy. One day the client tells the nurse, "The things they talk about in group don't really pertain to me." What is the nurse's most therapeutic response?

1. Confront the client with realistic feedback

2. Identify the client's stress-coping tolerance

3. Inform the client that he needs to get more involved

4. Ask the client what therapy he thinks would be more helpful

433. The practitioner prescribes a diet high in vitamin B$_1$ (thiamine) for a client with a long history of alcohol abuse. The nurse evaluates that the client understands the teaching about foods high in thiamine when the client states, "I will select something for each meal from among:

1. fish, aged cheese, and breads."

2. lean beef, organ meat, and nuts."

3. poultry, milk products, and eggs."

4. green vegetables, lentils, and citrus fruits."

434. A client being admitted for alcoholism reports having had alcoholic blackouts. The nurse identifies that an alcoholic blackout is best described as:

1. Fugue state resembling absence seizures

2. Fainting spells followed by loss of memory

3. Loss of consciousness lasting less than ten minutes

4. Absence of memory in relation to drinking episodes

435. During the intake interview at a mental health clinic, a client in withdrawal reveals to the nurse long-term, high-dose cocaine use. Which signs and symptoms support the conclusion that the client has been abusing cocaine for a prolonged time? Select all that apply.

1. _____ Sadness

2. _____ Euphoria

3. _____ Loss of appetite

4. _____ Impaired judgment

5. _____ Psychomotor retardation

436. A client with a history of methamphetamine use is admitted to the medical unit. What clinical manifestation does the nurse expect when assessing the client?

1. Constricted pupils

2. Intractable diarrhea

3. Increased heart rate

4. Decreased respirations

DRUG-RELATED RESPONSES

437. A practitioner prescribes venlafaxine (Effexor) for a client with the diagnosis of major depressive disorder who has been taking herbal medications. When discussing this medication with the client, the nurse should determine if the client is taking:

1. Ginseng

2. Valerian

3. Kava-kava

4. St. John's wort

438. Methylphenidate (Ritalin) is prescribed to treat a 7-year-old child's attention-deficit–hyperactivity disorder (ADHD). The nurse considers that methylphenidate is used in the treatment of this disorder in children for its:

1. Diuretic effect

2. Synergistic effect

3. Paradoxical effect
4. Hypotensive effect

439. A practitioner prescribes alprazolam (Xanax) 0.25 mg PO three times a day for a client with anxiety and physical symptoms related to work pressures. For what most common side effect of this drug should the nurse monitor the client?
   1. Drowsiness
   2. Bradycardia
   3. Agranulocytosis
   4. Tardive dyskinesia

440. A nurse determines that after administering alprazolam (Xanax) it is important to assess the client for side effects. Initially the nurse should:
   1. Measure urinary output
   2. Monitor the blood pressure
   3. Assess for abdominal distention
   4. Check the size of the pupils frequently

441. A client's parents ask about the treatment of their son who recently was diagnosed with schizophrenia. Before responding, the nurse considers that:
   1. Electroconvulsive therapy is more effective in treating schizophrenia than mood disorders
   2. Family therapy has not proven to be effective in the treatment of clients with schizophrenia
   3. Insight therapy has proven to be highly successful in the treatment of clients with schizophrenia
   4. Drug therapy, although not eliminating the underlying problem, reduces the symptoms of acute schizophrenia

442. A young adult being treated for substance abuse asks the nurse about methadone. The nurse responds that methadone is useful in the treatment of opioid addiction because it:
   1. Is a nonaddictive drug
   2. Has an effect of longer duration
   3. Does not produce a cumulative effect
   4. Carries little risk of psychological dependence

443. A client is started on chlorpromazine (Thorazine). To prevent life-threatening complications from the administration of this medication to an anxious, restless client, it is important that the nurse:
   1. Provide adequate restraint
   2. Monitor the client's vital signs
   3. Protect against exposure to direct sunlight
   4. Watch the client for extrapyramidal side effects

444. On the psychiatric unit, a client has been receiving high doses of haloperidol (Haldol) for 2 weeks. The client states, "I just can't sit still and I feel jittery." Which side effect does the nurse suspect that the client may be experiencing?
   1. Akathisia
   2. Torticollis
   3. Tardive dyskinesia
   4. Parkinsonian syndrome

445. In addition to hydration during alcohol withdrawal delirium, parenteral administration of lorazepam (Ativan) is prescribed for a client. The nurse identifies that this drug is given during detoxification primarily to:
   1. Prevent injury when seizures occur
   2. Enable the client to sleep better during periods of agitation
   3. Reduce the anxiety-tremor state and prevent more serious withdrawal symptoms
   4. Quiet the client and encourage cooperation by promoting acceptance of the treatment plan

446. A practitioner prescribes routine lithium levels to be performed. How many hours after the last dose of lithium should the nurse plan to obtain the blood specimen?
   1. 2 to 4
   2. 4 to 6
   3. 6 to 8
   4. 8 to 12

447. A client has been receiving lithium carbonate (Eskalith) for 3 days. The nurse checks the client's lithium level before administering the medication and finds it to be 0.3 mEq/L. The nurse should:
   1. Notify the practitioner
   2. Administer the medication
   3. Observe for adverse side effects
   4. Withhold the next dose of the medication

448. A depressed client is receiving paroxetine (Paxil). The nurse monitors this client for the side effects associated with this drug. Select all that apply.
   1. _____ Sexual dysfunction
   2. _____ Depressed respirations
   3. _____ Insomnia and restlessness
   4. _____ Hypertension or hypotension
   5. _____ Irregular menses or secondary amenorrhea

449. A client has recently been receiving a new neuroleptic drug and the nurse observes extrapyramidal effects. Which drug does the nurse anticipate will be prescribed to limit these side effects?
   1. Zolpidem (Ambien)
   2. HydrOXYzine (Vistaril)
   3. Dantrolene (Dantrium)
   4. Benztropine mesylate (Cogentin)

450. A nurse identifies that haloperidol (Haldol) is most effective for clients who exhibit behavior that is:
   1. Depressed
   2. Overactive
   3. Withdrawn
   4. Manipulative

451. A client who is taking lithium arrives at the mental health center for a routine visit. The client has slurred speech, has an ataxic gait, and complains of nausea. The nurse identifies that these signs and symptoms are:
   1. Related to low lithium levels
   2. Associated with cyclic mood disorders
   3. Often related to therapeutic lithium levels
   4. Probably associated with toxic levels of lithium

452. A client is admitted to the emergency department after ingesting a tricyclic antidepressant in an amount that is

30 times the daily recommended dose. What is the immediate treatment the nurse anticipates?

1. Administration of physostigmine as soon as possible
2. Closer monitoring to prevent further suicidal attempts
3. Gastric lavage with activated charcoal while supporting physiological functioning
4. Intravenous administration of an anticholinergic in response to changes in vital signs

453. A noncompliant, suspicious client with schizophrenia lives with an aging mother and attends an outreach group. The nurse concludes that the medication most appropriate for this client is:

1. Imipramine (Tofranil)
2. Isocarboxazid (Marplan)
3. Fluphenazine hydrochloride (Prolixin)
4. Fluphenazine decanoate (Prolixin Decanoate)

454. A client is started on fluphenazine decanoate (Prolixin Decanoate). What should the nurse emphasize when teaching the client about taking this medication?

1. Driving is forbidden
2. There will be a feeling of increased energy
3. Sunscreen should be used for outdoor activities
4. High blood pressure indirectly will be controlled

455. A client is brought by ambulance to the emergency department. The client's signs and symptoms are associated with opioid overdose. What should the nurse expect the practitioner to prescribe?

1. Naloxone
2. Methadone
3. Epinephrine
4. Amphetamine

456. The nurse should teach a client receiving isocarboxazid (Marplan) that failure to adhere to the dietary restrictions can result in:

1. Syncope
2. Bradycardia
3. Hypertensive crisis
4. Hyperglycemic episodes

457. A nurse is performing discharge teaching for a client who has been receiving disulfiram (Antabuse). What statement indicates to the nurse that the client understands the teaching concerning disulfuram?

1. "I must be careful to check over-the-counter medications."
2. "I can never take this medication at the same time as an antibiotic."
3. "I will not be able to eat aged cheeses while taking this medication."
4. "I should wait at least eight hours after taking this pill before drinking alcohol."

458. A client who is going to be discharged has been receiving risperidone (Risperdal) 3 mg three times a day. The nurse should teach the client that the medication:

1. Can be reduced if the client feels better at home
2. Can be discontinued after the client is discharged
3. May cause sedation if taken concurrently with alcohol
4. Should be taken early in the day to be sure they are not forgotten

459. A depressed client is started on citalopram hydrobromide (Celexa). Six days later the client tearfully comments to the nurse, "I'm taking an antidepressant but it is not working. I am hopeless." The most therapeutic response by the nurse is:

1. "You feel hopeless."
2. "It's easy to get discouraged."
3. "It takes about 2 to 3 weeks before it begins to relieve depression."
4. "Give it a little more time because it works more slowly in some people."

460. When talking with a client who has been receiving paroxetine (Paxil), the nurse identifies that more clarification is needed when the client states:

1. "I will be a little drowsy in the mornings."
2. "I'm expecting to feel somewhat better but I may need other therapy."
3. "I've been on the medication for 8 days now and I don't feel any better."
4. "I know I will probably have to take this medication for several months."

461. A client has been taking amoxapine (Asendin) for the past 3 months with no improvement. The practitioner prescribes phenelzine (Nardil) to be given additionally. The nurse should:

1. Question the prescription and withhold the medication
2. Ask the client about allergies to feathers before giving the first dose
3. Withhold the medication until a specimen for liver enzymes is drawn
4. Remind the client this medication should be taken with meals and milk products must be avoided

462. The practitioner prescribes a tricyclic antidepressant medication to decrease a suicidal client's depression. What factor should the nurse consider when initiating treatment with this type of medication?

1. Eating aged cheese may cause a hypertensive crisis
2. There may not be a noticeable improvement for 2 to 3 weeks
3. They must be given with milk to avoid gastrointestinal irritation
4. Blood specimens are required weekly for 3 months to check for therapeutic drug levels

463. A client has become increasingly depressed, and the practitioner prescribes an antidepressant. After 20 days of therapy, the client returns to the clinic. The client appears relaxed and smiles at the nurse. The most significant conclusion the nurse can draw from this behavior is that the client:

1. Wants to please the staff
2. Has resolved her conflicts
3. May be in denial of her problems
4. Is responding to the antidepressant therapy

464. A client is extremely depressed, and the practitioner prescribes a tricyclic antidepressant, imipramine

(Tofranil). The client asks the nurse what the medication will do. The nurse responds, "This medication will help:

1. "you forget why you are depressed."
2. "keep you alert and cure your insomnia."
3. "you feel better after taking it for several days."
4. "increase your appetite and make you feel better."

465. A client with an organic mental disorder becomes increasingly agitated and abusive. The practitioner prescribes haloperidol (Haldol). For what untoward effects should the nurse assess the client?
1. Jaundice and vomiting
2. Tardive dyskinesia and nausea
3. Parkinsonism and agranulocytosis
4. Hiccups and postural hypotension

466. A client with schizophrenia is given an antipsychotic drug. The nurse considers that of all the extrapyramidal effects associated with this type of medication, the one that requires the discontinuation of the drug is:
1. Akathisia
2. Tardive dyskinesia
3. Parkinsonian syndrome
4. Acute dystonic reaction

467. A client with the diagnosis of schizophrenia, paranoid type, has been receiving a phenothiazine drug. The day care center is planning a fishing trip. It is important that the nurse:
1. Provide the client with a sun screen ointment
2. Caution the client to limit exertion during the trip
3. Give the client an extra dose of medication to take after lunch
4. Take the client's blood pressure before allowing participation in the outing

468. A client with schizophrenia, undifferentiated type, is receiving a typical antipsychotic/neuroleptic. For which extrapyramidal effects should the nurse be alert?
1. Shuffling gait, tremors, and restlessness
2. Nausea, vomiting, and muscular cramps
3. Drowsiness, disorientation, and slurred speech
4. Tachycardia, urinary retention, and constipation

469. A practitioner prescribes haloperidol (Haldol) 10 mg PO twice a day for a client who is also receiving phenytoin (Dilantin) for control of epilepsy. When planning the client's care, the nurse considers that anticonvulsants may interact with haloperidol to:
1. Mask its therapeutic effect
2. Interfere with its absorption
3. Enhance its rate of metabolism
4. Potentiate its central nervous system depressant effect

470. Bupropion (Wellbutrin) has a unique side effect not shared by most other drugs of its class. The nurse should assess the client for which unique possible side effect of this drug?
1. Heart failure
2. Breast tumors
3. Tardive dyskinesia
4. Generalized seizures

471. A client has a bipolar disorder for which the practitioner prescribes a mood-stabilizing medication. The nurse completes a teaching session with a client concerning the medical regimen. Which client comment indicates to the nurse that further teaching is needed?
1. "I know I won't have to stay on this medication for too long."
2. "I realize that I will need to keep in touch with my physician."
3. "Taking medication without using other forms of therapy may not be as effective."
4. "Taking the medication is better than experiencing the highs and lows I have been having."

472. The nurse is teaching a client who is receiving an MAO inhibitor about dietary restrictions. Considering this drug, the nurse plans to caution the client to avoid:
1. Pork, spinach, and fresh oysters
2. Milk, grapes, and meat tenderizers
3. Cheese, beer, and products with chocolate
4. Leafy green vegetables, fresh apples, and ice cream

473. A client is receiving haloperidol (Haldol) for agitation, and the nurse is monitoring the client for side effects. Which response identified by the nurse is unrelated to an extrapyramidal tract effect?
1. Akathisia
2. Opisthotonos
3. Oculogyric crisis
4. Hypertensive crisis

474. A nurse considers that the blocking of dopamine by antipsychotic drugs can cause extrapyramidal side effects such as akathisia. Which client behaviors reflect the presence of akathisia?
1. Acute muscle spasms and torticollis
2. Bizarre facial and tongue movements
3. Motor restlessness, foot tapping, and pacing
4. Tremor, shuffling gait, drooling, and rigidity

475. A client who has schizophrenia is receiving a phenothiazine antipsychotic medication. Which serious client responses to the medication should the nurse immediately report to the practitioner? Select all that apply.
1. _____ Akathisia
2. _____ Shuffling gait
3. _____ Yellow sclerae
4. _____ Photosensitivity
5. _____ Involuntary tongue movements

476. A nurse is caring for a client with the diagnosis of schizophrenia who is started on fluphenazine decanoate (Prolixin Decanoate). What is the primary advantage of this medication?
1. There are no side effects
2. It has a long-lasting effect
3. It is safe to use during pregnancy
4. There is less need for laboratory monitoring

477. A client with schizophrenia, who is receiving an antipsychotic medication, develops a shuffling gate and tremors. The practitioner prescribes the anticholinergic medication benztropine (Cogentin) 2 mg daily. What

should the nurse assess the client for daily when administering these medications together?
1. Constipation
2. Hypertension
3. Increased salivation
4. Excessive perspiration

478. A client receiving the medication buspirone hydrochloride (BuSpar) is admitted to the hospital with the diagnosis of possible hepatitis. The nurse identifies that the client's sclerae look yellow. What should be the nurse's initial action?
1. Withhold the medication
2. Give the BuSpar with milk
3. Reduce the dosage of the medication
4. Ensure that the medication can be given parenterally

479. A client has been taking the prescribed dose of clozapine (Clozaril). The nurse should assess the client for which life-threatening side effect of this drug?
1. Polycythemia
2. Agranulocytosis
3. Hypertensive crisis
4. Pseudoparkinsonism

480. A nurse on a mental health unit administers a variety of antipsychotic medications. The nurse concludes that olanzapine (Zyprexa Zydis) has a distinct advantage over other antipsychotics because:
1. Extrapyramidal symptoms do not occur
2. Drug effects last weeks after administration
3. Dopamine is increased at receptor sites, decreasing psychotic behavior
4. Tablets disintegrate immediately in the mouth preventing tablet "cheeking"

481. A practitioner plans to have a client with the diagnosis of bipolar disorder continue taking lithium after discharge. The nurse identifies that the teaching about the medication plan is understood when the client states, "I know that this medication:
1. should be stopped if illness is suspected."
2. may need to be taken for the rest of my life."
3. causes no serious side effects when taken correctly."
4. will require me to increase the dosage at the beginning of a manic episode."

482. A client is receiving imipramine (Tofranil), a tricyclic antidepressant, for depression. The nurse assesses the client for side effects and adverse effects. Which adverse effect requires further assessment and possible medical intervention?
1. Dry mouth
2. Weight gain
3. Blurred vision
4. Urinary hesitancy

483. An antianxiety medication is prescribed for an extremely anxious client. The client states, "I'm afraid to take these pills because I heard they're addictive." The nurse teaches the client that antianxiety medications:
1. Rarely cause dependence when the dosage is controlled
2. May require increased dosages but rarely cause dependence

3. Usually result in psychologic but not physiologic dependence
4. Have the potential for physiologic and psychologic dependence

484. A client is prescribed a monoamine oxidase inhibitor. The nurse teaches the client about what foods to avoid when taking this medication. Select all that apply.
1. _____ Fresh fish
2. _____ Citrus fruits
3. _____ Aged cheese
4. _____ Ripe avocados
5. _____ Delicatessen meats

485. A client is prescribed sertraline (Zoloft), an antidepressant. What should the nurse include when preparing a teaching plan about the side effects of this drug?
1. Seizures
2. Agitation
3. Tachycardia
4. Agranulocytosis

486. A neuromuscular blocking agent is administered to a client before ECT therapy. At this time, the nurse should monitor the client for:
1. Seizures
2. Vomiting
3. Loss of memory
4. Respiratory difficulties

487. Considering the anticholinergic-like side effects of many of the psychotropic drugs, the nurse should encourage clients taking these drugs to:
1. Restrict their fluid intake
2. Eat a diet high in carbohydrates
3. Suck on sugar-free hard candies
4. Avoid products that contain aspirin

488. A client who has been taking the prescribed dose of zolpidem (Ambien) for 5 days returns to the clinic for a follow-up visit. When interviewing the client, the nurse identifies that the medication has been effective when the client says:
1. "I have less pain."
2. "I have been sleeping better."
3. "My blood glucose is under control."
4. "My blood pressure is coming down."

489. A nurse is administering hydrOXYzine (Vistaril) to a client. For which common side effects of this drug should the nurse monitor the client?
1. Ataxia and confusion
2. Drowsiness and dry mouth
3. Vertigo and impaired vision
4. Slurred speech and headache

490. The psychiatrist is concerned that one of the clients receiving haloperidol (Haldol) may be developing neuroleptic malignant syndrome. When assessing for this syndrome, for which clinical manifestations should the nurse monitor the client?
1. Jaundice and malaise
2. Tremors and seizures
3. Diaphoresis and hyperpyrexia
4. Dry skin and hyperbilirubinemia

491. A client is receiving an antipsychotic medication. When assessing for signs and symptoms of pseudoparkinsonism, the nurse should monitor the client for:
1. Drooling
2. Blurred vision
3. Muscle tremors
4. Photosensitivity

492. A client with a family history of diabetes is concerned about the effects of psychiatric medication on the endocrine system. Which psychotropic medication is most likely to cause metabolic syndrome?
1. Lithium (Carbolith)
2. Diazepam (Valium)
3. Alprazolam (Xanax)
4. Risperidone (Risperdal)

493. Naltrexone (Depade) is used to treat clients with substance abuse problems. In which situation does the nurse anticipate naltrexone to be administered?
1. Treat opioid overdose
2. Block the systemic effects of cocaine
3. Decrease the recovering alcoholic's desire to drink alcohol
4. Prevent severe withdrawal symptoms from antianxiety agents

494. A client asks the nurse how psychotropic medications work. The nurse should reply, "These medications:
1. decrease the metabolic needs of your brain."
2. increase the production of healthy nervous tissue."
3. affect the chemicals used in communication between nerve cells."
4. regulate the sensory input received from the external environment."

495. A male client who is taking clozapine (Clozaril) is seen by the nurse in the outpatient mental health clinic. The nurse interviews the client, sends a venous blood specimen to the laboratory, obtains the vital signs, and finally reviews all the collected information. Which complication associated with clozapine does the nurse suspect the client is experiencing?
1. Anemia
2. Agranulocytosis
3. Orthostatic hypotension
4. Neuroleptic malignant syndrome

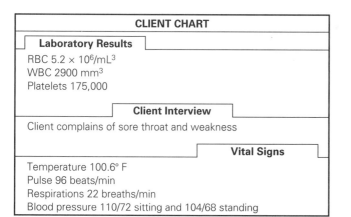

CLIENT CHART

Laboratory Results
RBC $5.2 \times 10^6/\text{mL}^3$
WBC 2900 mm^3
Platelets 175,000

Client Interview
Client complains of sore throat and weakness

Vital Signs
Temperature 100.6° F
Pulse 96 beats/min
Respirations 22 breaths/min
Blood pressure 110/72 sitting and 104/68 standing

496. A client with schizophrenia becomes severely agitated and the nurse is concerned for the safety of the client, other clients, and the nursing team. The practitioner prescribes haloperidol (Haldol) 2.5 mg IM stat. The vial of haloperidol states that each mL is equal to 5 mg. How much solution should the nurse administer?
Answer: _____ mL

497. The practitioner prescribes valproic acid (Depakene) 750 mg daily to be administered in 2 equally spaced doses. The medication is supplied as a syrup of 250 mg/5 mL. How much solution should the nurse administer per dose?
Answer: _____ mL

498. The practitioner prescribes methylphenidate (Ritalin) for a 7-year-old child recently diagnosed with ADHD. The prescription states, methylphenidate 10 mg PO once in the morning for 1 week and then 15 mg PO once in the morning for the second week. The medication is supplied as an oral solution of 5 mg/1 mL. How much solution should the nurse teach the child's mother to administer during the second week of therapy?
Answer: _____ mL

499. A young adult with a history of mental retardation and tonic-clonic seizures is admitted to a group home. Among the client's medications is an order for phenytoin (Dilantin) 125 mg PO three times a day. Phenytoin is supplied as an oral suspension of 25 mg/5 mL. How much solution should the nurse administer for each dose?
Answer: _____ mL

500. A client who has been taking a conventional antipsychotic for several days comes to the clinic complaining of neck spasms. The picture illustrates the client's physical status observed by the nurse. What extrapyramidal side effect has the client developed?

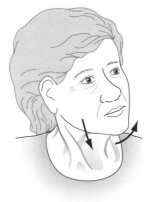

1. Torticollis
2. Tardive dyskinesia
3. Pseudoparkinsonism
4. Neuroleptic malignant syndrome

Additional review questions can be found on the enclosed companion CD.

MENTAL HEALTH NURSING
ANSWERS AND RATIONALES

NURSING PRACTICE

1. **2 Keeping the nursing staff informed indicates that housekeeping members are part of the health team and their input is valued; this will help keep lines of communication open.**
   1 This is not the responsibility of the housekeeping staff. Disregarding input from members of the health team does not promote collaboration.
   3 Client behaviors should never be disregarded. The housekeeping staff should notify a nursing team member if this behavior happens again.
   4 This type of record keeping is not the responsibility of the housekeeping staff.

2. **4 Expected outcomes are the desirable projected responses to therapeutic interventions that consider the client's present and potential capabilities; they are measurable and realistic.**
   1 Expected outcomes can be either short-term or long-term, not only long term.
   2 Variances occur when a client's response to interventions is different from what usually is expected.
   3 Expected client outcomes are a component of a clinical pathway; a clinical pathway is a written standardized process that identifies projected provider behaviors and interventions and expected client outcomes based on the client's diagnosis.

3. **4 Clients cannot select the members of the health care team when admitted to an inpatient setting that delivers care 24 hours a day 7 days a week.**
   1 This is included in the Client Bill of Rights.
   2 This is included in the Client Bill of Rights.
   3 This is included in the Client Bill of Rights.

4. **3 Autonomy is the ethical principle that respects the independence and self-determination of others. In this situation the nurse focuses on helping the client make a choice.**
   1 Justice is the ethical principle that requires all people to be treated fairly, regardless of gender, age, religion, diagnosis, marital status, or socioeconomic level.
   2 Veracity is the ethical principle that requires truthfulness.
   4 Beneficence is the duty to do good and promote the welfare of others.

5. **1 It is the responsibility of the psychiatrist, who is the primary care provider, to discuss the test results with the mother.**
   2 This is beyond the scope of the nurse's role.
   3 The mother should be referred to the psychiatrist, not the psychologist, because the psychiatrist is the leader of this health team.

4 Teaching about the tests should have been done before, not after, the tests were administered.

6. **2 Talking with colleagues who face or who have faced the same problems may provide constructive help with the situation.**
   1 This is an avoidance technique; feelings must be addressed.
   3 This does not address the needs of the nurse and may interfere with a productive nurse-client relationship.
   4 This does not address the needs of the nurse and may interfere with a productive nurse-client relationship.

7. **1 The client freely discussed her sexual history; it is necessary to document that she has been previously sexually active and the date of her last menstrual period. Documenting details of her past sexual activity is a violation of her rights.**
   2 Chief complaints and verbatim statements about the assault should be documented.
   3 It is essential that physical trauma be noted on a body map or by photographs when permission is granted.
   4 These are essential data that should be recorded on the medical record.

8. **3 An understanding and supportive approach to a colleague with burnout allows the individual to identify the problem; this intervention points out behavior.**
   1 This interferes with self-identification of the problem; also, the individual may get defensive.
   2 This is trying to solve a problem before the individual has an opportunity to share feelings or identify the problem.
   4 This is an accusatory approach and does not give the individual an opportunity to address the overtime or to express feelings.

9. **3 The type of care needed by the client requires trust in the caregiver, which develops more rapidly when there is a cooperative relationship.**
   1 Limiting staff time may place the client in jeopardy.
   2 The staff should not be put in the position of punishing the client; the client with dementia cannot be held responsible for uncooperative behavior.
   4 Clients with moderate dementia will not remember and learn from a reward system.

10. **2 When the nurse and client agree to work together, a contract should be established, and the length of the relationship should be discussed in terms of its ultimate termination.**
   1 The client may discuss termination during the working phase; however, the subject should initially be discussed during the orientation phase.
   3 Termination and discharge plans may be discussed more thoroughly during this phase, but the subject initially should be discussed during the orientation phase.

4 Termination and discharge plans may be discussed more thoroughly during this phase, but the subject initially should be discussed during the orientation phase.

11. **4 This will ensure that a thorough assessment of the family's needs is made and the appropriate assistance initiated.**

1 This is inadequate; in addition, household objects can serve as well as store-bought toys.

2 This can frighten the client and precipitate feelings of guilt.

3 This is premature and may or may not be necessary.

12. **1 Assessment is the first step of the nursing process and must be done before planning care.**

2 Nursing interventions follow assessment; high levels of anxiety interfere with interactions.

3 This technique may be used once the anxiety is reduced; assessment is the priority at this time.

4 This technique may be used once the anxiety is reduced; assessment is the priority at this time.

13. **2 Evaluation includes assessing the client's response to care, judging the effectiveness of the plan of care, and changing the plan as necessary.**

1 Planning includes the development of a plan that focuses on specific goals and actions unique to the client's needs.

3 Assessing entails collecting and reviewing objective and subjective data about the client's health status.

4 Implementation includes performing specific actions designed to achieve the stated goals.

14. **4 This verifies family and practitioner agreement and uses institutional policy developed by the ethics committee.**

1 The nurse should not accept this inappropriate order.

2 Neither the nurse nor the nursing supervisor should accept this inappropriate order.

3 The order must be in ink on the written record.

15. **1 Primary prevention is directed toward health promotion and prevention of problems.**

2 Tertiary prevention is focused on rehabilitation and the reduction of residual effects of illness.

3 Secondary prevention is related to early detection and treatment of problems.

4 There is no category of prevention called therapeutic prevention.

16. **4 To confront burnout, the individual must first identify stressors, coping strategies used, and effectiveness of these strategies.**

1 This may help, but prevention begins with knowing oneself and the effectiveness of one's coping strategies.

2 This may help prevent burnout, but it is not the first step in confronting the problem after it occurs.

3 This may help prevent burnout, but it is not the first step in confronting the problem after it occurs.

PERSONALITY DEVELOPMENT

17. **3 Displacement reduces anxiety by transferring the emotions associated with an object or person to another emotionally safer object or person.**

1 Projection is the attempt to deal with unacceptable feelings by attributing them to another.

2 Dissociation is an attempt by the person to detach emotional involvement or the self from an interaction or the environment.

4 Intellectualization is the use of facts or other logical reasoning rather than feelings to deal with the emotional effect of a problem; this is a form of denial.

18. **4 The nurse is using facts and knowledge to detach the self from the emotional effect of the client's problem and decrease the anxiety it is causing.**

1 Substitution is similar to displacement; this reduces anxiety by transferring the emotions associated with an object or person to another safer object or person.

2 Sublimation is the channeling of unacceptable thoughts or feelings into acceptable activity.

3 Identification is the unconscious imitation of the behavior of another, who is considered important, in an attempt to incorporate this important other into the self.

19. **1 Without the development of trust, the child has little confidence that the significant other will return; separation is considered abandonment by the child.**

2 Without identity, the individual will have a problem forming a social role and a sense of self; this results in identity diffusion and confusion.

3 Without initiative, the individual will experience the development of guilt and feelings of inadequacy.

4 Without autonomy, the individual has little self-confidence, develops a deep sense of shame and doubt, and learns to expect defeat.

20. **1 This is the developmental conflict that faces the preschool child; the child will feel guilty if initiative is stifled by others.**

2 This is the conflict of the school-age child.

3 This is not a developmental conflict identified by Erikson.

4 This is not a developmental conflict identified by Erikson.

21. **2 Major tasks of young adulthood are centered on human closeness and sexual fulfillment; lack of love results in isolation.**

1 This stage is associated with infancy.

3 This stage is associated with middle childhood.

4 This stage is associated with middle adulthood.

22. **2 Projection is the process of attributing one's own thoughts about one's self to others.**

1 Denial involves pushing out of awareness one's own thoughts, wishes, or feelings that are unacceptable to one's own self.

3 Introjection is the process of taking in someone else's values, beliefs, attitudes, or qualities.

4 Sublimation is the process of substituting a socially acceptable activity for one that is less so.

23. 2 **This is the task of the older adult; the client has difficulty accepting what life is and was; this results in feelings of despair and disgust.**

1 This is the task of the preschool child.

3 This is the task of the young adult.

4 This is the task of the adolescent.

24. 2 **This action will not call attention to the accident and will minimize the child's embarrassment.**

1 The child probably will be unable to accomplish this task without assistance; failure to complete the task can add to embarrassment.

3 This will add to the child's embarrassment.

4 This will add to the child's embarrassment.

25. 3 **Adolescence is a time of great upheaval and maturation. Before this maturational process is completed, adolescents act without thinking things through and are more concerned with their own needs, rather than the needs of others.**

1 The rapid and complex biological, social, and emotional changes during adolescence do not necessarily lead to these psychological responses.

2 The rapid and complex biological, social, and emotional changes during adolescence do not necessarily lead to these psychological responses.

4 The rapid and complex biological, social, and emotional changes during adolescence do not necessarily lead to these psychological responses.

26. 2 **According to Erikson, adolescents are struggling with identity vs. role confusion.**

1 This reflects part of the struggle for independence; it does not indicate failure to resolve the conflicts of adolescence.

3 Adolescents tend to be group oriented, not isolated; they struggle to belong, not to escape.

4 Adolescents may experiment with drug and alcohol use, but most of them do not become abusers.

27. 1 **Adolescents learn about who they are by assuming and experiencing a variety of roles; experimentation results in the retention or rejection of behavior and roles.**

2 This is not constructive; this does not allow for experimentation with a variety of roles.

3 Sublimation is not constructive and delays and interferes with the successful completion of the struggle to formulate one's identity.

4 This is not constructive; it does not allow for the development of independence.

28. 3 **This action fosters the development of an improved self-esteem.**

1 A problem does exist; their child is overeating.

2 Parents cannot avoid talking about the sibling, but should avoid any comparisons.

4 The child already is doing this, and it has diminished her self-esteem.

29. 3 **This is an achievable action that involves a personal goal; also it should bolster the adolescent's self-esteem.**

1 This may not improve the adolescent's self-esteem.

2 This may not improve the adolescent's self-esteem.

4 This may not improve the adolescent's self-esteem.

30. 3 **Compensation is replacing a weak area or trait with a more desirable one.**

1 Sublimation is rechanneling unacceptable desires and drives into those that are socially acceptable.

2 Transference is the unconscious tendency to assign to others in the present environment feelings and attitudes associated with another person.

4 Rationalization is the use of justification to make tolerable certain feelings, behaviors, and motives.

31. 4 **This demonstrates a movement toward peer group activity and interests; exercise demonstrates an interest in an improved physical condition.**

1 There are no data to indicate that school is a problem.

2 This does not demonstrate an increase in self-esteem.

3 This does not demonstrate an increase in self-esteem.

32. 3 **Erikson theorized that how well people adapt to the present stage depends on how well they adapted to the stage immediately preceding it, in this instance adulthood.**

1 This is the task of an earlier stage of development. Although Erikson believed that the strengths and weaknesses of each stage are present in some form in all succeeding stages, their influence decreases with time.

2 This is the task of an earlier stage of development. Although Erikson believed that the strengths and weaknesses of each stage are present in some form in all succeeding stages, their influence decreases with time.

4 This is the task of an earlier stage of development. Although Erikson believed that the strengths and weaknesses of each stage are present in some form in all succeeding stages, their influence decreases with time.

33. 4 **This encourages the client to accept what life is or was and helps avoid feelings of despair.**

1 Although this may be done by many older adults, it is not the task associated with Erikson's theory concerning older adults.

2 According to Erikson's developmental theory, this is the task of young adults.

3 This desire must come from the client.

34. 4 **The individual who can reflect back on life and accept it for what it was and is and who can adjust to and enjoy the changes retirement brings is**

less likely to develop health problems, especially stress-related health problems.

1 These changes may not be reversible.

2 Most emotionally healthy older individuals do not focus on these thoughts.

3 Dependency is often threatening to this age group.

35. 3 **An individual's ability to handle stress develops through experience with life; aging does not reduce this ability but often strengthens it.**

1 The senses of taste and/or smell are often diminished in the older individual.

2 Muscle or motor strength is diminished in the older individual.

4 Short-term memory is diminished in the older individual, while long-term memory remains strong.

36. 1 **Isolation is the separation of thought or memory from feeling.**

2 Splitting is the polarizing of positive and negative feelings.

3 Introjection is integrating the beliefs and values of another into one's own ego.

4 Compensation is making up for a real or imagined lack in one area by overemphasizing another.

THERAPEUTIC RELATIONSHIPS

37. 2 **Family therapy views the whole (Gestalt) within the context in which the emotional problems are occurring.**

1 Efficiency is not an adequate rationale for choosing this therapeutic approach.

3 This may or may not be true; an astute nurse can control manipulation and alliance within any group.

4 Promotion of truthfulness is a secondary gain achieved through this mode of therapy.

38. 1 **The client is in the anger or "why me" stage of grieving; encouraging the client to express feelings will help resolve them while moving toward acceptance.**

2 This is a judgmental response that may create a rift in the nurse-client relationship.

3 Suggesting that the client speak with a religious leader may precipitate guilt feelings and ignores the present concern.

4 This response does not reflect what the client said; people who are newly diagnosed with a chronic illness grieve for their loss of health.

39. 3 **If religious beliefs are a family concern, then the nurse should allow discussion of the family's thoughts and feelings on the subject.**

1 If religion is a family concern, its discussion should be encouraged, not limited.

2 The role of the nurse is to facilitate and listen, not to have a mutual discussion about religious beliefs.

4 The religious leader is not part of the family unit and can be invited only if requested by the family.

40. 1 **In behavior modification, positive behavior is reinforced and negative behavior is not reinforced or punished.**

2 This may be a part of the program, but it is not a major component.

3 This may be a part of the program, but it is not a major component.

4 This may be a part of the program, but it is not a major component.

41. 1 **Before therapy can begin, a trusting relationship must develop.**

2 A client with major depression does not have the impetus or energy to investigate new leisure activities.

3 This is not appropriate initially; a trusting one-to-one relationship must be developed first.

4 This will not be successful unless the client has developed a trusting, comfortable relationship with the nurse.

42. 1 **This response changes the subject; it is better to continue discussing the same subject.**

2 This is an acceptable response because it focuses on the client's implied feelings.

3 This is a therapeutic response because it asks the client to clarify and elaborate.

4 This is a therapeutic response because it asks the client to focus on more specific details.

43. 4 **Evaluation and termination are the foci of a discharge planning conference; it is important for the nurse to assist the family in viewing the hospitalization as a learning experience.**

1 This should have been done before the discharge conference, where evaluation and future planning are the foci.

2 This should have been done before the discharge conference, where evaluation and future planning are the foci.

3 This should have been done before the discharge conference, where evaluation and future planning are the foci.

44. 1 **Empathy is the projection of self into another's emotions to share the emotions and the other's state of mind; this technique helps the nurse understand the meaning and significance of the experience to the client.**

2 Sympathy is a shared expression of sorrow over a real or imagined loss.

3 Projection is an unconscious defense mechanism, not a therapeutic technique.

4 This does not require the nurse to project the self into the client's emotions but rather to accept the client and the emotions.

45. 3 **Focusing is indicated when communication is vague; the nurse attempts to concentrate or focus the client's communication on one specific aspect.**

1 Touch invades the client's space and will not help focus the client's communication.

2 Silence prolongs the rambling communication; the client needs to be focused.

4 Until the concern is identified and explored, summarizing is impossible.

46. 2 **This demonstrates that the nurse believes that what the client has to say is important; also, this encourages verbalization of feelings.**

1 This may increase feelings of worthlessness and persecution.

3 This will accomplish little; individuals cannot be talked out of feelings.

4 These are feelings, not information, and they cannot always be explained; this forces the client to further develop the delusional system.

47. 1 **Silence is a tool employed during therapeutic communication that indicates that the nurse is listening and receptive; it allows the client time to collect thoughts, gain control of emotions, or speak without hurrying.**

2 Silence should be comfortable and should not create pressure to talk.

3 Clients should feel that they have an opportunity to think about the interaction.

4 This will close communication.

48. 4 **This lets the client know the nurse is trying to understand; it increases the client's feeling of self-esteem and points out reality.**

1 Clients with schizophrenia have problems with associative links, and these same problems will occur regardless of the topic.

2 This statement cuts off communication and tells the client that the nurse will speak only if the client's communication makes sense.

3 This statement cuts off communication and tells the client that the nurse will speak only if the client's communication makes sense.

49. 4 **This response reflects the feelings being expressed at this time.**

1 Although this can be interpreted as an empathic response, it does not focus on the mother's major concern.

2 This avoids the issue; the fear may be that next time control may be lost and abuse may occur.

3 This does not address the real concern; the mother's argument may have been justified and the daughter's behavior should not be rewarded.

50. 1 **Recognizing the spouse's feelings and giving simple factual information help to allay anxiety.**

2 This discourages further verbalization of concerns and promotes feelings of isolation and helplessness.

3 This is an inappropriate statement, especially during this time of stress; it also gives little assurance to the client's spouse.

4 This is false reassurance and does not allow the spouse to verbalize anxieties or fears.

51. 4 **This statement addresses the reality that the client is on the mental health unit and offers assistance.**

1 On the basis of the information available, it is too early to make this decision.

2 This is a hostile statement that assumes the client is unable to follow the conversation.

3 This statement assumes the client is disoriented as to place; it sounds like the beginning of a lecture.

52. 4 **This response addresses the client's misconceptions about mental health services and the specific fear of being "crazy."**

1 This response ignores the feeling tones behind the client's statement and focuses on facts.

2 This response ignores the feeling tones behind the client's statement and focuses on facts.

3 This response ignores the feeling tones behind the client's statement and focuses on facts.

53. 4 **This response is optimistic and supportive and clarifies the purpose of the relationship.**

1 This statement diminishes the client's response and sets up a challenge; it does not foster a therapeutic relationship.

2 This statement diminishes the client's response and sets up a challenge; it does not foster a therapeutic relationship.

3 This statement diminishes the client's response and sets up a challenge; it does not foster a therapeutic relationship.

54. 2 **Unless the nurse answers the question, the client will continue to focus on the nurse rather than on the self; the nurse can best redirect after a brief answer.**

1 This moves the focus to the nurse's opinions rather than the client's feelings.

3 This moves the focus to the nurse's opinions rather than the client's feelings

4 This is not therapeutic; the client is being asked to share, and the nurse should also be willing to share.

55. 1 **Neurologic responses are slowed because of reduced sensory-receptor sensitivity.**

2 Excluding pathological processes, the personality will be consistent with that of earlier years.

3 There is no loss of intellectual ability unless there is a pathological problem.

4 Short-term, not long-term, memory is reduced because of a shortened attention span, delayed transmission of information to the brain, and perceptual deficits.

56. 1 **This response recognizes problems of the caregiver without a hint of blame for the admission; it opens the channel of communication.**

2 This response avoids the caregiver's concerns.

3 This is a hostile response that will place the caregiver on the defensive.

4 This is a hostile response that will place the caregiver on the defensive.

57. 1 **This response identifies the child's feelings and lets the child know the nurse understands them.**

2 This is an unrealistic response; the child probably is unable to express his feelings to peers; also, there is no way of predicting how his peers will respond.

3 This denies the child's feelings and offers little support.

4 This is unrealistic and the nurse cannot be sure that the child will lose weight or if weight loss will improve the child's athletic ability.

58. 4 **Commenting on the silence encourages exploration of what is happening in the group and the members' thoughts and feelings about it.**

1 Waiting indefinitely can result in increased anxiety and a power struggle between members and the leader, each determined to outwait the other.

2 Calling on specific members limits growth potential of the members; allowing the group to respond spontaneously increases growth potential.

3 Forcing responses instead of allowing spontaneous responses will decrease thoughtful exploration of what is happening.

59. 1 **When the group becomes united (cohesive) it enables clients to feel accepted, valued, and part of the group; this is the optimum time for the working phase to begin.**

2 Confrontation occurs later in the working phase of group process, not in the beginning.

3 Imitative behavior occurs later in the working phase of group process, not in the beginning.

4 Corrective recapitulation occurs later in the working phase of group process, not in the beginning.

60. 4 **This response focuses the client on the behavior and what the client is trying to achieve by such behavior; it also helps the client to see how such behavior affects others.**

1 The group members will not know what the client was trying to tell the nurse; only the client knows and should be asked directly.

2 This response uses a nondirective approach to attack the client.

4 This is an attacking, defensive response made without knowing what the client was attempting to accomplish.

61. 3 **New group leaders experience anxiety and insecurity, which limit their ability to mediate conflicts between members.**

1 This behavior is self-serving and disruptive to the group process.

2 This is often counterproductive, especially with regressed long-term clients who may decompensate when confronted with their behavior.

4 Long-term regressed clients need more help with communication than clients with acute problems.

62. 4 **The use of pronouns "we," "us," and "our" often indicates that group members experience a sense of belonging.**

1 Cohesive groups tend to accept and sometimes even protect disliked members.

2 Cohesive groups tend to resent new members.

3 This reflects lack of group cohesion; socialization may be superficial.

63. 4 **This is an open-ended nonjudgmental response that points out incongruity between the client's verbal and nonverbal communication.**

1 This will not help the client recognize the incongruity.

2 This will not help the client recognize the incongruity.

3 This will not help the client recognize the incongruity.

64. 2 **This response uses paraphrasing to restate the content of the client's statement; it encourages further communication.**

1 Feelings are personal and can really not be understood by others; this is an ineffective attempt to empathize and refocuses the attention on the nurse.

3 This response negates the client's feelings and changes the subject; the client needs to talk, and this response cuts off communication.

4 This response negates the client's feelings, makes feelings impossible to share, may make the client feel guilty for the feelings, and tells the client how to behave and feel.

65. 4 **Helping the client understand the meaning of the family member's behavior reduces the family member's emotional control over the client.**

1 This ignores the necessity of clarifying the family member's behavior.

2 Distraction is not a therapeutic way to deal with realistic feelings.

3 This is a temporary measure and does not reduce the emotional conflict with the family member.

66. 3 **Anger is a common feeling when people do not have control over decisions that affect them.**

1 There is no information that indicates this conclusion.

2 There is no information that indicates this conclusion.

4 There is no information that indicates this conclusion.

67. 2 **This response brings the client back to the current concern; in crisis therapy, time is limited and refocusing helps to use it in the most therapeutic manner.**

1 This statement is too pointed; although it is important to focus on reality, it should be done in a manner that does not belittle the client.

3 This statement is too blunt; the aim is to refocus the client on the current problem without being demeaning.

4 This statement encourages discussion of material not directly related to the crisis.

68. 1 **This allows the agitated, angry client time to regain self-control; telling the client that the nurse will return will decrease possible guilt feelings and**

implies to the client that the nurse cares enough to return.

2 This does not respect the client's feelings; it may decrease trust and increase feelings of anger, help-lessness, and hopelessness.

3 An agitated, angry client will not be able to accept a logical explanation.

4 Continued insistence may provoke increased anger and further loss of control.

69. 3 **The answer to this question will provide the nurse with an idea of the client's hopes and frustrations without being threatening or probing.**

1 This question is probing, disregards the client's complaints, and will provide little information for the nurse to use when planning care.

2 This question is probing, disregards the client's complaints, and will provide little information for the nurse to use when planning care.

4 This question is probing, disregards the client's complaints, and will provide little information for the nurse to use when planning care.

70. 2 **Before deciding how to decrease the client's fears of addiction, the nurse must explore the full extent of the client's knowledge and feelings about taking this medication.**

1 Information may or may not be helpful; the client's feelings are what must be addressed.

3 Although this eventually may be done, it is not the priority at this time.

4 Although this eventually may be done, it is not the priority at this time.

71. 4 **All behavior has meaning; before planning intervention, the nurse must try to understand what the behavior means to the client.**

1 Ignoring behavior does little to alter it, and it may even cause further acting-out.

2 Isolation may increase anxiety and precipitate more acting-out behavior.

3 The nurse cannot explain the meaning of the client's behavior; only the client can.

72. 3 **This is a technique that prevents misunderstanding so that both the client and the nurse can work toward a common goal in the therapeutic relationship.**

1 This technique does not provide for clarification or understanding.

2 This technique does not provide for clarification or understanding.

4 This technique does not provide for clarification or understanding.

73. 2 **The psychoanalytic model studies the unconscious and uses the strategies of hypnosis, dream interpretation, and free association as a means of releasing repressed feelings.**

1 The behaviorist model subscribes to the belief that the self and mental symptoms are viewed as learned behaviors that persist because they are consciously

rewarding to the individual; this model deals with behaviors on a conscious level of awareness.

3 The psychobiologic model views emotional and behavioral disturbances as stemming from a physical disease; abnormal behavior is directly attributed to a disease process; this model deals with behaviors on a conscious level of awareness.

4 The social-interpersonal model affirms that crucial social processes are involved in the development and resolution of disturbed behavior; this model deals with behavior on a conscious level of awareness.

74. 4 **Environmental (milieu) therapy aims at having everything in the client's surroundings geared toward helping the client.**

1 Role-playing is not a necessary ingredient of any type of therapy.

2 Neither natural treatments nor medications are a necessary part of environmental therapy.

3 Clients are strongly encouraged to be involved in various types of activities.

75. 4 **This response should limit anxiety; it identifies feelings and tells the client what will happen in the immediate future.**

1 This is threatening and provides false reassurance; it puts responsibility on the client and does not allow for the expression of feelings.

2 Being with other people in a strange environment will add more stress to the new and already frightening experience of hospitalization.

3 This may lead the client to think that the environment is unsafe, which can increase insecurity and anxiety.

76. Answer: 1, 4, 5

1 **This phase focuses on developing the client's problem-solving skills while addressing the areas in the client's life that are causing problems. The nurse helps clients to identify these topics for discussion.**

2 This behavior occurs during the orientation phase before trust is established.

3 This behavior occurs during the orientation phase before trust is established.

4 **Resistant behaviors usually are overcome by the working phase. By the working phase of a therapeutic relationship trust is established based on mutual respect.**

5 **Once trust is established the client will feel comfortable enough to express feelings; feelings of transference and countertransference usually awaken during the working phase of a therapeutic relationship.**

77. 2 **The stress of termination may precipitate fears of abandonment and the client may regress.**

1 The client is expressing fear, not thanks.

3 There are no data to suggest that the client is manipulating the nurse; the client's expression of apprehension is typical of someone in this situation.

4 The client's statement is not indicative of anything that should cause a delay in discharge but rather indicates anxiety over termination.

78. 4 **An explicit termination statement is most appropriate; offering an expression of well-wishes sets an optimistic, positive tone while maintaining the nurse-client relationship.**

1 A return of the physical contact should be avoided because it may precipitate anxiety in the client or may be interpreted as a desire to change the relationship from professional to personal.

2 Smiling and saying nothing may indicate acceptance of the physical exchange and blurs boundaries.

3 This response is nontherapeutic because it indicates an ongoing rather than a terminating relationship.

79. 3 **The client's inability to recall is an example of repression, which is the unconscious and involuntary forgetting of painful events, ideas, and conflicts.**

1 There is nothing to demonstrate that denial, an unconscious refusal to admit an unacceptable situation, exists.

2 There is nothing to demonstrate that regression, a return to an earlier, more comfortable developmental level, has occurred.

4 There is nothing to demonstrate that dissociation, the separation and detachment of emotional affect and significance from a particular idea, situation, or incident, has occurred.

80. 2 **Helping the client to understand the meaning of the parents' behavior can reduce the parents' emotional control over her.**

1 This is a temporary measure and does not reduce the emotional conflict with the parents.

3 Distraction is not a therapeutic way to cope with realistic feelings.

4 This ignores the necessity of clarifying her parents' behavior.

81. 4 **This goal is appropriate and measurable.**

1 This is not related to the client's problem; the priority for this client is to facilitate interaction with others.

2 Acting-out behavior is not inherent in the situation.

3 Acting-out behavior is not inherent in the situation.

82. 2 **Without an awareness of personal beliefs, the nurse unconsciously may stop listening if the client expresses actions and beliefs that contradict those of the nurse's.**

1 Although this may create some anxiety, usually it does not interfere with accurate listening.

3 Although this may create some anxiety, usually it does not interfere with accurate listening.

4 Although this may create some anxiety, usually it does not interfere with accurate listening.

83. 4 **If nurses are unaware of their biases about sexual assault, they will be unprepared to evaluate objectively and meet the client's needs.**

1 This may interrupt communication; information can be solicited later.

2 The nurse should be able to help this client without assistance.

3 Although this may be important, it is not the priority.

84. 1 **Value clarification is a technique that reveals individuals' values so that the individuals become more aware of them and their effect on others.**

2 This is not an outcome of value clarification.

3 This is not an outcome of value clarification.

4 This is not an outcome of value clarification.

85. 3 **The ability to discuss feelings about others and life situations is necessary for positive mental health.**

1 This is a long-term, not a short-term, goal.

2 This is a long-term, not a short-term, goal.

4 This is a long-term, not a short-term, goal.

86. 4 **When acceptance is reached the individual is beginning to withdraw; communication is simple, concise, and most often nonverbal.**

1 Kübler-Ross's research has shown that this stage usually needs verbal interventions and communication.

2 Kübler-Ross's research has shown that this stage usually needs verbal interventions and communication.

3 Kübler-Ross's research has shown that this stage usually needs verbal interventions and communication.

87. 3 **The client's goal is meaningful, and the nurse should do everything possible to help the client achieve it.**

1 There is no reason to attempt to move the client away from a meaningful goal despite its difficulty.

2 The evidence does not demonstrate that the client is in denial.

4 If the client wants to work toward a goal, the energy expenditure is justified.

88. 4 **An individual must feel a sense of control over self and the environment to feel secure, reduce anxiety, and function at an optimum level.**

1 Most emotionally ill people are too introspective to empathize with others.

2 Although some emotionally ill people will reject help, many are in pain and recognize they need psychological support. Some clients actively seek out care based on positive past experiences and the secondary gain of getting attention.

3 Many individuals with mental illness do not demonstrate observable signs of socially inappropriate behavior.

89. 2 **Families who are informed about the client's status can help with treatment goals and discharge planning.**

1 This may be a secondary gain but is not the primary purpose.

3 This may be a secondary gain but is not the primary purpose.

4 This may be a secondary gain but is not the primary purpose.

90. 3 **The client cannot be expected to accept or even respond to a plan that is incompatible with the family's lifestyle.**
    1 The family should not have to adjust to the nurse's biases; the nurse must self-identify biases and ensure that they do not interfere with nursing care.
    2 There is no evidence that misconceptions may occur.
    4 All individuals respond differently to situations.

91. 2 **When planning a group, the nurse must ensure that clients have similar needs to promote relationships and interactions; diverse needs do not foster group process.**
    1 Although important, this is not a primary consideration.
    3 Behavior and needs, rather than diagnoses, are of primary importance.
    4 This has little effect on group process.

92. 4 **The development of trust is the first step in developing a nurse-client relationship.**
    1 This is not the purpose; it provides a less stressful environment for the client to develop the belief that the staff is concerned and supportive.
    2 This cannot be achieved in several days; the ability to develop insight may take a lifetime or may never be accomplished.
    3 Not all clients with schizophrenia have bizarre, agitated behavior.

93. 1 **Regressed, long-term clients need structure and external controls to help organize their thought processes.**
    2 These clients need gentle assistance to deal with conflict situations.
    3 Most regressed long-term clients would be too anxious to assume a leadership role.
    4 Such experiences are beyond the capability or psychologic tolerance of these clients.

94. 1 **This is a necessary phase of group development because it helps members discover what they can expect from the leader and other members.**
    2 It is inappropriate to make this assumption at the first meeting.
    3 Group factions are unlikely to emerge in the first session; moreover, factions seldom emerge to control disruptive group behavior.
    4 The group has not yet developed to this phase; conflict resolution and management occur only in operating groups.

95. 1 **To achieve the greatest therapeutic value from a group session, the members must be involved in deciding what will be discussed.**
    2 By this response the nurse leader abdicates the leadership role and places the responsibility for the success of the group on its members.
    3 This response presents an extremely structured view of the purpose of a therapy group; the members must be involved in the selection of the topics to be discussed.

4 This response presents an extremely structured view of the purpose of a therapy group; the members must be involved in the selection of the topics to be discussed.

96. 2 **The nurse must accept the client's statement and beliefs as real to the client to develop trust and move into a therapeutic relationship.**
    1 Clients cannot be argued out of delusions.
    3 Medication should not be the initial approach.
    4 Redirecting the client's conversation whenever negative topics are brought up may make the client believe that these thoughts and feelings are being ignored.

97. 1 **The client has been able to function well up to this time, and the client's usual behavior and routines should be supported.**
    2 At this time the data presented do not identify this as a need.
    3 At this time the data presented do not identify this as a need.
    4 At this time the data presented do not identify this as a need.

DISORDERS FIRST EVIDENT BEFORE ADULTHOOD

98. 4 **Rationalization is the offering of an explanation to oneself or others to allay anxiety.**
    1 Denial involves avoiding the reality of a situation.
    2 Projection is blaming others for one's shortcomings.
    3 Regression is returning to an earlier more familiar mode of behavior.

99. 3 **Children who have experienced attachment difficulties with primary caregivers are not able to trust others and therefore relate superficially.**
    1 This is a possibility, but not a necessity for this diagnosis.
    2 The child probably will not cling or react when separated from the mother.
    4 Attachment will not occur with either parent.

100. 4 **Verbalization of negative feelings to others often can escalate and result in antisocial or acting-out behavior.**
    1 The environment must be consistent and predictable to limit manipulative behavior.
    2 This provides opportunities for the client to have some control.
    3 Consequences for unacceptable behavior can motivate individuals to act appropriately.

101. 4 **Unresponsiveness to the environment may be an indicator of severe childhood depression, autism, or possibly schizophrenia.**
    1 This may be seen in children without emotional problems as well as in those with emotional problems; this behavior alone does not indicate severe emotional problems.

2 This may be seen in children without emotional problems as well as in those with emotional problems; this behavior alone does not indicate severe emotional problems.

3 This may be seen in children without emotional problems as well as in those with emotional problems; this behavior alone does not indicate severe emotional problems.

102. 2 **This structured but nonthreatening statement avoids beginning with problems and may put the child at some ease, producing information that may be useful.**

1 This statement is too open and global; the child will probably not know how to answer this question or know where to begin.

3 The child may not know the answer to this question.

4 This question will probably produce an "I don't know" response; the focus should be on the child, not the mother.

103. 1 **Children have difficulty verbally expressing their feelings; acting-out behaviors, such as temper tantrums, may indicate an underlying depression.**

2 Adult and childhood depression may be manifested in different ways.

3 Childhood depression is not necessarily short and requires treatment.

4 Many conventional therapies for adults with depression, including medication, are effective for children with depression.

104. 1 **Tertiary prevention focuses on interventions that prevent complete disability or reduce the severity of a disorder or its associated disabilities.**

2 This is secondary prevention aimed at case-finding and early intervention.

3 This is primary prevention.

4 This is secondary prevention aimed at case-finding and early intervention.

105. 3 **This helps the child gain control by reducing stimuli while helping limit and prevent the use of tantrums by the child as an attention-getting behavior.**

1 This will probably increase the behavior associated with the tantrum.

2 Although ignoring the temper tantrum may sometimes help, it often forces the child to act out further; using time-out is more successful because the child is removed and both the parent and child have a cooling-off period.

4 Medication is not the treatment of choice.

106. 4 **One of the symptoms an autistic child displays is a lack of responsiveness to others; there is little or no extension to the external environment.**

1 Music is nonthreatening, comforting, and soothing for a child with this disorder.

2 Repetitive behavior provides comfort for a child with this disorder.

3 Repetitive visual stimuli, such as a spinning top, are nonthreatening and soothing for a child with this disorder.

107. 2 **Shortening the story nonjudgmentally limits the activity while supporting the child's self-esteem; the child cannot control his inattention and hyperactivity. The mother should select activities that are more interactive or interesting for the child to engage his attention.**

1 The child does not have a hearing problem and speaking louder will not change the behavior.

3 Inattention and hyperactivity cannot be controlled; this intervention may precipitate feelings of doubt, shame, and/or guilt and reinforce a low self-esteem.

4 This is unnecessary in this situation; therapeutic holding is used when a child is out of control and at risk for self-harm or violence toward others; it reassures the child that the adult is in control and promotes feelings of security and comfort.

108. 1 **The autistic child repeats sounds or words spoken by others.**

2 Stuttering is a speech disorder in which the same syllable is repeated, usually at the beginning of a word.

3 This is associated with neurological disorders, not autism.

4 Pressured speech is rapid, tense, and difficult to interrupt. This is associated with anxiety, not autism.

109. 4 **Children usually blame themselves for their parents' marital problems, believing that they are the reason one parent leaves.**

1 No data are presented to lead to this conclusion.

2 No data are presented to lead to this conclusion.

3 The child's response is not typical of anger.

110. 2 **Comparison over time is the only way for the nurse to accurately assess the mental status of a child.**

1 This may be unrealistic and biased. The nurse should consider the parents' description of behavior but should rely on personal assessment and observation over time.

3 The child's ability to discuss feelings is limited. In addition, the child's feelings are subjective symptoms that are known only by the child.

4 This can be threatening and may precipitate anxiety.

111. 2 **This is the family constellation as it is now constructed; without prior discussion and permission, an invitation to anyone else is an intrusion of privacy.**

1 In addition to needing the mother's permission to invite the father, the nurse must also include the child in family therapy.

3 The father cannot be invited without prior discussion with and permission of the mother.

4 The teacher is not part of the family constellation.

112. 3 **When all the members of a family blame one member for all their problems, scapegoating is occurring.**

1 There are no data to support identifying this pattern of relating.

2 There are no data to support identifying this pattern of relating.

4 There are no data to support identifying this pattern of relating.

113. 4 **This action sets a foundation for trust because it allows the child to see that the nurse cares.**

1 This is threatening at this stage of the relationship.

2 This is too infrequent to develop trust.

3 Although this is necessary, limit-setting does not support the development of a trusting relationship as much as providing support and emphasizing safety.

114. 4 **A behavior modification program tailored for and developed with the individual child is the most appropriate approach at this time.**

1 This may not be true. The child may not like school and may not think it is fun; having fun is not the purpose of school.

2 This serves no purpose and may be viewed by the child as a reward for behavior.

3 There are no data to indicate that the child is in need of special education.

115. 2 **The DSM-IV-TR reports an incidence of ADHD in about 3% to 7% of school-age children.**

1 This problem usually becomes evident around 6 to 7 years of age and is noted in at least two different settings (school and home).

3 Socioeconomic factors do not play a major role in the occurrence of this disorder.

4 Children with ADHD have less need for sleep than children without ADHD.

116. 2 **This intervention will be most successful because it provides a time period for the hyperactive child to regain control. It is neither a positive nor a negative reinforcement of acting-out behavior; it prevents injury to the other children.**

1 Ignoring the behavior may force the child to act out even more to gain attention.

3 This will not change the acting-out behavior.

4 This action rewards acting-out behavior by providing special attention.

117. 3 **This provides an opportunity for the team, the child, and the parents to interact in a therapeutic environment.**

1 It is too late; this should have been done much earlier.

2 This is not the responsibility of the nurse.

4 It is too late; this should have been done much earlier.

ANXIETY, SOMATOFORM, FACTITIOUS, AND DISSOCIATIVE DISORDERS

118. 1 **The identification of unhealthy habits or specific problems will allow the client to determine which additional coping skills need to be developed and practiced.**

2 A rehabilitation program is more appropriate for clients with psychotic or substance abuse disorders, not clients who are experiencing anxiety.

3 Further assessment is required before initiating the use of medication.

4 Although a consistent method for performing self-care is important, it is not the priority.

119. 1 **A primary gain is always the reduction of anxiety.**

2 This is related to a secondary gain.

3 This is unrelated to primary gains.

4 This is unrelated to primary gains.

120. 3 **Perceptual fields are a key indicator of anxiety level because the perceptual fields narrow as anxiety increases.**

1 This is not related directly to anxiety levels.

2 This is not related directly to anxiety levels.

4 This is not related directly to anxiety levels.

121. 1 **The client's statement is an example of the use of denial, a defense that blocks problems by unconsciously refusing to admit they exist.**

2 Projection is a defense that is used to deny unacceptable feelings and emotions and attribute them to others.

3 Sublimation is a defense that is used to substitute socially acceptable behavior for unacceptable instincts.

4 Displacement is a defense that is used to allow the shifting of feeling from an emotionally charged person or object to a safe, substitute person or object.

122. 2 **A compulsion is an uncontrollable, persistent urge to perform an act repetitively to relieve anxiety.**

1 An obsession is a persistent idea, thought, or impulse that cannot be eliminated from consciousness by logical reasoning.

3 The urge to perform a compulsive act is not under the client's control because avoiding the act increases anxiety.

4 Clients are compelled to perform these ritualistic behaviors; they are not trying to rebel.

123. 1 **Relaxation techniques refocus energy and eventually reduce physical and emotional stress.**

2 This is not always possible; forced quiet activity may increase stress and anger rather than reduce it.

3 This is not always possible; stress can develop from a variety of feelings stimulated by many situations.

4 This is not easy to identify; it is better to learn to deal with feelings once they develop.

124. 3 **Discussion of the feared object triggers an emotional response to the object.**

1 People with phobias generally acknowledge their existence.

2 Extreme fear is more of a problem than anger.

4 Distortion of reality related to the daily routine usually is not a problem for a person with a phobia.

125. 3 **The person transfers anxieties to activities or objects, usually inanimate objects, which are then avoided to decrease anxiety.**

1 Splitting is the compartmentalization of opposite affective states and the inability to integrate the positive and negative aspects of others or self.

2 Regression, the return to an earlier, more comfortable level of development, is not the defense mechanism used by someone with a phobia.

4 Conversion, the transferring of a mental conflict into a physical symptom, is not the defense mechanism used by someone with a phobia.

126. 1 **The most successful therapy for people with phobias involves behavior modification techniques using desensitization.**

2 Insight into the origin of the phobia will not necessarily help the client overcome the problem.

3 This may increase understanding of the phobia, but may not help the client to cope with the fear; there is no maladaptive thought process associated with phobias.

4 Psychoanalysis may increase understanding of the phobia, but may not help the client cope successfully with the unreasonable fear.

127. 2 **Experiencing the actual trauma in dreams or flashbacks is the major symptom that distinguishes posttraumatic stress disorders from other anxiety disorders.**

1 This usually is not associated with anxiety disorders.

3 This is more common with phobic disorders.

4 Although depression may be generated by discussion of the traumatic situation, the affect is usually exaggerated, not blunted.

128. 1 **The ability to connect feelings, thoughts, and actions, plus inattention for all but the anxiety-causing subject, are associated with a moderate level of anxiety.**

2 Severe anxiety is related to dissociation, selective inattention, and an inability to connect feelings, thoughts, and actions.

3 The development of mild or moderate anxiety is common in new situations because of apprehension related to the unknown.

4 There is insufficient information to come to this conclusion.

129. 2 **These actions make the environment as emotionally nonthreatening as realistically possible.**

1 All needs cannot be met; the person must learn how to cope with delaying gratification.

3 It is not possible or realistic to meet all of a person's requests.

4 Order in the environment is of less importance; providing a nonthreatening environment is the priority action.

130. 1 **Anxiety is a threat to the identity of the individual; the client is seeking assurance that the fear and panic being experienced will not mean loss of control.**

2 This is not evidence of insightfulness but a plea for help in reducing the anxiety.

3 The client is not exhibiting depression but severe anxiety and panic.

4 The client is not seeking the nurse's trust; the client is asking for help.

131. 1 **Mild and moderate levels of anxiety can be beneficial because they focus attention on the environment by attempting to ward off additional anxiety.**

2 Initially, anxiety increases physiological functioning; these functions decrease after prolonged anxiety because of exhaustion.

3 Automatic behavioral responses may hinder, rather than increase, an individual's awareness.

4 Ego defense mechanisms may hinder, rather than increase, an individual's awareness.

132. 3 **Because anxiety can be an interpersonal experience, it is contagious; the nurse then has a strong urge to get away.**

1 The desire to go off duty would not suddenly make the nurse uncomfortable.

2 This is possible, but not probable; the client is exhibiting anxiety, not hostility, at this time.

4 There is no indication that this or any other behavior encountered has been bizarre.

133. 2 **Freedom to ventilate feelings acts as a safety valve to reduce anxiety.**

1 The suppression of anger may increase the client's anxiety.

3 This is not therapeutic; it may increase the anxiety the client is feeling.

4 This may or may not be helpful; the client's family may provide support to the client.

134. 4 **The nurse should clarify if the spouse has discussed the child's visiting with the client before commenting further.**

1 This response assumes that the client has consented to the visit; this assumption may be incorrect.

2 This response assumes that the client has consented to the visit; this assumption may be incorrect.

3 This response makes an assumption that requires more data and discussion to validate.

135. 2 **The nurse's presence may provide the client with support and feelings of control.**

1 The client is too upset to respond; this question may lead to more anxiety.

3 The client is too distraught to sit; to be therapeutic the nurse should walk with the client, thus demonstrating concern.

4 The client is in a panic; anger is not primary, and there is no need to work off aggression.

136. 1 **Fear can be overwhelming; the nurse's presence provides protection from possible danger.**

2 The client's anxiety level is interfering with the ability to communicate; anxiety must be reduced first.

3 The client's anxiety level is so high that sufficient emotional energy to set parameters is not available.

4 This may increase the client's anxiety at this time.

137. 3 **This response helps the client focus on situations that precipitate frightening feelings, but not the attack itself.**

1 This response will not help the client focus on feelings.

2 This response will not help the client focus on feelings. Also "why" questions often make people feel defensive.

4 This is false reassurance; the nurse cannot guarantee that the feelings will not come back.

138. 1 **The client will be unable to concentrate or focus on the interview if anxiety is not reduced.**

2 This is not the priority at this time; anxiety must be reduced and the client's level of comfort increased.

3 The client will not rest until anxiety is reduced.

4 This is not the priority at this time; anxiety must be reduced and the client's level of comfort increased.

139. 1 **During a panic attack the attention span is shortened, making it difficult to follow long sentences. An authoritative voice lets the client know that the nurse is in control of the situation; the client is unable to set controls because of the anxiety level.**

2 This may increase the client's anxiety level further.

3 This may increase the client's anxiety level further.

4 Crying is an outlet and should not be discouraged; telling someone not to cry usually increases the crying and the anxiety.

140. 1 **Intellectually the person knows the compulsive acts are senseless but is unable to stop doing them because they control anxiety.**

2 This is an example of denial. Most people with compulsive behaviors are not in denial.

3 This is rationalization; obsessive-compulsive behavior usually is counterproductive, time consuming, and interferes with functioning.

4 This is an example of delusional thinking.

141. 2 **The ritual reduces anxiety; when not permitted to complete the ritual, a client with an obsessive-compulsive disorder will experience increased anxiety, frustration, and anger and may act out.**

1 The client is experiencing anxiety not related to a personality clash.

3 The client is experiencing anxiety not related to the nurse's manner.

4 The client is experiencing anxiety not related to an aggressive personality.

142. 3 **These are positive coping behaviors that can be used consciously to promote mental health.**

1 These are not healthy coping behaviors, and their frequent use can lead to distortions of reality. Also usually they are not under conscious control.

2 These are not healthy coping behaviors, and their frequent use can lead to distortions of reality. Also usually they are not under conscious control.

4 These are not healthy coping behaviors, and their frequent use can lead to distortions of reality. Also usually they are not under conscious control.

143. 4 **This demonstrates that the client feels comfortable enough to discuss the problems that motivated the behavior.**

1 This does not demonstrate a resolution of problems underlying the behavior.

2 Without discussion of the problems underlying the behavior, little is accomplished.

3 This does not demonstrate a resolution of problems underlying the behavior.

144. 1 **The development of confusion indicates that the client's ability to maintain equilibrium has not been achieved and that further disequilibrium is occurring.**

2 This does not indicate the plan needs to be changed unless the client's history demonstrates no prior use of this defense.

3 This does not indicate the plan needs to be changed unless the client's history demonstrates no prior use of this defense.

4 This is a positive response to the plan of care which does not need reassessment.

145. 3 **Members have not established trust and are hesitant to discuss problems; the behaviors observed reflect anxiety and insecurity.**

1 This can add to the anxiety and insecurity of group members.

2 These behaviors are expected in the early stage of group interaction.

4 This can add to the anxiety and insecurity of group members.

CRISIS SITUATIONS

146. 1 **Caplan's theory states that a crisis is an internal disturbance caused by a stressful event that alters the usual way of coping with a threat to the self; this temporarily disturbs the equilibrium of the person involved.**

2 This is not the definition of a crisis.

3 This is not the definition of a crisis; it is the assessment the nurse must make in the first phase of crisis intervention.

4 This is not the definition of a crisis but how a crisis is resolved.

147. 4 **Awareness of limitations and the ability to place oneself in another's situation are essential to being able to intervene effectively.**

1 This is not a necessary characteristic to help families with problems and many times it is impossible to achieve; this is not a prerequisite for understanding.

2 Although this may be helpful, it is not a priority and may confuse professional and social roles.

3 Although this may be helpful, it is not a priority and may confuse professional and social roles.

148. 4 **The data presented indicate developmentally related struggles and specific situations that are extremely stressful, resulting in the adolescent's use of projection as a defense. Multiple stresses can produce a crisis situation for the individual when past coping mechanisms are ineffective.**
 1 It is not the experience but the individual's response to the experience that determines a crisis.
 2 A crisis is not an age-related problem; a crisis results when the individual's past coping mechanisms are no longer effective for managing a present stressful situation.
 3 The individual's inability to cope indicates a crisis.

149. 2 **A crisis occurs when usual methods of coping are no longer effective and the individual is so overwhelmed that emotional distress and cognitive impairment result.**
 1 A crisis is precipitated by a known acute situation, not a situation that comes and goes.
 3 A crisis is precipitated by a known acute situation, not a situation that builds up slowly.
 4 Feeling tense, irritable, or uneasy is associated with anxiety. However, feelings associated with a crisis cause such severe disequilibrium that the individual is unable to concentrate or function.

150. 3 **A situational crisis is a sudden, unexpected event with which the individual is unable to cope using past coping behaviors; this time frame provides an opportunity for the individual to learn new coping behaviors.**
 1 This is too short a period of time for the individual to develop new, successful coping mechanisms.
 2 This is too short a period of time for the individual to develop new, successful coping mechanisms.
 4 This is longer than the expected time period within which a crisis should be resolved.

151. 2 **Personal internal strengths and supportive individuals are critical to the development of a crisis intervention plan; they must be explored with the client.**
 1 Although this information may be helpful, it is not essential; factors concerning the present situation are paramount.
 3 Identifying unconscious conflicts takes a long time and is inappropriate for crisis intervention.
 4 This is a goal of psychotherapy, not crisis intervention.

152. 4 **Any aspect of the treatment environment can be used to benefit the client in milieu therapy.**
 1 These are separate treatment modalities, not part of milieu therapy.
 2 This is part of behavioral modification, not milieu therapy.
 3 This is part of psychoanalytic, not milieu, therapy.

153. 3 **A crisis intervention group helps clients reestablish psychological equilibrium by assisting them to explore new alternatives for coping; it considers** realistic situations using rational and flexible problem-solving methods.
 1 This is not an immediate goal of crisis intervention.
 2 Clients are never given a solution; they are assisted to arrive at their own acceptable, workable solutions.
 4 It is not necessary for crisis intervention workers to be psychologists.

154. 4 **The client should be able to state specific behaviors that can be used to decrease self-destructive thoughts and actions; the client must be empowered.**
 1 This is ineffective because the client may end the conversation and remain suicidal.
 2 The nurse may gather data through the suicidal risk assessment tool, but the client may not have attained a catharsis; therefore, the dialogue should continue until a contract has been set or self-destructive behaviors have diminished.
 3 This is an indication that the nurse should help the client focus on life and not on suicide; the client has not yet attained a catharsis.

155. 3 **Although the client's facial expression suggests happiness, the client's tone of voice gives the message of anger; the behaviors are not congruent.**
 1 The data given do not support this assessment.
 2 The data given do not support this assessment.
 4 The data given do not support this assessment.

156. 4 **The client is using intellectual reasoning to block confronting the unconscious conflict and the stress of having to deal with his girlfriend's pregnancy.**
 1 There are no data that demonstrate that the client is projecting blame on anyone else.
 2 There are no data that demonstrate that the client is concentrating thoughts and emotions on his inner self.
 3 There are no data that demonstrate the shifting of emotions from an emotionally charged object or person to a neutral one.

157. 3 **A crisis is defined as a situation in which the client's previous methods of adaptation are inadequate to meet present needs.**
 1 A crisis is not necessarily related to the degree of stress; it occurs when past coping mechanisms are ineffective.
 2 This is not the immediate stress for which the client has no coping mechanism.
 4 This is not causing the crisis; the client's lack of coping mechanisms is the cause.

158. 4 **The crisis center nurse's main responsibility is to assist the client in using the problem-solving process; the client should be helped to explore alternative solutions and be given information regarding other agencies, facilities, and services.**
 1 Although the client's decision should be supported, this is a judgmental response.

2 This is not part of the immediate intervention during the crisis; the client may be encouraged to seek help later for other problems.

3 This is an option for which the client must take primary responsibility.

159. 1 **Intrinsic motivation is motivation that is stimulated from within the learner; it is most effective because the learner recognizes the need to know, is self-directed, and is ready to learn.**

2 This is stimulation from outside sources and is often ineffective; desire should come from within.

3 Operant conditioning is a form of therapy requiring reinforcement of desired behavior.

4 Behavior modification. is a form of therapy requiring reinforcement of desired behavior.

160. 2 **The client is grieving the loss of a fantasized child; talking about it is part of the typical grief reaction.**

1 The client is sad, not out of control or immobilized.

3 The client is coping with the loss effectively.

4 The client recognizes the loss but is lamenting what could have been.

161. 3 **The client's anger about the miscarriage is shifted to the staff and the hospital because she is unable to cope with her loss at this time.**

1 The client is neither ignoring nor refusing to recognize reality.

2 The client is not attributing unacceptable or undesirable thoughts or feelings to another.

4 The client is not using a behavior pattern opposite to what she feels.

162. 4 **The nurse should be sensitive to any cultural or religious beliefs that may help the parents cope with their grief.**

1 Immediately discussing this topic is insensitive to the parents' grief at this time.

2 Immediately discussing this topic is insensitive to the parents' grief at this time.

3 The parents are too involved with their own grief at this time to consider their other children's grief.

163. 1 **The parents must be involved with developing alternative methods to cope with the present crisis; this involves problem-solving techniques.**

2 This is aimed at insight and subsequent change in behavior and is not focused specifically on one problem.

3 This dictates to the parents rather than adding to their self-esteem by having them contribute to the solution.

4 The parents' feelings may be explored, but this is supplemental to the work of problem solving.

164. **Answer: 3, 5**

1 Abusive parents typically have an ill-developed nurturing role with little perception of their parenting inability.

2 Abusive parents are more concerned with their own needs than their child's.

3 **Abusive parents seek gratification for their own needs rather than their child's needs; they may**

even project blame for the abuse on their child and find it difficult to conceal their hostility.

4 Abusive parents are more concerned with their own needs than their child's.

5 **Abusive parents often delay obtaining help for their child's injuries; the behavior is precipitated by a concern to conceal the injury and a lack of concern for the child.**

165. 2 **If one child in the family is identified as being different by the parents or siblings, coupled with other signs of abuse, physical abuse should be suspected and further investigation is warranted.**

1 Taking a walk is helpful for both the mother and the child and does not indicate abuse.

3 This is an acceptable punishment for misbehavior.

4 Although this is demeaning, it is not physical abuse.

166. **Answer: 1, 2, 5**

1 **Feelings of being overwhelmed are symptomatic of crisis.**

2 **Crises cause increased levels of anxiety that lead to adaptations of emotional distress and cognitive impairment.**

3 Crises are acute situations, not situations that come and go; they are associated with feelings of being overwhelmed, not vague feelings of uneasiness.

4 Crises are acute situations that are precipitated by specific identifiable events.

5 **Crises occur when usual methods of coping are no longer effective.**

167. 2 **A history of high-lethality attempts at suicide confirms that the individual attempted suicide in the past and therefore may attempt to commit suicide in the future.**

1 Although the correlation between substance abuse, particularly alcohol, and suicide is high, this is of lesser concern at this time because of the client's incarceration.

3 Isolation from friends and co-workers is of less significance than having an unstable, dissatisfying life with family members or having a history of prior suicide attempts.

4 Although both of these events may cause stress, numerically they receive a lesser rating than having a history of multiple high-risk suicide attempts.

168. 4 **Displacement is a defense mechanism in which one's pent-up feelings toward others who are a threat are discharged on others who are less threatening.**

1 Idealization is attributing overstated positive characteristics to others.

2 Transference is a mechanism by which affects or emotional tones are shifted from one individual to another.

3 Manipulation is a mechanism by which individuals attempt to manage, control, or use others to suit their own purpose or to gain an advantage.

169. 2 **These underlying beliefs commonly precipitate trying to improve the child's behavior by physical consequences for behavior they consider unacceptable.**
     1 These parents usually do not admit their behavior, so they do not have a need to rationalize it.
     3 These parents offer many vague explanations of how the child was injured; rarely is the explanation detailed.
     4 This is an unusual request because the abusing parent usually does not ask to see the child.

170. 3 **Management of the abused child places protection of the child's total being above consideration for parents' rights or wishes.**
     1 Protecting the child, not promotion of parental attachment, is the priority at this time.
     2 Supervision may be necessary, but it is only part of maintaining the child's well-being.
     4 Teaching methods of discipline is not appropriate at this time.

171. 3 **By learning how the toddler's behavior provokes frustration, parents may develop more acceptable ways of responding.**
     1 Although these parents need to learn what behavior is appropriate for a given age level, it is most important that they learn how to respond appropriately to their toddler's inappropriate behavior.
     2 Punishment is an act of retribution, not an act of discipline.
     4 Negative behavior cannot be ignored, but should be handled appropriately.

172. 2 **This child will distrust any approach because approaches commonly result in pain; abused children remain alert in an attempt to ward off an attack.**
     1 This child will not be open to an approach by a stranger; basic trust of others does not develop in abused children.
     3 This child usually will not cry out; abused children learn not to expect comforting or soothing of pain by others.
     4 This child will be acutely aware of anyone coming near; abused children attempt to defend themselves by keeping alert to the possibility of attack.

173. Answer: 1, 2, 5
     1 **These children often have nonsexual needs met by this individual and are powerless to refuse; ambivalence results in self-blame and guilt.**
     2 **Anger may exist, especially toward the nonabusing parent who is not protecting the child.**
     3 Revenge may exist, but it is not the overwhelming feeling reported.
     4 Disbelief may exist, but it is not the overwhelming feeling reported.
     5 **These children often have nonsexual needs met by this individual and are powerless to refuse; ambivalence results in self-blame and guilt.**

174. 3 **This is an emotionally supportive response; it demonstrates that sharing this information is acceptable and provides hope that she will get help.**
     1 The client may draw the conclusion that her actions precipitated the father's behavior; the client needs support and this response may precipitate or increase feelings of guilt.
     2 This implies that the client does not know what she is talking about; the client needs support, whether the act is real or imagined.
     4 This is not a priority at this time and may interfere with future sharing; the client needs immediate emotional support.

175. 1 **This provides reassurance and support for the child.**
     2 Asking the child to make this decision at this time is nontherapeutic and may be threatening.
     3 Using the phrase "anything wrong down there" may cause the child to have negative feelings about the self.
     4 Depending on the mother's involvement, this may be threatening rather than supportive to the child.

176. 2 **This response will elicit further clarification of what the child means by "bad."**
     1 This is not helpful; it will do nothing to clarify the child's idea of what "bad" means or the child's feelings about what happened.
     3 The nurse must determine what the child means by the word "bad" before reflecting the term back to the child. Also questions that require a yes or no response do not promote expression of feelings.
     4 This is not a therapeutic response because the focus is on what the nurse thinks rather than on what the child thinks.

177. 3 **This revelation should be accepted as truthful and it should be investigated immediately so that emotional and physical care can be instituted; the student needs to feel safe and supported.**
     1 Accusations of incest rarely are used in this way.
     2 Although lying may be a way of calling attention to unmet needs, this particular type of lie is rare.
     4 Blaming a family member is not the usual way that teenagers attempt to explain a pregnancy.

178. Answer: 4, 1, 3, 2
     Treatment of physical injuries is always the priority of care. Further information about the client's history is needed to determine if she is in an abusive situation. Allowing the client to express her feelings in a safe environment establishes trust, which is the foundation of psychosocial interventions. Providing information about community resources will offer alternatives to remaining in the abusive situation.

179. 4 **Whatever action the client took to save her life was the right action; this statement supports the woman.**
     1 This is not therapeutic; the word "submit" in any form is emotionally charged and increases feelings of guilt.

2   This is not therapeutic; the word "submit" in any form is emotionally charged and increases feelings of guilt.

3   This leaves the client with the thought she could have done something else.

180. 1   **Because a sexual assault is a threat to the sense of control over one's life, some control should be given back to the client as soon as possible.**

2   This is an expected form of ventilating emotions; the client should be told that medication is available if desired.

3   This takes control away from the client; the client may view this as an additional assault on the body that increases feelings of vulnerability and anxiety and does not restore control.

4   This takes control away from the client; the client may view this as an additional assault on the body that increases feelings of vulnerability and anxiety and does not restore control.

181. 2   **Partners may themselves feel angry and abused; these feelings should be quickly and openly discussed.**

1   This should not be done yet; rape counselors work with the victim and partner together.

3   The partner's feelings must be resolved before the partner can help the client and the nurse may not fully know the wife's feelings.

4   This may be reassuring, but it leaves the partner alone to deal with feelings.

182. 2   **This is the most direct approach to ascertain if pills were ingested; the client usually will respond to this type of direct question.**

1   This does not provide useful information.

3   This is not an initial response; a determination first must be made regarding the number of pills taken.

4   This is appropriate later; it is not the priority now.

183. 1   **Anger at her husband for leaving her may make her feel guilty for having these feelings.**

2   Financial security may or may not be a problem for this client.

3   Loneliness will be something she will have to cope with later, depending on her support system; it is not an immediate problem.

4   Estrangement may be something she will have to cope with later; it is not an immediate problem.

184. 4   **Whether there is a suicide plan is a major criterion when assessing the client's determination to make another attempt.**

1   Although this may be important for planning future therapeutic approaches, this does not explore the potential for suicide, the priority at this time.

2   Although this may be important for planning future therapeutic approaches, this does not explore the potential for suicide, the priority at this time.

3   Although this may be important for planning future therapeutic approaches, this does not explore the potential for suicide, the priority at this time.

185. 1   **Suicide threats and gestures are a means of communicating anger, frustration, hopelessness, and despair to significant others and should always be taken seriously.**

2   Children have many means readily available; there are many common objects around the home and playground that can be used to commit suicide.

3   Although suicide is the second leading cause of death in the 15- to 24-year-old age group, children younger than age 6 do attempt suicide and some succeed.

4   A suicide attempt usually is self-destructive; it is not an attempt to manipulate or control others.

186. 3   **The parents are focusing their feelings about their child's prognosis on someone or something else, in this case each other.**

1   Denial is ignoring, avoiding, or refusing to recognize painful realities.

2   Projection is the attribution of one's own feelings to another person.

4   Compensation is making up for a perceived deficiency by emphasizing another feature perceived as an asset.

187. 2   **Reasonable limits are necessary because they provide security and help to keep the child's behavior within acceptable bounds.**

1   This is an unrealistic approach that allows the child to manipulate the situation.

3   This is an unrealistic approach that allows the child to manipulate the situation.

4   Relationships, not special privileges, should provide the necessary security.

188. 2   **Seeing their child as soon as possible will validate the death for them and initiate the grieving process.**

1   This will delay and prolong the grieving process; the response offers no explanation for waiting.

3   This is unnecessary; the parents have asked to see their child now.

4   It is more traumatic to wait and delay the reality of the death.

189. 1   **Deaths that are perceived as preventable cause more guilt for the mourners and therefore increases the intensity and length of the grieving process.**

2   It may prolong and intensify the mourning process but will not necessarily result in a pathological reaction.

3   The opposite usually is true.

4   It may prolong and intensify the mourning process but will not necessarily result in a pathological reaction.

190. 1   **This provides support until the individuals' coping mechanisms and personal support systems can be mobilized.**

2   This is not the role of the nurse.

3   The individuals, not the nurse, must mobilize their support systems.

4   The individuals need time before the full reality of the loss can be accepted.

191. 4 **Support is most important when coping with the crisis of death; the support system must be relied on for coping with the loss.**
   1 The client's age may play a role in coping, but it is not the most important factor.
   2 The timing may be important if death is just one of a multiplicity of stresses, but it is not the most important factor in helping a client cope.
   3 The socioeconomic status may be important in long-term planning, but it is not the most important factor in the grieving process.

192. 1 **Resolving a loss is a slow, painful, continuous process until a mental image of the dead person, almost devoid of negative or undesirable features, emerges.**
   2 This stage usually is dominated by a refusal to accept or comprehend the fact that a loved one has died.
   3 The reality of the death and its meaning as a loss, plus anger, dominate this stage.
   4 The various rituals of the funeral help to initiate the recovery or restitution stage.

193. 3 **Successful resolution means being able to remember the good as well as the bad qualities of the deceased and accepting them as part of being human.**
   1 Resolution involves working through feelings, not just accepting what occurred.
   2 Resolution does not mean forgetting but rather realistically remembering the past.
   4 This is an unhealthy response that can become pathological because of the unresolved feelings about the person's other qualities.

194. 3 **Discussing the partner and the partner's death will help the client work through the grief process.**
   1 This refocuses the client's attention away from addressing feelings; the client probably does not have the physical or emotional energy to get involved with group activities.
   2 The client must cope with the past and present before addressing the future.
   4 This refocuses the client's attention away from addressing feelings; the client probably does not have the physical or emotional energy to get involved with others.

195. 2 **Intervention is aimed at restoring equilibrium by helping the client develop new ways to cope and assisting with the exploration of available support systems.**
   1 Identification of the precipitating factors should have taken place during the assessment phase.
   3 Decreasing support systems will not lead to independence but will increase the client's vulnerability and precipitate feelings of abandonment.
   4 The client's perception may be distorted; the nurse should strive to help maintain a realistic perception.

196. 4 **Helping a client cope with unresolved grief involves assisting the client to express thoughts and** feelings about the lost object or person as a necessary part of grief work.
   1 This is too threatening; at this point the client needs therapeutic one-to-one interaction.
   2 This is the responsibility of the nurse; another client does not have the expertise to help this client.
   3 The current nonverbal behavior indicates that the client is dealing with feelings; an opportunity should be provided for a verbal exploration.

197. 3 **Insomnia, depressed mood, anxiety, and anorexia are common responses associated with coping with loss, especially the death of a spouse.**
   1 The client is communicating information about not "feeling right" since her husband's death.
   2 The client is communicating information about not "feeling right" since her husband's death.
   4 Eight months does not constitute a prolonged period of mourning and therefore her grieving is not impaired.

198. 2 **Such stimuli encourage the client to remain reality oriented; research has shown that competing stimuli are useful in controlling hallucinations.**
   1 This does not ensure that the client's needs will be met.
   3 This is not realistic and fosters greater dependency; it focuses on the client's inability to cope with the problem and increases the client's fear of being alone.
   4 This is not realistic and fosters greater dependency; it focuses on the client's inability to cope with the problem and increases the client's fear of being alone.

199. 2 **Anger is associated with one of the stages of dying; understanding the stages leading to the acceptance of death may help the family to accept the client's moods and anger.**
   1 Avoiding the situation reflects the stage of denial when reality of the situation is not acknowledged; anger is not common in this stage.
   3 There are not enough data to come to this conclusion.
   4 There are not enough data to come to this conclusion.

200. 4 **A starting point for working with all clients is ascertaining what is known, their understanding of their particular situation, and its meaning to them.**
   1 It is not merely understanding what death and the dying process means, but how the individual feels about the present situation.
   2 Encouraging conversation about the condition tends to decrease anxiety and is desirable.
   3 This meets the needs of others rather than the client, who is the priority concern.

201. 1 **This response is on a feeling level and therefore encourages the exploration of feelings.**
   2 This statement supports the negative feelings of worthlessness.

3 This response focuses on negative feelings; "why" questions are difficult and sometimes impossible to answer.

4 This statement will elicit a yes or no response and will not encourage the exploration of feelings.

202. 2 **It is important for the couple to discuss their feelings to maintain open communication and support each other.**

1 This action will not meet the needs of this couple; it focuses only on the husband's needs and ignores the partner's needs.

3 This action will not meet the needs of this couple; it focuses only on the wife's needs and ignores the partner's needs.

4 This may be useful in the future but probably is premature; they need to share their feelings with each other first.

203. 3 **The spouse is expressing the expected feelings of guilt associated with the death of a loved one; there usually is initial guilt over what might have been.**

1 There is no evidence to support this conclusion.

2 The spouse is expressing guilt, not shame.

4 There is no evidence to support this conclusion.

204. 4 **With this sedating medication, the individual does not face the reality of the loss and merely delays the onset of the pain associated with it. Because most support is available at the time of the death and the funeral, a benzodiazepine at this time denies the individual the opportunity to use this assistance.**

1 This classification of drugs does not magnify the risk of suicide.

2 This classification of drugs does not cause or prevent depression.

3 Although sedation and muscle relaxation initially may occur with these drugs, these are not the reasons they are not ordered.

205. 2 **Crying is an expression of an emotion that if not expressed increases anxiety and tension; the increased anxiety and tension use additional psychic energy and hinder coping.**

1 Crying does not relieve depression, nor does it help a client face reality.

3 This is not universally true. In most instances the client's defenses should not be taken away until they can be replaced by more healthy defenses. The nurse must interfere with behavior and defenses that may place the client in danger; the client's current behavior creates no threat to the client.

4 This is not always true. Many clients are embarrassed by what they consider to be a "show of weakness" and have difficulty relating to the individual who witnessed it. The nurse must do more than just accept the crying to strengthen the nurse-client relationship.

206. 4 **A starting point for working with all clients is ascertaining what is known, their understanding of their particular situation, and its meaning to them.**

1 It is not merely understanding what death means to the client, which is a philosophical discussion, but how the individual feels about the situation.

2 Encouraging conversation about the situation tends to decrease anxiety.

3 This is part of the plan of care, but it is secondary; coping behavior is the priority according to the data provided.

207. 4 **This response validates the client's feelings and encourages the client to look at the basis or reality of the expressed concern.**

1 This response ignores the client's statement; the client has already told the nurse the basis for the feelings.

2 This puts the responsibility for the husband's behavior on the client, who may not be able to handle it.

3 This may or may not be true and does not focus on the client's feelings.

DEMENTIA, DELIRIUM, AND OTHER COGNITIVE DISORDERS

208. 2 **The signs and symptoms associated with vascular dementia have an abrupt onset (days to weeks) because of the occlusion of small arteries or arterioles in the cortex of the brain. Dementia of the Alzheimer's type is associated with a gradual (years), progressive loss of function.**

1 Both vascular dementia and dementia of the Alzheimer's type are associated with this deficit in functioning.

3 Both vascular dementia and dementia of the Alzheimer's type are associated with this deficit in functioning.

4 Both vascular dementia and dementia of the Alzheimer's type are associated with this deficit in functioning.

209. 4 **Dementias, such as that of the Alzheimer's type, result from pathological changes of CNS cells producing deterioration that is long term and progressive. These changes involve cognitive, functional, and behavioral changes that reflect predictable stages (stage 1, mild; stage 2, moderate; and stage 3, severe). The duration of Alzheimer's disease is 3 to 20 years with an average of 10 years.**

1 Symptoms of delirium, not dementia, develop rapidly as a result of derangements of cerebral metabolism and neurotransmission.

2 Once CNS neurons are destroyed, remissions are uncommon.

3 Interpersonal events do not precipitate dementias.

210. 1 **Depression, which is common with dementia, can lead to disinterest in food.**

2 Uninhibited social behavior results from the lack of impulse control.

    3 Delusions and hallucinations are the result of perceptual/cognitive deficits, not alteration in mood.

    4 This is not related to mood.

211. **1** **This action will reduce the need for sleeping pills, which frequently add to the older client's confusion.**

    2 The family is not asking that the client be moved from the home; the nurse's focus should be to help reduce the confusion the client experiences at night, keep the client safe, and ease the burden on the family.

    3 Continually changing a cognitively impaired client's environment and routine will increase confusion and anxiety. This client needs a consistent environment with a set daily routine of activities, which provides structure and comfort.

    4 Restraints add to the client's confusion and tend to increase inappropriate behavior.

212. **2** **Confabulation, or the filling in of memory gaps with imaginary facts, is a defense mechanism used by people experiencing memory deficits.**

    1 Concretism is demonstrated by an inability to comprehend abstract concepts.

    3 Flight of ideas is demonstrated by thoughts and speech that jump from one topic to another with no obvious connection for either the speaker or the listener.

    4 Associative looseness is demonstrated by speech that is difficult to follow because the connections between the speaker's statements or train of thought are so loose that they are not obvious to the listener.

213. **4** **A moderate level of cognitive impairment because of dementia is characterized by increasing dependence on environmental and social structure and by increasing psychological rigidity with accentuated previous traits and behaviors.**

    1 Although paranoid attitudes, which are associated with hypervigilance, may be exhibited, the decrease in cognitive functioning, disorientation, and loss of memory usually does not lead to hypervigilance.

    2 With the decrease in impulse control that is associated with dementia, decreased, not increased, inhibition occurs.

    3 An enhancement of intelligence does not occur with dementia; initially, intellectual deterioration is subtle.

214. **3** **Dementia of the Alzheimer's type accounts for 80% of dementias in older adults; it may be due to a neurotransmitter deficiency and it is characterized by a steady decline in intellectual functioning, including memory deficits, disorientation, and decreased cognitive ability.**

    1 More than 90% of people with dementia of the Alzheimer's type are older than the age of 50.

    2 It is an organic, not functional, disorder.

    4 Dementia of the Alzheimer's type is difficult to diagnose and often is made when other etiologies for the dementia have been ruled out.

215. **Answer: 3, 4, 5**

    1 Depression does not cause memory deficits.

    2 A typical symptom of depression is loss of interest in food.

    3 **This is associated with depression because of low self-esteem.**

    4 **People who are depressed do not have physical or emotional energy; "I don't know" answers require little thought and/or decision making.**

    5 **People who are depressed do not have physical or emotional energy; "I can't remember" answers require little thought and/or decision making.**

216. **2** **Routines and familiarity with activities or the environment provide for a sense of security.**

    1 Change is not well tolerated; frustration and the inability to accomplish tasks lead to lowered self-esteem.

    3 Decreased physical capacity and attention span limit active participation; frustration can result.

    4 Challenging activities can be frustrating and can lead to hostility or withdrawal.

217. **3** **In stage 1, clients have a mild cognitive impairment with short-term memory loss; establishing a daily routine, posting it, and adhering to it provides a concrete, structured approach.**

    1 This may be required during stage 3 or the end of stage 2 if the daughter is unable to cope with the mother's functional and behavioral changes.

    2 In stage 1, clients can provide for their own basic activities of daily living such as bathing, dressing, and eating.

    4 These clients can make simple decisions in stage 1 and they have the right to make choices; an authoritarian approach may promote regression, anxiety, depression, and/or anger.

218. **3** **Clients with dementia have the greatest loss in the area of recent memory.**

    1 Memory of remote events usually remains fairly intact.

    2 Memory of remote events usually remains fairly intact.

    4 Memory of remote events usually remains fairly intact.

219. **3** **When the client is unable to perform a task, frustration occurs and results in more disorganized behavior.**

    1 Clients with disorientation and cognitive impairment may show little interest in unit activities, but should be included to the best of their ability. However, this does not address the client's disorganized behaviors.

    2 The client's disorientation is documented and will not change, although some day-to-day variations may occur; most important is the assessment of the client's ability to function.

    4 The client probably will never adjust any further.

220. **1** **This client needs toileting every 2 hours to prevent soiling; physically seating the client on the toilet**

often prevents accidents and negates the use of disposable pads or underwear.

2 The client has cognitive impairment, and reality orientation probably will be ineffective.

3 The client needs more than just supervision.

4 The client may be unable to control the incontinence and this response is demeaning.

221. 1 **This forces the client to find a common characteristic of two things, an ability that is the criterion for abstract thinking.**

2 This tests orientation, not abstract thinking.

3 This tests judgment, not abstract thinking.

4 This tests short-term memory, not abstract thinking.

222. 3 **A common sign of dementia is the loss of memory for recent events.**

1 Disorientation of self is not a common sign of dementia; disorientation to time and place is more common.

2 Recollection of past events is less impaired than that of recent events.

4 This is not as common as recent memory loss; if there are speech or language disturbances, this ability should be assessed.

223. 2 **Confabulation is used as a defense mechanism against embarrassment caused by a lapse of memory; the client fills in the blanks in memory by making up details, thus maintaining self-esteem.**

1 Regression is a defense mechanism in which the individual moves back to earlier developmental defenses; the client is not regressing at this time.

3 Although older adults fear being forgotten or losing others' affection, this is not the reason for confabulation.

4 Confabulation is not used to reminisce about past achievement.

224. 4 **This action maintains, for as long as possible, the client's remaining intellectual functions by providing an opportunity to use them.**

1 Although pain syndromes can occur in clients with dementia from AIDS, frequent pain assessment is not a priority; providing cognitive stimulation facilitates the use of nonpharmacological treatments for pain management as long as possible.

2 Remotivation is not always possible with extensive organic brain damage.

3 There are no data to indicate that the client needs custodial care at this time.

225. 2 **This client requires a structured environment, regardless of the cause of the behavior; this helps to provide a safe environment.**

1 This is important but is secondary to promotion of an environment conducive to safety and security.

3 A battery of screening tests probably will be used in an attempt to determine the cause of the dementia; however, provision for safety is necessary first.

4 This is important but is secondary to promotion of an environment conducive to safety and security.

226. 2 **The client needs constant reassurance because forgetfulness blocks previous explanations; frequent presence of staff members serves as a support system.**

1 This client will be unable to explain the reasons for his concerns.

3 The client will not be able to decode a written schedule; the client needs continual reassurance.

4 This client will not remember the explanation from one moment to the next.

227. 4 **Disoriented clients need assistance in how they direct their energy to limit inappropriate behaviors.**

1 The staff cannot prevent all gross motor activity; the client needs to use muscles but their use must be controlled.

2 Further deterioration usually cannot be prevented in this disorder.

3 Behavior modification methods do not work well with disoriented forgetful clients.

228. 1 **This approach assists the client with decision making; new situations may be stressful and lead to ambivalence.**

2 This will increase stress and possible feelings of guilt.

3 The client may perceive this as punishment; the client may not have the psychic energy or decision-making ability to get dressed without help.

4 This is not sharing decision making, and hurrying the client may lead to feelings of frustration and resentment.

229. 3 **Intellectual deterioration associated with dementia decreases interest in the environment.**

1 Diffuse impairment of brain tissue functioning results in fluctuations in the extremes of emotions; lability of mood is common with dementia.

2 Clients with dementia usually fluctuate between aggressive acting out and passive acceptance.

4 In clients with dementia, intellectual deterioration can result in behavior that mimics withdrawal.

EATING AND SLEEP DISORDERS

230. 4 **Amenorrhea results from endocrine imbalances that occur when fat stores are depleted.**

1 The client is dehydrated; edema is not expected.

2 Constipation, not diarrhea, may occur because of lack of fiber in the diet.

3 Hypotension, not hypertension, may occur because of dehydration.

231. Answer: 1, 2, 5

1 **Weight management moved into the mainstream in the 1950s and increased its momentum with the fitness industry in the 1980s and 1990s. In the new century, women are constantly bombarded by the media with products and programs that are designed to help them attain the perfect body, which for most women is unrealistic.**

2 Since the 1960s the trend in fashion has been toward thinness with fabrics that cling and styles that reveal the body. Print and movie media, including advertising dollars, focus on a thin, perfect ideal that is unattainable for most women.

3 Although some people with bulimia nervosa may eat fast food, the fast-food industry is unrelated to the etiology of anorexia nervosa or bulimia nervosa.

4 Although some people with an eating disorder may use over-the-counter medications, particularly laxatives, over-the-counter medications are unrelated to the etiology of eating disorders.

5 Several women's sports, such as gymnastics and figure skating, emphasize low body weights as does ballet. These demands may lead to eating disorders in girls and women who wish to compete.

232. 1 **These clients often hide food or force vomiting; therefore, they must be carefully observed.**

2 This is insufficient because these clients may induce vomiting after eating.

3 Fluid and electrolyte balance can become a problem for these clients and monitoring is required, but at this time it is the responsibility of the nurse, not the client, to do this.

4 These clients will not become involved in planning meals; this is a long-term goal.

233. 3 **The client's behavior has resulted in obtaining attention; it provides a sense of power and control.**

1 This reflects a disturbed perception about her body.

2 Although clients with anorexia nervosa are concerned about social acceptance, perfectionism, and achievement and may obtain high grades in school, this is not a secondary gain related to the eating behaviors associated with anorexia nervosa.

4 This is a result of starvation, not a secondary gain.

234. 4 **The client with anorexia nervosa denies the need for food or presence of hunger; the client with bulimia nervosa hides the behavior because there is recognition that the behavior is a problem.**

1 Clients with anorexia nervosa are more introverted and tend to avoid relationships.

2 Clients with anorexia nervosa are more introverted and tend to avoid relationships.

3 Clients with bulimia are at a greater risk for fluid and electrolyte problems because of the purging; clients with anorexia nervosa are more at risk for severe nutritional deficiencies.

235. 1 **This is the best initial response; it encourages additional ventilation of feelings.**

2 This is not necessarily true, and the response is somewhat threatening and nontherapeutic.

3 This is not therapeutic; also, this is false reassurance because the client may not feel better later.

4 This is not therapeutic; the client is verbally expressing feelings, and the behavior does not require medication at this time.

236. 3 **These are the major signs of anorexia nervosa; weight loss is excessive (15% of expected weight); nutritional deficiencies result in amenorrhea and a distended abdomen.**

1 Although pulse irregularities and alopecia are associated with anorexia, weight loss is excessive, not mild.

2 Although compulsive behaviors are common, excessive fears and nausea are not associated with anorexia nervosa.

4 Memory lapses are not associated with anorexia nervosa; excessive exercising and pulse irregularities are.

237. 1 **Eating and weight loss become the means of control to decrease anxiety related to perfectionistic thinking.**

2 Controlling oneself within the family seems to be more important than peer group acceptance.

3 Although this is true, the response of the client with anorexia nervosa falls outside the usual range.

4 Although the client with anorexia nervosa's fear of weight gain sometimes reaches delusional proportions, it is based on a belief that being fat is the problem that must be controlled.

238. 3 **Dental enamel erosion occurs from repeated self-induced vomiting.**

1 This is not associated with bulimia.

2 Often body image is disturbed and there is low self-esteem.

4 Habitual regurgitation of small amounts of undigested food (rumination) and reswallowing of food are not associated with bulimia; emptying of the stomach contents through the mouth (vomiting) is associated with bulimia.

239. 1 **Individuals with anorexia often display irritability, hostility, and a depressed mood.**

2 This is associated with individuals with autism.

3 These are associated with individuals with schizophrenia.

4 Clients with eating disorders usually are meticulous about dress and physical appearance; a disheveled appearance is more associated with clients with dementia or depression.

240. 2 **These children usually are severely malnourished and have severe fluid and electrolyte imbalances. Unless these imbalances are corrected, cardiac irregularities and death can occur.**

1 This is important, but it is not the priority at this time.

3 This is important, but it is not the priority at this time.

4 This is important, but it is not the priority at this time.

241. 3 **These clients have severely depleted levels of potassium and sodium because of their starvation diet and energy expenditure; these electrolytes are necessary for adequate cardiac functioning.**

1 Although this may occur, it is not the major health problem.

2 Although this may occur, it is not the major health problem.

4 Although this may occur, it is not the major health problem.

242. 4 **This is a nonthreatening, open-ended response that focuses discussion and leaves channels of communication open.**

1 Although this does not quite accuse the client of lying, it is a threatening response that questions the client's truthfulness.

2 Although this does not quite accuse the client of lying, it is a threatening response that questions the client's truthfulness.

3 Although this is a true statement this response does not encourage discussion.

243. 4 **Clients with bulimia nervosa have a history of eating as a response to strong internal feelings rather than as a response to the sensation of hunger.**

1 Clients with anorexia, not bulimia, often feel powerless and tend to use restrictive eating as a way to enhance a personal sense of control, not to control others.

2 Clients with bulimia nervosa usually eat excessive amounts of food when alone rather than with others. They know that their behavior is dysfunctional and attempt to hide it from others.

3 Binge eating usually is not associated with a woman's menstrual cycle.

244. 1 **Behavior modification programs are helpful treatment modes for many clients with anorexia nervosa.**

2 This is ineffective. The person with anorexia nervosa is more concerned with losing weight than with eating a balanced diet.

3 A well-balanced diet should be encouraged, but actual weight gain is critical and must be reinforced.

4 Although family therapy may be helpful, placing emphasis on the anorexia may reinforce the negative behavior. Also family therapy will not be a priority until the client gains weight.

245. 3 **It is most therapeutic for the staff to control food needs at this time, thus removing the parents from the struggle.**

1 This may be interpreted as accusatory and may precipitate or increase the parents' guilt.

2 This is nontherapeutic; it cuts off the parents from future involvement.

4 This continues the struggle between the parents and the client.

246. Answer: 1, 5

1 **A state of malnutrition with muscle wasting, weakness, and emaciation (cachexia) occurs with anorexia nervosa; clients usually are 15% to 30% below ideal body weight.**

2 Recurrent episodes of the rapid consumption of a large amount of food in a discrete period of time (binge eating) are associated with bulimia nervosa.

3 Constipation can occur with both anorexia nervosa and bulimia nervosa, usually because of a lack of adequate fluids and intestinal-stimulating foods.

4 Hypotension can occur with both anorexia nervosa and bulimia nervosa, usually because of dehydration.

5 **Many clients with anorexia nervosa exhibit psychological symptoms, including a lack of age-appropriate interest in sex and relationships.**

247. 3 **The client's security is increased by limit-setting; guidelines remove responsibility for behavior from the client and increase compliance with the regimen.**

1 The client needs limit-setting, not empathy.

2 Simply maintaining control is not therapeutic and increases the power struggle.

4 Emphasis on food and nutrition may establish a power struggle between the client and the nurse.

248. 3 **This action reinforces behaviors that assist in the achievement of specific goals.**

1 This is not included in a behavior modification program.

2 This is not included in a behavior modification program.

4 Clients talk freely about food; the problem is with ingestion, not discussion.

249. 2 **All food issues should be discussed with the nutritionist, thus removing a potential source of conflict between the nurse and client.**

1 This will accomplish little because the client's failure to eat is not based on food likes or dislikes.

3 This will increase the conflict between the nurse and client.

4 This may be self-defeating because a discussion of food will be the major focus of all nurse-client interactions.

250. 4 **By talking to the client on the telephone at mealtimes, the family is enabling the client to continue destructive behavior; the client and family must be included in discussion of and possible solutions to the problem.**

1 This is a punitive approach that does not address the underlying problem.

2 This is a behavior modification approach that may be used if talking to the family does not produce needed change.

3 This is a punitive approach that does not address the underlying problem.

251. 3 **This demonstrates a change in behavior as well as a positive approach to meals.**

1 The problem is not a lack of interest about food but a deliberate refusal to ingest food.

2 This is typical behavior of a client with anorexia nervosa.

4 This behavior is unrelated to the behavior that needs to be changed.

252. 2 Recovery necessitates major changes in self-esteem and body image, which require therapy over a long time.

1 This is too simplistic a response; anorexia nervosa is not a desire merely to lose weight.

3 Long-term therapy is required.

4 This is only one factor; the client must also be willing to work with the family and to accept the pain associated with change.

253. 4 The anorexic client feels out of control in most situations. The client needs to assume responsibility for treatment associated with this lifelong problem; input into planning and preparation gives some responsibility to the client as well as others in the family.

1 This is not a passing fad.

2 Close supervision takes away the client's responsibility in the treatment regimen and impedes the development of independence from the parents.

3 Close supervision takes away the client's responsibility in the treatment regimen and impedes the development of independence from the parents.

DISORDERS OF MOOD

254. 1 Eye contact reflects a willingness to be open and connect with another person; usually this occurs when trust exists.

2 Accompanying the nurse to the dining room may or may not indicate the presence of trust; this behavior may merely indicate the acceptance of an authority figure.

3 Responding to a question may or may not indicate the presence of trust; this behavior may merely indicate the acceptance of an authority figure.

4 Allowing others to provide for ADLs may or may not indicate the presence of trust; this behavior may merely indicate the acceptance of an authority figure.

255. 4 Limiting unnecessary interactions will decrease stimulation and thus agitation.

1 Constant client and staff contact increases stimulation and thus agitation.

2 Not all disturbed clients are suspicious. This client is unlikely to benefit from this discussion at this time.

3 This bombards the client's sensorium and increases agitation.

256. 3 Depression is characterized by feelings of hopelessness, helplessness, and despair, leaving little room for any pleasure; alteration in appetite (either decreased or increased) is common in depressed clients.

1 Although there is a narrowing of perception, rigidity is uncommon with depression.

2 Fatigue is continually present and does not alternate with a high energy level.

4 There is a loss of interest in socialization and little participation in activities of daily living.

257. 3 Depression usually is both emotional and physical, so a simple daily routine is the least stressful and least anxiety producing.

1 Too many stimuli increase anxiety in a depressed client.

2 A depressed client has limited interest in any activity; offering many may increase anxiety.

4 An extremely depressed client may be incapable of making even simple decisions.

258. 4 Depression is "contagious"; it affects the nurse as well as the client.

1 The client's lack of energy should not make nursing care difficult.

2 These clients usually do not offer negative responses; they offer no response.

3 The client's lack of energy should not make nursing care difficult.

259. 1 Because clients cannot be argued out of their feelings, it is best to initially accept what they say; it also encourages communication.

2 This delays discussing the client's feelings, and the client's low energy level may prevent involvement in activities.

3 This has little effect on the depressed client; it can increase depression.

4 The depressed client does very little talking and needs to be encouraged to communicate.

260. 2 Allowing the client to make decisions that can be handled helps improve confidence.

1 The client is depressed, and this can result in total inactivity.

3 This action will demoralize the client; also it is impossible for one individual to make all the decisions for another.

4 The client is depressed, and this can result in total inactivity.

261. 4 This action demonstrates to the client that the nurse feels the client is worth spending time with, and it helps restore and build trust.

1 This action is impossible to carry out on a regular basis unless the client is potentially suicidal.

2 This action does little to establish communication between the nurse and the client and might be threatening.

3 The depressed client may never get around to speaking to the nurse and, left alone, will withdraw even further.

262. 3 The fact that the nurse spends time with the client conveys a feeling of importance and helps build the client's self-esteem.

1 This places the client on the defensive and does not respond to the feelings of worthlessness communicated by the client.

2 This infers agreement with the client's statement that the client is not worthy; the nurse should stay to convey a sense of self-worth to the client.

4 This response may put the client on the defensive and cut off communication; the client responds better to actions than to words.

263. 2 **This response focuses on the client's feelings rather than the statement, and it serves to open channels of communication.**

1 This response asks the client to decide what is causing feelings; most people are unable to answer why they feel as they do.

3 This response simply echoes the client's statement and does not reflect feelings or stimulate further communication.

4 This response does nothing to stimulate further communication; in fact, it tells the client to talk about feelings with someone else.

264. 1 **This is a therapeutic approach that indicates an awareness of the client's feelings and encourages verbalization.**

2 Moralizing is a barrier to effective communication.

3 This conveys a judgmental or critical attitude toward the client.

4 This is diverting the client's attention to something other than feelings.

265. 3 **Working on the bulletin board with staff members involves minimal energy and decision making and is the least threatening activity.**

1 Playing a board game is too stressful an activity at this time and is a better intervention when self-esteem improves and depression lessens.

2 Singing karaoke is too stressful an activity because it requires energy and a positive self-esteem, which the client does not have at this time.

4 Selecting a movie is too stressful at this time and is a better intervention when self-esteem improves and depression lessens.

266. 2 **Group interaction provides a sense of belonging and fosters the assumption of responsibility.**

1 This is not ensured by group interaction.

3 This is not ensured by group interaction.

4 The group is not the best arena for the expression of repressed hostility.

267. 1 **The client will be most likely to eat if accompanied and encouraged by an individual with whom a trusting relationship has been established.**

2 This will not encourage the client to eat and will promote isolation.

3 This is inappropriate at this time; the client is not interested in maintaining health, nor is the client ready for any teaching.

4 This will be ineffective at this time; the client is too introspective to care.

268. 3 **Depressed clients demonstrate decreased social interaction because of a lack of psychic or physical energy. They tend to withdraw, speak in monosyllables, and avoid contact with others.**

1 This is not a common problem associated with the diagnosis of major depression.

2 This is not a common problem associated with the diagnosis of major depression. Hallucinations are associated with schizophrenic disorders.

4 Depressed clients commonly are negative and pessimistic, especially regarding their future.

269. 2 **Sharing painful feelings reduces the isolation and sense of uniqueness that feelings can cause; sharing of these feelings usually decreases depression.**

1 This will do little to decrease the client's sadness and does not consider the client's low level of energy.

3 This will do little to decrease the client's sadness and does not consider the client's low level of energy.

4 This may be important for the future, if a problem exists, but the sharing of painful feelings is more important than improving communication.

270. 1 **Some success is important to increase the client's self-esteem.**

2 This will support the client's feelings of uselessness.

3 The client, who is in a major depression, does not have the interest or energy to be involved in the decision-making process.

4 The client, who is in a major depression, does not have the interest or energy to act independently.

271. 3 **This therapeutic approach encourages expression of the client's feelings.**

1 This does not explore feelings, and the client may interpret it as a put-down.

2 Although this response appears empathic, it does not encourage an expression of feelings.

4 This question elicits a yes or no response rather than encouraging expression of feelings.

272. 4 **The best long-term goal is that the client attains a positive attitude about the self, others, and life in general; this indicates that treatment has been effective and discharge can occur.**

1 This is a short-term goal associated with a therapeutic milieu.

2 This is a short-term goal and an expected behavior on an inpatient unit.

3 This is an intermediate goal that helps the client focus on others; this goal is a step toward achieving long-term goals.

273. 1 **ECT is contraindicated in the presence of a brain tumor because the treatment causes an increase in intracranial pressure.**

2 There is no contraindication to ECT with this health problem.

3 There is no contraindication to ECT with this health problem.

4 There is no contraindication to ECT with this health problem.

274. 4 **The expression of these feelings may indicate that this client is unable to continue the struggle of life.**

1 These are not indications of potential suicide; the client is still responding to the world, not attempting to leave it.

2 These usually are not sufficient to precipitate a suicide attempt.

3 The client attempting suicide usually sees death as a release.

275. 3 **This is the most important assessment to make because suicide is a possibility with every depressed client.**

1 The client has already said this, and it responds to only part of the client's statement.

2 This is a philosophical approach that will not encourage discussion of feelings.

4 The client probably is unable to answer this question.

276. 1 **As the client's motivation and energy return, there is a greater threat that suicidal ideation will be acted out.**

2 There are no data regarding visitation rights; the priority concern is the greater risk for suicide.

3 Although this eventually will be done, the priority is to determine the potential for suicide.

4 Although this should be done, the greater risk of suicide takes precedence.

277. 3 **This statement provides clues that the client feels no one cares, so there is no reason the client should care. These feelings are common in depression.**

1 The clues presented do not lead to this conclusion.

2 The clues presented do not lead to this conclusion.

4 The clues presented do not lead to this conclusion.

278. **Answer: 3, 4, 5**

1 Although depressed clients may not have the energy to eat, this is not an initial priority.

2 An inability to concentrate is a common complaint of depressed clients, but it has not been linked to an increased risk for suicide.

3 **Some depressed clients demonstrate agitation rather then psychomotor retardation. Agitated clients are more likely to act impulsively, increasing the risk for self-harm.**

4 **Clients who have attempted suicide in the past are at risk for attempting suicide in the future.**

5 **Suicidal ideation may progress to suicide threats, gestures, or attempts.**

279. 4 **This is the correct description; the client had attained orgasm previously.**

1 Libido is sexual desire; it usually does not influence physiological response.

2 This is a nonexistent term; it is impossible to evaluate the quality of an orgasm.

3 This defines the disorder whereby the female has never attained an orgasm.

280. 1 **Decreased sexual desire is a major symptom of clinical depression. Other vegetative signs of depression include changes in bowel elimination, eating habits, and sleeping patterns.**

2 Although depression is often related to unmet dependency needs, the decreased sexual desire is associated with the depression, not the unmet dependency needs.

3 The sexual difficulties are associated with the depression, and the depression may be the major cause of marital stress, not the sexual difficulties. Also, there are no data indicating marital stress.

4 Role confusion, not identity confusion, usually is associated with depression.

281. 4 **This recognizes feelings and behavior; it encourages the client to share feelings and promotes trust, which is essential for a therapeutic relationship.**

1 Although these are important actions, they are not enough; nursing intervention with the client must be included.

2 Without verbal encouragement, the depressed client will not respond to this intervention.

3 This assumes too much and may be inaccurate; an indirect approach should be used.

282. 1 **A matter-of-fact approach helps avoid a cycle in which the nurse expresses concern to a client who feels unworthy, which increases feelings of unworthiness.**

2 Citing a hospital policy focuses on rules and regulations, which may exacerbate the client's negative personal feelings because he is breaking the rules.

3 This is a statement that the client may not be able to explain.

4 This response may increase feelings of unworthiness because it creates a gap between the nurse's estimate of the client and what the client feels.

283 3 **The suicidal client cannot think about a positive future; therefore, focusing on the future indicates improvement.**

1 Feeling like a burden to others reflects a low self-esteem, which also increases the risk for suicide.

2 Feeling alone reflects a perceived lack of support, which increases the risk for suicide.

4 Not being able to talk about feelings increases the risk for suicide because the client must be able to verbalize feelings to reduce anxiety, seek help, or engage in therapy.

284. 4 **As depression increases, thought processes become slower and verbal expression decreases due to lack of emotional energy.**

1 Elation is related to a bipolar disorder, manic episode; the affect of a depressed person usually is one of sadness or it may be blank.

2 Loose associations are related to schizophrenia, not depression.

3 Physical exhaustion is associated with a bipolar disorder, manic episode; decreased physical activity does not produce physical exhaustion.

285. 2 **This response demonstrates empathy; in addition, it focuses on the client's feelings.**

1 This can be answered yes or no; an open-ended response allows for more self-expression.

3 This response reflects only part of the content; it may be the least significant part of the client's statement.

4 "Why" questions should be avoided because people often do not know why they feel or behave the way they do; this question may cause defensiveness.

286. **4 During a manic episode hyperactivity and the inability to sit still long enough to eat are the causes of eating difficulties.**

1 Feelings of guilt do not precipitate eating difficulties in clients with the diagnosis of bipolar disorder, manic episode.

2 Clients in a manic episode of bipolar disorder have a need to avoid and therefore control anxiety associated with depression; they do not have a need to control others.

3 Clients in a manic episode of bipolar disorder have a need to avoid and therefore control anxiety associated with depression; they do not have a desire for punishment.

287. **2 During the manic phase of the illness, the client responds to everything in the environment; therefore, it is important that the room be quiet and restful to decrease stimulation.**

1 This is not an important consideration at this time for this client.

3 A room close to the nurse's desk is too stimulating because of its location.

4 This probably will increase both the client's and the roommate's behavioral acting out.

288. **3 The client in a manic episode of the illness often neglects basic needs; these needs are a priority to ensure adequate nutrition, fluid, and rest. The hyperactivity of mania creates an increased need for calories.**

1 Although the client needs to expend excess energy, physical exhaustion and dehydration are real possibilities during the manic episode of the illness.

2 This is counterproductive and punitive.

4 The client is unable to actively participate in group activities at this time.

289. **1 The client who is aggressive in groups must begin socialization in one-to-one interactions that are less stimulating and distracting.**

2 Promoting self-care avoids addressing behaviors in group and social situations.

3 The client may not be interested in or able to follow guidelines for appropriate conduct at this time.

4 The client may not be able to decrease his activity at this time and therefore it must be channeled appropriately.

290. **1 Because the plan does not meet the client's needs, it should be changed.**

2 The client has already let the staff know that finger foods are not wanted.

3 Continuing the plan will be frustrating for the client and the staff because the client's behavior indicates that snacks are not wanted.

4 When the client's needs are not being met, the plan should be changed immediately.

291. **Answer: 2, 3**

1 Touching can be threatening for many clients and should not be used indiscriminately.

2 **Structure tends to decrease agitation and anxiety and to increase the client's feelings of security.**

3 **Whether the individual is experiencing mania or depression nutritional needs must be met. The hyperactivity associated with mania interferes with the ability to sit still long enough to eat; hyperactivity requires an increase in the intake of calories for the energy expended.**

4 Conversations should be kept simple. The client with a bipolar disorder, either depressed or manic phase, may have difficulty following involved conversations about current affairs.

5 Clients with bipolar disorders are in contact with reality, so this activity will serve little purpose.

292. **4 Acting-out behavior may precipitate negative feelings toward the client. These individuals are acutely aware of others' feelings; perceived negative feelings may increase the client's hostility and inappropriate behavior.**

1 If the nurse's feelings are negative, increasing the time spent with the client will exaggerate problems for both the nurse and the client.

2 Placing the client in isolation may appear punitive rather than therapeutic.

3 Ignoring some minor acting-out behavior may be beneficial; however, limits usually need to be set to maintain the client's dignity and prevent escalation of inappropriate behavior.

293. **2 During a manic episode a client has an inflated self-esteem that replaces feelings with which the client cannot cope.**

1 This feeling is not associated with bipolar disorder, manic episode.

3 This feeling is not associated with bipolar disorder, manic episode.

4 This feeling is not associated with bipolar disorder, manic episode.

294. **3 During the manic phase when clients are unable to control their behavior they should be protected from embarrassing themselves or harming others.**

1 These clients are unable to deal with others' feelings; the client's own feelings are primary at this time. Also the statement is too general to communicate which behaviors are dysfunctional.

2 The client's behavior cannot be ignored because the client or others may be hurt if limits are not set.

4 This statement is critical of the client who is unable to respond differently at this time.

295. **2 During a manic episode clients attempt to keep active to prevent the feeling of depression from overtaking them; avoidance of their feelings, not**

food, is their priority, and they do not take the time to eat.

1 Feelings of grandeur have replaced unconscious feelings of unworthiness at this phase of the illness.

3 The manic phase is not characterized by a desire for punishment. These clients usually are not aware of unconscious feelings.

4 Clients in the manic phase do not control anxiety by the use of ritualistic behavior; ritualistic behavior is common in clients with an obsessive-compulsive disorder.

296. 1 **The excited, overactive client needs a calm environment; external stimulation causes further excitation.**

2 The client needs reduced, not increased, external stimulation.

3 The client needs reduced, not increased, external stimulation.

4 The client needs reduced, not increased, external stimulation.

297. 2 **A firm voice is most effective; the statement tells the client that it is the behavior, not the client, that is upsetting to others.**

1 Demanding that the client stop the current behavior is a useless action; the client is out of control and needs external control.

3 The client does not know what is precipitating the behavior, and the question will be frustrating.

4 This should be done if the client does not respond to firm limit-setting.

298. 1 **These individuals are acutely aware of what is happening and react strongly to environmental stimuli.**

2 These clients' symptoms are an attempt to avoid anxiety and do not cause embarrassment.

3 These clients are not out of contact with reality; in fact, they are continually reacting to it.

4 These individuals are unable to control acting-out behavior.

299. 4 **This response simply states a fact, specifically identifies positive behavior, and delivers praise without making demands.**

1 This puts the total responsibility for control on a client who needs external controls set.

2 This does not help the client separate the self from the behavior; it tells the client that acting-out behavior will result in rejection.

3 The client may not recall what happened yesterday and may not be able to compare the differences.

300. 1 **This distracts the client and provides for a controlled expenditure of energy without impinging on others.**

2 This is punitive and the client may react with increased activity.

3 The hyperactive client is unable to sit still long enough to play cards, and the activity will not allow for an expenditure of energy.

4 Logic will not necessarily interrupt the behavior; the nursing intervention needs to be more concrete.

301. 3 **The client with hypomanic symptoms cannot tolerate sitting still long enough to eat an adequate meal; handheld foods will help to meet the client's nutritional needs and do not require the client to sit down.**

1 This client will most likely ignore the tray.

2 Unworthy feelings are related to a depressive, not manic, episode.

4 It is unlikely that this client will understand or care about this information.

302. 4 **Antidepressants can induce rapid cyclic behaviors or the client may not be taking medications as prescribed; this statement elicits information in a nonchallenging, nonthreatening manner.**

1 This statement is challenging and is not focused on assessing the problem.

2 This question is not focused on the behavior manifested.

3 This statement does little to promote discussion with this client.

303. 3 **For the safety of the client and everyone on the unit, improvement in a client's level of self-control is essential before progressively reducing the degree of restraint and seclusion.**

1 Continuing intensive interaction at this time would not be productive and could cause the client's behavior to escalate.

2 The nurse's prime responsibility should be the client; staff members can assess other staff members.

4 Observing for side effects of medications is only one of the many components to be assessed when determining the client's level of self-control.

DISORDERS OF PERSONALITY

304. 3 **Clients with the diagnosis of schizoid personality disorder neither desire nor enjoy close relationships, prefer solitary activities, and demonstrate emotional coldness, detachment, and a flattened affect.**

1 These are typical of clients with the diagnosis of obsessive-compulsive personality disorder.

2 These are typical of clients with the diagnosis of dependent personality disorder.

4 These are typical of clients with the diagnosis of schizotypal personality disorder.

305. 2 **Acting-out is the process of expressing feelings behaviorally.**

1 The action is not exploitive because no evidence is provided to demonstrate that anyone has been used to get what the client wants.

3 The action is not manipulative because no evidence is provided to demonstrate that anyone has been influenced against his or her wishes.

4 The action is not disguising unacceptable feelings by expressing opposite emotions.

306. 1 **Imagery is a therapeutic approach used to facilitate positive self-talk; mental pictures under the control of and initiated by the client may correct faulty cognitions.**

  2 This is a useful general behavioral approach but is not a specific desensitization technique.

  3 This is a useful general behavioral approach but is not a specific desensitization technique.

  4 This is a useful general behavioral approach but is not a specific desensitization technique.

307. 1 **A discussion of the feared object will trigger an emotional response to the object.**

  2 Extreme fear is more of a problem than resentment.

  3 Clients with phobias generally have rigid impulse control.

  4 Distortion of reality is not a problem for a client with a phobia.

308. 4 **The client's expressed feelings are opposite and are an acceptable substitute for repressed antisocial feelings when facing the roommate.**

  1 The client's feelings are expressed to the nurse, not projected or attributed to others.

  2 The client expressed real feelings to the nurse and made no attempt to make an instinctual, socially unacceptable impulse into an acceptable behavior.

  3 The client did not mask covert hostility by overt compliance.

309. 3 **The mother's behavior sends two conflicting messages; one says "I care" and the other says "I don't care"; this behavior is often demonstrated by people with personality disorders.**

  1 If the mother were rejecting the daughter, she would not have brought a gift.

  2 There is no evidence of a projection of feelings.

  4 Passive-aggressive behavior is an indirect, rather than direct, expression of angry or hostile feelings.

310. 4 **This response demonstrates acceptance of the client and sets limits on the client's manipulative behavior.**

  1 This reinforces the client's statement that the evening staff is punishing her, which could cause splitting among the staff members.

  2 This response indicates that the nurse has been manipulated by the client.

  3 This is false reassurance; the nurse cannot make everything all right.

311. 2 **The establishment of trust between the client and nurse should be a prerequisite for using confrontation.**

  1 The last time medication was administered is not a significant factor in relation to the use of confrontation.

  3 Clients with the diagnosis of borderline personality disorder tend to be impulsive and egocentric and have difficulty being empathic toward others.

  4 Client self-awareness is not a prerequisite for the use of confrontation; the purpose of confrontation is to help the client become self-aware.

312. 4 **Sitting with the client indicates acceptance and demonstrates that the nurse feels the client is worthy of the nurse's time.**

  1 It is better to stay with the client quietly until control is regained; staying prevents a follow-through on the client's threat.

  2 This provides little comfort for the client.

  3 This may close off further communication.

313. 3 **The withdrawn pattern of behavior prevents the individual from reaching out to others for sharing; the isolation produces feelings of loneliness.**

  1 Feelings of anger may result in withdrawal, but withdrawal does not produce feelings of anger.

  2 Feelings of paranoia may result in withdrawal, but withdrawal does not produce these feelings.

  4 Repression is an unconscious defense whereby the individual excludes ideas, feelings, or situations from the conscious level of thought; this does not result from withdrawal.

314. 1 **Withdrawal provides a temporary defense against anxiety because it limits contact with reality and decreases the client's world.**

  2 Withdrawal does not accomplish this because feelings and anxieties are still present and little attempt is made to work through problems.

  3 Withdrawal does not accomplish this because feelings and anxieties are still present and little attempt is made to work through problems.

  4 Withdrawal does not accomplish this because feelings and anxieties are still present and little attempt is made to work through problems.

315. 1 **If this goal is met, the client's relationship with others should improve in all aspects, including sexual, as self-esteem and self-confidence improve.**

  2 Increasing insight may be helpful, but should not receive priority. The client may or may not have a sexual disorder.

  3 This goal is not appropriate at this time; examining these feelings is nonproductive until the client's self-esteem improves.

  4 Increasing the client's knowledge of sexual functioning may be done, but improving self-esteem should receive priority.

316. 4 **A conflict exists between wanting to be taken care of and wanting to be self-reliant; ambivalence fosters lowered self-esteem.**

  1 These do not relate to the behavior described; people usually do not alternate these emotions, which are at opposite ends of the spectrum.

  2 This is the developmental conflict of the infant, according to Erikson; it is not related to the behavior described.

  3 This is the developmental conflict of the young adult, according to Erikson; it is not related to the behavior described.

317. **2 In the early part of treatment, before new defenses are developed, enough time must be allowed for the client to complete the ritual to keep anxiety under control.**
1 The ritual is a defense that cannot be interrupted or delayed; it is used until new defenses are developed.
3 The ritual is a defense that cannot be interrupted or delayed; it is used until new defenses are developed.
4 The client probably will select the ritual, which will jeopardize the client's nutritional status. Forcing the client to make this choice may be perceived as punitive.

318. **1 Ritualistic behavior seen in this disorder is aimed at controlling feelings of anxiety and guilt by maintaining an absolute set pattern of action.**
2 Although the person with an obsessive-compulsive disorder may be angry and hostile, the feelings of anger and hostility do not precipitate the rituals.
3 Although the person with an obsessive-compulsive disorder may be embarrassed and ashamed as a result of performing the ritual, the basic feelings precipitating the rituals usually are feelings of anxiety and guilt.
4 Although the person with an obsessive-compulsive disorder may feel hopeless and powerless as a result of performing the ritual, the basic feelings precipitating the rituals usually are feelings of anxiety and guilt.

319. **2 This is the psychoanalytical explanation for the development of obsessive-compulsive symptomatology.**
1 Compulsive rituals commonly result in interference with activities of daily living and the individual becomes dysfunctional; rituals cannot be controlled.
3 This is the general description of phobias.
4 The client is unable to consciously stop the behavior because anxiety will become overwhelming if the ritualistic defense is not used. The behavior is not overwhelming because it limits anxiety.

320. **1 This limits the time lost to the ritual but still allows the ritual; until the underlying cause of anxiety can be dealt with, rituals should be allowed as much as possible.**
2 This provides for only one time period which probably will result in increased anxiety.
3 One ritual cannot be substituted for another; this will interfere with the performance of the original ritual and may result in overwhelming anxiety.
4 This is the client's decision; the nurse should not recommend this action.

321. **2 Paraphrasing encourages further ventilation of feelings and concerns by the client.**
1 This is a negative response that may increase the client's fears about being "crazy."
3 This provides false reassurance and implies that the client is out of control, which may increase fears.
4 This response denies the client's feelings.

322. **3 This validates the client's feelings and attempts to help the client problem solve.**
1 The client may or may not be exhausted, and the response gives advice, which should be avoided because it promotes dependency.
2 This response is judgmental and belittles the client.
4 Although this response attempts to validate the client's feelings, it also belittles the client because it implies that the children's behavior is acceptable and the client is unreasonable.

323. **1 The rituals used by a client with obsessive-compulsive disorder help control the anxiety level by maintaining a set pattern of action.**
2 The client cannot consciously control the ritual.
3 Rituals are used primarily to handle feelings of anxiety and generally are seen by the client as illogical; they provide few secondary gains.
4 Rituals are used primarily to handle feelings of anxiety and are a means of diverting attention from these feelings.

324. **3 This reflects a reenactment of the mother-child relationship; behavior vacillates between distancing to avoid engulfment and clinging to avoid being rejected.**
1 Shame often results from a struggle, but is not the focus of a conflicting fear.
2 Self-esteem and fear of hostility are outcomes, not the focus of a conflict.
4 Engulfment is part of the conflict, but interdependence is not a conflicting fear and may be a healthy balance of dependence and independence.

325. **1 The expectation is communicated that before the medication is given the client must first try to sleep.**
2 No data are given to indicate that the client is out of touch with reality, nor is this a form of reality testing.
3 No data are given to substantiate that the nurse is enforcing a rule to preserve a routine; in addition, it does not individualize care.
4 The nurse's response is not an attempt to condition behavior; it merely communicates an expectation.

326. **4 The client is angry and reacts impulsively; the action is unplanned and is not under the client's control.**
1 No data are provided to suggest that the client is out of contact with reality; the client is reacting to a real situation with anger.
2 There is no identifiable cluster of behaviors to suggest that the client has a violent personality.
3 There is no pattern of behavior to suggest an antisocial personality, which may or may not involve impulse control.

327. **1 The client is unable to control impulses at this time, so controls must be provided for the client; the nurse's behavior provides a role model.**
2 The client is not able to establish self-controls; freedom may be frightening to a client who is not in control.

3 This is not therapeutic; this probably will provoke more acting-out behavior.

4 This is not therapeutic; this probably will provoke more acting-out behavior.

328. 1 **Cluster A includes paranoid, schizoid, and schizotypal personality disorders. These clients are odd and eccentric and use strange speech, are angry, and have impaired relationships.**

2 Cluster C includes avoidant, dependent, and obsessive-compulsive personality disorders. These clients are anxious, fearful, tense, and rigid.

3 Cluster B includes antisocial, borderline, histrionic, and narcissistic personality disorders. These clients are dramatic, erratic, labile, impulsive, hostile, and manipulative.

4 Cluster B includes antisocial, borderline, histrionic, and narcissistic personality disorders. These clients are dramatic, erratic, labile, impulsive, hostile, and manipulative.

329. 2 **Both clients must be included in a discussion about this behavior to make certain that limits on future behavior are understood by both of them; this action also places controls on the manipulative behavior often used by clients with an antisocial personality disorder.**

1 This action will cause the clients to find another place to meet; the response sets no limits on behavior but only addresses the location of the behavior.

3 This action does not set any limits on behavior and puts a staff member in the policing role.

4 Although this may be necessary, the nurse must respond directly to the clients involved in this situation.

330. 4 **These are the most therapeutic parental actions; the client must be made accountable for behavior and must know that manipulation and acting-out will not be tolerated.**

1 This probably is a continuation of the parents' previous response to the client and proves to be of little value.

2 This may cause the client to continue to act out to test the limit of the parents' endurance.

3 These activities are outside the parents' control.

331. 3 **To prevent these behaviors the nurse must be steadfast and consistent in confronting unacceptable behaviors, protecting vulnerable clients, and enforcing the rules and policies of the unit.**

1 Observation is a passive approach that will neither protect the other clients nor foster the client's understanding of the behavior.

2 Although this will protect the other clients, it will not help the client begin to understand how others feel and react to his unacceptable behaviors.

4 These actions do not provide the client with feedback about unacceptable behaviors. Limiting contact with all other clients is punitive.

332. 2 **The nurse's response is not therapeutic because it does not recognize the client's needs but tries to make the client feel guilty for being demanding.**

1 Impulse control refers to a sudden driving force being constrained or held back.

3 Nothing in the nurse's statement achieves reality reinforcement; the nurse is defensive, not therapeutic.

4 Nothing in the nurse's statement sets limits; the nurse is defensive, not therapeutic.

333. **Answer: 4, 5**

1 Aloofness is associated with the schizoid personality.

2 Suspiciousness is associated with the paranoid personality.

3 Perfectionism is associated with the paranoid personality.

4 **People with antisocial personalities often are irresponsible, amoral, and dishonest, and do not learn from negative experiences.**

5 **People with antisocial personalities often can be charming and calculating when exploiting others; they show no remorse for hurting others and do not develop insight into predictable consequences.**

334. 4 **The expression of feelings by this individual demonstrates the development of some insight and a willingness to at least begin to look at underlying causes of behavior.**

1 This probably will have little meaning to the client.

2 This probably will have little meaning to the client.

3 This probably will have little meaning to the client.

335. 3 **A client with an antisocial personality disorder is charming on first contact; this charm is a manipulative ploy. These clients usually are bright and use their intelligence for self-gain.**

1 This behavior more closely applies to an individual with an obsessive-compulsive personality disorder.

2 The client with a borderline personality disorder self-mutilates when under stress; there is a fear of abandonment so that any relationship is better than no relationship.

4 This resembles the behavior of an individual with a paranoid personality, which includes suspiciousness and lack of trust.

336. 2 **Clients with an antisocial personality disorder need a consistent, united staff approach because they are experts in manipulation and exploitation; they can ignore rules and divide staff members.**

1 These clients do not need to be encouraged to interact with other people because they are forward in their approach to others.

3 A nurturing, forgiving tone will foster and increase manipulation, not decrease it.

4 Seclusion is an overreaction to manipulative behaviors; it implies punishment, which is not productive. Seclusion is used only when the client may injure self or others.

337. 3 **A dissociative identity disorder is a complex, multifaceted problem that requires long-term therapy to achieve integration of the personalities.**
  1 Each personality has the ability to deal openly with feelings, but the personalities need to be integrated.
  2 None of the personalities can be ignored because their presence must be dealt with before integration can occur.
  4 The multiple personalities do serve a protective purpose. If they did not serve a protective purpose, they would be abandoned.

SCHIZOPHRENIC DISORDERS

338. 2 **A delusion is a fixed false belief.**
  1 An illusion is a false sense interpretation of an external stimulus.
  3 Confabulation is the client's attempt to fill gaps in memory with imaginary events.
  4 An hallucination is a false sensory perception with no external stimulus.

339. 4 **These clients are threatened by reality; withdrawal from reality and the use of magical thinking reduce anxiety.**
  1 The loosening of associative links that occurs in schizophrenia makes this impossible.
  2 Clients with severe depression, not schizophrenia, may be preoccupied with suicidal thoughts.
  3 Clients with schizophrenia have low self-esteem and usually have feelings of guilt and self-blame.

340. 4 **A person with this disorder will not have adequate self-boundaries.**
  1 A weak ego and a negative self-perception are associated with schizophrenia.
  2 Low self-esteem is associated with schizophrenia because these people have inadequate ego defenses, lack of ego strengths, and distortions of reality.
  3 Concrete thinking is symptomatic of schizophrenia.

341. 4 **Loose associations are thoughts that are presented without the logical connections that are usually necessary for the listener to interpret the message.**
  1 Echolalia is the purposeless repetition of words spoken by others or repetition of overheard sounds.
  2 Neologisms are new meaningless words coined by the client, or new unique meanings given to old words.
  3 Flight of ideas is the rapid skipping from one thought to another; these thoughts usually have only superficial or chance relationships.

342. 1 **The presence of ego strengths is demonstrated by some level of adjustment before the occurrence of the precipitating event; these ego strengths can be used to help the client reorganize the personality.**
  2 This tends to contribute to a poor prognosis.
  3 This tends to contribute to a poor prognosis.
  4 This tends to contribute to a poor prognosis.

343. 2 **The usual age of onset of schizophrenia is adolescence or early adulthood.**
  1 Signs and symptoms usually do not appear this early.
  3 Signs and symptoms usually do not appear this early.
  4 Signs and symptoms usually do not appear this early.

344. 2 **Ideas of reference, seen with psychotic thinking, is a delusional belief that others are talking about the client.**
  1 Flight of ideas is the rapid thinking seen in clients in a manic state.
  3 Grandiose delusions are irrational beliefs that overestimate one's ability or worth.
  4 Thought broadcasting is the delusional belief that others can read one's thoughts.

345. 2 **Neologisms are words that are invented and understood only by the person using them.**
  1 Echolalia is the verbal repeating of exactly what is heard.
  3 Concretism is a pattern of speech characterized by the absence of abstractions or generalizations.
  4 Perseveration is a disturbed system of thinking manifested by repetitive verbalizations or motions, or persistent repetition of the same idea in response to different questions.

346. 3 **The client needs to feel comfortable in the environment before establishing enough trust to undress for showering; the nurse's statement allows the client to make the decision.**
  1 This statement can add to the client's anxiety and feelings of loss of control; also it can add to any delusional thoughts the client may have.
  2 This action can add to the client's anxiety and feelings of loss of control; also it can add to any delusional thoughts the client may have.
  4 This statement will not help the client's self-image, and it does not matter what other clients think.

347. Answer: 1, 3, 5
  1 **Bizarre behavior is associated with undifferentiated schizophrenia.**
  2 Extreme negativism is associated with catatonic schizophrenia.
  3 **Disorganized speech is associated with undifferentiated schizophrenia.**
  4 Persecutory delusions are associated with paranoid schizophrenia.
  5 **Auditory hallucinations are associated with undifferentiated schizophrenia.**

348. 3 **A somatic delusion is a fixed false belief about one's body.**
  1 Echolalia is the automatic and meaningless oral repetition of another's words or phrases.
  2 Hypochondriasis is a severe, morbid preoccupation with an unrealistic interpretation of real or imagined physical symptoms.
  4 Depersonalization is a feeling of unreality and alienation from oneself.

349. 1 **This explores more fully the client's ideas, experiences, or relationships; this response promotes communication.**
    2 Arguing about delusions increases anxiety and diminishes trust.
    3 This denies feelings and implies the client is wrong; it may cause the client to defend feelings further.
    4 This puts the blame on the client and implies the feelings are based on reality.

350. 2 **Failure to accept the client and the client's fears establishes a barrier to effective communication.**
    1 Today, mental health therapy is directed toward returning the client to the community as rapidly as possible.
    3 Electroconvulsive therapy (ECT) is not the treatment of choice for clients with schizophrenia.
    4 Family cooperation is helpful but not an absolute necessity.

351. 4 **Command hallucinations are auditory hallucinations that give verbal messages to do harm either to the self or others; giving an identity to the hallucinated voice increases the risk of compliance.**
    1 A delusion is a false belief held to be true even with evidence to the contrary.
    2 When a person has magical thinking, the individual believes that thinking about something can make it happen. Magical thinking is common in young children.
    3 The data do not indicate the client has regressed to a prior level of development.

352. 3 **These are classic behaviors exhibited by clients with a diagnosis of schizophrenia.**
    1 These are more commonly associated with dementia.
    2 These are more commonly associated with bipolar disorder, manic phase.
    4 These are more commonly associated with depression.

353. 2 **Word salad is an incoherent mixture of words.**
    1 Echolalia is a pathologic repeating of another's words or phrases.
    3 Confabulation is the unconscious filling in of memory gaps with imagined or untrue experiences.
    4 Flight of ideas is a speech pattern of rapid transition from topic to topic. The client's statement is too limited to be considered flight of ideas.

354. 2 **The client cannot reach out to others because of lack of trust. Withdrawal is used to defend against interpersonal threats, which results in isolation.**
    1 Chronic confusion and disorientation are not usually associated with this disorder. Illogical thinking and impaired judgment are associated with schizophrenia.
    3 Individuals with the diagnosis of schizophrenia often have personal boundary difficulties. They lack a sense of where their bodies end in relation to where others begin. Loss of ego boundaries can result in depersonalization and derealization.

    4 Most clients with schizophrenic disorders are not violent.

355. 4 **Any other approach will be threatening, increase anxiety, and probably result in a physical confrontation.**
    1 This will increase anxiety, not foster decision making.
    2 This will increase the client's anxiety and probably result in a physical confrontation.
    3 This will increase anxiety, not self-esteem.

356. 4 **A somatic delusion is a false belief that one has a disease or a physical defect.**
    1 A delusion about being a person of importance is a grandiose delusion.
    2 A delusion about death is a nihilistic delusion.
    3 A delusion that others are out to cause personal harm is a paranoid delusion.

357. 3 **Helping the client to develop feelings of self-worth will reduce the client's need to use pathological defenses.**
    1 Faith or the lack of faith is not the basic underlying problem but merely a symptom of it.
    2 Self-control or the lack of self-control is not the basic underlying problem but merely a symptom of it.
    4 Insight can develop only when the need to use the defense is reduced; this is a long-term goal.

358. 2 **By using the defense mechanism of projection, the client is attributing to others those personal feelings that are objectionable to the self.**
    1 No evidence is given to support an interpretation that redirection is being used.
    3 The client is not exploring emotionally charged reactions.
    4 There is no evidence to support this interpretation.

359. 2 **This response accepts the client at the client's present level and allows the client to set the pace of the relationship.**
    1 This approach to any client can be misinterpreted and may precipitate an aggressive response.
    3 This response asks the client to reach out to the nurse; in the therapeutic relationship the nurse must reach out to the client.
    4 Even if the client is too withdrawn to respond, the nurse's physical presence can be reassuring.

360. Answer: 1, 2
    1 **A lack of energy (anergy) is a negative symptom associated with schizophrenia type II.**
    2 **Inadequate grooming results from apathy and lack of energy and is a negative symptom associated with schizophrenia type II.**
    3 Illogical speech that reflects disorganized thinking is a positive symptom associated with schizophrenia type I.
    4 Ideas of reference, a thought process in which a person believes he or she is the object of environmental attention, is a positive symptom associated with schizophrenia type I.

5 Agitated, hostile, angry, and violent behaviors are positive symptoms associated with schizophrenia type I.

361. 2 This is an example of an olfactory hallucination, a sense of perception for which no external stimulus exists.

1 This is an example of a delusion of grandeur. A delusion is a fixed false belief held to be true by the person even with evidence to the contrary.

3 This is an example of a compulsion. A compulsion is a repetitive, intrusive urge to perform an act contrary to one's ordinary wishes or standards.

4 This is an example of an obsession. An obsession is an insistent, painful, intrusive idea, impulse, or emotion that arises from within and cannot be suppressed or ignored.

362. 1 Participating with one trusted individual gradually diminishes the need for withdrawal. It also allows for nonverbal communication.

2 This is not an appropriate initial activity because it requires a higher level of functioning than the other activities presented.

3 This activity fosters competition, which is not helpful at this time.

4 This will not increase socialization but rather will promote withdrawal.

363. 2 These ideas are not well connected and there is no clear train of thought. This is an example of loose association.

1 Word salad refers to incoherent expressions that contain jumbled words. This client's thoughts are coherent but not connected.

3 Thought blocking occurs when the client loses the train of thinking and ideas are not completed. Each of the client's thoughts is complete but not linked to the next thought.

4 These statements are reality based and not reflective of delusional thinking.

364. 1 This statement lets the client know the nurse sees her as a person and is willing to help her face a new experience.

2 This will do nothing to allay the client's anxiety about facing a new situation.

3 This is not true; even if the client does not like it, as part of the therapy program, she should be encouraged to go.

4 This will do nothing to allay the client's anxiety about facing a new situation.

365. 4 This is helpful in decreasing hallucinations because it provides another stimulus to compete for the client's attention.

1 This will foster and support the hallucinations.

2 This will foster and support the hallucinations.

3 Connections should be made to decrease the use of hallucinations.

366. 3 To function interpersonally with a group, these individuals must first develop a trusting one-to-one relationship.

1 These individuals need interaction to increase trust; they will not seek interactions without encouragement.

2 If forced, these individuals will be too fearful of the group to function in it or benefit by it.

4 Dependency can have an adverse effect on individuals with schizophrenia.

367. 1 Because the client is newly admitted, the nurse needs to do a thorough assessment before intervening.

2 This may eventually be done but it is not the priority.

3 This response assumes that the client is hallucinating. Because the client is newly admitted, further assessment is necessary first.

4 The client's behavior does not indicate the need for extra medication at this time. Some clients with schizophrenia have hallucinations throughout their lives.

368. 3 Projection is the common defense mechanism found in delusions. Projection is attributing to others one's own unacceptable feelings, impulses, or thoughts.

1 Splitting occurs when the individual fails to integrate the positive and negative qualities of the self or others into cohesive images and compartmentalizes opposite affective states.

2 Undoing is symbolically canceling out an experience.

4 Sublimation is the channeling of unacceptable impulses into constructive activities.

369. 4 The client truly believes the voices are real because they reflect the client's thoughts; the voices usually are accusatory and derogatory and therefore may be frightening.

1 Playing soft music after hallucinations have started will not be strong enough to compete for the client's attention.

2 This is too late; competing stimuli must be present to block the occurrence of hallucinations.

3 The client cannot be talked out of a hallucination.

370. 2 This helps the client explore underlying feelings and allows the client to understand the message the verbalizations are communicating.

1 This denies the client's feelings rather than accepting and working with them.

3 This focuses on the delusion itself rather than the feeling causing the delusion.

4 Attempting to divert the client denies feelings rather than accepting and working with them.

371. 3 This provides specific realistic feedback without rejecting the client.

1 This reply is defensive and insulting to the client.

2 This will most likely encourage more inappropriate communication.

4 Her behavior is the issue and switching assignments does not address this. The client may view this as rejection.

372. 2 **A broad opening encourages communication that may elicit the client's perception of the day's events.**
    1 This is premature.
    3 What is most important is the client's, not the parents', perception of what has occurred.
    4 This is premature; there are no data that indicate that the client may harm himself or others.

373. 2 **Ambivalence makes decision making difficult if not impossible; simple, easy-to-follow declarative statements limit the choices available for the indecisive client.**
    1 The client will be unable to interpret nonverbal communication and will experience increased confusion and indecision.
    3 This is inappropriate because the pressure to make choices may increase the client's ambivalence and discomfort.
    4 This is inappropriate because the pressure to make choices may increase the client's ambivalence and discomfort.

374. 1 **This response reflects the client's feelings and avoids focusing on the delusion.**
    2 This will not change the client's feelings because the belief is real to the client.
    3 This will not change the client's feelings because the other pitcher also may be perceived as poisoned.
    4 This will not change the client's feelings; the client will believe that the nurse was not really drinking the juice.

375. 4 **This approach gives the client and family an opportunity to discuss their feelings together and clarifies their expectations.**
    1 This is the nurse's responsibility and should not be passed to someone else.
    2 This is not the nurse's role; the family may never be reassured.
    3 This will do little to reassure the family.

376. 1 **The fetal position represents regressed behavior; regression is a way of responding to overwhelming anxiety.**
    2 This interpretation assumes that the nurse controls the client's behavior; the client is not responding to the nurse any differently than to anyone else who tries to establish reality contact.
    3 There are no data to substantiate this; further assessment is necessary to make this interpretation.
    4 There are no data to substantiate this; further assessment is necessary to make this interpretation.

377. 2 **This allows the client to work off energy without upsetting other clients.**
    1 This will isolate the client and should be used only as a last resort if the client presents an actual danger to himself or others.
    3 The client's present emotional state limits concentration and prevents interaction with others.
    4 The client's present emotional state limits concentration and prevents interaction with others.

378. 3 **This provides a stimulus that competes with and reduces hallucinations.**
    1 This is a direct question that the client probably cannot answer; also, it may increase anxiety.
    2 If the nurse waits for the client to stop hallucinating, there may be no chance for contact with this client.
    4 In addition to setting unrealistic standards, this response fails to recognize that the client believes the hallucinations are real.

379. 4 **Chronically ill clients with schizophrenia usually have a lack of social skills, so this topic is appropriate for this group.**
    1 Relaxation techniques can be helpful for anyone; however, this is not the most therapeutic focus for this group.
    2 Rational behavior therapy is helpful for clients coping with depression.
    3 Many chronically mentally ill clients have difficulty applying the concepts associated with being assertive.

380. 1 **By realistically rewarding the healthy behaviors, the nurse provides secondary gains and encourages the continued use of healthy behaviors.**
    2 This is important but will do little to increase the client's self-esteem.
    3 This is important but will do little to increase the client's self-esteem.
    4 This is important but will do little to increase the client's self-esteem.

381. 3 **This response validates the presence of the client's hallucinations without agreeing with them, which communicates acceptance, and can form a foundation for trust; it may help the client return to reality.**
    1 The client's contact with reality is too tenuous to explore this kind of analysis.
    2 This response demeans the client, which blocks a trusting relationship and future communication.
    4 This response is condescending and may impair future communication.

382. 2 **Auditory hallucinations are most troublesome when environmental stimuli are diminished and there are few competing distractions.**
    1 This is a time of relatively high, competing environmental stimuli.
    3 This is a time of relatively high, competing environmental stimuli.
    4 This is a time of relatively high, competing environmental stimuli.

383. 3 **The state in which the client feels unreal or believes that parts of the body are distorted is known as depersonalization or loss of personal identity.**
    1 This is not an example of a hallucination; a hallucination is a sensory experience for which there is no external stimulus.
    2 The client's statement does not indicate any feelings that others are out to do harm, are responsible for what is happening, or are in control of the situation.

4   The statement is not an example of autistic verbalization.

384. 1   This declarative statement invites the client to walk, and the client can comply without making a verbal decision. A client with schizophrenia is often ambivalent and decision making is difficult.
2   Withdrawn, apathetic clients probably will not internalize and/or appreciate rationales for interventions.
3   Saying that the voices want the client to exercise supports the client's hallucinations.
4   Withdrawn, apathetic clients probably will not internalize and/or appreciate rationales for interventions.

385. 2   Deciding on and directing activities for the client are needed until delirium and confusion clear.
1   This is false reassurance.
3   Clients who are delirious are unable to develop insight into their behavior.
4   This is not therapeutic and does not assist the client to develop insight.

386. 3   This statement depicts the cognitive disturbance called a delusion, which is a fixed set of false beliefs that cannot be corrected by reason.
1   An illusion is a misperception of an actual environmental stimulus.
2   A hallucination is a sensory experience, unrelated to external stimuli.
4   Neologisms are made-up words understood only by the speaker.

387. 1   Projection is a mechanism in which inner thoughts and feelings are projected onto the environment, seeming to come from outside the self rather than from within.
2   Regression is the use of a behavioral characteristic appropriate to an earlier level of development.
3   Repression is the involuntary exclusion of painful or conflicting thoughts from awareness.
4   Identification is the taking on of the thoughts and mannerisms of an individual who is admired or idealized.

388. 4   This statement recognizes the client's feelings and points out reality.
1   Although this is an empathic response, it does not point out reality; the word "trick" does not have the same connotation as "do me in."
2   This response reinforces the client's delusional system.
3   This does not focus on feelings and places the client on the defensive.

389. 3   The client is fearful and suspicious; the feeling of being in a powerful position helps the client cope with anxiety.
1   The client is not out of touch with self-identity; the real identity has been given an important role.
2   The client is not attempting to manipulate others. The client is compensating for feelings of inadequacy.

4   The client is compensating for feelings of inadequacy, not depression about his problems.

390. 1   Clients use a structured delusional system to justify and compensate for their feelings of worthlessness and low self-esteem.
2   Clients experiencing delusions of a paranoid nature are isolated and need contact with people to increase their contact with reality.
3   There are no data to indicate this client is not accepted by others.
4   This is not the purpose of the delusional system.

391. 4   This will help the client develop self-esteem and reduce the use of paranoid ideation.
1   Because people must function in a social environment, it is almost impossible to avoid placing some demands on others.
2   It is impossible to remove all stress in the environment.
3   This will succeed in supporting the client's ideas of persecution and may lower the client's self-esteem.

392. 2   Thoughts of being pursued by some powerful agent or agents because of one's special attributes or powers are fixed false beliefs and referred to as delusions of grandeur.
1   There is no evidence to indicate that a delusion of total or partial nonexistence is being used.
3   There is no evidence to indicate that a sensory-perceptual disturbance is present.
4   Delusions of grandeur usually are used to deny unconscious feelings of low self-esteem.

393. 3   The client's verbalization reflects feelings that others are blaming the client for negative actions.
1   There are no data that demonstrate the client has feelings of greatness or power.
2   There are no data that demonstrate the client is experiencing confusing misinterpretations of stimuli.
4   There are no data that demonstrate the client is hearing voices at this time.

394. 2   These clients are hypersensitive to external stimuli and respond with less anxiety to a minimally threatening environment.
1   This is too threatening an approach and interferes with the goals of therapy.
3   Focusing on delusional material will reinforce the delusional system.
4   This is not therapeutic; it may trigger suspiciousness and hostile outbursts.

395. 3   The recommended approach for working with suspicious clients is to allow them to set the pace for the relationship.
1   This may be perceived as threatening and add to feelings of paranoia.
2   This may be perceived as threatening and add to feelings of paranoia.
4   This may be perceived as threatening and add to feelings of paranoia.

396. 1 **Activities that require limited interpersonal contact are less threatening.**
    2 Group activities require interaction with other people, which is threatening to individuals with paranoid feelings.
    3 Group activities require interaction with other people, which is threatening to individuals with paranoid feelings.
    4 Individuals with schizophrenia, paranoid type, usually do not respond to an authoritarian approach because they do not trust others, particularly those who act in an aggressive manner.

397. 3 **Clients with paranoia often feel safer selecting foods from a cafeteria-type display that is prepared for the general population rather than eating from a tray specifically prepared for them.**
    1 This will not provide security because part of the food may still be viewed as poisoned.
    2 This will not provide security because part of the food may still be viewed as poisoned.
    4 This will not provide security because part of the food may still be viewed as poisoned.

398. 3 **This statement sets limits and provides support; hallucinations can be frightening and the nurse's presence provides support while not actually focusing on the hallucination.**
    1 This statement does not recognize the client's need for support and direction.
    2 This statement does not recognize the client's need for support and direction
    4 This statement makes a judgment with insufficient evidence and focuses on the hallucination; it fails to recognize the client's need for support and direction.

399. 2 **A nonconfrontational validation of reality is the most therapeutic response that one can provide for a delusional client.**
    1 Asking what the voices are saying enters into the client's delusion, which will strengthen the delusional system.
    3 Saying nothing is nontherapeutic because it does not interject reality into the incident.
    4 It is not therapeutic to directly challenge a client's delusion; it will not change the client's belief.

SUBSTANCE ABUSE

400. 4 **Because of cross-tolerance the client may need large doses of analgesia for pain relief.**
    1 Confronting the client is not the nurse's responsibility at this time.
    2 The client must be helped to recognize that a problem with drugs exists.
    3 This approach is ingenuous and may be perceived as condescending.

401. 1 **Denial is a method of resolving conflict or escaping unpleasant realities by ignoring their**
existence. The person denies that the drinking is out of control and causing problems.
    2 With projection the person faults another person for having unacceptable impulses, thoughts, or behaviors that are too uncomfortable to accept as one's own. Although projection is used by saying drinking is caused by other people's actions, this is not the most commonly used defense mechanism.
    3 With displacement the person transfers an emotion from one object, person, or situation to another, usually safer, object, person, or situation.
    4 With compensation the person makes up for personal inadequacies by emphasizing attributes to gain social approval.

402. 4 **The attempt to justify a behavior by giving it acceptable motives is an example of rationalization.**
    1 Sublimation is the substitution of a maladaptive behavior for a more socially acceptable behavior.
    2 Suppression is the intentional exclusion of things, people, feelings, or events from consciousness.
    3 Compensation is the attempt to emphasize a characteristic viewed as an asset to make up for a real or imagined deficiency.

403. 1 **Alcohol is a central nervous system depressant; these responses are the body's neurological adaptation to the withdrawal of alcohol.**
    2 Convulsions are not early signs of alcohol withdrawal; they do not occur before 48 to 72 hours of abstinence.
    3 These are late signs of severe withdrawal that occur with alcohol withdrawal delirium; tachycardia results from autonomic overactivity.
    4 Fever and diaphoresis may occur during prolonged periods of delirium and are a result of autonomic overactivity.

404. 2 **The nurse should remove the substance before the client or other clients have an opportunity to consume more alcohol.**
    1 The primary concern is not where the alcohol was obtained, but protecting the client from consuming more.
    3 Making the client feel guilty can increase the desire for more alcohol.
    4 The client may drink the remaining alcohol while the nurse documents the information and notifies the practitioner.

405. 2 **Motivation is necessary to assist the client in withstanding the pain of giving up a defense; internal motivation is more influential in facilitating change than any external factor.**
    1 Although having family support is important, internal motivation to change is the most important factor.
    3 This can be of assistance, but internal factors will have a greater effect on rehabilitation than external factors.
    4 Self-esteem will be useful if it precipitates abstinence behavior; however, people who are alcoholics commonly have low self-esteem.

406. 3 **A client with this disorder has a loss of memory and adapts to this by filling in areas that cannot be remembered with made-up information.**
  1 Ideas of grandeur do not occur with this type of dementia.
  2 The use of confabulation is not attention-seeking behavior; the individual is attempting to mask memory loss.
  4 This person is not coping with the diagnosis; when confabulating, the individual is attempting to mask memory loss.

407. 2 **This disorder is caused by a prolonged deficiency of vitamin B$_1$ (thiamine) and the direct toxic effect of alcohol on brain tissue.**
  1 This is unrelated to substance-induced persisting dementia caused by alcoholism.
  3 This is unrelated to substance-induced persisting dementia caused by alcoholism.
  4 This is unrelated to substance-induced persisting dementia caused by alcoholism.

408. 1 **Alcohol, by depressing the central nervous system and distorting or altering reality, reduces anxiety.**
  2 Alcohol depresses the central nervous system; it may cause lability of mood, impaired judgment, and aggressive actions rather than euphoria.
  3 Although alcohol is used as a social lubricant, alcoholics frequently drink in isolation. Also alcohol can lead to inappropriate and aggressive behavior that may impair social interaction.
  4 Alcohol depresses the central nervous system; amphetamines and cocaine are stimulants.

409. 3 **Alcohol withdrawal delirium, a life-threatening CNS response to alcohol withdrawal, occurs in 1 to 3 days when blood alcohol levels drop as alcohol is detoxified and excreted.**
  1 Jitteriness, nervousness, and insomnia may occur at this time; these are not life threatening.
  2 Nervousness, insomnia, nausea, vomiting, and increased BP and pulse may occur at this time; these are not life threatening.
  4 Withdrawal symptoms will begin to subside at this time; the risk for complications is diminished.

410. 1 **This response forces the client to face what going to AA meetings means to the client.**
  2 This focuses the client on negative aspects; also, the client may be unable to answer this question.
  3 This reinforces avoidance, which delays dealing with the problem; the client may never feel like going to AA meetings.
  4 Although this is true, it does not explore the client's feelings.

411. 3 **The central nervous system is affected by the abrupt withdrawal of alcohol intake, resulting in the classic responses indicated in the situation; they occur 1 to 3 days after the cessation of alcohol intake.**
  1 The information presented does not demonstrate the presence of impaired short-term or long-term memory.
  2 The information presented does not demonstrate the presence of hallucinations.
  4 There are insufficient data to identify dementia; impairment of thought processes, judgment, and intellectual abilities should continue for 3 weeks or longer to consider dementia as a diagnosis.

412. 2 **To maintain sobriety, alcoholics must forever alter patterns of behavior that have been reinforced and used for prolonged periods.**
  1 A return to drinking may cause a break in relationships, not increased attention.
  3 After a period of sobriety there is no known physiological need for alcohol.
  4 Alcoholics do not have character defects; drinking helps to blunt the pain of reality.

413. 2 **Clients who abuse alcohol characteristically have lowered self-esteem; therefore, it is important for the nurse to accept the person as an individual with value.**
  1 Although nurturing is important, this client must learn self-reliance.
  3 This probably is an old story to this client and will have a minimal positive effect.
  4 This action will not provide an atmosphere that can help the client withstand the stress of the detoxification program.

414. 4 **The client must learn to develop and use more healthful coping mechanisms if drinking is to be stopped. The responsibility is with the client because the client must do the changing.**
  1 Although confrontation may be helpful in breaking through denial, it alone does not foster increased responsibility for maintaining sobriety.
  2 Medications do not provide the motivation for change; this must come from within the client.
  3 This will tell the client what to expect but will not instill responsibility for change.

415. 1 **This statement identifies the feeling of ambivalence associated with admitting that a problem with alcohol exists; this occurs early in treatment.**
  2 This places the client on the defensive and interferes with communication.
  3 This places the client on the defensive and interferes with communication.
  4 This places the client on the defensive and interferes with communication.

416. 3 **This focuses on the client's feelings with a supportive, helpful approach.**
  1 This is a judgmental approach that alienates the client from the therapeutic process and prevents the establishment of a rapport.
  2 This is a judgmental approach that alienates the client from the therapeutic process and prevents the establishment of a rapport.

4 This intervention reinforces the client's denial and avoidance of the problem and implies that others are responsible for the drinking behavior.

417. **Answer: 3, 4, 5**
1 Polydipsia, excessive intake of oral fluids, is one of the signs associated with diabetes mellitus.
2 Hyperalertness, not drowsiness, may occur.
3 **As withdrawal from alcohol progresses autonomic hyperactivity occurs, resulting in profuse diaphoresis.**
4 **As withdrawal from alcohol progresses autonomic hyperactivity occurs, resulting in a heart rate greater than 100 beats per minute.**
5 **As withdrawal from alcohol progresses autonomic hyperactivity occurs, resulting in increased vital signs including temperature, pulse, respirations, and blood pressure.**

418. 4 **Clients must learn new lifestyles and coping skills to maintain sobriety.**
1 This is an unrealistic, unattainable plan.
2 This is judgmental, negative thinking that will lower self-esteem.
3 Abstinence is essential; social drinking is not an option.

419. 3 **Withdrawal from central nervous system depressants, such as barbiturates, is associated with more severe morbidity and mortality. Symptoms begin with anxiety, shakiness, and insomnia; within 24 hours convulsions, delirium, tachycardia, and death can occur.**
1 Withdrawal from heroin rarely is life threatening, but it does cause severe discomfort such as abdominal cramping and diarrhea.
2 Withdrawal from methadone rarely is life threatening, but it does cause severe discomfort such as abdominal cramping and diarrhea.
4 Withdrawal from amphetamines rarely is life threatening, but it causes severe exhaustion and depression.

420. 3 **A person with an addictive personality is unable to delay gratification; drugs help to blur reality and reduce frustrations.**
1 It is possible, but not easy; it requires a change in attitude and a deconditioning process.
2 Users of drugs are concerned with reality, and their drug use is an attempt to blur the pains of reality.
4 Intellectually these people may be aware of the dangers of drug addiction but emotionally cannot buy into the reality that it can happen to them.

421. **Answer: 1, 2, 3**
1 **Cocaine, an alkaloid stimulant, can precipitate anxiety, hypervigilance, euphoria, agitation, and anger.**
2 **The loss of appetite and increased metabolic rate associated with cocaine addiction both promote weight loss.**
3 **Cocaine is a stimulant that has cardiac effects such as tachycardia and dysrhythmias.**

4 This behavior is associated with barbiturate addiction.
5 This behavior is associated with other addictions such as alcohol and methadone.

422. 2 **There is no set of symptoms associated with cocaine withdrawal, only the depression that follows the high caused by the drug.**
1 Insomnia is more commonly associated with withdrawal from central nervous system depressants.
3 Disinhibition is commonly associated with alcohol intoxication.
4 Hyperactivity is more commonly associated with withdrawal from opioids or antianxiety drugs.

423. 4 **Cocaine is a chemical that when inhaled causes destruction of the mucous membranes of the nose.**
1 This problem is associated with alcoholic cirrhosis.
2 These problems are associated with alcoholic cirrhosis and are related to malnutrition, dehydration, and ascites.
3 These problems are associated with typical antipsychotic medications.

424. **Answer: 1, 2, 4, 3**
When opioids, which are CNS depressants, are withdrawn initially the client will experience a runny nose (rhinorrhea), tearing of the eyes (lacrimation), diaphoresis, yawning, and irritability. As withdrawal progresses a rebound hyperexcitability precipitates muscle twitching, restlessness, hypertension, tachycardia, temperature irregularities, tremors, and loss of appetite. Finally, flulike symptoms, insomnia, and yawning occur. Once withdrawal is complete the appetite returns, vital signs become stable, and other withdrawal signs and symptoms subside and eventually disappear.

425. 3 **The client is unconscious and unable to meet physical needs; a patent airway, breathing, and circulation are essential needs.**
1 Understanding and support are important once the client's physical condition has stabilized.
2 Maintaining a drug-free environment will be a priority later in the treatment program.
4 Establishing a therapeutic relationship will increase in importance once the client's physical condition has stabilized.

426. 1 **Opioids cause central nervous system depression, resulting in severe respiratory depression, hypotension, tachycardia, and unconsciousness.**
2 These findings, particularly the respirations, are not indicative of an overdose of an opioid.
3 These findings, particularly the respirations, are not indicative of an overdose of an opioid.
4 These findings, particularly the respirations, are not indicative of an overdose of an opioid.

427. 2 **Individuals often take drugs because they cannot deal with the pain of reality; the drug blurs the pain and reduces anxiety.**
1 Drugs increase dependency rather than foster independence.

3 Although this factor may encourage initial use by some adolescents, it is not the most common reason for their use.

4 The use of drugs fosters social isolation.

428. 2 **Stimulating the central nervous system with cocaine most commonly causes these responses, which can progress to fear, hallucinations, paranoid delusions, and violent behavior.**

1 Nausea is not a side effect. Euphoria, rather than fatigue, and loss of appetite, rather than hunger, are side effects.

3 These are not common side effects of cocaine use.

4 An increase in energy, rather than lethargy, occurs. Some cocaine users believe it maximizes sexual experiences, but there is no documentation of this physiologic response. Hormone imbalances are not common side effects.

429. 1 **Tolerance is a phenomenon that occurs in addicted individuals and increases the amount of drug needed to satisfy their need; the client should receive adequate analgesia postoperatively.**

2 Drug habituation is a mild form of psychological dependence; the individual develops a habit of taking the substance.

3 A physical addiction is related to biochemical changes in body tissues, especially the nervous system. The tissues come to require the substance for usual functioning.

4 Psychological dependence is emotional reliance on the substance to maintain a sense of well-being.

430. 1 **This allows the individual to use staff members as a support system and removes an opportunity to deny the problem.**

2 This supports and permits denial; both the individual and the staff know a problem exists, and the individual must cope with it.

3 This is a nonprofessional approach that is not therapeutic.

4 Although this may be part of a return-to-work contract, it is not necessarily therapeutic; it simply reduces legal risks.

431. 3 **This is a nonpunitive approach that attempts to help the nurse as an individual and as a professional.**

1 This may be necessary for long-term therapy but is not the initial approach.

2 This is a punitive nontherapeutic response that offers no chance for rehabilitation.

4 The client has an addiction problem; promises will not keep the client from abusing drugs.

432. 1 **The client is using denial to separate from group members and needs realistic feedback to prevent withdrawal.**

2 This will not help the client to become involved with the group.

3 This is inadequate; the client first needs to recognize that the problems being discussed are applicable.

4 The client is avoiding treatment. Asking about therapy preferences is not helpful.

433. 2 **These provide high levels of thiamine; other sources include legumes, whole and enriched grains, and lean pork.**

1 In this list, only fish is considered a source of thiamine.

3 In this list, only eggs are considered a source of thiamine; this list contains sources of protein.

4 In this list, only lentils (legumes) are considered a source of thiamine; most vegetables contain only traces of thiamine; citrus fruits provide vitamin C.

434. 4 **Although unclear, alcoholic blackouts appear to result from responses that central nervous system cells have to the substance.**

1 The individual does not have any type of seizure during the blackout.

2 Fainting is not associated with the blackout.

3 The individual loses memory but not consciousness.

435. Answer: 1, 5

1 **Although cocaine is an alkaloid stimulant, depressant effects such as a decreased mood, hypotension, and psychomotor retardation are associated with long-term, high-dose use.**

2 Cocaine is a stimulant, and this response is associated with cocaine intoxication, not prolonged high-dose cocaine use.

3 Cocaine is a stimulant, and this response is associated with cocaine intoxication, not prolonged high-dose cocaine use.

4 Cocaine is a stimulant, and this response is associated with cocaine intoxication, not prolonged high-dose cocaine use.

5 **Although cocaine is an alkaloid stimulant, depressant effects such as psychomotor retardation, hypotension, and a decreased mood are associated with long-term, high-dose use.**

436. 3 **Methamphetamine is a stimulant that causes the release of adrenaline which activates the sympathetic nervous system.**

1 The pupils will dilate, not constrict, because the sympathetic nervous system is activated.

2 Clients withdrawing from opioids, not methamphetamines, experience diarrhea.

4 The respirations will be increased, not decreased, because of the activation of the sympathetic nervous system.

DRUG-RELATED RESPONSES

437. 4 **When taking venlafaxine (Effexor), a selective serotonin reuptake inhibitor (SSRI), and St. John's wort concurrently, the client is at risk for serotonin syndrome. This syndrome is a drug-induced excess of intrasynaptic serotonin.**

1 Ginseng can precipitate a hypertensive crisis in clients taking a monoamine oxidase inhibitor.

2   Valerian (valerian root) can enhance sedation in clients taking a tricyclic antidepressant.

3   Kava-kava can increase the risk of dystonic reactions in clients taking an antipsychotic medication.

438. **3   Methylphenidate (Ritalin), a stimulant, has an opposite effect on hyperactive children; this action is as yet totally unexplained.**

1   Methylphenidate does not have this effect.

2   Methylphenidate does not have this effect.

4   Although methylphenidate has a hypotensive effect, this is not why it is given to hyperactive children.

439. **1   Alprazolam (Xanax), a benzodiazepine, potentiates the actions of GABA, enhances presympathetic inhibition, and inhibits spinal polysynaptic afferent pathways. Drowsiness, dizziness, and blurred vision are common side effects.**

2   Alprazolam may cause tachycardia, not bradycardia.

3   Agranulocytosis usually is a side effect of the antipsychotics in the phenothiazine, not benzodiazepine, group.

4   Tardive dyskinesia occurs after prolonged therapy with antipsychotic medications; alprazolam is an antianxiety medication, not an antipsychotic.

440. **2   Hypotension is a major side effect of alprazolam (Xanax) that occurs early in therapy.**

1   An alteration in urinary output is not a common side effect; however, urinary retention may occur after prolonged use.

3   This is not a common side effect; abdominal distention from constipation may occur after prolonged use.

4   Blurred vision, not dilated pupils, may occur. Dilated pupils associated with CNS depression are not a common side effect, although they may occur with overdose or prolonged use.

441. **4   Psychoactive drugs have been shown to be capable of interrupting the acute psychiatric process, making the client more amenable to other therapies.**

1   Electroconvulsive therapy (ECT) may be effective in treating depressed clients.

2   Family therapy is effective but is a long-term, costly therapy; signs and symptoms must be reduced before the client can participate.

3   Clients with schizophrenia usually have little insight into their problems. Confronting the client through insight therapy will increase anxiety.

442. **2   The duration of effect is 12 to 24 hours compared with other opioids, which have a 3- to 6-hour duration of effect.**

1   It is just as addictive but it controls the addiction and keeps the client out of the illicit drug market.

3   Methadone does produce a cumulative effect.

4   Physical as well as psychological dependence is possible, just as with other opioids.

443. **2   Tachycardia, hyperpyrexia and tachypnea are indications of neuroleptic malignant syndrome, which is a life-threatening complication.**

1   Restraints of any type may increase the client's anxiety and result in struggling and increased agitation.

3   Photosensitivity occurs most commonly when clients are taking large doses and are spending time outdoors in the sun, but it is not life threatening.

4   Tardive dyskinesia usually results from prolonged large doses of phenothiazines in susceptible clients, but it is not life threatening.

444. **1   Akathisia, a side effect of haloperidol (Haldol), develops early in therapy and is characterized by restlessness and agitation.**

2   Torticollis is characterized by a stiff neck (wry neck).

3   Tardive dyskinesia is characterized by gross involuntary movements of the extremities, tongue, and facial muscles that develop after prolonged therapy.

4   Pseudoparkinsonism is characterized by motor retardation, rigidity, and tremors; the reaction resembles Parkinson's syndrome but usually responds to decreasing the dose, the administration of an antidyskinetic medication, or discontinuation of the haloperidol.

445. **3   Lorazepam (Ativan) potentiates the actions of GABA, which reduces the anxiety and irritability associated with withdrawal.**

1   This drug helps to reduce the risk of seizures but does not prevent physical injury if a seizure occurs.

2   Although this benefit may occur, it is not the primary objective for using the drug.

4   The ability of the client to accept treatment depends on readiness to accept the reality of the problem.

446. **4   Lithium concentration is most stable at this time; absorption and excretion occur 8 to 12 hours after the last dose.**

1   Absorption and excretion rates vary; concentrations may be falsely higher at this time affecting the reliability of the readings.

2   Absorption and excretion rates vary; concentrations may be falsely higher at this time affecting the reliability of the readings.

3   Absorption and excretion rates vary; concentrations may be falsely higher at this time affecting the reliability of the readings.

447. **2   The level 0.3 mEq/L is below the therapeutic range of 0.5 to 1.5 mEq/L; therefore, the medication should be administered as prescribed to increase the serum drug level.**

1   There is no need to notify the practitioner because the level is still subtherapeutic.

3   Adverse side effects are not expected until the level exceeds the therapeutic range of 0.5 to 1.5 mEq/L.

4   There is no need to withhold the medication because the level is still subtherapeutic.

448. **Answer: 1, 3, 4**

1   **Genitourinary side effects of paroxetine (Paxil) include ejaculatory disorders, male genital disorders, and urinary frequency.**

2   This is associated with opioids that depress the central nervous system.

3 **Central nervous system side effects of paroxetine include insomnia, restlessness, dizziness, tremors, nervousness, and headache.**

4 **Cardiovascular side effects of paroxetine include hypertension, orthostatic hypotension, palpitations, and vasodilation.**

5 These are associated with tiagabine hydrochloride (Gabitril), an antiepileptic used for bipolar disorders.

449. 4 **Benztropine (Cogentin), an anticholinergic, helps balance neurotransmitter activity in the CNS and helps control extrapyramidal tract symptoms.**

1 Zolpidem (Ambien) is a sedative-hypnotic drug used for short-term insomnia.

2 HydrOXYzine (Vistaril) is a sedative that depresses activity in the subcortical areas in the CNS; it is used to reduce anxiety.

3 Dantrolene (Dantrium), a muscle relaxant, has a direct effect on skeletal muscle by acting on the excitation-contraction coupling of muscle fibers and not at the level of the CNS as do most other muscle relaxation drugs.

450. 2 **Haloperidol (Haldol) reduces emotional tensions, excessive psychomotor activity, panic, and fear. It is used for clients with thought disorders and hyperactivity.**

1 Clients exhibiting excited-depressed behavior do not respond well to haloperidol because it tends to increase the depression.

3 Haloperidol appears to have few stimulating effects for a withdrawn client and, in fact, increases feelings of lassitude and fatigue.

4 Haloperidol does not decrease manipulative behavior. Clients who are capable of manipulation usually do not exhibit behavior that involves overactivity, fear, and panic.

451. 4 **The classic signs and symptoms that indicate lithium toxicity include slurred speech, ataxia, nausea, and vomiting.**

1 When lithium levels are low the client presents with recurring signs and symptoms of the mood disorder.

2 These are not signs and symptoms of a mood disorder.

3 If lithium levels are within the therapeutic range, the client's mood is more stable; the client may experience GI symptoms, but will not experience slurred speech or an ataxic gait.

452. 3 **Gastric lavage with charcoal may help decrease the level of tricyclic antidepressant overdose. Supportive measures such as mechanical ventilation may be needed until the medical crisis passes.**

1 Physostigmine salicylate had been used in the past to promote improvement in consciousness. Now its use is contraindicated because it can cause bradycardia, asystole, and seizures in clients with tricyclic antidepressant toxicity.

2 Prevention of suicidal behavior is always advantageous; however, in this case, immediate emergency intervention is necessary.

4 Acetylcholine levels are depressed from the tricyclic antidepressant; anticholinergics are most effective in managing the side effects of antipsychotic/neuroleptic drugs, not tricyclic antidepressant drugs.

453. 4 **Fluphenazine decanoate (Prolixin Decanoate) is effective for noncompliant clients; it is an injectable form of the drug and lasts 3 to 4 weeks.**

1 Imipramine (Tofranil), a tricyclic antidepressant, is not appropriate for this client; it is administered to clients who are depressed.

2 Isocarboxazid (Marplan), a monoamine oxidase inhibitor (MAOI), is not appropriate for this client; it is administered to clients with mood disorders.

3 Fluphenazine hydrochloride (Prolixin) is a short-acting medication; it is not as effective as fluphenazine decanoate for a noncompliant client.

454. 3 **Extreme photosensitivity is a common side effect of fluphenazine decanoate (Prolixin Decanoate); use of sunscreens and avoidance of tanning is essential.**

1 Once the client's medication is adjusted and CNS response is noted, driving may be permitted; drowsiness usually subsides after the first few weeks.

2 This is untrue; energy usually is decreased.

4 Although this drug can cause postural hypotension, it does not consistently lower blood pressure.

455. 1 **This drug is an opioid antagonist that displaces opioids from receptors in the brain, reversing respiratory depression.**

2 This is a synthetic opioid that causes CNS depression; it will accelerate the effects of the overdose.

3 This drug will have no effect on respiratory depression related to the presence of an overdose of a narcotic.

4 Amphetamine is a stimulant, not an opioid antagonist.

456. 3 **Monoamine oxidase uptake is inhibited by the medication, increasing concentrations of endogenous epinephrine, norepinephrine, serotonin, and dopamine in CNS storage sites; high levels of these transmitters in the presence of tyramine (e.g., cheeses, herring, wine, sausages) can cause hypertensive crisis.**

1 This may be an adverse reaction to the drug but it is not related to drug-food interaction.

2 This may be an adverse reaction to the drug but it is not related to drug-food interaction.

4 This is not related to drug-food interactions.

457. 1 **Some over-the-counter medications contain alcohol and may trigger a reaction.**

2 Disulfiram (Antabuse) and antibiotics generally can be administered concurrently.

3 This is appropriate for clients receiving monoamine oxidase inhibitors (MAOIs).

4   Disulfiram is aversion therapy for clients who abuse alcohol. Eight hours after taking the medication adverse effects can still occur. These include severe nausea, vomiting, hypotension, headache, tachycardia, tachypnea, flushed face, bloodshot eyes.

458. 3   **Risperidone (Risperdal) potentiates the action of alcohol and can cause oversedation if the drug and alcohol are taken together.**
1   This medication should be taken consistently to prevent recurrence of symptoms and maintain therapeutic blood drug levels.
2   This medication should be taken consistently to prevent recurrence of symptoms and maintain therapeutic blood drug levels.
4   Medications should be taken as prescribed; taking them all at one time can interrupt the maintenance of a constant therapeutic blood level.

459. 3   **Informing the client about the expected response to the medication is factual information that may decrease the client's sense of hopelessness.**
1   Although empathic responses may be helpful, at this time the client needs information and reassurance based on fact.
2   Although empathic responses may be helpful, at this time the client needs information and reassurance based on fact.
4   Citalopram hydrobromide (Celexa) does not work more slowly in some people.

460. 3   **This is too short a period of time to expect a therapeutic response to an antidepressant; clients usually begin to feel a lightening of depression in approximately 14 to 20 days, with the full antidepressant effects being felt between 3 and 4 weeks.**
1   Drowsiness, fatigue, and insomnia are common side effects.
2   Medication alone may not be effective; some form of psychotherapy often is needed.
4   Clients usually remain on these medications for several months.

461. 1   **Amoxapine (Asendin) is a tricyclic antidepressant (TCA) and phenelzine (Nardil) is a monoamine oxidase inhibitor (MAOI); tricyclic antidepressants are contraindicated in concomitant use with monoamine oxidase inhibitors.**
2   Although checking for allergies is important, an allergy to feathers is not specific to MAOIs.
3   Blood tests are not done specifically before administering MAOIs.
4   Phenelzine does not have to be taken with food. Milk products, with the exception of aged cheeses and yogurt, may be eaten; products containing tyramine must be avoided.

462. 2   **These drugs do not produce an immediate effect; nursing measures must continue to decrease the risk of suicide.**
1   These food precautions are taken with MAO inhibitors.

3   These precautions are unnecessary.
4   This is not necessary; toxicity is not as prevalent a problem with tricyclic antidepressants as it is with medications such as lithium.

463. 4   **Improvement in mood can be seen in about 3 weeks with antidepressants.**
1   There are insufficient data to draw this conclusion.
2   It is unlikely that conflicts have resolved in such a short time.
3   Since the client has been depressed and sought treatment, it is unlikely she is in denial.

464. 4   **This drug creates a general sense of well-being, increases appetite, and helps lift depression. It blocks the reuptake of norepinephrine and serotonin into nerve endings, increasing their action in nerve cells.**
1   The client might not know the reason for depression, and the drug does not cause amnesia.
2   Side effects of imipramine (Tofranil) include drowsiness and insomnia. The situation does not indicate that the client is experiencing insomnia.
3   Symptomatic relief usually begins after 2 to 3 weeks of therapy.

465. 3   **The parkinsonian signs and symptoms are related to extrapyramidal tract effects, and agranulocytosis is related to bone marrow depression.**
1   Jaundice is an adverse reaction; vomiting is not.
2   Tardive dyskinesia is an adverse reaction; nausea is not.
4   The occurrence of orthostatic hypotension is low; hiccups usually do not occur.

466. 2   **Tardive dyskinesia is characterized by protrusion and vermicular movements of the tongue, chewing and puckering movements of the mouth, and a puffing of the cheeks. These adverse effects may or may not be reversible when the antipsychotic medication is withdrawn.**
1   Motor restlessness (akathisia) can be treated with an antiparkinsonian or anticholinergic drug while the antipsychotic medication is continued.
3   Parkinsonian-like symptoms can be treated with antiparkinsonian or anticholinergic drugs while the antipsychotic medication is continued.
4   An acute dystonic reaction can be treated with antiparkinsonian or anticholinergic drugs while the antipsychotic medication is continued.

467. 1   **Phenothiazines frequently cause a photosensitivity that can be controlled with sunscreens.**
2   Limiting activity is not a necessary precaution when taking phenothiazines.
3   The medication must be administered as prescribed.
4   Participating in the outing should not negatively affect the client's blood pressure.

468. 1   **These are common extrapyramidal signs (pseudoparkinsonism) that occur as side effects of neuroleptics; they usually are controlled with antiparkinsonian drugs.**

2 These are signs of lithium toxicity.

3 These are common side effects that occur with CNS depressants.

4 These are common side effects that occur with antidepressants.

469. **4 Antiseizure medications and haloperidol (Haldol) exert a synergistic CNS depressant effect.**

1 The effect is potentiated, not masked.

2 Anticonvulsants do not affect the absorption of haloperidol.

3 Anticonvulsants do not affect the metabolism of haloperidol.

470. **4 Bupropion (Wellbutrin) inhibits the reuptake of dopamine, serotonin, and norepinephrine and may cause seizures that can be life threatening; also it may cause headaches, agitation, sedation, tremors, and confusion.**

1 This condition is not a side effect of bupropion.

2 This condition is not a side effect of bupropion.

3 This can occur with the use of neuroleptics.

471. **1 This comment reveals that the client does not understand that the medication is necessary to prevent mood swings; long-term adherence to the pharmacological regimen is important for managing bipolar disorder.**

2 Regular medical visits are needed to ensure the best management of the illness.

3 Various cognitive and behavioral therapies provide support in coping with life's stressors.

4 Adherence to the medication regimen should eliminate the mood swings for most people with bipolar disorder.

472. **3 These foods are high in tyramine, which in the presence of an MAO inhibitor, can cause an excessive epinephrine-type response that can result in a hypertensive crisis.**

1 There is no relationship between these foods and this medication.

2 There is no relationship between these foods and this medication.

4 There is no relationship between these foods and this medication.

473. **4 A hypertensive crisis is not associated with extrapyramidal tract symptoms.**

1 Akathisia, characterized by restlessness and twitching or crawling sensations in muscles, is an extrapyramidal side effect.

2 Opisthotonos, characterized by hyperextension and arching of the back, is an extrapyramidal side effect.

3 Oculogyric crisis, characterized by the uncontrolled upward movement of the eyes, is an extrapyramidal side effect.

474. **3 These are signs of akathisia, which is an involuntary movement disorder characterized by an inability to sit still.**

1 Muscle spasms and pulling of the head to the side by neck muscles (torticollis) are related to acute dystonia.

2 These are associated with tardive dyskinesia.

4 These are signs of pseudoparkinsonism.

475. **Answer: 3, 5**

1 Akathisia is a common side effect that usually is alleviated by antiparkinsonian agents.

2 A shuffling gait is a common side effect that usually is alleviated by antiparkinsonian agents.

3 **Yellow sclerae are a sign of toxicity that has damaged the liver and necessitates withholding the drug.**

4 Photosensitivity is an expected side effect of the drug; the medication does not have to be withheld.

5 **Abnormal movements of involuntary muscle groups, particularly of the face, mouth, tongue, fingers, and toes, can occur after a prolonged period of dopamine blockade. Conversion to an atypical antipsychotic is warranted.**

476. **2 This medication can be taken every 2 weeks instead of every day.**

1 The side effects are the same as most other antipsychotic drugs.

3 The action of this drug during pregnancy is uncertain; animal studies have demonstrated an adverse effect on the fetus.

4 The side effects and the routine monitoring of the client's laboratory results are the same as for most other antipsychotic drugs.

477. **1 The anticholinergic activity of each drug is magnified, and adverse effects such as paralytic ileus may occur.**

2 Hypertension, not hypotension, occurs with anticholinergic medications.

3 Dryness of the mouth, not increased salivation, occurs with anticholinergic medications.

4. Decreased, not increased, perspiration occurs with anticholinergic medications.

478. **1 The medication should be stopped immediately because jaundice indicates possible liver damage, which prolongs elimination of the drug and may result in toxic accumulation.**

2 Milk does not change the effect of the drug.

3 The drug must be stopped, not reduced.

4 The drug is available only in an oral form; in addition, the route of administration will not influence the occurrence of toxic accumulation.

479. **2 Agranulocytosis occurs in 1% to 2% of clients receiving clozapine (Clozaril) and is potentially fatal; weekly blood counts are necessary.**

1 Polycythemia is not a side effect of Clozapine.

3 Clozapine may cause hypotension; hypertensive crisis is a side effect of MAOIs.

4 Pseudoparkinsonism may occur but it can be managed with anticholinergic medications.

480. 4 **Olanzapine (Zyprexa Zydis) is an oral disintegrating tablet that dissolves on contact with moisture.**
    1 Extrapyramidal effects are possible side effects of this medication.
    2 This medication must be administered daily.
    3 Olanzapine's action is unknown; it is believed to be a dopamine and serotonin type 2 antagonist. Increased dopamine at receptor sites increases psychotic behavior.

481. 2 **For clients with bipolar disorders, it has been shown that long-term lithium therapy flattens the highs of the euphoric episodes and minimizes the lows of the depressed episodes.**
    1 The practitioner should be notified before medication is stopped.
    3 The therapeutic level and the toxic level are very close, and serious side effects can occur.
    4 Clients should never adjust their own dosage of medication.

482. 4 **Urinary hesitancy and urinary retention are adverse effects of imipramine (Tofranil) that may require immediate medical intervention.**
    1 Dry mouth is a side effect of imipramine. This side effect usually decreases over time or can be managed through nursing interventions.
    2 Weight gain related to increased appetite is a side effect of imipramine. This side effect usually decreases over time or can be managed through nursing interventions.
    3 Blurred vision may occur as a side effect of imipramine. This side effect usually decreases over time or can be managed through nursing interventions.

483. 4 **Antianxiety medications have the potential for physiological and/or psychological dependence; the nurse should teach the client about both the advantages and disadvantages of taking this drug.**
    1 Physiological and/or psychological dependence can develop even when the dosage is controlled.
    2 Tolerance does develop and can lead to dependence.
    3 Both psychological and physiological dependence can develop.

484. Answer: 3, 4, 5
    1 Fresh fish does not need to be avoided while taking an MAO inhibitor. Dried, pickled, cured, fermented, and smoked fish should be avoided.
    2 Citrus fruits do not need to be avoided while taking an MAO inhibitor. Figs and bananas in large amounts should be avoided.
    3 **Foods high in tyramine, such as aged cheese, should be avoided when taking a monoamine oxidase inhibitor. When taking a monoamine oxidase inhibitor, tyramine can increase to an unsafe level and cause a life-threatening hypertensive crisis.**
    4 **Foods high in tyramine, such as ripe avocados, should be avoided when taking a monoamine oxidase inhibitor. When taking a monoamine oxidase**

inhibitor, tyramine can increase to an unsafe level and cause a life-threatening hypertensive crisis.
    5 **Delicatessen meats that are fermented, such as bologna, pepperoni, salami, and sausage, are high in tyramine and should be avoided when taking a monoamine oxidase inhibitor. When taking a monoamine oxidase inhibitor, tyramine can increase to an unsafe level and cause a life-threatening hypertensive crisis.**

485. 2 **Sertraline (Zoloft), a selective serotonin reuptake inhibitor (SSRI), inhibits neuronal uptake of serotonin in the central nervous system, thus potentiating the activity of serotonin. Central nervous system side effects of this drug include agitation, anxiety, confusion, dizziness, drowsiness, and headache.**
    1 Seizures are a side effect of clozapine (Clozaril), an antipsychotic, not sertraline, which is an antidepressant.
    3 Tachycardia is a side effect of tricyclic antidepressants, not sertraline, which is an SSRI antidepressant.
    4 A decrease in the production of granulocytes (agranulocytosis) causing a pronounced neutropenia is a side effect of clozapine, not sertraline, which is an antidepressant.

486. 4 **A neuromuscular blocker, such as succinylcholine (Anectine), produces respiratory depression because it inhibits contractions of respiratory muscles.**
    1 This medication does not cause seizures.
    2 Because the client is not permitted anything by mouth for 8 to 10 hours before the treatment, this is not a major problem.
    3 The loss of memory results from the ECT treatment, not from the neuromuscular blocking agent.

487. 3 **Hard candy may produce salivation, which helps alleviate the anticholinergic-like side effect of dry mouth that is experienced with some psychotropics. Dry mouth increases the risk for cavities; candy with sugar adds to this risk.**
    1 Fluids should be encouraged, not discouraged; fluids may alleviate the dry mouth.
    2 This is unnecessary.
    4 This is unnecessary.

488. 2 **Zolpidem (Ambien) is a sedative-hypnotic that produces CNS depression in the limbic, thalamic, and hypothalamic areas of the brain.**
    1 Zolpidem is not an analgesic medication.
    3 Zolpidem is not an antidiabetic medication.
    4 Zolpidem is not an antihypertensive medication.

489. 2 **This drug suppresses activity in key regions of the subcortical area of the CNS; it also has antihistaminic and anticholinergic effects.**
    1 These adaptations are not associated with hydrOXYzine (Vistaril).
    3 These adaptations are not associated with hydrOXYzine.

4 These adaptations are not associated with hydrOXYzine.

490. 3 **These are the classic signs of neuroleptic malignant syndrome, which is caused by neuroleptic-induced blockage of dopamine receptors.**
   1 These are side effects of haloperidol (Haldol), not neuroleptic malignant syndrome.
   2 These are side effects of haloperidol, not neuroleptic malignant syndrome.
   4 These are side effects of haloperidol, not neuroleptic malignant syndrome.

491. 3 **Drug-induced parkinsonism presents with the classic triad of adaptations associated with Parkinson's disease, which include rigidity, slowed movement (bradykinesia), and tremors.**
   1 The anticholinergic effects of antipsychotic medication cause dry mouth, not drooling. Neither side effect is related to pseudoparkinsonism.
   2 This is a side effect of anticholinergic, not antipsychotic, medications.
   4 This is a side effect of anticholinergic, not antipsychotic, medications.

492. 4 **Atypical antipsychotics, such as risperidone (Risperdal) can cause metabolic syndrome in which the client experiences weight gain and increases in cholesterol and triglyceride levels. Diabetes mellitus and diabetic ketoacidosis may occur between 5 weeks to 17 months after initiation of therapy.**
   1 Although lithium (Carbolith) may cause weight gain, it does not cause metabolic syndrome.
   2 Although diazepam (Valium) may cause weight gain, it does not cause metabolic syndrome.
   4 Although alprazolam (Xanax) may cause weight gain, it does not cause metabolic syndrome.

493. 3 **Naltrexone (Depade) is effective in reducing relapse among recovering alcoholics in conjunction with other types of therapy.**
   1 Naloxone (Narcan), not naltrexone, is used for opioid overdose.
   2 Naltrexone does not treat the effects of cocaine.
   4 Naltrexone is an opioid antagonist. It is not used for antianxiety agent withdrawal.

494. 3 **Most psychotropic medications affect neurotransmitters such as dopamine and norepinephrine, which enter the synapses between neurons, allowing them to signal each other.**
   1 Psychotropic medications do not work by changing the metabolic needs of the brain.
   2 Psychotropic medications do not increase the production of nervous tissue.
   4 Although there may be some effect on sensory input, this is because of the change in neurotransmitters.

495. 2 **Clozapine (Clozaril) can cause bone marrow suppression. The expected WBC value for an adult is 4500 to 10,000 mm³. The client has a reduction in WBCs, making the client vulnerable to infection.**

A fever with complaints of a sore throat and weakness support the conclusion that the client may have an infection.
   1 The RBC count does not indicate anemia. The expected range of RBCs for an adult male is 4.6 to $6.2 \times 10^6/\text{mL}^3$.
   3 The small change in the blood pressure from standing to sitting does not support the conclusion of orthostatic hypotension. Labile hypertension is associated with neuroleptic malignant syndrome.
   4 There are insufficient data to support this conclusion. Although tachycardia and tachypnea are associated with neuroleptic malignant syndrome, the client's fever would be more than 100.6° F. Additional characteristics of neuroleptic malignant syndrome include labile hypertension, diaphoresis, drooling, increased muscle tone, and decreased level of consciousness.

496. **The nurse should administer 0.5 mL.** Solve the problem by using ratio and proportion.

$$\frac{2.5 \text{ mg}}{5 \text{ mg}} \times \frac{1 \text{ mL}}{1 \text{ mL}}$$
$$5 \text{ x} = 2.5 \text{ mL}$$
$$\text{x} = 2.5 \div 5$$
$$\text{x} = 0.5 \text{ mL}$$

497. **The nurse should administer 7.5 mL per dose.** Solve the problem by using ratio and proportion.

$$750 \text{ mg} \div 2 = 375 \text{ mg per dose}$$
$$\frac{375 \text{ mg}}{250 \text{ mg}} \times \frac{\text{x mL}}{5 \text{ mL}}$$
$$250 \text{ x} = 1875$$
$$\text{x} = 1875 \div 250$$
$$\text{x} = 7.5 \text{ mL}$$

498. **The correct amount of solution to administer is 3 mL. Solve the problem by using ratio and proportion.**

$$\frac{15 \text{ mg}}{5 \text{ mg}} \times \frac{\text{x mL}}{1 \text{ mL}}$$
$$5 \text{ x} = 15$$
$$\text{x} = 15 \div 5$$
$$\text{x} = 3 \text{ mL}$$

499. **The correct amount of solution to administer at each dose is 25 mL of phenytoin (Dilantin). Solve the problem by using ratio and proportion.**

$$\frac{125 \text{ mg}}{25 \text{ mg}} \times \frac{\text{x mL}}{5 \text{ mL}}$$
$$25 \text{ x} = 625$$
$$\text{x} = 625 \div 25$$
$$\text{x} = 25 \text{ mL}$$

500. 1 **Torticollis is an acute dystonia that involves muscle spasms of the head and neck. Torticollis develops within 1 to 5 days after beginning therapy with a conventional antipsychotic.**

2 Tardive dyskinesia is involuntary repetitious tonic muscular spasms that involve the face, tongue, lips, limbs, and trunk. Tardive dyskinesia takes several months to years to develop after beginning therapy with a conventional antipsychotic.

3 Pseudoparkinsonism is an extrapyramidal tract response that includes masklike facies, shuffling gait, pill-rolling tremors, stooped posture, and drooling. Pseudoparkinsonism develops within several days to 1 month after beginning therapy with a conventional antipsychotic.

4 Neuroleptic malignant syndrome is a severe, potentially fatal (10%) response to conventional antipsychotics. It is believed to be caused by an acute reduction in brain dopamine activity precipitating hyperthermia, tachycardia, tachypnea, unstable blood pressure, hypertonicity, dyskinesia, incontinence, decreased level of consciousness, and pulmonary congestion. Neuroleptic malignant syndrome can occur during the first week of therapy, but often occurs later during therapy.

MENTAL HEALTH NURSING
QUIZ

1. A nurse teaches a client about the side effects and precautions associated with the typical antipsychotic haloperidol (Haldol). The nurse evaluates that the teaching is understood when the client states:
   1. "I will immediately report any diarrhea or vomiting to my doctor."
   2. "I will not eat any tyramine-containing foods while I'm taking this drug."
   3. "I'll avoid direct sunlight and use a sunscreen product when I go outdoors."
   4. "I'll maintain an adequate fluid intake because I may urinate more than usual."

2. A middle-age female client who has lost 20 pounds over the last 2 months cries easily, sleeps poorly, and refuses to participate in any family or social activities that she previously enjoyed. What is the most important nursing intervention?
   1. Provide the client with a high-calorie, high-protein diet
   2. Reduce the client's crying episodes by setting firm, consistent limits
   3. Assure the client that she will regain her usual function in a short time
   4. Allow the client to externalize her feelings, especially anger, in a safe manner

3. A client with the diagnosis of schizophrenia, paranoid type, is admitted to the hospital. The client says to the nurse, "I know they're spying on me in here, too. I'm not safe anywhere!" What is the most therapeutic response by the nurse?
   1. "Nobody's spying on you in here."
   2. "Why do you feel they'd want to follow you here?"
   3. "You don't feel safe anywhere, not even in the hospital?"
   4. "You are safe in the hospital; nothing can happen to you here."

4. A deeply depressed, withdrawn client remains curled up in bed and refuses to talk to the nurse. What should the nurse do initially to break through the client's withdrawal?
   1. Sit with the client for set periods of time each hour
   2. Touch the client gently on the arm when the opportunity arises
   3. Urge the client to participate in simple games with other clients
   4. Inform the client that going to the lounge is required in the daytime

5. A nurse is assessing an adolescent client with the diagnosis of schizophrenia, undifferentiated type. Which signs and symptoms should the nurse expect the client to experience?
   1. Paranoid delusions and hypervigilance
   2. Depression and psychomotor retardation
   3. Loosened associations and hallucinations
   4. Ritualistic behavior and obsessive thinking

6. A nurse is working with a couple and their two children. Their 14-year-old son has been in trouble at school because of truancy and poor grades. Their 16-year-old daughter is quiet and withdrawn and refuses to talk to her parents. The parents have had severe marital problems for the past 10 years. The priority nursing concern at this time is how the:
   1. Parents can set limits on their children's behavior
   2. Couple's marital problems are impacting on their children
   3. Son's behavior in school will impair his peer social relationships
   4. Daughter's withdrawn behavior limits her ability to talk with her friends

7. A nurse is working with an adolescent client diagnosed with conduct disorder. Which strategies should the nurse implement while working on the goal of increasing the client's ability to meet personal needs without manipulating others? Select all that apply.
   1. _____ Discuss how others can precipitate anxiety
   2. _____ Provide physical outlets for aggressive feelings
   3. _____ Establish a contract regarding manipulative behavior
   4. _____ Develop activities that provide opportunities for success
   5. _____ Encourage the client to verbalize negative feelings to others

8. When a disturbed client who has a history of using neologisms says to the nurse, "My lacket hss kelong mon," the nurse should respond by:
   1. Trying to learn the language of the client
   2. Telling the client that these words are not understood
   3. Communicating in simple terms directed toward the client
   4. Recognizing that the client needs a nurse who can understand the fantasies expressed

9. A disturbed male client, unprovoked, attacks another client. A short-term plan for this client should include:
   1. Placing the client in restraints or secluding the client
   2. Having the client sit with a staff member in whom he trusts
   3. Keeping the client actively participating in activities and in contact with reality
   4. Getting the client to apologize for the attack to the other client and to show remorse

10. The nurse anticipates that the medication that will be used to prevent symptoms of withdrawal in clients with a long history of alcohol abuse is:
    1. Lorazepam (Ativan)
    2. Phenobarbital (Luminal)
    3. Chlorpromazine (Thorazine)
    4. Methadone hydrochloride (Methadone)

11. A female nurse has been caring for a 75-year-old depressed woman who reminds her of her grandmother.

The nurse spends extra time with her every day and brings her home-baked cookies. The nurse's behavior reflects:
1. Affiliation
2. Displacement
3. Compensation
4. Countertransference

12. An older adult, accompanied by family members, is admitted to a long-term care facility with symptoms of dementia. During the admission procedure the initial statement by the nurse most helpful to this client is:
    1. "You are somewhat disoriented now, but do not worry. You will be all right in a few days."
    2. "Do not be frightened. I am the nurse, and everyone here in the hospital is here to help you."
    3. "I am the nurse on duty today. You are at the hospital. Your family can stay with you for a while."
    4. "Let me introduce you to the staff here first. In a short while I'll get you acquainted with our unit routine."

13. A nurse identifies that a 6-year-old child, who has attained an acceptable level of psychosocial development, has achieved Erikson's developmental conflicts related to trust, autonomy, and:
    1. Identity
    2. Industry
    3. Intimacy
    4. Initiative

14. The daycare treatment team and a client with an obsessive-compulsive personality disorder decide it will be therapeutic for the client to get a part-time job. On the day of the job interview, the client comes to the center very anxious and displays an increase in compulsive behaviors. The nurse's best response to these behavioral changes is:
    1. "I know you're anxious. However, make yourself go and try to conquer your fear."
    2. "You probably really don't want that job after all. I think you should think more about it."
    3. "The thought of this interview is making you very anxious. It seems you're not ready to work."
    4. "Going for your interview triggered some feelings in you. Describe what you're feeling at this time."

15. A group of clients from a psychiatric unit are going to a professional ballgame accompanied by staff members. The purpose of visits into the community under the supervision of staff members is to:
    1. Assist the clients in adjusting to stressors in the community
    2. Help the clients return to reality under controlled conditions
    3. Observe the clients' abilities to cope with a more complex society
    4. Broaden the clients' experiences by providing exposure to cultural activities

16. To foster a healthy grieving response to the birth of a stillborn child, the nurse's best acknowledgment of the mother's questions about the cause is:
    1. "You are young; wait and see, you'll have other children."

2. "You may be wondering if something you did caused this."
3. "This often happens when something is wrong with the baby."
4. "It's God's will; we have to have faith that it was for the best."

17. One day the nurse and a young adult client sit together and draw. The client draws a face with horns on top of the head and says, "This is me. I'm a devil." What is the nurse's best response?
    1. "I don't see a devil. Why do you see a devil?"
    2. "Let's go to the mirror to see what you look like."
    3. "When I look at you, I see an attractive person, not a devil."
    4. "You are not a devil. Why do you talk about yourself like that?"

18. A nurse anticipates that most clients with phobias will use the defense mechanisms of:
    1. Dissociation and denial
    2. Introjection and sublimation
    3. Projection and displacement
    4. Substitution and reaction formation

19. A nurse manager identifies that one of the nurses in ICU may be experiencing burnout. The nurse manager plans to help this nurse begin to confront the problem by:
    1. Transferring to another nursing care unit
    2. Choosing a nursing position on a low-stress unit
    3. Attending educational programs as often as possible
    4. Identifying personal responses to daily work stresses

20. A client with a history of sleeplessness, lack of interest in eating, and charging excessive purchases to charge accounts is seen in the mental health clinic. The adaptation that the nurse should expect the client to exhibit is:
    1. Depressed mood
    2. Increased insight into behavior
    3. Decreased psychomotor activity
    4. Intrusive involvement with environmental activities

21. A client leaves group therapy in the middle of the session. The nurse finds the client obviously upset and crying. The client tells the nurse that the group's discussion was too much to tolerate. The most therapeutic nursing action at this time is to:
    1. Request kindly but firmly that the client return to the group to work out conflicts
    2. Suggest that the client accompany the nurse to a quiet place so that they can talk about the situation
    3. Ask the group leader what happened in the group session and base intervention on this additional information
    4. Respect the client's right to decline therapy at this time and report the incident to the rest of the health team members

22. A client sits huddled in a chair and leaves it only to assume the fetal position in a corner. The nurse, observing this, identifies that this behavior is classified as:
    1. Reactive
    2. Regressive

3. Dissociative
4. Hallucinatory

23. When caring for a withdrawn, reclusive, psychotic client, the priority goal is for the client to develop:
   1. Trust
   2. Self-worth
   3. A sense of identity
   4. An ability to socialize

24. When reviewing the medications for a group of clients on a psychiatric unit, the nurse concludes that the pharmacotherapy for anxiety disorders is moving away from benzodiazepines and moving toward:
   1. Anticholinergics
   2. Lithium carbonate
   3. Antipsychotic medications
   4. Selective serotonin reuptake inhibitors

25. A nurse is caring for a client who has been experiencing delusions. According to psychodynamic theory, delusions are:
   1. A defense against anxiety
   2. The result of magical thinking
   3. Precipitated by external stimuli
   4. Subconscious expressions of anger

26. A nurse on the psychiatric unit is assigned to work with a male client who appears reclusive and distrustful of everyone. The nurse can help the client to develop trust by:
   1. Being prompt for their scheduled meetings
   2. Stating sincerely that the nurse cares about his feelings
   3. Handing the client medication and not watching to see if it is swallowed
   4. Listening attentively to his positive feelings and ignoring negative feelings

27. A female client in the terminal stage of cancer is admitted to the hospital in severe pain. The client refuses the prescribed intramuscular analgesic for pain because it puts her to sleep and she wants to be awake. One day, despite the client's objection, a nurse administers the pain medication saying, "You know that this will make you more comfortable." The nurse in this situation could be charged with:
   1. Assault
   2. Battery
   3. Invasion of privacy
   4. Lack of informed consent

28. A nurse, understanding the possible cause of alcohol-induced amnestic disorder, should take into consideration that the client is probably experiencing:
   1. Thiamine deficiency
   2. A reduced iron intake
   3. An increase in serotonin
   4. Riboflavin malabsorption

29. The day after the birth of their baby, the parents are upset to learn that the baby has a heart defect. At this time it is most helpful for the nurse to:
   1. Have the parents talk with other parents
   2. Explain the diagnosis in a variety of ways
   3. Encourage the expression of their feelings
   4. Assure the parents that surgery will correct the problem

30. An older client with vascular dementia has difficulty following simple directions for selecting clothes to be worn for the day. The nurse identifies that these problems are the result of:
   1. Receptive aphasia
   2. Impaired judgment
   3. Decreased attention span
   4. Clouding of consciousness

31. A nurse is creating a therapy group for low-functioning clients. Which client is the most appropriate member?
   1. 77-year-old man with anxiety and mild dementia
   2. 28-year-old man with bipolar disorder in a hypermanic state
   3. 52-year-old woman with alcoholism and an antisocial personality
   4. 38-year-old woman whose depression is responding to medication

32. During a well-baby visit, the parents complain that their 2-year-old daughter soils herself because she is lazy. The parents plan to make her wear her soiled clothing to teach her a lesson. The nurse is concerned about the potential for child neglect and abuse. Which nursing intervention is most therapeutic at this time?
   1. Have child protective services remove the daughter from the home
   2. Provide a toileting schedule and instruction about effective hygiene
   3. Refer the parents to classes on anger management and communication skills
   4. Teach the parents developmental milestones in relation to acceptable disciplining methods

33. During an interview of a client with a diagnosis of bipolar I disorder, manic episode, the nurse expects the client to demonstrate:
   1. Flight of ideas
   2. Ritualistic behaviors
   3. Associative looseness
   4. Auditory hallucinations

34. To therapeutically relate to parents who are known to have maltreated their child, the nurse must first:
   1. Recognize the emotional needs of the parents
   2. Identify personal feelings about child abusers
   3. Develop a trusting relationship with the child
   4. Gather information about the child's home environment

35. A young woman who has just lost her first job comes to the mental health clinic very upset and states, "Without warning, I just start crying without any reason." What should be the nurse's initial response?
   1. "Do you know what makes you cry?"
   2. "Most of us need to cry from time to time."
   3. "Crying unexpectedly can be very upsetting."
   4. "Are you having any other problems at this time?"

36. On the first day of the month a practitioner orders an antipsychotic medication for a client with schizophrenia. The initial dose is 25 mg once a day, which is to be titrated

in increments of 25 mg every other day to a desired dose of 175 mg daily. On what day of the month will the client reach the desired dose of 175 mg?
1. 7th
2. 9th
3. 13th
4. 15th

37. The nurse finds a client with schizophrenia lying under a bench in the hall. The client states, "God told me to lie here." What is the best response by the nurse?
   1. "I didn't hear anyone talking. Come with me to your room."
   2. "What you heard was in your head; it was your imagination."
   3. "Come to the dayroom and watch television. You will feel better."
   4. "God would not tell you to lie in the hall. God wants you to behave reasonably."

38. One day as the nurse sits next to a depressed client, the client states, "I want to tell you something but you must promise not to tell anyone." What is the best response by the nurse?
   1. "OK, I won't. It's good for you to talk about what's bothering you."
   2. "You can tell me if you want to. However, I cannot give you that promise."
   3. "I give you my promise not to tell anyone. What's the secret you want to tell me?"
   4. "You seem to be more depressed today. Why don't you tell me what you are thinking?"

39. A client who is a polysubstance abuser was mandated to seek drug and alcohol counseling. When working with the client, the nurse identifies several treatment goals. List in chronological order the outcome criteria for this client.
   1. Discusses effect of drug use on self and others
   2. Verbalizes that a substance abuse problem exists
   3. Explores the use of substances and problematic behaviors
   4. Expresses negative feelings about the present life situation
   Answer: _____

40. When working with clients who use manipulative, socially acting-out behaviors, the nurse should be:
   1. Strict, punishing, and restrictive
   2. Sincere, cautious, and consistent
   3. Supportive, accepting, and friendly
   4. Sympathetic, nurturing, and encouraging

41. A male client with the diagnosis of antisocial personality disorder takes a female nurse by the shoulders, suddenly kisses her, and shouts, "I like you." What is the most appropriate response by the nurse?
   1. "Thank you, I like you too."
   2. "I wish you wouldn't do that."
   3. "Don't ever touch me like that again. I don't like it"
   4. "Your behavior is inappropriate. Don't do that again."

42. A client with schizophrenia is started on an antipsychotic/neuroleptic medication. The nurse explains to a family member that this drug primarily is used to:

1. Keep the client quiet and relaxed
2. Control the client's behavior and reduce stress
3. Reduce the client's need for physical restraints
4. Make the client more receptive to psychotherapy

43. A client says, "Since my husband died, I have nothing to live for. I just want to die." The nurse hears the nursing assistant say, "Things will get better soon." The nurse identifies this response as:
   1. Offering advice
   2. Belittling the client
   3. Changing the subject
   4. Providing false reassurance

44. A young adult client is admitted to the hospital with a diagnosis of schizophrenia, paranoid type. The client has been saying, "The voices in heaven are telling me to come home to God." Initial nursing care should focus on the client's:
   1. Disturbed self-esteem
   2. Potential for self-harm
   3. Dysfunctional verbal communication
   4. Impaired perception of environmental stimuli

45. A recently hired nurse is caring for several clients on a mental health unit at a local community hospital. The nurse manager is evaluating the nurse's performance. What situation reflects that the nurse-client boundaries of the recently hired nurse are appropriate?
   1. The nurse shares with the entire treatment team vital information the client disclosed in a private session
   2. The nurse is often busy doing other tasks when the client and nurse are scheduled for a counselling session
   3. A client enters the therapeutic group late with the nurse's permission even though group rules say this is not allowed
   4. A client's overall behavior is significantly more independent and higher functioning on the days the nurse is not working

46. A nurse identifies that each time the practitioner or nurse manager visits a disturbed female client, she becomes extremely anxious. Today, after visiting with the practitioner, the client sits wringing her hands. What is the best initial response by the nurse?
   1. "How do you handle your anxiety?"
   2. "I notice that you are wringing your hands."
   3. "Tell me why you are afraid of authority figures."
   4. "Do you realize why you are wringing your hands?"

47. A female client with the diagnosis of obsessive-compulsive disorder attends a day treatment program. The client feels her hands are dirty and has a need to wash them 70 to 80 times a day. The client's hands are red and raw with some bleeding. An immediate nursing intervention for this client is to get the client to:
   1. Understand that her hands are not dirty
   2. Gain insight into her emotional problems
   3. Stop washing her hands so the skin will heal
   4. Limit the number of times she washes her hands

48. The nurse, when assessing the behavior of the parents of a physically maltreated child, expects that they:

1. Become irritable about having the history taken
2. Show concern about the child's medical condition
3. Give contradictory explanations about what happened
4. Present a detailed account of how the trauma occurred

49. An inpatient therapy group on a psychiatric unit has as its goal helping clients participate in life more fully by gaining insight and changing behavior. The nurse leader can best help the group achieve this goal by using a leadership style that is:
    1. Democratic and guiding
    2. Autocratic and directing
    3. Laissez-faire and observing
    4. Passive and nonconfrontational

50. The nurse explains to a nursing assistant that behavior usually is viewed and accepted as normal if it:
    1. Fits within standards accepted by one's society
    2. Helps the person to reduce the use of coping skills
    3. Expresses the individual's feelings and thoughts accurately
    4. Allows achievement of short-term and long-term goals by the individual

MENTAL HEALTH NURSING QUIZ
ANSWERS AND RATIONALES

1. 3 **Photosensitivity is a side effect of many antipsychotic medications.**
   1 These adaptations are side effects of lithium, not Haldol.
   2 Avoiding tyramine-containing foods is a precaution associated with MAO inhibitors, not Haldol.
   4 This is a precaution associated with lithium, not Haldol.
   Client Needs: Pharmacological and Parenteral Therapies; **Cognitive Level:** Analysis; **Integrated Process:** Teaching/Learning; **NP:** Evaluation

2. 4 **When a client exhibits adaptations related to depression, the greatest danger is self-inflicted injury when feelings, especially anger, are internalized.**
   1 There are not enough data to determine if the weight loss resulted from malnutrition.
   2 The client is unable to regulate this behavior at this time.
   3 This is false reassurance; this is not supportive of the client's feelings.
   Client Needs: Psychosocial Integrity; **Cognitive Level:** Application; **Integrated Process:** Caring; **NP:** Implementation

3. 3 **Rephrasing allows for further communication, expresses understanding, and does not belittle the client's feelings.**
   1 Presenting reality to the client at this time only raises anxiety and leads the client to defend the delusion.
   2 "Why" questions make a client defensive, and the wording implies that the client's delusion may be true.
   4 This is false reassurance; additionally, a suspicious client will not believe the nurse.
   Client Needs: Psychosocial Integrity; **Cognitive Level:** Analysis; **Integrated Process:** Caring; **NP:** Implementation

4. 1 **Sitting quietly with a severely withdrawn client can provide an opportunity for nonthreatening interaction.**
   2 Entering a withdrawn client's body space is intrusive and stressful; it often precipitates a need for further withdrawal.
   3 The client is unable to socialize with others at this time.
   4 Placing demands on the withdrawn client causes a sense of threat, increased anxiety, and a need for additional withdrawal.
   Client Needs: Psychosocial Integrity; **Cognitive Level:** Application; **Integrated Process:** Caring; **NP:** Planning

5. 3 **Loosened associations and hallucinations are the primary behaviors associated with a thought disorder such as schizophrenia.**
   1 Paranoid delusions and hypervigilance are more common in paranoid-type schizophrenia than in the undifferentiated type.
   2 Depression and psychomotor retardation are not characteristic of schizophrenia.

   4 Ritualistic behavior and obsessive thinking generally are associated with obsessive-compulsive disorders, not schizophrenia.
   Client Needs: Psychosocial Integrity; **Cognitive Level:** Analysis; **NP:** Assessment

6. 2 **The parents' ongoing marital problems appear to have interfered with their parental roles, resulting in their children's behavioral problems.**
   1 At this time the children need support, not limits.
   3 There are no data to support this diagnosis.
   4 There are no data to support this diagnosis.
   Client Needs: Psychosocial Integrity; **Cognitive Level:** Analysis; **NP:** Analysis

7. **Answer: 2, 3, 4**
   1 The opposite is true; clients with conduct disorders tend to generate stress for others.
   2 **Channeling energy to healthy physical activities can decrease violent behavior.**
   3 **A behavioral contract is used to reinforce problem solving and encourage the use of social skills.**
   4 **Successful experiences improve the client's self-esteem and should decrease the manipulative behavior.**
   5 Verbalization of negative feelings to others can often escalate and result in antisocial or acting out behavior.
   Client Needs: Psychosocial Integrity; **Cognitive Level:** Analysis; **Integrated Process:** Caring; **NP:** Planning

8. 2 **This is a simple statement that the client is not understood; it provides feedback and points out reality.**
   1 Neologisms have symbolic meaning only for the client.
   3 Although this should be done, it does not address the problem.
   4 There is no one other than the client who can understand the fantasies.
   Client Needs: Psychosocial Integrity; **Cognitive Level:** Application; **Integrated Process:** Communication and Documentation; **NP:** Implementation

9. 2 **The client needs someone with whom there is a working and trusting relationship; this individual must observe, protect, anticipate, and prevent the client from acting out on destructive impulses.**
   1 These eventually may be necessary to do, but they are too restrictive for an initial intervention.
   3 Although there is a need to be kept in touch with reality, the client may not be ready for participation.
   4 At this time the client cannot be held responsible for this behavior.
   Client Needs: Safety and Infection Control; **Cognitive Level:** Application; **Integrated Process:** Caring; **NP:** Planning

10. 1 **Lorazepam (Ativan) is most effective in preventing the signs and symptoms associated with withdrawal**

from alcohol. **It depresses the CNS by potentiating GABA, an inhibitory neurotransmitter.**

2 Phenobarbital (Luminal) is used to prevent withdrawal symptoms associated with barbiturate use.

3 Chlorpromazine (Thorazine), an antipsychotic medication, is not used for alcohol withdrawal.

4 Methadone hydrochloride (Methadone) is used to prevent withdrawal symptoms associated with opioid use.

Client Needs: Pharmacological and Parenteral Therapies; **Cognitive Level:** Analysis; **NP:** Planning

11. 4 **With countertransference the professional provider of care exhibits an emotional reaction to a client based on a previous relationship or on unconscious needs or conflicts.**

1 Affiliation is turning to others for support and help when stressed or conflicted.

2 Displacement is the discharge of pent-up feelings onto something or someone else that is less threatening than the original source of the feelings.

3 Compensation is attempting to balance deficiencies in one area by excelling in another area.

Client Needs: Psychosocial Integrity; **Cognitive Level:** Analysis; **NP:** Analysis

12. 2 **Familiarity with the environment and a self-introduction may help promote security and feelings of trust.**

1 This denies the client's feelings and provides false reassurance.

3 This statement denies feelings and is false reassurance because all personnel are not involved with the client.

4 A person under stress cannot assimilate much information; verbiage could lead to more confusion.

Client Needs: Psychosocial Integrity; **Cognitive Level:** Analysis; **Integrated Process:** Communication and Documentation; **NP:** Implementation

13. 4 **A 6-year-old child should have resolved the previous developmental conflicts of trust vs. mistrust (infancy) and autonomy vs. shame and doubt (toddlerhood). During the preschool years children learn to assume responsibility for themselves and their possessions as well as develop more socially acceptable behavior (initiative vs. guilt).**

1 Resolution of identity vs. role confusion occurs at adolescence.

2 Resolution of industry vs. inferiority does not occur until the end of the school-age years.

3 Resolution of intimacy vs. isolation occurs at adulthood.

Client Needs: Health Promotion and Maintenance; **Cognitive Level:** Comprehension; **NP:** Assessment

14. 4 **These behaviors are a defense against anxiety, which triggers old fears; the client needs support.**

1 This denies the client's overwhelming anxiety and lacks realistic support.

2 This is judgmental; an increase in anxiety does not necessarily mean the client does not want to attain the goal.

3 This is judgmental; the client should be encouraged to work through the concerns, not to avoid risk.

Client Needs: Psychosocial Integrity; **Cognitive Level:** Analysis; **Integrated Process:** Caring; **NP:** Implementation

15. 3 **The nurse's observations can help identify those clients who are ready to cope with outside stress and those who are not.**

1 Attendance at a ballgame will not accomplish this.

2 Attendance at a ballgame will not accomplish this.

4 There is nothing to indicate that any of these clients needed to broaden their cultural experiences.

Client Needs: Psychosocial Integrity; **Cognitive Level:** Application; **NP:** Planning

16. 2 **The mother must be helped to identify feelings.**

1 This is false reassurance; it does not encourage the client to explore feelings.

3 Many stillborn children are apparently free of any defects.

4 This answer is based on the nurse's religious beliefs; there is no indication that the client has the same beliefs; this closes off communication.

Client Needs: Psychosocial Integrity; **Cognitive Level:** Analysis; **Integrated Process:** Caring; **NP:** Implementation

17. 3 **This response points out reality while attempting to let the client understand that the nurse sees the client as a person of worth.**

1 This asks the client to explain feelings, which may be unrealistic.

2 The client may indeed view the self as a devil.

4 This is a somewhat belittling response; it cuts off communication.

Client Needs: Psychosocial Integrity; **Cognitive Level:** Analysis; **Integrated Process:** Caring; **NP:** Implementation

18. 3 **Clients with phobias cope with anxiety by placing it on specific persons, objects, or situations through the process of displacement and/or projection.**

1 The person with a phobia recognizes and admits the exaggerated fear as a real part of the self.

2 Neither introjection, whereby a person internalizes and incorporates the traits of another, nor sublimation, whereby socially acceptable behavior is substituted for unacceptable instincts, is related to phobic activity.

4 A less-valued object is not substituted for one more highly valued (substitution) nor are the expressed feelings opposite to the experienced feelings of fear (reaction formation).

Client Needs: Psychosocial Integrity; **Cognitive Level:** Analysis; **NP:** Analysis

19. 4 **Identification of work stressors in the environment, coping strategies used, and evaluating the effectiveness of these strategies are the first steps.**

1 This may help, but prevention begins with knowing oneself and the effectiveness of one's coping strategies.

2 Choosing a nursing position on a low-stress unit can help alleviate burnout, but it is not the first step in confronting the problem when it occurs.

3 Attending continuing education programs can help alleviate burnout, but this is not the first step in confronting the problem when it occurs.

Client Needs: Management of Care; **Cognitive Level:** Application; **Integrated Process:** Caring; **NP:** Planning

20. 4 **In an attempt to ward off depression, the client in the hyperactive phase of bipolar I disorder runs headlong into reality, becoming totally involved in everything that goes on in the environment.**

1 This is more indicative of a depressive episode.

2 During this phase, there is no insight into behavior.

3 The opposite occurs; psychomotor activity is greatly increased.

Client Needs: Psychosocial Integrity; **Cognitive Level:** Application; **NP:** Assessment

21. 2 **This approach incorporates the principles of starting where the client is and helping the client verbalize feelings; it also provides for additional data collecting.**

1 The client is not ready to do this.

3 This should be a later step, after the more appropriate nursing action is completed.

4 This accepts the client's right not to be forced back into the group; however, direct nursing intervention should be attempted at this time.

Client Needs: Psychosocial Integrity; **Cognitive Level:** Application; **Integrated Process:** Communication and Documentation; **NP:** Implementation

22. 2 **This behavior reflects the early fetal position; the individual curls up for both protection and security.**

1 The client's behavior is not in response to an observable stimulus.

3 The client's behavior does not indicate dissociation or depersonalization.

4 The client's behavior gives no indication of a hallucinatory pattern.

Client Needs: Psychosocial Integrity; **Cognitive Level:** Analysis; **NP:** Analysis

23. 1 **Trust is basic to all therapies; without trust a therapeutic relationship cannot be established.**

2 The development of self-worth is a long-term goal; developing trust is the priority.

3 There is nothing to indicate that the client does not have a sense of identity.

4 Although helping the client relate to others is a part of the treatment, it is not a priority goal at this time.

Client Needs: Psychosocial Integrity; **Cognitive Level:** Application; **Integrated Process:** Caring; **NP:** Planning

24. 4 **Selective serotonin reuptake inhibitors have better safety profiles and do not have the risk of substance abuse and tolerance.**

1 Anticholinergics are administered concurrently with antipsychotics to minimize extrapyramidal side effects.

2 Lithium carbonate is a drug used to treat bipolar disorder.

3 Antipsychotics are administered to clients with thought disorders.

Client Needs: Pharmacological and Parenteral Therapies; **Cognitive Level:** Analysis; **NP:** Analysis

25. 1 **Delusions are a way the unconscious defends the individual from real or imagined threats.**

2 Magical thinking is the belief that one's thoughts and behaviors can control situations and other people. For example, having bad thoughts about someone can cause that person to die. This type of thinking is found in young children but is pathological in adults.

3 Illusions are false interpretations of actual external stimuli.

4 Delusions are precipitated by feelings of anxiety, not anger.

Client Needs: Psychosocial Integrity; **Cognitive Level:** Comprehension; **NP:** Analysis

26. 1 **This helps the client to feel important enough for the nurse to remember their meeting and be on time.**

2 The client is distrustful of others and will probably not believe the nurse; caring is best demonstrated through behavior.

3 This is not only an unsafe practice but it may make the client feel that the nurse does not care enough to stay.

4 Feelings should never be ignored but should be accepted as important to the client.

Client Needs: Psychosocial Integrity; **Cognitive Level:** Application; **Integrated Process:** Caring; **NP:** Implementation

27. 2 **This is the intentional touching of one person by another without permission of the person being touched.**

1 This is an intentional act without touching that makes a person fearful or produces reasonable apprehension of bodily harm.

3 This refers to the right of clients to have their private affairs protected.

4 Informed consent applies to permission for procedures and treatments to be performed.

Client Needs: Management of Care; **Cognitive Level:** Analysis; **NP:** Evaluation

28. 1 **The deficiency of thiamine (vitamin B$_1$) is thought to be a primary cause of alcohol-induced amnestic disorder.**

2 This is unrelated to alcohol-induced amnestic disorder.

3 This is unrelated to alcohol-induced amnestic disorder.

4 This is unrelated to alcohol-induced amnestic disorder.

Client Needs: Psychosocial Integrity; **Cognitive Level:** Analysis; **NP:** Assessment

29. 3 **Parents need to express and deal with their feelings, then perhaps they can move toward other coping strategies.**

1 This does not focus on their present concern but could be useful sometime in the future.

2 This does not focus on the need presented by the parents.

4 This is premature and possibly false reassurance.

Client Needs: Psychosocial Integrity; **Cognitive Level:** Application; **Integrated Process:** Communication and Documentation; **NP:** Implementation

30. **1 Receptive aphasia interferes with interpreting and defining words in addition to following directions and selecting clothes.**

2 Following directions does not require skill in judgment or decision making.

3 The selection of clothes does not require an intact attention span.

4 Dementia does not cause a clouding of consciousness; delirium does.

Client Needs: Psychosocial Integrity; **Cognitive Level:** Analysis; **NP:** Analysis

31. **1 An older person with mild dementia and anxiety can participate in a low-functioning group where there is greater structure and staff direction.**

2 This client may be disruptive in a low-functioning therapy group.

3 This client may be disruptive in a low-functioning therapy group.

4 A depressed client who is responding to medication should be able to participate in a higher-functioning group.

Client Needs: Management of Care; **Cognitive Level:** Analysis; **NP:** Analysis

32. **4 The parents' expectation of accident-free toilet training by age 2 is developmentally unrealistic. Their methods of discipline can cause harm. Teaching them what to expect of their child and how to respond more appropriately is critical at this time.**

1 This intervention is unnecessary. This intervention is appropriate for more serious situations of child endangerment.

2 Although instruction on the importance of hygiene is helpful, the underlying issue is their choice of inappropriate discipline for a 2-year-old.

3 Anger management and communication skills are not the problems.

Client Needs: Health Promotion and Maintenance; **Cognitive Level:** Application; **Integrated Process:** Teaching/Learning; **NP:** Implementation

33. **1 This is a fragmented, pressured, nonsequential pattern of speech typically used during a manic episode.**

2 These are repetitive, purposeful, and intentional behaviors that are carried out in a stereotyped fashion; they are found in clients with obsessive-compulsive disorders.

3 This is the pattern of speech found in clients with schizophrenia; usual connections between words and phrases are lost to the listener and meaningful only to the speaker.

4 Hallucinations are false perceptions generated by internal stimuli; they are found in clients with the diagnosis of schizophrenia.

Client Needs: Psychosocial Integrity; **Cognitive Level:** Analysis; **NP:** Assessment

34. **2 Self-awareness is an essential element in providing support, understanding, and empathy to others.**

1 Meeting the emotional needs of these parents cannot be accomplished until an interpersonal relationship is established; to establish an interpersonal relationship with clients the nurse must first be aware of personal feelings.

3 Although this eventually should be done, this does not address the nurse's relationship with the parents.

4 Although important, these data do not take priority at this time.

Client Needs: Psychosocial Integrity; **Cognitive Level:** Application; **NP:** Assessment

35. **3 This response identifies the client's feelings.**

1 This is an unrealistic question; the cause of anxiety may not be known.

2 This response moves the focus away from the client.

4 This disregards the client's comment; it is a direct question that may impede communication.

Client Needs: Psychosocial Integrity; **Cognitive Level:** Analysis; **Integrated Process:** Communication and Documentation; **NP:** Implementation

36. **3 The client will reach the desired dose of 175 mg on the 13th day of the month; the 1st day is 25 mg, 3rd day is 50 mg, 5th day is 75 mg, 7th day is 100 mg, 9th day is 125 mg, 11th day is 150 mg, and 13th day is 175 mg.**

1 This is an incorrect calculation of when the desired dose of 175 mg will be reached.

2 This is an incorrect calculation of when the desired dose of 175 mg will be reached.

4 This is an incorrect calculation of when the desired dose of 175 mg will be reached.

Client Needs: Pharmacological and Parenteral Therapies; **Cognitive Level:** Application; **NP:** Planning

37. **1 The nurse is focusing on reality and trying to distract and refocus the client's attention.**

2 This statement is too blunt and belittling; this approach rarely is effective.

3 This is false reassurance; the nurse does not know that the client will feel better.

4 This may be interpreted as belittling or an attempt to convince the client that the behavior is irrational; it usually is ineffective.

Client Needs: Psychosocial Integrity; **Cognitive Level:** Analysis; **Integrated Process:** Caring; **NP:** Implementation

38. **2 By being honest, if a client tells the nurse something that should be shared, the nurse will not have to break a promise or risk harm to the client or others.**

1 Encouraging discussion is helpful, but putting oneself in the position of possibly having to break a promise is not therapeutic.

3 This puts the nurse in the position of maybe having to break a promise, which may destroy rapport and decrease trust.

4 This response ignores the client's statement and avoids the issue.

Client Needs: Management of Care; **Cognitive Level:** Analysis; **Integrated Process:** Communication and Documentation; **NP:** Implementation

39. **Answer: 2, 1, 4, 3**

Clients must first acknowledge that a substance abuse problem exists and creates chaos in their lives. The clients can then discuss the numerous ways that drug use has changed and controlled their lives. Assistance from the nurse may be required at this time for the client to express and process negative feelings. Finally, clients will require assistance establishing the relationship between substance use and their current lifestyle problems.

Client Needs: Psychosocial Integrity; **Cognitive Level:** Analysis; **NP:** Planning

40. **2 A sincere, cautious, and consistent attitude limits this individual's ability to manipulate both situations and staff members.**

1 This approach can create power struggles and can limit the development of a therapeutic nurse-client relationship.

3 When accepting the person, the nurse should not support negative behavior; a friendly attitude may encourage further problem behavior.

4 This may encourage clients to continue in their lifestyle rather than learn appropriate ways to relate to others.

Client Needs: Psychosocial Integrity; **Cognitive Level:** Analysis; **Integrated Process:** Caring; **NP:** Planning

41. **4 This accepts the client while rejecting and setting limits on the behavior the client is using.**

1 This encourages this type of behavior instead of setting limits.

2 This response makes it appear that it is the nurse's preference, not the client's behavior, that is the issue.

3 This response makes it appear that it is the nurse's preference, not the client's behavior, that is the issue.

Client Needs: Psychosocial Integrity; **Cognitive Level:** Analysis; **Integrated Process:** Communication and Documentation; **NP:** Implementation

42. **4 Antipsychotic/neuroleptic medications help control anxiety, improve cognition, and decrease acting-out behavior, making the client better able to participate in therapy.**

1 Although the medication may produce these effects, they are not the primary purpose of administration.

2 Although the medication may produce these effects, they are not the primary purpose of administration.

3 Although the medication may prevent the need for restraints, it is not the primary purpose of administration.

Client Needs: Pharmacological and Parenteral Therapies; **Cognitive Level:** Comprehension; **Integrated Process:** Teaching/Learning; **NP:** Implementation

43. **4 False reassurance is an effort to be supportive that often uses clichés and is not based on fact.**

1 Offering advice tells the client what to do; clients should be encouraged to problem solve.

2 Belittling statements demean the client or minimize client concerns.

3 The nursing assistant's statement did not change the subject.

Client Needs: Management of Care; **Cognitive Level:** Application; **NP:** Evaluation

44. **2 Client safety always is the priority over any other client need and command hallucinations increase the risk for injury.**

1 Although promoting a positive self-esteem is important, this is not a priority at this time.

3 There are no data to support the need to focus on the client's ability to verbally communicate.

4 Verbal hallucinations occur within the individual; they are not precipitated by an environmental stimulus.

Client Needs: Reduction of Risk Potential; **Cognitive Level:** Analysis; **NP:** Analysis

45. **1 The nurse is part of the treatment team and must share vital information with its members. Keeping secrets indicates over-involvement by a nurse.**

2 When the nurse is under-involved in the nurse-client relationship, respect and trust, which are necessary for therapy, do not develop. This is an example in which the nurse places other responsibilities over the commitment made to the client.

3 When a nurse becomes over-involved in the nurse-client relationship, the nurse may bend the rules for a specific client. This is detrimental to that client and other clients who see the preferential treatment.

4 When a nurse becomes over-involved in the nurse-client relationship, the nurse may foster regressive behaviors that make the client more dependent.

Client Needs: Management of Care; **Cognitive Level:** Analysis; **Integrated Process:** Communication and Documentation; **NP:** Evaluation

46. **2 The nurse is making an observation; bringing it to the attention of the client is an initial step in understanding that behavior.**

1 This is premature because the client may not even be aware of anxiety.

3 This is premature and does not allow for self-recognition of feelings.

4 This is requesting a response that the client probably is incapable of explaining.

Client Needs: Psychosocial Integrity; **Cognitive Level:** Analysis; **Integrated Process:** Communication and Documentation; **NP:** Implementation

47. **4 This action still permits the client to cope with feelings of anxiety while aiming to reduce skin damage.**

1 The anxiety is too great for the client to understand why handwashing is not necessary.

2 Recognition must precede the development of insight; neither can be done until the level of anxiety is reduced.

3 This will not allow the client any outlet for coping with extreme anxiety, which is the priority need at this time. The client will need to wash the hands sometimes, such as after toileting.
Client Needs: Psychosocial Integrity; **Cognitive Level:** Application; **Integrated Process:** Caring; **NP:** Planning

48. **3 In an attempt to block the hospital staff from discovering what happened, abusing parents often provide inconsistent accounts.**
1 This may or may not occur.
2 Abusing parents tend to show more concern about how the child's condition affects them than about how the child is affected.
4 Abusing parents tend to be vague about the details of the accident but maintain the child was accidentally injured.
Client Needs: Psychosocial Integrity; **Cognitive Level:** Application; **NP:** Assessment

49. **1 This type of leader stimulates, guides, and assists the group to develop its maximum potential by facilitating and balancing group forces.**
2 This type of leader makes most of the decisions and controls the group, thus limiting group growth potential.

3 This type of leader allows group members to take over the group; if there are no members with leadership skills, little is gained from the group.
4 This type of leader does not provide adequate leadership to make the group effective.
Client Needs: Psychosocial Integrity; **Cognitive Level:** Analysis; **Integrated Process:** Communication and Documentation; **NP:** Implementation

50. **1 An accepted practice in some parts of the world may well be considered abnormal behavior in others. Cultural context is necessary to understand behavior.**
2 Coping skills are behaviors that help people adapt to stress. Whether they are viewed as normal or not depends on their cultural context.
3 Accurate expressions of feelings may take the form of behaviors considered abnormal.
4 If the behavior were aggressive or destructive, even though it helped reach a goal, it cannot be considered normal.
Client Needs: Management of Care; **Cognitive Level:** Comprehension; **Integrated Process:** Teaching/Learning; **NP:** Implementation

CHAPTER 4

Childbearing and Women's Health Nursing

Review Questions

NURSING PRACTICE

1. A plan of care is created for a term small-for-gestational-age (SGA) neonate who was admitted to the neonatal intensive care unit (NICU). The goal was for the newborn to reach 5 pounds by a specified date. On the specified date the infant weighs 4 pounds, 2 ounces. What should the nurse do next?
   1. Increase the daily number of calories
   2. Change the goal to a more realistic number
   3. Reassess the problem before altering the plan
   4. Postpone the evaluation date for another month

2. A 17-year-old client, who is at 38 weeks' gestation, is being prepared for an emergency cesarean birth because there is an abruptio placentae and severe fetal compromise. The client received nalbuphine (Nubain) 10 mg IV 30 minutes ago. Because the client is too sedated to sign the consent form, the nurse should:
   1. Call the client's mother and request a verbal consent
   2. Proceed with the preparation and forgo written consent
   3. Have the surgeon and attending practitioner sign the consent form
   4. Sign the consent form and have the nurse manager countersign the form

3. A female client is scheduled for a hysterectomy. When discussing the preoperative preparation, the nurse identifies that the client has inadequate understanding of the surgery. What is the next nursing intervention?
   1. Describe the proposed surgery to the client
   2. Proceed with implementing the preoperative plan
   3. Notify the surgeon that the client needs more information
   4. Explain gently that she should have asked more questions

4. A client in labor is being prepared for a cesarean birth. What is the most important nursing intervention before anesthesia is administered?
   1. Prepare the abdomen
   2. Obtain informed consent
   3. Initiate an intravenous infusion
   4. Insert an indwelling urinary catheter

5. New parents are asked to sign the consent for their son to be circumcised. They ask for the nurse's opinion of the procedure. How should the nurse respond?

   1. "You should talk to the physician about this if you have any questions."
   2. "Let's talk about it because there are advantages and disadvantages."
   3. "It is a safe procedure and it is best for male infants to be circumcised."
   4. "Although it may be a somewhat painful experience for the baby, I would allow it if I were you."

6. A new mother tells the nurse that her baby "spits up" after each formula feeding. The nurse teaches her how to position her newborn after feedings. Following the next feeding the nurse observes that the mother positions the baby correctly. The nurse observed this activity to:
   1. Prepare a basic teaching plan
   2. Validate that learning has occurred
   3. Ascertain the mother's knowledge base
   4. Determine the mother's readiness to learn

7. The parents of a newborn tell the nurse that they do not want their infant's eyes treated with a prophylactic agent. How should the nurse respond?
   1. "This is really for the baby's good."
   2. "This is a legal requirement that must be done."
   3. "It is best that you discuss this with your pediatrician."
   4. "You'll have to sign an informed consent to refuse the treatment."

8. When obtaining informed consent for sterilization from a developmentally challenged adult client, the nurse must be sure that the:
   1. Parent or guardian signs the consent
   2. Client is able to explain what the procedure entails
   3. Client is able to comprehend the outcome of the procedure
   4. Parent or guardian has encouraged the client to make the decision

9. A client at 16 weeks' gestation arrives at the prenatal clinic for a routine visit. During the examination the nurse observes bruises on the client's face and abdomen. There are no bruises on her legs and arms. Further assessment is required to confirm:
   1. Domestic abuse
   2. Hydatidiform mole
   3. Excessive exercising
   4. Thrombocytopenic purpura

10. A nurse is teaching a prenatal class about infant safety. After the class several of the students are heard discussing what they had learned. The nurse identifies that the teaching is effective when one of the future parents states:
    1. "My mother has already made the cutest pillowcases for the baby's pillows."
    2. "I have just bought a new baby seat that can be strapped into the front seat of the car."
    3. "My mother can't believe that babies are supposed to sleep on their backs, not their stomachs."
    4. "I was given a baby tub at my shower that has a special safety strap that lets me leave the baby alone in it."

EMOTIONAL NEEDS RELATED TO CHILDBEARING AND WOMEN'S HEALTH

11. A 16-year-old girl at 28 weeks' gestation arrives at the prenatal clinic with her mother for a routine sonogram. Before the procedure, the girl requests that the nurse not reveal the fetus's gender if it should become apparent. Afterward the mother asks the nurse the sex of the fetus. Considering the mother-daughter relationship, the nurse's best response is:
    1. "That information is not available at this time."
    2. "I'm not allowed to divulge confidential information."
    3. "Your daughter asked me not to give that information to anyone."
    4. "The sex of the baby isn't the most important information to know at this time."

12. Because of the high discomfort level during the transition phase of labor, nursing care should be directed toward:
    1. Helping the client maintain control
    2. Decreasing the rate of intravenous fluid
    3. Administering the prescribed medication
    4. Having the client breathe in a uniform pattern

13. The nurse is caring for a client who is in the taking-in phase of the postpartum period. The area of health teaching that the client will be most responsive to is:
    1. Perineal care
    2. Infant feeding
    3. Infant hygiene
    4. Family planning

14. A postpartum adolescent mother confides to the nurse that she hopes her baby will be good and sleep through the night. What should the nurse plan to teach the client to do?
    1. Talk softly and cuddle her baby when crying occurs
    2. Keep her baby awake for longer periods during the day
    3. Ensure sleep by adding cereal to her baby's bedtime bottle
    4. Put a soft and brightly colored toy next to her baby at bedtime

15. The husband of a woman who had her fourth child 3 weeks ago states she has been irritable and crying since bringing her newborn home. The nurse tries to assist him in understanding the situation by stating that:
    1. Having four children is tiring and assistance may be needed
    2. His wife probably has postpartum blues and it will soon pass
    3. This behavior is common after birth and he should not be too concerned
    4. Women often express themselves by crying and he should allow her to continue

16. A client with mild preeclampsia is told that she must remain on bed rest at home. The client starts to cry and tells the nurse that she has two small children at home who need her. How should the nurse respond?
    1. "How do you plan to manage with getting child care help?"
    2. "Are you worried about how you will be able to handle this problem?"
    3. "You can get a neighbor to help out and your husband can do the housework in the evening."
    4. "You can prepare light meals and the children can go to nursery school a few hours each day."

17. What is the best nursing intervention to achieve the cooperation of an extremely anxious pregnant client during her first pelvic examination?
    1. Distract the client by asking her preference as to the sex of her infant
    2. Assist the practitioner so the client's examination can be completed quickly
    3. Explain the procedure and maintain eye contact while touching the client gently
    4. Encourage the client to squeeze the nurse's hand, close her eyes, and hold her breath

18. A pregnant client whose first child has Down syndrome is about to undergo an amniocentesis. The client tells the nurse that she does not know what she will do if this fetus has the same diagnosis. The client asks the nurse, "Do you think abortion is the same as killing?" How should the nurse respond?
    1. "Some people think this is what an abortion is."
    2. "No, I do not think so, but it is your decision to make."
    3. "I really can't answer that question. Are you ambivalent about abortion?"
    4. "I don't want to answer that question at this time. How do you feel about it?"

19. A client who has just given birth to an infant with Down syndrome tells the nurse that she could not possibly take a retarded child home and asks whether she should plan to place the child in an institution. Which response is the most appropriate at this time?
    1. "It must be difficult not to realize your vision of a perfect child."

2. "I understand how you feel. I will notify the nursery personnel of your decision."

3. "Give yourself time to get acquainted, and you will see that your baby may not be retarded."

4. "You should not make such a hasty decision because your baby is like any other baby right now."

20. A neonate is born with exstrophy of the bladder and the parents are upset. They are told that corrective surgery will be done as soon as possible. How can the nurse best help the parents at this time?

1. Teaching the parents about preoperative and post-operative care

2. Caring for the newborn in the same manner as any other newborn

3. Keeping the newborn as clean as possible to decrease the odor of urine

4. Reassuring the parents that after surgery their newborn will grow and develop without any after effects

21. A 4-day-old male with exstrophy of the bladder and ambiguous genitalia is in the neonatal intensive care unit (NICU). The everted bladder is inflamed and there is continual leaking of urine onto the surrounding skin. What is the nurse's initial concern when trying to support his mother?

1. Promote her acceptance of her baby as he is

2. Prepare her for the surgery her baby will require

3. Teach her how to care for her baby's urinary needs

4. Instruct her on ways she can meet her baby's emotional needs

22. A client with severe preeclampsia who was admitted to the high-risk unit anxiously asks the nurse, "Will my baby be all right?" How should the nurse respond?

1. "There is no way of telling at this time what the outcome will be."

2. "If you do what the physician tells you to do, everything will progress normally."

3. "The baby will probably be all right. Do you know that the amniotic fluid provides protection?"

4. "We will be monitoring your baby's condition continuously. Would you like to listen to the baby's heartbeat?"

23. A client in active labor is rushed from the emergency department to the labor and birth suite screaming, "Knock me out." Examination reveals that her cervix is 9 cm dilated. What should the nurse say while trying to calm her?

1. "I'll rub your back, which will help ease your pain."

2. "You will get a shot when you reach the birthing room."

3. "I'm sure you're in pain, but try to bear with it for the baby's sake."

4. "Medication may interfere with the baby's first breaths; try to bear the pain."

24. A preterm male newborn will be in the neonatal intensive care unit (NICU) for several weeks. The parents live about 100 miles away and say they can visit only every 2 weeks or so. What is most important for the nurse to do when planning care for this newborn and the family?

1. Plan for contact with the parents by sending e-mails with pictures of the infant

2. Focus on the infant's biophysical needs in view of his present critical condition

3. Refer the infant's parents to the social worker to arrange housing close to the hospital

4. Prepare a teaching plan to be given to the parents on the day of their infant's discharge

25. A nurse understands the stages of parental adjustment that follow birth of an at-risk infant who is in the neonatal intensive care unit (NICU). To better plan nursing care, nursing observations and assessments are based on the recognition that the:

1. Parents should be encouraged to visit their newborn within the first day of birth

2. Mother should not see the infant until she has completed the necessary grief work

3. Mother should be reunited with her infant as soon as possible to enhance adjustment

4. Nurse should wait until the parents request to see their newborn before suggesting a visit

26. A nurse in the neonatal intensive care unit (NICU) is showing a mother her preterm infant for the first time. The mother immediately starts to cry and refuses to touch her baby. What does this behavior represent?

1. A typical detachment behavior

2. An incomplete bonding behavior

3. An expected reaction to the situation

4. A negative reaction to the NICU environment

27. The parents of a preterm newborn visit the neonatal intensive care unit (NICU) for the first time. They are obviously overwhelmed by the amount of equipment and the tiny size of their baby. What is the nurse's most appropriate response to their reaction?

1. Placing the baby in the mother's lap

2. Showing the parents how to touch the baby

3. Explaining the purpose of the equipment being used

4. Discouraging the parents from staying too long on this first visit

28. When seeing her preterm infant son in the neonatal intensive care unit (NICU) for the first time, a mother exclaims, "My baby is so little. How will I ever care for him?" The nurse explains to the mother that she:

1. Will be encouraged to participate in his care as much as possible

2. Can watch his care to assist her in becoming familiar with the specific routines

3. Should find someone with preterm care training to help at home for the first week

4. Will be able to care for him in a special nursery for a few days before his discharge

29. On the third postpartum day, a client who had an unexpected cesarean birth is found crying when the nurse enters her room. She says, "I know my baby is fine, but I can't help crying. I wanted natural childbirth so much. Why did this have to happen to me?" The nurse responds knowing that:
    1. The client's feelings will pass after she has bonded with her infant
    2. The client is probably suffering from a postpartum depression and needs special care
    3. A cesarean birth may be a traumatic experience but most women know it is a possible outcome
    4. A woman's self-concept may be negatively affected by a cesarean birth, and the client's statement may reflect this

30. Before an amniocentesis both parents express anxiety about the fetus's safety during the test. Which nursing intervention will best promote the parents' ability to cope?
    1. Initiating a parent-practitioner conference
    2. Reassuring them that the procedure is safe
    3. Informing them about the procedure step by step
    4. Arranging for the father to be present during the test

31. A nurse determines that the husband of a client is reacting positively to his wife's pregnancy when, during the second trimester, he says:
    1. "I'm planning to take a part-time job because we'll need a larger apartment."
    2. "I'm so proud of my wife. I'm already digging a baseball diamond in our backyard."
    3. "I get so excited when I feel the baby kicking. I didn't realize how strong those little legs are."
    4. "I hope I'll be able watch my baby's birth. A childbirth movie was shown in class last night that sort of turned me off."

32. During labor a client tells the nurse that she and her husband are very concerned because the baby will be born 2 months early. How should the nurse respond?
    1. "You should be concerned; I feel for you."
    2. "If you are concerned; let's talk about it."
    3. "Try not to worry about it; just concentrate on your labor."
    4. "Don't worry; the care of preterm babies has greatly improved."

33. A client who is at 28 weeks' gestation and in active labor is crying. She says, "I just know this baby will die. What's the use of doing all this to save it?" The nurse concludes that the client is:
    1. Depressed and needs firm, positive support during labor
    2. Experiencing anticipatory grief and withdrawing from bonding
    3. In need of sedation to aid her in coping with the impending birth
    4. Demonstrating difficulty dealing with the birth by using the word "it"

34. What must the nurse assess first when planning to promote mother-infant attachment?
    1. Mother-infant interaction
    2. Mother-father interaction
    3. The infant's physical status
    4. The mother's ability to care for her infant

35. What common concern of the mother after an unexpected cesarean birth should the nurse anticipate?
    1. Postoperative pain
    2. Prolonged period of hospitalization
    3. Inability to assume the mothering role
    4. Sense of failure in the birthing process

36. A nurse is instructing a client to cough and deep breathe after an emergency cesarean birth. The client says, "Get out of here. Don't you know that I am in pain?" Which response is most effective?
    1. "I'm sure you are in pain. I'll come back later."
    2. "If you are unable to cough, try to take six very deep breaths."
    3. "Your pain is to be expected, but you must exercise your lungs."
    4. "I'll give you something for your pain. We can start the coughing tomorrow."

37. A client who had a cesarean birth seems upset. She has been having difficulty breastfeeding for 2 days and now asks the nurse to bring her a bottle of formula. What is the nurse's initial action?
    1. Obtaining the requested formula
    2. Administering the prescribed pain medication
    3. Assessing the client's breastfeeding technique
    4. Notifying the practitioner of the client's request to switch feeding methods

38. On the first postpartum day, a client whose infant is rooming-in asks the nurse to return her baby to the nursery and bring the baby to her only at feeding time. How should the nurse respond?
    1. "It seems you changed your mind about rooming-in."
    2. "I think you are having difficulty caring for the baby."
    3. "All right, I will inform the other nurses of your decision."
    4. "You must be tired. I'll bring the baby back at feeding time."

39. A client at 37 weeks' gestation gives birth to a healthy boy. When inspecting her newborn in the birthing room the client becomes concerned and asks, "What's this sticky white stuff all over him?" How should the nurse respond?
    1. "It's a secretion from the baby's fat cells and is called milia."
    2. "This is vernix. It helps protect the baby while he's in the uterus."
    3. "Your baby was born several weeks early and we expect to see this."
    4. "It's nothing to be concerned about. Most newborns are covered with it."

40. The mother of a pregnant teenager asks the nurse how her daughter could have been so foolish because birth

control had been discussed with her many times. How should the nurse respond?

1. "Apparently your daughter was not listening to you."
2. "You should have made sure her boyfriend understood birth control, too."
3. "Teenagers often fail to use birth control because they forget to discuss this with their sexual partner."
4. "Although teenagers can intellectually discuss birth control, they don't believe that they will become pregnant."

41. The mother of a newborn son tells the nurse that she is concerned about a circumcision because of the pain involved. What is the nurse's best response?

1. "A newborn's nerves are not mature enough to feel pain."
2. "It is such a short procedure that the pain will not last long."
3. "Your baby should have no memory of it even if there is pain."
4. "The practitioner will tell you how your baby's pain will be controlled."

42. Since her infant's birth, a woman has breastfed her now 6-month-old infant. The woman becomes hysterical after learning her husband has been seriously injured in an automobile accident. Culturally, this woman believes that emotional stress while breastfeeding can "sour the milk," and she indicates she must wean her infant immediately. What should the nurse do?

1. Instruct the mother about formula feeding
2. Explain to the mother that these beliefs are wrong
3. Provide the mother with books which indicate that the milk does not sour
4. Encourage the mother to take an antianxiety drug while continuing breastfeeding

43. A client in preterm labor does not respond to therapy, and birth seems imminent. The client begins to cry and says, "I'm so worried about my baby." Which is the nurse's best response?

1. "All of this must leave you very confused and frightened."
2. "Think positively; your anxiety will increase your contractions."
3. "You are receiving the best medical and nursing care available."
4. "This hospital has a neonatal unit; it can handle emergencies such as yours."

44. A 28-year-old woman is recovering from her third consecutive spontaneous abortion in 2 years. What is the most therapeutic nursing intervention for this client?

1. Focus on the client's physical needs
2. Encourage the client to verbalize her feelings about the loss
3. Remind the client that she will be able to become pregnant again
4. Encourage the client to think of herself, her husband, and their future

45. After a difficult labor a client gives birth to a 9-pound boy who dies shortly afterward. That evening the client tearfully describes to the nurse her projected image of her son and what his future may have been. What is the nurse's most therapeutic response?

1. "I guess you wanted a son very much."
2. "It must be difficult to think of him now."
3. "I am sure he would have been a wonderful child."
4. "If you dwell on this now your grief will be harder to bear."

46. The nurse is caring for a client who has a newborn with a neurological impairment. What is the most important nursing action?

1. Assisting the client with the grieving process
2. Performing frequent neurologic assessments of the newborn
3. Arranging for social services to discuss possible placement of the newborn
4. Obtaining a prescription for an antidepressant to help the client cope with the depressing news

47. The nurse is obtaining the history of a client in the third trimester who is visiting the prenatal clinic for the first time. She tells the nurse she has two toddlers at home, and their father abandoned the family last month. She adds that she doesn't know what to do. The nurse concludes that the client is:

1. Angry that the father has left
2. Overwhelmed by the situation
3. Ambivalent about her pregnancy
4. Denying the reality of her pregnancy

48. While a client in the prenatal clinic is dressing at the completion of her pelvic examination, she states, "Why must I be pregnant now? It's the wrong time." What is the nurse's most therapeutic response?

1. "This is a typical response to pregnancy."
2. "No time is ever the right time to be pregnant."
3. "You don't seem to be happy about this pregnancy."
4. "There are alternatives if you don't want to be pregnant."

49. A client had a mastectomy because of breast cancer. She is now receiving chemotherapy, which caused hair loss. The client states, "I feel like I have lost my sense of power." What is the nurse's best response?

1. "Hair does not empower a person."
2. "Losing power seems important to you."
3. "Knowledge is power; I will give you some pamphlets to read."
4. "Losing hair is common; it will grow back, so you should not worry."

50. A 49-year-old client is admitted with a diagnosis of cervical cancer. While obtaining her health history she tells the nurse, "I have not had a Pap smear for more than 5 years. I probably wouldn't be in the hospital today if I'd had those tests more often." How should the nurse respond?

1. "Please tell me why you waited so long."
2. "You feel like you've neglected your health."

3. "It's never too late to start taking care of yourself."
4. "Most women hate to have Pap smears done although it's really important."

51. A husband is sitting in the waiting room while his wife is getting her infertility prescription refilled by the clinic pharmacist. As the nurse sits down beside him he blurts out, "It's like there are three of us in bed—my wife, me, and the doctor." What feeling is reflected by this statement?
1. Guilt
2. Anger
3. Depression
4. Unworthiness

REPRODUCTIVE CHOICES

52. A client who is taking an oral contraceptive calls the nurse with concerns about side effects of the medication. Which adverse effect to this medication should alert the nurse to inform the client to immediately stop the contraceptive and contact the practitioner? Select all that apply.
1. _____ Nausea
2. _____ Weight loss
3. _____ Visual disturbances
4. _____ Persistent headaches
5. _____ Decreased blood pressure

53. A nurse is instructing a client who is taking oral contraceptives to increase her intake of dietary supplements. Which supplement should be increased?
1. Calcium
2. Vitamin C
3. Vitamin E
4. Potassium

54. A client who is visiting the family planning clinic has an oral contraceptive prescribed. As part of teaching the nurse plans to inform the client of the possibility of developing:
1. Cervicitis
2. Ovarian cysts
3. Fibrocystic disease
4. Breakthrough bleeding

55. What should a nurse include in the teaching plan for a couple who seek information about family planning?
1. Condoms must be held in place by the rim when withdrawing the penis from the vagina
2. Diaphragms are effective even when the partners choose not to utilize a spermicidal cream
3. When coitus interruptus is used, sperm cannot reach the ovum if the man withdraws before ejaculation
4. When periodic abstinence is used, the woman should have intercourse on days that she has an increase in temperature

56. A 28-year-old woman seeks advice about oral contraceptives from the nurse in her company health office. What should the nurse tell her if she is a smoker?
1. Oral contraceptives can cause thrombophlebitis
2. Oral contraceptives can be used with other methods

3. Some oral contraceptives can be used without concern
4. Some oral contraceptives are safe while others are not safe

57. A nurse at a women's health clinic identifies that client teaching regarding use of an oral contraceptive is understood when the client states, "I:
1. can stop the pill and try to get pregnant right away."
2. may miss two periods and not worry about being pregnant."
3. will put a baby's picture on my bathroom mirror, so I'll see it every morning."
4. am so glad we won't have to use condoms even if I miss just one pill during the month."

58. A nurse is counseling a client with type 1 diabetes who has requested contraceptive information. On which method of contraception should the nurse place the most emphasis?
1. Rhythm
2. Diaphragm
3. Oral contraceptive
4. Intrauterine device

59. A nurse in a family planning clinic determines that a client understands the discussion about using a cervical cap with a spermicide when the client states that after intercourse, a cervical cap must be left in place for at least:
1. 6 hours
2. 5 hours
3. 3 hours
4. 2 hours

60. A couple tells the nurse that they wish to use the rhythm method of birth control. The woman states that she menstruates every 32 days. What should the nurse teach the couple about when her ovulation probably occurs?
1. On the 14th day of the cycle
2. 10 days after the first day of bleeding
3. 14 days before the start of the next menses
4. 2 to 3 days after the last day of menstrual bleeding

61. The school nurse is teaching a group of 16-year-old girls about the female reproductive system. One student asks how long after ovulation it is possible for conception to occur. The nurse's most accurate response is based on the knowledge that an ovum is no longer viable after:
1. 12 hours
2. 24 hours
3. 48 hours
4. 72 hours

62. A client states that she wishes to use the calendar method of birth control. The nurse concludes that the client understands how to calculate the beginning of the fertile period when she states, "I will:
1. Subtract 11 days from the length of my longest cycle."
2. Subtract 18 days from the length of my shortest cycle."

3. Abstain from sexual intercourse after the 10th day of my cycle."

4. Abstain from intercourse from the 10th day prior to the middle of my average cycle."

63. When teaching a client about using a diaphragm as a form of contraception, the nurse should tell her that the diaphragm:
    1. May or may not be used with a spermicidal lubricant
    2. Should remain in place for at least six hours after intercourse
    3. Must be inserted with the dome facing down to be maximally effective
    4. Often appears puckered, but this will not interfere with its being effective

64. While a nurse is discussing methods of contraception with a client during her first visit to the woman's health clinic, the client expresses a desire to postpone her first pregnancy for at least 5 years. Her health history reveals that she currently smokes 1½ packs of cigarettes a day, has never been pregnant, and does not want to use a barrier method of contraception. Which method should the nurse anticipate the practitioner will recommend?
    1. A vaginal ring (NuvaRing)
    2. An intrauterine device (IUD)
    3. MedroxyPROGESTERone (Depo-Provera)
    4. Combined oral contraceptive pills (COCPs)

65. The nurse in a women's health clinic is counseling a 34-year-old client who has requested a prescription for oral contraceptives. The nurse determines that more discussion is necessary if the client's health history reveals:
    1. Anemia
    2. Depression
    3. Hypertension
    4. Dysmenorrhea

66. The nurse assesses a married 35-year-old client who is to undergo a tubal ligation to determine the client's possible emotional response to the procedure. A factor in the history that contributes most to the healthy resolution of any emotional problem associated with sterilization is that the client:
    1. Has a son and daughter and feels her family is complete
    2. Believes that the surgery will relieve her monthly dysmenorrhea
    3. Knows that her husband does not want her to have any more children
    4. Has just had a complicated birth and never wants to undergo another birth again

67. A couple at the prenatal clinic for a first visit tells the nurse that their 2-year-old child has just been diagnosed with cystic fibrosis. They state there is no family history of this disorder. They ask the nurse what the chances are for their having another child with cystic fibrosis. Based on the knowledge that this disorder has an autosomal recessive mode of inheritance, how should the nurse respond?

1. There is a 50% chance that this baby will also be affected
2. If this baby is male, there is a 50% chance of his being affected
3. If this baby is female, there is no chance of her being affected, but she will be a carrier
4. There is a 25% chance the baby will be affected, but a 50% chance that the baby will be a carrier

68. A woman in the family planning clinic has decided to use the diaphragm for contraception. What should the nurse teach her about using a diaphragm?
    1. Completely cover the outside of the diaphragm with spermicidal jelly or cream
    2. Douche within 1 hour after intercourse to enhance the effectiveness of the diaphragm
    3. Correct placement of the diaphragm allows an inch between the diaphragm and the vaginal wall
    4. Insert the diaphragm before intercourse and leave it in at least 6 hours after intercourse to kill all the sperm

69. A couple, married for 5 years, want to start a family. When talking with them the husband says, "Well, I guess we are going to have to jump into bed three or four times a day, every day until it works." What is the nurse's best response?
    1. Tell them to continue intercourse as usual until conception occurs
    2. Instruct them on the frequency and timing of intercourse to promote conception
    3. Discourage this because sperm production decreases with frequent sexual intercourse
    4. Agree that the frequency of intercourse must increase but twice daily is sufficient to promote conception

70. A female client with Hodgkin's disease is to start chemotherapy. She and her husband have been trying to have a child and are quite concerned when they learn that sterility may result. On what information should the nurse base the reply?
    1. Ova can be harvested and frozen for future use
    2. Chemotherapy is not radical enough to destroy ovarian function
    3. Ovarian function will be temporarily destroyed but will return in time
    4. Radiation can be substituted for chemotherapy to preserve ovarian function

71. A 16-year-old girl who has become sexually active asks the nurse, "What is the most effective way to prevent a pregnancy?" Which method of preventing pregnancy should the nurse tell her is most effective?
    1. Using birth control pills
    2. Using spermicidal foam
    3. Abstinence from sexual intercourse
    4. Having an intrauterine device inserted

72. A client asks the nurse what she should do if she forgets to take the pill one day. How should the nurse respond?
    1. "Take your pills as instructed."
    2. "Call your practitioner immediately."

3. "Continue as usual and there should not be a problem."

4. "On the next day take one pill in the morning and one before bedtime."

HEALTHY CHILDBEARING

73. At a client's first visit to the prenatal clinic, the nurse asks the client when she had her last menstrual period so the estimated date of birth (EDB) can be determined. The client responds, "January 21." Using Nägele's rule, what is the month and day of the client's EDB?
    1. October 21
    2. October 28
    3. November 21
    4. November 28

74. A client visiting the prenatal clinic for the first time tells the nurse that she has heard conflicting stories about sex during pregnancy and asks about continuing sexual activity. How should the nurse respond?
    1. "Intercourse should be discontinued after the second trimester."
    2. "This information can be given only by your obstetrician or nurse-midwife."
    3. "With an uncomplicated pregnancy, there are no limitations on sexual activity."
    4. "Sexual activity should be avoided during the first and last six weeks of pregnancy."

75. An active 19-year-old primigravida attends the prenatal clinic for the first time. She asks the nurse if she can continue playing tennis and go horseback riding while she is pregnant. How should the nurse reply?
    1. "Continue your usual activities as long as you are comfortable."
    2. "Horseback riding is acceptable, but only up to the last trimester"
    3. "Tennis is good exercise for you, but horseback riding is too strenuous."
    4. "Both of these sports have been found to be too strenuous for a pregnant woman."

76. At a client's first prenatal visit, the nurse-midwife performs a pelvic examination. The nurse states that the client's cervix is bluish purple, which is known as Chadwick's sign. The client becomes concerned and asks if something is wrong. The nurse replies, "This is expected and it:
    1. helps confirm your pregnancy."
    2. is not unusual even in women who are not pregnant."
    3. occurs because the blood is trapped by the pregnant uterus."
    4. is caused by increased blood flow to the uterus during pregnancy."

77. A client at 7 weeks' gestation tells the nurse in the prenatal clinic that she has been bothered by episodes of nausea, but no vomiting, throughout the day. What should the nurse recommend? Select all that apply.
    1. _____ Focus on and repeat a rhythmic chant
    2. _____ Sit upright for 30 minutes after meals

    3. _____ Take low-sodium antacids after meals
    4. _____ Drink carbonated beverages with meals
    5. _____ Eat small but frequent meals with dry crackers in between

78. A pregnant client is experiencing nausea and vomiting. The nurse determines that this discomfort:
    1. Is present during early pregnancy
    2. Will disappear when lightening occurs
    3. Is a common response to an unwanted pregnancy
    4. May be related to an increased human chorionic gonadotropin level

79. The nurse explains to a pregnant woman that absorption of medications taken orally during pregnancy may be altered as a result of:
    1. Delayed gastrointestinal emptying
    2. A reduced glomerular filtration rate
    3. Developing fetal-placental circulation
    4. Increasing secretion of hydrochloric acid

80. A client at her first visit to the prenatal clinic asks which immunization can be administered safely to a pregnant woman. What should the nurse reply?
    1. Rubella (measles)
    2. Rubeola (German measles)
    3. Inactivated poliovirus (IPV)
    4. Diphtheria, tetanus, pertussis (dTAP)

81. The nurse instructs a pregnant client about the sources of protein that assist in meeting the increased daily requirements during pregnancy. How many grams of protein should she eat each day?
    1. 65 grams
    2. 60 grams
    3. 55 grams
    4. 50 grams

82. A client at 8 weeks' gestation tells the nurse that she does not feel like making love to her husband since becoming pregnant and is concerned that her husband may not understand. What is the nurse's most appropriate response?
    1. "Was this a problem before your pregnancy?"
    2. "Why don't you feel like having intercourse?"
    3. "A decrease in libido is expected during the first trimester of pregnancy."
    4. "I'm sure your husband will understand that this feeling is related to your pregnancy."

83. A client at 10 weeks' gestation tells the nurse in the maternity clinic that she is worried because she is voiding frequently. How should the nurse respond?
    1. Recommend that she inform her practitioner
    2. Explain why this is expected in early pregnancy
    3. Tell the client not to worry because this is expected
    4. Collect the client's urine for a culture and sensitivity test

84. The nurse-midwife palpates the uterus of a client who is at 12 weeks' gestation and determines that it is enlarged and:
    1. Just above the symphysis pubis
    2. Buried deep in the pelvic cavity
    3. Three fingerbreadths above the symphysis pubis
    4. Causing noticeable bulging of the abdominal wall

85. A primigravida complains of morning sickness. What should the nurse plan to teach her?
    1. Increase her fluid intake
    2. Eat three small meals a day
    3. Increase the calcium in her diet
    4. Avoid long periods without food

86. The nurse discusses the recommended weight gain during pregnancy with a newly pregnant client, who is 5 feet, 3 inches tall and weighs 125 pounds, The nurse explains that to achieve the recommended weight gain at term, the client should weigh about:
    1. 150 pounds
    2. 140 pounds
    3. 135 pounds
    4. 130 pounds

87. A primigravida who is in her 7th week of gestation asks the nurse when she can expect to feel her baby move. The nurse replies that quickening usually occurs in the:
    1. 24th week
    2. 20th week
    3. 16th week
    4. 12th week

88. A pregnant client asks the nurse for information about toxoplasmosis during pregnancy. What should the nurse teach the client?
    1. Pork and beef should be thoroughly cooked before eating
    2. Toxoplasmosis is a disease that is most prevalent in foreign countries
    3. Raw shellfish are intermediary hosts and should be avoided during pregnancy
    4. Salad dressings made with mayonnaise should be avoided during the summer months

89. A pregnant client tells the nurse that she thinks she has developed an allergy because her nose is often very congested and she has difficulty breathing. How should the nurse reply?
    1. "It will help if you use a nasal decongestant at least twice a day."
    2. "It is common for women to develop allergies during pregnancy."
    3. "This is not normal; perhaps you have a chronic respiratory infection."
    4. "This is an expected occurrence; the increased hormones are responsible for the congestion."

90. The nurse should explain to the newly pregnant primigravida that the fetal heartbeat will first be heard with:
    1. A fetoscope around 8 weeks
    2. A fetoscope at 12 to 14 weeks
    3. An electronic Doppler after 17 weeks
    4. An electronic Doppler at 10 to 12 weeks

91. A client, who is at 10 weeks' gestation, returns for her second prenatal visit. She asks why she has to urinate so often. The nurse tells her that urinary frequency in the first trimester is:
    1. Caused by the baby's head descending into the uterus

2. Influenced by the enlarging uterus, which is still within the pelvis
3. Because the mother's kidneys filter more waste products excreted by the growing fetus
4. Mostly a psychological phenomenon that results from knowing that the pregnancy has occurred

92. A client at 10 weeks' gestation tells the nurse that she urinates more often now, without discomfort, and would like to know what to do. What does the nurse tell the client to do?
    1. Collect a clean catch specimen for testing
    2. Contact her practitioner as soon as possible
    3. Maintain increased fluid intake during the day
    4. Try to resist the urge to void as long as possible

93. What prenatal teaching is applicable for a client who is between 12 and 24 weeks' gestation?
    1. Infant care, travel to the hospital, and signs of labor
    2. Growth of the fetus, personal hygiene, and nutritional guidance
    3. Interventions for nausea and vomiting, urinary frequency, and anticipated care
    4. Danger signs of preeclampsia, relaxation breathing techniques, and signs of labor

94. A client in her second trimester is at the prenatal clinic for a routine visit. While listening to the fetal heart, the nurse hears a heartbeat at the rate of 136 in the right upper quadrant and also at the midline below the umbilicus. What are the sources of these 2 sounds?
    1. Heart rates of two fetuses
    2. Maternal and fetal heart tones
    3. Funic souffle and fetal heart rate
    4. Maternal heart rate with a uterine souffle

95. At a routine prenatal visit the sign or symptom that a healthy primigravida at 20 weeks' gestation will most likely report for the first time is:
    1. Quickening
    2. Palpitations
    3. Pedal edema
    4. Vaginal spotting

96. A client at 28 weeks' gestation has gained 13 pounds and tells the nurse in the prenatal clinic that she is glad she has not gained as much weight as her sister did during her pregnancy. How should the nurse respond?
    1. "Do you think you are getting fat?"
    2. "Are you trying to watch your figure?"
    3. "You have to eat right during pregnancy."
    4. "Tell me what you have been eating lately."

97. During a routine 32-week prenatal visit, a client tells the nurse that she has had difficulty sleeping on her back at night. What should the nurse advise the client about her position when she sleeps?
    1. Turn from side to side
    2. Try to sleep on her stomach
    3. Elevate the head of the bed on blocks
    4. Place two pillows under her knees while sleeping

98. A primigravida at 34 weeks' gestation tells the nurse that she is beginning to experience some lower back

pain. What should the nurse recommend that the client do? Select all that apply.

1. _____ Wear low-heeled shoes
2. _____ Wear a maternity girdle while awake
3. _____ Sleep flat on her back with her feet elevated
4. _____ Perform pelvic tilt exercises several times a day
5. _____ Take an acetaminophen (Tylenol) tablet at the start of back pain

99. A client at 35 weeks' gestation calls the prenatal clinic concerned that she has "not felt the fetus move as much as usual." The most appropriate recommendation by the nurse is to have the client call the clinic with the results after she has:
1. Drunk a glass of orange juice and timed 10 fetal movements
2. Sat in a tub filled with warm water and then timed 30 fetal movements
3. Walked for 15 minutes and checked if the fetus moved more frequently
4. Taken a nap and counted the number of fetal movements for 20 minutes

100. The nurse discusses fetal weight gain with a pregnant client. When does it usually show a marked increase?
1. During the third trimester
2. During the second trimester
3. At the end of the first trimester
4. At the beginning of the first trimester

101. What should the nurse emphasize in a class about childbirth?
1. Birth as a family experience
2. Labor without using analgesics
3. Education, exercise, and breathing techniques
4. Hydration, relaxation, and pain control during labor

102. A pregnant client, interested in childbirth education, asks how the Lamaze method differs from the Read method. What should the nurse explain about the Lamaze method?
1. It is an easier method to teach and learn
2. It requires extensive prenatal preparation
3. This is a natural approach based on childbirth without pain
4. This avoids the use of pain-relieving medications during labor

103. During a childbirth class the nurse evaluates that the women understand how to use effleurage correctly when they are observed:
1. Rocking gently on their knees
2. Practicing panting to avoid pushing during labor
3. Taking deep breaths before imagined contractions
4. Massaging their abdomens gently with their fingertips

104. Methods of relieving back pain are explained during a childbirth class. What activities identified by the client permit the nurse to conclude that the teaching is understood? Select all that apply.
1. _____ Tailor sitting
2. _____ Pelvic rocking

3. _____ Forward tilting
4. _____ Sacral pressure
5. _____ Kegel exercises

105. The nurse teaches a pregnant client about fetal growth and development. Which statement indicates that the client needs further teaching?
1. "Pregnant women need to drink more milk."
2. "Pregnant women need to eat more protein."
3. "The fetus gets nutrients from the amniotic fluid."
4. "The fetus gets oxygen from blood in the placenta."

106. The nurse is caring for four clients on the postpartum unit. Which client will most likely state that she is having difficulty sleeping because of afterbirth pains?
1. Multipara who has 3 children
2. Primipara whose newborn weighed 7 pounds
3. Primipara with effectively controlled diabetes
4. Multipara whose second child was small for gestational age

107. The nurse is teaching a prenatal breathing and relaxation class. What does the nurse suggest to best ease back discomfort during labor?
1. Clients should alternate lying on the back and side
2. Support persons should use back massage techniques
3. Support persons should use distraction techniques such as abdominal effleurage
4. Clients should assume the knee-chest position before and after assessments of the fetal heart rate

108. A client attending a prenatal class about nutrition tells the nurse that she is a strict vegetarian (vegan). What should the nurse encourage the client to eat that includes all the essential amino acids?
1. Macaroni and cheese
2. Whole grain cereals and nuts
3. Scrambled eggs and buttermilk
4. Brown rice and whole-wheat bread

109. A pregnant client who is a strict vegetarian (vegan) asks the nurse if there is anything special she should do in relation to her diet. What should the nurse recommend?
1. Taking a vitamin supplement daily
2. Eating at least 40 grams of protein a day
3. Drinking at least 1 quart of milk per day
4. Including specific nonanimal proteins in her daily diet

110. The nurse teaches a pregnant client why she needs a folic acid supplement. Which neonatal disorder does this prevent?
1. Phenylketonuria
2. Down syndrome
3. Neural tube defects
4. Erythroblastosis fetalis

111. When discussing dietary needs during pregnancy, a client tells the nurse that milk constipates her at times. What should the nurse teach the client?
1. Substitute a variety of cheeses for the milk
2. Replace fat-free or low-fat milk for whole milk

3. Increase intake of prenatal supplements and omit the milk

4. Treat constipation when it occurs and continue drinking milk

112. The nurse teaches a client about the increased need for vitamin A to meet rapid fetal tissue growth during pregnancy. Which nutrients should the nurse encourage the client to ingest to meet this increased need? Select all that apply.
    1. _____ Carrots
    2. _____ Citrus fruits
    3. _____ Fat-free milk
    4. _____ Sweet potatoes
    5. _____ Extra egg whites

113. The nurse teaches a client in early pregnancy about the need to increase her intake of complete proteins. The nurse asks the client to identify foods that contain these proteins. Which response indicates that she understands the teaching? Select all that apply.
    1. _____ Spinach and broccoli
    2. _____ Milk, eggs, and cheese
    3. _____ Beans, peas, and lentils
    4. _____ Fish, hamburger, and chicken
    5. _____ Whole grain cereals and breads

114. A newly married client visits the women's health clinic because she has not been feeling well. What indicates that the client may be pregnant?
    1. Her menses is a week late
    2. Her urine immunoassay test is positive
    3. She relates that she has urinary frequency
    4. She complains that she has nausea every morning

115. At a routine monthly visit, while assessing a client who is in her 26th week of gestation, the nurse identifies the presence of striae gravidarum. How is this condition described?
    1. Brownish blotches on the face
    2. Purplish discoloration of the cervix
    3. Reddish streaks on the abdomen and breasts
    4. Black line that is seen between the umbilicus and the mons veneris

116. The nurse is caring for a pregnant client who is having an ultrasound examination during the first trimester. Why is a sonogram done during the first trimester?
    1. Estimates fetal age
    2. Detects hydrocephalus
    3. Rules out congenital defects
    4. Approximates fetal linear growth

117. A pregnant client's blood test reveals an elevated alpha-fetoprotein (AFP) level. What condition does the nurse suspect this result indicates?
    1. Cystic fibrosis
    2. Phenylketonuria
    3. Down syndrome
    4. Neural tube defect

118. A 40-year-old primigravida is scheduled to have her first ultrasound scan. What should the nurse's instructions include?

1. Postponing breakfast until after the test
2. Drinking eight glasses of water before the test
3. Emptying the bladder immediately before the test
4. Inserting a suppository after arising on the day of the test

119. How does the nurse know that a client, at 40 weeks' gestation, is experiencing true labor?
    1. Cervical dilation
    2. Membranes rupture
    3. Fetal heart rate decreases
    4. Contractions become more intense

120. The nurse is interpreting the results of a nonstress test (NST) on a client at 41 weeks' gestation. After 20 minutes, which result is suggestive of fetal reactivity?
    1. Absent long-term variability
    2. Above average fetal baseline heart rate of 160
    3. No late decelerations associated with contractions
    4. Two accelerations of 15 beats per minute lasting 15 seconds

121. A client whose membranes have ruptured is admitted to the birthing unit. Her cervix is 3 cm dilated and 50% effaced. The amniotic fluid is clear and the fetal heart rate is stable. What does the nurse anticipate?
    1. Second stage of labor will be prolonged
    2. Delayed effacement will result in a difficult birth
    3. Birth of the fetus will probably occur within a day
    4. Stimulation of labor with an oxytocin infusion will be required

122. A primigravida at 36 weeks' gestation is admitted to the birthing room with ruptured membranes and a cervix that is 2 cm dilated and 75% effaced. What is the priority question the nurse should ask?
    1. "When is your expected date of birth?"
    2. "How have you planned to manage your labor?"
    3. "When was your last meal and what did you eat?"
    4. "How frequent are your contractions and how long do they last?"

123. When a client at 39 weeks' gestation arrives at the birthing suite she says, "I have been having contractions for 3 hours and I think my membranes have ruptured." What will the nurse do to confirm if the membranes have ruptured?
    1. Take the client's temperature
    2. Test the leaking fluid with nitrazine paper
    3. Obtain a clean-catch urine specimen and send it to the laboratory
    4. Place the client in the reverse Trendelenburg position and observe the vagina for leaking fluid

124. During labor the nurse encourages the client to void. The nurse considers that an overdistended urinary bladder during labor can:
    1. Predispose to uterine hemorrhage after birth
    2. Interfere with the assessment of cervical dilation
    3. Prevent the diagnosis of cephalopelvic disproportion
    4. Delay expulsion of the placenta after the birth of the neonate

125. When is the most appropriate time for the nurse to administer an opioid analgesic to a client in active labor?
    1. Between contractions
    2. When a contraction starts
    3. At the peak of a contraction
    4. Just before the end of a contraction

126. A client is admitted to the birthing room in active labor. The nurse determines that the fetus is in the left occiput posterior (LOP) position. At what point can the fetal heart be heard?
    1. a
    2. b
    3. c
    4. d

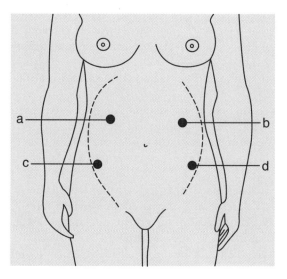

127. A nurse performs Leopold's maneuvers on a newly admitted client in labor. Palpation reveals a soft, firm mass in the fundus; a firm, smooth mass on the mother's left side; several knobs and protrusions on the mother's right side; and a hard, round movable mass in the pubic area with the brow on the right. Based on these findings, the nurse identifies that the fetal position is:
    1. LOA
    2. ROA
    3. LMP
    4. RMP

128. The fetus of a client in labor is in the left occiput posterior (LOP) position. What should the nurse advise the client's partner to do to alleviate some of the discomfort caused by this type of labor?
    1. Encourage the client to sleep whenever possible
    2. Instruct the client to take deeper breaths during contractions
    3. Apply pressure to the client's sacral area during a contraction
    4. Elevate the head of the client's bed to a semi-Fowler position

129. An expectant couple asks the nurse about the cause of low back pain during labor. The nurse replies that this pain occurs most often when the position of the fetus is:
    1. Breech
    2. Transverse
    3. Occiput anterior
    4. Occiput posterior

130. Which position does the nurse teach the client to avoid when experiencing back pain during labor?
    1. Sims position
    2. Supine position
    3. Right lateral position
    4. Left side-lying position

131. A woman at 40 weeks' gestation is having contractions. She is concerned whether she is in true labor. She states, "How will you know if I am really in labor?" What knowledge must the nurse have before responding?
    1. The cervix dilates and effaces in true labor
    2. The bloody show is the first sign of true labor
    3. Membranes rupture at the beginning of true labor
    4. Fetal movements lessen and become weaker in true labor

132. The teaching plan for a father who is acting as a coach during labor should include the information that it is best for him to:
    1. Leave the room periodically so that his wife can rest between contractions
    2. Let his wife know the progress she is making and that she is doing a good job
    3. Keep the conversation in the birthing room to a minimum so that his wife can concentrate
    4. Maintain his wife in the supine position so that fetal and uterine monitoring equipment will not be disturbed

133. The partner of a woman in labor is having difficulty timing the frequency of contractions and asks the nurse to review the procedure. How should the timing of contractions be performed?
    1. End of one contraction to the end of the next contraction
    2. End of one contraction to the beginning of the next contraction
    3. Beginning of one contraction to the end of the next contraction
    4. Beginning of one contraction to the beginning of the next contraction

134. A husband who is coaching his wife during labor demonstrates an understanding of the transition phase of labor when, as his wife starts to push with each contraction, he instructs her to:
    1. Take cleansing breaths before pushing
    2. Take quick, shallow breaths, and then blow
    3. Use slow rhythmic, diaphragmatic breathing
    4. Switch between accelerated and decelerated breathing

135. After a client has been in labor for 6 hours at home, she is admitted to the birthing room. The client is 5 cm

dilated and at −1 station. In the next hour her contractions gradually become irregular but are more uncomfortable. What does the nurse conclude?
1. The client is in false labor
2. The client has a full bladder
3. There is uterine dysfunction
4. There is a breech presentation

136. A client in active labor is admitted to the birthing room. A vaginal examination reveals the cervix is 6 to 7 cm dilated. Based on this finding, the nurse expects the:
1. Client may experience nausea and vomiting
2. Client's bloody show to become more profuse
3. Client will have uncontrollable shaking of her legs
4. Client's contractions to become more frequent and longer in duration

137. As the nurse inspects the perineum of a client who is in active labor, the client suddenly turns pale and says she feels as if she is going to faint even though she is lying flat on her back. What should the nurse do?
1. Turn her onto her left side
2. Elevate the head of the bed
3. Place her feet on several pillows
4. Give her oxygen via a face mask

138. A client in labor is admitted to the birthing room. The nurse's assessment reveals that the fetus is at −1 station. Where is the presenting part?
1. 1 cm above the ischial spines
2. 1 cm below the ischial spines
3. Visible at the vaginal opening
4. At the level of the ischial spines

139. During the assessment of a client in labor, the cervix is determined to be 4 cm dilated. What stage of labor does the nurse record?
1. First
2. Second
3. Prodromal
4. Transitional

140. A vaginal examination reveals that a client's cervix is 90% effaced and 6 cm dilated. The fetus's head is at station 0, and is in an ROA position. The contractions are occurring every 3 to 4 minutes, are lasting 60 seconds, and are of moderate intensity. What should the nurse record about the client's stage of labor?
1. Early first stage of labor
2. Transition stage of labor
3. Beginning second stage labor
4. Midway through first stage of labor

141. A nurse helps a client to the bathroom to void several times during the first stage of labor. This is done because a full bladder:
1. Is often injured during labor
2. May inhibit the progress of labor
3. Jeopardizes the status of the fetus
4. Predisposes the client to urinary infection

142. During labor a client begins to experience dizziness and tingling of her hands. What should the nurse instruct the client to do?

1. Breathe into her cupped hands
2. Pant during the next three contractions
3. Hold her breath with the next contraction
4. Use a fast, deep or shallow breathing pattern

143. A multigravida in active phase of labor states, "I feel all wet. I think I urinated." What should the nurse do first?
1. Give her the bedpan
2. Change the bed linens
3. Inspect her perineal area
4. Auscultate the fetal heart rate

144. A nurse assesses a primigravida who has been in labor for 5 hours. The fetal heart rate tracing is reassuring. Contractions are of mild intensity lasting 30 seconds and are 3 to 5 minutes apart. An oxytocin (Pitocin) infusion is prescribed. What is the priority nursing intervention at this time?
1. Checking cervical dilation every hour
2. Keeping the labor environment dark and quiet
3. Infusing oxytocin by piggybacking into the primary line
4. Positioning the client on the left side throughout the infusion

145. The nurse considers the pros and cons of external fetal monitoring versus internal fetal monitoring. What is one advantage of the external fetal monitor?
1. Simpler to read
2. Allows freedom of movement
3. Assesses the fetal heart rate more accurately
4. Prevents foreign material from entering the uterus

146. The nurse is caring for a client who is in the first stage of labor. The fetal heart rate monitor displays an irregular baseline with variability. What is the priority nursing intervention?
1. Administering oxygen
2. Notifying the practitioner
3. Changing the client's position
4. Continuing to monitor the client

147. During labor a client has an internal fetal monitor applied. The nurse should take action in response to a fetal heart rate that:
1. Remains at 140 beats per minute during contractions
2. Uniformly drops to 120 beats per minute with each contraction
3. Fluctuates from 130 to 140 beats per minute unrelated to contractions
4. Repeatedly drops abruptly to 90 beats per minute unrelated to contractions

148. A client in labor is receiving an oxytocin (Pitocin) infusion. What should the nurse do first when repetitive late decelerations of the fetal heart rate are observed?
1. Administer oxygen
2. Place the client on the left side
3. Discontinue the oxytocin infusion
4. Check the client's blood pressure

149. Although a client in labor is prepared and plans to participate in the labor and birth process, she states that she is in severe discomfort. The nurse administers the

prescribed butorphanol (Stadol). During which phase of labor is the safest time for the nurse to administer this medication?
1. Early phase
2. Active phase
3. Transition phase
4. Expulsion phase

150. A client's membranes rupture and the nurse identifies the presence of a prolapsed umbilical cord. The nurse alerts another nurse, who calls the practitioner. Place the following nursing interventions in the order in which they should be performed.
1. Check the fetal heart rate
2. Administer oxygen by face mask
3. Move the presenting part off the cord
4. Place client in the Trendelenburg position
    Answer: _____

151. A vaginal examination reveals that a client in labor is 7 cm dilated. Soon afterward she becomes nauseated, has the hiccups, and has an increase in bloody show. What phase of labor does the nurse determine the client is entering?
1. Latent phase of labor
2. Active phase of labor
3. Transition phase of labor
4. Early active phase of labor

152. Nursing assessment of a client in labor reveals that she is entering the transition phase of the first stage of labor. Which clinical manifestations support this conclusion?
1. Facial redness and an urge to push
2. Bulging perineum, crowning, and caput
3. Less intense and less frequent contractions
4. Increased bloody show, irritability, and shaking

153. How can the nurse best manage a client's care during the transition phase of labor?
1. Decrease the fluid intake
2. Help the client maintain control
3. Administer the prescribed opioid medication
4. Encourage the client to breathe in simple patterns

154. What is a priority nursing intervention for a laboring client with a sudden prolapse of the umbilical cord protruding from the vagina?
1. Preparing the client for surgery
2. Gently replacing the cord in the vaginal vault
3. Checking the fetal heart rate every 15 minutes
4. Starting oxygen at 10 L per minute via a tight facemask

155. While having contractions every 2 to 3 minutes lasting from 60 to 90 seconds, a client complains of severe rectal pressure. What should the nurse do?
1. Assess for change in the fetal heart rate
2. Inspect the client's perineum for bulging
3. Determine when the client's labor began
4. Verify whether the membranes have ruptured

156. A client in labor states that she feels an urge to push. After a vaginal examination, the nurse determines that the cervix is 7 cm dilated. Which breathing pattern does the nurse encourage the client to use?

1. Expulsion breathing
2. Rhythmic chest breathing
3. Continuous blowing-breathing
4. Accelerated-decelerated breathing

157. A primigravida at term is admitted to the birthing room in active labor. Later, when the client is 8 cm dilated, she tells the nurse that she has the urge to push. The nurse instructs her to pant-blow at this time because pushing can:
1. Prolapse the cord
2. Rupture the uterus
3. Cause cervical edema
4. Lead to a precipitous birth

158. A client's membranes rupture during the transition phase of labor and the amniotic fluid appears pale green. What nursing care should the nurse give the newborn immediately after birth?
1. Stimulate crying
2. Administer oxygen
3. Put a moist saline dressing on the cord stump
4. Provide for suctioning the oropharynx as the head emerges

159. When doing her shallow, rapid breathing during transition, a client in labor experiences tingling and numbness of her fingertips. The nurse encourages her to breathe into:
1. A paper bag
2. An oxygen mask
3. A compressed air mask
4. An incentive spirometer

160. A nurse is caring for a client in the first stage of labor and an external fetal heart monitor is in place. What do the tracings indicate?
1. Fetal tachycardia
2. Early accelerations
3. Variable decelerations
4. Inadequate long-term variability

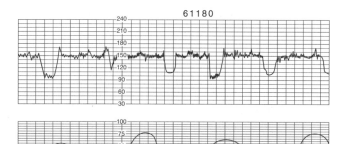

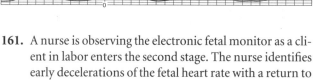

161. A nurse is observing the electronic fetal monitor as a client in labor enters the second stage. The nurse identifies early decelerations of the fetal heart rate with a return to the baseline at the end of each contraction. What does this usually indicate?
1. Maternal diabetes
2. Fetal cord prolapse

3. Maternal hypotension

4. Fetal head compression

162. A local anesthetic is administered to a client as second stage labor begins. What response does the nurse anticipate?

1. Fewer contractions

2. Depressed respirations

3. Decreased blood pressure

4. Accumulated respiratory secretions

163. The cervix of a client in labor is fully dilated and 100% effaced. The fetal head is at +3 station, the fetal heart rate ranges from 140 to 150 beats per minute, and the contractions are 2 minutes apart lasting 60 seconds. What does the nurse expect to observe when inspecting the perineum?

1. Small tears in the perineum

2. Greenish-yellow amniotic fluid

3. Enlarging areas of caput with each contraction

4. Increasing amounts of amniotic fluid with each contraction

164. A pregnant woman arrives in the emergency department crying, "My baby is coming!" The nurse identifies that the fetus's head is crowning and birth is imminent. What should the nurse do to support the baby's head?

1. Apply suprapubic pressure

2. Distribute fingers evenly around the head

3. Place a hand firmly against the mother's perineum

4. Maintain firm pressure against the anterior fontanel

165. A client gives birth to an 8-pound baby. Ten minutes after the birth, the placenta has not yet separated. What is the next nursing intervention?

1. Applying fundal pressure

2. Administering a second dose of oxytocin

3. Continuing to assess the client for signs of separation

4. Preparing a consent form for manual removal of the placenta

166. Five minutes after a birth the nurse-midwife assesses that the client's placenta is separating. What indicates that this is occurring?

1. Uterine fundus relaxes

2. Umbilical cord lengthens

3. Abdominal pain becomes severe

4. Vaginal seepage of blood is continuous

167. One hour after a birth a nurse palpates a client's fundus to determine if involution is taking place. The fundus is firm, in the midline, and two fingerbreadths below the umbilicus. What should the nurse do next?

1. Encourage the client to void

2. Notify the practitioner immediately

3. Massage the uterus and attempt to express clots

4. Continue periodic assessments and record the findings

168. What is the primary outcome for client care in the third stage of labor?

1. Absence of discomfort

2. Firmly contracted uterine fundus

3. Efficient fetal heart beat-to-beat variability

4. Maternal respiratory rate within the expected range

169. A nurse caring for a client who gave birth to a healthy neonate evaluates the client's uterine tone 8 hours later. How does the nurse determine that the uterus is involuting appropriately?

1. Amount of lochia rubra is moderate

2. Numerous clots are passed vaginally

3. Bleeding from the episiotomy has stopped

4. Uterine cramps are absent during breastfeeding

170. After a cesarean birth a nurse performs fundal checks every 15 minutes. During one check the nurse determines that the fundus is soft and boggy. What is the priority nursing action at this time?

1. Elevate the client's legs

2. Massage the client's fundus

3. Increase the client's oxytocin drip rate

4. Examine the client's perineum for bleeding

171. After giving birth, the mother's vital signs are T, 99.3° F (37.4° C); P, 80 regular and strong; R, 16 slow and even; and BP, 148/92 mm Hg. Which vital sign should the nurse monitor more frequently?

1. Pulse

2. Respirations

3. Temperature

4. Blood pressure

172. In the second hour after giving birth a client's uterus is firm, above the level of the umbilicus, and to the right of midline. What is the most appropriate nursing action?

1. Have the client empty her bladder

2. Observe for signs of retained secundines

3. Massage the uterus vigorously to prevent hemorrhage

4. Explain to the client that this is a sign of uterine stabilization

173. The nurse is caring for a group of postpartum clients. What places a client at increased risk for postpartum hemorrhage?

1. Breastfeeding in the birthing room

2. Receiving a pudendal block for the birth

3. Having a third stage of labor that lasts 10 minutes

4. Giving birth to a baby weighing 9 pounds, 8 ounces

174. During the fourth stage of labor, about 1 hour after giving birth, a client begins to shiver uncontrollably. What should the nurse do?

1. Cover the client with blankets to alleviate this typical postpartum sensation

2. Check vital signs because the client may be experiencing hypovolemic shock

3. Monitor the client's blood pressure because shivering may cause it to elevate

4. Obtain an order for increasing the IV fluid infusion to restore the client's fluid reserves

175. A primipara gave birth 12 hours ago. Although an ice bag has been applied to her perineal area, the client continues to complain of rectal pressure causing excruciating pain in the area of the episiotomy. What does the nurse conclude is the cause of the client's pain?

1. Multiple hemorrhoids

2. Low tolerance to pain

3. Hematoma in the perineal area

4. Infection at the episiotomy site

176. What does the nurse anticipate that a primipara with a second-degree laceration and repair is most likely to develop during the postpartum period?
    1. Posterior vaginal varicosities
    2. Difficulty voiding spontaneously
    3. Delayed onset of milk production
    4. Maladaptive bonding with the newborn

177. A nurse teaches a postpartum client how to care for her episiotomy at home. What statement indicates to the nurse that the client understands the priority instruction?
    1. "I should discontinue the sitz baths once I am in my own home."
    2. "I must not climb up or down stairs for at least 3 days after discharge."
    3. "I should continue the sitz baths 3 times a day if it makes me feel better."
    4. "I must continue perineal care after I go to the bathroom until everything is healed."

178. Twelve hours after a spontaneous birth a client's temperature is 100.4° F. What does the nurse suspect caused this temperature elevation?
    1. Mastitis
    2. Dehydration
    3. Puerperal infection
    4. Urinary tract infection

179. Twenty-four hours after an uncomplicated labor and birth a client's CBC reveals a WBC count of 17,000/mm³. How should the nurse interpret this WBC count?
    1. Usual decrease in white blood cells
    2. Expected response to the process of labor
    3. Acute sexually transmitted viral infection
    4. Bacterial infection of the reproductive system

180. A primipara about to be discharged with her newborn asks the nurse many questions regarding infant care. What phase of maternal adjustment does this behavior illustrate?
    1. Let-down
    2. Taking-in
    3. Taking-hold
    4. Early parenting

181. A nurse is giving discharge instructions to a new mother. What is the most important instruction to help prevent postpartum infection?
    1. "Don't take tub baths for at least six weeks."
    2. "Wash your hands before and after changing your sanitary napkins."
    3. "Douche with a dilute antiseptic solution twice a day and continue for a week."
    4. "Tampons are better than sanitary napkins for inhibiting bacteria in the postpartum period."

182. Before discharge, a breastfeeding postpartum client and the nurse discuss methods of birth control. The client asks the nurse, "When will I begin to ovulate again?" How should the nurse respond?

    1. "You should discuss this at your first clinic visit."
    2. "Ovulation will occur after you stop breastfeeding."
    3. "Ovulation may occur before you begin to menstruate."
    4. "I really can't tell you because everyone is so different."

183. On the third postpartum day a nurse is preparing a breastfeeding mother of twins for discharge. Which statement by the client indicates there is a potential problem?
    1. "I've been urinating large amounts ever since I gave birth."
    2. "My lochia is bright red with small brown clots the size of my thumb."
    3. "My breasts feel full, heavy, and tingly before I breastfeed the babies."
    4. "I hope I will stop being so hungry because I don't want to gain weight."

184. The nurse in the postpartum unit is teaching self-care to a group of new mothers. What color does the nurse teach them the lochial discharge will be on the fourth postpartum day?
    1. Dark red
    2. Deep brown
    3. Pinkish brown
    4. Yellowish white

185. A client gives birth to a 7-pound, 2-ounce baby and has decided to breastfeed. What should the nurse tell the client to expect regarding breastfeeding?
    1. Lochial flow will increase
    2. Weight loss will occur rapidly
    3. Involution of her uterus will be delayed
    4. Application of heat to her breasts is contraindicated

186. A new mother who has begun breastfeeding asks for assistance with removing the baby from her breast. What should the nurse teach her?
    1. "Pinch the baby's nostrils gently to help release the nipple."
    2. "Let the baby nurse as long as desired without interruption."
    3. "Pull your nipple out of the baby's mouth when the baby falls asleep."
    4. "Insert your finger in the corner of the baby's mouth to break the suction."

187. A statement by a breastfeeding mother that indicates that the nurse's teaching about stimulating the let-down reflex has been successful is, "I will:
    1. take a cool shower before each feeding."
    2. drink a couple of quarts of fat-free milk a day."
    3. wear a snug-fitting breast binder day and night."
    4. apply warm packs and massage my breasts before each feeding."

188. A client's nipples become sore and tender as a result of her newborn's vigorous sucking. What should the nurse recommend that the mother do to alleviate the soreness? Select all that apply.
    1. _____ Apply ice packs before each feeding
    2. _____ Formula feed the baby for a few days

3. _____ Take the prescribed analgesic medication

4. _____ Expose the nipples to air several times a day

5. _____ Apply hydrogel pads to the nipples after each feeding

189. A client who has been breastfeeding her newborn every 3 hours develops sore nipples. What should the nurse teach her about decreasing nipple soreness?
  1. Using breast shields at each feeding
  2. Washing with mild soap when cleansing the nipples
  3. Changing the baby's breastfeeding position for each feeding
  4. Allowing just the edge of the nipple to be placed in the baby's mouth

190. A new mother wishes to breastfeed her infant and asks the nurse whether she needs to alter her diet. How should the nurse respond?
  1. "Eat as you have been doing during your pregnancy."
  2. "Drink a lot of milk and the added calcium will help you make milk."
  3. "Your body produces the milk your baby needs as a result of the vigorous sucking."
  4. "You'll need greater amounts of the same foods you've been eating and more fluids."

191. A client arrives at the clinic with swollen, tender breasts and flulike symptoms. A diagnosis of mastitis is made. What does the nurse plan to do?
  1. Assist her to wean the infant gradually
  2. Teach her to empty her breasts frequently
  3. Review breastfeeding techniques with her
  4. Send a sample of her milk to the laboratory for testing

192. What should the nurse teach a formula-feeding mother about breast engorgement when it occurs?
  1. Wear a tightly-fitted brassiere
  2. Take two aspirin every 4 hours
  3. Cease drinking milk for 2 weeks
  4. Apply warm compresses to her breasts

193. The nurse is teaching a client, who is formula feeding her infant, how to care for her engorged breasts. The statement that indicates that the client understands the teaching is, "I am:
  1. wearing a well-fitting, tight brassiere."
  2. drinking 10 glasses of liquid every day."
  3. expressing milk from my breasts every 4 hours."
  4. letting warm water run over my breasts when I am showering."

HIGH-RISK PREGNANCY

194. A primigravida with pregestational type 1 diabetes is at her first prenatal visit. When discussing changes in insulin needs during pregnancy and after birth, the nurse explains that based on the client's blood glucose levels, she should expect to increase her insulin dosage. Between which weeks of gestation is this expected to occur?
  1. 10th and 12th weeks of gestation
  2. 18th and 22nd weeks of gestation

  3. 24th and 28th weeks of gestation
  4. 36th and 40th weeks of gestation

195. During her first visit to the prenatal clinic a client tells the nurse that she has a cat and is responsible for changing the cat's litter box. The client asks if doing this will be harmful to her or the fetus. How should the nurse reply?
  1. "Cat litter is not harmful during pregnancy."
  2. "Exposure to cat litter for short periods of time is not harmful."
  3. "There are several factors that determine a person's response to the toxins in cat litter."
  4. "Fetal abnormalities are associated with exposure to cat litter, even after minimal contact."

196. During their first visit to the prenatal clinic, a couple asks the nurse whether the woman should have an amniocentesis for genetic studies. Which factor indicates that an amniocentesis should be performed?
  1. Recent history of drug abuse
  2. Family history of genetic problems
  3. More than 3 prior spontaneous abortions
  4. Older than 30 years of age at time of first pregnancy

197. A client at her first visit to the prenatal clinic states that she has missed three menstrual periods and thinks she is carrying twins because her abdomen is so large. She now has a brownish vaginal discharge. Her blood pressure is elevated, indicating that she may have gestational hypertension. What condition does the nurse suspect the client may have?
  1. Renal failure
  2. Placenta previa
  3. Hydatidiform mole
  4. Abruptio placentae

198. A client with pregestational type 1 diabetes is being counseled on what to expect during her recently confirmed pregnancy. Which statement indicates that the client needs further education?
  1. "I can expect that my baby will be larger than average."
  2. "My blood glucose levels may be lower during my first trimester."
  3. "Additional insulin may be needed in the second half of my pregnancy."
  4. "Drinking more water will decrease my risk of getting a urinary tract infection."

199. A pregnant client who has type 2 diabetes and a history of three miscarriages is scheduled for a contraction stress test. Before the test she begins to cry when answering the nurse's questions about her previous pregnancies. She states, "I know it's my diabetes. This baby will never live. It's all my fault." What is the nurse's best response?
  1. "I understand that this must be very stressful for you."
  2. "Diabetes is a difficult disease to manage during pregnancy."
  3. "This baby will live because it is being very closely monitored."
  4. "I know you're worried, although getting upset can alter test findings."

200. The nurse in the prenatal clinic determines the fundal height of a healthy multipara, at 16 weeks' gestation, to be one fingerbreadth above the umbilicus. What should the nurse do next?
    1. Assess for two distinct fetal heart rates
    2. Ascertain birth weights of her other children
    3. Inform the client that she may be mistaken about her due date
    4. Instruct the client about appropriate weight gain during pregnancy

201. A nurse is teaching a prenatal class about smoking during pregnancy. What neonatal consequence of maternal smoking should the nurse include in the teaching?
    1. Low birthweight
    2. Facial abnormalities
    3. Chronic lung problems
    4. Hyperglycemic reactions

202. A client has a diagnosis of an unruptured tubal pregnancy. Which assessments correlate with this diagnosis? Select all that apply.
    1. _____ Firm, rigid abdomen
    2. _____ Referred shoulder pain
    3. _____ Unilateral abdominal pain
    4. _____ History of a sexually transmitted infection
    5. _____ Ecchymotic blueness around the umbilicus

203. The nurse teaches a client who is to have an amniocentesis that ultrasonography will be performed just before the procedure to determine the:
    1. Gestational age of the fetus
    2. Amount of fluid in the amniotic sac
    3. Position of the fetus and the placenta
    4. Location of the umbilical cord and the placenta

204. A client is to have an amniocentesis at 38 weeks' gestation to determine fetal lung maturity. What lecithin/sphingomyelin ratio (L/S ratio) is adequate for the nurse to conclude that the fetus's lungs are mature enough to sustain extrauterine life?
    1. 2:1
    2. 1:1
    3. 1:4
    4. 3:4

205. What is the priority nursing care after an amniocentesis?
    1. Giving perineal care
    2. Encouraging fluids every hour
    3. Changing the abdominal dressing
    4. Monitoring for signs of uterine contractions

206. The nurse explains to a pregnant client undergoing a nonstress test that the test is a way of evaluating the condition of the fetus by comparing the fetal heart rate with:
    1. Fetal lie
    2. Fetal movement
    3. Maternal blood pressure
    4. Maternal uterine contractions

207. What should be included in the nursing care for a client at 41 weeks' gestation who is to have a contraction stress test (CST)?

    1. Having the client empty her bladder
    2. Placing the client in a supine position
    3. Informing the client about the need for cesarean birth
    4. Preparing the client for insertion of an internal monitor

208. A nurse is caring for a client at 42 weeks' gestation, who is having a contraction stress test (CST). What does a positive test indicate?
    1. Placenta has stopped growing
    2. Fetal lungs have not yet matured
    3. Amniotic fluid is meconium stained
    4. Function of the placenta has diminished

209. Laboratory studies reveal that a pregnant client's blood type is O and she is Rh positive. Problems related to incompatibility may develop in her infant if the infant is:
    1. Rh negative
    2. Type A or B
    3. Born preterm
    4. Type O and Rh positive

210. A 16-year-old primigravida who appears to be at or close to term arrives at the emergency department stating that she is in labor and complaining of pain continuing between contractions. The nurse palpates the abdomen, which is firm with no signs of relaxation. What problem does the nurse conclude the client is experiencing?
    1. Placenta previa
    2. Precipitous birth
    3. Abruptio placentae
    4. Breech presentation

211. A client who is pregnant for the first time and is carrying twins is scheduled for a cesarean birth. What should preoperative teaching include?
    1. Frequent ambulation is begun within 24 hours
    2. Discharge from the hospital occurs in 5 to 7 days
    3. Enemas are required for effective bowel movements
    4. Sponge baths are taken until incisional healing is complete

212. A 40-year-old multigravida's pregnancy is confirmed at 8 weeks' gestation. She states, "I can't wait another 2 months for an amniocentesis to find out whether my baby has a chromosomal anomaly like my first child." The nurse responds that she can have a chorionic villi sampling between the 10th and 12th weeks because if it is performed before this time:
    1. It can cause fetal anomalies
    2. The results are not as accurate
    3. The information it provides is inadequate
    4. It must be done using laparoscopic surgery

213. Which clients are at the highest risk for developing a postpartum infection?
    1. Women who require catheterization after voidings that are less than 75 mL
    2. Women who have lost at least 350 mL of blood during the birthing process

3. Primiparas who have given birth to an infant weighing more than 8.5 pounds
4. Multiparas who have hemoglobin levels of 11 grams at the time of admission

214. A client who is having a difficult labor is diagnosed with cephalopelvic disproportion. Which medical order should the nurse question?
1. Maintain NPO status
2. Start peripheral IV of ¼ NS
3. Record fetal heart tones every 15 minutes
4. Piggyback another 10-unit bag of oxytocin (Pitocin)

215. What is the priority nursing intervention for a client who has just given birth to her fifth child?
1. Palpating her fundus frequently because she is at risk for uterine atony
2. Offering her fluids because multiparas generally lose more fluid during labor
3. Assessing her bladder tone because she is at increased risk for urinary tract infection
4. Performing passive range-of-motion exercises on her extremities because she is at risk for thrombophlebitis

216. The nurse is caring for a group of postpartum clients. Which one should the nurse monitor most closely?
1. Primipara who had an 8-pound newborn
2. Grand multipara who just had her sixth child
3. Primipara who received 50 mcg of IV fentanyl during her labor
4. Multipara whose placenta was expelled 5 minutes after the birth

217. A client had a cesarean birth 4 hours ago. What is the major nursing intervention at this time?
1. Promoting dietary intake
2. Promoting bowel function
3. Relieving gaseous distention
4. Relieving postoperative pain

218. A client who had a cesarean birth is unable to void 3 hours after the removal of an indwelling catheter. How can the nurse evaluate whether the client's bladder is distended?
1. Catheterizing the client for residual urine
2. Palpating the client's suprapubic area gently
3. Determining if the client is experiencing suprapubic pain
4. Asking the client whether she still feels the urge to urinate

219. On her first visit to the prenatal clinic a client with rheumatic heart disease asks the nurse if she will have special nutritional needs. What supplements in addition to the regular pregnancy diet and prenatal vitamin and minerals will she need? Select all that apply.
1. _____ Iron
2. _____ Calcium
3. _____ Folic acid
4. _____ Vitamin C
5. _____ Vitamin B$_{12}$

220. What is the nursing action, during the postpartum period, that has the highest priority for a client with class I heart disease?

1. Promoting early ambulation
2. Observing for signs of cardiac decompensation
3. Assessing the mother's emotional reaction to the birth
4. Instructing the mother about activity levels during the postpartum period

221. A client at 28 weeks' gestation with previously diagnosed mitral valve stenosis is being evaluated in the clinic. Which sign or symptom indicates that the client is experiencing cardiac difficulties?
1. Systolic murmur
2. Heart palpitations
3. Syncope on exertion
4. Displaced apical pulse

222. While a client at 30 weeks' gestation is being examined in the prenatal clinic, the nurse identifies a respiratory rate of 26, blood pressure of 100/60, diaphragmatic tenderness, and a reported increased urinary output. Which finding indicates that the client may be experiencing a complication?
1. Urinary output
2. Blood pressure
3. Respiratory rate
4. Diaphragmatic tenderness

223. A client is diagnosed with placenta previa and asks the nurse what this means. What is the nurse's best response?
1. "It is premature separation of a normally implanted placenta."
2. "The placenta is not implanted securely in place on the uterine wall."
3. "It is premature aging of a placenta that is implanted in the uterine fundus."
4. "The placenta is implanted in the lower uterine segment, covering part or all of the cervical opening."

224. A client with frank vaginal bleeding is admitted to the birthing unit at 30 weeks' gestation. The admission data include BP, 110/70; P, 90; R, 22; FHR, 132; uterus, nontender; contractions, none; membranes, intact. Based on this information, what problem does the nurse suspect this client has?
1. Preterm labor
2. Uterine inertia
3. Placenta previa
4. Abruptio placentae

225. A nurse in the high-risk prenatal unit admits a client at 35 weeks' gestation with a diagnosis of complete placenta previa. What is the most appropriate nursing intervention at this time?
1. Apply a pad to the perineal area
2. Have oxygen available at the bedside
3. Allow bathroom privileges with assistance
4. Educate the client regarding the intensive care nursery

226. A nurse gently performs Leopold's maneuvers on a client with a suspected placenta previa. What does the nurse expect from this assessment?

1. Fetal head is firmly engaged
2. Small fetal parts are difficult to palpate
3. Fetal presenting part is high and floating
4. Uterus is hard and tetanically contracted

227. A client is admitted with a marginal placenta previa. What should the nurse have available?
    1. One unit of freeze-dried plasma
    2. Vitamin K for intramuscular injection
    3. Two units of typed and screened blood
    4. Heparin sodium for intravenous injection

228. A client arrives in the birthing unit from the emergency department with blood running down both legs. What is the primary intervention?
    1. Assessing fetal heart tones
    2. Observing for a prolapsed cord
    3. Starting an intravenous infusion
    4. Inserting a uterine pressure catheter

229. A client who at 24 weeks' gestation is admitted to the high-risk unit with a diagnosis of preeclampsia. She has a seizure. What is the nurse's immediate action?
    1. Turn the client's head to the side
    2. Check the client for an imminent birth
    3. Place an airway into the client's mouth
    4. Observe for bleeding from the client's vagina

230. A pregnant client is admitted with abdominal pain and heavy vaginal bleeding. What is the priority nursing action?
    1. Administering oxygen
    2. Elevating the head of the bed
    3. Drawing blood for a hematocrit
    4. Giving an intramuscular analgesic

231. A nurse is caring for pregnant clients in the high-risk unit. In what disorder is stimulation of labor contraindicated?
    1. Diabetes mellitus
    2. Mild preeclampsia
    3. Total placenta previa
    4. Premature rupture of the membranes

232. A nurse is teaching a pregnant client with sickle cell anemia about the importance of taking supplemental folic acid. Folic acid is important for this client because it:
    1. Lessens sickling of RBCs
    2. Prevents vaso-occlusive crises
    3. Decreases oxygen needs of cells
    4. Compensates for a rapid turnover of RBCs

233. The laboratory blood tests of a client at 10 weeks' gestation reveal that she has anemia. The client refuses iron supplements. The nurse teaches her that the best source of iron is liver. What other foods does the nurse encourage her to eat? Select all that apply.
    1. _____ Tofu
    2. _____ Chicken
    3. _____ Canned ham
    4. _____ Broiled halibut
    5. _____ Ground beef patty

234. A pregnant client with sickle cell anemia visits the clinic each month for a routine examination. What additional assessment should be made at each visit?

1. Signs of hypothyroidism
2. Evidence of pyelonephritis
3. Symptoms of hypoglycemia
4. Presence of hyperemesis gravidarum

235. A client in labor is admitted with a suspected breech presentation. For what occurrence should the nurse be prepared?
    1. Uterine inertia
    2. Prolapsed cord
    3. Imminent birth
    4. Precipitate labor

236. The nurse is caring for a client whose fetus is in a breech presentation. Suddenly the membranes rupture and meconium appears in the vaginal introitus. The nurse realizes that this:
    1. Indicates that the cord will prolapse
    2. Is evidence of fetal heart abnormalities
    3. Is a common occurrence in breech presentations
    4. Requires immediate notification of the practitioner

237. A client in labor is admitted to the birthing unit. Assessment reveals that the fetus is in a footling breech presentation. What should the nurse consider about breech presentations when caring for this client?
    1. Severe back discomfort will occur
    2. Length of labor usually is shortened
    3. Cesarean birth probably will be necessary
    4. Meconium in the amniotic fluid is a sign of fetal hypoxia

238. A client's membranes ruptured 20 hours before admission. She was in labor for 24 hours before giving birth. The nurse plans to monitor her closely. For which postpartum complication is she at highest risk?
    1. Infection
    2. Hemorrhage
    3. Uterine atony
    4. Amniotic fluid embolism

239. A pregnant client has a history of multiple preterm births followed by neonatal deaths. What is the danger sign that the nurse must teach the client to report?
    1. Leg cramps
    2. Pelvic pressure
    3. Nausea after 11 AM
    4. No fetal movement at 12 weeks

240. A multipara whose membranes have ruptured is admitted in early labor. Assessment reveals a breech presentation, cervical dilation at 3 cm, and fetal station at −2. For what complication should the nurse assess when caring for this client?
    1. Vaginal bleeding
    2. Urinary tract infection
    3. Prolapse of the umbilical cord
    4. Meconium in the amniotic fluid

241. A client is admitted to the emergency department at 34 weeks' gestation with trauma and significant bleeding from the leg. What is the priority intervention after determining fetal well-being?
    1. Obtaining the client's vital signs
    2. Offering the client emotional support

3. Placing the client in a left lateral position

4. Drawing the client's blood for laboratory screening

242. When entering the room of a client in active labor to answer the call light, the nurse identifies that the client is ashen gray, is clutching her chest, and is dyspneic. What should the nurse do after pressing the emergency light in the client's room?

1. Administer oxygen by face mask

2. Check for rupture of the membranes

3. Begin cardiopulmonary resuscitation

4. Increase the rate of intravenous fluids

243. A pregnant client with a history of preterm labor is at home on bed rest. What instructions should a teaching plan for this client include?

1. Place blocks under the foot of the bed

2. Sit upright with several pillows behind the back

3. Lie on the side with the head raised on a small pillow

4. Assume the knee-chest position at regular intervals throughout the day

244. A nurse is caring for a client with a history of treatment for preterm labor during this pregnancy. The client now is at 33 weeks' gestation. With regard to sexual intercourse, the nurse should explain that it is:

1. Allowed if penile penetration is not deep

2. Permitted unless there is vaginal discomfort

3. Limited to once a week to decrease contractions

4. Eliminated to prevent stimulation of uterine activity

245. A client who is in the first trimester is being discharged after a week of hospitalization for hyperemesis gravidarum. She is to be maintained at home with rehydration infusion therapy. What is the priority nursing activity for the home health nurse?

1. Determining fetal well-being

2. Monitoring for signs of infection

3. Assessing for signs of electrolyte imbalances

4. Teaching about changes in nutritional needs during pregnancy

246. A client with type 1 diabetes is scheduled for an amniocentesis at 36 weeks' gestation. She asks the nurse why this is done so late in her pregnancy. What should the nurse consider before responding?

1. Fetus's age can be calculated

2. Fetal lung maturity can be evaluated

3. Vaginal birth will be performed if fetal size permits

4. Cesarean birth can be performed before labor begins

247. A nurse is caring for a client with type 1 diabetes on her first postpartum day. What changes in the client's insulin requirements does the nurse expect?

1. Slowly decrease

2. Quickly increase

3. Suddenly decrease

4. Usually remain unchanged

248. What assessment finding should the nurse consider a concern in a client at 35 weeks' gestation?

1. Frequent painless urination

2. Painful intermittent contractions

3. Increased fetal movement after eating

4. Lower back pain that results in insomnia

249. A client who had tocolytic therapy for preterm labor is being discharged. What instructions should the nurse include in the teaching plan?

1. Restrict fluid intake

2. Limit daily activities

3. Monitor urine for protein

4. Avoid deep-breathing exercises

250. A client at 34 weeks' gestation is receiving terbutaline (Brethine) subcutaneously. Her contractions increase to every 5 minutes, and her cervix dilates further to 4 cm. The tocolytic is discontinued. What is the priority nursing care during this time?

1. Promoting maternal-fetal well-being during labor

2. Reducing the anxiety associated with preterm labor

3. Supporting communication between the client and her partner

4. Assisting the client and her partner with the breathing techniques needed as labor progresses

251. A client who is in labor is admitted 30 hours after her membranes ruptured. For what condition does the nurse anticipate that the client is most at risk?

1. Cord prolapse

2. Placenta previa

3. Chorioamnionitis

4. Abruptio placentae

252. The husband of a client in labor asks what the indentation is on his wife's abdomen. The nurse identifies that it is a retraction ring (Bandl's ring). What is the next nursing action?

1. Explain to him what it means and notify the practitioner

2. Advise him that his wife is starting to enter the second stage of labor

3. Inform him that it is a sign that the fetus is descending in the birth canal

4. Tell him that this indentation is expected and reflects the strength of the contractions

253. A client at 35 weeks' gestation is admitted to the birthing unit with a small amount of bright red vaginal bleeding without contractions. What should the nurse do after placing the client in bed?

1. Check fetal heart tones

2. Obtain an amniotomy pack

3. Take the client's vital signs

4. Perform a vaginal examination

254. A client's membranes rupture spontaneously during the latent phase of the first stage of labor, and the fluid is greenish brown. What does the nurse conclude?

1. Infection is present

2. Cesarean birth is necessary

3. Precipitate birth is imminent

4. Fetus may be compromised in utero

255. While a multiparous client is in active labor her membranes rupture spontaneously, and the nurse observes

a loop of umbilical cord protruding from her vagina. What is the priority nursing action?
1. Monitoring the fetal heart rate
2. Covering the cord with a saline dressing
3. Pushing the cord back into the vaginal vault
4. Holding the presenting part away from the cord

256. A pregnant client's history reveals opioid abuse. What is the nurse's initial plan for providing pain relief measures during labor?
   1. Scheduling pain medication at regular intervals
   2. Administering the medication only when the pain is severe
   3. Avoiding the administration of medication unless it is requested
   4. Recognizing that less pain medication will be needed compared with other women in labor

257. What are the signs and symptoms of withdrawal that the nurse identifies in a postpartum client with a history of opioid abuse?
   1. Paranoia and evasiveness
   2. Extreme hunger and thirst
   3. Depression and tearfulness
   4. Irritability and muscle tremors

258. A client in labor, who is 4 cm dilated, is admitted to the birthing room. An electronic fetal monitor is applied. Which assessment should alert the nurse to notify the practitioner?
   1. Contractions every 4 minutes that last 50 seconds
   2. Contractions every minute that last for 120 seconds
   3. Fetal heart rate accelerations at the beginning of a contraction
   4. Fetal heart rate decelerations to 110 BPM before the peak of a contraction

259. A client in the 38th week of gestation develops a slight increase in blood pressure. The practitioner advises her to remain in bed at home in a side-lying position. The client asks why this is important. What is the nurse's response about the advantage of this position?
   1. Increases blood flow to the fetus
   2. Decreases intra-abdominal pressure
   3. Elevates the mean arterial pressure
   4. Prevents the development of thromboses

260. A nurse is caring for a client who is admitted with a tentative diagnosis of placenta previa. What procedure usually confirms this diagnosis?
   1. Laparoscopy
   2. Nonstress test
   3. Amniocentesis
   4. Ultrasound exam

261. A client is admitted to the birthing unit with uterine tenderness and minimal, dark red vaginal bleeding. She has a marginal abruptio placentae. The priority assessment includes fetal status, vital signs, skin color, and urine output. What additional assessment is essential?
   1. Fundal height
   2. Obstetric history
   3. Time of the last meal
   4. Family history of bleeding disorders

262. A pregnant client is diagnosed with gestational hypertension. She tells the nurse that she has been following the recommended pregnancy diet. What should the nurse teach her about her diet at this time?
   1. Limit proteins
   2. Change nothing
   3. Restrict sodium
   4. Increase carbohydrates

263. A client at 36 weeks' gestation arrives at the prenatal clinic for a routine examination. The nurse identifies that the client's blood pressure has increased from 102/60 to 134/88 and is concerned she may be developing mild preeclampsia. What other sign of mild preeclampsia does the nurse anticipate?
   1. Proteinuria of 1+
   2. Mild ankle edema
   3. Episodes of dizziness on arising
   4. Weight gain of 2 pounds in 2 weeks

264. In her 30th week of gestation, a 16-year-old primigravida whose usual blood pressure is 120/70 mm Hg has a blood pressure of 130/88 mm Hg. She is admitted to the birthing unit and says, "I don't know why the doctor is so worried about my blood pressure. According to a book I have, it's normal." The nurse should respond, "Your:
   1. physician is being cautious."
   2. blood pressure is high for your age group."
   3. blood pressure is increased according to pregnancy guidelines."
   4. textbook is for older women who have higher blood pressures."

265. A nonstress test is scheduled for a client with preeclampsia. During the nonstress test the nurse concludes that if nonperiodic accelerations of the fetal heart rate occur with fetal movement, it probably indicates:
   1. Fetal well-being
   2. Fetal head compression
   3. Uteroplacental insufficiency
   4. Umbilical cord compression

266. A nurse admits a client with preeclampsia to the high-risk prenatal unit. What is the next nursing action after the vital signs have been obtained?
   1. Call the practitioner
   2. Check the client's reflexes
   3. Determine the client's blood type
   4. Administer the prescribed intravenous normal saline

267. A client at 36 weeks' gestation is admitted to the high-risk unit because she gained 5 pounds in the previous week and there is a pronounced increase in blood pressure. What is the initial intervention in the client's plan of care?
   1. Preparing for an imminent cesarean birth
   2. Providing a dark, quiet room with minimal stimuli
   3. Initiating intravenous furosemide to promote diuresis
   4. Administering calcium gluconate to lower the blood pressure

268. What should the nurse assess before continuing the administration of IV magnesium sulfate therapy to a client with preeclampsia?
    1. Temperature and respirations
    2. Plantar reflexes and urinary output
    3. Urinary glucose and specific gravity
    4. Level of consciousness and funduscopic appearance

269. A client with preeclampsia is admitted to the labor and birthing suite. Her blood pressure is 130/90 and she has 2+ protein in her urine and edema of the hands and face. For which signs or symptoms should the nurse assess to determine if the client may be developing HELLP syndrome? Select all that apply.
    1. _____ Headache
    2. _____ Constipation
    3. _____ Abdominal pain
    4. _____ Vaginal bleeding
    5. _____ Flulike symptoms

270. A client with severe preeclampsia is admitted to the high-risk unit, and the nurse starts an IV infusion of magnesium sulfate. How is magnesium sulfate classified and what is the mechanism that makes it effective?
    1. Hypotensive that relaxes smooth muscles
    2. Cholinergic that increases the release of acetylcholine
    3. Muscle relaxant that decreases the severity of uterine contractions
    4. Central nervous system depressant that blocks neuromuscular transmissions

271. A nurse on the high-risk unit assesses a client admitted with severe preeclampsia. The client has audible crackles in the lower left lobe, slight blurring of vision in the right eye, generalized facial edema, and epigastric discomfort. Which client adaptation indicates the potential for a seizure?
    1. Audible crackles
    2. Blurring of vision
    3. Epigastric discomfort
    4. Generalized facial edema

272. An infusion of oxytocin is administered to a client for induction of labor. After several minutes the uterine monitor indicates contractions lasting 100 seconds with a frequency of 130 seconds. What is the next nursing action?
    1. Discontinue the infusion
    2. Check the fetal heart rate
    3. Slow the oxytocin flow rate
    4. Turn the client onto her left side

273. An amniotomy is performed to stimulate labor in a client who is at 42 weeks' gestation. Place the nursing care in order of priority.
    1. Check the fetal heart rate tracings.
    2. Evaluate the client for signs of an infection.
    3. Assess the characteristics of the amniotic fluid.
    4. Observe the perineum for umbilical cord prolapse
    Answer: _____

274. A client with a history chof phenylketonuria (PKU), who was maintained on a low-phenylalanine diet until

9 years of age, is pregnant. What is most important for the nurse to discuss with this client?
    1. The infant may be mentally retarded because of her history of PKU
    2. Reinstitution of the low-phenylalanine diet will protect her baby from the disorder
    3. The fetus is not at risk prenatally but will require immediate care at birth to prevent PKU
    4. Phenylalanine should be avoided even when not pregnant so that her body is able to support a pregnancy

275. A nurse provides a list of foods to avoid to a breastfeeding client with phenylketonuria. Which nutrient is in the foods on this list?
    1. Lactose
    2. Glucose
    3. Fatty acids
    4. Amino acids

276. A client at 6 weeks' gestation who has type 1 diabetes is attending the prenatal clinic for the first time. The nurse explains that during the first trimester insulin requirements may decrease because:
    1. Body metabolism is sluggish in the first trimester
    2. Morning sickness may lead to decreased food intake
    3. Fetal requirements of glucose in this period are minimal
    4. Hormones of pregnancy increase the body's need for insulin

277. A nurse who is teaching a prenatal class is asked why infants of mothers with diabetes (IDM) are larger than those who do not have diabetes. On what information about pregnant women with diabetes should the nurse base the response?
    1. Taking exogenous insulin stimulates fetal growth
    2. Consuming more calories covers the insulin secreted by the fetus
    3. Extra circulating glucose causes the fetus to acquire fatty deposits
    4. Fetal weight gain increases due to the common response of maternal overeating

278. A nurse is teaching a pregnant client with type 1 diabetes at her first visit to the clinic how to minimize fetal/neonatal complications. What is the most important action that the client should take?
    1. Exercise daily
    2. Adhere to the prescribed diet
    3. Adhere to the management plan
    4. Keep the scheduled appointments

279. In her 37th week of gestation, a client with type 1 diabetes has an amniocentesis to determine fetal lung maturity. The L/S ratio is 2:1, phosphatidylglycerol is present, and creatinine is 2 mg/dL. What conclusion should the nurse draw from this information?
    1. A cesarean birth will be scheduled
    2. A birth must take place immediately
    3. The fetus need not be monitored any longer
    4. The newborn should be free from respiratory problems

280. A nurse is caring for a group of postpartum clients. Which client is at the highest risk for disseminated intravascular coagulation?
    1. Gravida III with twins
    2. Gravida V with endometriosis
    3. Gravida II who had a 9-pound baby
    4. Gravida I who had an intrauterine fetal death

281. A nurse is assessing a postpartum client for signs of an impending hemorrhage secondary to lacerations of the cervix. What other assessment is important, in addition to monitoring for a firm uterus?
    1. Decrease in pulse rate
    2. Increase in blood pressure
    3. Persistent muscular twitching
    4. Continuous trickling of blood

282. A client at 36 hours' postpartum is being treated with subcutaneous enoxaparin (Lovenox) for left calf deep vein thrombosis. Which client adaptation is of most concern to the nurse who is monitoring the client?
    1. Dyspnea
    2. Pulse rate of 62
    3. Blood pressure of 136/88
    4. Positive left leg Homans' sign

283. A nurse places fetal and uterine monitors on the abdomen of a client in labor. When observing the relationship between the fetal heart rate and uterine contractions, the nurse identifies four late decelerations. What condition is most frequently associated with late decelerations?
    1. Head compression
    2. Maternal hypothyroidism
    3. Uteroplacental insufficiency
    4. Umbilical cord compression

284. A client who has undergone a cesarean birth because of the presence of active genital herpes is transferred to the postpartum unit. Which isolation precautions does the nurse plan to institute?
    1. Enteric
    2. Droplet
    3. Contact
    4. Airborne

285. A client with an abruptio placentae had an emergency cesarean birth. Subsequently the nurse observes that there is bloody urine in the indwelling catheter collection bag. What impending problem does the nurse suspect the client has?
    1. Incisional nick in the bladder
    2. Urinary infection from the catheter
    3. Uterine relaxation with increased lochia
    4. Disseminated intravascular coagulopathy

286. Two hours after giving birth, a client's physical assessment includes BP 86/40; TPR 98/100/22; fundus firm, four fingerbreadths above umbilicus; small spots of lochia rubra on perineal pad; and distended bladder. After a urinary catheterization the client's fundus remains firm and four fingerbreadths above the umbilicus. What should the nurse do next?

    1. Catheterize the client again
    2. Palpate the client's fundus every 2 hours
    3. Notify the client's practitioner immediately
    4. Recheck the client's vital signs in 30 minutes

287. A primigravida at 39 weeks' gestation is admitted to the high-risk unit with an acute infection and is to have labor induced. In what sequence should the nurse implement the practitioner's orders?
    1. Initiate monitoring via an electronic fetal/maternal monitor
    2. Start oxytocin (Pitocin) 30 units in 1000 mL of D_5W per protocol
    3. Call the anesthesia department to evaluate the client for an epidural
    4. Give the client a 2-gram loading dose of ampicillin (Omnipen) followed by 1 gram every 4 hours

    Answer: _____

NORMAL NEONATE

288. A new mother exclaims to the nurse, "My baby looks like a conehead!" How should the nurse respond?
    1. "Are you disappointed in how your baby looks?"
    2. "Don't worry, your baby's head will be round in a few days."
    3. "Is there anyone in your family whose head shape is similar to your baby's?"
    4. "This often happens as the baby's head moves down the birth canal the bones move for easier passage."

289. In specific situations, gloves are used when handling newborns whether they are HIV positive or not. When is it unnecessary for the nurse to wear gloves while caring for newborns?
    1. Offering a feeding
    2. Changing the diaper
    3. Giving an admission bath
    4. Suctioning the nasopharynx

290. At 1 minute after birth the nurse identifies that an infant is crying, has a heart rate of 140, has blue hands and feet, resists the suction catheter, and keeps the legs flexed and the arms extended. What Apgar score should the nurse assign for this infant?
    1. 6
    2. 7
    3. 8
    4. 9

291. Where is the best area for the nurse to assess adequate tissue oxygenation in a neonate born of black parents?
    1. Heels and buttocks
    2. Upper tips of the ears
    3. Nail beds on the hands and feet
    4. Mucous membranes of the mouth

292. Immediately after birth, what is the first nursing intervention for the newborn with a 1 minute Apgar score of 7?
    1. Administer oxygen
    2. Perform a brief physical assessment

3. Dry and place in a warm environment
4. Cut the umbilical cord and attach a clamp

293. When checking a newborn's reflexes, the nurse is unable to elicit one reflex response that is often absent in neonates born vaginally in the breech presentation. How should the nurse attempt to elicit this response?
    1. Move the thumb along the sole of the foot
    2. Stroke the ulnar surface of the hand and fifth finger lightly
    3. Touch the skinfold of the mouth and cheek on the same side
    4. Hold in the upright position while pressing the feet flat on the crib mattress

294. During a newborn assessment a nurse identifies the absence of the red reflex in the eyes. The nurse should:
    1. Notify the practitioner
    2. Rinse the eyes with sterile saline
    3. Expect edema to subside within a few days
    4. Conclude that this is a result of the prescribed eye prophylaxis

295. An assessment of a newborn includes the differentiation between cephalhematoma and caput succedaneum. When making this assessment, the nurse identifies that the newborn with caput succedaneum has scalp edema that:
    1. Becomes ecchymotic
    2. Crosses the suture line
    3. Increases after several hours
    4. Is tender in the surrounding area

296. A nurse identifies a right cephalhematoma on an otherwise healthy 1-day-old newborn. What should the nurse teach the parents at the time of discharge?
    1. How to observe for signs of jaundice
    2. To lower the feedings to every 3 hours
    3. How to assess the fontanels for tenseness
    4. To record the number of wet diapers during the first 24 hours

297. How should the nurse assess a newborn's grasp reflex?
    1. Put direct pressure along the sole of the newborn's foot
    2. Jar the crib and watch the movement of the newborn's hands
    3. Press examining fingers against the palms of the newborn's hands
    4. Hold the body upright and allow the newborn's feet to touch a surface

298. Shortly after birth, the nurse instills erythromycin ophthalmic ointment into the newborn's eyes. The father asks why an antibiotic is needed because the mother does not have an infection. The nurse explains that it is mandatory in the United States because it protects the newborn from developing eye infections. What are these eye infections?
    1. Chlamydia and gonorrhea
    2. Syphilis and toxoplasmosis
    3. Rubella and retrolental fibroplasia
    4. Cytomegalovirus and varicella zoster

299. Two hours after birth a newborn develops an area of soft swelling in the left parietal region. Where should the nurse find the area of involvement?
    1. Over the eyes
    2. Behind the ears
    3. In back of the head
    4. On the top of the skull

300. During the physical assessment of a recently born neonate, the nurse palpates the infant's femoral pulses. For which cardiac defect is the nurse assessing?
    1. Atrial septal defect
    2. Coarctation of the aorta
    3. Patent ductus arteriosus
    4. Ventricular septal defect

301. Immediately after birth, a newborn is dried before being placed in skin-to-skin contact with the mother. What type of heat loss does this intervention prevent?
    1. Radiation
    2. Convection
    3. Conduction
    4. Evaporation

302. What does the nurse do to elicit the Moro reflex during a newborn assessment?
    1. Turns the infant's head quickly to one side
    2. Strokes the infant's back alongside the spine
    3. Jars the infant's bassinet suddenly but gently
    4. Taps the infant's bridge of the nose briskly but lightly

303. Parents of a newborn are concerned about the pinpoint red dots on their infant's face and neck. How should the nurse respond?
    1. They are obstructed sebaceous glands
    2. They are excessive superficial capillaries
    3. The cause is a decreased vitamin K level in the newborn
    4. The cause is an increased intravascular pressure during birth

304. A newborn's total body response to noise or movement is often distressing to the parents. What should the nurse tell the parents this response represents?
    1. A reflex that is expected in the healthy newborn
    2. A reflex that remains for the newborn's first year
    3. An autonomic reflex indicating that the newborn is hungry
    4. An autonomic reflex indicating the newborn's basic insecurity

305. The nurse determines that in the healthy full-term neonate, heat production is accomplished by:
    1. Oxidizing fatty acids
    2. Shivering when chilled
    3. Metabolizing brown fat
    4. Increasing muscular activity

306. A nurse is planning to use a newborn's foot to obtain blood for the required newborn metabolic testing. What part of the foot is the best site to use for the puncture?
    1. Big toe
    2. Foot pad
    3. Inner sole
    4. Outer heel

307. After the birth of her daughter, a mother tells the nurse, "I was told that my baby has to have an injection of vitamin K. She's so small to be getting a shot. Why does she have to have it?" How should the nurse respond?
    1. "Your baby needs the injection to help her develop red blood cells."
    2. "An injection of vitamin K will help prevent your baby from becoming jaundiced."
    3. "Newborns are deficient in vitamin K. This treatment will protect your baby from bleeding."
    4. "A newborn's blood clots extremely rapidly. This injection will help decrease the clotting time."

308. When performing a discharge assessment on a two-day-old neonate, a large amount of meconium is expelled. What does the nurse conclude about this occurrence?
    1. Precursor of newborn diarrhea
    2. Common finding in two-day-old neonate
    3. Pathological condition of the digestive system
    4. Immaturity of the autonomic nervous system

309. The nurse is assessing a newborn for developmental dysplasia of the hip (DDH). Where does the nurse look for extra skinfolds?
    1. Calf muscles
    2. Popliteal area
    3. Back of the thigh
    4. Lower portion of the abdomen

310. A nurse is performing the Ortolani test on a newborn. Which finding indicates a positive result?
    1. Dorsiflexion then fanning
    2. Hypertonia and jitteriness
    3. An arched back and crying
    4. An audible click on abduction

311. What should the nurse discuss with new parents to help them prepare for infant care?
    1. Allowing crying time to help develop the lungs
    2. Establishing a set feeding schedule to promote a steady weight gain
    3. Counting the number of wet diapers daily to determine adequate hydration
    4. Learning specific behaviors involving states of wakefulness to promote positive interactions

312. During the second reactive period a newborn becomes more alert and responsive and there is an increase in mucus production and gagging. What should the nurse do first?
    1. Report this finding
    2. Administer nasal oxygen
    3. Lower the head of the cribette
    4. Remove secretions from the pharynx

313. While inspecting her newborn, a mother asks the nurse if her baby has flat feet. How should the nurse respond?
    1. "Flat feet are more common in children than adults."
    2. "It is difficult to assess because the feet are so small."
    3. "There may be a bone defect that needs further assessment."
    4. "Infants' feet appear flat because the arch is covered with a fat pad."

314. Which does the nurse conclude is related directly to an infant's survival in the neonatal period?
    1. Gestational age and birthweight
    2. Reproductive history of the mother
    3. Parental health habits and social class
    4. Adequacy of the mother's prenatal care

315. A nurse assesses a newborn 1 minute after birth. The body is pink with blue extremities, the heart rate is 122, the legs are withdrawn when the soles are flicked, the respirations are easy with no evidence of distress, and the arms and legs are flexed and vigorously moving. What Apgar score should the nurse document in the newborn's medical record?
    1. 7
    2. 8
    3. 9
    4. 10

316. A newborn weighing 9 pounds, 14 ounces has a cesarean birth because of cephalopelvic disproportion. The Apgar score was 7 at 1 minute and 9 at 5 minutes. What should the nurse do after the initial physical assessment?
    1. Administer oxygen by hood
    2. Determine the blood glucose level
    3. Pass a gavage tube for a formula feeding
    4. Transfer the newborn to the neonatal intensive care unit

317. A 1-day-old newborn has just had a thick, greenish-black stool. The nurse determines that this is the first stool. What should the nurse do next?
    1. Document the stool in the infant's record
    2. Assess the infant for an intestinal obstruction
    3. Send the stool to the laboratory as per protocol
    4. Notify the practitioner that a tarry stool has been passed

318. A client gives birth to a full-term male with an 8/9 Apgar score. What should the immediate nursing care of this newborn include?
    1. Identifying the infant, assessing respirations, and keeping him warm
    2. Applying an antibiotic to the eyes, administering vitamin K, and bathing him
    3. Aspirating the oropharynx, rushing him to the nursery, and stimulating him often
    4. Weighing him, placing him in a crib, and waiting until the mother is ready to hold him

319. A client gives birth to a full-term newborn with an 8/9 Apgar score. List the initial nursing care in order of their priority?
    1. Place in heated crib
    2. Perform physical assessment
    3. Apply identification band to mother and infant
    4. Instill antibiotic prophylaxis and administer vitamin K
    Answer: _____

320. On her first postpartum day, a client asks the nurse if her baby had a test for phenylketonuria (PKU) yet. How should the nurse reply?

1. "The test will not be done until your baby reaches 10 pounds."
2. "The test will not be done today because newborns have sluggish circulation."
3. "The test will not be done until your baby has had enough milk for the results to be accurate."
4. "The test will not be done today because a newborn's liver does not produce enough enzymes before 7 days."

321. A newborn who has remained in the hospital because the mother had a cesarean birth is to be tested for phenylketonuria (PKU) on the morning of discharge. What should the nurse explain to the mother about the purpose of PKU testing?
    1. Tests for thyroid deficiency
    2. Detects possible retardation
    3. Measures protein metabolism
    4. Identifies chromosomal damage

322. On the second day of life, minutes after drinking 2½ ounces of formula, a newborn regurgitates about half an ounce. The mother states, "My baby spits up after every feeding." What should the nurse do next?
    1. Reassure the mother that many babies spit up some milk at first
    2. Suggest that she hold her baby upright for 30 minutes after feeding
    3. Feed a small amount of fresh formula when the baby returns to the nursery
    4. Teach the mother how to prop the baby in an infant seat for 1 hour after feeding

323. A newborn male is circumcised. What post-circumcision plan of care for her son alerts the nurse that the mother requires additional teaching?
    1. There will be frequent diaper changes
    2. Practitioner will be called if there is excessive bleeding
    3. Tub bath will be given starting on the day after the circumcision
    4. Petrolatum gauze will be applied to the penis with each diaper change

324. A newborn male is being discharged 4 hours after having had a circumcision. What should the nurse instruct the mother to do?
    1. Apply the diaper loosely for several days
    2. Give a crushed baby aspirin if there is irritability
    3. Check for bleeding every two hours during the first day home
    4. Call the practitioner if there is whitish exudate around the glans

325. A new mother asks the nurse why her baby seems to have a bowel movement after every feeding. When preparing a response to explain why this is an expected occurrence the nurse determines that it indicates an adequate:
    1. Fluid intake
    2. Cardiac sphincter
    3. Pancreatic amylase level
    4. Gastrocolic reflex response

326. Phenylketonuria (PKU) testing is performed on a newborn. The nurse plans to explain to the mother the purpose of this screening test. What does this test determine?
    1. If the infant is positive for PKU
    2. If the mother is a carrier for PKU
    3. The risk for the mother developing PKU later
    4. The risk for the infant developing PKU when older

327. When changing her newborn's diaper a new mother notes a reddened area on the infant's buttock and reports it to the nurse. What should the nurse do next?
    1. Have nursery staff members change the infant's diaper
    2. Use both lotion and powder to protect the involved area
    3. Request that the practitioner prescribe a topical ointment
    4. Encourage the mother to cleanse the area and change the diaper more often

328. A newborn develops jaundice 72 hours after birth. What should the nurse explain to the parents is the probable cause of the jaundice?
    1. An allergic response to the feedings
    2. The physiologic destruction of fetal red blood cells
    3. A temporary bile duct obstruction commonly found in newborns
    4. The seepage of maternal Rh-negative blood into the neonate's bloodstream

329. A community health nurse visits an infant who was born at home 24 hours ago. When assessing the infant the nurse identifies slight jaundice of the face and trunk. What should the nurse do next?
    1. Plan for immediate admission to the hospital
    2. Obtain a practitioner's order for a bilirubin level
    3. Document this expected finding in the infant's record
    4. Arrange for the infant to have phototherapy in the home

330. At a male newborn's first encounter with his mother the nurse encourages her to undress him. The mother strokes him with her whole hand and while looking at him intently says, "He feels so velvety, and he is going to be just as good looking as his daddy." The baby is alert and responsive while gazing at his mother. What is the nurse's assessment of this first mother-infant encounter?
    1. Early parenting behavior
    2. Neonatal attachment behavior
    3. Newborn consummatory behavior
    4. Overprotective parenting behavior

331. What should the nurse do to help parents proceed with bonding behaviors immediately after birth?
    1. Assess for typical parenting techniques
    2. Demonstrate desired behaviors to the parents
    3. Postpone foot printing the newborn until later in the day
    4. Delay administering the antibiotic to the newborn's eyes

332. After her baby's birth a client wishes to begin breast-feeding. How can the nurse assist the client at this time?
    1. Give the infant a bottle first to evaluate the sucking reflex
    2. Position the infant to grasp the nipple to express colostrum
    3. Leave the infant and parents alone to promote attachment behaviors
    4. Touch the infant's cheek adjacent to the nipple to elicit the rooting reflex

333. The nurse is helping a mother breastfeed her newborn. What is the best indication that the newborn has achieved an effective attachment to the breast?
    1. Tongue is securely on top of the nipple
    2. Mouth covers most of the areolar surface
    3. Loud sucking sounds are heard during the 15 minutes spent at each breast
    4. Vigorous sucking occurs for 5 minutes spent at each breast before falling asleep

334. The nurse assures a breastfeeding mother that one way she will know that her infant is getting an adequate supply of breast milk is if the infant gains weight. What behavior does the infant exhibit if an adequate amount of milk is being ingested?
    1. Has several firm stools daily
    2. Voids six or more times a day
    3. Spits out a pacifier when offered
    4. Awakens to feed about every four hours

335. A mother is breastfeeding her newborn. She asks when she can switch the baby to a cup. The nurse concludes that the mother understands the teaching about feeding when she says she will start to introduce a cup after the baby reaches:
    1. 4 months
    2. 6 months
    3. 12 months
    4. 16 months

336. A mother who is formula feeding her 1-month-old infant asks the nurse whether any vitamin or mineral supplements are required. The nurse bases the reply on the knowledge that infants who are fed with ready-to-use formula do require a supplement. What supplement is required?
    1. Iron
    2. Fluoride
    3. Vitamin K
    4. Vitamin B$_{12}$

337. A nurse teaches a new mother about neonatal weight loss in the first 3 days of life. What does the nurse explain is the cause of this weight loss?
    1. An allergy to formula
    2. A hypoglycemic response
    3. Ineffective feeding techniques
    4. Excretion of accumulated excess fluids

338. What should the nurse recommend to a new mother when teaching her about the care of the umbilical cord area?

1. Remove the cord clamp only after the cord stump has separated
2. Leave the area untouched or clean with soap and water then pat dry
3. Smooth ointment or baby lotion around the cord after the sponge bath
4. Wrap an elastic bandage snugly around the waist area over the cord site

339. On admission to the nursery a newborn is observed experiencing cold stress. What is the nurse's goal at this time?
    1. Minimize shivering
    2. Prevent hyperglycemia
    3. Limit oxygen consumption
    4. Prevent metabolism of fat stores

HIGH-RISK NEONATE

340. A mother asks the neonatal nurse why her infant must be monitored for hypoglycemia when her type 1 diabetes was in excellent control during her pregnancy. How should the nurse respond?
    1. "Newborns' glucose levels drop after birth so we are especially cautious with your baby because of your diabetes."
    2. "Newborns' pancreases produce increased amounts of insulin during the first day of birth so we are checking to see if hypoglycemia has occurred."
    3. "Babies of mothers with diabetes do not have a large supply of glucose stores at birth, so it is difficult for them to maintain their blood glucose levels within an acceptable range."
    4. "Babies of mothers with diabetes have a higher than average insulin level because of the excess glucose received from their mothers during pregnancy, so their glucose level may drop."

341. In her 36th week of gestation, a client with type 1 diabetes has a 9-pound, 10-ounce infant by cesarean birth. For which condition should the nurse monitor when caring for this infant of a diabetic mother (IDM)?
    1. Meconium ileus
    2. Physiologic jaundice
    3. Respiratory distress syndrome
    4. Increased intracranial pressure

342. A client at 24 weeks' gestation is admitted in early labor. What should the nurse consider regarding this client's problem?
    1. If contractions are regular, labor cannot be stopped effectively
    2. Birth at this gestational age usually results in a severely compromised neonate
    3. Attempts will be made to sustain the pregnancy for 2 or 3 more weeks to ensure neonatal survival
    4. Infants born at 30 to 34 weeks' gestation have a low morbidity rate because of advances in neonatal health care

343. A male born at 28 weeks' gestation weighs 2 pounds, 12 ounces. What does the nurse expect to observe when performing an assessment?
    1. Staring eyes
    2. Absence of lanugo
    3. Descended testicles
    4. Transparent red skin

344. A nurse is assessing a newborn of 33 weeks' gestation. Which sign alerts the nurse to notify the practitioner?
    1. Flaring nares
    2. Acrocyanosis
    3. Heartbeat of 140 per minute
    4. Respirations of 40 per minute

345. A client expresses a desire to breastfeed her preterm infant who is in the neonatal intensive care unit (NICU). How should the nurse respond?
    1. Tell the client that this is not possible because the infant will be fed by gavage
    2. Discourage the client because of the time and effort it will take to pump her breasts
    3. Support the client's decision and explain that her infant may be unable to finish breastfeeding because of exhaustion
    4. Explain to the client that breast milk is inadequate for a preterm infant because it does not contain all the necessary nutrients

346. A nurse assesses that a newborn is in respiratory distress. Which signs confirm this assessment? Select all that apply.
    1. _____ Crackles
    2. _____ Cyanosis
    3. _____ Wheezing
    4. _____ Tachypnea
    5. _____ Retractions

347. A neonate at 34 weeks' gestation is admitted to the neonatal intensive care unit. The nurse reviews the medical record and obtains the neonate's vital signs. What objective should the nurse designate as the priority?
    1. Oxygenation will remain adequate
    2. Weight will increase by 30 grams per day
    3. Body temperature will increase to 98.6° F
    4. Heart rate will recover to an acceptable range

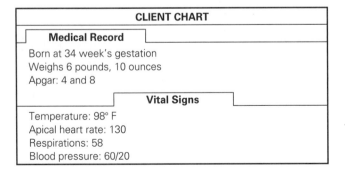

CLIENT CHART

Medical Record

Born at 34 week's gestation
Weighs 6 pounds, 10 ounces
Apgar: 4 and 8

Vital Signs

Temperature: 98° F
Apical heart rate: 130
Respirations: 58
Blood pressure: 60/20

348. Respiratory acidosis is confirmed in a neonate with respiratory distress syndrome when the nurse identifies that the laboratory report reveals:
    1. A pH of 7.35
    2. A potassium level of 4.6 mEq/L
    3. An increased $Paco_2$ of 55 mm Hg
    4. An arterial O_2 pressure of 80 mm Hg

349. A nurse is assessing a newborn. Which sign should the nurse report?
    1. Temperature of 97.7° F
    2. Pale pink, rust-colored stain in the diaper
    3. Heart rate that decreases to 115 beats per minute
    4. Breathing pattern with recurrent sternal retractions

350. A preterm newborn is given oxygen via hood. What should the plan of care include for this neonate?
    1. Ensuring that the oxygen is continuously warmed and humidified
    2. Assessing that the infant's skin and mucous membranes remain bright pink
    3. Monitoring the oxygen level in the hood every 4 hours and oxygen saturation continuously
    4. Informing the parents that oxygen will be given at 4 L per minute and therefore blindness is not a risk

351. Phototherapy is ordered for a preterm neonate with hyperbilirubinemia. Which nursing intervention is appropriate to reduce the potentially harmful side effect of the phototherapy?
    1. Covering the trunk to prevent hypothermia
    2. Using shields on the eyes to protect them from the light
    3. Massaging vitamin E oil on the skin to minimize drying
    4. Turning after each feeding to reduce exposure of each surface area

352. What should be included in the teaching plan for a mother of a newborn with exstrophy of the bladder?
    1. Maintaining sterility of the exposed bladder
    2. Measuring output from the exposed bladder
    3. Protecting the skin surrounding the exposed bladder
    4. Applying a pressure dressing to the exposed bladder

353. What is an appropriate nursing intervention for a neonate with respiratory distress syndrome (RDS)?
    1. Avoid handling to conserve energy
    2. Position to promote respiratory efforts
    3. Assess for congenital birth defects to enable early treatment
    4. Set incubator ten degrees below body temperature to prevent shivering

354. Why is it important for the nurse to know the infant's gestational age and how it compares with the birthweight?
    1. Potential problems may be identified
    2. Infants lose weight during the first few days of life
    3. Infant's weight must be included on the admission record
    4. Health insurance companies need this information for evaluating benefits

355. After an emergency cesarean birth, a neonate born at 35 weeks' gestation is admitted to the neonatal intensive care unit (NICU). The neonate has a

Silverman-Anderson score of 6. What nursing intervention is needed?
1. Monitoring cardiac status
2. Assessing neurological reflexes
3. Ensuring increased caloric intake and fluids
4. Administering respiratory support and observation

356. A client has a cesarean birth. The nurse monitors the newborn's respirations because infants experiencing a cesarean birth are more prone to atelectasis. Why does this occur?
1. The rib cage is not compressed, then released during birth
2. The sudden change in temperature at birth causes aspiration
3. There is usually oxygen deprivation following a cesarean birth
4. There is no gravity during the birth that promotes drainage from the lungs

357. What characteristic does the nurse anticipate in an infant born at 32 weeks' gestation?
1. Ear pinnae spring back when folded
2. Palms and soles have definite creases
3. Areolae and nipples are barely visible
4. Square window sign shows a zero-degree angle

358. When assessing a newborn the nurse observes the following findings: arms and legs slightly flexed; skin smooth and transparent; abundant lanugo on the back; slow recoil of pinnae; and few sole creases. What complication does the nurse anticipate based on these findings?
1. Polycythemia
2. Hyperglycemia
3. Postmaturity syndrome
4. Respiratory distress syndrome

359. A client with chronic hypertension and superimposed preeclampsia gives birth, at 39 weeks' gestation, to a 4-pound, 12-ounce infant. What condition does the nurse anticipate when assessing this infant?
1. Prematurity
2. Cardiac anomalies
3. Respiratory infection
4. Intrauterine growth restriction

360. A neonate born at 39 weeks' gestation is small for gestational age (SGA). What commonly occurring problem should the nurse anticipate when planning care for this infant?
1. Anemia
2. Hypoglycemia
3. Protein deficiency
4. Calcium deficiency

361. A small-for-gestational-age (SGA) newborn has just been admitted to the nursery. Nursing assessment reveals a high-pitched cry, jitteriness, and irregular respirations. With what condition are these signs associated?
1. Hypervolemia
2. Hypoglycemia

3. Hypercalcemia
4. Hypothyroidism

362. Which sign indicates to the nurse that a neonate is preterm?
1. Flexion of extremities
2. Absent femoral pulses
3. Positive Babinski reflex
4. Numerous superficial veins

363. What should cause the nurse to suspect that a preterm neonate who is receiving gastric feedings may have necrotizing enterocolitis (NEC)?
1. Large amounts of residual formula
2. Increased number of explosive stools
3. Several severe bouts of projectile vomiting
4. Circumoral pallor during the feeding process

364. What does the nursing care for an infant with necrotizing enterocolitis (NEC) include?
1. Diluting the formula mixture
2. Measuring abdominal girth every 2 hours
3. Giving half-strength formula by gavage feeding
4. Administering oxygen 10 minutes before each feeding

365. During the assessment of a preterm neonate the nurse determines that the infant is experiencing hypothermia. What should the nurse do?
1. Rewarm gradually
2. Notify the practitioner
3. Assess for hyperglycemia
4. Record skin temperature hourly

366. What should the nurse do when an apnea monitor sounds an alarm 10 seconds after cessation of respirations?
1. Assess for changes in skin color
2. Use tactile stimuli on the chest or extremities
3. Check the monitor for signs of a malfunction
4. Resuscitate with a face mask and an Ambu bag

367. What characteristic should the nurse identify in a preterm neonate that may be a potential nutrition problem?
1. Inadequate sucking reflex
2. Diminished metabolic rate
3. Rapid digestion of formula
4. Increased absorption of nutrients

368. A nurse is caring for a preterm infant who is receiving oxygen therapy. What should the nurse do in an attempt to prevent retinopathy of prematurity (ROP)?
1. Covering the neonate's eyes with a shield
2. Placing the neonate in an elevated side-lying position
3. Assessing the neonate every hour with a pulse oximeter
4. Supporting the neonate's respirations while providing minimal oxygenation

369. A nurse instills an antibiotic ophthalmic ointment into a newborn's eyes. What condition does this medication prevent?
1. Herpetic ophthalmia
2. Retrolental fibroplasia

3. Ophthalmia neonatorum

4. Hemorrhagic conjunctivitis

370. The parents of a preterm infant are preparing to take their baby home. What should the nurse do to evaluate the parents' competency in infant care?

1. Ask the parents what they plan to do at home

2. Determine rationales behind the parents' actions

3. Observe the parents while they are giving care to their infant

4. Demonstrate care before having the parents give a return demonstration

371. What does the nurse expect the size of a newborn to be if the mother had inadequately controlled type 1 diabetes during her pregnancy?

1. Average for gestational age, term

2. Small for gestational age, preterm

3. Large for gestational age, postterm

4. Large for gestational age, near term

372. A nurse who is monitoring the blood glucose levels of an infant of a diabetic mother (IDM) identifies a blood glucose level of 48 mg/dL. What should the nurse do?

1. Check the cord serum glucose level

2. Initiate oral feedings of 10% dextrose in water

3. Secure an order for an IV infusion of 50% dextrose

4. Continue to monitor the blood glucose for another day

373. A newborn's birth was prolonged because the shoulders were very wide. With which reflex does the nurse anticipate a problem?

1. Moro

2. Plantar

3. Babinski

4. Stepping

374. What characteristic does the nurse expect in a newborn of a mother with diabetes?

1. Irritability

2. Flushed skin

3. Hyperreflexivity

4. High-pitched cry

375. A newborn whose mother has type 1 diabetes is receiving a continuous infusion of fluids with glucose. What should the nurse do when preparing to discontinue the IV?

1. Decrease the rate slowly

2. Monitor for metabolic alkalosis

3. Withhold oral feedings for 4 to 6 hours

4. Check for elevated blood glucose levels every 1 to 2 hours

376. A client had a rubella infection (German measles) during the fourth month of pregnancy. At the time of the infant's birth, the nurse places the newborn in the isolation nursery. What type of infection control precautions should the nurse institute?

1. Enteric

2. Contact

3. Droplet

4. Standard

377. A nurse is caring for a preterm neonate with physiological jaundice who requires phototherapy. What is the action of this therapy?

1. Stimulates the liver to dispose of the bilirubin

2. Breaks down the bilirubin into a conjugated form

3. Facilitates the excretion of bilirubin by activating vitamin K

4. Dissolves the bilirubin, allowing it to be excreted by the skin

378. A newborn is being treated with phototherapy for hyperbilirubinemia. What is the nurse's role when providing phototherapy?

1. Turning the infant every 2 hours

2. Placing a diaper over the naked infant

3. Maintaining the infant on daily 24-hour phototherapy

4. Applying a sterile gauze pad on the infant's umbilical stump

379. When doing a newborn assessment of a male infant after a scheduled cesarean birth, the nurse identifies that the infant's head circumference is 4 cm smaller than his chest. What does this finding indicate?

1. Expected in male newborns

2. Predicted after cesarean birth

3. Larger than average chest size

4. Smaller than average head size

380. A nurse in the newborn nursery is monitoring an infant for jaundice related to ABO incompatibility. What blood type does the mother usually have to cause this incompatibility?

1. A

2. B

3. O

4. AB

381. A nurse takes into consideration that the effect PKU has on the infant's development will depend on:

1. Blood phenylalanine levels in utero

2. Excessive levels of epinephrine at birth

3. Diagnosis within the first 2 days after birth

4. Adherence to a corrective diet instituted early

382. A nurse is caring for a 3-week-old infant who was admitted with untreated phenylketonuria (PKU). How should the nurse document the odor of the infant's urine?

1. Fishy

2. Ammoniacal

3. Mousy or musty

4. Aromatic or pungent

383. A nurse assesses a newborn and observes central cyanosis. What type of congenital heart defect usually causes central cyanosis?

1. Shunting of blood from right to left

2. Shunting of blood from left to right

3. Obstruction of blood flow from the left side of the heart

4. Obstruction of blood flow between left and right sides of the heart

384. A new mother's laboratory results indicate the presence of cocaine and alcohol. Which craniofacial characteristic

indicates to the nurse that the newborn has fetal alcohol syndrome (FAS)? Select all that apply.
1. _____ Thin upper lip
2. _____ Wide-open eyes
3. _____ Small upturned nose
4. _____ Larger than average head
5. _____ Smooth vertical ridge in the upper lip

385. Twelve hours after birth, a nurse observes that the neonate is hyperactive and jittery, sneezes frequently, has a high-pitched cry, and is having difficulty sucking. Further assessment reveals increased deep tendon reflexes and a decreased Moro reflex. What problem does the nurse suspect?
    1. Cerebral palsy
    2. Neonatal syphilis
    3. Fetal alcohol syndrome
    4. Opioid drug withdrawal

386. A male newborn has been exposed to HIV in utero. Which finding supports the diagnosis of HIV infection in the newborn?
    1. Delay in temperature regulation
    2. Continued bleeding after circumcision
    3. Hypoglycemia within the first day of birth
    4. Thrush that does not respond readily to treatment

387. A nurse in the newborn nursery receives a call from the emergency department that a woman with active herpes virus lesions gave birth in a taxicab while coming to the hospital. What does the nurse, who is planning care, consider about the transmission of the herpes virus?
    1. Contact precautions are necessary
    2. It occurs during sexual intercourse
    3. It can be acquired during a vaginal birth
    4. Protection is provided via maternal immunity

388. An infant had surgery for repair of a myelomeningocele. For which early sign of impending hydrocephalus should the nurse monitor the infant?
    1. Frequent crying
    2. Bulging fontanels
    3. Change in vital signs
    4. Difficulty with feeding

389. A newborn with a myelomeningocele is transferred immediately from the birthing room to the neonatal intensive care unit (NICU). What is the first nursing intervention?
    1. Assess for paralysis
    2. Start antibiotic prophylaxis
    3. Provide routine newborn care
    4. Apply a sterile saline dressing

390. A newborn is diagnosed with a diaphragmatic hernia. What is the immediate nursing intervention after the neonate is admitted to the neonatal intensive care unit (NICU)?
    1. Hydrating the infant with isotonic enemas
    2. Limiting formula feedings to small amounts
    3. Placing the infant in the Trendelenburg position
    4. Providing gastric decompression via nasogastric tube

391. A client in labor, who is at term, is admitted to the birthing room. The fetus is in the left occiput posterior (LOP) position. Her membranes rupture spontaneously. What observation requires the nurse to notify the practitioner immediately?
    1. Greenish amniotic fluid
    2. Shortened intervals between contractions
    3. Clear amniotic fluid with specks of mucus
    4. Decreased fetal heart rate at the beginning of contractions

392. The mother of a newborn with exstrophy of the bladder tells the nurse that the doctor said her child may develop an unusual gait when learning to walk. What does the nurse tell the mother is the cause of waddling gait?
    1. Genu varum
    2. Tibial torsion
    3. Subluxation of the femur
    4. Separation of the pubic bones

393. A newborn male is admitted to the nursery. He weighs 10 pounds, 2 ounces, which is 2 pounds more than the birth weight of any of his siblings. What should the nurse do in relation to the baby's weight?
    1. Document the findings
    2. Place him in a heated crib
    3. Delay starting oral feedings
    4. Perform serial glucose readings

394. A preterm newborn appears to have a strong sucking reflex. How should the nurse plan to feed the infant to prevent respiratory embarrassment?
    1. Via a nasogastric feeding tube
    2. Every 4 to 6 hours with a special nipple
    3. Every 2 to 3 hours with diluted formula
    4. With small amounts of formula at each feeding

395. A client at 43 weeks' gestation has just given birth to an infant with typical postmaturity characteristics. Which postmature signs does the nurse identify? Select all that apply.
    1. _____ Cracked and peeling skin
    2. _____ Long scalp hair and fingernails
    3. _____ Red, puffy appearance of face and neck
    4. _____ Vernix caseosa covering back and buttocks
    5. _____ Creases on entire soles of feet and palms of hands

396. What does the nurse expect concerning the alveoli in the lungs of a 28-week-gestation neonate?
    1. They have a tendency to collapse with each breath
    2. There usually is a sufficient supply of pulmonary surfactant
    3. Although apparently mature they cannot absorb adequate oxygen
    4. Oxygen is not released into the circulation because they overinflate

397. An infant is admitted to the nursery after a difficult shoulder birth. For what condition should the nurse assess this newborn?
    1. Facial paralysis
    2. Cephalhematoma

3. Brachial plexus injury

4. Spinal cord syndrome

398. The mother of a neonate with Down syndrome visits the clinic 1 week postpartum. She explains to the nurse that she is having problems feeding her baby. What is the probable cause of these feeding difficulties?

1. Receding jaw

2. Brain damage

3. Tongue thrust

4. Nasal congestion

399. Which assessment leads a nurse to suspect that a newborn with a spinal cord lesion has increased intracranial pressure? Select all that apply.

1. _____ Irritability

2. _____ High-pitched cry

3. _____ Depressed fontanels

4. _____ Decreased urinary output

5. _____ Ineffective feeding behavior

400. A client is admitted in active labor at 39 weeks' gestation. During the initial examination the nurse identifies multiple red blister-like lesions on the edge of the client's vaginal orifice. After speaking to the practitioner and receiving orders, the priority nursing action should be to:

1. Begin the IV antibiotic

2. Prepare for a cesarean birth

3. Take a smear of the lesion for testing

4. Document the need for double gloving

REPRODUCTIVE PROBLEMS

401. During their initial visit to the fertility clinic a couple tells the nurse that after 2 years of unprotected intercourse they have not been able to conceive. A physical examination reveals that neither person has an abnormality. At their next visit the nurse informs them that laboratory data indicate an adequate quantity and quality of sperm. What question should the nurse ask now?

1. "Do you use any lubrication during intercourse?"

2. "Can both of you reach orgasm at the same time?"

3. "What type of birth control did you use in the past?"

4. "Are you consistent in the manner in which you have intercourse?"

402. A client at 16 weeks' gestation is being treated for *Trichomonas vaginalis*. Which statement best indicates to the nurse that the client has learned measures to prevent a recurrence?

1. "After having sex I will insert a vaginal suppository."

2. "My partner must get treated before we have sex again."

3. "I will urinate immediately after having sexual intercourse."

4. "Douching immediately after sexual intercourse will help protect me."

403. While a client is being prepared for surgery because of a ruptured tubal pregnancy, the client complains of feeling lightheaded. Her pulse is rapid, and her color is pale. What condition does the nurse suspect the client has?

1. Shock

2. Anxiety

3. Infection

4. Hyperoxia

404. A client who is admitted for surgery for a ruptured tubal pregnancy tells the nurse that she has shoulder pain. The nurse concludes that the pain is caused by:

1. Anxiety about the diagnosis

2. Cardiac changes from hypovolemia

3. Blood accumulation under the diaphragm

4. Rebound tenderness from the ruptured tube

405. What is a nurse's most important concern when caring for a client with a ruptured tubal pregnancy?

1. Infection

2. Hypervolemia

3. Protein deficiency

4. Diminished cardiac output

406. A client calls the nurse-midwife in the prenatal clinic complaining of sharp shooting pains in the lower abdomen and vaginal spotting. She is met at the emergency department of the hospital and a diagnosis of ruptured tubal pregnancy is made. At what stage of the pregnancy does the nurse suspect the initial symptoms began?

1. At 16 weeks' gestation

2. Immediately after implantation

3. About 6 weeks into the pregnancy

4. Toward the end of the second trimester

407. A nurse genetic counselor is working with a couple, each of whom is a carrier of an autosomal recessive disorder. Which statement indicates that the couple understood the teaching about this disorder?

1. "Most of our children will have the disorder."

2. "None of our children will have the disorder."

3. "There is a 1 in 4 chance of having a child with the disorder."

4. "There is a 1 in 2 chance of having a child with the disorder."

408. The nurse in a genetic counseling center determines that a disorder with a 50% occurrence rate in both males and females is:

1. X-linked recessive

2. Autosomal recessive

3. Autosomal dominant

4. Chromosomal trisomy

409. A client has a child with Tay-Sachs disease and wants to become pregnant again. She tells the nurse, "I'm worried it will happen again." How should the nurse respond?

1. "Did you discuss this with your physician?"

2. "Perhaps you should think about genetic counseling."

3. "Can you remember if Tay-Sachs occurred before in your family?"

4. "It is a rare disease that is statistically improbable to happen again."

410. A client who had a child with Tay-Sachs disease is pregnant and is to have an amniocentesis to determine if the fetus has the disease. The nurse counsels her to plan for the procedure at the optimum time during her pregnancy. When is the best time?
    1. 6 to 8 weeks' gestation
    2. 14 to 16 weeks' gestation
    3. 18 to 20 weeks' gestation
    4. 22 to 24 weeks' gestation

411. A female client who is undergoing infertility testing is taught how to examine her cervical mucus. After listening to the instructions the client says, "That sounds gross. I don't think I can do it." What does the nurse conclude from this statement?
    1. The client is unduly fastidious
    2. The client feels that having a baby is not that important
    3. Some women are uncomfortable touching their genitals
    4. Some women are afraid that they are the cause of the infertility

412. A couple is concerned about the risks associated with an in vitro fertilization embryo transfer (IVF-ET). What risk should the nurse's response include?
    1. Embryonic HIV
    2. Tubal pregnancy
    3. Congenital anomalies
    4. Hyperemesis gravidarum

413. A client comes to the fertility clinic for a hysterosalpingography using radiopaque contrast material to determine whether her fallopian tubes are patent. When preparing for the test, the nurse explains to the client that she:
    1. Will receive a local anesthetic and the pain will lessen
    2. Will have to rest in bed for 8 hours after the test is completed
    3. May have some persistent shoulder pain for 14 hours after the test
    4. May become nauseated during the test, but the nausea will subside

414. Because an infertility workup involves both partners, a male client is to have a semen analysis. What should the nurse include as part of his instructions?
    1. Obtain the specimen upon awakening
    2. Use a condom to collect the semen specimen
    3. Ejaculate at least 4 hours before collection to ensure a pure specimen
    4. Deliver the specimen to the laboratory within 2 hours of obtaining it

415. On a return visit to the fertility clinic, a couple has requested fertility drugs because, despite having a 28-day menstrual cycle and temperature readings that demonstrate an ovulatory pattern, the female has been unable to conceive. What should the nurse explain to the couple?
    1. A laparoscopy will be scheduled
    2. An endometrial biopsy will be required
    3. A fertility medication will be prescribed
    4. An examination of semen will be needed

416. A client at 12 weeks' gestation arrives in the prenatal clinic complaining of cramping and vaginal spotting. A pelvic examination reveals that the cervix is closed. Which probable diagnosis should the nurse expect?
    1. Missed abortion
    2. Inevitable abortion
    3. Incomplete abortion
    4. Threatened abortion

417. A client at 10 weeks' gestation phones the prenatal clinic to report that she is experiencing some vaginal bleeding and abdominal cramping. The nurse arranges for her to go to the local hospital. The vaginal examination reveals that her cervix is 2 cm dilated. What probable diagnosis should the nurse expect?
    1. Septic abortion
    2. Inevitable abortion
    3. Threatened abortion
    4. Incomplete abortion

418. A client is to have a vacuum curettage abortion because of a fetal demise at 16 weeks' gestation. The practitioner prescribes a dinoprostone (Cervidil) suppository to initiate softening, effacement, and dilation of the cervix (ripening). What should the nurse teach the client about the procedure?
    1. "General anesthesia will be used to insert the suppository."
    2. "There will be copious bleeding for several hours after the abortion."
    3. "Temperature of more than 100° F is common for the first 24 to 48 hours."
    4. "After insertion of the suppository you should lie flat in bed for 15 minutes."

419. A client is being discharged after a first-trimester aspiration abortion. Which statement indicates to the nurse that the instructions are understood?
    1. "I will be able to have sex in 4 to 5 days."
    2. "I can substitute tampons for sanitary pads after 24 hours."
    3. "I can expect my menstrual period to resume in 2 to 3 weeks."
    4. "I will call you if I must change my pad more than once in 4 hours."

420. A client who is pregnant for the first time expels the products of conception at 12 weeks' gestation. The client's blood type is Rh negative. What should the nurse anticipate concerning the administration of Rho(D) immune globulin (RhoGAM)?
    1. RhoGAM is not necessary if the fetus died in utero
    2. Administer RhoGAM immediately after the miscarriage
    3. Administer RhoGAM within 72 hours after the miscarriage
    4. RhoGAM will not be needed because the gestation was less than 20 weeks

421. A client at 18 weeks' gestation visits the prenatal clinic stating she still is very nauseated and vomits frequently.

Physical examination reveals that she has a brown vaginal discharge and her blood pressure is 148/90. What condition does the nurse suspect the client is experiencing?

1. Dehydration
2. Choriocarcinoma
3. Hydatidiform mole
4. Threatened abortion

422. After the removal of a hydatidiform mole, the nurse monitors the client's laboratory data during a follow-up visit. The nurse identifies that a prolonged elevation of the serum human chorionic gonadotropin (hCG) level is a danger sign. What condition is a possible outcome?

1. Uterine rupture
2. Choriocarcinoma
3. Hyperemesis gravidarum
4. Disseminated intravascular coagulation

WOMEN'S HEALTH

423. A 13-year-old adolescent whose menses began 2 years ago complains of lower abdominal pain midway between each period. How should the nurse respond to the adolescent?

1. It requires a physical examination
2. This usually occurs when menses first begin
3. It usually disappears when there is regular ovulation
4. This is a common occurrence known as mittelschmerz

424. During a pelvic examination of a 24-year-old woman, the nurse suspects a vaginal infection because there is a white curdlike vaginal discharge. What other assessment supports a fungal vaginal infection?

1. A foul odor
2. An itchy perineum
3. An ischemic cervix
4. A forgotten tampon

425. A client is receiving antibiotics and antifungal medications to treat a recurring vaginal infection. What should the nurse encourage the client to do to compensate for the effect of these medications?

1. Eat yogurt daily
2. Avoid spicy foods
3. Drink more fruit juices
4. Take a multivitamin every day

426. What statement helps the nurse determine that a woman with genital herpes (HSV-2) s her self-care related to this infection?

1. "When I have a baby, I don't want a cesarean."
2. "I can have sex as soon as the herpes sores have healed."
3. "When I finish the acyclovir prescription I will be cured."
4. "I must be careful when I have sex because herpes is a lifelong problem."

427. A 16-year-old high school student is referred to a community health center by a local hotline because of the fear of contracting herpes. The teenager is upset and shares this information with the community health center nurse. What should be the nurse's initial response?

1. "Let me get a brief health history now."
2. "Try not to worry until you know if you have herpes."
3. "You sound worried; let me make arrangements to have you examined."
4. "Herpes has received too much attention in the media; let's be realistic."

428. A 16-year-old adolescent has a steady boyfriend with whom she is having sexual relations. She asks the nurse how she can protect herself from contracting HIV. What should the nurse advise her to do?

1. Ask her partner to withdraw before ejaculating
2. Make certain their relationship is monogamous
3. Insist that her partner use a condom when having sex
4. Seek counseling about various contraceptive methods

429. A 16-year-old adolescent arrives at the clinic complaining of increased vaginal discharge, intermittent vaginal bleeding, excessive bleeding when menstruating, and pain in the lower abdomen. She relates an active sexual history with multiple partners. What disease does the nurse suspect the client has?

1. Herpes
2. Syphilis
3. Gonorrhea
4. Toxoplasmosis

430. A nurse is assessing a female client who is suspected of having primary syphilis. What sign of primary syphilis does the nurse expect the client to exhibit?

1. Flat wartlike plaques around the vagina and anus
2. An indurated painless nodule on the vulva that is draining
3. Glistening patches in the mouth covered with a yellow exudate
4. A maculopapular rash on the palms of the hands and soles of the feet

431. A client who has syphilis tells the nurse that it must have been contracted from a toilet seat. The nurse knows that this cannot be true because the causative agent of syphilis is:

1. Immobilized by body contact
2. Chelated by wood and plastic
3. Inactivated when exposed to a dry environment
4. Destroyed when exposed to a warm environment

432. A young client tells the nurse that her mother complains about having dysmenorrhea and asks the nurse what this means. How should the nurse describe dysmenorrhea?

1. Cessation of menstrual periods
2. Spotting between menstrual periods
3. Uterine pain during the menstrual period
4. Scant bleeding at the time of an expected menstrual period

433. A woman arrives at the women's health clinic complaining of frequency and burning pain when urinating. The

diagnosis is a urinary tract infection. What is important for the nurse to encourage the client to do?

1. Void every two hours
2. Record fluid intake and urinary output
3. Pour warm water over the vulva after voiding
4. Wash the hands thoroughly after urinating and defecating

434. A nurse is teaching a woman how to perform breast self-examination. Which statement indicates that the client needs further teaching?

1. "I examine my breasts about a week after my period starts."
2. "I have been looking for dimpling as well as checking for lumps."
3. "My breasts are so tender right before my period that I hate doing it."
4. "My grandmother examines her breasts on the first Monday of each month."

435. A nurse is teaching a class of premenopausal women how to perform breast self-examination correctly. When is the best time of the month for breast self-examination?

1. When ovulation occurs
2. The first day of every month
3. The day that the menses begins
4. About a week after menses ends

436. What does the nurse teach a client to do when performing breast self-examination?

1. Squeeze the nipples to examine for discharge
2. Use the right hand to examine the right breast
3. Place a pillow under the shoulder opposite the examined breast to raise it
4. Compress breast tissue to the chest wall with the palm of the hand to palpate for lumps

437. What factor identified by the nurse in a client's history places the client at an increased risk for breast cancer?

1. Early menopause
2. Low-income background
3. Delayed onset of menarche
4. Late beginning of childbearing

438. A client at 40 weeks' gestation visits the prenatal clinic. The nurse, knowing that this may be the client's last prenatal visit, performs a breast examination. What adaptation does the nurse identify that requires further assessment?

1. Darkening of the nipple areolae
2. Nodularity in an outer quadrant
3. Clear fluid leaking from a nipple
4. Prominence of the superficial veins

439. A nurse is assessing a 38-year-old female client who was admitted for a biopsy of a lump in her right breast. Which finding may indicate a malignancy?

1. A soft mass that is movable and nontender
2. Hard, hot, reddened areas that are tender and painful
3. Multiple bilateral lesions that are well delineated and movable
4. A lesion in the upper, outer quadrant that is poorly delineated and nonmobile

440. A client who recently was told by her practitioner that she has extensive metastatic carcinoma of the breast, tells the nurse that she believes an error has been made. She states that she does not have breast cancer, and she is not going to die. The nurse determines that the client is experiencing the stage of death and dying known as:

1. Anger
2. Denial
3. Bargaining
4. Acceptance

441. A client who had a mastectomy because of breast cancer returns to her room on the unit. What does the primary nurse anticipate?

1. Drainage container will be kept level with the affected arm
2. Affected arm will be abducted at the shoulder with the elbow extended
3. Hand and elbow of the affected arm will be elevated above the shoulder
4. Elbow and shoulder of the affected arm will be elevated with the hand resting on the abdomen

442. A client who had a lumpectomy of the breast is to have radiation therapy. What should the nurse do at the client's first visit to the surgeon's office after the surgery?

1. Provide a protective skin lotion
2. Assess the extent of wound healing
3. Teach sterile technique for skin care
4. Demonstrate how to dispose of urine safely

443. After 2 weeks of radiation therapy for cancer of the breast a client develops some erythema over the area being radiated. The area is sensitive but not painful. She states that she has been using tepid water and a soft washcloth when cleansing the area and applying an ice pack three times a day. What does the nurse conclude from this information?

1. Further teaching on skin care is necessary
2. No other intervention is needed at this time
3. The radiation team should be notified of this problem
4. Health teaching on the side effects of radiation is needed

444. A 28-year-old woman is diagnosed with cancer of the left breast. A simple mastectomy is performed at the insistence of the client. What should the plan of care include immediately after surgery?

1. Changing the client's pressure dressing as necessary
2. Inviting a member of Reach to Recovery to visit the client
3. Placing the client in the semi-Fowler position with the left arm elevated
4. Waiting for a cessation of drainage before the client resumes any activity

445. What is most important to teach a client who had a mastectomy before she leaves the hospital?

1. Why a breast prosthesis is necessary
2. Which of the more strenuous activities to curtail

3. What household tasks to avoid that require stretching

4. Why self-examination of the remaining breast is important

446. A client has a modified radical mastectomy because of a malignant tumor of the breast. What does the nurse plan to teach the client during the early postoperative period?

1. Keep the arm in an elevated position

2. Observe the incision site for redness and bleeding

3. Maintain a high Fowler position with the affected arm on a pillow

4. Perform range-of-motion exercises including flexion and abduction of the affected arm

447. When a client who had a mastectomy returns from surgery, a dressing and a portable wound drainage system to the axillary area are in place. The nurse observes an excessive amount of serosanguineous drainage on the mastectomy dressing. What is the nurse's next action?

1. Notifying the surgeon

2. Applying a pressure dressing

3. Checking the function of the drainage system

4. Using additional pillows to elevate the affected arm

448. A client at the women's health clinic complains of swelling of the labia and throbbing pain in the labial area after sexual intercourse. For what condition does the nurse anticipate the client will be treated?

1. Urethritis

2. Bartholinitis

3. Vaginal hematoma

4. Inflamed Skene's glands

449. An older female client tells the nurse in the clinic that she has a cystocele, which was diagnosed a year ago. She has urinary frequency and burning on urination. She asks, "The doctor wanted me to have surgery for the cystocele last year, but I can manage using peripads. It won't hurt not to have surgery, will it?" How should the nurse respond?

1. "Not really, but it should be done."

2. "Yes, you are risking kidney damage."

3. "Yes, you are risking bowel obstruction."

4. "Not really, but you will be more comfortable."

450. A female client having presurgical testing prior to a total abdominal hysterectomy says to the nurse, "When I have this surgery I know my husband will never come near me." The nurse's best initial response is, "You're:

1. underestimating his love for you."

2. wondering about the effect on your sexual relations."

3. worried that the surgery will change how others see you."

4. concerned about how your husband will respond to your surgery."

451. A woman is admitted for a hysterectomy and bilateral salpingo-oophorectomy. The nurse reviews the client's gynecological history. What condition does the client have that causes the nurse to anticipate an abdominal, rather than a vaginal, hysterectomy?

1. Prolapsed uterus

2. Large uterine fibroids

3. Mild dysplasia of the cervical os

4. Urinary incontinence when coughing

452. A client who is recovering from a total abdominal hysterectomy calls out to every nursing staff member who passes by the door and asks them to do or get something. The nurse can best manage this behavior by:

1. Having one staff member approach the client regularly and spend time talking with her

2. Closing the door to the room so the client cannot see the staff members as they pass by the room

3. Informing the client that one staff member will come in frequently and answer any questions she may have

4. Arranging for a variety of staff members to take turns going into the room to see whether the client has any requests

453. During the discharge conference with a client who had a hysterectomy the nurse includes instructions for avoiding the thromboembolic phenomena that can occur as a complication. What should these instructions include?

1. Avoid sitting for long periods of time

2. Limit fluids to less than 2000 mL per day

3. Have a blood coagulation test every 2 weeks

4. Continue with hormone replacement therapy

454. The nurse is planning care for an older woman who is admitted for a vaginal hysterectomy and an anterior and posterior repair of the vaginal wall. What should the nurse tell the client to expect in the immediate postoperative period?

1. Placement of a pessary

2. Insertion of a rectal tube

3. Use of a douche periodically

4. Presence of a urinary catheter

455. Four days after a vaginal hysterectomy a client calls the follow-up service and tells the nurse that she has a yellowish-green vaginal discharge. The nurse advises the client to return to the clinic for an evaluation. What does the nurse need to assess when a vaginal infection is suspected? Select all that apply.

1. _____ Abdominal pain

2. _____ Urinary frequency

3. _____ Rising temperature

4. _____ Decreased pulse rate

5. _____ Decreased blood pressure

456. After a vaginal hysterectomy and an anterior and posterior repair of the vaginal wall a client is returned to her room. What does the nurse include in the plan of care for this client?

1. Check vaginal packing

2. Elevate lower extremities

3. Observe dressing for bleeding

4. Start sitz baths tomorrow morning

457. During discharge teaching, a client who had a hysterectomy states, "After this surgery, I don't expect to be

interested in sex anymore." What should the nurse consider before responding?

1. Many women incorrectly equate hysterectomy with loss of libido
2. Surgically forced menopause usually results in a decreased sex drive
3. Loss of estrogen that results from this surgery will cause most women to experience a decrease in libido
4. Body image changes that occur after this surgery prevent many women from resuming sexual activity

458. A 35-year-old client is scheduled for a vaginal hysterectomy. She asks the nurse about the changes she should expect after surgery. How should the nurse respond?

1. "You will stop ovulating."
2. "A surgical menopause is predicted immediately."
3. "Sexual intercourse will be uncomfortable when resumed."
4. "A hysterectomy does not affect the chronological age when menopause usually occurs."

459. A young sexually active client at the family planning clinic is advised to have a Papanicolaou (Pap) smear. She has never had a Pap smear before. What should the nurse include in the explanation of this procedure?

1. Pap smears can detect cancer of the cervix
2. Vaginal bleeding is expected after a Pap smear
3. Colposcopy will be used to visualize the cervix
4. Scraping the cervix is the most uncomfortable part

460. A client is admitted with a diagnosis of stage 0 cervical cancer (carcinoma in situ). What does the nurse emphasize while helping the client to understand her diagnosis and prognosis?

1. Five-year survival rates for this cancer are nearly 100% with early treatment
2. Radiation therapy is as successful as surgery in the treatment of this type of cancer
3. Cancer has probably extended into the vaginal wall and may require a radical hysterectomy
4. Stage 0 indicates that the cancer is invasive and may require surgery in addition to radiation therapy

461. What should be included in the nursing care immediately after a sexual assault?

1. Obtaining the assault history from the client
2. Informing the police before the client is examined
3. Having the client void a clean-catch urine specimen
4. Testing the client's urine for seminal alkaline phosphatase

462. A nurse is interviewing a female client who is tentatively diagnosed with cystitis, pending laboratory results. The nurse anticipates that the causative agent of the cystitis is *Escherichia coli*. The nurse anticipates this microorganism because it:

1. Thrives in the kidneys
2. Is a virulent bacterium
3. Inhabits the intestinal tract
4. Competes with fungi for host sites

463. When performing a routine physical assessment on a client who is postmenopausal the nurse identifies that the client has enlarged breasts with galactorrhea. For what blood hormone level does the nurse expect the client to be tested?

1. Prolactin
2. Estrogen
3. Oxytocin
4. Progesterone

464. A nurse in a campus health clinic is assessing the female students for risk factors associated with the future development of osteoporosis. What factors are included in this assessment? Select all that apply.

1. _____ Cigarette smoking
2. _____ Moderate exercise
3. _____ Use of street drugs
4. _____ Familial predisposition
5. _____ Inadequate intake of dietary calcium

DRUG-RELATED RESPONSES

465. A client at 31 weeks' gestation is admitted in preterm labor. She asks the nurse if there is any medication that can help stop the contractions. What is the nurse's response?

1. "An oxytocic."
2. "An analgesic."
3. "A corticosteroid."
4. "A beta-adrenergic."

466. While receiving betamimetic (tocolytic) therapy for preterm labor the client begins to have muscle tremors and signs of nervousness. The client states, "My heart is racing." The nurse identifies that the client's pulse rate is 110 beats per minute and regular. What should the nurse do next?

1. Discontinue the medication as per protocol
2. Notify the practitioner that preterm labor has restarted
3. Obtain the client's laboratory results for electrolyte levels
4. Reassure the client that these are expected side effects of the medication

467. Ten minutes after administering nalbuphine (Nubain) via IV piggyback to a primigravida in active labor, the nurse observes a fetal heart rate of 132 with minimal variability. The client states that the pain is more tolerable and she is able to use her breathing techniques more effectively. Contractions continue every 2 to 3 minutes and are of 60 seconds' duration. What is the nurse's next action?

1. Reposition the client on the left side to increase placental perfusion
2. Administer oxygen via mask to minimize apparent fetal compromise
3. Have an opioid antagonist available to be administered to the infant at the time of birth
4. Document the findings, including the decreased fetal heart rate variability as a result of the opioid infusion

468. A multipara is admitted to the birthing room in active labor. Her vital signs are temperature, 98° F; pulse, 70 beats per minute; respirations, 18 per minute; and blood pressure, 126/76. A vaginal examination reveals a cervix that is 90% effaced and 7 cm dilated with the vertex presenting at 2+ station. The client is complaining of pain and asks for medication. Which medication should be avoided because it may cause respiratory depression in the newborn?
1. Naloxone (Narcan)
2. Lorazepam (Ativan)
3. Meperidine (Demerol)
4. Promethazine (Phenergan)

469. A client is receiving an epidural anesthetic during labor. For which side effect should the nurse monitor the client?
1. Hypertension
2. Urinary retention
3. Subnormal temperature
4. Decreased level of consciousness

470. A practitioner prescribes penicillin G benzathine suspension (Bicillin L-A) 2.45 million units for a client with a sexually transmitted infection (STI). The medication is available in a multidose vial of 10 mL in which 1 mL = 300,000 units. How many mL should the nurse administer?
Answer: _____mL

471. A client who is at 33 weeks' gestation has contracted gonorrhea and is prescribed probenecid (Benemid) and penicillin therapy. Which statement indicates to the nurse that the client understands the action of probenecid?
1. "My allergy to penicillin is minimized."
2. "The side effects of the disease are reduced."
3. "My immune defense mechanisms are more active."
4. "The amount of penicillin in my blood is increased."

472. A pregnant client with an infection tells the nurse that she has taken tetracycline (Tetracyn) for infections on other occasions and prefers to take it now. The nurse tells the client that tetracycline is avoided when treating an infection in pregnant women because it:
1. Affects breastfeeding adversely
2. Influences the fetus' teeth buds
3. Causes fetal allergies to the medication
4. Increases the fetus' tolerance to the medication

473. A 24-year-old thin woman who runs 10 miles weekly asks the nurse for advice about preventing osteoporosis. Which vitamin and other dietary supplement should the nurse recommend?
1. E and ginseng tea
2. B and ginkgo biloba
3. D and calcium citrate
4. C and glucosamine/chondroitin

474. A client is taking progesterone oral contraceptives (minipills). The nurse instructs the client to take one pill daily during the:
1. Five days of the ovulatory cycle
2. Latter part of the ovulatory cycle

3. First week of the menstrual cycle
4. Entire time of the menstrual cycle

475. A nurse evaluates that a client understands the most common side effects of estrogen in oral contraceptives when the client says, "I should notify the physician when I:
1. stop having menstrual periods."
2. feel depressed and lack energy."
3. experience nausea and vomiting."
4. have very light menstrual periods."

476. A nurse is teaching a client about the oral contraceptive prescribed by the practitioner. Which condition identified by the client indicates understanding about when the drug should be stopped immediately and the practitioner notified?
1. Chest pain
2. Menorrhagia
3. Mittelschmerz
4. Increased leukorrhea

477. A pregnant client with iron deficiency anemia is prescribed a daily iron supplement. What nutrient should the nurse suggest that the client include in her diet to potentiate the effect of the iron supplement?
1. Biotin
2. Lecithin
3. Vitamin C
4. Vitamin B complex

478. A 39-year-old woman who is Rh negative is seen by her primary care provider during the first trimester of pregnancy. Which week of gestation should the nurse teach the client that Rho(D) immune globulin (RhoGAM) will be administered?
1. 12 weeks
2. 28 weeks
3. 36 weeks
4. 40 weeks

479. What should the nurse explain to a newly pregnant client with cardiac disease?
1. Palpitations are expected as pregnancy progresses
2. Other cardiac medications will be substituted for digoxin
3. Maintenance dosages of cardiac medication probably will increase
4. Prophylactic penicillin administration is not safe during pregnancy

480. A nurse is caring for a pregnant client with thrombophlebitis. Which anticoagulant medication may be prescribed? Select all that apply.
1. _____ Heparin (Hep-Lock)
2. _____ Clopidogrel (Plavix)
3. _____ Warfarin (Coumadin)
4. _____ Enoxaparin (Lovenox)
5. _____ Acetylsalicylic acid (Acuprin)

481. A postpartum client developed a deep vein thrombosis and an IV infusion of heparin therapy was instituted 2 days ago. Her activated partial thromboplastin time (aPTT) is now 98 seconds. What should the nurse do?

1. Increase the intravenous rate of heparin
2. Interrupt the infusion and notify the practitioner of the aPTT result
3. Document the result on the medical record and re-check the aPTT in four hours
4. Call the practitioner to obtain a prescription for a low-molecular weight heparin

482. To halt preterm labor, a client is started on terbutaline (Brethine). For which side effect of this medication should the nurse monitor the client?
1. Bradycardia
2. Hyperkalemia
3. Widening pulse pressure
4. Hypotonic uterine contractions

483. Immediately after the third stage of labor a nurse administers the prescribed oxytocin (Pitocin) infusion. Why is this medication administered?
1. For contraction of the uterus
2. To lessen uterine discomfort
3. To aid in the separation of the placenta
4. For the stimulation of breast milk production

484. A client in labor is receiving an oxytocin (Pitocin) infusion. For which adverse reaction from prolonged administration should the nurse monitor the client?
1. Change in affect
2. Hyperventilation
3. Water intoxication
4. Elevated temperature

485. A client with severe preeclampsia is receiving 2 g/hr of IV magnesium sulfate. For what should the nurse assess to confirm the effectiveness of this therapy?
1. Elevated blood pressure
2. Excessive urinary output
3. Decreased respiratory rate
4. Diminished knee-jerk reflex

486. A nurse administers the prescribed intravenous dose of magnesium sulfate to a client with severe preeclampsia. What adverse effect should the nurse address when evaluating the client's response to the medication?
1. Visual blurring
2. Epigastric pain
3. Fetal tachycardia
4. Respiratory depression

487. When a client is receiving an intravenous infusion of magnesium sulfate, the nurse should have its antidote readily available. Which antidote should be available?
1. Protamine sulfate
2. Calcium gluconate
3. Sodium bicarbonate
4. Naloxone hydrochloride

488. A nurse is teaching a breastfeeding client about medications that are safe and unsafe to take. Which medication is contraindicated?
1. Heparin (Hep-Lock)
2. Propylthiouracil (PTU)
3. Gentamicin (Garamycin)
4. Diphenhydramine (Benadryl)

489. A nurse is caring for a client with severe preeclampsia who is receiving magnesium sulfate. What side effects indicate that the serum magnesium level may be excessive? Select all that apply.
1. _____ Knee-jerk reflex is +1
2. _____ Urine output is 100 mL/hr
3. _____ Blood pressure is 140/90 mm Hg
4. _____ Apical pulse is 80 beats per minute
5. _____ Respiratory rate is 11 breaths per minute

490. A client at 32 weeks' gestation is admitted in active labor. Her cervix is effaced and 4 cm dilated. Betamethasone (Celestone) 12 mg IM is prescribed. What should the nurse tell the client about why the medication is given?
1. Cervical dilation is increased
2. Fetal lung maturity is accelerated
3. Risk of a precipitous birth is reduced
4. Potential for maternal hypertension is minimized

491. A nurse is caring for a newborn suspected of drug addiction. What should the nurse do to most accurately confirm that the newborn is addicted?
1. Examine the mother's arms for needle marks
2. Monitor the newborn closely for the first 48 hours
3. Check the mother's medication record for the previous 24 hours
4. Collect the newborn's urine by applying a collection bag to obtain a sample for testing

492. A preterm infant is started on digoxin (Lanoxin) and furosemide (Lasix) for persistent patent ductus arteriosus. Which nursing assessment provides the best indication of the effectiveness of the furosemide?
1. Pedal edema is reduced
2. Digoxin toxicity is avoided
3. Fontanels appear depressed
4. Urine output exceeds fluid intake

493. What antidote to the side effects of terbutaline (Brethine) should a nurse have available?
1. Levodopa (L-Dopa)
2. Furosemide (Lasix)
3. Ritodrine (Yutopar)
4. Propranolol (Inderal)

494. A nurse administers two serial IM injections of betamethasone (Celestone) to a woman at 32 weeks' gestation, who is admitted in preterm labor. The nurse determines that this medication is given to:
1. Stop the process of labor
2. Increase placental perfusion
3. Facilitate fetal lung maturity
4. Reduce intensity of contractions

495. A client with systemic lupus erythematosus (SLE) is at 39 weeks' gestation. What does the nurse anticipate regarding this client?
1. Large-for-gestational age newborn
2. Postpartum dialysis may be necessary
3. More prominent butterfly-shaped rash
4. Salicylate therapy will be discontinued

496. A client with a large fetus is to have a pudendal block during the second stage of labor. What does the nurse

plan to instruct the client about the effectiveness of the block? Select all that apply.

1. _____ Contractions will decrease
2. _____ Perineal pain will not be felt
3. _____ Bladder sensation may be lost
4. _____ Episiotomy may not be needed
5. _____ Bearing down reflex will be diminished

497. Before the administration of Rho(D) immune globulin (RhoGAM) the nurse reviews the laboratory data of a pregnant client. Which blood type and Coombs' test result must a pregnant woman have to receive RhoGAM after giving birth?
    1. Rh positive and Coombs' positive
    2. Rh negative and Coombs' positive
    3. Rh positive and Coombs' negative
    4. Rh negative and Coombs' negative

498. During a prenatal visit a nurse explains to a client who is Rh negative when Rho(D) immune globulin (Rho-GAM) will be administered to her. When is the best time to administer RhoGAM?
    1. Within 72 hours after birth if the infant is Rh positive
    2. Weekly during the 9th month if the mother is a multipara
    3. Immediately after birth if the infant's Coombs' test is positive
    4. During the second trimester if an amniocentesis indicates a problem

499. A client at 30 weeks' gestation is admitted in preterm labor. An IV solution of the tocolytic agent ritodrine (Yutopar) is started. The nurse prepares to administer an IM injection of betamethasone (Celestone). The client asks why betamethasone is being administered. The nurse responds, "It:
    1. enhances uterine relaxation."
    2. prevents fetal hypoglycemia."
    3. stimulates fetal lung maturity."
    4. counteracts adverse reactions."

500. Vitamin K 0.5 mg is prescribed for a newborn. The vial on hand is labeled 1 mL = 2 mg. How many mL should the nurse administer?
    Answer: _____ mL

Additional review questions can be found on the enclosed companion CD.

CHILDBEARING AND WOMEN'S HEALTH NURSING ANSWERS AND RATIONALES

NURSING PRACTICE

1. **3 Before further intervention, the reason for the inadequate weight gain should be evaluated. Evaluation should take place before changing the plan or altering the goal.**
   1 This intervention is premature.
   2 This intervention is premature.
   4 This is unsafe; the reason for the lack of goal attainment must be identified.

2. **3 The data indicate a life-threatening emergency, and if the client is unable to sign an informed consent it is the legal responsibility of the surgeon and the health care provider to sign the consent form so that further injury to the client and her fetus may be prevented.**
   1 There is not enough time to obtain a verbal consent.
   2 It is illegal to perform the surgery without a signed consent.
   4 Legally, a nurse is not allowed to countersign an informed consent unless the client has signed it first.

3. **3 Legally, the person performing the surgery is responsible to inform the client adequately; the nurse may clarify information, witness the client's signature and cosign the consent form.**
   1 This is beyond the scope of nursing practice.
   2 The nurse may face criminal charges of assault and battery if proceeding when there is a lack of informed consent.
   4 This places blame on the client; it is the responsibility of the surgeon to impart the vital information required for consent.

4. **2 This is the priority before anesthesia is administered. Anesthesia depresses the central nervous system and the client cannot participate in decision making.**
   1 This can be done later; it is not the priority.
   3 This can be done later; it is not the priority.
   4 This can be done later; it is not the priority.

5. **2 This response permits exploration of the parents' wishes and leads to assisting them in making their own decision.**
   1 This response blocks further discussion; the nurse can answer some of the questions and refer those that cannot be answered to the practitioner.
   3 This is a value judgment; it denies the parents' right to decide.
   4 This response might frighten the parents; it denies the parents their power of decision.

6. **2 A return demonstration can validate that desired learning has taken place from earlier teaching.**
   1 Teaching was already done and now must be evaluated.
   3 This is not necessary; a return demonstration provides feedback for evaluation.
   4 This is not necessary; a return demonstration provides feedback for evaluation.

7. **4 This is the required intervention when legally mandated eye treatment is refused.**
   1 This denies the parents' desires and implies wrongdoing on their part.
   2 The parents have the right to refuse but must indicate their refusal on an informed consent form.
   3 This is shifting the responsibility to the pediatrician.

8. **3 The client must be intellectually competent; that is, able to comprehend the outcome of the procedure to give informed consent.**
   1 This avenue may be pursued after the client is deemed unable to provide informed consent. The parent or guardian must be designated by the court to perform this function.
   2 This may be unrealistic for this client; it is more important for the client to demonstrate that the outcome of the procedure is understood.
   4 The client should be free from the influence of others who might press to have the procedure performed. This is an individual decision by a client who is capable of making this decision.

9. **1 Domestic abuse is more likely to intensify during pregnancy and the attacks usually are directed toward the pregnant woman's abdomen.**
   2 A hydatidiform mole may be manifested by an unusually enlarged uterus for gestational age, hypertension, nausea and vomiting, and vaginal bleeding, not bruises on the face and abdomen.
   3 Excessive exercise may cause cardiovascular or pulmonary problems. It will not result in bruising.
   4 Thrombocytopenic purpura and other bleeding disorders are manifested by bruises and petechiae on many areas of the body surface, not just the face and abdomen.

10. **3 Research demonstrates that placing an infant on the back reduces the incidence of sudden infant death syndrome (SIDS).**
    1 Pillows in an infant's crib can cause suffocation.
    2 It is unsafe to strap an infant seat into the front seat of a car.
    4 Infants can drown in a very small amount of water in a tub; it is unsafe to leave an infant alone in a tub.

EMOTIONAL NEEDS RELATED TO CHILDBEARING AND WOMEN'S HEALTH

11. **1 This response supports the client's right to confidentiality without antagonizing the client's mother.**
    2 Although this response protects the client's right to confidentiality, it may disrupt the relationship between the client and her mother.
    3 Although this response protects the client's right to confidentiality, it may disrupt the relationship between the client and her mother.
    4 This is a judgmental, nontherapeutic statement.

12. **1 This is the most difficult phase of labor, and the client needs encouragement and support to cope.**
    2 Fluids should be increased at this time because of the increase in metabolism.
    3 Medication at this time is contraindicated because it can depress the newborn at birth.
    4 Breathing patterns should be complex, not uniform, at this time because they require a high level of concentration that helps to distract the client.

13. **1 During the taking-in phase a woman is primarily concerned with being cared for and being cared about.**
    2 This is best taught during the taking-hold phase of postpartum adjustment.
    3 This is best taught during the taking-hold phase of postpartum adjustment.
    4 This is not a primary concern during the immediate postpartum period.

14. **1 The mother needs to learn the realities of infant behaviors and how to cope with them; holding and talking to her infant are consoling measures.**
    2 It is unhealthy to disrupt a neonate's sleep pattern.
    3 The infant is too young to be given cereal.
    4 At this age a toy is not meaningful and is an inadequate substitute for parental attention.

15. **1 This statement acknowledges the situation and suggests a possible solution to the problem.**
    2 Postpartum blues occurs earlier; this may be postpartum depression and should not be dismissed lightly.
    3 This response is not only false reassurance, but it does not address the problem that is evident in the situation.
    4 This is stereotyping and nontherapeutic.

16. **1 This response addresses the problem directly while providing an opportunity for the client to examine her options. The therapeutic regimen includes bed rest and peace of mind; these can best be achieved if the children are cared for adequately.**
    2 This explores feelings without including a therapeutic regimen.
    3 This is giving solutions rather than exploring the situation with the client.
    4 Complete bed rest has been prescribed, and the suggested plan assumes that the client is able to afford nursery school for her children.

17. **3 Doing this will help the client relax and will lessen discomfort.**
    1 This may distract the client but will not produce relaxation.
    2 The client may become more anxious if the procedure is hurried.
    4 This may make the client more anxious; holding the breath causes tightening of the perineum.

18. **3 This response is nonjudgmental; it permits the client to identify her own feelings.**
    1 This is judgmental; it does not give the client the opportunity to express her feelings.
    2 This is judgmental; it gives the nurse's opinion on a moral question for the client.
    4 This response leaves the burden of the decision to the client without offering assistance.

19. **1 This is a nonjudgmental response that encourages exploration of feelings.**
    2 This response identifies the client's feelings but cuts off communication because it ends the discussion.
    3 This is a judgmental response that questions the mother's decision making and deals only with the present.
    4 This is a judgmental response that questions the mother's decision making and deals only with the present.

20. **2 The nurse's role modeling of the acceptance of the infant, even with the newborn's altered physical appearance, can help the parents to adjust.**
    1 This teaching is appropriate later; the parent's first need to deal with their feelings regarding the newborn's appearance.
    3 The parents' current major adjustment concern is the appearance of the infant; odor is secondary.
    4 This is false reassurance; there are no guarantees related to the outcome of the surgery.

21. **1 Before learning to care for her newborn emotionally and physically, the mother needs to begin to accept him as he is.**
    2 It is too soon to prepare the mother for the impending surgery. The priority at this time is to accept her baby.
    3 This concern is important but if the mother first accepts the infant with the defect, teaching will be more effective
    4 The mother will be better able to meet her baby's emotional needs after she has accepted him.

22. **4 This reassures the client of the fetus's well-being and the fact that the nurse will be monitoring the fetus's status.**
    1 This response does not provide the mother with reassurance of the fetus's status or that anything is being done to monitor the fetus.
    2 This provides false reassurance; following instructions does not guarantee a healthy newborn.
    3 This provides false reassurance; amniotic fluid makes the umbilical cord less vulnerable but does not protect against other causes of fetal compromise.

23. 4 **Analgesia crosses the placental barrier; because birth is imminent, it can cause respiratory depression in the newborn.**

1 The client is exhibiting fear and panic; a back rub at this time will not be effective and probably will be rejected.

2 This is incorrect information and provides false reassurance.

3 Although this is an empathic response, an explanation as to why medication cannot be given is more appropriate.

24. 1 **This intervention promotes bonding.**

2 Although the infant's physical condition is a priority, the nurse must not overlook the psychosocial aspects of care.

3 Such planning may be unrealistic because the parents may have work and family responsibilities.

4 Postponing teaching until discharge limits its effectiveness; this action does not give the parents time to demonstrate an understanding of and competence with skills that will be needed.

25. 3 **When the mother is emotionally prepared she should be reunited with her newborn at the first opportunity.**

1 There is no magic about the first 24 hours; some mothers are too ill or both parents may be too frightened to see their baby that soon.

2 Grief work will go on for an extended period and has no relationship to when the infant is seen.

4 Some parents may be too frightened to ask to see their baby; the nurse can prepare the parents and then suggest a visit.

26. 3 **To cry in this situation is a typical response. It is not unusual to be frightened about touching a small preterm infant and the nurse should provide support while encouraging the mother to do so.**

1 Bonding does not have a detachment behavior phase; the behavior indicates apprehension in a difficult situation.

2 This is not incomplete bonding but fear in a difficult situation.

4 This reaction to her newborn is more complex than merely fear of the NICU.

27. 2 **Parent-infant bonding follows a natural progression involving touch; touching helps the parent overcome fear and initiates the bonding process.**

1 The mother may not be ready for this step on her first contact and the newborn may not be well enough to be moved.

3 The parents are not ready for explanations about the equipment in their present state of anxiety.

4 This may make the parents feel unwelcome and set a negative tone for future visits

28. 1 **By participating in her infant's care, the mother will gain confidence in her own ability to meet her infant's needs.**

2 Watching the provision of care by others may only increase the client's sense of inadequacy.

3 There is no need for a specialist to care for the infant after discharge.

4 The mother should be involved with infant care as early as possible, not just a few days before discharge.

29. 4 **The client's response is appropriate to the situation reflecting disappointment in not achieving her goal; in addition, this is the time "postpartum blues" occur.**

1 This may or may not occur; there is no indication that the feeling will pass or that bonding is involved.

2 The client's statement is not indicative of depression.

3 With rising cesarean rates across the United States, most women know that a cesarean birth is a real possibility. However, knowing this does not negate the disappointment the client feels for not reaching her goal.

30. 3 **Giving the parents information about what to expect during the procedure will help to allay their fears and encourage their cooperation.**

1 The nurse should be able to provide information and interpretation of procedures for clients; delay in answering their questions may increase clients' concerns.

2 An amniocentesis is a low-risk procedure, but some complications may occur.

4 If the father is uninformed, viewing the procedure may increase his anxiety, even though his presence may be comforting to the mother.

31. 3 **During the second trimester the big event is palpation of movement. The husband's reaction indicates enthusiasm for the progress of the pregnancy.**

1 This is true of the first trimester when the father becomes concerned about the future needs of his expanded family.

2 This is true of the first trimester when the father expresses excitement over confirmation of pregnancy and his virility.

4 It is too early to predict the father's response to childbirth.

32. 2 **This response encourages the client to verbalize concerns; verbalization is an outlet for discharging tension.**

1 This response reinforces the client's fears; it conveys sympathy, not empathy.

3 This response denies the client's feelings and cuts off communication.

4 This response denies the client's feelings and gives false reassurance.

33. 2 **Anticipatory grief is expected with a potential loss; ventilation of feelings should be encouraged.**

1 Gentle, not firm, support is required to help the client cope with potential grieving; maintaining a positive attitude may provide false reassurance.

3 This delays the client's adaptation to the possible loss; it is more desirable to allow the client to

ventilate feelings and work through the anticipatory grieving process.

4 The use of the word "it" is not relevant; this refers to the fetus and is an expression of the grieving process.

34. 1 The extent and quality of the mother-infant interaction is believed to be a predictor of positive or negative attachment behaviors.

2 Although this is assessed, it is not as significant as mother-infant interaction.

3 Although this is assessed, it is not as significant as mother-infant interaction.

4 Although this is assessed, it is not as significant as mother-infant interaction.

35. 4 An unplanned cesarean birth can result in guilt, disappointment, anger, and a sense of failure as a woman.

1 This is not usually a common concern.

2 The hospital stay is not exceptionally prolonged; the client usually is discharged within 2 to 4 days.

3 Mothers who have had a cesarean birth can assume the mothering role to the same degree as women who have had a vaginal birth.

36. 2 This is important because deep breathing aids in fully expanding the alveoli and prevents stasis of pulmonary secretions.

1 This postpones needed pulmonary exercises, which may result in atelectasis and retained respiratory secretions.

3 This response avoids the problem; it states a fact and does not allow the client a sense of control.

4 Although this response is empathic, it postpones needed pulmonary exercises, which may compromise the client's respiratory status.

37. 3 The nurse should assess the client to determine why she is having difficulty with breastfeeding. She may be uncomfortable or in need of assistance with her breastfeeding technique.

1 Immediately providing the formula without assessing the situation does not meet the client's needs at this time.

2 Pain may be a factor in the client's frustration with breastfeeding, but this should be determined as a result of the assessment process.

4 This is premature. It is the nurse's responsibility to assess the situation and arrive at a solution in collaboration with the client.

38. 1 This opens communication and allows the client to verbalize thoughts and feelings.

2 This is judgmental; there are not enough data to make this assumption.

3 This does not give the client the opportunity to verbalize feelings and needs.

4 This ignores the client's needs and cuts off communication.

39. 2 A factual response will allay the mother's concern. Vernix caseosa is a cheesy white substance that

covers the fetus. Vernix caseosa protects the fetus from the amniotic fluid while in utero; most of it disappears by 40 weeks' gestation.

1 Milia are white pinpoint dots (sebaceous glands) on the newborn's nose, chin, and forehead that disappear within a few weeks.

3 The nurse should explain only what vernix is; referring to the infant as preterm may unnecessarily alarm the mother.

4 This is not answering the mother's question nor is it abundant on neonates born at term.

40. 4 Teenagers are capable of cognitively understanding the risk of unprotected sex but often believe themselves invulnerable, which leads to risk-taking behaviors.

1 This response does not help the mother to understand her daughter's behavior and may precipitate increased hostility toward the daughter.

2 This may precipitate feelings of guilt and does not help the mother to understand her daughter's behavior.

3 Sexual activity may be impulsive, which is not conducive to a discussion; also, adolescents who are developing their sense of sexuality may feel too insecure to raise this discussion.

41. 4 Each health care provider has a protocol for relieving the pain caused by the circumcision; the parent has the right to be informed before signing the consent form.

1 Newborns do feel pain, although their nervous systems are not yet mature enough to localize it.

2 The mother is concerned about her newborn's pain irrespective of the duration of the procedure.

3 Although the infant may have no memory of the pain, this does not address the mother's concern adequately.

42. 1 The nurse should teach the mother how to formula feed because cultural beliefs are deeply ingrained and it is unlikely at this time that the nurse can change the client's mind.

2 This is a judgmental response that does not recognize the client's beliefs or feelings. It is not therapeutic to contradict the client, especially when the alternative to breastfeeding will not harm the mother or infant.

3 This is a judgmental response that does not recognize the client's beliefs or feelings. This is not therapeutic.

4 Antianxiety medications are contraindicated when breastfeeding.

43. 1 Focusing on the mother's feelings permits her to express fears and concerns.

2 This answer will frighten the client and cut off further communication.

3 This is subjective and cuts off further communication.

4 This answer will frighten the client and cut off further communication.

44. **2 This intervention demonstrates understanding of grief work; the nurse should first help the client resolve the current problem.**
    1 Although this is important, it focuses only on a part of the necessary interventions; the client needs help to cope with her loss.
    3 This does not demonstrate understanding of the grieving process; the present loss must be dealt with before moving on to future plans.
    4 This does not demonstrate understanding of the grieving process; the present loss must be dealt with before moving on to future plans.

45. **2 This response uses empathy; the nurse is attempting to show understanding of the client's feelings.**
    1 This is nontherapeutic reassurance; the nurse has no way of knowing this.
    3 This switches the focus away from the client, whose needs should be met at this time.
    4 This denies the client's feelings; it implies that the client should curb painful emotions.

46. **1 Grieving is expected and necessary whenever a newborn is born less than healthy.**
    2 More data are needed to come to this conclusion; frequency of assessments depends on the severity and type of the neurological problem.
    3 This may be done later, but it is not the priority at this time.
    4 This may delay the client's ability to actively participate in dealing with feelings.

47. **2 Because of the critical home situation, this client is experiencing multiple stressors that may cause difficulty with coping.**
    1 There are no data to support this conclusion.
    3 There are no data to support this conclusion.
    4 The client is attending the prenatal clinic, which indicates that she is aware of reality and is not in denial.

48. **3 This is a reflective statement that opens the door for the client to express her feelings.**
    1 This is not a common reaction of most pregnant women.
    2 This response dismisses the client's concern; it may close the door for further discussion.
    4 Exploring abortion is premature. There are insufficient data for this response.

49. **2 This response provides an opportunity for the client to discuss feelings.**
    1 This statement is confrontational, which may cut off further communication.
    3 This response dismisses the client's concern and does not promote the client's further verbalization of feelings.
    4 This response dismisses the client's concerns and cuts off further communication.

50. **2 This indicates recognition of expressed feelings; a nondirective response encourages verbalization.**

1 This ignores the client's present emotional needs; direct statements frequently do not elicit feelings and may cut off communication.
3 This is a judgmental response because it implies that the client has been negligent.
4 Although this is a true statement, this response ignores the client's present emotional needs.

51. **2 Anger is a coping strategy that allows a person to gain a sense of control over life; the husband feels a loss of control over the spontaneity of his intimate relationship with his wife because intercourse is based on administration of the medications.**
    1 There is no evidence that the client is feeling guilty.
    3 The client is not withdrawing or expressing sadness, dejection, or lethargy.
    4 There is no evidence of the client feeling undeserving of an intimate relationship.

REPRODUCTIVE CHOICES

52. **Answer: 3, 4**
    1 Nausea is an expected side effect and does not require notification of the practitioner.
    2 Weight gain, not weight loss, may occur because of edema.
    3 Visual disturbances, such as a partial or complete loss of vision or double vision, may indicate neuro-ocular lesions, which are associated with the use of oral contraceptives.
    4 Persistent headaches may indicate hypertension, which can occur with the use of contraceptives.
    5 The client may develop hypertension, not hypotension.

53. **2 Oral contraceptives can affect the metabolism of certain vitamins, particularly vitamin C; supplementation may be required.**
    1 It is unnecessary to increase the intake of calcium when taking oral contraceptives.
    3 There is no clinical evidence that links oral contraceptives and a deficiency of vitamin E.
    4 There is no interrelationship between oral contraceptives and dietary intake of potassium.

54. **4 This commonly occurs when women start using oral contraceptives; it is midcycle bleeding and if it persists, the dosage should be changed.**
    1 There is no evidence that this is related to the use of oral contraceptives.
    2 There is no evidence that this is related to the use of oral contraceptives.
    3 There is no evidence that this is related to the use of oral contraceptives.

55. **1 Unless the condom is held, it can be displaced, allowing the sperm to enter the vagina.**
    2 Spermicidal cream is needed because the diaphragm may be displaced during intercourse.
    3 Sperm can be deposited at the beginning of intercourse without the man being aware of it.

4　When the woman has an increase in her basal temperature, she is most fertile and should avoid intercourse.

56. 1　**Studies have shown that women who smoke at least a pack of cigarettes a day are more prone to cardiovascular problems such as thrombophlebitis.**

2　This is not necessary if there are no contraindications; oral contraceptives are effective if used alone.

3　There are no "safe" oral contraceptives for all women; women at risk should be informed of the potential consequences.

4　There are no "safe" oral contraceptives for all women; women at risk should be informed of the potential consequences.

57. 3　**This acts as a reminder that the oral contraceptive must be taken every day.**

1　A woman should wait 2 to 3 months after stopping the oral contraceptive pill before attempting pregnancy.

2　If two consecutive menstrual cycles are missed the client should stop the contraceptive pill and perform a pregnancy test.

4　The client should use a barrier method of contraception for the first month of pill use and if a pill is missed to help prevent conception.

58. 2　**This is the preferred method for clients with diabetes because there are no physiological side effects.**

1　This requires dedication, self-control, and a strong desire to avoid pregnancy; it is not as effective as a diaphragm.

3　Oral contraceptives have a diabetogenic effect; they alter carbohydrate metabolism, and insulin dosage must be adjusted.

4　Because of the possibility of perforation, this method increases the risk of infection for women who have diabetes.

59. 1　**The cervical cap used in conjunction with a spermicide that remains active for 6 hours provides the most effective contraceptive result.**

2　The chemical barrier will not be capable of destroying all the sperm in such a short period of time.

3　The chemical barrier will not be capable of destroying all the sperm in such a short period of time.

4　The chemical barrier will not be capable of destroying all the sperm in such a short period of time.

60. 3　**In a regular cycle, ovulation occurs 14 days before the onset of the next menses.**

1　This occurs in a woman who menstruates every 28 days.

2　This is too early in the cycle.

4　This is too early in the cycle.

61. 2　**The ovum is viable for about 24 hours after ovulation, and if not fertilized before this time it degenerates.**

1　The ovum is viable longer than 12 hours.

3　The ovum is viable for a shorter length of time than this.

4　The ovum is viable for a shorter length of time than this.

62. 2　**The fertile period is determined by subtracting 18 days from the length of the shortest cycle to determine the first unsafe day and subtracting 11 days from the length of the longest cycle to determine the last unsafe day.**

1　This is how the last day, not the first day, of the unsafe period is determined.

3　This is true only if the shortest cycle is 28 days; the date depends on a calculation based on the length of the woman's shortest and longest cycles.

4　The longest and shortest cycles are used, not the average length of a cycle.

63. 2　**The diaphragm should remain in place for at least 6 hours after intercourse because the spermicidal jelly or cream requires this amount of time to be effective.**

1　The diaphragm must always be used with a spermicide to be effective.

3　The diaphragm may be inserted with the dome facing either up or down and still be effective.

4　Puckering, especially near the rim, may indicate thin spots that can rupture during intercourse; the diaphragm should be replaced if puckering is identified.

64. 3　**MedroxyPROGESTERone (Depo-Provera) is a long acting, progestin-only contraceptive that is less likely to cause cardiovascular problems in women who smoke than contraceptives containing estrogen.**

1　This contraceptive contains estrogen and is not recommended for women who smoke.

2　An intrauterine device (IUD) usually is not recommended for nulliparous women.

4　This contraceptives contains estrogen and is not recommended for women who smoke.

65. 3　**One of the side effects of oral contraceptives is hypertension; therefore, they are contraindicated for a woman who already has hypertension.**

1　This is not a contraindication for women who want to take oral contraceptives.

2　This is not a contraindication for women who want to take oral contraceptives.

4　Oral contraceptives may be prescribed for women with menstrual difficulties such as dysmenorrhea.

66. 1　**Many couples in their 30s who are happy with their family and feel their family is complete choose sterilization as their method of contraception.**

2　Sterilization via tubal ligation should have no effect on dysmenorrhea because hormonal influence does not change.

3　The decision for sterilization should not be made by others, only by the woman herself.

4 Decisions regarding sterilization should not be made during pregnancy or in the immediate post-partum period and especially if the client is stressed.

67. 4 **According to Mendelian law, because both parents are carriers, this baby has a 50% chance of being a carrier, a 25% chance of having the disease, and a 25% chance of being unaffected.**
1 This may occur with an X-linked inheritance, or in autosomal dominant inheritance patterns, but not in autosomal recessive inheritance when both parents are carriers.
2 This occurs in an X-linked inheritance pattern.
3 This occurs in an X-linked inheritance pattern.

68. 4 **This is important information; removing the diaphragm too early may allow for some still motile sperm to ascend into the uterus.**
1 Spermicidal jelly should be applied inside the dome so that it is directly over the cervical os.
2 Douching should not be done at all, especially while the diaphragm is in place because it will wash away some of the spermicidal jelly; also it interferes with the normal flora of the vagina.
3 Correct placement of the diaphragm affords a close fit from vaginal wall to vaginal wall while covering the cervix.

69. 2 **Instructing the couple to have intercourse four times a week with at least 12 to 24 hours between ejaculations will increase the chance of conception and will correct the client's misconceptions in a nonthreatening manner.**
1 This is too vague; specific instructions should be given in a nonthreatening manner.
3 To openly discourage the partner without providing instruction may be harmful to the relationship between the couple themselves or the couple and the nurse.
4 Twice daily intercourse is too frequent because it does not allow enough time between ejaculates for adequate spermatogenesis.

70. 1 **Women in the childbearing years should be informed of all options available to preserve the ability to reproduce.**
2 Chemotherapy can depress or destroy ovarian functioning.
3 Destroyed ovarian function cannot be reversed; it is permanent.
4 Both radiation and chemotherapy can destroy ovarian function.

71. 3 **Absence of sexual intercourse is the most effective form of birth control (100% effective) because the egg and sperm do not come into contact with one another.**
1 The oral contraception pill has a high, but not perfect (97% to 99%), effective rate when used correctly.
2 This is a fairly effective (82% to 98%) means of preventing pregnancy; effectiveness depends on correct, consistent use.

4 This is a fairly effective (94% to 99%) means of preventing pregnancy but it is contraindicated for nulliparas.

72. 4 **The client should make up for the missed pill by taking two the next day; taking one in the morning and one in the evening lessens the chance of the client becoming nauseated.**
1 This response does not tell the client what to do if a pill is missed; missing one pill can alter hormone levels and predispose the client to becoming pregnant.
2 It is unnecessary to call the practitioner unless other problems are identified.
3 This is wrong advice; missing one pill may alter hormone levels and predispose the client to pregnancy.

HEALTHY CHILDBEARING

73. 2 **October 28. Nägele's rule for determining the estimated date of birth (EDB) is to subtract 3 months from the first day of the last menstrual period and add 7 days and 1 year.**
1 According to Nägele's rule this is an incorrect calculation; this EDB is too early.
3 According to Nägele's rule this is an incorrect calculation; this EDB is too late.
4 According to Nägele's rule this is an incorrect calculation; this EDB is too late.

74. 3 **Although there are no limitations on sexual activity, as the pregnancy progresses the client and her partner may need some guidance in altering positions to make sexual activity more comfortable.**
1 Intercourse may be continued throughout the entire pregnancy if there are no complications.
2 Sex information can be given by a professional nurse; it is not necessary to refer this client to another care provider.
4 This is unnecessary if the cervical plug is still in place and the membranes are intact.

75. 1 **Any regular activity that was typical before pregnancy can be continued in pregnancy if there are no complications such as bleeding, cramps, or pain.**
2 It is not necessary to stop riding after the second trimester unless the woman is uncomfortable or it is otherwise contraindicated.
3 A woman used to riding horses can continue; no exercise is too strenuous if it was done consistently before pregnancy.
4 Both activities are acceptable as long as the woman is accustomed to doing them.

76. 4 **This response identifies the normalcy of Chadwick's sign and provides a simple explanation of the cause; women often need reassurance that the physical changes associated with pregnancy are expected.**

1 This answers part of the question but fails to explain why it occurs.

2 Chadwick's sign is a probable sign of pregnancy; it is not seen in nonpregnant women.

3 There is no free blood circulating in the uterus during pregnancy.

77. **Answer: 1, 5**

1 **Focusing helps mitigate odors, tastes, and thoughts that may cause nausea.**

2 Sitting upright after meals will help decrease heartburn but not nausea.

3 Prescribed low-sodium antacids may be taken between meals later in pregnancy to promote relief from heartburn.

4 Carbonated beverages may or may not help, but women should be advised to take fluids between, not with meals.

5 **Avoiding an empty stomach decreases the occurrence of nausea associated with pregnancy.**

78. 4 **Increased levels of human chorionic gonadotropin (hCG) may cause nausea and vomiting, but the exact reason for this is unknown.**

1 Some pregnant women do not experience nausea and vomiting.

2 Lightening occurs at the end of the third trimester; nausea and vomiting usually cease at the end of the first trimester.

3 Nausea and vomiting are unrelated to whether the pregnancy is desired or unwanted.

79. 1 **There is reduced GI motility during pregnancy because of the high level of placental progesterone and displacement of the stomach superiorly and of the intestines laterally and posteriorly; absorption of some medications, vitamins, and minerals may be increased.**

2 The glomerular filtration rate increases during pregnancy and is unrelated to the absorption of medications.

3 Developing fetal-placental circulation is unrelated to the absorption of medications.

4 The amount of gastric secretion is somewhat lower in the first and second trimesters but increases dramatically in the third trimester; neither decreased nor increased gastric secretions affect medication absorption.

80. 3 **The inactivated poliovirus (IPV) may be given because it is a killed virus vaccine and will not have a teratogenic effect on the fetus.**

1 This vaccine consists of an attenuated live virus that may be teratogenic to the fetus and is contraindicated during pregnancy.

2 This vaccine consists of an attenuated live virus that may be teratogenic to the fetus and is contraindicated during pregnancy.

3 This vaccine consists of an attenuated live virus that may be teratogenic to the fetus and is contraindicated during pregnancy.

81. 2 **The Food and Nutrition Board of the National Academy of Sciences recommends that a pregnant woman consume 60 grams of protein daily to meet the needs of pregnancy.**

1 65 grams of protein is the recommended daily intake of protein for a breastfeeding (lactating) woman.

3 55 grams of protein is less than the recommended daily intake of protein for a pregnant woman.

4 50 grams of protein is the recommended daily intake of protein for a healthy nonpregnant woman. This does not meet the protein needs of a pregnant woman.

82. 3 **Often there is a decrease in sexual desire in the first trimester, probably related to nausea and vomiting; if couples are informed about this, they are less likely to become distressed.**

1 Calling the situation a problem can cause more anxiety. The client has already stated this began with pregnancy.

2 The client is asking the nurse for information; the client may be unable to answer this question.

4 This does not tell the client why this feeling is occurring; furthermore it offers false reassurance.

83. 2 **The client should be given accurate information. Urinary frequency is caused by the pressure of the enlarging uterus on the bladder. Until 12 to 14 weeks the uterus is in the pelvic cavity. It then rises into the abdominal cavity and urinary frequency diminishes.**

1 It is unnecessary to refer the client to the practitioner. Urinary frequency is an expected adaptation during the first and last trimesters of pregnancy.

3 Telling the client not to worry is demeaning because it implies that the client is not capable of understanding an explanation.

4 It is not necessary to plan for a culture and sensitivity test because the routine urinalysis done at each visit will indicate if an infection is present.

84. 1 **At 12 weeks' gestation the enlarging uterus begins to rise out of the pelvis and is palpable just above the symphysis pubis.**

2 During the early weeks of gestation the uterus remains in the pelvic cavity.

3 Usually this occurs at about 16 weeks' gestation.

4 This occurs later than 12 weeks' gestation when the fundus has risen completely out of the pelvis and enters the abdominal cavity.

85. 4 **Fasting results in hypoglycemia, which can cause nausea; in addition, the developing fetus should not be deprived of nutrients for any length of time.**

1 Fluids need not be increased but should be consumed between meals.

2 This intake is insufficient to meet the nutritional needs of both mother and fetus.

3 Increasing calcium intake will not relieve nausea.

86. 1 **This is within the recommended weight gain of at least 25 pounds for a woman who was of average weight for her height before pregnancy.**
    2 This is less than the recommended weight gain for a woman who is average weight for her height before pregnancy.
    3 This is less than the recommended weight gain for a woman who is average weight for her height before pregnancy.
    4 This is less than the recommended weight gain for a woman who was of average weight for her height before pregnancy.

87. 2 **Most primigravidas feel movement by the 20th week of gestation.**
    1 This is very late to feel initial movement; lack of movement by the 24th week should be investigated.
    3 Multiparas may feel movement this early, but for most primigravidas movement is felt between 18 and 20 weeks.
    4 Twelve weeks is too early to feel movement.

88. 1 **This avoids the possibility of ingesting the cyst stage of the toxoplasma protozoa in inadequately cooked meat.**
    2 Even though this disease is more prevalent in foreign countries, it occurs in the United States and its prevention should be addressed.
    3 This is not related to toxoplasmosis.
    4 This is not related to toxoplasmosis.

89. 4 **Increased estrogen and progesterone levels during pregnancy cause increased vascularization and resultant congestion of mucous membranes.**
    1 Nasal decongestants are not advised during pregnancy; clients should consult their practitioner before using any medication.
    2 It is not common for women to develop allergies during pregnancy.
    3 This is expected because of the higher estrogen and progesterone levels during pregnancy.

90. 4 **The fetal heartbeat can be heard with an electronic Doppler between 10 and 12 weeks' gestation.**
    1 This is too early for the heartbeat to be heard with a fetoscope; a fetoscope cannot pick up the fetal heartbeat before the 17th week.
    2 This is too early for the heartbeat to be heard with a fetoscope; a fetoscope cannot pick up the fetal heartbeat before the 17th week.
    3 The fetal heartbeat can be heard at least 5 weeks earlier with an electronic Doppler.

91. 2 **The uterus remains in the pelvis until the second trimester, placing pressure on the bladder.**
    1 The fetus is in the uterus; this is too early for the uterus to descend, which occurs in the latter stages of pregnancy and can cause urinary frequency at that time.
    3 Fetal waste products are very slight at this time and do not influence urinary frequency.
    4 Frequency is a physiological, not a psychological, sign of early and late pregnancy.

92. 3 **During pregnancy the need for water is increased; it is related to the elevated metabolic rate and expanded blood volume.**
    1 This is unnecessary because there is no indication of a urinary tract infection.
    2 Urinary frequency is expected during the first and third trimesters of pregnancy and it is unnecessary to inform the practitioner.
    4 The bladder needs to be emptied often to prevent urinary stasis and cystitis, which can result in an ascending infection into the kidneys.

93. 2 **The issue of pregnancy is resolved by the time the client is in the second trimester. Awareness of the fetus as an individual and the body changes of pregnancy lead the client to desire to learn about fetal growth, body changes, and nutrition.**
    1 This information is appropriate for the last trimester.
    3 This information is appropriate for the first trimester.
    4 This information is appropriate for the last trimester.

94. 3 **The funic souffle is blood rushing through the fetal umbilical cord and is therefore the same rate as the fetal heart rate.**
    1 Twins will have different heart rates.
    2 The maternal heart rate should be much slower than the fetal heart rate.
    4 The uterine souffle is blood moving through the maternal side of the placenta and is the same as the mother's heart rate, which should be less than 100.

95. 1 **The recognition of fetal movement commonly occurs in primigravidas at 16 to 18 weeks' gestation; it is felt about 2 weeks earlier in multigravidas.**
    2 Palpitations should not occur in the healthy primigravida.
    3 Pedal edema may occur at the end of the pregnancy as the gravid uterus presses on the femoral arteries, impeding circulation. Immediate follow-up care is required when it occurs this early in the pregnancy.
    4 Vaginal spotting at this time requires immediate follow-up care.

96. 4 **Before the nurse can determine the adequacy of weight gain it is necessary to determine the client's current dietary intake.**
    1 This may prevent further exploration of the diet because the client may answer yes or no.
    2 This may prevent further exploration of the diet because the client may answer yes or no.
    3 This assumes the client is not eating properly.

97. 1 **The side-lying position will relieve back pressure; also it promotes uterine perfusion and fetal oxygenation.**
    2 At 32 weeks' gestation the abdomen is too distended to lie in the prone position.
    3 Elevating the head of the bed will not relieve back pressure; it is used to limit GERD. Lying on the

back is contraindicated because it puts pressure on the vena cava, resulting in hypotension and utero-placental insufficiency.

4 Pillows are contraindicated because they place pressure on the popliteal area, which compresses the venous circulation, increasing the risk of thrombophlebitis.

98. **Answer: 1, 4**
1 **Low heeled shoes help maintain her center of gravity to counterbalance the gravid uterus.**
2 A maternity girdle is not recommended routinely.
3 Sleeping in this position decreases venous return, impedes respirations, and puts pressure on the vena cava which can cause uteroplacental insufficiency.
4 **Pelvic tilt exercises help relieve lower backaches, are easily learned, and can be done without any equipment.**
5 Medication should be avoided during pregnancy; prescribing medications is beyond the scope of nursing practice.

99. 1 **Drinking orange juice can increase fetal movement. Fetal kick counts, either the number counted in 30 minutes or the length of time it takes for 10 kicks to occur, are the accepted methods of assessing for the appropriate amount of fetal movement.**
2 Sitting in a tub of warm water may help the client be more sensitive to fetal movements, but it is unnecessary to time 30 kicks.
3 Walking may increase fetal movements but accuracy regarding the timing of the movements is needed to make an adequate assessment.
4 Lying quietly may increase the sensitivity to fetal movements, but they must be counted for 30 minutes for an accurate assessment.

100. 1 **During the third trimester the fetus is laying down fat deposits and gaining the most weight.**
2 There is fetal weight gain throughout pregnancy, but it is most marked in the third trimester.
3 There is fetal weight gain throughout pregnancy, but it is most marked in the third trimester.
4 There is little fetal weight gain during this period of organ development.

101. 3 **The objective of childbirth classes is to adequately prepare parents for childbearing.**
1 This is only part of the class content.
2 This is not an absolute; most childbirth methods inform parents that analgesics are available if necessary.
4 This is only part of the class content.

102. 2 **There is much to be learned and practiced so that the client can vary the breathing and relaxation techniques through the stages of labor.**
1 The Read method can be quickly taught to an "unprepared" woman in labor.
3 The Read method focuses on naturalness and denial of pain.
4 Medication use is acceptable if required.

103. 4 **Effleurage is a gentle massage of the abdomen that is effective during the first stage of labor because it distracts the client from the discomfort of the contractions.**
1 This is the pelvic rock; it is used during pregnancy to relieve backache.
2 This is a technique of breathing.
3 This is a technique of breathing.

104. **Answer: 2, 3, 4**
1 Tailor sitting aids in relaxing the muscles of the pelvic floor.
2 **Pelvic rocking eases the tension in the muscles of the lumbar region. Lumbar pain during pregnancy results from the changes in posture as the uterus grows.**
3 **Forward tilting eases the tension in the muscles of the lumbar region. Lumbar pain during pregnancy results from the changes in posture as the uterus grows.**
4 **Applying the heel of the hand to the laboring client's sacral area (counterpressure) helps to relieve the back discomfort associated with a fetus in the occiput posterior position.**
5 Kegel exercises strengthen the muscles of the pelvic floor.

105. 3 **The amniotic fluid is a protective environment; it does not provide nutrition; the fetus depends on the placenta, along with the umbilical blood vessels, for obtaining nutrients and oxygen.**
1 This indicates that the client understands the teaching.
2 This indicates that the client understands the teaching.
4 This indicates that the client understands the teaching.

106. 1 **A multipara's uterus tends to contract and relax spasmodically, even if the uterine tone is effective, resulting in pain that may require an analgesic for relief.**
2 A primipara's uterus usually remains in the contracted state unless the newborn is large for gestational age (LGA). However, she is less likely to have afterbirth pains requiring an analgesic than a multipara.
3 If a client's diabetes is controlled during pregnancy she is not likely to give birth to a large infant.
4 Although a multipara might have afterbirth pains even with a small newborn, the pain probably will be mild because the uterus was not fully stretched.

107. 2 **The fetus exerts pressure against the spine during labor; back massage provides counterpressure, which eases the discomfort.**
1 The back-lying position is contraindicated because the weight of the fetus compresses the vena cava, decreasing the flow of blood to the placenta.
3 Although abdominal effleurage can be a distractor during labor, it will not relieve back discomfort.
4 The knee-chest position will not relieve back pain during labor.

108. 2 **This combination provides a complete protein for vegans because they do not eat foods from animal sources, which contain all the essential amino acids.**
    1 This combination provides a complete protein and is acceptable to ovo-lacto-vegetarians, who eat milk, eggs, and cheese, but is not acceptable to vegans.
    3 Eggs are a complete protein but are not acceptable to vegans, only to ovo-lacto-vegetarians, who eat milk, eggs, and cheese.
    4 These are both unrefined grains but together they do not provide a complete protein.

109. 4 **A conglomerate of incomplete proteins (vegetable proteins) can result in a combination that contains all the essential amino acids; the client must be taught which vegetables, nuts, and fruits to include in her daily diet that will supply all the essential amino acids.**
    1 Although important, the intake of optimum dietary nutrients is the priority.
    2 The pregnant client should be consuming at least 60 grams of protein daily.
    3 Strict vegetarians do not drink milk. Calcium is found in some vegetables and calcium supplements are available.

110. 3 **A folic acid supplement (0.4 mg/day) greatly reduces the incidence of fetal neural tube defects.**
    1 This is a genetic disorder that cannot be prevented by the action of folic acid.
    2 This is a genetic disorder that cannot be prevented by the action of folic acid.
    4 This is related to the Rh factor and is not prevented by folic acid.

111. 4 **Unless a lactose intolerance is present, the client should drink milk; eating dried fruits and high-fiber foods and increasing fluids and activity will aid in lessening constipation.**
    1 These can cause constipation.
    2 These can cause constipation.
    3 Megadoses of vitamins can be harmful; prenatal vitamins are not a substitute for milk.

112. Answer: 1, 4
    1 **Carrots provide the precursor pigment carotene, which the body converts to vitamin A.**
    2 These contain a very small amount of vitamin A precursor.
    3 This contains only about half the needed vitamin A precursor.
    4 **Sweet potatoes baked in the skin contain large amounts of carotene, which the body converts to vitamin A.**
    5 These do not contain any vitamin A precursor.

113. Answer: 2, 4
    1 Plant proteins are incomplete proteins.
    2 **These animal proteins are complete proteins containing all nine indispensable (essential) amino acids.**

3 Plant proteins are incomplete proteins.
    4 **These animal proteins are complete proteins containing all nine indispensable (essential) amino acids.**
    5 These are incomplete proteins; also, comparatively small amounts of protein are contained in these foods.

114. 2 **A probable sign of pregnancy is a positive urine pregnancy test because it is 95% accurate in detecting pregnancy; the basis for this test is the presence of human chorionic gonadotropin (hCG) in the urine.**
    1 This is a presumptive sign of pregnancy; there are many other causes of amenorrhea.
    3 This is a presumptive sign of pregnancy; there are other causes of frequency, such as urinary tract infection.
    4 This is a presumptive sign of pregnancy. Nausea can occur during the first trimester because of the secretion of hCG; there are many causes of nausea other than the hormones secreted in early pregnancy.

115. 3 **This is a description of striae gravidarum; they occur from the stretching of the breast and abdominal skin.**
    1 This is chloasma.
    2 This is Chadwick's sign.
    4 This is linea nigra.

116. 1 **Measurement of the crown-rump length (CRL) is useful in approximating fetal age in the first trimester.**
    2 This cannot be detected during the first trimester.
    3 Ultrasonography is used to detect structural defects in the second trimester.
    4 It is too early to determine this.

117. 4 **Elevated levels of alpha-fetoprotein in pregnant women have been found to reflect open neural tube defects such as spina bifida and anencephaly.**
    1 This is a genetic defect; it is not associated with alpha-fetoprotein levels.
    2 A Guthrie test soon after ingestion of formula can determine if the infant has PKU.
    3 This is a chromosomal defect that is associated with low alpha-fetoprotein levels.

118. 2 **A full bladder raises the uterus above the pelvis, providing a better visual field of its contents.**
    1 It is not necessary to arrive for the test with an empty stomach.
    3 The bladder should not be emptied until after the test.
    4 It is not necessary to evacuate the bowel before the test.

119. 1 **The markers for true labor are cervical dilation and/or effacement.**
    2 It is not uncommon for membranes to rupture before true labor begins.
    3 A change in the fetal heart rate does not indicate true labor; the rate may be slowing because the fetus is resting or fetal compromise is occurring.

4   The client's perception of the intensity of contractions is not an indication of true labor. Because of admission to the hospital and loss of diversionary activities, the client may perceive the contractions as becoming more intense.

120. 4   **The criteria for fetal reactivity in a healthy fetus are as follows: 2 or more accelerations of 15 beats per minute lasting 15 seconds in a 20-minute period; normal baseline rate; and long-term variability amplitude of 10 or more beats per minute.**

1   Absent long-term variability is an ominous sign that must be addressed.

2   An above-average baseline heart rate is acceptable up to 160 beats per minute. An increasing baseline heart rate is a sign of maternal infection.

3   Contractions are not expected with a nonstress test; early, late, or variable fetal heart rate decelerations are associated with uterine contractions.

121. 3   **In an uneventful full term pregnancy, birth usually occurs within 24 hours after membranes have ruptured. If the birth does not occur within this timeframe, both the mother and fetus will be exposed to sepsis and labor probably will be stimulated by the practitioner.**

1   There is no relationship between ruptured membranes and the second stage of labor.

2   There are no data that indicate that effacement is delayed.

4   Although this may be done eventually, it is too early to anticipate that labor will be stimulated.

122. 4   **The priority is to assess the progress of labor so that the nurse can plan care.**

1   This question should be asked, but it is not the priority.

2   This question should be asked, but it is not the priority.

3   This question should be asked, but it is not the priority.

123. 2   **The nitrazine paper will turn dark blue if amniotic fluid is present; it remains the same color if urine is present.**

1   Temperature assessment is not specific to ruptured membranes at this time; vital signs are part of the initial assessment.

3   Although this may be done as part of the initial assessment, a urine test is unrelated to leaking amniotic fluid.

4   This will not confirm rupture of the membranes.

124. 1   **An overdistended urinary bladder prevents the uterus from contracting after birth; contraction of the uterus constricts blood vessels, preventing hemorrhage.**

2   A digital examination to assess vaginal dilation does not require an empty urinary bladder to be accurate.

3   An overdistended urinary bladder may impede descent but does not interfere with this diagnosis.

4   This does not interfere with the third stage of labor.

125. 2   **When an analgesic is administered at the beginning of a contraction, the uterine muscle tension increases resistance to the absorption of the medication, thereby slowing its passage through the placenta to the fetus.**

1   This is the most relaxed state of the uterine muscle, thereby increasing the rate of the opioid's passage through the placenta to the fetus.

3   Although this will decrease the rate of the opioid's passage through the placenta, it is not the time of maximum resistance.

4   There will be minimum resistance to the opioid's passage through the placenta at this time.

126. 4   **Fetal heart sounds are heard through the fetus's back. When the position of the fetus is in the left occiput posterior (LOP) or left occiput anterior (LOA), the fetal heart sounds are located in the left lower quadrant of the mother.**

1   The fetus will be in the right sacrum anterior (RSA) position if the fetal heart tones are heard in this area.

2   The fetus will be in the left sacrum anterior (LSA) position if the fetal heart tones are head in this area.

3   The fetus will be in the right occiput posterior (ROP) position if the fetal heart tones are head in this area.

127. 1   **The fetus is in a left occiput anterior position because the buttock (firm mass) is in the fundus, the back is on the left, the small parts are on the right, and the head is flexed, indicating an anterior occiput.**

2   The right occiput anterior will reveal the back on the right side and the cephalic prominence on the left side; the occiput will be anterior.

3   The left mentum posterior will reveal cephalic prominence and the back on the same side, indicating an extended head and chin presentation.

4   The right mentum posterior will reveal the back and cephalic prominence on the same side (right), indicating an extended head and chin presentation.

128. 3   **Pressure on the sacral area during a contraction provides counterpressure to the gravitational force of the fetal head in the occiput posterior position.**

1   This may promote relaxation but will not relieve the back pain caused by the force of the head during a contraction.

2   This will not help to alleviate the back pain caused by the force of the fetal head during a contraction.

4   This may aggravate the back pain because it increases the pressure of the fetal head on the sacral area.

129. 4   **A persistent occiput posterior position causes intense back pain because of fetal compression of the sacral nerves.**

1   This position is not associated with back pain.

2   This position is not associated with back pain.

3   This is the most common fetal position and generally it does not cause back pain.

130. 2 **Low back pain is aggravated when the mother is in the supine position because of increased fetal pressure on the sacral nerves.**
   1 The Sims' position relieves back pain during labor, but it may not be as comfortable as the other lateral positions.
   3 This position relieves back pain during labor.
   4 This position relieves back pain during labor.

131. 1 **The major difference between true and false labor is that true labor can be confirmed by verifying dilation and effacement of the cervix.**
   2 Bloody show can occur before or after true labor begins.
   3 The membranes may rupture before or after labor begins.
   4 Fetal movements continue unchanged throughout labor.

132. 2 **Identifying progress and providing encouragement motivate the client and promote a positive self-concept.**
   1 A client in active labor should have continuous partner support unless it is specifically contraindicated.
   3 There are no data to indicate which phase of labor the client is in; diversion is preferred during early labor.
   4 Lying flat on her back may induce supine hypotension; side-lying should be encouraged to promote venous return. The electronic monitoring equipment will not be disturbed when in the side-lying position.

133. 4 **The frequency of contractions is noted from the beginning of one contraction to the beginning of the next; this is the point of reference for one contraction cycle.**
   1 The beginning, not the end, of a contraction is the starting point to time the frequency of contractions.
   2 This is the interval between contractions.
   3 This is too long a time frame and will result in inaccurate information.

134. 2 **This is done to prevent pushing because full dilation has not yet occurred.**
   1 This is not done until full dilation; it can cause cervical edema and may tire the mother.
   3 This is done early in the first stage of labor; it is ineffective in the transition phase.
   4 This is done in the middle of the first stage of labor.

135. 2 **A full bladder can impede the forces of labor and it must be emptied before any other assessment can be made.**
   1 The client's cervix is dilating, and therefore she is in true, not false, labor.
   3 Before this conclusion is considered, the client's bladder should be emptied to relieve the pressure of the bladder on the uterus; the client should then be observed to determine whether regular contractions have resumed.
   4 This should have been established during the admission examination.

136. 4 **This is a description of the contractions as labor progresses through the active portion of the first stage of labor.**
   1 This adaptation occurs in the transition phase of the first stage of labor.
   2 This adaptation occurs in the transition phase of the first stage of labor.
   3 This adaptation occurs in the transition phase of the first stage of labor.

137. 1 **The client is experiencing supine hypotension, which is caused by the gravid uterus compressing the large vessels; side-lying will relieve the pressure, increase venous return, improve cardiac output, and raise blood pressure.**
   2 Raising the head of the bed will not relieve uterine compression of large vessels.
   3 Elevating her feet will not relieve uterine compression of large vessels.
   4 Oxygen administration will not relieve uterine compression of large vessels.

138. 1 **Station −1 signifies that the fetal head is 1 cm above the ischial spines and has not reached the vaginal canal.**
   2 When the fetal head is 1 cm below the ischial spines it is at station +1.
   3 When the fetal head is visible at the vaginal opening it is at station +4.
   4 When the fetal head is level with the ischial spines it is at station 0.

139. 1 **The first stage of labor is from 0 cervical dilation to full cervical dilation (10 cm).**
   2 This is the stage from full cervical dilation to delivery.
   3 This is the stage before cervical dilation begins.
   4 This is the last phase of the first stage of labor from 8 cm dilation to 10 cm dilation.

140. 4 **The cervix is 90% effaced and 6 cm dilated during the active phase of the first stage of labor.**
   1 When the cervix is 6 cm dilated, the individual is beyond the early stage of labor.
   2 The transition is not a stage of labor; it is the last phase of the first stage of labor which begins when the cervix is 8 cm dilated.
   3 The second stage of labor begins when the cervix is fully dilated and 100% effaced.

141. 2 **A full bladder encroaches on the uterine space and impedes the descent of the fetal head.**
   1 The bladder can become atonic but is not physically damaged during the course of labor.
   3 A full bladder may lead to prolonged labor but generally it does not jeopardize fetal status as long as adequate placental perfusion continues.
   4 A full bladder during labor does not predispose the client to an infection.

142. 1 **These symptoms indicate respiratory alkalosis because the client probably is hyperventilating; breathing into cupped hands promotes rebreathing of carbon dioxide.**
    2 This may cause the client to hyperventilate further.
    3 This will not improve the client's respiratory alkalosis.
    4 This may cause the client to hyperventilate further.

143. 3 **Inspection of the perineum is done to determine if rupture of the membranes has occurred and if the umbilical cord has prolapsed.**
    1 This is not a priority.
    2 This is not the priority; it is done eventually if the membranes have ruptured.
    4 The fetal heart rate should be assessed after it is established that the membranes have ruptured and the cord has not prolapsed.

144. 3 **Piggybacking the oxytocin (Pitocin) infusion permits its discontinuation of the medication, if necessary, while permitting the vein to remain open via the primary IV.**
    1 Cervical dilation is checked when there is believed to be a change, not on a regular basis.
    2 Unless specifically requested by the client, there is no reason to maintain this environment.
    4 Although this intervention is recommended, it is not the primary concern at this time; there are no data to indicate maternal hypotension.

145. 4 **External fetal monitoring does not require the insertion of a probe into the head of the fetus. Internal monitoring requires the insertion of a probe into the fetal head inside the uterus, thus placing the mother and fetus at greater risk for infection.**
    1 The monitoring strips are the same.
    2 Each time the client with external monitoring moves, the baseline may need to be adjusted.
    3 Internal monitoring tends to be more accurate because the recording is not affected by the mother's movements.

146. 4 **This is an expected occurrence caused by the interplay between the sympathetic and parasympathetic nervous systems.**
    1 There is no need for this intervention because this is an expected response.
    2 There is no need for this intervention because this is an expected response.
    3 There is no need for this intervention because this is an expected response.

147. 4 **This fetal heart rate change is known as variable-type decelerations. This is indicative of umbilical cord compression that if left uncorrected may lead to fetal compromise; interventions are directed at improving umbilical circulation.**
    1 This is not an unusual finding and therefore does not require nursing intervention.
    2 These are recurrent early decelerations, a result of fetal head compression during a contraction. They are a benign reflex response requiring no immediate intervention.
    3 This is an expected variation of the fetal heart rate reflecting a well-oxygenated fetal nervous system.

148. 3 **The infusion should be stopped because it is the likely source of fetal compromise.**
    1 This may not be necessary if late decelerations stop with other interventions.
    2 This should be done after the oxytocin infusion is discontinued.
    4 This can be done, but it is not the priority.

149. 2 **Respiratory depression of the newborn will not occur if the medication is given at this time; it should not be given when birth is expected to occur within 2 hours.**
    1 The level of pain during this phase can usually be managed by other strategies such as breathing techniques or diversion; giving an opioid early in labor may slow the progress of labor.
    3 An opioid should be avoided within 2 hours of birth; giving it to a client in the transition phase can cause respiratory depression in the newborn.
    4 Giving the medication when birth is imminent is contraindicated because it may cause respiratory depression in the newborn; the mother's level of consciousness will be altered as well, making it difficult to cooperate with pushing efforts.

150. Answer: 3, 4, 2, 1
    If cord compression is allowed to continue, fetal hypoxia results in central nervous system damage or death; therefore, manual elevation of the presenting part is the priority. Then the client should be placed in the Trendelenburg position, which allows gravity to reduce pressure on the cord. The nurse should then administer oxygen because this will increase the amount of oxygen being perfused to the fetus. Finally, assessing the fetal heart rate obtains information to evaluate the fetus's response to the nursing interventions.

151. 3 **This is the most difficult phase of labor. It is characterized by restlessness, irritability, nausea, and increased bloody show; this phase continues from 8 to 10 cm dilation.**
    1 The latent phase is early labor (1 to 4 cm dilation). It is relatively easy to tolerate and the client generally is in control and not too uncomfortable.
    2 The active phase lasts from about 6 to 8 cm dilation. It is difficult but is not accompanied by nausea, irritability, and increasing bloody show.
    4 The early active phase lasts from about 4 to 6 cm dilation. It is difficult but is not accompanied by nausea, irritability, and increasing bloody show.

152. 4 **These are some of the classic signs of the transition phase of the first stage of labor. The increase in bloody show is related to the complete dilation of the cervix, the irritability is related to the intensity of contractions, and the shaking is believed to be a vasomotor response.**

1 These are associated with the start of the second stage of labor.

2 This signals that birth is imminent.

3 This may signal uterine hypotonicity, which can occur throughout the first stage of labor.

153. 2 **This phase is the most difficult part of labor, and the client needs encouragement and support to cope.**

1 Fluid management does not depend on the stage of labor.

3 An opioid at this time will depress the newborn's respirations and is contraindicated.

4 Breathing patterns should be complex and should require a high level of concentration to distract the client.

154. 1 **The fetus's life is in jeopardy and a cesarean birth must take place immediately.**

2 The cord is never handled because it can go into spasm and block the fetal blood supply.

3 This is not the priority; the client must be prepared for an emergency cesarean birth.

4 This is not the priority; the client must be prepared for an emergency cesarean birth.

155. 2 **All signs indicate impending birth; the perineum should be inspected for the appearance of caput.**

1 Assessment of fetal status is important; however, the nurse must first determine if birth is imminent.

3 This is important to know, but it does not address the client's complaint.

4 This is important to know, but it does not address the client's complaint.

156. 3 **A continuous blowing-breathing pattern overcomes the urge to push; pushing before 10 cm may traumatize the cervix.**

1 Expulsion breathing (pushing) should not be encouraged until the cervix is fully dilated; doing it too early may cause cervical trauma and fatigue.

2 This type of breathing is used in the early active phase of labor for relief of discomfort; it is not used to overcome the desire to push.

4 This breathing pattern is not effective in overcoming the urge to push.

157. 3 **The head cannot emerge when the cervix is not fully dilated. Pushing in this situation can cause cervical edema, predisposing the client to cervical lacerations.**

1 A prolapsed cord usually is associated with rupture of the membranes before the head is fully engaged; it occurs more frequently in multiparas.

2 A ruptured uterus may be caused by hypertonic uterine dysfunction or excessive oxytocic stimulation.

4 A precipitous birth results from sudden, rapid labor and an uncontrolled birth.

158. 4 **The color of the amniotic fluid is indicative of meconium staining; the practitioner must**

therefore prepare for the potential fetal aspiration of meconium.

1 The newborn should not be stimulated to cry until the airway is cleared of meconium.

2 Oxygen is administered only after a patent airway is established and if needed.

3 This is unnecessary because there is no indication that umbilical cord blood or a transfusion is needed.

159. 1 **The client is hyperventilating. Using a paper bag helps the client to rebreathe carbon dioxide, which corrects respiratory alkalosis.**

2 The client needs to elevate the carbon dioxide, not the oxygen, level.

3 Compressed air does not enhance the rebreathing of carbon dioxide.

4 An incentive spirometer is used to improve lung expansion, not to rebreathe carbon dioxide.

160. 3 **Variable decelerations are illustrated by a sudden decrease in the FHR below the baseline, lasting about 15 seconds and then returning to baseline within 2 minutes; they are caused by compression of the umbilical cord. If they occur during the first stage of labor, resolution usually occurs when the mother is repositioned from one side to the other.**

1 Fetal tachycardia is not reflected in this illustration.

2 Early accelerations are transitory and are not evident in this illustration.

4 Inadequate long-term variability is not reflected in this illustration.

161. 4 **Early decelerations are expected occurrences as the fetal head passes through the birth canal; the fetal heart rate returns to baseline quickly, indicating fetal well-being.**

1 The data do not indicate that the mother has diabetes.

2 Variable decelerations occur with umbilical cord compression, not prolapse.

3 This will cause late decelerations because of fetal hypoxia.

162. 3 **Mild reactions occur because of vasodilation from direct action of these medications on maternal pelvic blood vessels; vertigo, dizziness, and hypotension may occur.**

1 The progress of labor is not affected by a local anesthetic administered during the second stage of labor.

2 A local anesthetic does not affect the respiratory center in the central nervous system.

4 This is not caused by a local anesthetic administered during the second stage of labor.

163. 3 **The client should be pushing with each contraction; with the head at +3 station each push will bring more of the caput into view at the vaginal opening.**

1   It is too early for the perineum to be stretched to the point of tearing; if this should occur later, an episiotomy may be performed.

2   Meconium is discoloring the amniotic fluid; it is an unexpected finding that may indicate that the fetus is at risk.

4   There are decreased, not increased, amounts of amniotic fluid at the end of labor.

164. 2   **This will prevent rapid change in intracranial pressure after the birth of the head.**

1   This maneuver will not assist in the birth of the head; it is used if shoulder dystocia occurs during the birth process.

3   This may interfere with the birth and injure the fetus.

4   This may injure the fetus; gentle pressure over the entire head is the safest action.

165. 3   **The third stage of labor (from birth to expulsion of the placenta) may last as long as 30 minutes and still be within acceptable limits.**

1   This is an outmoded procedure; it may cause eversion of the uterus.

2   Oxytocin is not administered before the expulsion of the placenta.

4   At the time of admission the client signed a consent form that covers all the stages of labor.

166. 2   **As the placenta separates and descends down the uterus, the cord descends down the vaginal canal, thus appearing to lengthen.**

1   The fundus contracts and becomes rounded and firmer.

3   The client may feel a contraction, but it is not as uncomfortable as the painful contractions at the end of the first stage of labor.

4   Continual seepage occurs when there is hemorrhaging; a large sudden gush of blood heralds placental separation.

167. 4   **Immediately after birth the uterus is 2 cm below the umbilicus; during the first several postpartum hours the uterus will rise slowly to slightly above the level of the umbilicus. These findings are expected and they should be recorded.**

1   This is unnecessary; if the bladder is full, the uterus will be higher and pushed to one side.

2   This is unnecessary; involution is occurring as expected.

3   Massage is used when the uterus is soft and "boggy"; when the uterus is firm and the expected size, it is not necessary to attempt to express clots.

168. 2   **The third stage of labor is from the birth of the baby to the birth of the placenta; a firmly contracted uterus is desired to minimize blood loss.**

1   Providing comfort is a desirable goal but is secondary to the life-threatening possibility of hemorrhage associated with a boggy uterus.

3   This is a concern in the first and second stages of labor; it is no longer applicable after the fetus is born.

4   The maternal respiratory rate may vary above or below this range.

169. 1   **Red, distinctly blood-tinged vaginal flow (lochia rubra) is expected during the first few postpartum days; involution is progressing as it should.**

2   Clots indicate uterine atony, which prevents involution of the uterus.

3   The status of the episiotomy is unrelated to the status of the uterus.

4   Uterine cramps during breastfeeding are evidence that the uterus is involuting appropriately.

170. 2   **Gentle massage stimulates muscle fibers and results in firming the tone of the fundus; it also helps expel any clots that may be interfering with contraction of the fundus.**

1   Elevating the client's legs will increase return of blood from the extremities, but it will not improve the tone of the client's fundus.

3   This will be done if massaging the uterus is ineffective.

4   This should not be the first action at this time; gentle massage to contract the fundus is the priority.

171. 4   **This blood pressure is elevated; intervention may be necessary.**

1   This is within expected limits.

2   This is within expected limits.

3   This is a slight elevation, which is consistent with the physiology of the birthing process.

172. 1   **A full bladder elevates the uterus and displaces it to the right. Even though the uterus feels firm, it may relax enough to foster bleeding. Therefore, the bladder should be emptied to improve uterine tone.**

2   This may be done if emptying the bladder does not rectify the situation. If parts of the placenta, umbilical cord, or fetal membranes are not fully expelled during the third stage of labor, their retention limits uterine contraction and involution; a boggy uterus and bleeding may be evident.

3   Vigorous massage tires the uterus, and even with massage the uterus is unable to contract over a full bladder.

4   This is not a sign of uterine stabilization; the uterus will not remain contracted over a full bladder.

173. 4   **Chances of postpartum hemorrhage are five times greater with large infants because uterine contractions may be impaired after the birth.**

1   Early breastfeeding will stimulate uterine contractions and lessen the chance of hemorrhage.

2   This does not contribute to postpartum hemorrhage because the anesthetic for a pudendal block does not affect uterine contractions.

3   This is a short third stage; a prolonged third stage of labor, 30 minutes or more, may lead to postpartum hemorrhage.

174. 1   **There are several theories as to why chilling occurs; one theory is that it is caused by vasomotor instability resulting from fetus to mother transfusion during placental separation; comfort**

measures such as warm blankets or fluids are indicated.

2 Although the vital signs should be monitored during the fourth stage of labor, they are not being monitored because of the shivering, which is an expected response to the birth.

3 Changes in blood pressure are unexpected.

4 Shivering is not a sign of dehydration.

175. 3 **Pain becomes excruciating with hematoma development at the episiotomy site because of pressure on surrounding nerve endings. This pain is not relieved by the application of ice because ice only reduces edema formation around the incision.**

1 There are no data to indicate the presence of hemorrhoids.

2 There are no data to indicate that the client has a low pain tolerance.

4 It is too early to assume that an infection has developed; pyrexia and local signs of infection support this conclusion.

176. 2 **Voiding will be difficult because of periurethral edema and discomfort.**

1 This rarely occurs with primiparas, even when pushing during a prolonged second stage of labor.

3 A second-degree laceration is unrelated to lactation.

4 A second-degree tear is unrelated to bonding and attachment.

177. 4 **Prevention of infection is the priority.**

1 It is not necessary to stop sitz baths as long as they provide comfort.

2 Stair climbing may cause some discomfort but is not detrimental to healing.

3 This provides comfort, but is not the priority.

178. 2 **A client's temperature may be elevated to 100.4° F (38° C) within the first 24 postpartum hours as a result of dehydration and expenditure of energy during labor.**

1 Mastitis may develop after breastfeeding is established and mature milk is present.

3 An infection usually begins with a fever of 100.4° F or more on 2 successive days, excluding the first 24 postpartum hours.

4 Urinary tract infections usually become evident later in the postpartum period.

179. 2 **During the postpartum period, leukocytosis (WBC count of 15,000 to 20,000/mm³) is expected and related to the physical exertion experienced during labor and birth.**

1 This is not a drop in the WBC count because the usual postpartum white blood cell count is between 15,000 and 20,000/mm³.

3 This is an expected response to the physical exertion of labor and birth, not an infection.

4 This is an expected response to the physical exertion of labor and birth, not an infection.

180. 3 **This phase begins about the second or third postpartum day and involves concern about being a "good" mother; the new mother is most receptive to teaching at this time.**

1 This is not related to bonding. The let-down reflex refers to the flow of milk in response to suckling and is caused by the release of oxytocin from the posterior pituitary.

2 This is the first period of adjustment to parenthood. It includes the first 2 postpartum days; the mother is passive and dependent and preoccupied with her own needs.

4 The behavior described refers to the "taking-hold" phase of bonding. Early parenting involves many behaviors, of which "taking-hold" is only one.

181. 2 **Infection is most commonly transmitted through contaminated hands.**

1 Tub baths are permitted.

3 Douching is contraindicated.

4 Tampons are contraindicated in the postpartum period until the cervix is completely closed. Tampons promote infection when used too early.

182. 3 **If the client is breastfeeding, ovulation and fertility can occur before menstruation resumes.**

1 It is the nurse's responsibility to answer the client's questions.

2 Ovulation can occur while breastfeeding because the process of follicular maturation begins when prolactin levels decrease.

4 This response evades the question. There are general guidelines that the nurse can share with the client.

183. 2 **This indicates subinvolution and needs further assessment.**

1 This is the expected postpartum diuresis.

3 This is the influence of the posterior pituitary hormone, oxytocin, that causes the let-down reflex, which is expected before each feeding.

4 An increased appetite is expected when breastfeeding, especially twins.

184. 3 **Lochia serosa is the expected vaginal discharge around the third to tenth postpartum day; it is pinkish to brownish and consists of serous exudate, shreds of degenerating decidua, erythrocytes, leukocytes, cervical mucus, and numerous microorganisms.**

1 Lochia rubra is the expected vaginal discharge on the first 2 to 3 postpartum days; it is dark red and consists of epithelial cells, erythrocytes, leukocytes, shreds of decidua, and occasionally fetal meconium, lanugo, and vernix caseosa.

2 Lochia is never a dark brown.

4 Lochia alba is the expected vaginal discharge that begins about 10 days postpartum and persists for 1 to 2 weeks; it is a creamy or yellowish color and consists of leukocytes, decidual cells, epithelial cells, fat, cervical mucus, cholesterol crystals, and bacteria.

185. 1 **Breastfeeding stimulates oxytocin release and uterine contractions, resulting in increased lochial flow.**
    2 Weight loss may occur slowly for the breastfeeding mother because of her increased nutritional and caloric needs.
    3 The increased levels of oxytocin and subsequent uterine contractions will enhance involution.
    4 Heat is not contraindicated, and the client may take warm showers. Heat is used if the mother experiences problems such as engorgement or sore nipples.

186. 4 **This measure is painless and will avert damage to the mother's nipple.**
    1 This is somewhat cruel; breaking suction with a finger is less traumatic.
    2 The mother may need to remove the baby from the breast before the baby is ready to let go, and the mother should be taught how to do this.
    3 Pulling without first breaking the suction may traumatize the nipple.

187. 4 **This dilates milk ducts, promotes emptying of the breasts, and stimulates further lactation.**
    1 This will contract the milk ducts and interfere with the let-down reflex.
    2 A large consumption of milk products is not required to stimulate the production of milk.
    3 Breast binders may inhibit lactation; they fool the body into thinking that milk secretion is no longer needed.

188. Answer: 4, 5
    1 Ice packs are used to relieve the discomfort caused by engorged breasts, not sore nipples; if applied before a feeding, the let-down reflex is inhibited.
    2 If kept from the breast for a prolonged period, the infant may become accustomed to the bottle and not wish to breastfeed again; in addition, absence of suckling will inhibit lactation.
    3 Analgesic medication may relieve discomfort but will not help toughen the nipples.
    4 **Exposure of the nipples to air dries the nipples by evaporation; exposure also tends to harden the nipples, making them less tender.**
    5 **Hydrogel pads create a moist, healing environment.**

189. 3 **If the infant's position is changed for each feeding, the infant will exert pressure on different areas of the nipples while sucking, thus decreasing the possibility of soreness from constant pressure on one site.**
    1 Persistent use of nipple shields does not foster effective breastfeeding; the rubber nipple of the shield may cause infant "nipple confusion."
    2 The nipples should not be washed with soap because soap can cause further irritation.
    4 The entire nipple and surrounding areolar tissue should be in the infant's mouth.

190. 4 **Compared with the prenatal diet, the diet for lactation requires an increased intake of all food groups, vitamins, and minerals, plus increased fluid to replace that lost with milk secretion.**
    1 Breastfeeding mothers need an additional 200 to 500 calories and 5 grams of protein per day more than during pregnancy to maintain adequate milk production.
    2 The client needs additional calories, not just additional milk.
    3 This response does not address the mother's concern; optimum nutrition is necessary to produce an adequate milk supply.

191. 2 **Emptying the breasts limits engorgement because engorgement causes pressure and tenderness in an already tender site.**
    1 Breastfeeding should be continued; it is not only unnecessary but also unwise to remove the infant from breastfeeding. Sucking keeps the breasts empty, limits engorgement, and reduces pain.
    3 Learning is difficult when the client is in pain; this may be done eventually after the client has some relief from pain.
    4 The milk culture may be negative because the infection may be limited to the connective tissue of the breast.

192. 1 **This is like binding the breasts; it reduces pain and prevents further engorgement.**
    2 Medication will reduce pain but will not prevent further engorgement.
    3 Milk and fluids should not be restricted.
    4 Cold compresses will prevent further engorgement in the non-breastfeeding mother.

193. 1 **Wearing a well-fitting tight brassiere gives the body the message that milk production is not needed.**
    2 Non-breastfeeding mothers do not need extra fluids; 8 glasses of fluid per day is recommended for healthy adults.
    3 If the client expresses milk from her breasts, she is stimulating milk production and this will not relieve engorgement.
    4 Warm water running over the breasts will promote vasodilation, leading to emptying of the breasts, which promotes further milk production.

HIGH-RISK PREGNANCY

194. 3 **At the end of the second trimester and the beginning of the third trimester, insulin needs increase because there is increased maternal resistance to insulin.**
    1 During the earlier part of pregnancy, fetal demands for maternal glucose may lead to a tendency toward hypoglycemia.
    2 During the earlier part of pregnancy, fetal demands for maternal glucose may lead to a tendency toward hypoglycemia.

4 During the last weeks of pregnancy, maternal resistance to insulin decreases and insulin needs decrease accordingly.

195. 3 **Among the factors that can precipitate a teratogenic fetal response are exposure to the teratogen, intensity of the exposure, and maternal/fetal genetic predisposition.**
1 Exposure to cat feces containing oocysts of *Toxoplasma gondii* can cause maternal toxoplasmosis, which may be transmitted to the fetus.
2 The length of maternal exposure is but one variable in determining if the fetus will be affected.
4 The length of maternal exposure is but one variable in determining if the fetus will be affected.

196. 2 **One of the specific reasons to perform an amniocentesis is to diagnose genetic problems.**
1 This is not a reason for performing this invasive procedure.
3 This is not a reason for performing this invasive procedure.
4 An amniocentesis is no longer done routinely if the client is an older primigravida; a sonogram is done first.

197. 3 **Fifteen percent of the women with gestational hypertension during the first trimester develop hydatidiform mole.**
1 Renal failure is an unlikely complication unless the hypertension becomes severe or there was preexisting hypertension.
2 The client's adaptations are not associated with placenta previa. Placenta previa is a hemorrhagic condition that creates problems in the third trimester.
4 Premature separation of the placenta is associated with uterine bleeding, uterine hypertonicity, abdominal pain, and a boardlike abdomen; usually it occurs in the last trimester.

198. 1 **The infant of a diabetic mother (IDM) should not be larger than average if the client maintains glycemic control during the pregnancy.**
2 This is a true statement, and the client does not require further education.
3 This is a true statement, and the client does not require further education.
4 This is a true statement, and the client does not require further education.

199. 1 **The nurse empathizes with the client and keeps the lines of communication open without being judgmental.**
2 This response does not address the client's feelings and may increase anxiety.
3 This is false reassurance; close monitoring does not guarantee a live baby.
4 This response denies the client's right to emotions and may evoke more feelings of guilt about her obstetric history.

200. 1 **Twins should be suspected with a more rapid increase in fundal height than expected; the nurse should assess for two distinct heartbeats.**
2 Fundal height, not the size of the fetus, should alert the nurse to suspect a multiple pregnancy.
3 This cannot be determined until ultrasonography is done.
4 Weight gain does not influence the height of the fundus.

201. 1 **Smoking during pregnancy causes a decrease in placental perfusion, resulting in newborns who are small for gestational age (SGA).**
2 Facial abnormalities and developmental restriction may occur if the woman ingests alcoholic drinks during pregnancy and the infant has fetal alcohol syndrome (FAS).
3 Smoking during pregnancy and chronic lung problems in newborns are not related.
4 Maternal smoking may result in a small for gestational age neonate; these neonates may experience hypoglycemia, not hyperglycemia.

202. Answer: 3, 4
1 This is not expected if the tube has not ruptured; it occurs after the rupture of a tubal pregnancy.
2 This occurs as a result of diaphragmatic irritation caused by blood in the peritoneal cavity after a tubal pregnancy ruptures, not before.
3 **Pain usually occurs at the location of the affected tube before it has ruptured.**
4 **An STI is related to pelvic inflammatory disease; this increases the likelihood that the tubes will be affected, resulting in a tubal pregnancy.**
5 Ecchymotic blueness around the umbilicus (Cullen sign) indicates hematoperitoneum in a ruptured intra-abdominal ectopic pregnancy.

203. 3 **The position of the fetus and placenta is located by ultrasonography to avoid trauma from the needle during the amniocentesis.**
1 Although ultrasonography can be used to determine gestational age, this is not its purpose just before an amniocentesis.
2 This is not the purpose of ultrasonography just before an amniocentesis.
4 The position of the placenta and fetus, not just the cord and the placenta, is needed for safe introduction of the needle.

204. 1 **The lecithin concentration increases abruptly at 35 weeks, reaching a level that is twice the amount of sphingomyelin, which decreases concurrently.**
2 At about 30 to 32 weeks' gestation, the amounts of lecithin and sphingomyelin are equal, indicating lung immaturity.
3 This ratio does not reflect fetal lung maturity.
4 This ratio does not reflect fetal lung maturity.

205. 4 **It is possible that stimulation of the uterus resulting from the amniocentesis may cause uterine contractions.**

1 This is not necessary because an amniocentesis is not done via the vagina.

2 This is irrelevant because the amount of amniotic fluid is not influenced by fluid ingestion.

3 This is not necessary because the needlestick site seals immediately.

206. 2 **In a healthy well-oxygenated fetus the heart rate increases with fetal movement; there should be accelerations of 15 beats with fetal movement.**

1 This is not a part of the evaluation of the fetus in the nonstress test.

3 This is not a part of the evaluation of the fetus in the nonstress test.

4 This is used in the contraction stress test (CST).

207. 1 **Once the test is initiated the client will require continuous electronic monitoring and will be confined to bed; contractions are more uncomfortable with a full bladder.**

2 The client should be in the semi-Fowler position to avoid supine hypotension.

3 This discussion is premature, causing unnecessary anxiety; however, a cesarean birth may be necessary if the results of the test are positive.

4 Only external monitoring is done because there is no indication that the membranes have ruptured.

208. 4 **During a CST uterine blood flow to the placenta decreases. When there is too great a decrease, fetal hypoxia and late decelerations occur, reflecting diminished placental function.**

1 Although this may cause fetal problems, a CST cannot determine this.

2 The CST cannot determine fetal lung maturity; this is determined by an amniocentesis.

3 The CST cannot determine this because amniotic fluid is not obtained.

209. 2 **An ABO incompatibility may develop even in first-born infants because the mother has antibodies against the antigens of the A and B blood cells; these antibodies are transferred across the placenta and produce hemolysis of the fetal RBCs; if the infant were AB, an incompatibility may also occur.**

1 Problems will not occur if the mother is Rh positive and the infant is Rh negative.

3 A preterm birth will not produce an incompatibility; it may intensify problems if an incompatibility exists.

4 If the infant is the same type and has the same Rh factor as the mother, there is no incompatibility.

210. 3 **This indicates premature placental separation; the classic signs are abdominal rigidity, a tetanic uterus, and dark red bleeding.**

1 This occurs with a low-lying placenta and is manifested by painless bright red bleeding.

2 Information on cervical effacement, dilation, and station is required before coming to this conclusion.

4 Fetal presentation is not related to the client's signs and symptoms.

211. 1 **Early postoperative ambulation helps prevent postpartum complications such as thrombophlebitis and constipation.**

2 Clients usually are discharged by the third or fourth postpartum day.

3 A bowel movement can occur spontaneously if early ambulation and adequate fluids are ingested.

4 Clients are permitted to shower within 48 hours.

212. 1 **The American College of Obstetricians and Gynecologists recommends that a chorionic villi sampling (CVS) should not be performed before 9 weeks' gestation and should be performed between 10 to 12 weeks. If performed before 9 weeks' gestation it has the potential of interfering with organogenesis.**

2 The test, if successfully performed, is 100% accurate.

3 The test, if successfully performed, is 100% accurate and it provides enough information for a diagnosis.

4 A laparoscopic procedure is not necessary because CVS is performed either by transcervical catheter aspiration or transabdominal needle aspiration.

213. 1 **Repeated catheterizations for residual urine increase the chance of introducing bacteria and promoting its growth.**

2 A loss of 250 to 500 mL of blood is considered acceptable.

3 The size of the newborn does not predispose the mother to postpartum infection.

4 This does not reflect the highest risk for infection; a hemoglobin of 11 grams is at the low end of the acceptable range.

214. 4 **When there is cephalopelvic disproportion, a cesarean birth is indicated; infusing oxytocin (Pitocin) at this time may result in fetal compromise and uterine rupture.**

1 The NPO status is appropriate in anticipation of a cesarean birth.

2 A peripheral IV is needed not only for hydration but as a venous access if IV medications become necessary.

3 The client probably has an electronic monitor recording the FHR and uterine contractions; these assessments should be documented regularly according to hospital protocol.

215. 1 **Because of the client's multiple parity, postpartum uterine involution may be ineffective.**

2 Primiparas, not multiparas, become more dehydrated because their labors are usually longer.

3 There is no evidence of an increased risk for a urinary tract infection; routine assessment of bladder tone should be performed.

4 Clients are encouraged to ambulate soon after birth; it is too soon to be concerned about the effects of immobility.

216. 2 **A grand multipara is a woman who had at least 6 births. Multiple parity contributes to an increased incidence of uterine atony because the**

uterine muscle may not contract effectively, thus leading to postpartum hemorrhage.

1 A primipara should maintain a well-contracted uterus because with only one pregnancy the uterus usually maintains its tone.

3 50 mcg of fentanyl is not considered excessive for a primipara and will not contribute to uterine atony.

4 A multipara is a woman who has given birth to at least 2 children. The birth of the placenta 5 minutes after birth of the neonate is expected and does not affect uterine tone.

217. 4 **As with any abdominal surgery, pain is a major postoperative problem during the first 24 hours after cesarean birth.**

1 Oral intake is not a priority concern.

2 Promoting bowel function is not a priority concern.

3 Gaseous distention is more likely to occur later.

218. 2 **Palpation will indicate if bladder distention is present. The increased intra-abdominal space available after birth can result in bladder distention without discomfort.**

1 Assessment should be done first.

3 The increased intra-abdominal space available after birth can result in bladder distention without discomfort.

4 Trauma to the area makes surrounding organs atonic; the client may have a full bladder and not feel the urge to void.

219. Answer: 1, 3

1 **Because pregnant women with heart disease are more prone to anemia, there may be an additional need for iron.**

2 If the pregnant client with heart disease is eating the recommended pregnancy diet and taking prenatal vitamin and mineral supplements, there is no additional need for calcium.

3 **Because pregnant women with heart disease are more prone to anemia, there may be an additional need for folic acid.**

4 If the pregnant client with heart disease is eating the recommended pregnancy diet and taking prenatal vitamin and mineral supplements, there is no additional need for vitamin C.

5 If the pregnant client with heart disease is eating the recommended pregnancy diet and taking prenatal vitamin and mineral supplements, there is no additional need for vitamin B_{12}.

220. 2 **Cardiac decompensation may occur because of the increased circulating blood volume during the early postpartum period, which requires increased cardiac functioning.**

1 Although important, observation for cardiac decompensation is the priority.

3 Although important, observation for cardiac decompensation is the priority.

4 Although instructions are an essential component of care, at this time they are not the priority.

221. 3 **Syncope on exertion is a definitive sign of cardiac decompensation; cardiac output is not meeting cellular oxygen needs.**

1 This may occur in a healthy pregnant woman because of the displacement of the heart, caused by the enlarging uterus that shifts the contents of the thoracic cavity and the increased blood volume and cardiac output.

2 This may occur in a healthy pregnant woman because of the displacement of the heart, caused by the enlarging uterus that shifts the contents of the thoracic cavity and the increased blood volume and cardiac output.

4 This may occur in a healthy pregnant woman because of the displacement of the heart, caused by the enlarging uterus that shifts the contents of the thoracic cavity and the increased blood volume and cardiac output.

222. 3 **The increased respiratory rate is one sign of cardiac decompensation; cardiac output and increased blood volume peak during the second trimester, and signs and symptoms of cardiac disease become prominent at this time.**

1 Oliguria, not increased urine output, accompanied by edema of the face, legs, and fingers is a sign of cardiac complications.

2 The client's blood pressure is within the expected range for a pregnant woman.

4 Diaphragmatic tenderness is a vague symptom that is not related to heart disease.

223. 4 **This is the accepted definition of placenta previa.**

1 This occurs in abruptio placentae.

2 This occurs in abruptio placentae.

3 This may not lead to placenta previa but will place the fetus in jeopardy.

224. 3 **A nontender uterus and bright red bleeding are classic signs of placenta previa; as the cervix dilates the overlying placenta separates from the uterus and begins to bleed.**

1 There is no information to indicate that the client is in labor.

2 There is no indication that the client had contractions that have now ceased.

4 The classic adaptations to abruptio placentae are pain and a rigid boardlike abdomen; dark red blood may or may not be present.

225. 2 **If hemorrhage should occur, oxygen is needed to prevent maternal and fetal compromise.**

1 A perineal pad is not necessary; close monitoring is required.

3 The client admitted with a complete placenta previa usually is on complete bed rest.

4 It is too soon to discuss the neonatal intensive care unit (NICU); this may be unnecessary.

226. 3 **With a low-implanted placenta (placenta previa) the presenting part may have difficulty entering the pelvis.**

1 Engagement is difficult with a low-lying placenta.

2 Placenta previa does not make it difficult to palpate small fetal parts.

4 This occurs with abruptio placentae.

227. 3 **A sudden, severe hemorrhage may occur because of the location of the placenta near the cervical os; blood should be ready for administration to prevent shock.**

1 Freeze-dried plasma is not used in this situation.

2 Adults manufacture their own vitamin K, and an injection will not help to prevent bleeding from the placenta.

4 Giving heparin sodium is contraindicated in the presence of hemorrhage.

228. 1 **The priority is to determine fetal viability; this will determine the next intervention.**

2 Observing for a prolapsed cord is not the priority.

3 An intravenous line will be inserted, but it is not the priority.

4 Inserting a pressure catheter might increase the bleeding; it will not yield useful information.

229. 1 **This will allow saliva to drain out of the mouth by gravity, which will help to maintain a patent airway.**

2 Although birth may be imminent, the priority is to maintain a patent airway.

3 This is contraindicated because it may cause an injury.

4 Observing the client's vagina is not the priority, nor is bleeding an expected response to a seizure.

230. 1 **These adaptations indicate blood loss; to compensate for decreased cardiac output, oxygen is given to maintain the well-being of both mother and fetus.**

2 This will decrease blood flow to the vital centers in the brain.

3 This is not the priority.

4 This may mask abdominal pain and sedate an already compromised fetus. Also it requires a practitioner's prescription.

231. 3 **A total placenta previa requires a cesarean birth; early intervention helps ensure a healthy neonate and mother.**

1 This is a complication that may necessitate an early birth to ensure a healthy neonate and mother.

2 This is a complication that may necessitate an early birth to ensure a healthy neonate and mother.

4 Induction of labor is indicated if the fetus is at term because prolonged rupture of membranes can lead to maternal and/or fetal sepsis.

232. 4 **Folic acid is needed to produce heme for hemoglobin.**

1 Folic acid supplementation does not reduce sickling.

2 Folic acid supplementation will not prevent vaso-occlusive crisis. Adequate oxygenation and hydration help prevent vaso-occlusive crisis (painful episode).

3 There is no change in needs; sickling decreases the oxygen-carrying capacity of hemoglobin.

233. Answer: 1, 5

1 **Tofu contains 3 mg of iron per 3 ounces.**

2 White meat chicken contains 0.9 mg of iron per 3 ounces; dark meat chicken contains 1.2 mg of iron per 3 ounces.

3 Canned ham contains 0.8 mg of iron per 3 ounces.

4 Broiled halibut contains 0.91 mg of iron per 3 ounces.

5 **A ground beef patty contains 2.2 mg of iron per 3 ounces.**

234. 2 **Pregnant clients with sickle cell anemia are particularly vulnerable to infections, especially of the genitourinary tract; the examination of urine specimens should be performed frequently.**

1 Hypothyroidism affects 1 in 1500 women during pregnancy; women with sickle cell anemia are not at any higher risk for hypothyroidism than the general population.

3 Women with sickle cell anemia are not at an increased risk for this problem during pregnancy.

4 Women with sickle cell anemia are not at an increased risk for this problem during pregnancy.

235. 2 **The feet or buttocks are not effective in blocking the cervical opening, and the cord may slip through and be compressed.**

1 Uterine inertia may result from fatigue or cephalopelvic disproportion; it is not related to fetal position.

3 When a fetus is in the breech presentation the labor usually is long and difficult.

4 Rapid dilation and precipitate labor can occur with infants in cephalic positions as well.

236. 3 **This occurs because pressure on the fetal abdomen from the contractions forces meconium from the bowel.**

1 Cord prolapse is not an absolute, but it may occur if the presenting part does not fill the pelvic cavity.

2 Fetal heart abnormalities are identified by auscultation or continuous electronic fetal monitoring, not by the presence of meconium.

4 This is unnecessary; it is caused by pressure on the fetal abdomen during contractions when the fetus is in the breech presentation.

237. 3 **A cesarean birth may be performed when the fetus is in the breech presentation because there is an increased risk of morbidity and mortality.**

1 Vertex presentations in the occiput posterior position usually cause back pain.

2 Labors usually are longer with a fetus in the breech presentation because the buttocks are not as effective as the head as a dilating wedge.

4 Meconium is a common finding in the amniotic fluid of a client whose fetus is in a breech presentation because contractions compress the fetal intestinal tract causing release of meconium.

238. 1 **When the membranes rupture, microorganisms from the vagina may travel into the embryonic**

sac, causing chorioamnionitis. **The longer the time between the rupture of the membranes and the birth, the greater the risk for infection. The temperature should be assessed every 1 to 2 hours and an elevation to 100.4° F (38° C) should be reported.**

2 If there are no other complications, this is not expected.

3 If there are no other complications, this is not expected.

4 This is not likely to occur when the membranes rupture before birth because the fluid exits via the vagina rather than being forced upward.

239. 2 **Pelvic pressure or a feeling that the fetus is pushing down is one symptom of preterm labor and should be taught to the client so that she can seek care immediately.**

1 Leg cramps are not a danger sign of preterm labor.

3 Nausea is not a danger sign of preterm labor.

4 Fetal movement is not felt until approximately 16 weeks.

240. 3 **A breech presentation provides for a greater space between the cervix and the fetal sacrum than a vertex presentation. When the client is a multipara, the muscle tone of the cervix may be relaxed; thus the umbilical cord may prolapse and become compressed, leading to fetal hypoxia and potential fetal demise.**

1 Unless there were other complications, vaginal bleeding is not expected.

2 A urinary tract infection is not related to a breech presentation.

4 As the fetal sacrum is compressed during labor, meconium might be expelled; this is not a fetal life-threatening concern with a breech presentation.

241. 3 **The left lateral position will increase placental perfusion, which may be compromised because of the significant bleeding.**

1 Obtaining the client's vital signs is not the priority.

2 Although emotional support is important, preventing fetal and maternal compromise is the priority.

4 Although important, it is not the priority.

242. 1 **The client is exhibiting signs and symptoms of an amniotic fluid embolism; increasing oxygen intake is essential.**

2 The client is experiencing an emergency situation; checking for rupture of membranes is irrelevant at this time.

3 The client is breathing and conscious; CPR is not indicated, but it may be necessary if her condition worsens.

4 It is not necessary to increase the IV fluid rate, although the present rate should be maintained.

243. 3 **Bed rest keeps the pressure of the fetal head off the cervix. The side-lying position keeps the gravid**

uterus from impeding blood flow through major vessels, thus maintaining uterine perfusion.

1 The Trendelenburg position is used when the cord is prolapsed or the client is in shock.

2 Sitting up in bed increases pressure on the cervix; this may lead to further dilation.

4 This may aid in relieving pressure of the fetus on the cervix, but it will not enhance uterine perfusion.

244. 4 **Prostaglandins in semen may stimulate labor, and penile contact with the cervix may increase myometrial contractility.**

1 Sexual intercourse may cause labor to progress.

2 Sexual intercourse may cause labor to progress.

3 Sexual intercourse may cause labor to progress.

245. 3 **Rehydration fluids contain only saline and dextrose; if the client continues to vomit, she will lose electrolytes.**

1 Monitoring the fetus is not the priority. Early in the pregnancy the mother's well-being will be reflected by the fetus.

2 Although there is danger of infection when an IV is in place, monitoring for it is not the priority.

4 Teaching about nutritional needs is a nontherapeutic nursing action while the client is still vomiting.

246. 2 **A test of the amniotic fluid can determine the fetus's lung maturity; this determination can assist with the timing of a scheduled birth.**

1 This is done with ultrasonography.

3 The size of the fetus cannot be determined by amniocentesis; it may be approximated by palpation or sonographic measurements.

4 Cesarean births are not done routinely on women with diabetes unless a vaginal birth is ruled out.

247. 3 **Insulin requirements may decrease suddenly during the first 24 to 48 postpartum hours because the endocrine changes of pregnancy are reversed.**

1 Insulin requirements suddenly, not slowly, decrease because of the rapid physiologic changes occurring when the postpartum period starts.

2 Insulin requirements decrease, not increase, during the postpartum period.

4 Insulin requirements of women with diabetes fluctuate throughout pregnancy and decrease suddenly during the postpartum period.

248. 2 **Painful contractions at this time may indicate preterm labor or the presence of preparatory contractions (formerly called Braxton-Hicks contractions), although preparatory contractions may be painless or painful. The client's painful intermittent contractions must be assessed further to distinguish between the two.**

1 Frequent urination is common during the last trimester because of the pressure of the enlarging fetus; painful urination may indicate a urinary tract infection.

3 Fetal movements usually increase after the mother eats.

4 Difficulty sleeping and lower back pain are both common adaptations during the third trimester.

249. 2 **Although it has not been proven that bed rest limits preterm labor, it is often recommended; activities are restricted to bathroom privileges and movement to a daytime resting area.**

1 Fluid intake should not be restricted; hydration should be maintained.

3 Monitoring the urinary protein level is included in the care of a client with preeclampsia, not preterm labor.

4 Deep-breathing exercises do not influence preterm labor.

250. 1 **Labor is continuing, and the promotion of the well-being of the client and fetus is the priority nursing care during this period.**

2 This addresses one aspect of this client's needs; the priority is maternal/fetal well-being.

3 This addresses one aspect of this client's needs; the priority is maternal/fetal well-being.

4 This addresses one aspect of this client's needs; the priority is maternal/fetal well-being.

251. 3 **The risk of developing chorioamnionitis (intra-amniotic infection) is increased with prolonged rupture of the membranes; foul-smelling fluid is a sign of infection.**

1 A prolapsed cord usually occurs shortly after the membranes rupture, not 1½ days later.

2 This is an abnormally implanted placenta; it is unrelated to ruptured membranes.

4 Premature separation of the placenta is unrelated to ruptured membranes.

252. 1 **Bandl's ring is a pathological retraction ring; there is a ridge around the uterus at the junction of the upper and lower uterine segments. The upper segment is distended and thin and the lower segment is thick; it is a sign of impending uterine rupture.**

2 Although the ring may occur during the second stage of labor, it is not a sign that the second stage of labor is beginning.

3 A retraction ring impedes the progress of labor; it is associated with premature rupture of the membranes, dystocia, and prolonged labor.

4 A retraction ring is pathological; it is not expected.

253. 1 **Because there is vaginal bleeding, the priority nursing action is ascertaining whether a viable fetus is present.**

2 This is contraindicated; bright red bleeding is suggestive of placenta previa.

3 This is the next nursing action after fetal well-being is determined.

4 This is contraindicated; bright red bleeding is suggestive of placenta previa.

254. 4 **Greenish-brown amniotic fluid is a sign of meconium in utero, which may indicate that the fetus is compromised.**

1 There is not enough information to arrive at this conclusion.

2 This may be necessary if the fetal heart rate becomes nonreassuring, then a cesarean birth will help ensure a viable newborn.

3 Meconium-stained amniotic fluid is not an indication for an imminent birth during the latent phase of labor.

255. 4 **This must be done immediately to maintain cord circulation and prevent the fetus from becoming anoxic.**

1 The priority is maintaining cord circulation; although monitoring is important, it does not alter the emergency.

2 Keeping the cord moist is secondary; keeping pressure off the cord is the priority.

3 The cord should not be touched because it increases pressure on the cord and further reduces oxygen to the fetus.

256. 1 **This client will have lower tolerance for pain and greater need for pain relief.**

2 Larger doses may be needed if this is done.

3 Delays increase anxiety and discomfort, and larger doses are needed.

4 Individuals who abuse drugs need more medication than do others because of tolerance to the addictive drug.

257. 4 **The earliest sign of opioid withdrawal is CNS overstimulation.**

1 These are related to opioid drug abuse, not opioid withdrawal.

2 These have no relation to opioid withdrawal; most postpartum women are hungry and thirsty.

3 These are not specific to people who abuse opioids.

258. 2 **These contractions are too frequent and prolonged for a client who is only 4 cm dilated; the client may become exhausted, which will compromise the fetus.**

1 This is an expected finding and does not need further intervention.

3 This is an expected finding and does not need further intervention.

4 This is an expected finding and does not need further intervention.

259. 1 **This position decreases blood pressure and moves the gravid uterus off the great vessels of the lower abdomen, which increases venous return, improves cardiac output, and promotes kidney and placental perfusion.**

2 The side-lying position does not influence intra-abdominal pressure.

3 While on bed rest the blood pressure decreases.

4 The side-lying position does not prevent thromboses. Bed rest and immobility may increase the risk of developing thromboses.

260. 4 **This is a noninvasive, relatively harmless way to visualize the location of the placenta.**

1 This is an invasive surgical procedure that is not used for this purpose.

2 This provides information about the status of the fetus, not the location of the placenta.

3 This is an invasive procedure that is used to remove amniotic fluid for fetal assessment.

261. 1 **It is vital that a baseline measurement be obtained because increasing fundal height is a sign of concealed hemorrhage.**

2 This is an appropriate assessment, but it is not a priority at this critical time.

3 This is an appropriate assessment, but it is not a priority at this critical time.

4 This is an appropriate assessment, but it is not a priority at this critical time.

262. 2 **The recommended diet for a client with gestational hypertension is the same as that recommended for a normotensive pregnant client.**

1 Protein intake should be increased during pregnancy.

3 Pregnant clients with gestational hypertension should not restrict their sodium intake.

4 Pregnant clients with gestational hypertension should not increase their carbohydrate intake over the recommended amount.

263. 1 **Preeclampsia is characterized by an elevated BP and proteinuria.**

2 This is commonly seen in the third trimester; it is known as physiological edema. Although no longer a diagnostic criterion for preeclampsia, edema, evidenced by excessive weight gain or edema of the hands and face, may support the diagnosis.

3 This may occur in the third trimester because the enlarged uterus impedes venous return, causing supine hypotension.

4 This weight gain is expected during the third trimester.

264. 3 **An increase of 30 mm Hg in the systolic reading or an increase of 15 mm Hg in the diastolic reading indicates hypertension during pregnancy.**

1 This is false reassurance.

2 This response may cause anxiety and elevate the blood pressure even more.

4 There is not enough information about the book to draw this conclusion.

265. 1 **Nonperiodic accelerations with fetal movement indicate fetal well-being.**

2 Early decelerations are associated with fetal head compression.

3 Late decelerations are associated with uteroplacental insufficiency.

4 Variable decelerations are associated with cord compression.

266. 2 **The client is exhibiting signs of preeclampsia. The presence of hyperreflexia indicates central nervous system irritability, a sign of a** worsening condition. **This assessment will help direct the practitioner to appropriate interventions while alerting the nurse to the possibility of seizures.**

1 Although the practitioner will be called, a complete assessment should be done first to obtain the information needed.

3 Determining the client's blood type is not necessary at this time; assessment of the neurological status is the priority.

4 An IV may be started after the assessment, but a more dilute saline solution will be prescribed.

267. 2 **Increasing cerebral edema may predispose the client to seizures; therefore, stimuli of any kind should be minimized.**

1 It is too early to plan for a cesarean birth; other therapies will be tried first.

3 The client probably will receive IV magnesium sulfate to prevent a seizure, not furosemide to promote diuresis.

4 Magnesium sulfate will be used; calcium gluconate is its antidote.

268. 2 **An adequate urinary output, an indicator of effective renal function, is necessary to prevent toxicity because magnesium sulfate is excreted by the kidneys. Signs of magnesium sulfate toxicity include absent patellar reflexes and reduced respirations; therefore these assessments are essential.**

1 Although reduced respirations may indicate magnesium sulfate toxicity, deviations in temperature are not relevant.

3 These are urine tests; they are not relevant to magnesium sulfate therapy.

4 These are assessments that may indicate worsening preeclampsia; they are not determinants of responses to magnesium sulfate therapy.

269. Answer: 1, 3, 5

1 **Headache is a symptom of increasing severity of preeclampsia and HELLP syndrome.**

2 Constipation is not related to preeclampsia.

3 **Abdominal pain is a symptom of increasing severity of preeclampsia and HELLP syndrome.**

4 Vaginal bleeding is not related to preeclampsia.

5 **Flulike symptoms are related to increasing severity of preeclampsia and HELLP syndrome.**

270. 4 **Eclamptic seizures may be prevented by giving IV magnesium sulfate, which is a CNS depressant.**

1 Although magnesium sulfate is a neuromuscular sedative that relaxes smooth muscles and decreases BP, it is not considered an antihypertensive and is not given for that purpose.

2 Magnesium sulfate is considered a CNS depressant that decreases, not increases, the quantity of acetylcholine.

3 Decreased uterine contractions are not associated with magnesium sulfate administration.

271. 3 **Epigastric discomfort suggests liver edema; it is an ominous symptom that indicates an impending seizure.**
    1 Audible crackles indicate pulmonary edema; although they are a sign of severe preeclampsia they are not as definitive as epigastric pain.
    2 Blurred vision is a sign of retinal edema; although it is a sign of severe preeclampsia it is not as definitive as epigastric pain.
    4 Although generalized facial edema is a sign of severe preeclampsia it is not as definitive as epigastric pain.

272. 1 **Contractions lasting too long and occurring too frequently can lead to fetal hypoxia; stopping the oxytocin infusion should stop the contractions, thus increasing the oxygen flow to the fetus.**
    2 The fetal heart rate should be monitored, but this is not the priority.
    3 Oxytocin (Pitocin) will continue to promote uterine contractions; this is unsafe because the prolonged, frequent contractions decrease oxygen flow to the fetus.
    4 This will promote placental perfusion, but it is not the priority at this time.

273. **Answer: 4, 1, 3, 2**
    As fluid gushes out of the amniotic sac, it may carry the umbilical cord out of the birth canal before the presenting part. This should be assessed for first because it is an emergency and immediate intervention is necessary to prevent fetal harm.
    The status of the fetus should be assessed next; there may be temporary tachycardia, but bradycardia and variable decelerations are signs of fetal compromise and emergency action must be taken. The amniotic fluid should be assessed next. It should be clear and not foul smelling; if it is green and/or foul smelling, fetal and maternal well-being may be compromised and medical interventions may be necessary. Finally, the maternal vital signs, particularly the temperature, should be taken routinely. After the amniotic sac is pierced there is danger of microorganisms ascending the vaginal canal, and fetal and maternal well-being may become compromised.

274. 2 **The fetus is at risk for retardation prenatally from a buildup of metabolites in the PKU-affected mother if the prescribed diet is not followed.**
    1 This will not occur if a low phenylalanine diet is maintained by the mother.
    3 The fetus is at risk for mental retardation if the maternal diet is not low in phenylalanine; also, the infant can inherit PKU via an autosomal recessive gene.
    4 The client should restart a phenylalanine-restricted diet when planning to become pregnant and continue it throughout pregnancy.

275. 4 **PKU is an inborn error of metabolism involving an inability to metabolize phenylalanine, an essential amino acid.**
    1 This is metabolized in those with PKU.
    2 This is metabolized in those with PKU.
    3 This is metabolized in those with PKU.

276. 2 **Morning sickness, a common occurrence during pregnancy, contributes to decreased food intake; the insulin dosage must be reduced to prevent hypoglycemia.**
    1 The body's metabolism increases during pregnancy because the needs of the fetus as well as the mother must be met.
    3 Rapid organogenesis requires large amounts of glucose.
    4 During the first trimester blood glucose levels are reduced and glycemic control is enhanced; glycemic control is more difficult to maintain later in the pregnancy.

277. 3 **It is difficult to maintain maternal normoglycemia throughout pregnancy; excess glucose passes into the fetus, where it is converted to fat.**
    1 The problem is excess glucose, which is why exogenous insulin must be administered.
    2 Although all pregnant women consume extra calories to meet the increased metabolism associated with pregnancy, fetal insulin does not pass from the fetus to the mother.
    4 This is a stereotypical statement; not all clients with diabetes overeat.

278. 3 **Therapeutic management involves a comprehensive plan that includes diet, exercise, regulation of insulin dosage based on frequent blood glucose testing, and scheduled medical supervision.**
    1 This is too limited; this alone will not limit fetal/neonatal complications.
    2 This is too limited; this alone will not limit fetal/neonatal complications.
    4 This is too limited; this alone will not limit fetal/neonatal complications.

279. 4 **These test results confirm fetal lung maturity and the neonate should be free from major respiratory problems.**
    1 These test results are not related to the need for a cesarean birth.
    2 There is no indication of fetal compromise; an immediate vaginal or cesarean birth is not necessary.
    3 Further fetal monitoring will be necessary in the future, as with any pregnancy.

280. 4 **Intrauterine fetal death is one of the risk factors for developing disseminated intravascular coagulation (DIC); other risk factors are abruptio placentae, amniotic fluid embolism, sepsis, and liver disease.**
    1 A multiple pregnancy is not a risk factor for DIC.
    2 Endometriosis is not a risk factor for DIC.
    3 A large infant is not a risk factor for DIC.

281. 4 **The trickling of blood indicates continuous bleeding. Close monitoring is required and intervention is necessary if signs of hemorrhagic shock appear.**

1 The pulse becomes very rapid, but not until a significant amount of blood is lost.

2 Blood pressure is normotensive; it usually does not drop significantly until a large amount of blood is lost.

3 This is not a sign of impending hemorrhage.

282. 1 **A complication of deep vein thrombosis is a pulmonary embolism; dyspnea is a significant sign that should be reported immediately.**

2 A low pulse rate is common for several days after birth because of the cardiovascular changes that occur during the early postpartum period.

3 This blood pressure is not significant for a client with a deep vein thrombosis.

4 Checking for Homans' sign is contraindicated because the clot may be dislodged.

283. 3 **Late decelerations are suggestive of fetal hypoxia and occur when there is uteroplacental insufficiency.**

1 Head compression results in early decelerations; this is considered benign.

2 Hypothyroidism is unrelated to late decelerations.

4 Umbilical cord compression results in variable decelerations.

284. 3 **Contact precautions include wearing a gown, mask, and gloves; these protect the nurse from the virus; the client should be in a private room.**

1 The Centers for Disease Control (CDC) guidelines for isolation precautions do not include enteric precautions as a category.

2 These precautions are not necessary for a person with genital herpes.

4 These precautions are not necessary for a person with genital herpes.

285. 1 **During an emergency cesarean birth the urinary bladder may be nicked while attempting to reach the uterus.**

2 Bleeding associated with a urinary tract infection is unlikely to develop so soon after a birth.

3 Lochia is expelled from the vagina, not the bladder.

4 With DIC there would be bleeding from other sites such as the incision and the IV, not just the bladder.

286. 3 **The practitioner should be notified because the increased height of the uterus may be due to accumulation of blood in the uterus from internal hemorrhaging. Also the blood pressure is low and the pulse is rapid, and this may indicate impending shock.**

1 Another intervention will delay the immediate, urgent response that is needed.

2 The client may be hemorrhaging; an immediate, urgent response is needed.

4 The client may be hemorrhaging; an immediate, urgent response is needed.

287. Answer: 1, 4, 3, 2

The priority is to continually monitor the response of the fetal heart rate to maternal contractions. Administering the ampicillin (Omnipen) is necessary for fetal safety. Calling the anesthesia department next allows time for a response before severe discomfort ensues or birth becomes imminent. Starting the oxytocin (Pitocin) infusion should be the last step because the maternal-fetal response to the stimulation of labor is not yet known and preparedness is essential.

NORMAL NEONATE

288. 4 **This is accurate information. The mother needs information that is straightforward and understandable.**

1 This is an assumed reflection of the mother's feelings and does not address her concern; the nurse should recognize the mother is disappointed and offer an explanation.

2 This may add to the mother's anxiety because the reason for the infant's appearance has not been explained.

3 The shape of the newborn's head is most likely the result of "molding." As the baby's head moves down the birth canal the bones move for easier passage of the head through the birth canal. It will take several days to determine if the head is malformed. This response may add to the mother's anxiety.

289. 1 **Standard precautions do not include the use of gloves for feeding.**

2 Wearing clean gloves for diaper changes in all newborns is a standard protocol.

3 Clean gloves should be worn for all admission baths because the nurse will be exposed to blood and amniotic fluid.

4 Clean gloves should be worn when suctioning an infant.

290. 3 **The Apgar score is 8; 1 point is deducted for lessened muscle tone (the baby's arms do not flex) and 1 point for acrocyanosis, which is manifested by bluish hands and feet.**

1 This is too low a score.

2 This is too low a score.

4 This is too high a score.

291. 4 **Lack of skin pigmentation on the surfaces of the mucous membranes makes this the best area to assess this neonate's tissue oxygenation.**

1 These are usually highly pigmented areas and the buttocks often have Mongolian spots.

2 The tips of the ears will indicate the skin color later in life.

3 Because most neonates' hands and feet have acrocyanosis, the nailbeds may be cyanotic as well.

292. 3 **Preventing heat loss conserves the newborn's oxygen and glycogen reserves; this is a priority.**

1 Warming the infant will reduce cyanosis if no respiratory obstruction is present.

2 This is important but not a priority; assessment should be delayed until the infant is warm.

4 This can be done after provisions are made to prevent heat loss.

293. 4 **This action elicits the stepping response, which is absent when paresis is present or in neonates born vaginally in the breech presentation.**

1 This should elicit the Babinski reflex, which is unrelated to a vaginal breech birth.

2 This should elicit the digital response reflex, which is unrelated to a vaginal breech birth.

3 This should elicit the rooting response reflex, which is unrelated to a vaginal breech birth.

294. 1 **An absence of the red reflex may be indicative of congenital cataracts. The red reflex is elicited by shining the light of an ophthalmoscope into the newborn's eyes and observing a reddish circle.**

2 Rinsing the eyes will not affect the red reflex.

3 The red reflex or its absence is not related to the edema that may occur after eye prophylaxis.

4 The absence of the red reflex is not related to eye prophylaxis.

295. 2 **This is the sign that differentiates between these two conditions; with caput succedaneum the swelling crosses the suture line, and it does not with cephalhematoma.**

1 Bruising can occur with either condition.

3 The swelling decreases in size; if the swelling increases, the newborn will have to be observed for signs of increased intracranial pressure.

4 Pain is not associated with either condition.

296. 1 **Bilirubin is a yellow pigment derived from the hemoglobin released with the breakdown of red blood cells as the hematoma resolves. Signs of jaundice should be reported.**

2 This action is not specific for a healthy neonate with a cephalhematoma.

3 This action is not specific for a healthy neonate with a cephalhematoma.

4 This action is not specific for a healthy neonate with a cephalhematoma.

297. 3 **This action should elicit the grasp reflex of the newborn's hands.**

1 This action will cause the toes to hyperextend with dorsiflexion of the big toe (Babinski reflex).

2 This action will elicit symmetric abduction and extension of the arms with the thumb and forefingers forming a C, followed by adduction of the arms, and finally a return of the arms to a relaxed position (Moro reflex).

4 This action will elicit alternating flexion and extension of the feet that simulates walking (stepping reflex).

298. 1 **The antibiotic ointment is administered prophylactically to prevent the development of ophthalmia neonatorum, which can be contracted during a vaginal birth if the mother has gonorrhea or chlamydia or both infections.**

2 Syphilis and toxoplasmosis are contracted by the fetus in utero, not during birth.

3 Rubella is contracted by the fetus in utero. The term "retrolental fibroplasia" has been replaced by the term "retinopathy of prematurity," which is a complex disorder that affects the retinal vessels of preterm infants, causing blindness.

4 Cytomegalovirus and varicella zoster are contracted by the fetus in utero during various stages of pregnancy, not during birth.

299. 4 **The parietal areas behind the frontal bone form the top sides of the cranial cavity. A swelling in one of these areas that does not cross the suture line is a cephalhematoma.**

1 The frontal area is the area over the eyes.

2 The temporal area is the area behind the ears.

3 The occipital area is the area at the back of the head.

300. 2 **Coarctation of the aorta results in diminished or absent femoral pulses.**

1 An atrial septal defect has no effect on the volume of peripheral circulation (minimal shunting occurs in the newborn period).

3 A patent ductus arteriosus has minimal effect on the volume of peripheral circulation (left-to-right shunt).

4 A ventricular septal defect has minimal effect on the volume of peripheral circulation (left-to-right shunt).

301. 4 **Evaporative heat loss is a result of the conversion of moisture into vapor, which is avoided when the newborn is dried.**

1 Radiation is the loss of heat to colder solid surfaces not in direct contact.

2 Convective heat loss is a result of contact of the exposed skin with cooler surrounding air currents.

3 Conductive heat loss is a result of direct skin contact with a cold solid object.

302. 3 **Sudden movement causes the startle response (Moro reflex) that begins with extension and abduction of the extremities with a C shape formed by the index finger and thumb, followed by flexion and adduction of extremities, and ending with return of the arms to a relaxed position.**

1 Turning the infant's head quickly to one side elicits the asymmetric tonic neck reflex that simulates the fencing position.

2 Stroking the infant's back alongside the spine elicits trunk incurvation or the Galant reflex.

4 Tapping the infant's bridge of the nose briskly but lightly causes the eyes to close tightly. This is the Glabellar, not Moro, reflex.

303. 4 **Pressure exerted during the birth process causes increased intravascular pressure, which may result in petechiae caused by capillary rupture.**

1 These are milia, which are white, not red; they are benign.

2 Superficial capillaries are intact capillaries. They are distinguished from petechiae if they disappear when the area is blanched.

3 Bloody stools or oozing from the umbilicus is the most common sign of vitamin K deficiency, not pinpoint red dots on an infant's face and neck.

304. 1 **This is the Moro reflex, which indicates an intact nervous system.**
   2 The Moro reflex is present up to the third to sixth month of life; if it persists there may be a neurologic disturbance.
   3 The Moro reflex has no relationship to hunger.
   4 The Moro reflex is an involuntary response to environmental stimuli.

305. 3 **This metabolic process releases energy and increases heat production in the newborn.**
   1 Fatty acids are byproducts of the breakdown of brown fat.
   2 Shivering is the mechanism of heat production for an adult, not for a newborn.
   4 This will not be successful unless there is an abundance of brown fat.

306. 4 **The site of the outer heel is well perfused and heals quickly.**
   1 This area is an inappropriate site to use to obtain a blood specimen from a newborn.
   2 This area is an inappropriate site to use to obtain a blood specimen from a newborn.
   3 This area is an inappropriate site to use to obtain a blood specimen from a newborn.

307. 3 **The absence of intestinal flora in the newborn results in low levels of vitamin K, causing a transient blood coagulation deficiency; an injection of vitamin K is given prophylactically to infants on the day of birth.**
   1 Vitamin K has no effect on erythropoiesis.
   2 Vitamin K is important for the synthesis of the clotting factor in the liver, but it will not prevent jaundice.
   4 Newborns have a blood coagulation deficiency; the blood clots more slowly, not more quickly.

308. 2 **Meconium is passed usually during the first several days of life.**
   1 Meconium has no relationship to the pathological state of diarrhea.
   3 Passing meconium is desired in the newborn in that it indicates patency of the colon and a perforate anus.
   4 Although the newborn's autonomic nervous system is not fully developed at birth, gastrointestinal function is adequate to meet digestive, absorption, metabolic, and elimination needs.

309. 3 **With developmental dysplasia of the hip there are extra skinfolds on the affected thigh as a result of the displacement of the head of the femur in the acetabulum.**
   1 There are no extra folds in this area in developmental dysplasia of the hip.
   2 There are no extra folds in this area in developmental dysplasia of the hip.
   4 There are no extra folds in this area in developmental dysplasia of the hip.

310. 4 **As the head of the femur moves within the acetabulum, sometimes there is an audible click when there is developmental dysplasia of the hip.**
   1 This is associated with the Babinski test.
   2 This is a neurological finding.
   3 This is opisthotonic posturing.

311. 4 **This information assists parents to understand the unique features of their newborn and promotes interaction and care during periods of wakefulness.**
   1 A healthy infant's lungs are developed at birth.
   2 It is best that infants be on a demand feeding schedule, not a routine schedule. Demand feeding provides for individuality; healthy infants gain weight steadily.
   3 This is a form of overprotection; healthy infants are not prone to dehydration.

312. 4 **An increase in mucus production is expected during the second reactive period; mucus should be removed either by swiping the oral cavity with a gloved finger or via the use of an aspiration device.**
   1 Reporting this finding is unnecessary; identifying and treating human responses is within the scope of nursing practice.
   2 Oxygen administration is useless if mucus is blocking the respiratory passages.
   3 Although lowering the head of the cribette may help secretions drain, the newborn cannot remove secretions that block respirations.

313. 4 **A fat pad covers the arch in newborns and infants; the arch develops when the child begins to walk.**
   1 Flat feet are no more common in children than in adults.
   2 The size of the feet is not relevant; arch development is related to walking.
   3 Flat feet are not associated with deformities of the bones.

314. 1 **Adaptation to the extrauterine environment is largely dependent on the functional capacity of vital organ systems, which is established during intrauterine development; this is measurable in terms of gestational age and weight.**
   2 Although the reproductive history of the mother may influence health, it is not critical to neonatal survival.
   3 Although parental health habits and social class may influence health, they are not critical to neonatal survival.
   4 Although adequacy of the mother's prenatal care may influence the mother's health and therefore the fetus's health, it is not as critical to neonatal survival as is another option.

315. 3 **One point was removed from the Apgar score because the extremities are blue.**
   1 This score is too low and does not reflect the status of the newborn.
   2 This score is too low and does not reflect the status of the newborn.
   4 This score is too high and does not reflect the status of the newborn.

316. 2 **This simple measure will detect hypoglycemia in this large-for-gestational-age (LGA) infant.**
  1 There are no data that indicate a need for oxygen.
  3 Formula will not be given at this time, and there are no data that indicate a need for gavage feeding.
  4 The situation does not indicate the need for transfer of the newborn to the NICU. The Apgar scores demonstrate that this infant is adapting to extrauterine life.

317. 1 **The neonate's first stool is thick and greenish-black and is called meconium; it is an expected occurrence that should be documented.**
  2 This stool is expected; there is no reason to suspect intestinal obstruction.
  3 Meconium stool on the first day of life is expected and does not require further examination.
  4 Meconium is not indicative of bleeding; meconium contains bile and other waste products produced by the fetus; it does not require notification of the practitioner.

318. 1 **Establishing a patent airway, diminishing cold stress, and identification of the newborn are the priorities.**
  2 Application of eye prophylaxis and administration of vitamin K are often delayed to allow the parents to bond with the infant; a bath at this time will increase the risk of cold stress.
  3 These measures are appropriate for a compromised newborn; an 8/9 Apgar score is indicative of a healthy newborn.
  4 These nursing interventions are not the priority care for a newborn.

319. **Answer: 1, 3, 2, 4**
  The newborn's thermoregulation mechanism is immature and an exogenous heat source is needed. Once the Apgar score has confirmed a healthy newborn and the infant is warm, the next step is to identify both mother and infant using bands with the same numbers. The newborn is now ready to be protected from contracting ophthalmia neonatorum and *Chlamydia* with an antibiotic, and hemorrhagic disease of the newborn with vitamin K.

320. 3 **The test cannot be done until the newborn has ingested a high phenylalanine (formula or breast milk) diet for at least 48 hours.**
  1 The test can be done at any weight; the important factor is ingestion of milk for at least 48 hours to obtain a reading.
  2 This is not the reason why the test is not being done at this time.
  4 Measurable enzymes are produced after the infant has ingested milk for at least 48 hours.

321. 3 **Phenylalanine, an essential amino acid necessary for growth and development, cannot be metabolized in infants with PKU; early diagnosis and treatment may prevent mental retardation.**
  1 This is done at the same time as PKU testing, but there is no relationship between thyroid deficiency and PKU.
  2 Recognition and treatment of PKU early in life can help prevent, not detect, mental retardation.
  4 Chromosomal damage cannot be detected with a PKU test.

322. 2 **Holding the infant upright enables gravity to move the feeding through the pyloric sphincter, which minimizes regurgitation.**
  1 Although it is common for infants to regurgitate, this response will not enhance mothering skills.
  3 The infant has had enough formula and does not require more during this feeding.
  4 A newborn should not be propped after feeding because pressure of the abdomen on the stomach puts pressure on the esophagus, which can precipitate regurgitation.

323. 3 **The newborn should not be submerged in a tub. The penis should be gently cleaned with clear, warm water; in addition, sponge baths are given until the cord stump detaches.**
  1 The diaper should be changed frequently to prevent irritation from the urine.
  2 There should be minimal bleeding; excessive bleeding requires immediate attention.
  4 Petrolatum gauze prevents the diaper from adhering to the operative site.

324. 1 **Applying the diaper loosely is done to avoid pressure on the circumcised area because the glans remains tender for 2 to 3 days.**
  2 Aspirin may prolong clotting and is contraindicated in children because of its relationship to Reye syndrome. Acetaminophen and comfort measures may be prescribed.
  3 The caregiver should check for bleeding every hour for the first 12 hours after the circumcision.
  4 Whitish exudate around the glans is expected and does not indicate an infectious process.

325. 4 **The gastrocolic reflex is stimulated when the newborn's stomach begins to fill with fluid; this causes an increase in peristalsis resulting in the passage of stool during or after a feeding.**
  1 Six to 10 voidings a day of pale straw-colored urine are indicative of adequate fluid intake, not the frequency of bowel movements.
  2 The cardiac sphincter is unrelated to bowel movements; the cardiac sphincter, located between the esophagus and the stomach, is immature in the newborn and is the reason for the newborn's tendency to regurgitate some of the feedings.
  3 Although pancreatic amylase is a digestive enzyme, it does not stimulate bowel movements after feedings.

326. 1 **The major purpose of this screening test is to determine if the infant has phenylketonuria (PKU), which can be detected after the infant has started ingesting milk.**

2 This is not the objective of the test for PKU.

3 Epidemiological information is a purpose of genetic screening; in this instance the most important determination is whether or not the infant has PKU.

4 Risk for later development of the disorder is not the purpose of PKU testing; it is to determine if the neonate has the disorder.

327. 4 **Frequent cleansing and diaper changing will limit the presence of irritating substances.**

1 Having the nurses change the diaper may lower the mother's self-esteem.

2 Powder and lotion will cake and retain moisture in the area.

3 This is a nursing, not a medical, problem.

328. 2 **After birth, fetal erythrocytes hemolyze, releasing bilirubin into the circulation, which the immature liver cannot metabolize as rapidly as it is produced, resulting in physiological jaundice.**

1 Jaundice is not an allergic response.

3 Bile duct obstruction, which is not common in newborns, is not the cause of the jaundice.

4 The newborn and mother have independent circulations and Rh-negative blood does not enter the fetus's bloodstream. A problem can occur if the mother is sensitized because her antibodies can enter the fetal circulation.

329. 2 **Jaundice that appears within 24 hours may be indicative of a pathological process; if the bilirubin level is elevated, intervention is required.**

1 Jaundice is not an indication for admission unless accompanied by a very high serum bilirubin level.

3 Physiologic jaundice does not appear until 72 hours after birth; this observation in 24 hours indicates pathologic hyperbilirubinemia.

4 The infant may require phototherapy after further assessment, but this is not the first action.

330. 1 **This is typified by the touch that shows maternal bonding; attachment is manifested when the newborn is compared to the father.**

2 Attachment behaviors in the neonate are defined as grasping and sucking the nipple.

3 Consummatory behaviors in the newborn are coordinated sucking and swallowing.

4 The mother's behavior does not demonstrate overprotection.

331. 4 **The parents need an opportunity for close eye-to-eye contact during the first hour. Prophylactic eye medications may irritate the newborn's eyes, preventing them from opening.**

1 Assessment is appropriate but will not facilitate parent-newborn bonding; favorable conditions for bonding should be provided before assessment.

2 The nurse should assess, not demonstrate, behavior at this time.

3 Footprinting should be done immediately to ensure proper identification of the newborn.

332. 4 **Stimulating the rooting reflex effectively encourages the newborn to turn toward the breast in preparation for suckling.**

1 Giving the neonate a bottle may interfere with learning to accept the breast.

2 For milk to be expressed the infant must grasp the entire areola, which contains the secretory ducts.

3 At first the mother should be supervised to help ensure a successful experience.

333. 2 **Effective attachment involves covering most of the areolar surface of the breast with the newborn's mouth; effective attachment helps compress the milk glands.**

1 The nipple must be on top of the newborn's tongue.

3 Loud sucking sounds indicate inadequate attachment.

4 The newborn should suckle for a longer period; the newborn may be sucking only on the nipple.

334. 2 **The presence of at least six to eight wet diapers each day indicates sufficient breast milk intake.**

1 Several firm stools daily may indicate an inadequate amount of fluid ingestion; the stools of breastfeeding neonates should be soft to loose.

3 Spitting out a pacifier is not an indication of adequate milk consumption; some infants need extra sucking stimulation.

4 Awakening to feed every four hours is not a reliable indicator of adequate breast milk intake; sleep patterns vary.

335. 2 **At about 6 months of age infants are able to swallow independently of sucking, and a cup can be introduced.**

1 Introducing a cup at 4 months is inappropriate because the infant does not have the ability to swallow independently of sucking at this age.

3 Between 9 and 12 months of age, infants can swallow four or five times consecutively and hold and carry a cup to the mouth; introduction of a cup at age 6 months makes the weaning easier at 9 to 12 months of age.

4 Sixteen months is too late to introduce a cup; by this time the child has teeth, and sucking on a bottle promotes the development of caries as well as a preference for milk over solid foods.

336. 2 **Unless fluoridated water is used by the manufacturer, fluoride supplementation of 0.25 mg daily is required.**

1 Commercial formulas are iron fortified.

3 The supply of vitamin K is adequate after the first week of life.

4 Vitamin B_{12} is unnecessary; it may be needed if the mother is a vegetarian and is breastfeeding.

337. 4 **Early weight loss occurs because excess fluid is lost, not body mass.**

1 Weight loss is expected; there are no data to support an allergic response.

2 Weight loss is not related to hypoglycemia.

3 Neither breast nor formula feeding will prevent the 10% weight loss that is expected in the first few days of life.

338. 2 **Healing is optimal when the area is left alone or, if needed, is washed with mild soap and water and then gently dried.**

1 The cord clamp is removed when the cord stump is dry, usually at 24 hours.

3 Ointment and other emollients will keep the cord moist; rapid drying of the cord is preferred.

4 This prevents the cord from drying and provides a dark, warm, moist medium for growth of organisms.

339. 4 **If the newborn is cold there is an increased brown fat metabolism (nonshivering thermogenesis), which elevates fatty acids in the blood, predisposing to acidosis.**

1 Newborns do not shiver.

2 Hypoglycemia, not hyperglycemia, can occur because the newborn's glycogen reserves are depleted rapidly when under stress.

3 Although oxygen consumption increases during cold stress, it is not the priority; increased fat metabolism is more serious.

HIGH-RISK NEONATE

340. 4 **An infant of a diabetic mother (IDM) produces higher levels of insulin in response to the elevated maternal glucose levels; after birth it takes several hours for the newborn to adjust to the loss of the maternal glucose.**

1 Healthy newborns' glucose levels do not drop significantly after birth.

2 Newborns' pancreases usually do produce more insulin as a response to maternal glucose levels, but this response is not specific to the IDM.

3 IDMs have the same glucose stores as other newborns; their responses to the loss of maternal glucose levels differ.

341. 3 **A 36-week old, large-for-gestational-age (LGA) infant of a mother with diabetes (IDM) may have immature lung tissue, which predisposes to respiratory distress.**

1 Meconium ileus is suggestive of cystic fibrosis, which is unrelated to maternal diabetes.

2 Physiologic jaundice is manifested about 24 hours after birth when fetal red blood cells begin to hemolyze; this is unrelated to maternal diabetes.

4 Increased intracranial pressure may be associated with birth injury or hydrocephalus; it is unrelated to maternal diabetes.

342. 2 **Morbidity and mortality rates of preterm neonates are highest between 24 and 26 weeks' gestation; complications include immature lung tissue, altered cardiac output, patent ductus arteriosus, intraventricular hemorrhage, necrotizing enterocolitis, and infections.**

1 Based on the status of cervical effacement and dilation a decision can be made to try to halt labor with the use of tocolytic medications and limited activity.

3 If possible, the pregnancy should be maintained past 37 weeks' gestation.

4 Neonates born at 34 weeks' gestation are still at high risk.

343. 4 **Transparent red skin is expected because of the absence of subcutaneous fat tissue.**

1 Preterm infants born nearer to term have open, staring eyes.

2 Preterm infants generally are born with large amounts of lanugo that begins to thin just before term and by 40 weeks is found only on the shoulders, back, and upper arms.

3 The preterm infant's scrotum is small and the testicles usually are high in the inguinal canal.

344. 1 **Preterm neonates are prone to respiratory distress; flaring nares are a compensatory mechanism in a neonate with respiratory distress syndrome (RDS) that attempts to lessen resistance of narrow nasal passages and increase oxygen intake.**

2 Acrocyanosis is not related to respiratory distress but is caused by vasomotor instability; this is an expected occurrence in the newborn.

3 A heartbeat of 140 beats per minute is an expected finding in the newborn.

4 Respirations of 40 breaths per minute is an expected finding in the newborn.

345. 3 **The mother should be given an opportunity to breastfeed, knowing that it will be terminated if the infant becomes exhausted. If the infant cannot breastfeed, the mother's breasts can be pumped and the breast milk used for gavage feedings.**

1. There is no indication of a plan to feed the infant by gavage.

2 Time and effort are insufficient reasons to discourage pumping the breasts.

4 Breast milk provides optimum nutrition, protects the infant from necrotizing enterocolitis, and provides antibodies.

346. Answer: 2, 4, 5

1 Crackles occur in the healthy newborn.

2 **Cyanosis occurs because of inadequate oxygenation.**

3 Wheezing in the newborn is benign.

4 **Tachypnea is a compensatory mechanism to increase oxygenation.**

5 **Retractions occur in an effort to increase lung capacity.**

347. 1 **At 34 weeks' gestation the respiratory system is not fully developed; adequate oxygenation is the priority. Newborn respirations range from 30 to 60/minute.**

2 A weight gain of 30 grams is too rapid a weight increase; 20 to 25 grams per day is expected at this gestational age.

3 A temperature of 98° F (36.7° C) is adequate for a newborn; increasing it to 98.6 ° F (37° C) is not necessary at this time.

4 The heart rate of a newborn is 110 to 160 beats per minute; a heart rate of 130 is within the expected range.

348. 3 **In respiratory acidosis, the pH decreases and the carbon dioxide level increases.**

1 This is within the expected range of 7.32 to 7.49 for a neonate.

2 This is within the expected range of 3.5 to 5 mEq/L.

4 The arterial oxygen level may or may not change with acidosis.

349. 4 **This breathing pattern is indicative of respiratory distress; the expected pattern is abdominal with synchronous chest movement.**

1 This is within the expected range of 97.6° F (36.4° C) to 99° F (37.2° C) for a newborn.

2 This is caused by uric acid crystals from the immature kidneys; it is a common occurrence.

3 This is within the expected range of 110 to 160 beats per minute for a newborn.

350. 1 **The oxygen must be warmed and humidified to avoid hypothermia and drying of the mucous membranes.**

2 Bright pink skin and mucous membranes may indicate an excessively high arterial oxygen level, which predisposes to retinopathy of prematurity.

3 Oxygen levels are monitored every 1 to 2 hours and are adjusted in response to the infant's condition.

4 Blindness develops with excessive arterial oxygen levels, which can occur at any percentage of oxygen.

351. 2 **The lights used for phototherapy can damage the infant's eyes, and eye shields are standard equipment.**

1 Maximum effectiveness is achieved when the infant's entire skin surface is exposed to the light.

3 Vitamin E oil is contraindicated because it can cause burns as well as result in an overdose of the vitamin.

4 The infant should be turned every 2 hours irrespective of feeding times so that all body surfaces are exposed to the light and no single body surface is overexposed.

352. 3 **Constant drainage of urine on the skin promotes excoriation and infection; it must be protected.**

1 Sterility is impossible to maintain because of the constant leakage of urine.

2 Output will be difficult to measure because of the constant leakage of urine.

4 A pressure dressing is contraindicated because it will traumatize the exposed bladder.

353. 2 **Positioning with the head slightly hyperextended and changing the position every 1 to 2 hours helps to drain respiratory secretions; this will increase oxygenation by enhancing respiratory efforts.**

1 Extensive handling is not desired, but infants do need to be touched.

3 All newborns are assessed for congenital birth defects, not just those with RDS.

4 This temperature is too low; it may exacerbate the respiratory distress.

354. 1 **A preterm, small-for-gestational-age (SGA) infant is at risk for problems not seen in the term small-for-gestational-age infant because of immaturity. This information will help the nurse to anticipate potential problems and aim interventions at prevention.**

2 The infant will lose weight, but the comparison of birthweight and gestational age is important for planning appropriate nursing measures.

3 The information is documented in the infant's record, but this is not the overriding reason for obtaining the data.

4 The health insurance company needs this information, but this is not the overriding reason for obtaining the data.

355. 4 **The Silverman-Anderson score is an index of neonatal respiratory distress.**

1 This score does not reflect cardiac function.

2 This score does not reflect neurological status.

3 This score does not reflect caloric needs.

356. 1 **The release, following compression of the chest during a vaginal birth, is the mechanism for expansion of the newborn's lungs; because this does not occur during a cesarean birth, lung expansion may be incomplete and atelectasis may result.**

2 Temperature change is not implicated in aspiration.

3 The infant is monitored closely to prevent oxygen deprivation.

4 Gravity can be used to promote drainage from the lungs after a cesarean birth by holding the newborn's head lower than the chest.

357. 3 **Breast tissue is not palpable in a newborn of less than 33 weeks' gestation.**

1 The ear pinnae spring back in an infant at 36 weeks' gestation.

2 Creases in the palms and on the soles of the feet are not clearly defined until after the 37th week of gestation.

4 A zero-degree square window sign is present in an infant at 40 to 42 weeks' gestation.

358. 4 **The assessment findings are indicative of a preterm infant; therefore, the nurse should monitor the infant for signs of respiratory distress syndrome.**

1 Preterm large-for-gestational-age (LGA) infants may develop polycythemia, but there are no data to indicate the infant is LGA.

2 Preterm infants may become hypoglycemic, not hyperglycemic.

3 The neonate is preterm, not postterm.

359. 4 **The pathological changes of maternal chronic vascular disease cause uteroplacental insufficiency;**

vasospasms diminish fetal oxygenation and nutrition, which lead to slow fetal growth.

1 Prematurity is defined as gestational age of less than 37 weeks.

2 There is no greater incidence of cardiac anomalies in infants with intrauterine growth restriction.

3 There is no greater incidence of infection in infants with low birthweight; however, they may have lowered resistance to infection.

360. **2 Hypoglycemia is common in newborns who are small for gestational age because of malnutrition in utero; the nurse can detect this with a blood glucose test and notify the practitioner.**

1 Polycythemia, not anemia, is more likely to occur.

3 Although a protein deficiency may occur, it is not life threatening at this time.

4 Although hypocalcemia may occur, it is not as common as hypoglycemia.

361. **2 SGA infants may exhibit hypoglycemia, especially during the first 2 days of life because of depleted glycogen stores and inhibited gluconeogenesis.**

1 These are not signs of hypervolemia. Hypervolemia usually is the result of excessive intravenous infusion. It is unlikely that a full-term SGA infant will need IV supplementation.

3 Hypercalcemia is uncommon in newborns.

4 These signs are unrelated to hypothyroidism; signs of hypothyroidism are difficult to identify in the newborn.

362. **4 Numerous superficial veins are observed in the preterm infant because of the lack of subcutaneous fat deposits.**

1 Flexion of the extremities is the posturing of healthy term infants; preterm infants usually posture with extremities extended and flaccid.

2 Absent femoral pulses are indicative of coarctation of the aorta, a congenital heart defect that is not related to gestational age.

3 A positive Babinski reflex is expected in the full-term, not preterm, newborn.

363. **1 Primary manifestations of NEC are feeding intolerance, increased gastric residual of undigested formula, and bile-stained emesis.**

2 This occurs with diarrhea; stools in infants with NEC are generally reduced in number and contain glucose and blood.

3 This occurs with hypertrophic pyloric stenosis.

4 This may occur with a cardiac anomaly, not NEC.

364. **2 Prolonged gastric emptying occurs with NEC; an increase in abdominal girth of greater than 1 cm in 4 hours is significant and needs immediate intervention.**

1 Formula feedings are stopped and the infant is given parenteral therapy.

3 Formula feedings are stopped and the infant is given parenteral therapy.

4. This will have no therapeutic value for an infant with NEC.

365. **1 Gradually rewarming an infant experiencing cold stress is essential to avoid compromising the infant's cardiopulmonary status.**

2 It is not necessary to notify the practitioner. It is the nurse's responsibility to rewarm the infant.

3 Infants experiencing cold stress will become hypoglycemic because glycogen and glucose are metabolized to maintain the core temperature.

4 Skin temperatures should be taken at least every 15 minutes until stable.

366. **2 The nurse applies tactile stimulation after validating that respirations are absent; this action may be sufficient to reestablish respirations in the high-risk neonate with frequent episodes of apnea.**

1 Assessment will not interrupt the period of apnea; respirations must be reestablished immediately.

3 The monitor should be assessed for proper functioning before use.

4 These measures are too invasive and aggressive for initial intervention; gentle stimulation should be attempted first.

367. **1 The reflexes and muscles of sucking and swallowing are immature; this may result in oral feedings that are ineffectual and exhausting.**

2 The metabolic rate is increased because of fatigue and growth needs.

3 The digestive process is slow, especially in the ability to digest lipids.

4 Absorption of nutrients is decreased because the gastrointestinal tract is immature.

368. **4 Retinopathy of prematurity (ROP) is a complex disease of the preterm infant; hyperoxemia is one of the numerous causes implicated. Oxygen therapy is maintained at the lowest level necessary to support respiratory status. If the oxygen concentration needs to be increased to maintain life, then ROP may not be preventable.**

1 Using a shield over the neonate's eyes will not prevent the development of ROP.

2 Positioning does not prevent ROP.

3 Assessment of the neonate every hour with a pulse oximeter alone will not prevent ROP. If the pulse oximeter results are within an acceptable range, oxygen concentration can be reduced.

369. **3 Ophthalmia neonatorum is caused by gonorrheal and/or chlamydial infections present in the vaginal tract. It is preventable by prophylactic use of an antibiotic ophthalmic ointment applied to the neonate's eyes.**

1 Herpes affects the neonate systemically.

2 Retrolental fibroplasia (retinopathy of prematurity) occurs from prolonged exposure to an oxygen concentration that is too high.

4 Hemorrhagic conjunctivitis usually is caused by rapid expulsion of the fetus's head from the vagina.

370. 3 **Observing the care that the parents actually give the infant provides direct validation of their skill and comfort levels.**

1 This action is helpful for providing anticipatory guidance but it is a small part of a competency evaluation.

2 Although this is helpful in identifying empirical knowledge, it does not test the parents' skill or comfort level.

4 This does not provide enough evidence of the parents' competency.

371. 4 **Newborns of diabetic mothers may be large for gestational age (LGA) because hyperglycemia in the mother precipitates hyperinsulinism in the fetus, resulting in excess deposits of fetal fat; they usually are born at or before term.**

1 Although these newborns generally are born at term, usually they are large, not average, for gestational age.

2 These newborns are large, not small, for gestational age. Diabetic mothers with advanced vascular and renal disease may have infants that are small for gestational age.

3 Because of the risk for fetal death, women with diabetes should give birth before the 40th week of gestation, either via induction of labor or if necessary by cesarean birth.

372. 4 **This is within the expected blood glucose level for a neonate (40 to 60 mg/dL) and requires no measures other than continued monitoring for the next 24 hours.**

1 Heel sticks are adequate for monitoring the blood glucose levels of a neonate.

2 Oral feedings of 10% dextrose in water are administered if the neonate's blood glucose level is low.

3 Administering 50% dextrose intravenously will cause hyperglycemia in the neonate.

373. 1 **A difficult birth because of broad fetal shoulders may result in a fractured clavicle, as evidenced by a knot or lump, limited arm movement, and a unilateral Moro reflex.**

2 Plantar reflex is unrelated to a difficult birth caused by a fetus with broad shoulders.

3 Babinski reflex involves the feet; it is not related to a difficult birth caused by a fetus with broad shoulders.

4 Stepping reflex involves the feet; it is not related to a difficult birth caused by a fetus with broad shoulders.

374. 2 **Infants of diabetic mothers (IDMs) are polycythemic and therefore appear flushed; the mechanism underlying this phenomenon is unknown.**

1 These infants generally are placid.

3 These infants are limp, not hyperreflexive.

4 A high-pitched cry is a sign of CNS involvement, which is not expected in an IDM.

375. 1 **Decreasing IV glucose slowly is necessary to prevent a hypoglycemic response.**

2 Metabolic alkalosis will not occur with discontinuation of the glucose infusion.

3 Withholding oral feedings while withdrawing IV glucose may result in hypoglycemia.

4 Hyperglycemia is unlikely to occur when decreasing the IV glucose because blood glucose levels will decrease.

376. 3 **Because the virus is found in the respiratory tract and the urine, isolation is necessary; rubella is spread by droplets from the respiratory tract.**

1 Enteric precautions is an outdated term; the techniques used with this precaution are incorporated under contact precautions.

2 The techniques used with contact precautions are incorporated under standard precautions.

4 The use of standard precautions alone is unsafe; additional precautions must be implemented to protect the nurse from droplet transmitted infection.

377. 2 **Phototherapy changes unconjugated bilirubin in the skin to conjugated bilirubin bound to protein, permitting excretion via the urine and feces.**

1 Phototherapy does not affect liver function; the liver does not dispose of bilirubin.

3 Vitamin K is necessary for prothrombin formation, not bilirubin excretion.

4 The bilirubin is not excreted via the skin.

378. 1 **The infant's position is changed every 2 hours to expose all skin surfaces to the phototherapy for maximum effect.**

2 The infant should be kept nude for maximum exposure to the lights.

3 The infant may be removed from the lights for feeding and the eye patches removed to assess the eyes for irritation.

4 The lights will dry the cord more quickly, which is a desired effect.

379. 4 **The head circumference usually is 2 cm larger than the chest; a head circumference 4 cm smaller than the chest may indicate microcephaly.**

1 According to growth charts, the range of head circumference for boys is just slightly (1.25 cm) larger than the chest.

2 Molding does not occur with cesarean birth; therefore, the head should be about 2.5 cm larger than the chest at birth.

3 The expected ratio of head to chest circumference indicates that the chest is too small, not too large, for the head size.

380. 3 **Mothers with type O blood have anti-A and anti-B antibodies that are transferred across the placenta. This is the most common incompatibility because the mother is type O in 20% of all pregnancies.**

1 This usually is not a problem.

2 This usually is not a problem.

4 This usually is not a problem.

381. 4 **Adherence to the diet is necessary for optimal physical growth with little or no adverse effects on**

mental development; a diet that is instituted late will not reverse brain damage.

1 The fetus does not have an excessive level of phenylalanine. Although PKU can be detected in the fetus via genetic studies, excessive levels of phenylalanine first become measurable several days after the neonate starts feeding.

2 Epinephrine levels are decreased, not increased. Tyrosine, an amino acid produced by the metabolism of phenylalanine is absent in PKU; tyrosine is needed to form epinephrine.

3 Two days after birth is too soon to make a diagnosis. Detection cannot occur until the infant has taken milk or formula that contains phenylalanine for 24 hours and metabolites accumulate in the blood. Behaviors indicating mental retardation and CNS involvement usually are evident by about 6 months of age in the untreated infant.

382. 3 **The term "phenylketonuria" is derived from phenylpyruvic acid, which gives urine a mousy, musty odor.**

1 This odor is not present with phenylketonuria.

2 This odor is not present with phenylketonuria.

4 This odor is not present with phenylketonuria.

383. 1 **Right-to-left shunts result in inadequate perfusion of blood; not enough blood flows to the lungs for oxygenation.**

2 Left-to-right shunts result in too much blood flowing to the lungs; blood is adequately perfused.

3 Left-sided obstruction to the flow of blood results in decreased peripheral pulses, not cyanosis.

4 This usually occurs with patent ductus arteriosus. There should be no shunting of blood between the right and left sides of the heart after the ductus arteriosus has closed. If the ductus remains open, the shunting is from left to right and cyanosis is not a factor.

384. Answer: 1, 3, 5

1 **The abnormal facies associated with fetal alcohol syndrome includes a thin upper lip (vermilion), which is distinctive in these infants.**

2 Infants with FAS have small eyes with epicanthic folds.

3 **The abnormal facies associated with fetal alcohol syndrome includes a small upturned nose, which is distinctive in these infants.**

4 Infants with FAS have microcephaly (head circumference less than the tenth percentile).

5 **The abnormal facies associated with fetal alcohol syndrome includes a smooth vertical ridge (philtrum) in the upper lip, which is distinctive in these infants.**

385. 4 **These signs are indicative of withdrawal from an opioid with typical changes occurring in the central nervous system; the newborn should be monitored during the first 24 to 48 hours.**

1 The signs of cerebral palsy usually are manifested later in infancy.

2 The signs of syphilis are a low-grade fever with copious serosanguineous discharge from the nose.

3 The signs of fetal alcohol syndrome are growth deficiencies in length, weight, and head circumference, and distinctive facies.

386. 4 **Thrush, an oral infection caused by *Candida albicans*, is an opportunistic infection that may be indicative of HIV infection.**

1 Delay in temperature regulation is more frequently associated with immaturity of the hypothalamus.

2 Bleeding after a circumcision is associated with a bleeding disorder such as hemophilia.

3 Hypoglycemia usually is associated with the infant of a diabetic mother (IDM).

387. 3 **Herpesvirus can be fatal to a newborn, and the infant should be admitted to the neonatal intensive care unit (NICU).**

1 Although this is a true statement it is not relative to meeting the needs of this neonate who was exposed to the herpesvirus during the birthing process.

2 Although this is a true statement it is not relative to meeting the needs of this neonate who was exposed to the herpesvirus during the birthing process.

4 Although this is a true statement it is not relative to meeting the needs of this neonate who was exposed to the herpesvirus during the birthing process.

388. 2 **After closure, spinal fluid may accumulate and reach the brain, increasing intracranial pressure and causing the fontanels to bulge.**

1 Frequent crying may be a typical pattern for the neonate; it does not of itself indicate changes in intracranial pressure.

3 Changes in vital signs are not among the early signs of increasing intracranial pressure in an infant.

4 Difficulty with feeding can indicate changes in intracranial pressure but is not one of the first signs.

389. 4 **Applying a sterile saline dressing helps prevent infection while keeping the membranes moist.**

1 Although assessing for paralysis should be done, it is not the priority.

2 Antibiotics are not given prophylactically.

3 This newborn needs more than just routine care because of the outpouching of the meninges.

390. 4 **When a diaphragmatic hernia is present, the intra-abdominal pressure must be minimized; this is accomplished by the use of gastric decompression.**

1 Hydrating the infant with isotonic enemas is not beneficial.

2 These infants are not fed orally; intravenous fluids are given with careful measurement of electrolytes and intake and output to guide replacement therapy.

3 The Trendelenburg position is contraindicated; the abdominal organs will increase pressure on the diaphragm.

391. 1 **Greenish amniotic fluid indicates the presence of meconium and is considered a sign that the fetus is compromised.**
    2 Shortened intervals between contractions should occur as labor progresses.
    3 Clear amniotic fluid with specks of mucus describes the expected amniotic fluid.
    4 Decreased fetal heart rate at the beginning of contractions is an early deceleration caused by fetal head compression; it is benign.

392. 4 **The incomplete fetal bladder development may interfere with development of the pelvis.**
    1 Genu varum (bowlegs) can be congenital or caused by rickets; it is not related to exstrophy of the bladder.
    2 Tibial torsion is a rotation of the tibia and is unrelated to exstrophy of the bladder.
    3 Subluxation of the femur is a form of hip dislocation and is unrelated to exstrophy of the bladder.

393. 4 **Large newborns may be the result of gestational diabetes; it is necessary to check the neonate for hypoglycemia because maternal glucose is no longer available.**
    1 The nurse should do more than document the findings; the practitioner should be notified after the serial glucose levels are determined.
    2 This is indicated if the temperature is low and the newborn needs additional warmth.
    3 The infant may be hypoglycemic and require the glucose in an oral feeding immediately.

394. 4 **This prevents the neonate's stomach from becoming too distended and pressing upward against possibly compromised lungs.**
    1 A nasogastric feeding tube will not prevent respiratory embarrassment. The infant with a strong sucking reflex should be fed with a nipple, otherwise the sucking reflex will diminish.
    2 Four to 6 hours is too long between feedings; preterm infants should be fed every 2 to 3 hours because it takes this long for the preterm infant's stomach to empty.
    3 Preterm infants need the full caloric value of formula.

395. Answer: 1, 2, 5
    1 **Dry, peeling skin is related to decreased vernix and prolonged immersion in amniotic fluid.**
    2 **Abundant scalp hair and long fingernails are characteristics of postmaturity. These are typically found in a term newborn who is 2 to 3 weeks old.**
    3 These are not signs of postmaturity; newborns of diabetic mothers usually have this appearance.
    4 Vernix is found on a newborn at about 38 weeks' gestation and disappears after 40 weeks' gestation.
    5 **These creases are typical of full-term maturity; preterm newborns have few sole and palm creases.**

396. 1 **This occurs because of a lack of pulmonary surfactant to overcome surface tension in the alveoli.**

    2 Surfactant is present in sufficient amounts when the birth is closer to term.
    3 Fetal alveoli mature closer to term at about 35 to 36 weeks.
    4 The alveoli tend to collapse and may stay collapsed resulting in atelectasis.

397. 3 **Brachial plexus paralysis (Erb-Duchenne palsy) is the most common injury associated with dystocia related to a shoulder presentation; it is caused by pressure and traction on the brachial plexus during the birth process.**
    1 The newborn's face is not involved with a shoulder presentation.
    2 Cephalhematoma is a soft-tissue injury of the head and is not related to a shoulder dystocia.
    4 Spinal cord syndrome is associated with a breech presentation and is not related to shoulder dystocia.

398. 3 **Tongue extrusion, a reflex response to the tip of the tongue being touched, is characteristic of infants with Down syndrome and interferes with feeding; this reflex disappears at approximately 4 months of age.**
    1 A receding jaw does not interfere with sucking.
    2 Down syndrome is caused by a chromosomal defect, not brain damage; the feeding problem is related to the chromosomal defect.
    4 Nasal congestion is not a characteristic associated with newborns with Down syndrome.

399. Answer: 1, 2, 5
    1 **Pressure on the cerebral structures influences the central nervous system, resulting in irritability.**
    2 **A high-pitched cry is common in neonates with increased intracranial pressure.**
    3 The fontanels are bulging, not depressed, with increased intracranial pressure.
    4 Decreased urinary output is related to dehydration and kidney problems, not increased intracranial pressure.
    5 **Ineffective feeding behavior is typical of neonates with increased intracranial pressure.**

400. 2 **The lesions are probably a herpes infection, which can be fatal to the newborn if it is transmitted during a vaginal birth.**
    1 Herpes is a viral infection that does not respond to antibiotics.
    3 A client in active labor will give birth vaginally before the test results of the smear become available.
    4 Standard precautions should be used; double gloving is unnecessary.

REPRODUCTIVE PROBLEMS

401. 1 **Some lubricants act as a spermicide; they should be avoided, or only a recommended one should be used.**
    2 A female orgasm is not necessary for conception; achieving simultaneous orgasms is not relevant.

3 The type of birth control used 2 years prior to trying to conceive is not relevant at this time; some hormonal contraceptives should be discontinued 6 to 18 months before trying to conceive.

4 Consistency in the manner of intercourse usually is not relevant to conception, although a change in position may be recommended.

402. 2 **The male should be treated to prevent the infection from passing back and forth between him and his sexual partner.**

1 Inserting a vaginal suppository after having sex is an ineffective remedy and will not prevent a recurrence.

3 The organism usually is present in the partner's urogenital tract; voiding will not prevent a recurrence.

4 A douche is not recommended either during pregnancy or in the nonpregnant state.

403. 1 **Hemorrhage can result from a ruptured tubal pregnancy and shock can ensue.**

2 Although the client may be very anxious, the signs and symptoms are those of hemorrhagic shock.

3 There are no data, such as fever or rising white blood cell count, to support the conclusion that the client has an infection.

4 The data do not include information related to respiratory patterns leading to hyperventilation and hyperoxia resulting in respiratory alkalosis.

404. 3 **Any blood from the rupture will accumulate, causing phrenic nerve irritation and pain.**

1 Shoulder pain is not a response to anxiety; it is a typical symptom of phrenic nerve irritation.

2 The cardiac changes caused by hypovolemia do not cause shoulder pain.

4 A ruptured tube can cause rebound tenderness in the abdomen, not the shoulder.

405. 4 **The bleeding is causing decreased circulating blood volume and therefore there is a decreased cardiac output.**

1 Infection may occur later but it is not a problem at this time.

2 There will be hypovolemia, not hypervolemia, because of a decrease in circulating blood volume due to hemorrhage.

3 There are no data to justify the conclusion that the client has a protein deficiency.

406. 3 **At this time the fallopian tube is unable to expand to the size of the growing products of conception.**

1 Tubal pregnancies are unable to advance to this stage because of the tube's inability to expand with the growing products of conception.

2 The size of the fertilized egg at this time is minuscule and will cause no problem.

4 Tubal pregnancies are unable to advance to this stage because of the tube's inability to expand with the growing products of conception.

407. 3 **According to Mendelian genetic theory, when both parents are carriers of an autosomal recessive disorder there is a 25% probability that a child will have the disorder.**

1 There is a 25% probability that a child will have this disorder. This statement indicates that the couple does not understand Mendel's theory of probability.

2 When both partners are carriers there is a 50% probability that a child will be a carrier and a 25% probability that a child will have the disorder.

4 If one of the parents has the disorder there is a 50% probability that a child will have the disorder.

408. 3 **An autosomal dominant disorder is caused by one defective dominant gene passed to an offspring by a parent with the gene and the disorder.**

1 An X-linked recessive disorder usually occurs in males; it is not an autosomal disorder.

2 The chance of having this disorder is 25% if both parents carry the same recessive gene.

4 A chromosomal disorder relates to a defective chromosome, not a defective gene.

409. 2 **This response informs the client of the need for genetic counseling and gives her an option for decision making.**

1 This shifts the responsibility to the practitioner; the nurse should be involved in teaching about resources.

3 This response does not address the client's concern and changes the focus of the discussion.

4 Although the disease is rare in the general population, it is an inherited autosomal recessive disorder and there is a 25% probability that it can occur again in the same family.

410. 2 **An amniocentesis is done at this time because a therapeutic abortion can be legally and safely performed if desired by the parents.**

1 This is too early to perform an amniocentesis because the uterus has not ascended into the abdomen and there is little amniotic fluid present.

3 Although an amniocentesis and therapeutic abortion can be performed at this time, it is preferred that they are done as early as possible.

4 This is too late; the parents should not delay an amniocentesis if they are considering a therapeutic abortion.

411. 3 **Some women find it emotionally stressful to handle their genitals and discharges.**

1 The data do not support this conclusion.

2 The data do not support this conclusion.

4 The data do not support this conclusion.

412. 2 **There is an increased risk of tubal pregnancy with IVF-ET.**

1 There is not an increased risk for embryonic HIV with IVF-ET.

3 There is not an increased risk for congenital anomalies with IVF-ET.

4 There is not an increased risk for hyperemesis gravidarum with IVF-ET.

413. 3 **This is referred pain from passage of the contrast medium through the tubes; it usually is indicative of tubal patency.**
   1 An anesthetic is not given; the client's complaint of pain can be managed with position change and mild analgesics.
   2 The client can resume usual activities as soon as the test is over.
   4 The client usually does not experience nausea and/or vomiting.

414. 4 **This is necessary to keep the sperm viable for determining sperm count and viability.**
   1 The specimen can be collected at any time.
   2 Rubber solvents and preservatives may affect the semen specimen.
   3 This may result in an inadequate specimen.

415. 4 **Because the client has an ovulatory cyclic pattern, the infertility may be a result of a seminal factor; the partner's semen should be examined before more extensive studies or treatments are begun.**
   1 A laparoscopy is an invasive procedure that may be needed after all noninvasive tests are completed and the cause of the infertility remains undetermined.
   2 An endometrial biopsy is an invasive procedure that may be needed after all noninvasive tests are completed and the cause of the infertility remains undetermined.
   3 After all diagnostic and treatment options are exhausted, a fertility medication may be prescribed if it is determined that the medication will enhance the probability of conception.

416. 4 **Because the cervix is closed, the abortion is threatened.**
   1 The lifeless products of conception are retained with a missed abortion.
   2 Once the cervix is dilated the abortion is inevitable.
   3 Portions of the products of conception will have to be passed for a diagnosis of incomplete abortion.

417. 2 **Once cervical dilation has begun, the abortion is classified as inevitable.**
   1 In this type of abortion the cervix is dilated and there is bleeding; also, the discharge is malodorous.
   3 Bleeding and cramping may be present, but the cervix is still closed in a threatened abortion.
   4 The products of conception have been partially expelled with an incomplete abortion.

418. 4 **Remaining supine for 10 to 15 minutes permits the suppository to remain in place while it melts to body temperature.**
   1 General anesthesia is unnecessary when inserting a dinoprostone suppository.
   2 The bleeding that occurs after this abortion usually is equivalent to a heavy menstrual period. Excessive bleeding or cramping should be reported to the practitioner.
   3 A temperature more than 100° F (37.8° C) is a danger sign and the practitioner should be notified.

419. 4 **This indicates that the bleeding is excessive and the practitioner should be notified.**
   1 Although instructions vary among health care providers, sexual intercourse usually may be resumed in 1 to 3 weeks.
   2 Although instructions vary among health care providers, tampons usually are contraindicated for 3 days to 3 weeks.
   3 The menstrual period usually resumes in 4 to 6 weeks.

420. 3 **Rho(D) immune globulin (RhoGAM) should be given within 72 hours after a miscarriage or birth to have an effect on future pregnancies.**
   1 RhoGAM is always indicated at the termination of a pregnancy, whether it is at term or before term and whether the fetus is alive or dead.
   2 It is not necessary to administer RhoGAM this early.
   4 RhoGAM is always indicated at the termination of a pregnancy, whether it is at term or before term and whether the fetus is alive or dead.

421. 3 **A hydatidiform mole, in which chorionic villi degenerate into grapelike vesicles, causes these signs and symptoms.**
   1 Although vomiting may cause dehydration, this conclusion ignores the vaginal discharge and hypertension.
   2 Choriocarcinoma is a sequel to a hydatidiform mole; the hCG blood level is monitored for 1 year after removal of the mole. If the hCG blood level decreases to the expected range and remains there for 1 year, the client can plan another pregnancy.
   4 Although a vaginal discharge is related to a threatened abortion, an elevated blood pressure and severe nausea and vomiting are not.

422. 2 **Human chorionic gonadotropin (hCG) increases shortly after the onset of pregnancy, peaks at the end of the second month, then decreases and is sustained at a lower level until the end of pregnancy; a continued elevation indicates retained trophoblastic tissue and possible choriocarcinoma.**
   1 Uterine rupture is characterized by persistent, localized abdominal pain; it does not have a higher incidence in women with hydatidiform mole.
   3 Hyperemesis gravidarum cannot occur after termination of a pregnancy.
   4 Disseminated intravascular coagulation is manifested by shock, bleeding, a low platelet count, and elevated PT and PTT levels; it does not have a higher incidence in women with hydatidiform mole.

WOMEN'S HEALTH

423. 4 **Mittelschmerz is pain that sometimes occurs at the time of ovulation when the ovum erupts from the follicle.**

1 The pain is mild, cyclic, and characteristic of mittelschmerz; it does not require further evaluation.

2 When menses first begin the girl is anovulatory and does not experience the pain known as mittelschmerz.

3 The pain probably will occur more often in the future when ovulation is well established.

424. 2 **This type of vaginal discharge usually occurs with candidiasis, a fungal infection; pruritus is the most common symptom.**

1 An odorous, frothy greenish discharge occurs with trichomoniasis, a protozoal infestation.

3 Ischemia of the cervix is not associated with candidiasis; candidiasis causes vaginal and cervical inflammation.

4 A forgotten tampon may cause a bacterial, not fungal, vaginitis.

425. 1 **Yogurt contains *Lactobacillus acidophilus*, which replaces the intestinal flora destroyed by antibiotics.**

2 This is not relevant to antibiotics or intestinal flora.

3 This is not relevant to antibiotics or intestinal flora.

4 This is not relevant to antibiotics or intestinal flora.

426. 4 **Genital herpes (HSV-2) is characterized by remissions and exacerbations; it cannot be cured.**

1 Most pregnant women with HSV-2 have children by cesarean birth to prevent the newborns from contracting the disease while passing through the vagina.

2 Clients should abstain from sex until 10 days after the lesions heal.

3 Herpes can be controlled, not cured.

427. 3 **This response immediately identifies the client's fear as real and offers a service to meet the need for information about the client's physical status.**

1 This response ignores the client's concern and focuses on the nurse's need to complete the task of obtaining a health history.

2 This response minimizes the client's concern about having a sexually transmitted infection.

4 This response minimizes the client's concern and implies that the client is being unrealistic.

428. 3 **A condom covers the penis and contains the semen when it is ejaculated; semen contains a high percentage of HIV in infected individuals.**

1 Pre-ejaculatory fluid carries the HIV in an infected individual.

2 Although a monogamous relationship is less risky than having multiple sexual partners, if one partner is HIV positive, the other person is at risk for acquiring the HIV.

4 The client is not asking about various contraceptive methods. Most contraceptives do not provide protection from the HIV.

429. 3 **The client has signs and symptoms indicative of pelvic inflammatory disease (PID), which is a complication of gonorrhea.**

1 Herpes is noted for its painful lesions on the genitals; there are no data to indicate the presence of these lesions.

2 The client does not have the signs and symptoms associated with syphilis.

4 The client does not have the signs and symptoms associated with toxoplasmosis.

430. 2 **This is a description of a chancre, which is the initial sign of syphilis.**

1 These are condylomata, which are typical of the secondary stage of syphilis.

3 This is typical of the secondary stage of systemic involvement, which occurs from 2 to 4 years after the disappearance of the chancre.

4 This is typical of the secondary stage.

431. 3 **A dry environment inactivates the *Treponema pallidum*, making it incapable of causing disease.**

1 The organism is transferred by sexual contact; warm, moist body contact supports growth of the organism.

2 Nothing chelates this organism.

4 A warm, moist environment supports the growth of the organism.

432. 3 **This is the correct definition of dysmenorrhea.**

1 This occurs with menopause and during pregnancy.

2 This is bleeding that occurs at any time other than during the menstrual period; there may or may not be pain.

4 This may occur if the client is taking an oral contraceptive or in the first month or two of pregnancy.

433. 4 **This medical aseptic technique should limit the spread of microorganisms and help prevent future urinary tract infections if incorporated into the client's health practices.**

1 This is unnecessary, but the client should be encouraged to void when the urge occurs.

2 Intake and output need not be measured.

3 This is unnecessary for cystitis; it may be used as a part of perineal care for other problems.

434. 3 **Breast self-examination should be performed about a week after menstruation when the breasts are less engorged and tender.**

1 This is when menstruating women should examine their breasts.

2 Dimpling may occur when a tumor attaches to the skin or underlying tissues and therefore should be reported.

4 After menopause, selection of a specific time each month for breast self-examination reduces the possibility of forgetting.

435. 4 **Breast engorgement has abated at this time, limiting lumps that may occur because of fluid accumulation.**

1 Breast engorgement begins before ovulation and does not subside until several days after menses ends; engorgement interferes with accurate palpation.

2 Inaccurate assessment may result because examination occurs at different times of the menstrual cycle; accurate comparisons may not be made from month to month.

3 Breast engorgement begins before ovulation and does not subside until several days after menses ends; engorgement interferes with accurate palpation.

436. 1 **Serous or bloody discharge from the nipple is pathological and must be reported.**

2 The right hand should examine the left breast because this allows the flattened fingers to palpate the entire breast including the tail (upper, outer quadrant toward the axilla) and axillary area.

3 A small pillow or rolled towel should be placed under the scapula of the side being examined because it helps to raise the chest wall and spread and flatten out breast tissue.

4 The flat part of the fingers, not the palm or fingertips, should be used for palpation.

437. 4 **Advanced age at birth of a first child is one of the risk factors for malignancy of the breast because of prolonged exposure to unopposed estrogen.**

1 This is not considered a risk factor.

2 This is not considered a risk factor.

3 This is not considered a risk factor.

438. 2 **Although nodularity of the breasts may occur during pregnancy as a response to increased hormone levels, the greatest number of malignant tumors are located in the tail of Spence area, and further assessment is needed.**

1 Increased levels of melanotropin, secreted by the anterior pituitary gland, cause darkening of the nipple areolae in all pregnant women.

3 High levels of luteal and placental hormones stimulate the production of colostrum and there may be leakage from one or both nipples at the end of pregnancy; it is a benign occurrence.

4 There is an increased blood supply to the breasts causing vein engorgement; these blood vessels become visible as pregnancy progresses.

439. 4 **Most breast malignancies are painless, fixed, and in the upper outer quadrant; painful, mobile lesions usually are benign.**

1 These findings are suggestive of a lipoma.

2 These findings are suggestive of a lactation breast abscess.

3 These findings are suggestive of fibrocystic benign breast tumors.

440. 2 **The client has difficulty accepting the inevitability of death and is attempting to deny the reality of it.**

1 In the anger stage the client strikes out with the "why me" and the "how could God do this" type of statements. The client is angry at life and still angrier to be removed from it by death.

3 In this stage the client attempts to bargain for more time. The reality of death is no longer denied, but the client attempts to manipulate and extend the remaining time.

4 In the acceptance stage the client accepts the inevitability of death and peacefully awaits it.

441. 3 **This position supports venous return by gravity and promotes mobility of the arm.**

1 The container should be lower, not level, with the affected arm; although portable wound drainage systems work by negative pressure, gravity assists the flow of drainage.

2 Abduction may put unnecessary stress on the suture line at this time; slight flexion of the elbow promotes functional alignment.

4 When the hand is positioned lower than the elbow and shoulder venous stasis and edema of the hand may occur.

442. 2 **Radiation will interfere with wound healing if initiated too soon; inadequate healing should be reported to the practitioner.**

1 Topical preparations should not be used unless prescribed.

3 Sterile technique is not necessary unless there is a break in the skin.

4 Urine or other excreta of a client receiving radiation to the breast area are not affected by the radiation.

443. 1 **Further teaching is needed because extremes of temperature should be avoided; ice constricts blood vessels, interfering with circulation.**

2 Continued application of cold is contraindicated because it may cause tissue damage.

3 Erythema is an expected reaction; however, pain, vesicle formation, or sloughing of tissue requires intervention.

4 The knowledge deficit relates to skin care, not the side effects of radiation therapy.

444. 3 **The semi-Fowler position and elevation of the arm on the affected side minimize edema related to the inflammatory process.**

1 Pressure dressings are rarely used because portable wound drainage systems are used to remove accumulated fluid from the operative site.

2 A member from Reach to Recovery will not visit on the day of surgery; the visit will probably be made in the client's home.

4 Activities of daily living that permit only slight flexion of the elbow and avoid abduction of the arm on the affected side are permitted.

445. 4 **Clients who have cancer of one breast are at risk for development of cancer in the other breast.**

1 A breast prosthesis is not used until healing has occurred.

2 Most clients can resume full activity as strength returns.

3 Stretching activities are considered helpful in regaining full movement.

446. 1 **Elevation promotes drainage by gravity and reduces the risk of developing lymphedema.**

2 This is not the responsibility of the client at this time.

3 A high-Fowler's position keeps the arm in a dependent position, thus limiting venous return and promoting lymphedema.

4 Abduction, moving the arm away from the body, increases tension on the suture line and is contraindicated at this time.

447. 3 **If the tubing is patent and negative pressure is present, the wound should be free of exudates.**

1 Drainage is expected; it is the nurse's responsibility to maintain the drainage system.

2 Pressure dressings are not used with portable wound drainage systems because the latter are effective in removing interstitial fluid.

4 Although elevating the arm may facilitate drainage, it is not the priority in relation to the data presented.

448. 2 **The Bartholin glands are located beneath the vaginal vestibule; if cysts form and they become infected they cause labial, vaginal, or pelvic pain particularly during or after intercourse (dyspareunia).**

1 Urethritis causes painful urination.

3 A vaginal hematoma causes swelling in the vaginal wall, not the labia.

4 Skene's glands are located in the urethra, not the labia.

449. 2 **A cystocele is a herniation of the bladder through the vaginal wall because of weakened pelvic structures; the herniated bladder does not empty effectively and urinary stasis, chronic infection, and renal failure can develop.**

1 The surgery improves bladder function and prevents renal failure; it is needed.

3 Bowel obstruction is a complication of a rectocele, not cystocele.

4 Although corrective surgery will reduce perineal pressure, its primary purpose is to improve bladder function and prevent complications.

450. 4 **This is an open-ended response that encourages further discussion without focusing on an area that the nurse, not the client, feels is the problem.**

1 This response denies the client's feeling and can cause feelings of guilt for questioning the partner's love.

2 This is too specific; the nurse does not have enough information to come to this conclusion.

3 This response shifts the focus from the client's voiced concerns; the client specifically referred to her husband, not others.

451. 2 **Attempting to remove a uterus with large uterine fibroids vaginally can cause trauma, resulting in hemorrhage.**

1 Vaginal hysterectomy is indicated for prolapsed uterus because the uterus is usually collapsed into the vagina.

3 A hysterectomy is not the treatment of choice for mild cervical dysplasia; when a hysterectomy is necessary, the vaginal route is preferred.

4 Urinary incontinence when coughing may be related to stress incontinence, which does not require a hysterectomy.

452. 1 **This action provides continuity and demonstrates to the client that the nursing staff is concerned; frequent contact reduces the client's need to call staff members.**

2 This will increase the client's anxiety and the need for more contact with staff members.

3 Telling the client is not the same as doing it; the client will not believe that staff members will come in frequently to talk.

4 This will not provide continuity of care.

453. 1 **Sitting for long periods leads to pooling of blood in the pelvic area, predisposing the client to thrombus formation.**

2 Fluids should be increased to 3000 mL daily to decrease blood viscosity, which can lead to thrombus formation.

3 Blood coagulation tests are not done routinely because clotting elements usually are not disturbed by a hysterectomy.

4 Hormone replacement therapy is not considered unless the client is premenopausal and an oophorectomy was performed.

454. 4 **After surgery the urethral orifice may be distorted and edematous; a urinary retention catheter keeps the bladder empty, limiting pressure on the operative site.**

1 A pessary placed in the vagina is used for a displaced uterus; following an anteroposterior repair (colporrhaphy), vaginal packing is used to support the surgical repair.

2 A rectal tube is used for abdominal distention caused by flatulence; it rarely is necessary.

3 A cleansing douche may be ordered before, not after, surgery.

455. Answer: 1, 3

1 **A pelvic infection is suspected. A characteristic of this is abdominal pain.**

2 Urinary frequency is associated with cystitis, not a vaginal discharge associated with a pelvic infection.

3 **A rising temperature is a sign of infection.**

4 An increase, not decrease, in pulse rate is expected because the metabolic rate increases in the presence of an elevated temperature.

5 An increase, not decrease, in blood pressure is expected because the metabolic rate increases in the presence of an elevated temperature.

456. 1 **Vaginal packing supports the repair and provides slight pressure to prevent bleeding; the packing should be checked for possible bleeding.**

2 Elevating the legs is unnecessary; leg exercises and a gradual increase in ambulation are encouraged to prevent pulmonary emboli.

3 There is no dressing, only vaginal packing and a sanitary pad.

4 Sitz baths are not instituted until the packing is removed; an ice pack and/or a heat lamp may be used to promote comfort.

457. 1 **The uterus often is erroneously believed necessary for a satisfying sexual life.**

2 Sexuality should not be diminished, particularly because the fear of pregnancy no longer exists.

3 Although estrogen levels are reduced, libido is influenced by psychological as well as hormonal factors.

4 Although body image changes can interfere with sexuality, this is not an expectation for most women.

458. 4 **As the term "hysterectomy" implies, only the uterus is removed and the ovaries remain; therefore, the client will experience menopause during the same years as all women who have functioning ovaries.**

1 The client will ovulate because the ovaries are not removed with a hysterectomy.

2 The client has not had an oophorectomy; therefore, the client will not experience a surgical menopause.

3 There should be no discomfort if there is an appropriate period of healing before resuming sexual intercourse.

459. 1 **Pap smears can detect cancer of the cervix by screening for atypical as well as cancerous cells.**

2 Scraping the cells can cause a few drops of blood to be expelled; vaginal bleeding does not occur.

3 A colposcopy is not part of a routine Pap smear procedure.

4 Insertion of the speculum usually is the most uncomfortable part of the test.

460. 1 **With carcinoma in situ the epithelium is eroded and replaced by rapidly dividing neoplastic cells. There is no distinct tumor; with treatment the prognosis is excellent.**

2 Preinvasive lesions of the cervix are treated with cryotherapy, laser therapy, or loop electrosurgical excision procedure (LEEP). Radiation therapy is used for invasive cervical cancer.

3 Stage II involves the vaginal wall; stage 0 is preinvasive.

4 Stages I to IV are considered invasive by increasing degrees; stage 0 is preinvasive. Treatment is based on the staging.

461. 1 **This routine screening for information provides a basis for assessing trauma; in a younger client it also is necessary to assess the risk for pregnancy.**

2 Examination may precede reporting; the decision to report is mandated by law.

3 Urination may wash away spermatic or bloody evidence.

4 A test for seminal acid phosphate, not seminal alkaline phosphatase, is performed.

462. 3 ***E. coli* is commonly found in the bowel and, because of anatomical proximity and possibly**

careless hygiene after bowel movements, may spread to the urethra.

1 *E. coli* is not found in the kidneys.

2 *E. coli* is no more virulent than other infective agents.

4 *E. coli* does not compete with fungal organisms for host sites.

463. 1 **Prolactin is a hormone that is produced and secreted by the anterior pituitary. A pituitary tumor is the most probable cause of elevated prolactin levels that result in lactation not associated with childbirth or nursing (galactorrhea).**

2 If the client is taking oral contraceptives estrogen levels will increase, causing galactorrhea in some women; this client is postmenopausal.

3 The production of oxytocin is not related to the occurrence of galactorrhea.

4 The production of progesterone is not related to the occurrence of galactorrhea.

464. Answer: 1, 4, 5

1 **Cigarette smoking is a high-risk behavior associated with an increased incidence of osteoporosis in later life.**

2 Moderate exercise is not considered a risk factor for the development of osteoporosis, although a sedentary life style is.

3 Use of street drugs is not considered a risk factor for osteoporosis.

4 **Familial predisposition is considered a risk factor for the development of osteoporosis.**

5 **Inadequate calcium intake during the premenopausal years is a risk factor for the development of osteoporosis after menopause.**

DRUG-RELATED RESPONSES

465. 4 **Beta-adrenergic medications are tocolytic agents that may halt labor, although only temporarily. Other tocolytics that may be used are magnesium sulfate, prostaglandin inhibitors, and calcium channel blockers.**

1 Oxytocin is a hormone that is secreted by the posterior pituitary gland; it stimulates contractions and is released after birth to initiate the let-down reflex.

2 Analgesics do not halt preterm labor.

3 Corticosteroids do not halt labor; they are used during preterm labor to accelerate fetal lung maturity, when birth is likely to occur within 24 to 48 hours.

466. 4 **Betamimetics have the unpleasant side effects of nervousness, tremors, and palpitations; clients should be informed that these side effects are expected.**

1 If contractions are lessened and the maternal heart rate is less than 120 and regular, the medication is performing as expected and does not need to be discontinued.

2   Muscle tremors and palpitations are not signs and symptoms of preterm labor.

3   Electrolyte levels are unrelated to these side effects of the tocolytic agent.

467. **4**   **A common side effect of an opioid analgesic is decreased fetal heart rate variability. Because the fetal heart rate and the length and duration of the contractions remain stable and the analgesic appears to be effective, the only nursing action is to document the findings.**

1   Repositioning the client is not necessary because the data do not indicate decreased placental perfusion.

2   It is not necessary to administer oxygen because the data do not indicate fetal compromise.

3   Naloxone (Narcan), an opioid antagonist, may need to be administered to the newborn, but the present data do not indicate that this is necessary.

468. **3**   **Meperidine (Demerol) is an opioid that can cause respiratory depression in the neonate if administered less than 4 hours before birth.**

1   Naloxone (Narcan) is an opioid antagonist that reverses the effects of respiratory depression in the newborn.

2   Lorazepam (Ativan) is a sedative; it does not cause respiratory depression in the newborn, but it does not relieve pain by itself.

4   Promethazine (Phenergan) is a tranquilizer; it does not cause respiratory depression in the newborn. Promethazine does not relieve pain by itself.

469. **2**   **Anesthesia blocks the sensory pathways so that the mother does not sense bladder distention and may be unable to void.**

1   Hypotension, not hypertension, is a side effect of epidural anesthesia.

3   An epidural anesthetic does not influence body temperature.

4   A decreased level of consciousness occurs with general anesthesia, not epidural anesthesia; general anesthesia is used when there is an emergency.

470.   **Answer: 8.2 mL.** Use ratio and proportion:

$$2,450,000 \text{ units} : 300,000 \text{ units} = x \text{ mL} : 1 \text{ mL}$$
$$300,000 \, x = 2,450,000$$
$$x = 8.2 \text{ mL}$$

471. **4**   **Probenecid (Benemid) reduces renal tubular excretion of penicillin.**

1   This is unrelated to the concomitant administration of penicillin and probenecid.

2   This is unrelated to the concomitant administration of penicillin and probenecid.

3   This is unrelated to the concomitant administration of penicillin and probenecid.

472. **2**   **Tetracycline (Tetracyn) has an affinity for calcium; if used during tooth bud development it may cause discoloration of teeth.**

1   Tetracycline does not adversely affect breastfeeding.

3   Tetracycline does not cause fetal allergies to the medication.

4   Tetracycline does not increase the fetus's tolerance to the medication.

473. **3**   **All women, except those who are pregnant or lactating, should ingest between 1000 and 1300 mg of calcium daily; if the client is unable to ingest enough calcium in food, then supplements of calcium and vitamin D are recommended.**

1   These supplements do not help prevent osteoporosis.

2   These supplements do not help prevent osteoporosis.

4   These supplements maintain cartilage and connective tissue integrity but they do not help prevent osteoporosis.

474. **4**   **Maintenance of serum progesterone levels keeps cervical mucus thick and hostile to sperm at all times.**

1   This is inaccurate information; the pill must be taken throughout the menstrual cycle.

2   Progesterone oral contraceptives (Minipills) must be taken throughout the cycle; combined estrogen and progesterone oral contraceptives are taken during the second, third, and fourth weeks of the cycle.

3   Fertility drugs are often taken during the first part of the cycle to encourage ovulation, not for contraception.

475. **3**   **Nausea and vomiting are related to excessive amounts of estrogen; these usually can be controlled by reducing the dosage.**

1   When taking oral contraceptives containing estrogen, breakthrough bleeding is more common than amenorrhea.

2   Depression and lethargy are related to both excessive estrogen and excessive progesterone, but are not common side effects.

4   Hypomenorrhea is caused by estrogen deficiency.

476. **1**   **Oral contraceptives should be discontinued with the presence of any symptom related to a pulmonary embolus.**

2   Menorrhagia, painful menstruation, is a side effect related to excessive amounts of estrogen; immediate discontinuance of the oral contraceptive is unnecessary.

3   Mittelschmerz, pain at the time of ovulation, does not occur if the client is taking an oral contraceptive.

4   Increased leukorrhea may be a sign of infection, not a side effect of oral contraceptives.

477. **3**   **Iron absorption is pH dependent; therefore, iron should be taken with a source of ascorbic acid to enhance duodenal absorption.**

1   Biotin is unrelated to the absorption of iron.

2   Lecithin is unrelated to the absorption of iron.

4   Vitamin B complex is unrelated to the absorption of iron.

478. 2 **Rho(D) immune globulin (RhoGAM) adminis-tration during the 28th week of gestation limits an active antibody response in an Rh-negative woman exposed to the positive blood of the fetus.**
    1 Week 12 is too early in the pregnancy to administer Rho(D) immune globulin (RhoGAM).
    3 Rho(D) immune globulin is given at 28, not 36, weeks in the pregnancy as a preventive measure.
    4 Rho(D) immune globulin is given at 28, not 40, weeks in the pregnancy as a preventive measure.

479. 3 **During the second and third trimesters the blood volume and cardiac output increase, placing a greater workload on the heart. Women with preexisting heart disease may require larger doses of cardiac medication to prevent cardiac decompensation.**
    1 Palpitations can occur when the heart rate reaches 120 beats per minute. A heart rate of more than 100 beats per minute may be an indicator of cardiac decompensation; further assessment is required and treatment instituted.
    2 Digoxin (Lanoxin) is a category C medication and is prescribed during pregnancy.
    4 Penicillin is a category B medication and is relatively safe to take during pregnancy.

480. **Answer: 1, 4**
    1 **Heparin (Hep-Lock) can be used during pregnancy because it does not cross the placental barrier and will not cause hemorrhage in the fetus.**
    2 Clopidrogrel (Plavix) is a platelet aggregation inhibitor. It is not used for thrombophlebitis; it is used to reduce the risk of brain attack, TIA, unstable angina, and myocardial infarction.
    3 Warfarin (Coumadin) crosses the placental barrier causing hemorrhage in the fetus.
    4 **Enoxaparin (Lovenox) does not cross the placental barrier; its classification for pregnancy is B.**
    5 Acetylsalicylic acid (Acuprin) is a platelet aggregation inhibitor and is not recommended during pregnancy (D category).

481. 2 **Heparin should not be given because 98 seconds is almost 3 times the normal time it takes a fibrin clot to form (25 to 36 seconds) and prolonged bleeding may result; the therapeutic range for heparin is 1½ to 2 times the normal range. The practitioner should be notified.**
    1 Heparin must not be increased; the client already has received too much.
    3 This is unsafe. Continuing the infusion may result in hemorrhage.
    4 The medication does not have to be changed; it should be stopped temporarily until the aPTT is within the therapeutic range.

482. 3 **A widening pulse pressure is a side effect of terbutaline.**
    1 Tachycardia, not bradycardia, only occurs.
    2 Hypokalemia, not hyperkalemia, is a potential side effect.
    4 The purpose of terbutaline is to halt contractions, not make them weaker.

483. 1 **Oxytocin (Pitocin) given after the third stage of labor will stimulate the uterus to contract and remain contracted.**
    2 Oxytocin does not have an analgesic effect.
    3 Oxytocin is administered after the placenta is expelled (third stage of labor).
    4. Prolactin, not oxytocin, stimulates milk production.

484. 3 **Oxytocin (Pitocin) has an antidiuretic effect, acting to reabsorb water from the glomerular filtrate.**
    1 Oxytocin does not alter the client's affect.
    2 Hyperventilation is caused by inappropriate breathing patterns, not by prolonged use of oxytocin.
    4 Fever occurs with infection or dehydration, not with prolonged administration of oxytocin.

485. 4 **Magnesium sulfate is used to depress CNS irrita-bility; diminished reflexes indicate the medica-tion's effectiveness.**
    1 Magnesium sulfate is a CNS depressant; a decrease in blood pressure, an increase in urinary output, and diminished reflexes indicate that the magnesium sulfate is effective.
    2 Magnesium sulfate is not a diuretic; it acts as an anticonvulsant.
    3 Decreased respiratory rate is a sign of toxicity.

486. 4 **Respiratory depression is a late indicator of toxic-ity; if the respiratory rate decreases below 12 per minute the infusion should be discontinued.**
    1 Visual blurring is associated with worsening of preeclampsia, which may lead to a seizure; it is not a toxic effect of the magnesium sulfate.
    2 Epigastric pain is associated with worsening of preeclampsia, which may lead to a seizure; it is not a toxic effect of the magnesium sulfate.
    3 The fetal heart rate is not affected by the infusion of magnesium sulfate.

487. 2 **Calcium gluconate will reverse the central nervous system depressant action of magnesium sulfate.**
    1 Protamine sulfate is the antidote for heparin toxicity.
    3 Sodium bicarbonate counteracts acidosis.
    4 Naloxone hydrochloride is an opiate antagonist.

488. 2 **The concentration of propylthiouracil (PTU) excreted in breast milk is 3 to 12 times higher than its level in maternal serum; this may cause agranu-locytosis or goiter in the infant.**
    1 Heparin (Hep-Lock) is not excreted in breast milk.
    3 The amount of breast milk excretion of gentamicin (Garamycin) is unknown, but it can be given to infants directly without adverse effects.
    4 Diphenhydramine (Benadryl) is excreted in breast milk, but it does not adversely affect the infant when therapeutic doses are given to the mother.

489. Answer: 1, 5

1 **A knee-jerk reflex that is +1 is a manifestation of hyporeflexia; it is a possible indication of magnesium sulfate toxicity.**

2 A urinary output that is 100 mL/hr is an adequate urinary output; a urinary output of less than 30 mL/hr indicates inadequate excretion of magnesium sulfate and the potential for toxicity.

3 The maternal blood pressure is not directly related to magnesium sulfate administration or toxicity; however, if the blood pressure decreases, it indicates treatment is effective.

4 A pulse rate of 80 beats per minute is an expected pulse rate; it is not indicative of toxicity.

5 **A respiratory rate of 12 breaths per minute is a cause for concern; fewer than 12 breaths per minute is a sign of magnesium sulphate toxicity.**

490. 2 A steroid such as betamethasone (Celestone) or dexamethasone (Decadron) administered to the mother crosses the placenta and promotes lung maturity in the fetus.

1 Steroids do not cause an increase in cervical dilation.

3 Steroids do not reduce the risk of a precipitous birth.

4 Steroids do not minimize the potential for maternal hypertension.

491. 4 This is the most reliable method to confirm newborn addiction.

1 Examining the mother's arms for needle marks will not determine the amount of drugs the mother used or the last time the drug was taken.

2 The priority is to determine if the newborn is addicted before clinical signs of withdrawal occur.

3 It is the mother's drug habit that is important, not the prescribed medications she received the previous day.

492. 4 This is the expected outcome. If output exceeds intake, it indicates that the infant is diuresing from the effect of the furosemide (Lasix).

1 Although it is important to assess whether pedal edema is reduced, this is subjective; intake and output measurements are objective.

2 Furosemide can cause hypokalemia, which can precipitate digoxin toxicity; it is not given to prevent digoxin toxicity.

3 Depressed fontanels are not the desired outcome; this indicates dehydration, which can occur with excessive diuresis.

493. 4 Propranolol (Inderal) is a beta-blocking agent that reverses the uterine inhibitory responses and cardiovascular effects of terbutaline (Brethine).

1 Levodopa (L-dopa) is not an antidote for terbutaline; it is used for Parkinson's disease.

2 Furosemide (Lasix) is a diuretic; it will not reverse the cardiovascular effects indicated.

3 Ritodrine (Yutopar) may cause responses similar to those of terbutaline; it is sometimes used to halt premature labor because it inhibits beta-2 receptors.

494. 3 Corticosteroids stimulate surfactant production; they also have been shown to reduce the incidence of intraventricular hemorrhage.

1 Betamethasone (Celestone) does not affect the labor process.

2 Betamethasone does not increase placental perfusion.

4 Betamethasone does not affect the intensity of contractions.

495. 4 Salicylate therapy is used because clients with SLE have an increased risk for thrombus formation; as the time of birth approaches salicylate therapy should be discontinued to reduce the possibility of bleeding in the newborn.

1 There is a greater probability that the newborn will be small for gestational age.

2 There is no need for dialysis during the postpartum period.

3 The butterfly-shaped rash that can occur with SLE does not become more prominent during late pregnancy.

496. Answer: 2, 5

1 The block anesthetizes the perineum, not the cervix or the body of the uterus.

2 **The block provides anesthesia to the perineum and therefore pain is not felt.**

3 The block affects only the perineum, not the bladder.

4 The block does not influence the decision of whether or not to have an episiotomy.

5 **Although the bearing-down reflex is lessened, muscle control is not affected and the client is able to bear down with contractions.**

497. 4 Rho(D) immune globulin (RhoGAM) is given to an Rh-negative mother after birth if the infant is Rh positive and the Coombs' test reveals that the mother was not previously sensitized (negative).

1 An Rh-positive mother will not develop antibodies to a fetus who is either Rh positive or Rh negative; therefore, a Coombs' test is not performed.

2 An Rh-negative mother with a positive Coombs' test indicates that she has Rh-positive antibodies; therefore, Rho(D) immune globulin is not given because it will not be effective.

3 An Rh-positive mother will not develop antibodies to a fetus who is either Rh positive or Rh negative; therefore, a Coombs' test is not performed.

498. 1 Rho(D) immne globulin (RhoGAM) is given to an Rh-negative mother after birth if the infant is Rh positive and the mother was not previously sensitized.

2 RhoGAM is administered once after birth if the mother was not previously sensitized.

3 The infant's Coombs' test result does not influence the timing of the RhoGAM administration.

4 A small dose of RhoGAM may be given prophylactically in the 28th week of gestation if there is

a minimal increase in the antibody titer. If there is a significant increase in the antibody titer, an amniocentesis is performed. Treatment of the fetus is dependent on the results of the amniocentesis.

499. **3**   **Betamethasone (Celestone) is a glucocorticoid that the National Institutes of Health recommends for all women in preterm labor between 28 and 32 weeks' gestation, unless there is a medical condition that specifically contraindicates its use (e.g., cord prolapse or abruptio placentae). It stimulates the release of enzymes that produce lung surfactant, which promotes fetal lung maturity.**

   1   Betamethasone is not given to enhance uterine relaxation caused by ritodrine (Yutopar).

   2   Although ritodrine may cause fetal hyperglycemia and neonatal hypoglycemia, betamethasone is not given to prevent these side effects.

   4   Betamethasone is not given to counteract adverse reactions to ritodrine.

500.   **Answer: 0.25 mL.** Solve for x by using ratio and proportion.

$$0.5 \text{ mg} : x \text{ mL} = 2 \text{ mg} : 1 \text{ mL}$$
$$2x = 0.5$$
$$x = 0.5 \div 2$$
$$x = 0.25 \text{ mL}$$

Additional review questions can be found on the enclosed companion CD.

CHILDBEARING AND WOMEN'S HEALTH NURSING
QUIZ

1. A pregnant client who has asthma is expected on the unit for induction of labor. What medication should the nurse question when evaluating newly written practitioner's prescriptions?
   1. Albuterol inhaler
   2. Epidural anesthesia
   3. IV D_5W with piggyback oxytocin (Pitocin)
   4. Prostaglandin E2 (Prostin E2) vaginal suppository

2. A client with severe preeclampsia is receiving magnesium sulfate therapy. What is the priority nursing assessment when monitoring this client's response to therapy?
   1. Urinary output
   2. Respiratory rate
   3. Deep tendon reflexes
   4. Level of consciousness

3. A pregnant woman arrives in the emergency department on a stretcher via an ambulance. During the assessment the nurse observes that the fetus's head has emerged. How should the nurse assist the mother in the birth of her fetus's anterior shoulder?
   1. Gently guiding the head downward
   2. Gradually flexing the head toward the maternal thigh
   3. Gently putting pressure on the head by pulling upward
   4. Gradually extending the head above the maternal symphysis pubis

4. The nurse assesses a newborn using the Apgar score. At 1 minute after birth the newborn has a heart rate of 120, slow and irregular respirations, weak cry, some flexion of extremities, and a pink body with blue extremities. What number does the nurse document for the 1 minute Apgar score?
   1. 4
   2. 5
   3. 6
   4. 7

5. During the initial assessment of a dark-skinned neonate the nurse observes several dark round areas on a newborn's buttocks. How should this observation be documented?
   1. Stork bites
   2. Forceps marks
   3. Mongolian spots
   4. Ecchymotic areas

6. Pregnant women with cardiac problems must be assessed frequently. Which adaptation does the nurse suspect is the result of early decompensation?
   1. Hemoptysis
   2. Tachycardia
   3. Increasing fatigue
   4. Generalized edema

7. What breathing technique does the nurse instruct a pregnant woman to use as the fetus's head crowns on the perineum?
   1. Deep chest
   2. Open glottis
   3. Rapid shallow
   4. Accelerated-decelerated

8. A nurse in the neonatal intensive care unit (NICU) is assessing visiting parents for behaviors that might indicate a difficulty with bonding. The nurse determines that intervention may be helpful to the parents who are:
   1. Visiting other babies in the NICU
   2. Touching their baby with their fingertips
   3. Discussing equipment being used for their baby
   4. Asking numerous questions about their baby's condition

9. What is the safest and most reliable birth control method that the nurse should recommend to a client with type 1 diabetes?
   1. Vaginal sponge
   2. Oral contraceptive
   3. Rhythm method with a condom
   4. Diaphragm with a spermicidal gel

10. A couple seeking genetic counseling are heterozygous carriers of Tay-Sachs disease. They ask the nurse what the chances are for each of their children inheriting the disease. The nurse responds that the probability is:
    1. 0%
    2. 25%
    3. 50%
    4. 100%

11. A 20-year-old developmentally disabled woman is a resident in a group home. She has had four abortions in the past 2 years, and the agency supervisor recommends that she be sterilized. It is obvious that the client is unable to exercise informed consent for sterilization. The nurse understands that the procedure cannot be performed without legal consent from the:
    1. Next of kin
    2. Court-appointed individual or group
    3. Agency designated to perform the abortion
    4. Organization or agency licensed to administer the group home

12. During the discharge examination of a 2-day-old newborn, the nurse observes an edematous area confined to the right side of the scalp. How should the nurse document this condition?
    1. Molding
    2. Hydrocephalus
    3. Cephalhematoma
    4. Caput succedaneum

13. A client had a fourth-degree perineal laceration during the birth of her neonate. What should the nurse recommend to protect the area from additional trauma?
    1. Take sitz baths at least three times each day
    2. Apply a premoistened anesthetic pad to the area

3. Prevent straining at stool by administering an enema
4. Encourage a high-fiber diet with increased fluid intake

14. A 24-year-old client complains to the nurse in the women's health clinic that her breasts become tender before her menstrual period. What should the nurse recommend that the client do 1 week before an expected menses?
   1. Take salt tablets daily
   2. Increase protein intake
   3. Eliminate daily exercise
   4. Decrease caffeine intake

15. A client who is a mother for the first time appears anxious about her new parenting role. The nurse recommends that she join the new mothers support group at the local YWCA. Which type of prevention is this?
   1. Tertiary
   2. Primary
   3. Secondary
   4. Therapeutic

16. A client who suspects that she is 6 weeks pregnant appears mildly anxious as she is waiting for her first obstetric appointment. What mild symptom of anxiety does the nurse expect this client to experience?
   1. Dizziness
   2. Breathlessness
   3. Abdominal cramps
   4. Increased alertness

17. A nurse is counseling a pregnant client who is a vegetarian. What should the nurse plan to do to ensure optimum nutrition during the pregnancy?
   1. Refer the client to a dietician to help plan her daily menu
   2. Encourage the client to join a group that teaches nutrition
   3. Counsel the client that she needs to include meat in her diet at least once daily
   4. Advise the client that it is unhealthy to continue a vegetarian diet during her pregnancy

18. A client in her 30th week of gestation is in preterm labor, and the practitioner prescribes betamethasone (Celestone). The client asks the nurse why she is receiving this drug. As a basis for the response the nurse takes into consideration that it:
   1. Prevents chorioamnionitis."
   2. Increases uteroplacental exchange."
   3. Promotes neonatal pulmonary maturity."
   4. Treats fetal respiratory distress syndrome."

19. A nurse is caring for a pregnant woman in active labor, who is lying in bed in the high Fowler position. Epidural anesthesia and an oxytocin (Pitocin) infusion were started 45 minutes ago. The client complains of feeling lightheaded and nauseated. What should the nurse do after reviewing the client's admission data, vital signs, and present status?
   1. Interrupt the oxytocin infusion
   2. Give the client oxygen via a facemask
   3. Place the client in a flat side-lying position
   4. Notify the practitioner that the fetus is experiencing distress

---

CLIENT CHART

Admission Data

Cervix: 6 cm dilated and 80% effaced
Contractions: 4 minutes apart, 60 seconds' duration
Fetal heart rate: 146 with episodic accelerations

Maternal Vital Signs

Admission VS: T, 98.8° F; P, 88 regular rhythm; R, 20, regular; BP, 132/86
Present VS: T, 99° F; P, 76, regular rhythm; R, 18, regular; BP, 110/68

Present Status

Cervix: 7 cm dilated and 80% effaced
Contractions: 3 minutes apart, 70 seconds' duration
Fetal heart rate: 118 with early decelerations

---

20. A nurse teaches a woman who is planning to breastfeed how to relieve breast engorgement. The nurse determines that further teaching is necessary when the woman states she will:
   1. Manually express breast milk
   2. Breastfeed the infant less frequently
   3. Apply warm compresses to both breasts
   4. Place cold compresses on the breasts just after breastfeeding

21. A 16-year-old primigravida at 32 weeks' gestation is admitted to the high-risk unit. Her blood pressure is 170/110 mm Hg and she has 4+ proteinuria. She gained 50 pounds during the pregnancy and her face and extremities are edematous. What complication, which occurs in the latter part of pregnancy, does the nurse identify?
   1. Eclampsia
   2. Severe preeclampsia
   3. Chronic hypertension
   4. Gestational hypertension

22. A client at 36 weeks' gestation is admitted to the high-risk unit with the diagnosis of severe preeclampsia and antiseizure therapy is instituted. A fetal monitor and an electronic blood pressure machine are applied. What complication of severe preeclampsia requires frequent monitoring of the blood pressure?
   1. Brain attack
   2. Hemorrhage
   3. Precipitous labor
   4. Disseminated intravascular coagulation

23. The school nurse discusses herpes genitalis as part of a high school sex education program. The nurse instructs the students that herpes genitalis is:
   1. Painless in women
   2. Curable with antibiotics
   3. Transmitted via fomites such as toilet seats
   4. Responsible for local as well as systemic reactions

24. A client with a history of endometriosis has abdominal surgery to remove adhesions. What should this client's postoperative plan of care include?
   1. Encouraging the client to ambulate in the hallway
   2. Elevating the client's lower extremities by gatching the bed

3. Assisting the client to dangle her legs over the side of the bed

4. Maintaining the client on bed rest until the dressings are removed

25. The nurse is teaching a sex education course to high school students. What should the nurse teach them about why gonorrhea is difficult to control? Select all that apply.
    1. _____ Symptoms of the disease are vague
    2. _____ Screening blood tests are expensive
    3. _____ The incubation period is relatively short
    4. _____ Causative organisms have become resistant to treatment
    5. _____ Diagnostic tests for the causative organism are not yet available

26. When a nurse who is carrying a newborn to the mother enters the room, a visitor asks to hold the infant. The visitor is sneezing and coughing. What is most important for the nurse to do?
    1. Give the infant to the mother
    2. Have the visitor step outside the room
    3. Verify the infant's and the mother's identification bands
    4. Ask the visitor if the coughing and sneezing are caused by a cold

27. A nurse is planning to teach a new mother about breastfeeding. What should the nurse consider before preparing the client to breastfeed?
    1. Oxytocin stimulates milk production
    2. Suckling stimulates the release of oxytocin
    3. Estrogen stimulates the secretion of lactogenic hormones
    4. Placental separation stimulates the release of progesterone

28. A client arrives in the birthing room with the fetal head crowning. Birth is imminent. What should the nurse tell the client to do?
    1. Push forcefully
    2. Turn to the left side
    3. Use the pant-breathing pattern
    4. Assume the knee-chest position

29. A mother is inspecting her newborn girl for the first time. The infant's breasts are edematous and there is a pink vaginal discharge. How should the nurse respond when the mother asks what is wrong?
    1. "You seem very concerned. I don't see anything unusual."
    2. "Your baby appears to have a problem. I'll notify the pediatrician."
    3. "The swelling and discharge will go away. It's nothing to worry about."
    4. "The swelling and discharge are expected. They're a response to your hormones."

30. Examination of a client in active labor reveals fetal heart sounds in the right lower quadrant. The head is in the anterior position, is well flexed, and is at the level of the ischial spines. What fetal position should the nurse document?
    1. ROA, 0 station
    2. LOP, −2 station
    3. ROP, −3 station
    4. LOA, +1 station

31. A client had a dilation and curettage (D&C) after an early miscarriage (spontaneous abortion). The nurse finds her crying later in the day. What is the most appropriate statement by the nurse?
    1. "This must be a very hard experience for you to deal with."
    2. "You will have other children to take the place of the one you lost."
    3. "Of course you are sad now, but at least you know you can get pregnant."
    4. "I know how you feel, but when a woman miscarries it is usually for the best."

32. A woman in labor with her third child is 7 cm dilated and the fetal head is at station +1. Her membranes rupture. What should the nurse do first?
    1. Notify the practitioner
    2. Observe the vaginal opening for a prolapsed cord
    3. Reposition the client on a sterile towel on her left side
    4. Check the fetal heart rate while observing the color of the amniotic fluid

33. A postpartum client is being prepared for discharge. The laboratory report indicates that she has a white blood cell count of 16,000/dL. What is the next nursing action?
    1. Check with the nurse manager to see if the client can go home
    2. Reassess the client for signs of infection by taking her vital signs
    3. Delay the client's discharge until the practitioner performs a complete examination
    4. Place the report in the client's record because this is an expected postpartum finding

34. The nurse is caring for a client, who in the third trimester, is to have an amniocentesis. What should the nurse do to prepare the client for this test?
    1. Instruct her to void immediately before the test
    2. Tell her to assume the high Fowler position before the test
    3. Encourage her to drink three glasses of water before the test
    4. Advise her to take nothing by mouth for several hours before the test

35. A newborn is admitted to the nursery and is classified as small for gestational age (SGA). What is the priority nursing intervention for this infant?
    1. Test the infant's stools for occult blood
    2. Monitor the infant's blood glucose levels
    3. Place the infant in the Trendelenburg position
    4. Compare the infant's head circumference to the chest circumference

36. A newborn's discharge from the hospital is being delayed because of a rising reticulocyte count. The infant's mother, who is being discharged, asks the nurse why her baby must stay. The nurse's response is based on an understanding that the infant needs to be observed for:
    1. Bacterial infection
    2. Significant jaundice

3. Bleeding tendencies

4. Adequate oxygenation

37. A 17-year-old client tells the nurse that her sister had an ectopic pregnancy about 3 months ago and had to have her fallopian tube removed. The nurse determines that this young woman needs additional information when she states:

1. "Pelvic infections can cause this to happen."

2. "This kind of thing can happen to my sister again."

3. "I guess I'll have to wait a while to become an aunt."

4. "My sister is lucky because she won't have a period again."

38. A client is admitted to the high-risk prenatal unit with the diagnosis of placenta previa. What should the nurse instruct the client to do?

1. Breathe deeply to ensure that the fetus gets oxygen

2. Keep movement to a minimum to diminish bleeding

3. Remain on her back to minimize pressure on the cervix

4. Lie on her side to avoid putting pressure on the vena cava

39. A nurse concludes that a positive contraction stress test (CST) may be indicative of potential fetal compromise. A CST is positive when during contractions the fetal heart rate shows:

1. Late decelerations

2. Early accelerations

3. Variable decelerations

4. Prolonged accelerations

40. A 24-year-old client is admitted at 40 weeks' gestation. The cervix is 5 cm dilated and is 100% effaced, and the presenting part is at station 0. The nurse assesses that the fetal heart tones are just above the umbilicus. What does the nurse document as the fetus's presentation?

1. Face

2. Brow

3. Breech

4. Shoulder

41. Epidural anesthesia is administered to a pregnant woman in labor. What client response to this medication is of most concern to the nurse?

1. Tachycardia

2. Hypotension

3. Decreased urine production

4. Precipitous second stage of labor

42. Which nursing assessment is most important for a large-for-gestational-age (LGA) infant of a diabetic mother (IDM)?

1. Temperature less than 98° F

2. Heart rate of 110 beats per minute

3. Blood glucose level less than 40 mg/dL

4. Bilirubin increasing during the first 24 hours

43. What is an important nursing intervention when a client is receiving IV magnesium sulfate for preeclampsia?

1. Limiting IV fluid intake

2. Preparing for a possible precipitous birth

3. Maintaining a quiet, darkened environment

4. Obtaining magnesium gluconate as an antagonist

44. A few weeks after discharge, a postpartum client develops mastitis and telephones for advice concerning breastfeeding. The nurse notifies the practitioner to have antibiotics prescribed. What should the nurse recommend that the client do?

1. Wean the infant from the breast

2. Start formula feedings immediately

3. Breastfeed often to keep the breasts empty

4. Apply ice packs to suppress milk production

45. A woman at 39 weeks' gestation, whose membranes have ruptured at home, arrives at the clinic to be evaluated. Assessment reveals mild irregular contractions 10 to 15 minutes apart and a fetal heart rate of 186 beats per minute auscultated between contractions. Based on this assessment what does the nurse conclude?

1. The fetus is not at risk

2. A precipitous birth is imminent

3. This is a response to an infection

4. A further assessment is necessary

46. A nurse assesses that a 1-day-old newborn has a heart rate of 138 beats per minute. What is the best nursing action at this time?

1. Document the heart rate

2. Rewrap the infant quickly

3. Place the infant in a heated crib

4. Assess the heart rate again in an hour

47. A preterm newborn is placed in the neonatal intensive care unit (NICU). What is the first concern that the nurse anticipates for this infant's mother?

1. Fear of touching the infant

2. Failure to bond with the infant

3. Inability to provide breast milk for the infant

4. Anxiety that the father may not accept the infant

48. A nurse is assessing a newborn with exstrophy of the bladder. What other defect associated with exstrophy of the bladder is of concern to the nurse?

1. Absence of one kidney

2. Congenital heart disease

3. Pubic bone malformation

4. Tracheoesophageal fistula

49. A 60-year-old woman is to have a total abdominal hysterectomy for noninvasive endometrial cancer. The nurse anticipates the client may have difficulty adjusting emotionally to this type of surgery. What is the most common reason for this difficulty?

1. Loss of femininity

2. Body image changes

3. Diminished sexual desire

4. Slow postmenopausal recovery

50. A client had a blood pressure of 90/50 during her first visit to the prenatal clinic. At 34 weeks' gestation her blood pressure is now 120/76. The nurse concludes that this can occur because of:

1. The presence of chronic hypertension

2. The possible development of preeclampsia

3. An increased stroke volume during the third trimester

4. An expected rise in blood pressure as pregnancy progresses

CHILDBEARING AND WOMEN'S HEALTH NURSING QUIZ ANSWERS AND RATIONALES

1. **4 A side effect of prostaglandin E₂ (Prostin E₂) is bronchoconstriction, which may cause a bronchospasm in clients with asthma.**
   1 Albuterol inhalers may be used as needed.
   2 This medication is not contraindicated for pregnant clients with asthma.
   3 This medication is not contraindicated for pregnant clients with asthma.
   Client Needs: Pharmacological and Parenteral Therapies; **Cognitive Level:** Analysis; **NP:** Implementation

2. **2 Respiratory depression occurs with toxic levels of magnesium sulfate; calcium gluconate should be readily available to counteract toxicity.**
   1 Although this is an important assessment, it is not the priority.
   3 Although this is an important assessment, it is not the priority.
   4 Although this is an important assessment, it is not the priority.
   Client Needs: Pharmacological and Parenteral Therapies; **Cognitive Level:** Application; **NP:** Evaluation

3. **1 After the newborn's head has externally rotated, the nurse gently guides the head downward for the birth of the anterior shoulder.**
   2 This is contraindicated.
   3 This is contraindicated.
   4 This is contraindicated.
   Client Needs: Health Promotion and Maintenance; **Cognitive Level:** Application; **NP:** Implementation

4. **3 According to the Apgar scoring scale: heart rate above 120 = 2, respirations below 30 = 1, some flexion of extremities = 1, weak cry = 1, blue extremities = 1; these numbers total 6. Each category on the Apgar scale is assigned a 2, with 10 being the highest possible Apgar score.**
   1 This number is too low and does not reflect an accurate assessment of this newborn.
   2 This number is too low and does not reflect an accurate assessment of this newborn.
   4 This number is too high and does not reflect an accurate assessment of this newborn.
   Client Needs: Reduction of Risk Potential; **Cognitive Level:** Analysis; **NP:** Assessment

5. **3 Mongolian spots are bluish-black areas of pigmentation commonly found on the back and buttocks of dark-skinned newborns; they are benign and fade gradually over time.**
   1 Stork bites are short red marks commonly found near the base of the neck of newborns.
   2 Forceps marks are red and have a distinctive imprint on the face and head matching the configuration of the instrument.
   4 These are not ecchymotic areas; ecchymosis is the extravasation of blood into subcutaneous tissue.

   Client Needs: Health Promotion and Maintenance; **Cognitive Level:** Application; **Integrated Process:** Communication and Documentation; **NP:** Analysis

6. **3 This is one of the early signs of decompensation resulting from an increased cardiac workload.**
   1 This is a later sign of cardiac decompensation that is associated with pulmonary edema.
   2 This is a later sign of cardiac decompensation and may be accompanied by other signs of heart failure.
   4 This is a later sign of cardiac decompensation and may be accompanied by other signs of heart failure.
   Client Needs: Physiological Adaptation; **Cognitive Level:** Application; **NP:** Analysis

7. **2 Breathing with the glottis open prevents the Valsalva maneuver, thus limiting the strong urge to push and allows for a more controlled birth of the head.**
   1 This is not helpful in overcoming the urge to push; this is used during the latent phase of the first stage of labor.
   3 This breathing pattern does not help to control the birth of the fetus.
   4 This is not helpful in overcoming the urge to push; this is used during active labor when the cervix is 3 to 7 cm dilated.
   Client Needs: Health Promotion and Maintenance; **Cognitive Level:** Application; **Integrated Process:** Teaching/Learning; **NP:** Implementation

8. **1 By visiting other babies in the NICU the parents are avoiding interacting with their own infant. The parents need assistance to begin bonding.**
   2 Touching an infant with the fingertips is early bonding behavior.
   3 By discussing the equipment at the bedside they are addressing their infant's needs, which is an early bonding behavior.
   4 Asking questions about their baby's condition reflects bonding with the infant
   Client Needs: Psychosocial Integrity; **Cognitive Level:** Application; **NP:** Assessment

9. **4 A diaphragm with a spermicidal gel, if used correctly, offers a low risk for conception, has a high degree of reliability, and is the safest contraceptive method for a person with type 1 diabetes.**
   1 A vaginal sponge can be used by women with type 1 diabetes, but it is less reliable than the diaphragm with spermicidal gel.
   2 Even a low-dose oral contraceptive increases the risk for vascular complications; women with type 1 diabetes are already at risk for vascular complications.
   3 The rhythm method is not reliable because menses during the postpartum and lactation periods are often irregular; condoms can fail and must be used correctly and consistently throughout sexual intercourse.

NP: Nursing process.

Client Needs: Health Promotion and Maintenance; **Cognitive Level:** Application; **Integrated Process:** Teaching/Learning; **NP:** Implementation

10. **2 Because Tay-Sachs disease is an autosomal recessive disorder, the probability of one of their offspring inheriting this disorder is 25%.**
    1 This occurs if one parent is a Tay-Sachs carrier and the other does not have the gene.
    3 This occurs if one parent is heterozygous and the other is homozygous; however, this does not occur because children with Tay-Sachs disease do not live long enough to reproduce.
    4 This does not occur because children with Tay-Sachs disease do not live long enough to reproduce.

    Client Needs: Health Promotion and Maintenance; **Cognitive Level:** Application; **Integrated Process:** Teaching/Learning; **NP:** Implementation

11. **2 In the United States each state has its own restrictions; the approval of a court-appointed individual or group is required to give legal consent.**
    1 This does not meet the legal requirements for granting consent. The states have an obligation to oversee the best interests of the mentally disabled, and the court must be involved.
    3 This does not meet the legal requirements for granting consent. The states have an obligation to oversee the best interests of the mentally disabled, and the court must be involved.
    4 This does not meet the legal requirements for granting consent. The states have an obligation to oversee the best interests of the mentally disabled, and the court must be involved.

    Client Needs: Management of Care; **Cognitive Level:** Comprehension; **NP:** Planning

12. **3 Cephalhematoma is a collection of blood beneath the periosteum of the skull bone; the blood mass does not cross the suture line and is confined to one side of the head. It reabsorbs within 3 to 6 weeks.**
    1 Molding is overlapping of the cranial bones or shaping of the fetal head to accommodate and conform to the bony and soft parts of the mother's birth canal during labor; it resolves within 3 days.
    2 Hydrocephalus is an enlargement of the entire head (macrocephaly) caused by an abnormal enlargement of the cerebral ventricles and skull, which results from an obstruction in the flow of cerebral spinal fluid.
    4 Caput succedaneum is an edematous swelling of the scalp that extends across the suture line; it resolves within 3 to 4 days.

    Client Needs: Health Promotion and Maintenance; **Cognitive Level:** Application; **Integrated Process:** Communication and Documentation; **NP:** Implementation

13. **4 Fluid intake and fiber help promote soft stools and defecation. Promoting defecation is a priority because a fourth-degree laceration impinges on the** rectal sphincter. Constipation will further traumatize the rectum.
    1 Although sitz baths relieve pain and promote healing, they do not prevent additional trauma.
    2 Although anesthetic pads relieve pain, they do not prevent additional trauma.
    3 An enema would cause additional trauma to the rectum and is contraindicated.

    Client Needs: Health Promotion and Maintenance; **Cognitive Level:** Application; **Integrated Process:** Teaching/Learning; **NP:** Implementation

14. **4 The client is exhibiting one symptom of premenstrual syndrome (PMS); eliminating food and beverages containing caffeine can limit breast swelling.**
    1 Salt intake should be reduced premenstrually to limit the development of edema.
    2 Increasing protein intake is unnecessary if the client is eating a nutritious diet.
    3 Exercise should be increased premenstrually to help reduce the symptoms of PMS.

    Client Needs: Health Promotion and Maintenance; **Cognitive Level:** Application; **Integrated Process:** Teaching/Learning; **NP:** Implementation

15. **2 Primary prevention focuses on health promotion and illness prevention.**
    1 Tertiary prevention focuses on rehabilitation and the reduction of residual effects.
    3 Secondary prevention focuses on early detection and treatment.
    4 There is no type of prevention that is specifically known as therapeutic; however, all types of prevention should be therapeutic.

    Client Needs: Management of Care; **Cognitive Level:** Analysis; **NP:** Planning

16. **4 Increased alertness is an expected common behavior that occurs in new or different situations when a person is mildly anxious.**
    1 This is a common sign of moderate to severe anxiety.
    2 This is a common sign of moderate to severe anxiety.
    3 This is a common sign of moderate to severe anxiety.

    Client Needs: Psychosocial Integrity; **Cognitive Level:** Application; **NP:** Assessment

17. **1 The dietician can give the client specific information that would help her plan nutritious meals. Specific foods, such as nuts and soy products, can be substituted for meat or animal-related products.**
    2 The client may know healthy nutrition; this client needs help to adapt the vegetarian diet to meet pregnancy needs.
    3 This ignores the client's beliefs and lifestyle; a nutritious vegetarian diet is available during pregnancy.
    4 This ignores the client's beliefs and lifestyle; a nutritious vegetarian diet is available during pregnancy.

    Client Needs: Management of Care; **Cognitive Level:** Application; **Integrated Process:** Communication and Documentation; **NP:** Planning

18. 3 **Betamethasone (Celestone), a corticosteroid, accelerates lung maturity and reduces intravascular hemorrhage and necrotizing enterocolitis in the preterm neonate if given 24 hours before birth.**
    1 Chorioamnionitis is treated with antibiotic therapy; this problem may occur if the membranes rupture prematurely and birth does not occur within 24 hours.
    2 Corticosteroids do not have an effect on uteroplacental exchange.
    4 The neonate, not the fetus, develops respiratory distress syndrome (RDS); if betamethasone is given to the mother 24 hours before a preterm birth, the severity and incidence of RDS in the neonate should decrease.
    Client Needs: Pharmacological and Parenteral Therapies; **Cognitive Level:** Comprehension; **Integrated Process:** Communication and Documentation; **NP:** Implementation

19. 3 **The client's blood pressure has decreased, causing supine hypotension. Lying flat will maintain the client's head at the same level as the heart, enabling more oxygenated blood to reach the brain, thus relieving the symptoms of lightheadedness and nausea. The side-lying position promotes placental perfusion.**
    1 The contractions and fetal heart rates are within the expected range. Interrupting the oxytocin (Pitocin) infusion is counterproductive and will prolong the labor.
    2 If the client continues to feel lightheaded after the position change, oxygen administration is the next nursing action.
    4 The fetal heart rates are within the expected range. Episodic accelerations occur during fetal movement and are indications of fetal well-being. Early decelerations occur in response to fetal head compression and are a benign finding.
    Client Needs: Pharmacological and Parenteral Therapies; **Cognitive Level:** Analysis; **NP:** Implementation

20. 2 **Frequent nursing empties the milk ducts, thus relieving engorgement.**
    1 Manual expression initiates milk flow, empties the ducts, and relieves engorgement.
    3 Warmth will dilate ducts and facilitate flow of milk, thus relieving engorgement.
    4 If the breasts remain engorged immediately after breastfeeding, cold compresses help relieve the discomfort.
    Client Needs: Health Promotion and Maintenance; **Cognitive Level:** Application; **Integrated Process:** Teaching/Learning; **NP:** Evaluation

21. 2 **With severe preeclampsia, arteriolar spasms cause hypertension and decreased arterial perfusion of the kidneys. Decreased perfusion to the kidneys causes an alteration in the glomeruli, resulting in oliguria and proteinuria, and retention of sodium and water, resulting in edema.**
    1 Eclampsia is characterized by seizures; there are no data to indicate that the client is having or has had seizures.
    3 Chronic hypertension is hypertension diagnosed before pregnancy or before 20 weeks' gestation. If hypertension diagnosed during pregnancy for the first time persists beyond the postpartum period, it also is considered chronic hypertension.
    4 Gestational hypertension is hypertension that occurs during mid-pregnancy for the first time and without proteinuria; it is definitively diagnosed when the hypertension resolves 12 weeks postpartum.
    Client Needs: Physiological Adaptation; **Cognitive Level:** Analysis; **NP:** Analysis

22. 1 **The likelihood of a brain attack increases with rising blood pressure readings.**
    2 The degree of hypertension is not associated with hemorrhage.
    3 The course of labor is not affected by blood pressure changes except in the presence of abruptio placentae.
    4 Fluctuations in blood pressure do not affect the status of clotting factors.
    Client Needs: Physiological Adaptation; **Cognitive Level:** Analysis; **NP:** Evaluation

23. 4 **Fever, malaise, and headache may accompany local reactions.**
    1 Vesicles on genitalia rupture, causing painful ulcerations.
    2 Herpes is of viral origin; there is no cure, and antibiotics are ineffective.
    3 Most transmissions occur through intimate sexual contact with acute or healing lesions.
    Client Needs: Health Promotion and Maintenance; **Cognitive Level:** Application; **Integrated Process:** Teaching/Learning; **NP:** Implementation

24. 1 **Muscle contraction during ambulation improves venous return, which prevents venous stasis and thrombus formation.**
    2 Gatching the bed places pressure on the popliteal spaces, limiting venous return and increasing the risk of thrombus formation.
    3 Dangling the legs places pressure on the popliteal spaces, limiting venous return and increasing the risk of thrombus formation.
    4 Bed rest is associated with venous stasis, which increases the risk of thrombus formation.
    Client Needs: Reduction of Risk Potential; **Cognitive Level:** Application; **Integrated Process:** Teaching/Learning; **NP:** Planning

25. **Answer: 1, 3**
    1 Many clients are asymptomatic.
    2 There is no effective readily available blood test for gonorrhea.
    3 The incubation period is 3 to 5 days.
    4 Gonorrhea responds well to treatment; however, at times back-up secondary medications have to be used.
    5 Urethral/vaginal smears or cultures are specific for the identification of the gonococcal organism.

Client Needs: Health Promotion and Maintenance; **Cognitive Level:** Analysis; **Integrated Process:** Teaching/Learning; **NP:** Implementation

26. **2 Protection of newborns from unnecessary exposure to microorganisms is the priority.**
    1 This should not be done until the mother and newborn's identification bands are verified.
    3 This should be done after the visitor leaves the room.
    4 This discussion should take place outside the room. The visitor should be asked to leave if indications of an infection are present.
    Client Needs: Safety and Infection Control; **Cognitive Level:** Application; **NP:** Implementation

27. **2 Suckling or nipple stimulation precipitates the release of oxytocin, which initiates the let-down reflex.**
    1 The hormone prolactin stimulates milk production.
    3 Estrogen inhibits the secretion of lactogenic hormones.
    4 Placental separation initiates the hormonal changes of the postpartum period.
    Client Needs: Health Promotion and Maintenance; **Cognitive Level:** Comprehension; **NP:** Planning

28. **3 Panting will slow the process so the nurse can support the head as it is born.**
    1 Pushing will speed the birth, which may injure both mother and fetus.
    2 This will have no effect on the progress of the second stage of labor and it is difficult to accomplish when the fetal head is crowning.
    4 This will have no effect on the progress of the second stage of labor and it is difficult to accomplish when the fetal head is crowning.
    Client Needs: Health Promotion and Maintenance; **Cognitive Level:** Application; **Integrated Process:** Communication and Documentation; **NP:** Implementation

29. **4 This response emphasizes that these findings are expected and explains why they occur; this may relieve the client's anxiety.**
    1 This response denies that there is anything to explain to the mother and it is somewhat belittling.
    2 Calling the pediatrician is not necessary; these findings are expected.
    3 This comment tells the mother that the findings are expected, but offers no explanation and is somewhat belittling.
    Client Needs: Health Promotion and Maintenance; **Cognitive Level:** Application; **Integrated Process:** Communication and Documentation; **NP:** Implementation

30. **1 The fetal heart is in the right quadrant; therefore, the fetus's head and back are on the right side. The head is engaged and is at 0 station.**
    2 In this position the fetal heart should be heard on the left side; at station −2 the head is mobile.
    3 The information states that the head is anterior and flexed; at −3 station the head is mobile.
    4 In this position the fetal heart should be heard on the left side; at +1 station the head is engaged below the ischial spines.

Client Needs: Health Promotion and Maintenance; **Cognitive Level:** Analysis; **Integrated Process:** Communication and Documentation; **NP:** Analysis

31. **1 This acknowledges the validity of the grief and provides the client with an opportunity to talk if she wishes.**
    2 Other children cannot and should not be substituted for a lost fetus.
    3 Getting pregnant is not the issue; this statement belittles the lost fetus.
    4 The nurse cannot know how the client feels. This comment is patronizing and diminishes the significance of the lost fetus.
    Client Needs: Psychosocial Integrity; **Cognitive Level:** Application; **Integrated Process:** Caring; **NP:** Implementation

32. **4 Fetal well being is the priority. The fetal heart rate will reflect the fetus's response to the occurrence of ruptured membranes and the color of the amniotic fluid will reveal if there is meconium staining.**
    1 This is necessary if the nurse's assessments reveal fetal compromise.
    2 Although important, it is not the priority; the fetal head is engaged at station +1.
    3 While positioning the client on the left side promotes placental perfusion, it is not the priority. A sterile pad is not needed.
    Client Needs: Health Promotion and Maintenance; **Cognitive Level:** Application; **NP:** Implementation

33. **4 Leukocytosis (15,000 to 20,000 mm³ WBC) typically occurs during the postpartum period as a compensatory defense mechanism.**
    1 There is no need for further intervention because the client is exhibiting an expected postpartum leukocytosis.
    2 There is no need for further intervention because the client is exhibiting an expected postpartum leukocytosis.
    3 There is no need for further intervention because the client is exhibiting an expected postpartum leukocytosis.
    Client Needs: Reduction of Risk Potential; **Cognitive Level:** Application; **Integrated Process:** Communication and Documentation; **NP:** Implementation

34. **1 This is done to prevent injury to the bladder as the needle is introduced into the amniotic sac.**
    2 The supine position with a hip roll under the right hip is the preferred position to place the client during this procedure.
    3 This will fill the bladder, making it vulnerable to injury as the needle is inserted into the amniotic sac. This is advised if the amniocentesis is performed early during pregnancy.
    4 There is no reason to withhold food or fluid because the test does not involve the gastrointestinal tract.
    Client Needs: Reduction of Risk Potential; **Cognitive Level:** Application; **Integrated Process:** Communication and Documentation; **NP:** Implementation

35. **2 SGA infants are prone to hypoglycemia because they have little subcutaneous fat or glycogen stores.**
    1 Intestinal bleeding is not common in SGA infants.
    3 This has no therapeutic value for SGA infants.
    4 Hydrocephalus or microcephaly is not characteristic of SGA infants.
    Client Needs: Reduction of Risk Potential; **Cognitive Level:** Application; **NP:** Assessment

36. **2 A rising reticulocyte count indicates accelerated erythropoietic activity that may reflect increased RBC destruction; increased RBC destruction increases the bilirubin level, causing jaundice.**
    1 With an infection the sedimentation rate or WBCs, not the reticulocytes, is elevated.
    3 Although the reticulocyte count may be elevated with chronic blood loss, there are no data to indicate the infant is bleeding.
    4 This test does not reflect respiratory functioning.
    Client Needs: Reduction of Risk Potential; **Cognitive Level:** Application; **NP:** Analysis

37. **4 Removing a fallopian tube will not halt menses; endometrial proliferation and shedding will occur as long as the ovaries and uterus are present.**
    1 Pelvic infections can lead to constriction of fallopian tubes, and a fertilized ovum may become trapped.
    2 There is evidence that clients who have had one tubal pregnancy have a high probability of having another tubal pregnancy.
    3 Pregnancy should be delayed 6 to 12 months after a tubal pregnancy.
    Client Needs: Health Promotion and Maintenance; **Cognitive Level:** Application; **Integrated Process:** Teaching/Learning; **NP:** Evaluation

38. **4 The side-lying position decreases pressure on the vena cava from the gravid uterus, ensuring adequate oxygenation of the fetus.**
    1 Without proper positioning, breathing techniques will be less effective.
    2 Although the client will probably have an order for bed rest, she is allowed to move.
    3 Lying on the back will increase pressure on the vena cava, further compromising the fetus.
    Client Needs: Physiological Adaptation; **Cognitive Level:** Application; **Integrated Process:** Teaching/Learning; **NP:** Implementation

39. **1 The fetus with a borderline cardiac reserve will demonstrate hypoxia by a decreased heart rate when there is minimal stress, making the CST positive.**
    2 Accelerations are not defined as early, late, or prolonged.
    3 These are nonuniform drops in FHR before, during, or after a contraction; variable decelerations during a CST do not make the test positive.
    4 Accelerations are not defined as early, late, or prolonged.
    Client Needs: Reduction of Risk Potential; **Cognitive Level:** Application; **NP:** Analysis

40. **3 In the breech presentation, the fetal head is in the fundal portion of the uterus; the chest or back is at or above the umbilicus, where fetal heart tones can be heard.**
    1 In the vertex presentation, the head is the presenting part; the chest and back are in lower quadrants, where the fetal heart is heard.
    2 The brow presentation is a type of cephalic presentation, where the fetal head is partially extended; the fetal heart is heard in the lower abdomen, not above the umbilicus.
    4 In the shoulder presentation, the fetal heart usually is heard in the midabdominal region.
    Client Needs: Health Promotion and Maintenance; **Cognitive Level:** Analysis; **Integrated Process:** Communication and Documentation; **NP:** Analysis

41. **2 Regional anesthesia lowers the blood pressure, which places both mother and fetus in jeopardy.**
    1 The blood pressure, not the heart rate, is affected first.
    3 The client may not have the sensation to void but the amount of urine in the bladder does not decrease because a regional block does not affect the kidneys.
    4 Epidural anesthesia does not shorten the second stage of labor.
    Client Needs: Pharmacological and Parenteral Therapies; **Cognitive Level:** Application; **NP:** Evaluation

42. **3 At birth, circulating maternal glucose is removed; however, the infant of a diabetic mother (IDM) still has a high level of insulin and may develop rebound hypoglycemia.**
    1 The temperature-regulating ability of an IDM is similar to that of a healthy neonate, unless the IDM is preterm.
    2 This heart rate is within the expected range for a newborn. After transition, the newborn's heart rate should be 130 to 140 beats per minute.
    4 Pathologic jaundice is associated with hemolytic diseases such as Rh and ABO incompatibilities and sepsis, not maternal diabetes.
    Client Needs: Physiological Adaptation; **Cognitive Level:** Application; **NP:** Assessment

43. **3 A quiet, darkened room helps to reduce stimuli, which is essential for limiting or preventing seizures.**
    1 IV infusions are not limited. Infusions are monitored closely and usually are maintained at a volume of 125 mL/hr.
    2 Precipitous birth is not a usual side effect of magnesium therapy.
    4 Calcium gluconate, not magnesium gluconate, is the antagonist for magnesium sulfate and should be on hand if signs of toxicity appear.
    Client Needs: Pharmacological and Parenteral Therapies; **Cognitive Level:** Application; **NP:** Implementation

44. **3 This keeps the breasts as empty as possible, limiting pressure within the ducts, thereby reducing pain.**

Also, milk stasis and exacerbation of the infection can be prevented.

1 Weaning will cause stasis of milk ducts and increase the fullness of the breasts at this time, thereby increasing pain.

2 Alternatives should be tried first; breastfeeding should be continued.

4 Ice packs will suppress milk production and impede breastfeeding.

Client Needs: Health Promotion and Maintenance; **Cognitive Level:** Application; **Integrated Process:** Teaching/Learning; **NP:** Implementation

45. 4 **The fetal heart rate should be 110 to 160; an FHR of 186 is tachycardic and further evaluation is necessary.**

1 The fetus may be at risk because an FHR of 186 is above the expected range of 110 to 160 beats per minute.

2 Based on the data the client is in early labor.

3 Although fetal tachycardia is associated with infection, there may be other causes.

Client Needs: Health Promotion and Maintenance; **Cognitive Level:** Analysis; **NP:** Analysis

46. 1 **This is within the expected range of 130 to 140 beats per minute for the heart rate of a newborn.**

2 This is not necessary.

3 This is not necessary.

4 This is not necessary.

Client Needs: Health Promotion and Maintenance; **Cognitive Level:** Application; **Integrated Process:** Communication and Documentation; **NP:** Implementation

47. 1 **The fear stems from the size and frailty of the newborn and the overwhelming environment of the intensive care area; parents should be encouraged to touch and handle their infant when possible.**

2 Bonding is possible and can be enhanced when the fear of touching has been overcome.

3 The breasts can be pumped and the milk administered via gavage feedings.

4 Although this may be a concern, it is not the most common initial concern.

Client Needs: Psychosocial Integrity; **Cognitive Level:** Application; **Integrated Process:** Caring; **NP:** Assessment

48. 3 **Incomplete formation of the pubic bone is associated with exstrophy of the bladder.**

1 This is not associated with exstrophy of the bladder.

2 This is not associated with exstrophy of the bladder.

4 This is not associated with exstrophy of the bladder.

Client Needs: Physiological Adaptation; **Cognitive Level:** Comprehension; **NP:** Assessment

49. 1 **Removal of the uterus may produce changes in how some women view themselves sexually because it is a reproductive organ.**

2 Although this may occur, it is more likely to occur with surgery that has obvious external changes.

3 The libido of a postmenopausal woman probably will not be altered unless there are concerns about sexuality.

4 A 60-year-old otherwise healthy woman should have an uneventful recovery.

Client Needs: Psychosocial Integrity; **Cognitive Level:** Application; **NP:** Analysis

50. 2 **During the second trimester the blood pressure usually decreases, and it stays lower for the remainder of the pregnancy; an increase in systolic pressure of 30 mm Hg and diastolic pressure of 15 mm Hg warrants close observation for preeclampsia.**

1 The client's baseline blood pressure was low, suggesting that the increase in blood pressure is pregnancy related (gestational hypertension).

3 This physiological change does not cause a rise in blood pressure.

4 An increase in blood pressure of this amount, at 34 weeks' gestation, is not expected.

Client Needs: Health Promotion and Maintenance; ;**Cognitive Level:** Analysis; **NP:** Analysis

Child Health Nursing

Review Questions

NURSING PRACTICE

1. A 16-year-old adolescent, her 1-month-old infant, and the infant's grandmother come to the emergency department saying that the infant accidentally fell down the stairs. What should the nurse consider when obtaining legal consent for the infant's treatment?
   1. Consent is postponed because this is an emergency
   2. Responsibility rests with the mother who should sign the consent
   3. Decisions are made by family court because the mother is a minor
   4. Signature on the consent form must be obtained from the grandmother

2. An infant is scheduled for emergency surgery. The nursing history reveals that the mother is 13 years old and the father is 16 years old. The infant's father and the paternal grandmother, who cares for the baby, are at the bedside. Legally, who can provide informed consent at this time?
   1. Paternal grandmother
   2. Hospital administrator
   3. Sixteen-year-old father
   4. Thirteen-year-old mother

3. What is the nurse's primary responsibility when there is the suspicion that a child is abused?
   1. Treat the child's traumatic injuries
   2. Protect the child from future abuse
   3. Confirm the child's suspected abuse
   4. Have the child examined by the practitioner

4. What is the most appropriate approach for the school nurse to take concerning children who are given medications while in school?
   1. Assure the children that their privacy will be respected
   2. Teach each class about taking medications in the school setting
   3. Encourage the children to tell their friends that they are taking a medication
   4. Ask teachers to answer questions when other students ask about medications given in school

5. A 10-year-old boy who is about to begin chemotherapy for acute myelogenous leukemia (AML) tells the nurse that he is old enough to refuse treatment. What is the nurse's most appropriate response?
   1. "You seem frightened. Let's talk about it."
   2. "Your parents have given their consent. I have to begin."
   3. "Your age prevents you from refusing treatment. You need to be 18 years old."
   4. "You are old enough. You're also old enough to know you need the chemotherapy."

6. A community health nurse makes a home visit to the mother of a 13-year-old boy who is disabled and who has three siblings younger than 6 years old. The nurse observes that the 6-month-old sister lies quietly in her crib, rarely smiles or vocalizes, and barely has her basic needs attended. What is the priority nursing action?
   1. Teach the disabled brother how to play with his sister
   2. Discuss how the mother can be assisted with caring for the infant
   3. Encourage the mother to buy appropriate toys for the infant's age level
   4. Explain that without stimulation the infant's growth and development will be affected

7. A 6-year-old boy is sent to the school nurse on a below-freezing snowy day because he arrived without a coat, wearing shorts, a T-shirt, and sandals. What is the first nursing intervention?
   1. Call Child Protective Services
   2. Provide a warm liquid to drink
   3. Assess for the presence of frostbite
   4. Ask the child who helped him dress

8. A teacher's aide in a kindergarten class informs the school nurse that a male student said that his mother beat him and he has bruises on the back and shoulders. What is the initial nursing action?
   1. Notify Child Protective Services
   2. Report this information to the principal
   3. Call the parents to arrange a conference
   4. Assess the child for the presence of bruises

9. An infant is admitted to the hospital with gastroenteritis. The infant vomits shortly after admission. Following standard precautions, what protective equipment should the nurse wear when cleaning the infant after the vomiting episode?
   1. Mask
   2. Gown
   3. Face shield
   4. Pair of gloves

GROWTH AND DEVELOPMENT

10. A mother brings her 9-month-old infant to the clinic. The nurse is familiar with the mother's culture and knows that belly binding to prevent extrusion of the umbilicus is a common practice. The nurse accepts the mother's cultural beliefs but is concerned for the infant's safety. What variation of belly binding does the nurse discourage?
    1. Coin in the umbilicus
    2. Tight diaper over the umbilicus
    3. Binder that encircles the umbilicus
    4. Adhesive tape across the umbilicus

11. A nurse is performing a neurological assessment of a 7-month-old infant. What reflex should the nurse be able to elicit?
    1. Moro
    2. Babinski
    3. Tonic neck
    4. Palmar grasp

12. A nurse is teaching a class about behavioral expectations of infants and children to a group of parents. The nurse includes those behaviors expected of 8-month-old infants. Select all that apply.
    1. _____ Stranger anxiety
    2. _____ Playing peek-a-boo
    3. _____ Drinking from a cup
    4. _____ Removing some clothing
    5. _____ Standing by holding on to furniture

13. An infant who weighed 7.5 pounds at birth now weighs 15 pounds at 1 year. The nurse concludes that this infant's weight gain:
    1. Suggests possible maternal neglect
    2. Reflects the expected growth curve
    3. Signifies an inadequate weight gain
    4. Indicates insufficient dietary protein

14. A nurse is assessing a 1-year-old infant. What behavior does the nurse expect? Select all that apply.
    1. _____ Jumps with both feet
    2. _____ Attempts climbing stairs
    3. _____ Explores away from the parent
    4. _____ Communicates in simple sentences
    5. _____ Builds a tower consisting of several blocks

15. A nurse is assessing a 15-month-old girl at the well-child clinic. The nurse determines that further education about toddler development is necessary when the mother says, "She:
    1. is always trying to get out of her car seat."
    2. cries when I leave her at the daycare center."
    3. gets into everything with toys scattered everywhere."
    4. has a temper tantrum every time I put her on the potty chair."

16. The nurse manager of a home health care agency is teaching a group of nursing assistants about pica. Which age group is most likely to engage in this practice?
    1. Toddlers
    2. Older adults
    3. Preschoolers
    4. Pregnant women

17. What is a nurse's most appropriate response when asked about spanking as a disciplinary technique?
    1. "Effectiveness depends on the child's age."
    2. "Spanking is strongly suggestive of negative role modeling."
    3. "Spanking may be the only option when no other technique works."
    4. "Research studies have shown it to be an effective disciplinary technique."

18. A 6-week-old infant grasps a rattle placed in the hand. The mother is impressed with this skill. What should the nurse teach the mother about this behavior?
    1. This is the palmar grasp reflex and is expected at this age
    2. This is the pincer grasp, which disappears within several months
    3. Grasping is a voluntary behavior usually observed in older infants
    4. Grasping is an atypical behavior and further evaluation is required

19. A nurse is trying to soothe a 2-month-old who is crying. What is the best way to soothe a young infant?
    1. Offer the infant a bottle of diluted juice
    2. Hold and rock the infant in a quiet room
    3. Change the diaper before returning the infant to the crib
    4. Wrap a blanket around the infant and place in a supine position

20. The mother of a 3-month-old infant asks the nurse in the well-baby clinic what toys to give her child. What is the nurse's response? Select all that apply.
    1. _____ Push-pull toy
    2. _____ Stuffed animal
    3. _____ Metallic mirror
    4. _____ Colorful mobile
    5. _____ Large plastic ball

21. Which behavior does the nurse expect when observing a 5-month-old infant?
    1. Picking up a toy and putting it into the mouth
    2. Waving the fists and dropping toys placed in the hands
    3. Exploratory searching when an object is hidden from view
    4. Simultaneously kicking the legs while batting the hands in the air

22. A mother tells the nurse that her 7-month-old infant has just started sitting without support. The nurse teaches the mother that this:
    1. Is expected developmental behavior at this age
    2. Is an indication that walking will begin within 2 months
    3. Reflects infants in the upper 10% of physical development
    4. Indicates a possible developmental delay requiring further evaluation

23. A nurse counsels a mother of an 8-month-old infant to be sure the floors are free of small objects when her child is crawling. What is the rationale for this instruction?
    1. Sharp objects can injure the fragile skin of an infant
    2. Eight-month-old infants hide small objects, making them difficult to locate
    3. Floors may cause infections in infants when they pick up and mouth objects
    4. Eight-month-old infants pick up small objects and place them into their mouths

24. A nurse teaches a mother about appropriate play for an 8-month-old infant. Which of the mother's suggestions indicate that the teaching was understood? Select all that apply.
    1. _____ Textured book
    2. _____ Modeling clay
    3. _____ Stuffed animal
    4. _____ Play telephone
    5. _____ Hanging mobile

25. A nurse in the child health clinic is assessing a 9-month-old infant. What developmental findings does the nurse expect? Select all that apply.
    1. _____ Enjoys push-pull toys
    2. _____ Sits steadily without support
    3. _____ Feeds self with a baby spoon
    4. _____ Responds to simple commands
    5. _____ Has a vocabulary of two words

26. A nurse is teaching a class to parents about keeping medications and household cleaning supplies out of the reach of toddlers. The nurse explains that this is necessary because toddlers:
    1. Have increased appetites
    2. Are developing a sense of taste
    3. Have a high level of oral activity
    4. Are rebelling against parental authority

27. A nurse assesses that a 22-month-old child uses 2- or 3-word phrases (telegraphic speech), has a vocabulary of about 20 words, and often uses the word "me." The nurse concludes the child's language development is:
    1. Delayed
    2. Advanced
    3. Appropriate
    4. Pathological

28. A nurse must administer a medication by injection to a 2-year-old whose parent is not present. What is the most therapeutic approach for the nurse to use?
    1. Avoid telling the child beforehand, give the injection, and then cuddle the child
    2. Demonstrate how an injection is given, tell the child why it is needed, and then gather the equipment
    3. Give a doll the injection, encourage the child to give the doll an injection, and then give the the injection
    4. Warn the child about the injection just before administering it, say it is OK to cry, and then comfort the child

29. A father expresses concern that his 2-year-old daughter has become a "finicky eater" and is eating less. How should the nurse respond?
    1. "Your daughter has become manipulative."
    2. "She probably is experiencing the stress of a typical two year old."
    3. "She may have an eating problem requiring a referral to a specialist."
    4. "Your daughter's behavior is expected in response to her slower growth."

30. The mother of a 2-year-old girl expresses concern that her daughter's growth rate has slowed. What should the nurse explain to the mother about the growth of toddlers?
    1. "This growth pattern is typical at this age."
    2. "Toddlers are too busy exploring their world to eat."
    3. "This growth pattern cannot be interpreted for another year."
    4. "Toddlers usually lose their taste for foods they liked when younger."

31. Several 3-year-old girls in the day care center are having a tea party with their dolls. The center's nurse concludes that this behavior is:
    1. Evidence of abstract thought
    2. Appropriate make-believe play
    3. Inappropriate exclusion of boys
    4. Maladaptive use of magical thinking

32. A mother in the postpartum unit expresses concern that her 3-year-old daughter will be jealous of her new brother. What should the nurse suggest?
    1. Ignore negative comments that the daughter makes about the baby
    2. Allow the daughter to stay with her baby brother when the mother rests
    3. Explain in simple terms why the mother must spend more time with the baby
    4. Bring home a new baby doll for the daughter when her baby brother is brought home

33. During a routine visit to the child health clinic, the parent of a 3-year-old girl reports, "My daughter is still sucking her thumb." What is the nurse's best response?
    1. "She will stop when she is ready."
    2. "You can buy a bitter liquid for her thumb."
    3. "Is she being teased by her friends in nursery school?"
    4. "Do you want me to recommend a child psychologist?"

34. The parents of a 3-year-old tell the nurse that their child is afraid to sleep alone because of monsters under the bed. They ask for suggestions. What should the nurse recommend?
    1. Tell the child that monsters do not exist
    2. Allow the child to sleep with the parents temporarily
    3. Look under the bed and say, "I don't see any monsters."
    4. Leave a small light on at night and state, "Monsters aren't allowed in the house."

35. A nurse is planning to foster independence in a group of 4-year-old children. What self-care skill does the nurse expect 4-year-old children to be capable of performing?
   1. Parting and combing hair
   2. Putting on a shirt and buttoning it
   3. Cutting meat using a fork and knife
   4. Slipping into shoes and tying shoelaces

36. A nurse is assessing a 4-year-old child. What age-appropriate language skills does the nurse expect the child to have achieved? Select all that apply.
   1. _____ Uses appropriate grammar
   2. _____ Uses 6- and 8-word sentences
   3. _____ Asks the meaning of new words
   4. _____ Pronounces the sounds CH and TH
   5. _____ Has a vocabulary of 150 to 200 words

37. During a clinic visit a 4-year-old girl suddenly yells, "Don't sit on Erin!" The parent whispers that Erin is an imaginary friend. What should the nurse include in the teaching plan for this child's family?
   1. Referral to classes on parenting
   2. Special instructions for discipline
   3. Increasing peer social interaction for the daughter
   4. Referral to a child psychologist regarding the imaginary friend

38. When talking with a 4-year-old child, a nurse identifies that the child is shy and stutters. What does stuttering in a 4-year-old child indicate?
   1. Speech impediment
   2. Emotional problems
   3. Typical preschooler speech
   4. Delay in neural development

39. A 4-year-old child is being prepared for a myringotomy in the ambulatory care unit. What should the nurse do when the child is called to go to the operating room?
   1. Remove the child's toys
   2. Allow the child to climb onto the gurney
   3. Have the parents accompany the child to the operating suite
   4. Ask the parents to leave before giving the preoperative sedative

40. A school nurse is teaching a group of parents about age-related issues of 5-year-old children. What should the nurse include as a major concern of children of this age?
   1. Fear of separation
   2. Anxiety about body integrity
   3. Apprehensive regarding strangers
   4. Threats to their dependency needs

41. A 5-year-old child is brought to the child health clinic for a routine visit, and the nurse observes the child interacting with other children. What type of play does the nurse expect of the child?
   1. Team
   2. Parallel
   3. Initiative
   4. Cooperative

42. A nurse is evaluating whether a 5-year-old child is displaying appropriate behaviors for this age. What developmental findings does the nurse expect? Select all that apply.
   1. _____ Enjoys imitative play
   2. _____ Engages in ritualistic games
   3. _____ Makes up rules for a new game
   4. _____ Asks for a pacifier when uncomfortable
   5. _____ Plays near others quietly but not with them

43. A Girl Scout leader arrives at the hospital's emergency department with a 7-year-old child who may have a broken ankle. The history reveals that the child fell about 1 mile from the camp while on a hike with the scout leader and four other 7-year-olds. The nurse asks if all the children are safely back in camp. Assuming that the scout leader acted appropriately, the nurse expects the scout leader to respond, "I:
   1. left the girls and brought the injured child to the hospital."
   2. sent two of the girls back to camp and had them ask for help."
   3. carried the injured girl and led the rest of the girls back to camp."
   4. stayed with the injured girl and sent the four other girls back to camp for help."

44. A 12-year-old child is to be bedridden at home for several weeks after orthopedic surgery. What activity should the nurse encourage the parents to plan?
   1. Drawing pictures
   2. Playing card games
   3. Watching television
   4. Continuing schoolwork

45. What is the most appropriate communication strategy for the nurse working with adolescents in a clinic in a large city health center?
   1. Relating on a peer level
   2. Using typical teenage language
   3. Establishing a relationship over time
   4. Having discussions in concrete terms

46. Parents of a boy born with hypospadias ask the nurse at what age the repair of this congenital defect is performed. What is the most appropriate response by the nurse?
   1. Shortly after birth
   2. Between 4 and 5 years of age
   3. Just before the onset of puberty
   4. After 6 months and before 1 year of age

47. A 4-month-old infant is admitted to the pediatric unit. How does the primary nurse expect the infant to behave when approached?
   1. Smile socially in recognition of the nurse's face
   2. Cry when the nurse approaches for the first time
   3. Reach out to the nurse for the attention that is being offered
   4. Cling to the mother when the nurse tries to establish contact

48. The mother of a 7-month-old infant who is to be catheterized to obtain a sterile urine specimen expresses fear that this procedure may emotionally traumatize her baby. How should the nurse respond?

1. "I will obtain a clean-catch specimen instead."
2. "You have a legal right to refuse the catheterization."
3. "The procedure will not be emotionally traumatic at this age."
4. "Your child's catheterization takes priority over your concern."

49. A 6-month-old infant is admitted to the pediatric unit with a diagnosis of failure to thrive. The birth weight was 7 pounds. Based on growth and development charts, how many pounds does the nurse conclude that the infant should weigh?
    1. 12
    2. 14
    3. 18
    4. 22

50. A 1-year-old infant is brought to the pediatric clinic for the first time. During the assessment the nurse suspects there is a developmental delay. What developmental milestone should have been achieved by this age?
    1. Saying six words
    2. Standing without support
    3. Responding to peek-a-boo
    4. Building a tower of two cubes

51. The parents of an 18-month-old toddler are anxious to know why their child has experienced several episodes of acute otitis media. What should the nurse explain to the parents about why toddlers are prone to middle ear infections?
    1. Immunological differences between adults and young children
    2. Structural differences between eustachian tubes of younger and older children
    3. Functional differences between eustachian tubes of younger and older children
    4. Circumference differences between middle ear cavity size of adults and young children

52. A nurse is teaching the parents of an 18-month-old child the procedure for instilling ear drops. How should this procedure be done?
    1. Cleanse ear canal before instilling the drops
    2. Apply medicated ear wicks after instilling the drops
    3. Pull pinna up and back after drop insertion to promote disbursement of the drops
    4. Pull pinna down and back to straighten the auditory canal before insertion of the drops

53. A 2-year-old boy who has fallen from a tree tells his parents and the nurse, "Bad, bad tree." The nurse concludes that the child is within the cognitive developmental norm of Piaget's:
    1. Concrete operations
    2. Concept of reversibility
    3. Preconceptual operations
    4. Sensorimotor development

54. A 2½-year-old girl whose older sibling recently died has started hitting her mother and refusing to go to bed at night. The nurse explains to the mother that her daughter probably is:

1. Fearing dying while sleeping
2. Attempting to get more parental attention
3. Reacting appropriately to the family's grieving
4. Displaying behavior that is typical of the stage of autonomy

55. A 3-year-old child is hospitalized with nephrotic syndrome. The child has oliguria and generalized edema. What factor does the nurse identify that will have the greatest effect on the child's adjustment to hospitalization?
    1. Lack of parental visits
    2. Inability to select a variety of foods
    3. Response of peers to the edematous appearance
    4. Willingness to participate in cooperative play activities

56. An IV catheter is to be inserted into a 3-year-old toddler's peripheral vein. As local topical anesthetic is applied, the toddler starts to cry and asks if it is going to hurt. How should the nurse respond?
    1. "Yes, it may hurt, but not for very long."
    2. "Maybe it will hurt, but remember big children don't cry."
    3. "Yes, it may hurt, but if you hold still it won't hurt too much."
    4. "It will hurt a little, but I'm good at getting the needle into your arm."

57. A nurse is caring for a 4-year-old child in the pediatric unit. What does the nurse expect concerning the behavior of a preschooler during hospitalization?
    1. Refusing to cooperate with nurses during the parents' absence
    2. Demonstrating despair if the parents do not visit at least once a week
    3. Crying when the parents leave and return, but not during their absence
    4. Avoiding interacting and playing with peers in the playroom if other parents are present

58. How should a nurse assess a 4-year-old child with abdominal pain?
    1. Ask the child to point to where it hurts
    2. Auscultate the child's abdomen for bowel sounds
    3. Observe the position and behavior while the child is moving
    4. Question the parents about their child's eating and bowel habits

59. A nurse plans care of 4-year-old hospitalized children based on their developmental level. What is these children's major vulnerability?
    1. Separation anxiety
    2. Altered family roles
    3. Intrusive procedures
    4. Enforced dependency

60. What nursing intervention best meets the developmental needs of hospitalized preschool-age children?
    1. Help them learn to read
    2. Play simple games with them

3. Encourage visits from family members
4. Provide materials for simulating activities

61. A nurse is caring for a 4-year-old child whose arm is immobilized. What play activity is most appropriate for this child?
    1. Watching television
    2. Cutting out paper dolls
    3. Solving jigsaw puzzles
    4. Looking at comic books

62. What play activity should the nurse provide for a 4-year-old child on bed rest?
    1. Finger painting on blank sheets of paper
    2. Using crayons to color in a coloring book
    3. Engaging in a checker game with an adult
    4. Playing dominos with a school-age roommate

63. What is the most appropriate toy for the nurse to give a 6-year-old child on complete bed rest?
    1. Game of checkers
    2. Set of building blocks
    3. Game of ball and jacks
    4. Coloring book and crayons

64. A 6-year-old child is in the acute phase of nephrotic syndrome. The mother asks the nurse about play activities for her child. What should the nurse suggest? Select all that apply.
    1. _____ Hula hoop
    2. _____ Video games
    3. _____ Large puzzles
    4. _____ Stuffed animal
    5. _____ Children's books

65. A 7-year-old boy who is about to have an IV inserted cries out that he is afraid of IVs. What is the nurse's most therapeutic response?
    1. "Tell me what frightens you."
    2. "It's just a little prick in the arm."
    3. "You are a big boy; this will hardly hurt."
    4. "Come on; there's no reason to be afraid."

66. A school nurse is asked to screen children in a third-grade class for head lice. Based on 8-year-olds' developmental level, how should the nurse first address the class?
    1. Describe what head lice are and how they look
    2. Teach the importance of daily frequent hair washing and not to share combs
    3. Explain that every student must be checked because head lice are spread easily
    4. Tell them that if they have head lice the rest of the family will become infected

67. An 8-year-old child is being prepared for surgery the next day. How should the nurse present preoperative instructions to this child?
    1. Repeat instructions often
    2. Provide time for needle play
    3. Use several abstract examples
    4. Focus on simple anatomical diagrams

68. A school nurse is teaching a class of school-age children about bicycle safety. The nurse identifies a child who needs further teaching when the child states, "I will always wear a helmet and:
    1. ride with traffic facing me."
    2. walk my bike to cross busy streets."
    3. keep as close to the curb as possible."
    4. stay in a single file when I ride with my friends."

69. A 15-year-old girl with a history of allergies develops chronic sinusitis. The mother tells the nurse that she thinks her daughter is becoming a hypochondriac. What is the nurse's best response?
    1. Describes the complications of chronic sinusitis
    2. Examines the underlying causes of hypochondriasis
    3. Discusses the developmental behaviors of adolescents
    4. Explains the concept of transference of her fears to the daughter

70. An adolescent who has had type 1 diabetes for 5 years stops adhering to the therapeutic regimen. Considering the client's developmental level, the nurse concludes that the behavior is a reflection of a:
    1. Need for attention
    2. Struggle for identity
    3. Denial of the diabetes
    4. Regression related to the illness

71. A nurse is caring for a 15-year-old adolescent who is receiving chemotherapy for leukemia. The nurse expects that adolescents with health problems are most concerned about:
    1. Missing time at school
    2. Limiting social activities
    3. Being dependent while enjoying the sick role
    4. Feeling different regarding changes in body image

72. An adolescent who has sickle cell anemia is recovering from a painful episode. What does the nurse suspect is the priority issue for this adolescent?
    1. Restriction of movement during periods of arthralgia
    2. Separation from family during periods of hospitalization
    3. Alteration in body image resulting from skeletal deformities
    4. Interruption of education as a result of multiple hospitalizations

EMOTIONAL NEEDS RELATED TO HEALTH PROBLEMS

73. A 3-year-old child's parents have been unable to visit since the child was admitted to the hospital. The toddler has become quiet and withdrawn. To best help the child at this time, the nurse should:
    1. Bring the child a stuffed animal to cuddle
    2. Contact the parents to encourage them to visit the child
    3. Encourage the child to play games with the other children
    4. Assign the same nurse to care for the child whenever possible

74. A 9-year-old boy recently is told he must stay in the hospital for at least 2 weeks. The nurse finds him crying and unwilling to talk. What is the priority nursing care at this time?
    1. Assure him that his illness is not permanent
    2. Distract him to prevent further embarrassment
    3. Arrange for him to receive tutoring immediately
    4. Provide privacy to allow him to express feelings

75. A 30-month-old boy who was transferred to a regional hospital has not seen his parents for 2 weeks. He now responds to the staff with friendliness and affection. When his mother visits he turns away from her and ignores her. What should the nurse explain to the mother?
    1. "Your little boy has adapted so well; he loves all of us and is so happy."
    2. "Your little boy misses you very much; give him time and he'll reach for you."
    3. "Toddlers usually cry when they see their mothers; your little boy is so mature."
    4. "Toddlers have such short memories; that's why your little boy doesn't remember you."

76. While caring for a terminally ill child the nurse identifies that the parent's visits have become less frequent. What should the nurse do to resolve this situation?
    1. Ask the parents why they are visiting so seldom
    2. Accept the parent's need to maintain a distance at this time
    3. Explain to the parents why visiting is so important to their child
    4. Suggest to the parents that they visit more often while spending less time at each visit

77. The parents of a critically ill child constantly blame each other for their child's illness. What parental response suggests that the nurse's intervention was successful?
    1. Father brings the child expensive gifts
    2. Parents promise the child a trip to an amusement park
    3. Parents make an appointment with a family counselor
    4. Mother assumes the blame for ignoring the child's complaints

78. The parents of an infant with a congenital heart anomaly are told their child's diagnosis. They appear overwhelmed and anxious. What nursing intervention will best help the parents cope with their grief?
    1. Explaining the diagnosis in a variety of ways
    2. Encouraging the parents to express their feelings
    3. Recommending that the parents talk with other parents
    4. Offering assurance that surgery probably will correct the problem

79. An infant is admitted to the intensive care unit with multiple injuries. When the adolescent mother sees her infant for the first time, she cries out, "I didn't mean to hurt her." What should the nurse do first?

1. Notify Child Protective Services
2. Encourage the mother's family to visit and comfort her
3. Offer support by saying, "This must be difficult for you."
4. Respond by saying, "You caused your baby's injury and you feel guilty."

80. The mother of an infant with meningitis is concerned that if she stays with her infant at the hospital her toddler at home will feel neglected. How should the nurse respond?
    1. "Has anything happened to make you feel this way?"
    2. "It's so important to spend your time here with the baby."
    3. "Try to divide your time evenly between the two children."
    4. " Can you arrange with someone to stay here when you are at home?"

81. A nurse is assessing the family dynamics of a suspected abusive family. What behavior is expected? Select all that apply.
    1. _____ Child cringes when approached
    2. _____ Child has unexplained healed injuries
    3. _____ Parents are overly affectionate toward the child
    4. _____ Child lies still while surveying the environment
    5. _____ Parents give detailed accounts of the child's injuries

82. A 7-year-old girl arrives at the school health office in tears. She tells the nurse that several of her classmates teased her. What is the nurse's most therapeutic response?
    1. "Tell me more about it."
    2. "Has this happened before?"
    3. "Were they boys or girls who teased you?"
    4. "This happens to everyone at some time or another."

83. A child who survived a near-drowning episode is in critical condition. At one point the child smiles and the eyes open, prompting the mother to say to the nurse, "Look, I think my child will get better now." How should the nurse respond?
    1. "This is a very good sign."
    2. "Try to get your child to hold your hand."
    3. "God must have been watching over your child."
    4. "Everything is being done to help your child recover."

84. A toddler who was physically abused is admitted to the pediatric unit. What behavior does the nurse expect when approaching the child?
    1. Smiles readily when anyone enters the room
    2. Is wary of physical contact initiated by anyone
    3. Begins to cry when anyone approaches the bedside
    4. Pays little attention to anyone standing at the bedside

85. A home health nurse is caring for children in a family that is economically deprived. Which characteristic is most common to those living in poverty?
    1. Open expression of anger
    2. Long-term feeling of powerlessness
    3. Willingness to postpone gratification
    4. Compliance with health recommendations

86. A female client who had physically abused her son is receiving treatment to control her behavior. Which statement indicates that the client has developed insight into her behavior as a parent?
    1. "I promise that I won't get so angry when my son causes trouble again."
    2. "If my son gets straightened out, we should not have these type of problems."
    3. "I think the root of the problem is when my husband comes home after drinking."
    4. "If I feel angry at my son again, I'm going to need a pillow in the bedroom to punch."

87. A 19-month-old boy who has been in the hospital for 2 weeks becomes increasingly withdrawn and mute. What is the most appropriate nursing action?
    1. Offer distracting toys
    2. Move him into a room with other children
    3. Encourage the parents to stay with him as much as possible
    4. Provide sensory stimulation by assigning different nurses to care for him

88. During the course of treatment a toddler is to receive an intramuscular injection. What is the priority nursing intervention that should be included in the plan of care?
    1. Distracting the toddler's attention with a toy car
    2. Telling the parents exactly what will be done to the toddler
    3. Giving the toddler the choice of having the injection now or later
    4. Involving the parents in comforting the toddler after the injection

89. What is the primary nursing objective for a child recently diagnosed with celiac disease?
    1. Prevent celiac crisis and resulting problems
    2. Minimize complications from respiratory involvement
    3. Teach the parents to establish a diet that promotes optimum growth
    4. Help the parents and child adjust to the long-term dietary restrictions

90. A nurse is preparing an intramuscular injection to be administered to a 3-year-old child. What approach is the most therapeutic?
    1. "This might hurt and it's important that you be still."
    2. "You are afraid of getting a shot because of the pain."
    3. "Another nurse is here to help me give you the injection."
    4. "Act like a big child and we can be done as quickly as possible."

91. A 4-year-old child with a new colostomy is to be discharged in several days. What should the nurse teach the parents about their child's home care?
    1. Performing colostomy care
    2. Restricting daily fluid intake
    3. Instituting dietary restrictions
    4. Encouraging unrestricted activity

92. A 4-year-old boy with Reye syndrome is beginning to show signs of recovery. The intracranial pressure has receded, the vital signs are stable, the fever has subsided, and urinary output is within an acceptable range for the child's weight and fluid intake. What should the nurse tell the parents about their son's recovery?
    1. "The illness has resolved."
    2. "Your son is out of danger now."
    3. "Your son seems free of complications."
    4. "The recovery is now progressing as hoped."

93. A 5-year-old child is admitted to the pediatric unit for an appendectomy. What question should the nurse ask to determine what the child thinks is the reason for hospitalization?
    1. "Why did you come to the hospital?"
    2. "Have you brought any toys with you?"
    3. "Did your parents tell you why you are here?"
    4. "Do you know you are going to have an operation?"

94. A 5-year-old girl is receiving a course of chemotherapy. One day the nurse observes the child crying. The child tells the nurse, "All my hair is gone and everyone stares at me." What is the nurse's best response?
    1. "Let's take the hair off your doll so you two will look alike."
    2. "Let's ask your mother to bring in a hat for you to wear until your hair grows back."
    3. "You just think that everyone is staring at you because you feel funny without your hair."
    4. "You shouldn't have to look at yourself without hair so I'm going to take this mirror out of your room."

95. A 5-year-old child newly arrived from Latin America attends a nursery school where everyone speaks English. The child's mother tells the nurse that her child is no longer outgoing and is very passive in the classroom. What is the probable reason for the child's behavior?
    1. Social immaturity
    2. Undergoing culture shock
    3. Experiencing discrimination
    4. Disinterest in school activities

96. After treatment for Lyme disease, a child expresses fear of going camping again because of the ticks. What is the nurse's best response?
    1. "Tell me more about your fears about camping."
    2. "Frequent checks for ticks will help prevent an infection."
    3. "Just think of all the fun you'll be missing if you don't go to camp."
    4. "It's hard to believe you're afraid to go camping just because of a tick."

97. A 6-year-old boy is receiving chemotherapy for a neuroblastoma, stage IV. He had his first chemotherapy session last week and arrives with his mother for this week's session. How should the nurse greet the child?
    1. "Its time for your next dose."
    2. "Did you vomit afterward last time?"
    3. "There are only three more sessions."
    4. "How did you feel after your last treatment?"

98. A 12-year-old child is admitted to the pediatric unit with a diagnosis of meningococcal meningitis. Three days after admission the child is afebrile and asymptomatic but appears sad and cries frequently. How should the nurse assist the child to verbalize thoughts and feelings?
    1. Ask the child what seems to be the trouble
    2. Encourage the parents to speak with their child
    3. Show the child some photos of hospitalized children and have the child tell stories about them
    4. Have the child watch videotapes about sick children and answer any questions that the child may have

99. A nurse assesses that a newly diagnosed adolescent with type 1 diabetes has sufficient knowledge of the disorder. What is the next nursing action?
    1. Set goals with the client
    2. Develop a rapport with the client
    3. Teach the client how to give insulin injections
    4. Instruct the client how to monitor blood glucose

100. A 16-year-old with full-thickness burns of the entire right arm states, "I'll never be able to use my arm again. I'll be scarred forever." What is the nurse's best initial response?
    1. "Think about how lucky you are. You are still alive."
    2. "Minimizing scarring is the goal of the entire professional staff."
    3. "Being worried is understandable, but it is really too early to tell."
    4. "Try not to worry. Concentrate on doing your range-of-motion exercises."

BLOOD AND IMMUNITY

101. The mother of a 6-week-old infant asks the nurse at the pediatric clinic why, with the exception of hepatitis B, her baby's immunizations will not begin until 2 months of age. How should the nurse respond?
    1. Vaccines cause disease in younger infants' bodies
    2. Younger infants rarely are exposed to infectious diseases
    3. Insufficient antibodies are produced by younger infants' spleens
    4. Maternal antibodies interfere with younger infants' antibody production

102. A 4-month-old infant is to receive the second DTaP immunization. The nurse reviews the infant's medical history before administering the vaccine. What information in the infant's history will influence the decision whether to administer the vaccine?
    1. Allergy to eggs
    2. Lactose intolerance
    3. Infectious dermatitis
    4. High fever after the first dose

103. Before administering the first series of immunizations to a 2-month-old infant, the nurse tells the mother that reactions may occur. What are the characteristics of these reactions?
    1. Local or systemic and usually mild
    2. Often serious and may require hospitalization
    3. Sometimes cause ulceration at the injection site
    4. May be responsible for permanent neurological damage

104. A nurse administers the first series of immunizations to a 2-month-old infant. The nurse instructs the mother that if the site becomes inflamed, she should give the prescribed acetaminophen (Tylenol). What else should the nurse instruct the mother to do?
    1. Place a warm compress on the area
    2. Put a witch hazel compress on the site
    3. Give a cool sponge bath for 15 minutes
    4. Apply an ice pack to the area for 2 minutes

105. A nurse is teaching a mother about the immunization schedule for her baby. Between which months of age should the measles vaccine be given?
    1. 2 and 5
    2. 6 and 8
    3. 9 and 11
    4. 12 and 15

106. A father questions the nurse about the immunization schedule for his 15-month-old toddler who is being treated for acute lymphoid leukemia. What vaccine is contraindicated for a child receiving chemotherapy?
    1. Hib (influenza)
    2. HepB (hepatitis B)
    3. MMR (measles, mumps, rubella)
    4. DTaP (diphtheria, tetanus, acellular pertussis)

107. A hospitalized 3-year-old child with leukemia is receiving chemotherapy. The mother tells the nurse that her child is asking for fried chicken. How should the nurse respond?
    1. Fried foods might cause nausea and vomiting during chemotherapy
    2. Any food that is requested should be given because the child needs calories
    3. Coatings on foods to be fried can irritate the child's mouth and may cause bleeding
    4. Foods from outside should not be brought to the unit because of the potential for infection

108. A 13-month-old child is having a lumbar puncture to confirm a diagnosis of bacterial meningitis. During the procedure the nurse observes that the spinal fluid is cloudy. What does this finding indicate?
    1. Healthy spinal fluid
    2. Increased glucose level
    3. Elevated white blood cell count
    4. Rising number of red blood cells

109. A mother tells the nurse that she is concerned about her 8-month-old baby's diet because the infant will eat only mashed potatoes and drink only milk. The nurse anticipates that this diet will result in a deficiency of:
    1. Iron
    2. Vitamins
    3. Potassium
    4. Amino acids

110. A 1-year-old child is diagnosed with nutritional iron deficiency anemia. What nursing interventions are important when caring for an infant with iron deficiency anemia? Select all that apply.
    1. _____ Conserving the infant's energy
    2. _____ Protecting the infant from infection
    3. _____ Teaching the parents about nutrition
    4. _____ Telling the parents to offer small, frequent feedings
    5. _____ Instructing the parents to increase the amount of milk offered

111. A nurse is teaching the mother of an 18-month-old toddler with iron deficiency anemia about her child's dietary needs. What foods should the nurse suggest for inclusion in the child's diet?
    1. Pumpkin pie
    2. Seedless grapes
    3. Slices of a whole apple
    4. Gingerbread molasses cookies

112. A child with leukemia is to continue taking predniSONE (Meticorten) at home. The nurse discovers that the child's sibling is home from school with chickenpox. What knowledge will affect the nurse's discharge plan?
    1. The child must be immunized before going home
    2. Chickenpox can be fatal to individuals with leukemia
    3. An individual receiving prednisone is immune to chickenpox
    4. Prevention of direct contact between siblings permits discharge to the home

113. A 4-year-old child is admitted to the pediatric unit for a tonsillectomy. During preoperative planning a nurse reviews the child's laboratory report. Which value is of most significance in this situation?
    1. Potassium level
    2. Coagulation studies
    3. Red blood cell count
    4. Erythrocyte sedimentation rate

114. On return to the pediatric unit after a tonsillectomy, a nurse identifies that a 4-year-old child is swallowing frequently. What is the probable cause of this response?
    1. Pharyngeal edema
    2. Postoperative bleeding
    3. Tenacious oral secretions
    4. Increased saliva production

115. A 4-year-old child is admitted to the pediatric unit with a tentative diagnosis of acute lymphocytic leukemia (ALL). What signs and symptoms does the nurse expect when obtaining the health history and performing a physical assessment? Select all that apply.
    1. _____ Edema
    2. _____ Alopecia
    3. _____ Anorexia
    4. _____ Insomnia
    5. _____ Petechiae

116. A nurse obtains a health history from the parents of a toddler who is admitted to the pediatric unit with the diagnosis of acute lymphocytic leukemia (ALL). What problems does the nurse expect the parents to report? Select all that apply.
    1. _____ Loss of appetite
    2. _____ Sores in the mouth
    3. _____ Paleness of the skin
    4. _____ Inability to fall asleep
    5. _____ Purplish spots on the skin

117. To confirm a tentative diagnosis of leukemia a bone marrow aspiration and biopsy are to be performed on a 4-year-old boy. The nurse gives an age-appropriate explanation of the procedure to the child. What else is involved in caring for this child?
    1. Telling the child that there will be pressure without pain
    2. Explaining to the child that he will sleep during the procedure
    3. Placing the child in the semi-Fowler position supported by pillows
    4. Asking the child to hold some nonsterile equipment during the test

118. A 3-year-old child with sickle cell anemia is admitted to the child health unit during a painful episode. Splenomegaly is identified. The nurse explains to the parents that splenomegaly usually is:
    1. Common in infancy
    2. Difficult to palpate in children
    3. Initiated by vaso-occlusive crisis
    4. Most evident during late childhood

119. A toddler is admitted with an acute infection and dehydration. There is a prescription for an IV antibiotic to be piggybacked to a continuous hydration solution. During the administration of the antibiotic the child becomes restless, flushes, and begins to wheeze. What should the nurse do? Place the nurse's actions in order of their priority.
    1. Notify the practitioner
    2. Stop the antibiotic infusion
    3. Assess the respiratory status
    4. Maintain the hydration infusion
    Answer:_____

120. A 10-year-old child who has sickle cell anemia is admitted to the hospital with a vaso-occlusive painful episode. The nurse manager plans to place the child in the same room as a child with the diagnosis of:
    1. Pneumonia
    2. Thalassemia
    3. Acute pharyngitis
    4. Chronic osteomyelitis

121. A child with sickle-cell anemia is admitted to the pediatric unit during a vaso-occlusive crisis (painful episode). What does the nurse conclude about why the crisis occurred?
    1. Severe depression of the circulating thrombocytes
    2. Diminished red blood cell production by the bone marrow
    3. Pooling of blood in the spleen that results in splenomegaly
    4. Blockage of small blood vessels with clumped red blood cells

122. A child who was hospitalized for a vaso-occlusive crisis (painful episode) is to be discharged. What should the nurse include when reviewing the child's discharge instructions with the parents?
    1. Play outdoors to get adequate sunshine
    2. Participate in active sports to increase endurance
    3. Increase fluid intake 2 times the usual amount to promote hemodilution
    4. Place ice packs on the joints for 15 minutes every 4 hours in an attempt to limit pain

123. After being bitten by a rabid dog, a child is to receive a series of antirabies inoculations. The nurse who is to administer the injections should consider that rabies is a:
    1. Viral infection characterized by seizures and difficulty swallowing
    2. Bacterial infection characterized by encephalopathy and opisthotonos
    3. Bacterial infection characterized by septicemia and bone deterioration
    4. Viral infection characterized by immunosuppression and opportunistic infections

124. A nurse in the pediatric clinic plans to administer a booster immunization for polio to a child. Which vaccine should the nurse administer?
    1. Hib
    2. IPV
    3. OPV
    4. DTaP

125. A nurse is assessing a child with the diagnosis of hemophilia. In what part of the body does the nurse expect bleeding to occur?
    1. Brain
    2. Joints
    3. Intestines
    4. Pericardium

126. When providing care to a child with leukemia a nurse observes blood on the pillowcase and several bloody tissues. What blood component value on the child's laboratory results should the nurse verify?
    1. Platelets
    2. Neutrophils
    3. Erythrocytes
    4. Lymphoblasts

127. A home health nurse teaches a father how to provide oral care for his child who is receiving chemotherapy. The nurse observes a return demonstration and identifies that he needs further teaching when he attempts to use:
    1. A cotton swab
    2. Mild toothpaste
    3. Saline mouthwash
    4. An electric toothbrush

128. A nurse is caring for a child who is receiving chemotherapy to treat leukemia. What is the priority nursing action?
    1. Promoting optimum growth and development
    2. Using techniques to minimize risk of infection
    3. Encouraging food that will improve nutritional status
    4. Providing emotional support for the child and family members

129. A child with leukemia who is receiving chemotherapy is susceptible to rectal ulcerations. What should the nurse recommend to the parents that will lessen the severity of this problem?
    1. Encourage lying on the abdomen when in bed
    2. Have the child wear cotton underpants at night
    3. Apply rectal ointments liberally four times a day
    4. Clean the child's perianal area after each bowel movement

130. A child with leukemia is to be discharged home on a protocol that includes several antineoplastic medications. What should the nurse plan to teach the parents?
    1. Use an electric toothbrush to provide meticulous oral care
    2. Limit their child's contact with peers to avoid being exposed to infections
    3. Withhold the antineoplastic medications when vomiting occurs to prevent additional episodes
    4. Notify the practitioner if the child has a temperature of 100° F to obtain an antibiotic prescription

131. A nurse is teaching the parents of a 5-year-old girl who is to continue chemotherapy at home. What statement indicates that the parents understand the discharge instructions?
    1. "She will be allowed to eat food at her own pace."
    2. "We will plan for structured play activities each day."
    3. "She will be encouraged to rinse her mouth with mouthwash."
    4. "We will protect her from coming into contact with children her age."

132. A child who just completed a cycle of chemotherapy is to be discharged home. What is the priority intervention the nurse should teach the parents about caring for their child at home?
    1. Purchase a wig
    2. Ensure adequate rest
    3. Offer sufficient fluids
    4. Perform thorough handwashing

133. A nurse is caring for a child with AIDS. The nurse teaches the parents that children with AIDS are more prone to infection than adults with AIDS because:
    1. Immune systems of children produce insufficient antibodies
    2. Children are exposed to more pathogens each day than are adults
    3. AIDS virus attacks children's immune systems through different mechanisms
    4. Adults have had more exposure to pathogens over time, thereby producing more antibodies

134. What precautions should a nurse use when caring for a child who is HIV positive?
    1. Droplet
    2. Contact

3. Airborne

4. Standard

135. A child with thalassemia (Cooley anemia) is being discharged from the hospital. What should the nurse include in the instructions to the parents?
 1. Minimize risk of infection
 2. Offer frequent iron-rich meals
 3. Encourage increased fluid intake
 4. Restrict activity allowing only quiet play

136. A child with a puncture wound on the sole of the foot is brought to the emergency department. Because of a language barrier the caregiver cannot provide a clear history of previous tetanus immunizations. Tetanus immunoglobulin (TIG) is prescribed by the practitioner. The nurse explains to the caregiver that this medication is given because it:
 1. Produces lifelong passive immunity to tetanus
 2. Confers short-term passive defense against tetanus
 3. Induces long-lasting active protection from tetanus
 4. Stimulates the production of antibodies to fight tetanus

137. One of the aims of therapy for a child with sickle cell anemia is the prevention of the sickling phenomenon, which is responsible for the pathological sequelae. What should the plan of care include to minimize the potential for a sickling episode?
 1. Provide an iron-rich diet
 2. Ensure hemoconcentration
 3. Enforce periods of quiet play
 4. Promote adequate oxygenation

138. The mother of a 13-year-old child who has sickle cell anemia tells the nurse that the family is going camping by a lake this summer. She asks what activities are appropriate for her child. Which activity should the nurse suggest?
 1. Swimming in the lake
 2. Soccer with the family
 3. Climbing the mountain trails
 4. Motorboat rides around the lake

139. A nurse evaluates that the teaching about sickle cell anemia is understood when an adolescent with the disorder states, "I know that symptoms will appear when I:
 1. drink less fluid."
 2. have fewer thrombocytes."
 3. decrease the iron in my diet."
 4. have fewer white blood cells."

140. A nurse is teaching a 12-year-old child about a bone marrow aspiration. What statement indicates that the preadolescent needs further explanation about the procedure?
 1. "I will need to rest after the procedure."
 2. "My hip will be sore after the procedure is completed."
 3. "There will be a tight dressing to put pressure on the area."
 4. "The doctor will inject a needle into the center of one of my hip bones."

141. An adolescent visits the allergy clinic because of seasonal environmental allergies. Blood is drawn for testing. Which laboratory finding indicates to the nurse that an allergic response is in progress?
 1. Decreased platelet count
 2. Elevated eosinophil level
 3. Elevated lymphocyte count
 4. Decreased immunoglobulin level

142. A 16-year-old male student who was injured while skateboarding arrives in the emergency department with a deep laceration on his leg. He does not remember when he received his last tetanus immunization. The nurse explains that tetanus immunoglobulin (TIG) and tetanus toxoid are required because:
 1. Neither medication is effective alone
 2. Both eliminate the need for additional medications
 3. Different mechanisms are used to stimulate the immune response
 4. Tetanus toxoid minimizes the risks related to the tetanus immunoglobulin

143. A nurse confirms that a 9-month-old infant's immunization schedule is up-to-date. Which immunization will the infant receive at 15 months of age?
 1. Hepatitis B
 2. Polio vaccine
 3. Tetanus toxoid
 4. Measles, mumps, and rubella

CARDIOVASCULAR

144. An infant is admitted to the pediatric unit with the diagnosis of heart failure. What should the nurse include in the infant's plan of care?
 1. Increase fluid intake
 2. Position flat on the back
 3. Offer small frequent feedings
 4. Measure head circumference

145. A 2-month-old infant with the diagnosis of heart failure is discharged with a prescription for digoxin (Lanoxin) 0.05 mg PO every 12 hours. The bottle of digoxin is labeled 0.05 mg/mL. What vessel should the nurse teach the mother to use when administering the medication?
 1. Nipple
 2. Calibrated syringe
 3. Plastic measuring spoon
 4. Bottle with an ounce of water

146. A 2-month-old girl is admitted to the pediatric unit in heart failure. The practitioner orders nothing by mouth and semi-Fowler position. How should the nurse obtain the infant's weight?
 1. Weigh the infant quickly in the supine position
 2. Ask the mother for the infant's most recent weight
 3. Have the mother hold the infant, weigh them both, and then subtract the weight of the adult
 4. Place the infant in an infant seat, observe the weight, and then subtract the weight of the seat

147. A nurse is caring for an infant with heart failure. What treatment does the nurse anticipate for this infant?
    1. Open heart surgery
    2. Multiple operations during childhood
    3. Medications that are specific for infants and children
    4. Medications that are prescribed for both children and adults

148. A parent asks the nurse, "The doctor said my baby has pulmonic stenosis. What does that mean?" How should the nurse respond?
    1. "What else did your doctor say?"
    2. "Your baby has a heart problem."
    3. "Are you concerned about your baby?"
    4. "I'll page your doctor so that you can discuss this again."

149. A 3-month-old infant is admitted to the pediatric unit with a diagnosis of tetralogy of Fallot. The nurse's assessment reveals that the infant's weight has declined from the 25th percentile to the 5th percentile. The nurse concludes that the probable reason for this inadequate weight gain is:
    1. Cyanosis resulting in cerebral changes
    2. Decreased arterial oxygen level resulting in polycythemia
    3. Pulmonary hypertension resulting in recurrent respiratory infections
    4. Inadequate oxygen perfusion leading to activity intolerance resulting in diminished energy to nurse

150. A nurse is caring for a child with tetralogy of Fallot. What clinical finding should the nurse expect when assessing this child?
    1. Slow respirations
    2. Clubbing of fingers
    3. Subcutaneous hemorrhages
    4. Decreased red blood cell count

151. An infant with tetralogy of Fallot becomes cyanotic and dyspneic after a crying episode. In what position should the nurse place the infant to relieve the cyanosis and dyspnea?
    1. Knee-chest
    2. Orthopneic
    3. Lateral Sims
    4. Semi-Fowler

152. A nurse teaches the parents of an infant with a cardiac defect how to detect impending heart failure. What should the parents identify as an early sign?
    1. Increased heart rate   *Tachycardia*
    2. Distended neck veins
    3. Decreased respirations
    4. Increased urinary output

153. A complete blood count is ordered for a 5-month-old infant with tetralogy of Fallot. What does the nurse expect when reviewing the laboratory results?
    1. Anemia
    2. Polycythemia   *↑ production of RBCs, response to hypoxemia*
    3. Agranulocytosis
    4. Thrombocytopenia

154. An infant with a cardiac defect is fed in the semi-Fowler position. After the nurse feeds and burps the infant and changes the infant's position, the infant has a bowel movement and almost immediately becomes cyanotic, diaphoretic, and limp. Which activity probably caused the infant's response?
    1. Burping
    2. Feeding
    3. Position change
    4. Bowel movement   *Homie pooped so hard he vagulled*

155. A 1-month-old infant with a ventricular septal defect (VSD) is examined in the cardiology clinic. What sign related to this disorder does the nurse expect when assessing this infant?
    1. Bradycardia at rest
    2. Activity-related cyanosis
    3. Bounding peripheral pulses
    4. Murmur at the left sternal border

156. A 4-year-old child from a third world country is admitted to the pediatric unit for surgery to correct a congenital heart defect. The mother asks the nurse why her child squats after exertion. The nurse responds, in language the mother understands, that this position:
    1. Reduces muscle aches   *Tetralogy*
    2. Enhances the pull of gravity
    3. Decreases the cardiac workload
    4. Facilitates blood return to the heart

157. A 5-year-old child with a ventricular septal defect is scheduled for a cardiac catheterization. The parents ask the nurse why this test is done. Before replying, the nurse takes into consideration that it:
    1. Identifies the specific location of the defect
    2. Confirms the presence of a pansystolic murmur
    3. Determines the degree of cardiomegaly present
    4. Establishes the presence of ventricular hypertrophy

158. A 3½-year-old child returns to the room after a cardiac catheterization. What is the priority nursing intervention after this procedure?
    1. Encouraging early ambulation
    2. Monitoring the insertion site for bleeding
    3. Comparing the blood pressure in each extremity
    4. Restricting fluids until the blood pressure stabilizes

159. An infant with a congenital heart defect returns to the unit after a cardiac catheterization. The nurse manager is observing a nurse newly assigned to the unit. Which nursing intervention should the nurse manager interrupt?
    1. Offering fluids and foods as tolerated
    2. Performing range-of-motion exercises
    3. Monitoring the apical pulse for rate and rhythm
    4. Assessing the pulses distal to the catheterization site

160. A child who had a cardiac catheterization is being discharged. What should the nurse include in the discharge instructions to the parents?
    1. Limit fluid intake for 3 days to prevent nausea
    2. Give sponge baths for 3 days to prevent infection

3. Return to the clinic in 5 days to have the pressure dressing removed
4. Apply ice compresses every 20 minutes on the first day to lessen edema

161. A 4-month-old infant who has a congenital heart defect develops heart failure and is exhibiting marked dyspnea at rest. The nurse determines that this finding can be attributed to:
1. Anemia
2. Hypovolemia
3. Pulmonary edema
4. Metabolic acidosis

162. The mother of a 5-month-old infant with heart failure questions the necessity of weighing her baby every morning. The nurse's response is based on the fact that this daily information is important in determining:
1. Fluid retention
2. Kidney function
3. Nutritional status
4. Medication dosage

163. A nurse is reviewing the laboratory values of a child with rheumatic heart disease. Which finding does the nurse conclude is related to this condition?
1. Negative C-reactive protein
2. Increased reticulocyte count
3. Positive antistreptolysin titer
4. Low erythrocyte sedimentation rate

164. A 5-year-old child returns to the pediatric intensive care unit (PICU) after cardiac surgery. The child has a left chest tube attached to water-seal drainage, an IV of D5 ½ NS at 4 mL/hr, and a double-lumen nasogastric tube to continuous suction. The child is attached to a cardiac monitor and has a left chest dressing. What is the priority nursing intervention?
1. Obtain vital signs
2. Test for level of consciousness
3. Measure drainage from both tubes
4. Determine suction pressure of the nasogastric tube

165. A child has open heart surgery to repair a cardiac defect. The practitioner informs the parents that antibiotics are required before any dental work is performed. Later the parents ask the nurse why this is necessary. When responding, the nurse incorporates the fact that this is done to prevent:
1. Gingivitis
2. Pericarditis
3. Myocarditis
4. Endocarditis

ENDOCRINE

166. A nurse is teaching a young adolescent with type 2 diabetes about nutritional needs. Which statement demonstrates that the adolescent understands what was taught?
1. "I may eat low-fat, low-calorie candy bars."
2. "Regular soft drinks are better than diet ones."
3. "It's okay for me to eat one slice of pizza at a party."
4. "My fasting blood sugar should be no higher than 150."

167. What should a nurse emphasize when teaching lifelong management of type 1 diabetes to an adolescent?
1. Soaking the feet in hot water each day
2. Inspecting both feet frequently for signs of trauma
3. Drying the feet thoroughly after a bath by rubbing with a towel
4. Treating minor cuts on the feet with an antiseptic such as iodine

168. An adolescent who was admitted to the hospital with ketoacidosis is stable and receiving Novolin R subcutaneously. One hour after its administration the nurse enters the room and observes that the adolescent is diaphoretic and irritable. What is the nurse's first intervention?
1. Delay the client's lunch tray
2. Provide a glass of low-fat milk
3. Obtain a blood glucose reading
4. Cover the client with a light blanket

169. A 12-year-old child with type 2 diabetes is scheduled for abdominal surgery. Which factors are most important for the nurse to consider during the postoperative period? Select all that apply.
1. _____ Infection will probably occur at the operative site
2. _____ Ketoacidosis frequently occurs later in the postoperative period
3. _____ Blood glucose levels will increase because of the stress of surgery
4. _____ Urine test results are the most useful gauge for monitoring diabetic control after surgery
5. _____ Diabetic control maintained without insulin before surgery will not be effective during the postoperative period

170. A 14-year-old teenager with type 1 diabetes wants to go for a pizza after a volleyball game. The teenager asks the school nurse whether this is permissible on the insulin-diet-exercise regimen prescribed. How should the nurse respond?
1. "Fast foods are unhealthy, especially for teenagers with diabetes."
2. "It would be best if you ate at home, where your diet can be controlled."
3. "Go with your friends but make an effort to eat something other than pizza."
4. "I will teach you how to determine the amount of carbohydrates in different fast foods."

171. A nurse in a child health clinic is obtaining the health history of a 5-year-old boy who was just diagnosed with type 1 diabetes. When planning care the nurse anticipates that this child:
1. will feel different from friends and classmates.
2. will initially deny the fact that he has diabetes.
3. must develop skills to test blood glucose and report findings.

4. Must receive continual health teaching based on cognitive ability

172. A nurse is reviewing the laboratory report of a child with type 1 diabetes. What test is considered the most accurate when evaluating the effectiveness of diet and insulin therapy over time?
    1. Blood pH
    2. Serum protein levels
    3. Serum glucose levels
    4. Glycosylated hemoglobin

173. A child with type 1 diabetes, whose diabetes has been controlled for several years, is admitted in ketoacidosis. What does the nurse suspect is a precipitating cause of this episode of ketoacidosis?
    1. Infection
    2. Increased exercise
    3. Recent weight loss
    4. Overdose of insulin

174. A child with type 1 diabetes is admitted to the pediatric unit in ketoacidosis. What sign of ketoacidosis does the nurse expect to identify when assessing the child?
    1. Sweating
    2. Hyperpnea
    3. Bradycardia
    4. Hypertension

175. A nurse plans to teach a 7-year-old child recently diagnosed with type 1 diabetes how to give insulin injections. What should be included in the first lesson? Select all that apply.
    1. _____ Explaining why insulin is needed
    2. _____ Offering an illustrated booklet to read at home
    3. _____ Inviting the child's friends to participate in the lesson
    4. _____ Providing a syringe for the child to practice manipulating
    5. _____ Seeking a return demonstration of how to give an injection using a doll

176. A 9-year-old child with type 1 diabetes has a history of erratic blood glucose readings. On a day the child visits the clinic, the child is observed sneaking food and trying to talk the mother into providing sweets. The child complains of feeling hypoglycemic. What is the priority nursing action?
    1. Draw blood for a pH
    2. Give a cup of orange juice
    3. Obtain a blood glucose level
    4. Ask the child when food was last eaten

177. A child with type 1 diabetes who is learning disabled has difficulty measuring the required insulin dose. The child frequently draws up 42 units of insulin instead of the prescribed 24 units. What is the most appropriate intervention to ensure dosage safety?
    1. Have the child write the number on paper before filling the syringe
    2. Give the child a tuberculin syringe, which has different units of measure

3. Teach the child to use a magnifying glass to read the numbers on the syringe
4. Provide the child with a preset syringe that was developed for the visually impaired

178. An adolescent is diagnosed with type 1 diabetes. The nurse plans to teach the adolescent that dietary control and exercise can help regulate the disorder. What additional information should the nurse include in the teaching plan? Select all that apply.
    1. _____ Insulin therapy
    2. _____ Prophylactic antibiotics
    3. _____ Blood glucose monitoring
    4. _____ Oral hypoglycemic agents
    5. _____ Adherence to the treatment regimen

179. A 17-year-old student with type 1 diabetes asks the nurse which hormone causes the blood glucose level to rise. When responding the nurse should include that liver glycogenolysis is stimulated by a hormone secreted by the islets of Langerhans. This hormone is:
    1. ACTH
    2. Insulin
    3. Glucagon
    4. Epinephrine

180. A nurse is planning to teach a newly diagnosed child with type 1 diabetes about self care. Based on the assessment of what the child knows about diabetes, what is the next nursing intervention?
    1. Teaching the child how to perform blood glucose testing
    2. Developing a sequence of goals with the child and parents
    3. Instructing the child on how to administer insulin injections
    4. Establishing a trusting relationship with the child and parents

181. A nurse is caring for a child with type 1 diabetes and identifies that the child is experiencing an episode of hyperglycemia. What assessments led the nurse to this conclusion? Select all that apply.
    1. _____ Irritability
    2. _____ Headache
    3. _____ Diaphoresis
    4. _____ Increased thirst
    5. _____ Deep, rapid breathing

182. An unconscious 16-year-old adolescent with type 1 diabetes is brought to the emergency department. The adolescent's blood glucose level is 742 mg/dL. What finding does the nurse expect during the initial assessment?
    1. Pyrexia
    2. Hyperpnea
    3. Bradycardia
    4. Hypertension

183. What should the nurse emphasize when teaching insulin self-administration to a 10-year-old child recently diagnosed with diabetes?
    1. Wash the hands before preparing the insulin injection

2. Shake the bottle of insulin thoroughly before drawing up the dose
3. Alternate the sites of the insulin injections among the four extremities
4. Rub the injection site briskly for half a minute after giving the injection

184. A nurse plans to teach a child with type 1 diabetes, who is receiving both insulin lispro (Humalog) and insulin glargine (Lantus) daily, how to self-administer the insulin. What should the child do when learning to give the injections?
1. Alternate the sites until the best one to use is found
2. Self-administer the injections after being taught the technique
3. Draw up the insulin glargine first and then draw up the insulin lispro
4. Learn to use the needle and syringe by practicing on an insulin pad first

185. An 8-year-old child is receiving insulin glargine (Lantus) before breakfast. What is the most appropriate information for the nurse to give the parents concerning a bedtime snack?
1. Offer a snack to prevent hypoglycemia during the night
2. Provide a snack if signs of hyperglycemia become evident
3. Avoid a snack because the child is being treated with a long-acting insulin
4. Keep a snack at the bedside if the child should get hungry during the night

FLUIDS AND ELECTROLYTES

186. A 4-month-old infant is brought to the emergency department after 2 days of diarrhea. The infant is listless and has sunken eyeballs, a depressed anterior fontanel, and poor tissue turgor. The infant's breathing is deep, rapid, and unlabored. The mother states that there have been liquid stools and no obvious urine output. What problem does the nurse conclude that the infant is experiencing?
1. Kidney failure
2. Mild dehydration
3. Metabolic acidosis
4. Respiratory alkalosis

187. A 5½-month-old infant is admitted to the pediatric unit with a fever and a history of vomiting for 48 hours. What assessments are most helpful in developing a plan of care? Select all that apply.
1. _____ Vital signs
2. _____ Tissue turgor
3. _____ Daily weights
4. _____ Urinary output
5. _____ Neurological status

188. A mother arrives in the emergency department with her severely dehydrated infant. After being treated aggressively, the infant is rehydrated and ready to be discharged. What is the priority concern that the nurse should include in the teaching plan for the mother?
1. Importance of a well-balanced diet
2. Potential hazards of dehydration in infants
3. Maintaining cleanliness of feeding utensils
4. Effect of antibiotics on viral gastroenteritis

189. A dehydrated 15-month-old toddler is admitted to the pediatric unit with a diagnosis of intractable diarrhea. After several days of treatment the child is evaluated. Which finding indicates to the nurse that the child is no longer dehydrated?
1. Heart rate has increased
2. Blood pressure has decreased
3. Capillary refill time has increased
4. Urine specific gravity has decreased

190. A nurse is caring for a severely dehydrated infant. After adequate kidney function is confirmed, potassium is added to the intravenous rehydration solution. It is to be infused at 15 mL/kg of body weight every 24 hours. The infant weighs 13 pounds. What does the nurse calculate for the infant's intravenous fluid intake per day?
Answer: _____ mL

191. During the hourly assessment of the infusion rate of a child's IV the nurse discovers that the IV did not deliver the ordered amount during the last hour. What should the nurse do first?
1. Increase the flow rate
2. Notify the practitioner
3. Inspect the infusion setup
4. Give the child a glass of juice

192. A severely dehydrated infant admitted to the pediatric unit is too lethargic to receive oral rehydration therapy (ORT). An intravenous infusion is started. What is the nurse's primary responsibility?
1. Monitoring the prescribed rate of flow
2. Cuddling the infant during the infusion
3. Documenting the changes in the infant's behavior
4. Explaining the purpose of the infusion to the parent

193. A nurse is caring for an infant with gastroenteritis and diarrhea. What should the nurse evaluate to determine the magnitude of the infant's fluid loss?
1. Tissue turgor
2. Hematocrit value
3. Moistness of mucous membranes
4. Weight compared with prior weight

194. A dehydrated 2-month-old infant with a history of diarrhea is admitted to the pediatric unit. Oral rehydration therapy (ORT) is instituted. What is the most accurate method for monitoring the infant's hydration status?
1. Counting wet diapers
2. Obtaining daily weights
3. Measuring intake and output
4. Checking tissue turgor of the abdomen

195. A 3-week-old infant who has been vomiting for 3 days is admitted to the pediatric unit with a diagnosis of hypertrophic pyloric stenosis (HPS). What essential

information should the nurse identify during the admission procedure?
1. Character and amount of vomitus
2. Size and shape of the abdominal mass
3. Time of the last feeding, type of formula, and amount taken
4. Tissue turgor, respiratory status, amount and appearance of last voiding

196. A nurse is caring for an infant with hypertrophic pyloric stenosis (HPS). A pyloromyotomy is scheduled. Which pathophysiological modification must be addressed before this surgery can be performed safely?
1. Hydration must be restored
2. Serum chloride levels must be restored
3. Fluid and electrolyte imbalances must be corrected
4. Malnutrition and respiratory problems must be corrected

197. A nurse is caring for a toddler with the diagnosis of nephrotic syndrome. What is the best indicator of fluid balance in this toddler?
1. Daily weights
2. Urinary output
3. Abdominal girth
4. Improved appetite

198. Monitoring vital signs, particularly the blood pressure and the rate and quality of the pulse, is essential to detect physiological adaptations in a child with nephrotic syndrome. Which clinical manifestation should the nurse detect based on these vital signs?
1. Heart failure
2. Hypovolemia
3. Pulmonary embolus
4. Increased serum potassium

199. A 6-month-old infant, weighing 15 pounds, is admitted with a diagnosis of dehydration. There is a prescription for oral rehydration therapy (ORT) 4 mL/kg of Pedialyte over 4 hours. What is the approximate amount of fluid the infant should ingest during the 4 hours?
1. 28 mL
2. 32 mL
3. 38 mL
4. 42 mL

200. A nurse who is assigned to care for a 6-month-old infant with diarrhea is reviewing the infant's medical history, assessment findings, laboratory reports, and practitioner prescriptions. The infant's weight is 15½ pounds (7 kg). There is a prescription for potassium chloride to be added to the IV fluids. What assessment finding signals the nurse to question this prescription?
1. Incessant crying
2. Inadequate tissue turgor
3. Urinary output of 4 mL over 2 hours
4. Oral fluid intake of 12 mL over 8 hours

201. A nurse is admitting a 2-year-old toddler to the emergency department who ingested half of a bottle of aspirin tablets. What is the etiology of the metabolic acidosis caused by aspirin toxicity?

1. Deep rapid breathing
2. Higher pH of gastric contents
3. Rapid absorption of salicylate
4. Increased renal excretion of bicarbonate

202. A nurse is planning care for a toddler who has ingested aspirin. What assessment warrants close monitoring because its increase can result in further complications?
1. Blood pressure
2. Abdominal girth
3. Body temperature
4. Serum glucose level

203. An infant with a diagnosis of failure to thrive has been on enteral feedings for 3 days. All feedings have been retained, but the skin and mucous membranes are dry and the infant has lost weight. What should the nurse do based on these findings?
1. Notify the practitioner
2. Document the assessment findings
3. Increase the fluid component in the feeding
4. Increase the calorie component of the feeding

204. A nurse is caring for a 3-week-old infant with hypertrophic pyloric stenosis (HPS) who is severely dehydrated. What finding does the nurse expect when assessing the infant?
1. Weight loss of 5%
2. Severe allergic reactions
3. Depressed anterior fontanel
4. Urine specific gravity of 1.014

205. After surgery for the repair of a myelomeningocele an infant develops diarrhea and metabolic acidosis with a decreased urinary output. Based on the infant's status, what prescription does the nurse anticipate?
1. Isotonic saline
2. Sodium lactate
3. Serum albumin
4. Potassium chloride

206. What is the priority nursing action when a 3-month-old infant is receiving IV fluids via a scalp vein?
1. Restrain the infant's arms when no one is present
2. Monitor for infiltration behind the infant's occiput
3. Check both of the infant's pupils for dilation every hour
4. Tell the parents why they cannot hold the infant during IV therapy

207. A 5-month-old infant who weighs 12 pounds, 4 ounces (5.6 kg) is receiving 8 ounces of full-strength formula every 4 hours between 8 AM and midnight. Based on the recommended caloric intake of 108 calories/kg/day, what does the nurse conclude about the amount of formula ingested?
1. Meets recommended requirements
2. Exceeds recommended requirements
3. Falls below the amount recommended
4. Not enough data to determine the correct amount

208. The mother of an infant with a congenital heart defect, who was admitted to the pediatric unit with heart failure, questions why her baby must be weighed each

morning. The nurse explains that the baby's treatment is based on changes in daily weights. What complication can be prevented if treatment is successful?

1. Renal failure
2. Fluid retention
3. Digitalis toxicity
4. Protein malnutrition

209. A nurse teaches the parents of a 4-year-old child, weighing 33 pounds (15 kg), about their child's fluid needs. Instructions include that a child should receive 100 mL/kg/24 hours for the first 10 kg and then 50 mL/kg/24 hours for the next 10 kg. Which statement concerning their child's daily fluid intake indicates that the parents understand the teaching?

1. Two quarts are needed
2. Eight small glasses are enough
3. Ten 4-ounce servings are required
4. Four 6-ounce glasses are recommended

210. A child with Reye syndrome is receiving an intravenous solution of 10% glucose and mannitol (Osmitrol) to reduce cerebral edema. For which complication resulting from this therapy should the nurse monitor the child?

1. Overhydration
2. Seizure activity
3. Acute heart failure
4. Hypovolemic shock

211. An IV of D5W/0.45 NS is infusing when a child returns to the pediatric unit from surgery. The postoperative orders do not indicate the desired rate of infusion. What is the most appropriate action for the nurse to take?

1. Reduce the flow rate to keep the vein open and obtain an order
2. Adjust the flow rate to the 5 mL/hr the child was receiving before surgery
3. Maintain the present flow rate and call the nurse in the operating room to verify the rate
4. Regulate the flow rate to 25 mL/hr until the practitioner arrives for follow-up observation

212. What is the priority nursing intervention for a young infant who has an IV after receiving abdominal surgery?

1. Administering oral fluids
2. Limiting handling by parents
3. Weighing diapers after each voiding
4. Maintaining patency of the intravenous infusion

213. A nurse discusses dietary instructions with the parents of a child who has acute glomerulonephritis. The nurse teaches the parents the nutrients that are restricted. Select all that apply.

1. _____ Fats
2. _____ Sodium
3. _____ Glucose
4. _____ Potassium

214. A 30-month-old child is seen in the pediatric clinic after recovering from roseola. The child had temperatures of more than 102° F for 3 days. Assessment reveals that the child is moderately dehydrated and weighs 25 pounds. Oral rehydration therapy (ORT) is prescribed for 1 day. It is to be given in 2- to 3-ounce doses in addition to the fluids that the child usually drinks. The next day the mother calls the clinic to report how much fluid the child consumed.

Breakfast: 2 oz ORT, ½ cup orange juice, ½ cup milk in cereal
Snack: 3 oz ORT with cookies
Lunch: 1 cup chicken/vegetable/noodle soup with crackers
Snack: 3 oz ORT with cookies
Dinner: Refused ORT, ½ cup apple juice with dinner
Bedtime: 2 oz ORT with ice cream and cookies

What was the child's total intake in ounces for the day?

1. 30
2. 16
3. 42
4. 24

215. A 6-year-old child with glomerulonephritis has a fluid restriction of 600 mL in 24 hours. How can the nurse help the child cope with this limitation?

1. Withhold fluids from 7 PM to 7 AM
2. Divide fluids equally among each shift
3. Allow fluids as desired until limit is reached
4. Offer fluids in medicine cups throughout waking hours

216. A critically ill child develops Kussmaul respirations. The nurse suspects an increasing acid-base imbalance related to:

1. Metabolic alkalosis from an increase in base bicarbonate
2. Respiratory alkalosis from an excess carbon dioxide output
3. Respiratory acidosis from an accumulation of carbon dioxide
4. Metabolic acidosis from a concentration of cations in body fluids

217. In the immediate period after admission to the burn unit with severe burns, a 5-year-old child requests a drink of milk. What is the most appropriate nursing intervention?

1. Give ice chips as desired
2. Permit milk if it has been iced
3. Maintain NPO for 24 to 48 hours
4. Limit oral fluid to 15 mL every 4 hours

218. A child is brought to the emergency department with partial- and full-thickness burns of the extremities. The practitioner writes multiple orders. What nursing action is the priority?

1. Administering oxygen
2. Inserting a urinary catheter
3. Giving prescribed pain medication
4. Starting an IV with a large-bore catheter

219. An adolescent is hospitalized with multiple internal injuries after an automobile collision. The adolescent is being kept NPO and is receiving an IV infusion at 125 mL/hr and an antibiotic reconstituted in 10 mL of

normal saline every 6 hours (1 AM, 4 PM, 1 PM, 4 AM). What is the intake from 7 AM to 3 PM?
1. 1000 mL
2. 1010 mL
3. 1020 mL
4. 1030 mL

220. A nurse is caring for a child with severe dehydration and its associated acid-base imbalance. What compensatory mechanism within the body is activated to counteract the effects of the child's acid-base imbalance?
1. Profuse diaphoresis
2. Elevated temperature
3. Increased respiratory rate
4. Renal retention of hydrogen ions

221. The nurse manager of the infection control service is teaching a class for nurses regarding the care of young children with viral-related diarrhea. What therapy should the nurse manager recommend?
1. BRAT diet until after the diarrhea has stopped
2. Antiviral agent until the prescription is completed
3. Oral rehydration therapy until fluid balance is restored
4. Antidiarrheal agent after each stool until stools become formed

222. A child with acute glomerulonephritis has fluid intake restricted to the previous day's output plus 40 mL. The child's output in the past 24 hours was 140 mL. From 3 PM to 11 PM the child is to receive one third of the total daily fluid permitted. How much fluid should the nurse provide for the evening intake?
1. 60 mL
2. 70 mL
3. 80 mL
4. 90 mL

223. A nurse is planning care for a child with respiratory acidosis. What is the sequence of events that occurs in the child's respiratory response to acidosis? Place the physiological responses in the order in which they occur.
1. Increased pH
2. Hyperventilation
3. Decreased blood H^+ ions
4. Increased CO_2 elimination
Answer_____

GASTROINTESTINAL

224. An infant with a cleft lip is fed with a special nipple. What should the nurse teach the parents about feeding their infant to minimize regurgitation?
1. Offer a thickened formula
2. Burp frequently during a feeding
3. Place in an infant seat when feeding
4. Position on the side with the bottle propped

225. What is the primary focus of preoperative nursing care for an infant with a cleft lip?
1. Avoiding crying
2. Modifying feeding

3. Preventing infection
4. Minimizing handling

226. A nurse is caring for a 1-month-old infant who had surgery to repair a cleft lip. What should the nurse use to facilitate feeding during the immediate postoperative period?
1. Soft nipple
2. Plastic spoon
3. Feeding syringe
4. Nasogastric tube

227. A nurse is feeding an infant with a recent surgical repair of a cleft lip. What does the nurse plan to do for the infant just after each feeding?
1. Burp several times
2. Rinse the suture line
3. Place on the abdomen
4. Hold for several minutes

228. A nurse is caring for an infant during the immediate postoperative period after surgical repair of a cleft lip. What is the priority nursing action for this infant?
1. Keep restrained
2. Minimize crying
3. Oxygenate frequently
4. Handle as little as possible

229. An infant vomits after feedings and starts to lose weight. Galactosemia is diagnosed. The nurse explains to the parents that galactosemia is an inherited autosomal recessive disorder that results in an:
1. Intolerance to grains
2. Error in carbohydrate metabolism
3. Inability to metabolize an essential amino acid
4. Absence of parasympathetic ganglion cells in the colon

230. What dietary information should the nurse include in the teaching plan for parents of an infant with galactosemia? Select all that apply.
1. _____ Eliminate milk
2. _____ Substitute meat for eggs
3. _____ Provide soybean-based formulas
4. _____ Avoid baby cereals containing wheat flour
5. _____ Give prescribed pancreatic enzyme capsules with meals

231. The mother of an infant diagnosed with hypertrophic pyloric stenosis (HPS) states that she has never heard of this disorder and asks many questions. What should the nurse emphasize when responding?
1. "Surgery will not be necessary."
2. "This disorder has an excellent prognosis."
3. "Special feedings will be necessary for several months."
4. "This disorder is caused by an inborn error of metabolism."

232. A 3-week-old infant is admitted with a tentative diagnosis of hypertrophic pyloric stenosis (HPS). Before performing the admission assessment of the abdomen the nurse bicycles the infant's legs. How does this help the nurse's assessment?

   1. Relaxes abdominal muscles
   2. Detects weak abdominal muscles
   3. Enables palpation of abdominal contour
   4. Improves assessment of abdominal rebound
233. A nurse is assessing a 1-month-old infant suspected of having hypertrophic pyloric stenosis (HPS). Using the following figure, select the area where the nurse expects to palpate an olive-shaped mass:
   1. a
   2. b
   3. c
   4. d

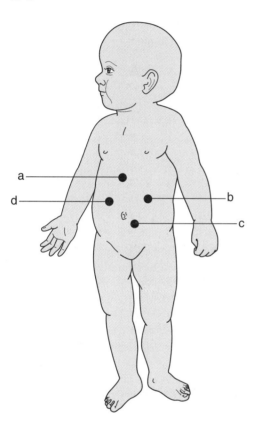

234. The mother of an infant with hypertrophic pyloric stenosis (HPS) asks the nurse many questions about the problem. What information should the nurse convey when answering these questions?
   1. Surgery usually is necessary
   2. Chromosomal mutation is the cause
   3. Slow feeding will be required for several months
   4. Dietary restrictions must be maintained throughout childhood
235. A 4-week-old infant is diagnosed with hypertrophic pyloric stenosis (HPS) and is scheduled for surgery. Oral feedings usually are initiated a few hours after surgery. What does the nurse expect the practitioner to prescribe initially?
   1. Electrolyte solution
   2. Full-strength formula
   3. Half-strength formula
   4. Cereal-thickened water

236. An infant who had surgery for hypertrophic pyloric stenosis (HPS) is being bottle fed by the mother. What should the nurse teach the mother about care after a feeding to decrease the chance of the infant vomiting?
   1. Rock for 20 minutes
   2. Place in an infant seat
   3. Keep awake for 20 minutes
   4. Position flat on the right side
237. A mother who is visiting the pediatric clinic with her 10-month-old son tells the nurse how pleased she is with her chubby infant. She states, "Look how much weight he has gained even though he drinks only orange juice. He won't drink any milk." How should the nurse respond?
   1. "He is a little overweight."
   2. "Let's talk about his nutrition."
   3 "Is he getting an iron supplement?"
   4. "Why is he drinking only orange juice?"
238. A nurse in the pediatric clinic is performing a physical assessment on a 15-month-old toddler. What finding indicates that a disorder may be present?
   1. Anterior fontanel is still palpable
   2. Liver is palpated 3 cm below the costal margin
   3. Respiratory abdominal movements are observed
   4. Apical pulse rate of 104 beats per minute is auscultated
239. Before administering a nasogastric feeding to a preterm infant the nurse aspirates a small amount of residual fluid from the stomach. What is the nurse's next action?
   1. Return the aspirate and withhold the feeding
   2. Discard the aspirate and give the full feeding
   3. Return the aspirate and subtract the amount of the aspirate from the feeding
   4. Discard the aspirate and add an equal amount of normal saline to the feeding
240. A nurse is preparing an infant for insertion of a nasogastric tube. List the steps of the procedure in the order they should be performed.
   1. Insert the tube
   2. Aspirate stomach contents
   3. Wash hands before opening package
   4. Use the tube to measure from ear to nose to stomach
   Answer_____
241. A 2-month-old infant is to have a nasogastric tube inserted. The nurse expects that:
   1. A pacifier will be offered to lessen gagging and allow easier insertion of the tube
   2. Gastric contents will not appear in the tube if the infant is receiving nothing by mouth
   3. The tube will be passed a distance equal to the length from the chin to the tip of the sternum
   4. Coughing, irregular breathing, and slight cyanosis will occur during introduction of the tube
242. A nurse just completes feeding a young child via a nasogastric tube. In what position should the child be placed to help retain the feedings and avoid aspiration?

1. Supine
2. Semi-Fowler
3. Trendelenburg
4. Left side-lying

243. A 6-week-old infant has the diagnosis of gastroesophageal reflux. What should the nurse teach the parents when discussing their infant's care?
    1. Feeding cereal with a spoon
    2. Providing formula thickened with cereal
    3. Placing the infant in an infant seat after feedings
    4. Explaining changes in care after surgical repair of the esophageal defect

244. For what complication should a nurse monitor an infant with gastroesophageal reflux?
    1. Bowel obstruction
    2. Increased hematocrit
    3. Respiratory problems
    4. Abdominal distention

245. A mother asks why her 2-year-old toddler's cleft palate was not repaired at the time the cleft lip was repaired. How should the nurse respond?
    1. "Waiting leaves time for other birth defects to be detected and corrected."
    2. "The cleft lip was so disfiguring that surgery was done as quickly as possible."
    3. "Your surgeon prefers to separate the operations to minimize potential complications."
    4. "The palate usually is repaired before a child starts to speak and some surgeons prefer to wait up to two years."

246. Elbow restraints are ordered for an 18-month-old toddler who just had surgery for a cleft palate. The nurse explains to the parents that the restraints are used to prevent:
    1. Playing with unsterile toys
    2. Rolling to a supine position
    3. Putting fingers into the mouth
    4. Removing the nasogastric tube

247. A toddler who had a cleft palate repair is now able to tolerate fluids. What should the nurse use to offer the toddler fluids?
    1. Small cup
    2. Soft nipple
    3. Bulb syringe
    4. Teflon-coated spoon

248. An infant is admitted to the pediatric unit with gastroenteritis and dehydration. The nurse determines that the parents understand the teaching about contact precautions when they state, "We should wash our hands and then:
    1. put on a mask when we are holding the baby."
    2. weigh the diaper each time we change the baby."
    3. keep the door to the baby's room closed most of the time."
    4. change our gloves each time we change the baby's diaper."

249. After receiving and tolerating an oral rehydration solution (Pedialyte) because of dehydration from diarrhea,

a 20-month-old toddler improves and a regular diet is started. What foods should the nurse suggest the parents offer their child? Select all that apply.
1. _____ Poached eggs
2. _____ Creamed soup
3. _____ Strained carrots
4. _____ Vanilla pudding
5. _____ Animal crackers

250. The mother of a 4-month-old infant weighing 11 pounds (5 kg) asks the nurse how much formula is required per day now that her baby is weaned from the breast. The recommended caloric intake is 108 kcal/kg and the formula contains 20 calories per ounce. How many ounces of formula a day should the nurse tell the mother to give to her infant?
    1. 21 ounces
    2. 27 ounces
    3. 33 ounces
    4. 39 ounces

251. A nurse teaches the mother of a young child which foods are the best sources of thiamine, a B complex vitamin. What nutrient should the nurse include in the teaching plan that is high in thiamine?
    1. Eggs
    2. Fruits
    3. Whole grains
    4. Green leafy vegetables

252. A nurse is caring for a child who had a laparoscopic appendectomy. What interventions should the nurse document on the child's clinical record? Select all that apply.
1. _____ Intake and output
2. _____ Measurement of pain
3. _____ Tolerance to low-residue diet
4. _____ Frequency of dressing changes
5. _____ Presence or absence of bowel sounds

253. The mother of a 2-year-old child calls her neighbor, who is a nurse, exclaiming that her child just ate some automatic dishwasher powder. What should the nurse tell the mother to do first?
    1. Give syrup of ipecac
    2. Wash the child's lips
    3. Call the poison control center
    4. Offer burnt toast with some milk

254. A toddler who swallowed drain cleaner is hospitalized for observation because of the risk for vomiting and aspiration. Over the next 24 hours the child does not exhibit any respiratory distress and does not vomit. At discharge the nurse emphasizes that the parents should monitor their child for the onset of:
    1. Tonic-clonic seizures
    2. Yellow-tinged sclera
    3. Gagging and vomiting
    4. Abdominal pain and diarrhea

255. A nurse is giving discharge instructions to the parents of a 5-year-old child who is recovering from surgery. What food should the nurse recommend that will ensure maintenance of a positive nitrogen balance?

1. Orange slices
2. Bacon sandwich
3. Hamburger on a bun
4. Chicken soup with carrots

256. The nurse epidemiologist of a large urban hospital is called to the pediatric unit to provide information about an outbreak of diarrhea caused by *Salmonella*. Which common foods does the nurse suspect are the cause of the outbreak? Select all that apply.
    1. _____ Ice cream
    2. _____ Raw carrots
    3. _____ Hamburgers
    4. _____ Soft-boiled eggs
    5. _____ Toasted cheese sandwich

257. A nurse is reviewing the orders for a child with diarrhea caused by a *Salmonella* infection. Which practitioner order should the nurse question?
    1. Stool for occult blood
    2. Oral rehydration therapy
    3. Bismuth subsalicylate (Kaopectate), 2 teaspoons after each stool
    4. Acetaminophen (Tylenol), 15mg/kg for temperature above 101° F

258. A neonate with an imperforate anus undergoes a colostomy. In which positions should the nurse place the infant during the postoperative period? Select all that apply.
    1. _____ Prone
    2. _____ Trendelenburg
    3. _____ Supine with head of crib elevated
    4. _____ Side-lying with head of crib elevated

259. A nurse is caring for preterm infants in the neonatal intensive care unit (NICU). The nurse anticipates that these infants may develop an intestinal obstruction associated with:
    1. Meconium ileus
    2. Imperforate anus
    3. Duodenal atresia
    4. Necrotizing enterocolitis

260. After several episodes of intermittent abdominal pain and vomiting a 5-month-old infant is admitted to the pediatric unit. A diagnosis of intussusception is made. What is the priority nursing assessment that assists in confirming the diagnosis?
    1. Auscultating for bowel sounds
    2. Listening for high-pitched crying
    3. Measuring fluid intake and output
    4. Observing characteristics of stools

261. A nurse bases the plan of care for a 15-month-old toddler with celiac disease on the pathophysiology of the disorder, which is characterized by an:
    1. Inability to metabolize gluten
    2. Absence of the enzyme phenylalanine
    3. Excessive amount of salt in the sweat glands
    4. Increase in the viscosity of mucous secretions

262. A nurse is obtaining a health history from the mother of a 15-month-old toddler with celiac disease. Specific to

celiac disease, the nurse expects the mother to indicate that her toddler:
    1. Has bulky, foul, frothy stools
    2. Drinks large amounts of fluid
    3. Is irritable throughout the day
    4. Voids strong, concentrated urine

263. The nurse is counseling the parents of a young child with a recently confirmed diagnosis of celiac disease. The parents ask how the diagnosis was confirmed. Before responding the nurse considers that the child's jejunal biopsy result indicated:
    1. Small areas of fatty plaques
    2. Atrophic changes in the mucosal wall
    3. Irregular areas of superficial ulcerations
    4. Diffuse degenerative fibrosis of the acini

264. The laboratory report of a child with celiac disease reveals that the child has anemia. What does the nurse suspect are the most likely causes of the anemia? Select all that apply.
    1. _____ Lack of gluten in the diet
    2. _____ Inadequate caloric intake
    3. _____ Absence of intrinsic factor
    4. _____ Incomplete absorption of iron
    5. _____ Incomplete absorption of folic acid

265. Discharge planning for a toddler newly diagnosed with celiac disease includes instructions related to dietary restrictions. What foods should the nurse recommend? Select all that apply.
    1. _____ Oatmeal
    2. _____ Ice cream
    3. _____ Rice cakes
    4. _____ Corn crisps
    5. _____ Whole-wheat toast

266. A nurse in the pediatric clinic is reviewing the health history of a 6-year-old child with celiac disease who has been on the dietary regimen for 6 months. What evaluation criterion does the nurse use to assess the child's adherence to the diet?
    1. Formed bowel movements
    2. Ability to handle stressful situations
    3. Understanding of the disease process
    4. Knowledge of foods allowed on the diet

267. A nurse is teaching the mother of a toddler with celiac disease the specific foods allowed on the gluten-free diet. What essential information should the nurse help the mother to understand?
    1. Corn flour is not included in the diet
    2. Labels of prepared foods must be read carefully
    3. Caloric intake is increased to compensate for a deficiency of proteins
    4. Gluten-free diets are discontinued when affected children start kindergarten

268. A nurse evaluates that teaching is effective when the mother of a child on a low-residue diet states that she will serve her child:
    1. Frankfurter on a roll
    2. Ripe peaches with ice cream

3. Peanut butter and jam on white bread

4. Scrambled eggs and toasted white bread

269. The mother of an 11-month-old infant who just had surgery to create a temporary colostomy is concerned about care at home. What instructions about care of the colostomy should the nurse include in the teaching plan?

   1. Empty and rinse the bag whenever necessary

   2. Limit diarrhea by restricting milk and milk products

   3. Irrigate the colostomy with as much water as possible

   4. Report slight bleeding from the stoma site immediately

270. A nurse in the pediatric clinic is examining a child suspected of having enterobiasis (pinworm). For which first sign of an infestation should the nurse assess the child?

   1. Anal itching

   2. Scaly skin patches

   3. Maculopapular rash

   4. Bald spot on the head

271. A nurse in the pediatric clinic is advising the mother of a toddler who has a pinworm infestation. What should the nurse teach the mother about caring for her child during and after treatment? Select all that apply.

   1. _____ How to identify pinworm eggs

   2. _____ Strategies to avoid reinfection

   3. _____ Need for medication for the entire family

   4. _____ Importance of handwashing before eating

   5. _____ Reason for obtaining stool specimens from the child

272. The mother of a 30-month-old toddler who was treated for pinworm infestation is taught how to prevent a recurrence. Which statement by the mother indicates that the teaching is effective? Select all that apply.

   1. _____ "I will keep the cat off my child's bed."

   2. _____ "I will disinfect my child's room every 2 days."

   3. _____ "The family's sheets will be washed every day."

   4. _____ "The school nurse must be told to have the toilets cleaned."

   5. _____ "I will remind family members to take the medication again in 2 weeks."

273. A 2-year-old boy living on a farm is diagnosed with *Ascaris lumbricoides* (roundworm). The nurse teaches the mother about the transmission of these parasites. What statement indicates that the mother needs further teaching?

   1. "The rest of the family will not need the medicine."

   2. "My little boy cannot play in the fields until he gets older."

   3. "The vegetables must be well cooked before the family eats them."

   4. "Everyone's bedding will have to be washed daily in soapy water."

274. The mother of a 2-year-old toddler tells the nurse that her child frequently is constipated. The nurse asks the mother how she handles the child's toileting. Which response indicates to the nurse that the mother requires further discussion?

1. "My child drinks a lot of fluids."

2. "I give my child high-fiber foods."

3. "My child has one bowel movement a day."

4. "I schedule my child's toileting before each meal."

275. The mother of a 6-year-old boy tells the nurse in the pediatric clinic that her son has become incontinent of his stool. The nurse plans to assess the child to determine the cause of his encopresis. In what order should the nurse perform the assessments?

   1. Bowel habits

   2. Nutrition history

   3. Psychosocial factors

   4. Physical examination

   Answer_____

276. A school nurse is teaching a unit on nutrition to a sixth-grade class. Why should the nurse include that eating in fast-food restaurants should be limited?

   1. Eating is rushed

   2. Portions are too large

   3. Food is high in calories

   4. Sanitary conditions are inadequate

INTEGUMENTARY

277. A nurse in the pediatric clinic is teaching a mother how to care for her infant who has eczema. What is most important for the nurse to teach the mother?

   1. Ensuring physical growth

   2. Identifying causative factors

   3. Providing adequate hydration

   4. Preventing secondary infections

278. A nurse is teaching skin and basic care to the mother of a 6-month-old infant with eczema. Which statement indicates that the mother needs further teaching?

   1. "I must be careful not to cut my baby's nails short."

   2. "I gave my baby's woolen blankets to my nephew."

   3. "My baby should not be given whole-milk products."

   4. "My baby will need a new wardrobe of cotton clothing."

279. A nurse in the pediatric clinic is taking a health history of a toddler with an exacerbation of eczema. What are the nurse's priority assessments of the child? Select all that apply.

   1. _____ Increase in appetite

   2. _____ Wearing cotton clothes

   3. _____ Toleration of new foods

   4. _____ Exposure to a viral infection

   5. _____ Recent contact with someone with eczema

280. A preschool child is diagnosed with atopic dermatitis. The nurse emphasizes that the child should be discouraged from scratching. The child's mother asks why scratching should be prevented. The nurse responds, "Scratching:

   1. causes lesions to become more contagious."

   2. spreads dermatitis to other areas of the body."

   3. results in skin breaks that can lead to infection."

   4. produces changes that are precursors to skin cancer."

281. During an infant's routine visit to the pediatric clinic the nurse identifies white patches adhering to the mucosa of the infant's mouth. What is the initial action by the nurse?
    1. Swipe a patch to obtain a specimen for a culture
    2. Scrape off the patches with a tongue blade or cotton swab
    3. Record the finding and continue with the physical examination
    4. Tell the mother to cleanse the mouth thoroughly after each feeding

282. A 3-month-old infant hospitalized with severe diarrhea has an excoriated diaper area. The mother becomes concerned when she discovers that the nurse has left her infant without a diaper. What is the nurse's explanation for this action?
    1. Exposing the excoriated areas helps to reduce the fever
    2. Cleansing the skin followed by air-drying reduces excoriation
    3. Air-drying the perineal area prevents the diaper from sticking to the skin
    4. Leaving the area exposed allows for observation of when the infant stools

283. A nurse is caring for an infant who just had surgery for a cleft lip. In which position should the nurse place the infant?
    1. Prone
    2. Low Fowler
    3. Left side-lying
    4. Caregiver's shoulder

284. The mother of a male infant who just had a cleft lip repair tells the nurse, "My baby seems restless. May I hold him?" What information influences the nurse's response?
    1. Holding may meet needs and reduce tension on the suture line
    2. Sedation limits activity and decreases tension on the suture line
    3. Handling may increase irritability, causing tension on the suture line
    4. Arm movements cannot be controlled, placing tension on the suture line

285. A nurse in the pediatric clinic receives a call from the mother of a 12-month-old infant who has a fever, runny nose, cough, and white spots in the mouth for 3 days. A rash has developed that started on the face and now has spread to the whole body. Which communicable infection does the nurse suspect the child has?
    1. Rubella
    2. Rubeola
    3. Pertussis
    4. Varicella

286. A school nurse is teaching a group of parents about the early signs of rubeola (measles). What sign related to rubeola should alert the parents to seek medical help?

    1. Macular rashes
    2. Scaly skin patches
    3. Bald patches on the scalp
    4. Generalized vesicular skin lesions

287. The mother of a child recovering from varicella (chickenpox) calls the nurse in the pediatric clinic asking how the child's itching can be relieved. What should the nurse suggest?
    1. Have the child wear mittens
    2. Rub an antibiotic ointment on the lesions
    3. Use wet to dry saline dressings over the oozing vesicles
    4. Pat the lesions while applying the prescribed calamine lotion

288. A woman and her children, who have not received immunizations for childhood diseases, immigrate to the United States. Before being immunized, one of the children acquires varicella (chickenpox). The nurse teaches the mother that varicella is:
    1. Communicable until all the vesicles are dry
    2. Still communicable even when dry scabs remain
    3. No longer communicable after the fever has subsided
    4. Not communicable while vesicles are surrounded by a red areola

289. A 10-year-old child has sustained partial-thickness burns on the anterior surfaces of both arms and hands and the upper half of the chest. Based on the grading system of the American Burn Association, the nurse estimates the total body surface area (TBSA) involved. What is the approximate body area affected?
    1. 17%
    2. 12%
    3. 20%
    4. 15%

290. A child is admitted to the burn unit with partial-thickness burns of both arms and the chest. What information about burns should guide the nurse's plan of care?
    1. Burns are extremely painful and disfiguring
    2. Some grafting of the burned area is necessary
    3. Pressure dressings and prolonged hydrotherapy are required
    4. Spontaneous epithelial regeneration occurs within several weeks

291. A child with partial-thickness burns on 21% of the total body surface area (TBSA) progresses from the emergent phase to the acute phase of burn care. What is the most important nursing intervention at this time?
    1. Recording intake and output
    2. Monitoring for signs of infection
    3. Instituting a pain management plan
    4. Maintaining a high nutritional intake

292. A child who has successfully completed the emergent (resuscitative) phase of treatment for a severe burn injury is started on a high-protein, high-calorie diet. Which snacks should the nurse encourage between meals? Select all that apply.
    1. _____ Crackers and cheese
    2. _____ White bread and honey

3. _____ Orange juice and cookies
4. _____ Banana pudding and whipped cream
5. _____ Frozen yogurt and chocolate sprinkles

293. A nurse is caring for a child with severe burns who has extensive eschar formation on the arms. What is the priority nursing intervention?
    1. Removing blisters
    2. Checking radial pulses
    3. Maintaining respiratory isolation
    4. Performing range-of-motion exercises

294. A child who had full-thickness burns is to have skin grafts. The nurse explains to the child's parents that for permanent grafts the child must have:
    1. Steroids
    2. Autografts
    3. Homografts
    4. Immunosuppressives

295. A nurse is changing the dressing on a child with severe burns. What basic principles of surgical asepsis must the nurse consider? Select all that apply.
    1. _____ A paper field must remain dry to be considered sterile
    2. _____ Sterile items held below the waist are considered sterile
    3. _____ A one-inch border around a sterile field is considered contaminated
    4. _____ Sterile objects in contact with clean objects are considered contaminated

296. A nurse is caring for a preschool-age child with leukemia who is receiving chemotherapy and is suspected of having a fever. What factors should the nurse consider before taking this child's temperature? Select all that apply.
    1. _____ Skin sensor temperatures are not accurate past infancy
    2. _____ Rectal temperatures are too upsetting for this age group
    3. _____ Oral temperatures are accurate for children with leukemia
    4. _____ Tympanic temperatures are not accurate when a fever is suspected
    5. _____ Rectal temperatures are avoided to reduce the risk of rectal trauma

297. A child is receiving radiation therapy for a brain tumor. What should the nurse include in the skin care for this child?
    1. Apply baby oil to the head
    2. Cleanse the head with water
    3. Wash the head with mild soap
    4. Rinse soap from the head under a shower

298. A nurse teaches a teenager who is receiving chemotherapy about the need for special mouth care because of the potential for lesions. The nurse evaluates that the instructions are understood when the teenager says, "I will:
    1. brush my teeth with baking soda."
    2. use mouthwash to rinse my mouth."
    3. swish my mouth out with hydrogen peroxide."
    4. use a soft-bristled toothbrush to clean my teeth."

299. The mother of a kindergartner tells the nurse that her daughter is constantly scratching behind her ears. The nurse suspects pediculosis capitis (head lice). What does the nurse expect to identify when performing a physical assessment?
    1. Small grayish-brown threadlike lines
    2. Scaly patches within areas of alopecia
    3. Streaked blisters surrounding a larger one
    4. White spots attached to the base of hair shafts

300. A school nurse is teaching a group of parents about pediculosis capitis (head lice). What common secondary infection does the nurse teach the parents to identify?
    1. Eczema
    2. Impetigo
    3. Cellulitis
    4. Folliculitis

301. A nurse is teaching the parents of a 5-year-old child about the application of permethrin 5% cream (Elimite) for scabies. The nurse teaches them to apply the medication:
    1. Before each meal and rinse it off in 1 hour
    2. At bedtime and wash it off the next morning
    3. After bathing and rinse it off after 15 minutes
    4. Each morning for a week and wash it off the last day

302. A child recently returned from a 3-day-camping trip during the spring vacation. The child has a rash, chills, and a low-grade fever and is taken to the clinic by the parents. What are the most important data for the nurse to assess when taking the child's history? Select all that apply.
    1. _____ Date of return to school
    2. _____ Sports played on camping trip
    3. _____ Proneness to allergic reactions
    4. _____ Duration of signs and symptoms
    5. _____ Recent exposure to poison oak or ivy

303. When a 12-year-old boy who received several tick bites on a camping trip becomes ill he is told that he may have Lyme disease. He asks the nurse, "What is Lyme disease?" How should the nurse respond?
    1. "You are concerned. Tell me what you want to know."
    2. "The infection is caused by a spirochete. It can be cured with penicillin."
    3. "The tick bites gave you an infection. There is medication that will treat it."
    4. "You sound upset. Don't worry, we have medicine that will make you better."

304. The mother of an adolescent asks the nurse, "What is the best way to remove a tick from the skin?" How should the nurse respond?
    1. "Touch the tick with a lighted cigarette."
    2. "Remove the tick carefully with tweezers."
    3. "Pour ammonia over the tick and it will shrivel up."
    4. "Spray the tick with insect repellent and it will fall off."

305. A 10-year-old boy arrives with his mother at the emergency department after being bitten by a stray dog. There is a bleeding soft tissue injury on the inner aspect of the left forearm. What is the priority nursing action?
1. Ask the mother if her son is allergic to horse serum
2. Assess the injury, vital signs, and past health history
3. Inoculate the child with human rabies immuno-globulin
4. Notify the police department to capture and test the dog

NEUROMUSCULAR

306. A nurse is caring for a 9-month-old infant who was admitted to the pediatric unit with a tentative diagnosis of meningitis. A lumbar puncture is performed. The nurse explains to the parents that the primary reason this procedure is performed is to:
1. Determine the causative agent
2. Identify the presence of blood
3. Reduce the intracranial pressure
4. Measure the spinal fluid glucose level

307. A nurse is preparing an infant for a lumbar puncture. In what position should the nurse hold the infant?
1. Sitting with the buttocks at the table's edge and the head flexed
2. Prone with the head extended over the table's edge and the extremities mummified
3. Lateral recumbent with the back at the table's edge and the head and legs extended
4. Side-lying with the back at table's edge and the head flexed with the knees brought to the chin

308. A nurse is caring for an infant with meningitis. When the nurse extends the baby's leg, the hamstring muscles go into spasm. What positive sign or reflex is the infant exhibiting?
1. Kernig sign
2. Babinski reflex
3. Chvostek sign
4. Cremasteric reflex

309. A child is admitted to the pediatric unit with a diagnosis of meningococcal meningitis. The nurse concludes that isolation:
1. Is unnecessary during the incubation period
2. Is required for 7 to 10 days until the fever subsides
3. Will be unnecessary after the diagnosis is confirmed
4. Will be necessary for 24 to 72 hours after initiating antibiotic therapy

310. A nurse places a child with bacterial meningitis in isolation with droplet precautions. What is the purpose of these precautions?
1. They separate the child from noninfected people
2. The infectious process is interrupted as quickly as possible
3. The child is protected from developing a secondary infection

4. They prevent the development of a hospital-acquired infection

311. How can a nurse best soothe a hospitalized infant who appears to be in pain?
1. Feed the infant
2. Hold the infant
3. Play soft music in the room
4. Provide a quiet environment

312. The mother of an infant with Down syndrome asks the nurse what is the cause of the disorder. Before responding the nurse considers that the genetic factor of Down syndrome results from:
1. Intrauterine infection
2. X-linked genetic disorder
3. Autosomal recessive gene
4. Extra chromosomal material

313. A nurse is caring for an infant with Down syndrome. What does the nurse anticipate is the most common serious anomaly associated with this disorder?
1. Renal disease
2. Hepatic defects
3. Congenital heart disease
4. Endocrine gland malfunction

314. A nurse is caring for an infant with a myelomeningocele. What does the nurse expect this infant to have that differentiates it from an infant with a meningocele?
1. Enlarged head
2. Sac over the lumbar area
3. Affected lower extremities
4. Infection of the spinal fluid

315. A nurse is caring for an infant who had surgery to correct a myelomeningocele. What assessment provides data about a potential major complication for this infant?
1. Daily weights
2. Fluid output every 8 hours
3. Blood pressure every 12 hours
4. Daily head circumference measurements

316. A nurse is assessing a 3-week-old infant admitted to the pediatric unit with hydrocephalus. What finding identifies a complication requiring immediate attention?
1. Tense anterior fontanel
2. Uncoordinated eye/muscle movement
3. Larger head circumference than chest circumference
4. Inability to support the head while in the prone position

317. An infant with a myelomeningocele is scheduled for surgery to close the defect. Which nursing action best facilitates parent-child relationships in the preoperative period?
1. Encouraging the parents to stroke their infant
2. Allowing the parents to hold their infant in their arms
3. Referring the parents to the Spina Bifida Association of America
4. Teaching the parents to use special techniques when feeding the infant

318. A 3-month-old infant has a ventriculoperitoneal (VP) shunt inserted. What should the nurse include in the infant's plan of care?
   1. Keep the infant in the prone position
   2. Apply sterile, moist dressings to the incision
   3. Observe for signs of cerebrospinal fluid leakage
   4. Teach the parents signs of increased intracranial pressure

319. The parents of a child who has a right ventriculoperitoneal (VP) shunt for hydrocephalus are taught about postoperative positioning. The nurse evaluates that they understand the teaching when they state, "We will place our baby lying:
   1. in the position that provides the most comfort."
   2. on the back with a small support beneath the neck."
   3. on the abdomen with the head turned to the left side."
   4. flat on the left side with the head and back supported."

320. The nurse assesses a 5-year-old child after a shunt procedure that was performed to correct increased intracranial pressure. Which finding is of most concern?
   1. Marked irritability
   2. Complaints of pain
   3. Temperature of 99.4° F
   4. Pulse of 100 beats per minute

321. On the day after surgery for insertion of a ventriculoperitoneal shunt for hydrocephalus, an infant's temperature increases to 103° F. The nurse immediately notifies the practitioner. What is the next nursing action?
   1. Cover the infant with a bath blanket
   2. Sponge the infant with tepid alcohol
   3. Reassess the infant's temperature in several hours
   4. Record the infant's temperature in the medical record

322. A nurse is teaching the parents of an infant with cerebral palsy how to provide optimum care. What should the nurse include in the teaching?
   1. Focus on cognitive rather than motor skills
   2. Maintain immobility of the limbs with splints
   3. Preserve muscle tone to prevent joint contractures
   4. Continue offering a special formula to limit gagging

323. An infant is diagnosed with cerebral palsy several months after birth. When the infant is 10 months old the mother comes to the pediatric clinic because the child has developed slow, writhing movements. The nurse explains that slow, writhing movements are characteristically associated with the type of cerebral palsy known as:
   1. Ataxic
   2. Spastic
   3. Dystonic
   4. Athetoid

324. A nurse is concerned about helping the parents of an infant with cerebral palsy to set long-term goals for the family. These goals should be set with the understanding that:
   1. Cognitive impairments require special education
   2. Progressive deterioration requires future institutionalization

   3. Unknown extent of the disability requires continual adjustments
   4. Diminished immune responses require protection from infection

325. While in the playroom a 7-year-old child has a twitching of the right arm and leg that progresses to a generalized tonic-clonic seizure. What is the nurse's initial action?
   1. Take other children to their rooms
   2. Insert an airway into the child's mouth
   3. Move toys and furniture away from the child
   4. Position the child on the back and place a pillow under the head

326. A nurse is caring for a child who has a tonic-clonic seizure. How should the nurse describe the clonic phase?
   1. Generalized rigidity
   2. Loss of consciousness
   3. Spasmodic body jerking
   4. Tremors of upper extremities

327. A 4-year-old child is admitted to the pediatric neurological service with a seizure disorder. Shortly after admission, while in bed, the child has a generalized seizure. What nursing actions are most appropriate? Select all that apply.
   1. _____ Assess the seizure
   2. _____ Take the child's vital signs
   3. _____ Turn the child onto the side
   4. _____ Pull the padded side rails up
   5. _____ Initiate oxygen administration

328. The mother of a 2-year-old child tells the nurse that she is concerned about her child's vision. What behavior when the child is tired leads the nurse to suspect the child has strabismus?
   1. One eyelid droops
   2. Both eyes look cloudy
   3. One eye moves inward
   4. Both eyes blink excessively

329. A nurse in the pediatric clinic is assessing a child with strabismus. What is one of the major goals for the surgical correction of this child's disorder?
   1. Improve appearance
   2. Avoid need for glasses
   3. Prevent legal blindness
   4. Restore peripheral vision

330. A nurse is assessing a 3-year-old child with a tentative diagnosis of lead poisoning. What clinical finding supports this diagnosis?
   1. Epistaxis
   2. Clumsiness
   3. Excessive salivation
   4. Decreased pulse rate

331. A nurse is teaching dietary management to the parents of a child who is receiving chelation therapy to treat lead poisoning. What should be included in the discussion of the dietary plan?
   1. Maintain a low salt diet
   2. Ensure adequate fluid intake

3. Avoid refined sugar and flour
4. Offer high-calorie and low-protein foods

332. After oral surgery the dentist writes a prescription for pain medication for an 18-month-old child. Which medication should the nurse question?
1. Tylenol
2. Codeine
3. Percodan
4. Morphine

333. An 8-year-old child is admitted to the emergency department with signs and symptoms of Reye syndrome. What information from the child's history is most important for the nurse to obtain in light of the child's diagnosis?
1. Recent rash
2. Tonsillitis attacks
3. Recent viral infection
4. Recurrent high fevers

334. A child is diagnosed with Reye syndrome. The parents ask the nurse for information about this disorder. The nurse responds that it is:
1. A genetic disorder
2. A bacterial infection
3. An encephalopathy of unknown etiology
4. An acute illness primarily affecting the brain

335. A 6-year-old child comes to the well-child clinic for a routine examination. The nurse identifies black lines on the teeth at the gum line. What does the nurse conclude is the possible cause of this finding?
1. Perthes disease
2. Lead poisoning
3. Salicylate toxicity
4. Tetracycline administration

336. A nurse suspects that a 7-month-old infant who is brought to the well-baby clinic for the first time may have a hearing deficit. What behavior leads the nurse to come to this conclusion?
1. Mother says the infant is unable to learn the word Mama
2. Infant does not always turn the head when called by name
3. Infant fails to demonstrate a Moro reflex in response to hand clapping
4. Mother says the infant stopped making verbal sounds about a month ago

337. A nurse is obtaining the health history of a 7-month-old boy who has had repeated episodes of otitis media. What question should be included in the interview with the mother?
1. "Please describe your son's feeding patterns."
2. "Tell me how often your son has had otitis media."
3. "What medicine do you give your son for the otitis media?"
4. "Do any of your children other than your son have this problem?"

338. A nurse is explaining a myringotomy procedure to a child's parents. The nurse includes that the incision:

1. Takes several days to heal, leaving some scar tissue
2. Provides immediate relief of pressure in the middle ear
3. Widens the perforation in the eardrum, allowing for drainage
4. May result in permanent perforation of the tympanic membrane

339. What should the nurse suggest to help parents promote the effectiveness of their child's myringotomy procedure?
1. Count how frequently the child swallows
2. Position the child with the affected ear down
3. Observe the child for bleeding from the ear that had surgery
4. Administer pain medication when the child awakens in the morning

340. The nurse is planning to give discharge instructions to the parents of a child who had a myringotomy. The nurse tells them about the most common complications associated with this surgery. Select all that apply.
1. _____ Lack of drainage
2. _____ Increasing ear pain
3. _____ Bleeding from the ear
4. _____ Moderate hearing loss
5. _____ Low-grade temperature

341. A child who had an adenoidectomy arrives at the practitioner's office for a follow-up visit. What other adaptations to the surgery should the nurse assess in addition to hearing? Select all that apply.
1. _____ Swallowing
2. _____ Sense of taste
3. _____ Sense of smell
4. _____ Speech sounds

342. What is most important for a nurse to teach the parents of a child with Duchenne muscular dystrophy to do for their child?
1. Maintain a high-calorie diet
2. Institute seizure precautions
3. Restrict the use of larger muscles
4. Perform range-of-motion exercises

343. The nurse is counseling the parents of a 12-year-old child with Duchenne muscular dystrophy about problems that may develop during adolescence. What body system does the nurse expect might be affected?
1. Neurological
2. Integumentary
3. Gastrointestinal
4. Cardiopulmonary

344. A 4-year-old girl with a brain tumor diagnosed as an astrocytoma is admitted to the pediatric unit. The nurse performs a physical assessment while the child is lying in the supine position. During the assessment the child states that her head hurts and begins to cry. What does the nurse conclude is the probable cause of the headache?

1. Hunger from fasting until blood tests are completed
2. Separation anxiety that manifests in physical symptoms
3. Increased intracranial pressure caused by blood pooling in the head
4. Mutilation anxiety which is most common in children of this age-group

345. A child is admitted to the pediatric unit with the diagnosis of a brain tumor. During breakfast the child vomits, and the nurse concludes that the vomiting was caused by increasing intracranial pressure. What are the nurse's priority interventions? Select all that apply.
    1. _____ Refeed breakfast
    2. _____ Notify the practitioner
    3. _____ Request a reevaluation
    4. _____ Administer the prescribed antiemetic
    5. _____ Increase the intravenous infusion rate

346. After a 4-year-old child has a craniotomy the nurse performs a neurological assessment that includes level of consciousness, pupillary activity, and reflex activity. What else should the nurse include in this assessment?
    1. Blood pressure
    2. Motor function
    3. Rectal temperature
    4. Head circumference

347. A child is about to be admitted to the pediatric intensive care unit (PICU) after surgery for removal of a brain tumor. The nurse manager should intervene immediately when the child's nurse:
    1. Places a hypothermia blanket at the bedside
    2. Adjusts the bed to the Trendelenburg position
    3. Obtains electronic equipment for monitoring the vital signs
    4. Secures a pump to administer the ordered intravenous fluids

348. The day after brain surgery a 9-year-old child with type 1 diabetes develops a temperature of 103° F. What does the nurse suspect is the probable cause of the fever?
    1. Children with diabetes usually develop an infection after surgery
    2. High temperatures are expected in children after surgical procedures
    3. Cerebral edema after brain surgery exerts pressure on the hypothalamus
    4. Excessive viscid secretions resulted in inadequate respiratory ventilation

349. A nurse in the emergency department is caring for a 9-year-old child suspected of having a spinal cord injury after falling off a bicycle. What is the initial nursing action?
    1. Place the child's head on a pillow for support
    2. Immobilize the child's spine to limit additional injury
    3. Log-roll the child to check for lacerations on the back
    4. Move the child onto a firm stretcher for transport to the x-ray department

350. An 8-year-old boy is diagnosed with a mild concussion and is to be discharged home. The mother is instructed to check her child for responsiveness every 2 hours and to wake him up for this assessment after he goes to sleep. She telephones the nurse that she is afraid to allow him to go to sleep. How should the nurse respond? Select all that apply.
    1. _____ "You can bring him to the hospital before bedtime, if you prefer."
    2. _____ "If your son becomes difficult to awaken, bring him to the hospital."
    3. _____ "There is no need to worry because your son is past the critical period."
    4. _____ "Awakening your son throughout the night should alert you to any change."

351. A child is brought to the emergency department after sustaining a blow to the head while playing football. The nurse performs a neurological assessment to determine if the child has an acute head injury. What should the nurse assess first?
    1. Ocular signs
    2. Muscular strength
    3. Level of consciousness
    4. Injuries to the scalp area

352. The mother of a 7-year-old boy arrives at the emergency department with her son. The history reveals that he hit his head after falling from his tree house and he saw stars. Later, he complains of a headache and feeling sick to his stomach. The nurse assesses his motor responses by evaluating his ability to:
    1. Draw a picture
    2. Balance on one foot
    3. Squeeze the nurse's hand
    4. Walk slowly around the room

353. A 12-year-old child is admitted to the hospital for observation after receiving a head injury. Twelve hours after the injury the child has none of the signs or symptoms of a head injury. What is the nurse's priority intervention at this time?
    1. Monitoring level of consciousness every hour
    2. Promoting rest by creating a quiet environment
    3. Questioning about the circumstances that led to the injury
    4. Administering the prescribed opioid for complaints of a headache

354. A nurse is teaching a class for staff members working in a group home about the cognitive development of children with mental retardation. What concept can these children probably learn the fastest?
    1. Love vs. hate
    2. Life vs. death
    3. Large vs. small
    4. Right vs. wrong

355. What should the nurse suggest when parents ask what to do about their preschooler's stuttering?
    1. Speak clearly and do not complete the child's sentences

2. Avoid looking at the child when there is difficulty forming words

3. Help the child by supplying the correct word when there is a block

4. Stop the conversation and tell the child to speak slowly when starting again

RESPIRATORY

356. What is the priority nursing intervention for a 6-month-old infant with bronchiolitis?
    1. Discouraging parental visits to conserve energy
    2. Monitoring skin color, anterior fontanel, and vital signs
    3. Wearing gown, cap, mask, and gloves when giving care
    4. Promoting stimulating activities to meet developmental needs

357. A nurse is reviewing the orders for a 2-year-old child who is admitted to the pediatric unit with acute laryngotracheobronchitis (croup). What is the rationale for the order to administer oxygen via a nasal cannula?
    1. Congeals mucous secretions and relieves dyspnea
    2. Decreases the effort required for breathing and allows for rest
    3. Triggers the cough reflex and facilitates expectoration of mucus
    4. Liquefies mucous secretions and makes them easier to expectorate

358. A child is admitted to the emergency department with a diagnosis of acute spasmodic laryngitis (spasmotic croup). After the spasms subside the child is ready to be discharged. What should the nurse teach the parents to do at home to help prevent another croup episode?
    1. Perform postural drainage
    2. Discourage before bedtime snacks
    3. Use a cool mist vaporizer in the child's room
    4. Demonstrate to the child how to expel air after inspiration

359. The parents of a 3-year-old child who has recurrent attacks of acute spasmodic laryngitis (spasmodic croup), asks the nurse why this happens to their child. The best rationale for the nurse to convey why this is a disorder of young children is that they:
    1. Have small airways
    2. Are mouth breathers
    3. Have immature immune systems
    4. Are prone to upper respiratory infections

360. When providing nursing care to children, the nurse takes into consideration that in the child, as in the adult, respiratory patterns are controlled by the:
    1. Medulla
    2. Cerebellum
    3. Hypothalamus
    4. Cerebral cortex

361. A nurse is preparing to suction a child with a tracheostomy tube. What nursing action will limit trauma to the trachea?
    1. Hyperoxygenating before the procedure
    2. Instilling sterile saline before suctioning
    3. Using negative pressure when inserting the suction catheter
    4. Selecting a suction catheter half the diameter of the tracheostomy tube

362. A toddler is admitted to the pediatric unit with a temperature of 103.5° F, a runny nose, and a productive cough. Respiratory secretion specimens are sent for culture and sensitivity tests. Standard precautions are followed until the results are known. What other precautions should the nurse include?
    1. Droplet
    2. Contact
    3. Airborne
    4. Neutropenic

363. A nurse is caring for a newborn with a diaphragmatic hernia who has impaired gas exchange. What does the nurse identify as the etiology of the infant's decreased gas exchange?
    1. Incarcerated hernia
    2. Decreased oxygen intake
    3. Increased basal metabolic rate
    4. Excessive respiratory secretions

364. A nurse is caring for an infant who had surgery to repair a diaphragmatic hernia. What is the best position for the nurse to place the infant?
    1. Semi-Fowler in an infant seat
    2. Side-lying onto the unoperated side
    3. Prone with the head turned to the side
    4. Supine with the head of the bed elevated

365. An infant with a diaphragmatic hernia had corrective surgery. What nursing assessment indicates that the infant's respiratory condition has improved?
    1. Cessation of crying
    2. Reduction of blood pH to 7.31
    3. Retention of 1 ounce of formula
    4. Auscultation of breath sounds bilaterally

366. An infant who had an open repair of a fractured sternum now has a chest tube. What should the nurse explain to the parents concerning the chest tube?
    1. The infant will not feel any discomfort
    2. It is inserted to drain the chest cavity of air
    3. The tube was inserted in case of an emergency
    4. It will be removed when the infant tolerates feedings

367. After returning from surgery an infant suddenly becomes cyanotic. What is the nurse's priority intervention?
    1. Check vital signs
    2. Administer oxygen
    3. Suction the nasopharynx
    4. Place in the side-lying position

368. A child in the pediatric intensive care unit (PICU) is on a ventilator. One of the nurses asks what should be done

when condensation collects in the ventilator tubing. How should the nurse manager respond?

1. Notify the physician's assistant
2. Decrease the amount of humidity
3. Empty the fluid and reconnect the tubing to the ventilator
4. Measure the fluid and mark it on the intake and output record

369. A nurse in the pediatric intensive care unit is assessing a 6-month-old infant with bronchiolitis. What physiological responses to this lower respiratory tract infection does the nurse expect? Select all that apply.
    1. _____ Wheezing
    2. _____ Bradycardia
    3. _____ Sternal retractions
    4. _____ Increased breath sounds
    5. _____ Prolonged expiratory phase

370. A child who was rescued from a burning building is admitted to the burn unit with a diagnosis of smoke inhalation. For what complication should the nurse monitor?
    1. Systemic infection
    2. Tracheobronchial edema
    3. Posttraumatic stress disorder
    4. Generalized adaptations to stress

371. A 10-year-old child who was rescued from a house fire is brought to the emergency department with burns of the extremities. When assessing the child, what finding is of most concern to the nurse?
    1. Elevated temperature
    2. Increasing activity level
    3. Burns around the mouth
    4. Edema distal to the burns

372. A nurse in the pediatric clinic is teaching the parents of children with asthma about allergens, such as insects, that contribute to an asthmatic episode. What insect is the most common allergen for children prone to asthma?
    1. Spider
    2. Centipede
    3. Carpenter ant
    4. Household cockroach

373. A nurse in the pediatric clinic is assessing an 8-year-old child who has had asthma since infancy. What clinical finding requires immediate intervention?
    1. Barrel chest
    2. Audible wheezing
    3. Heart rate of 105 beats per minute
    4. Respiratory rate of 30 breaths per minute

374. An 8-year-old boy with asthma is being taught breathing exercises. The nurse uses several techniques in a play situation. The child does a repeat demonstration for the nurse. Which technique indicates that the child needs further teaching?
    1. Moving a cotton ball when inhaling
    2. Singing songs that have long phrases

3. Puffing through a straw to move small items
4. Blowing through a plastic pipe to make soap bubbles

375. A nurse instructs the parents of a child with asthma how to reduce the allergens in the child's bedroom. The mother tells the nurse what she plans to do to make the room hypoallergenic. Which plan indicates that further teaching is needed?
    1. Removing a stuffed animal collection
    2. Storing off-season clothing in another room
    3. Covering the mattress with a plastic slipcover
    4. Using flat outdoor carpeting to cover hardwood floors

376. An 8-year-old child with a history of asthma is brought to the emergency department because of respiratory distress. The nurse immediately places the child in a bed with the head of the bed elevated and administers oxygen via a facemask. The practitioner performs a physical assessment, writes orders, and admits the child to the pediatric unit. Which order should the nurse carry out first?
    1. Administer the nebulizer treatment to facilitate breathing
    2. Obtain a blood specimen to send to the laboratory for tests
    3. Notify the respiratory therapist to perform chest physiotherapy
    4. Send a requisition to central supply for an incentive spirometer

---

CLIENT CHART

Practitioner Orders

Bed rest
Complete blood count
SMA 12
Albuterol (Proventil) 2.5 mg via nebulizer, one dose
Chest physical therapy bid
Incentive spirometer
Referral to allergist
Oxygen via mask @ 8L/min

Physical Assessment

Dyspnea, flaring of nares, productive cough (frothy, clear, gelatinous sputum), wheezing. Child indicates shortness of breath, chest discomfort, headache, and feeling tired.

Vital Signs

Temp 99.8° F (oral)
Pulse 90 beats/minute
Resp 30 breaths/minute
BP 120/78

---

377. A child admitted to the hospital with a diagnosis of status asthmaticus appears to be improving. What is the most objective way for the nurse to evaluate the child's response to therapy?
    1. Auscultate breath sounds
    2. Monitor respiratory pattern
    3. Assess lips for decreased cyanosis
    4. Evaluate peak expiratory flow rate

378. A nurse is planning to teach the parents of a child recently diagnosed with cystic fibrosis about why the child has respiratory problems. What should the nurse consider about the underlying pathophysiology?
    1. Airway irritability causes spasms
    2. Lung parenchyma becomes inflamed
    3. Excessively thick mucus obstructs airways
    4. Endocrine glands secrete surplus hormones

379. A nurse performs cupping, percussion, and postural drainage every 4 hours for a 6-month-old infant with cystic fibrosis. When is the best time for scheduling chest physiotherapy?
    1. Just before feedings
    2. During each feeding
    3. Midway between feedings
    4. Immediately after every feeding

380. A nurse is discussing the need for genetic counseling with a male teenager who has a sibling with cystic fibrosis (CF). Which test, identified by the teenager as necessary for him to undergo, indicates that he understands the genetic counseling?
    1. Chest x-ray
    2. Gene analysis
    3. Sweat chloride
    4. Chromosomal assay

381. A nurse is caring for a child with cystic fibrosis who was admitted to the pediatric unit with pneumonia. What potential consequence of repeated infections should the nurse consider when caring for this child?
    1. Increased irritability
    2. Development of diabetes
    3. Impaired academic ability
    4. Depression of bone marrow

382. A nurse anticipates that when administering routine oxygen therapy to a child, the oxygen:
    1. Should be labeled as flammable
    2. Is warmed before administration
    3. Concentration is closely monitored
    4. May be administered without an order

383. What is the best method for the nurse to teach a 4-year-old child about deep breathing before surgery?
    1. Provide a pamphlet with pictures
    2. Have the child blow a cotton ball across a table
    3. Have the child practice using an incentive spirometer
    4. Show a videotape of children doing deep breathing exercises

384. A child who just returned to the pediatric unit after surgery is drowsy. What should the nurse do to maintain an airway?
    1. Have a tongue blade available
    2. Use nasotracheal suction routinely
    3. Keep the child in the supine position
    4. Place the child in a side-lying position

385. A nurse is caring for an adolescent in the postanesthesia care unit (PACU). What action should the nurse take to ensure accuracy of a pulse oximeter reading?

    1. Place the probe on a finger or earlobe
    2. Fasten the probe to the abdomen or thigh
    3. Attach the probe to a different finger for each measurement
    4. Apply the probe, then wait ten minutes before obtaining a reading

386. A child survives a near-drowning episode in a cold pond. What factor does the nurse identify that will have the greatest effect on the child's prognosis?
    1. Hypoxia
    2. Hyperthermia
    3. Emotional trauma
    4. Aspiration pneumonia

387. A 10-year-old child who is developmentally delayed and blind must be fed all meals. The child has problems swallowing and frequently chokes and coughs during the feeding. What technique should the nurse use when feeding this child?
    1. Hold the child in an upright position and use a soft-tipped bulb syringe
    2. Place the child in the supine position and turn the child's head to the right
    3. Seat the child in a wheelchair, give small bites of food with metal tableware, and encourage participation
    4. Prop the child in a semi-sitting position, provide chopped food, and place it in the child's mouth with plastic tableware

388. A nurse in the pediatric clinic is examining the throat of a 5-year-old child. The tongue blade is placed to the side of the child's tongue. The nurse uses this technique to prevent:
    1. Injuring the rear teeth
    2. Eliciting the gag reflex
    3. Obstructing the airway
    4. Interfering with the visual field

389. A 10-month-old boy is in a restaurant with his parents and grandparents. The grandfather places several pieces of bread on the high chair tray for the infant. A nurse sitting nearby sees the infant gag, become red-faced, then turn cyanotic. With permission from the family, the nurse holds the child with the head downward and:
    1. Gives the infant five back blows
    2. Sweeps the infant's mouth with a finger
    3. Performs five abdominal thrusts on the infant
    4. Initiates the head-tilt-chin-lift maneuver on the infant

REPRODUCTIVE AND GENITOURINARY

390. A 4-year-old child with nephrotic syndrome is admitted to the pediatric unit. What clinical finding does the nurse expect when assessing this child?
    1. Severe lethargy
    2. Dark, frothy urine
    3. Chronic hypertension
    4. Flushed, ruddy complexion

391. A 3-year-old child is admitted to the pediatric unit with a diagnosis of nephrotic syndrome. The child has

ascites, oliguria, respirations of 40 per minute, and a recent weight gain of 10 pounds. What nursing intervention may help lessen the child's respiratory difficulty?
1. Providing 6 small meals daily
2. Maintaining a well-ventilated room
3. Ensuring bed rest in the low-Fowler position
4. Administering oxygen at 2 L per minute by mask

392. A 6-year-old child is admitted to the pediatric unit with a diagnosis of nephrotic syndrome. What should the plan of care include during the acute phase?
1. Offering a low-protein diet
2. Encouraging fluids every hour
3. Promoting frequent position changes
4. Providing time for active play periods

393. Which roommate should the nurse manager assign to a 4-year-old boy who was admitted to the pediatric unit with nephrotic syndrome?
1. 3-year-old boy with impetigo
2. 2-year-old boy with pneumonia
3. 5-year-old girl with thalassemia
4. 4-year-old girl with conjunctivitis

394. What should a nurse include in the plan of care for a child with nephrotic syndrome?
1. Providing meticulous skin care
2. Restricting fluids to four ounces each shift
3. Offering a diet low in carbohydrates and protein
4. Sending blood to the laboratory for typing and crossmatching

395. A nurse is giving discharge instructions to the parents of a boy with nephrotic syndrome. What parental statement about their child's care indicates that more instructions are needed?
1. "Any gain in weight is expected."
2. "Prednisone will be given with meals."
3. "We plan to test his urine for albumin."
4. "We will check his eyelids every morning."

396. A boy with nephrotic syndrome is in remission for several months. One day the mother calls the clinic to report that for the past week her child's skin has a muddy pale appearance, his appetite is poor, and he has been unusually tired after school. Based on the mother's description, what does the nurse suspect?
1. Impending renal failure
2. Excessive activity at school
3. Development of a viral infection
4. Nonadherence to the medication protocol

397. A nurse in the pediatric clinic is planning care for a 7-year-old boy with enuresis. What is an appropriate short-term goal for this child?
1. Groin rash will resolve in 1 week
2. Continence will continue throughout night
3. Time between voidings will increase by 1 hour
4. Self-esteem enhancement will occur when given praise

398. An infant is born with exstrophy of the bladder. What practitioner's order does the nurse expect to protect the exposed bladder until surgery is performed?

1. Antibacterial ointment
2. Pediatric urine collector
3. Warm moist compresses
4. Sterile nonadherent dressings

399. After surgical repair of a urinary tract malformation a child is to be discharged with an indwelling catheter. The nurse teaches the parents the necessary interventions if urine does not appear in the drainage bag for 1 hour or more. Place the interventions in the order that they should be performed.
1. Offer more fluids
2. Call the practitioner
3. Check for blocked drainage tubing
4. Press on the abdominal wall just above the bladder
Answer_____

400. The parents of a toddler who is admitted to the pediatric unit for surgery to correct hypospadias ask the nurse when this defect happened. The nurse responds that it usually occurs during the period of fetal development in the:
1. First 12 weeks
2. Third trimester
3. Second 16 weeks
4. Implantation phase

401. What should the plan of care include for a newborn with hypospadias?
1. Preparing the infant for insertion of a cystostomy tube
2. Explaining to the parents the genetic basis for the defect
3. Keeping the infant's penis wrapped with petrolatum gauze
4. Giving the parents reasons why a circumcision should not be done

402. An 8-month-old infant had a surgical correction for hypospadias. What is a priority nursing intervention during the postoperative period?
1. Ensure that privacy is maintained
2. Minimize pain with adequate analgesia
3. Restrict fluid intake until stent is removed
4. Gradually increase the time that the urinary catheter is clamped

403. A nurse is caring for a child with chordee and the parents ask why corrective surgery is necessary. Before responding the nurse considers that in adulthood if the chordee is not surgically corrected he will be at increased risk for:
1. Renal failure
2. Testicular cancer
3. Testicular torsion
4. Sexual dysfunction

404. A mother brings her 6-year-old child to the pediatric clinic stating that the child has not been feeling well, is weak and lethargic, and has a poor appetite, headaches, and smoky-colored urine. What additional information should the nurse obtain that will aid in making a diagnosis?

    1. Rash on palms and feet

    2. Pain in shoulders and knees

    3. Recent weight loss of 2 pounds

    4. Strep throat within the past 2 weeks

405. A child is admitted to the pediatric unit with a tentative diagnosis of acute glomerulonephritis. What does the nurse expect the laboratory report to reveal?

    1. Low sedimentation rate

    2. Increased serum complement

    3. Elevated antistreptolysin O titer

    4. Decreased blood urea nitrogen level

406. A nurse is assessing a child admitted to the pediatric unit with acute poststreptococcal glomerulonephritis (APSGN). What specific signs and symptoms does the nurse expect? Select all that apply.

    1. _____ Anorexia

    2. _____ Glycosuria

    3. _____ Hypotension

    4. _____ Periorbital edema

    5. _____ Elevated creatinine level

407. The mother of an 8-year-old child with the diagnosis of acute poststreptococcal glomerulonephritis (APSGN) is concerned that a 4-year-old sibling might be developing the disorder. When preparing to explain the disease process the nurse knows that it is caused by:

    1. A systemic infection causing clots in the small renal tubules

    2. A factor that is unknown and therefore is difficult to prevent

    3. An immune complex disorder occurring after a group A beta-hemolytic streptococcal infection

    4. An autosomal recessive trait with an increased probability that a sibling will develop the disease

408. A 10-year-old child with acute glomerulonephritis (AGN) is selecting foods for dinner from a menu. Which foods should the nurse encourage?

    1. Baked potato, meat loaf, banana, and pretzels

    2. Baked ham, bread and butter, peaches, and milk

    3. Corn on the cob, baked chicken, rice, apple, and milk

    4. Hot dog on a bun, potato chips, dill pickle slices, and brownie

409. A nurse who is caring for a child with acute glomerulonephritis assesses the child for cerebral complications. What signs and symptoms does the nurse identify that indicate cerebral involvement?

    1. Headache, drowsiness, and vomiting

    2. Generalized edema, anorexia, and restlessness

    3. Anuria, temperature greater than 103°F, and confusion

    4. Cardiac decompensation, heart rate of 114 beats per minute, and vomiting

410. A child treated for acute glomerulonephritis has improved and is soon to be discharged. What should the nurse plan to offer the parents in preparation for the discharge?

    1. Samples of no-added-salt diets for the child to continue at home

    2. Suggestions about activities to keep the child mobile for longer periods

    3. Instructions as to when the child should return for a workup for a kidney transplant

    4. Phone numbers to reach the nurse on the unit so that the parents can call if there are any questions

411. Which clinical findings indicate to the nurse that a child may have nephrotic syndrome (NS) rather than acute glomerulonephritis (AGN)? Select all that apply.

    1. _____ Lethargy

    2. _____ Gross hematuria

    3 _____ Generalized edema

    4. _____ Massive proteinuria

    5. _____ Unchanged blood pressure

412. A nurse anticipates that surgery will be needed for an 18-month-old child with undescended testes because:

    1. Psychological damage is limited

    2. Maturation of testes starts at age 7

    3. Future malignancy may be prevented

    4. Puboscrotal ring is more elastic at age 2

413. A nurse is assessing a child with vesicoureteral reflux. What clinical finding does the nurse expect to identify?

    1. Dysuria

    2. Oliguria

    3. Glycosuria

    4. Proteinuria

414. A 3-year-old child is admitted to the pediatric unit with a tentative diagnosis of Wilms tumor. The nurse obtains the child's health history from the parents. What does the child's history reveal that will aid in establishing the diagnosis?

    1. Periorbital edema

    2. Projectile vomiting

    3. Abdominal swelling

    4. Low-grade temperature

415. A 4-year-old child with Wilms tumor has a nephrectomy. What essential information should the nurse plan to teach the parents?

    1. Prepare for a kidney transplant

    2. Restrict the child's intake of sodium

    3. Maintain the child's fluid restrictions

    4. Recognize signs of a urinary tract infection

416. A nurse is caring for a child with a diagnosis of glomerulonephritis. The child's urinary output decreases to <100 mL every 24 hours, the creatinine clearance is 60 mL per minute, and there is an irregular apical pulse. A diagnosis of acute renal failure is made. Blood is drawn for testing. Which serum level is most significant?

    1. Sodium 126 mEq/L

    2. Bilirubin 0.3 mg/dL

    3. Creatinine 1.3 mg/dL

    4. Potassium 6.1 mEq/L

417. A child in renal failure who had the creation of an arteriovenous fistula access begins hemodialysis three times a week. The nurse teaches the mother the specific care her child needs. What statement indicates that further teaching is necessary?

1. "I'll offer more drinks in warm weather."
2. "I should call the clinic if vomiting or diarrhea occurs."
3. "I'll check the pulse at the wrist of both arms every day."
4. "I can take the blood pressure on the arm with the fistula."

418. A child with chronic kidney disease is receiving peritoneal dialysis. For what complication associated with this treatment should the nurse monitor the child?
    1. Petechiae
    2. Abdominal bruit
    3. Cloudy return dialysate
    4. Elevated blood glucose levels

419. A 7-year-old child must remain quietly in bed while having peritoneal dialysis. What activity is most appropriate for the nurse to plan for this child?
    1. Learning to play chess
    2. Constructing a model airplane
    3. Working multiple-piece puzzles with another child
    4. Using a large sponge ball to play catch with a roommate

420. A nurse in the adolescent clinic is obtaining a health history of a 16-year-old male with a complaint of a thick urethral discharge. What is the most appropriate nursing action to help confirm a tentative diagnosis of gonorrhea?
    1. Assess the temperature for a fever
    2. Collect a urine sample for a urinalysis
    3. Draw blood for a complete blood count
    4. Obtain a urethral specimen for a culture

421. A nurse in the adolescent clinic is assessing a teenager with a tentative diagnosis of primary syphilis. What is an early sign of this infection?
    1. Rash
    2. Genital lesion
    3. Genital discharge
    4. Multiple gummatous lesions

422. A 16-year-old male asks the nurse about the use of condoms. He states, "I have used condoms in the past but I'm not sure I'm using them correctly." What should be included as part of the teaching plan about condoms?
    1. Vaseline should be used as a lubricant
    2. They must be positioned after an erection has occurred
    3. They should be fitted against the tip of the penis, leaving no space at the end
    4. Withdrawal after ejaculation should be delayed until the penis becomes flaccid

SKELETAL

423. A 3-month-old infant with developmental dysplasia of the hip (DDH) is placed in a Pavlik harness. The home care nurse observes the infant sleeping without the harness. The mother explains that her baby will not sleep with the harness on. How should the nurse respond?

    1. Assure her that the harness can be removed during a short nap
    2. Encourage her to reapply the harness after her baby falls asleep
    3. Explain to her the importance of the harness being worn continuously
    4. Instruct her to eliminate one of the daily naps thus reducing the time out of the harness

424. What statement by the mother of a 6-week-old girl leads the nurse to assess the infant for the presence of a skeletal abnormality?
    1. "She seems to want to sleep curled up."
    2. "It's hard to put the diaper between her legs."
    3. "Her feet look flat when I put booties on her."
    4. "When I try to stand her up her legs won't straighten."

425. A nurse is assessing an infant suspected of having developmental dysplasia of the hip. What does the nurse expect the infant's orthopedic status to reveal?
    1. Apparent shortening of one leg
    2. Limited ability to adduct the affected leg
    3. Narrowing of the perineum with an anal stricture
    4. Inability to palpate movement of the femoral head

426. A nurse is assessing an 18-month-old toddler who is suspected of having developmental dysplasia of the left hip. In what position should the nurse place the toddler to elicit the Trendelenburg sign?
    1. Standing on the affected leg
    2. Supine with the back arched
    3. Side-lying on the unaffected side
    4. Sitting upright with the legs separated

427. Six weeks after birth an infant is diagnosed with developmental dysplasia of the hip. The nurse explains to the parents the benefits of early treatment. What is the rationale for corrective measures being instituted immediately?
    1. Mobility will be delayed if correction is postponed
    2. Traction is effective if it is used before toddlerhood
    3. Infants are easier to manage in spica casts than are toddlers
    4. Infants' cartilaginous hip joints promote molding of the acetabulum

428. A 2-year-old child with developmental dysplasia of the hip has a spica cast applied. The mother asks the nurse how to keep the cast clean. How should the nurse respond?
    1. "Tuck a folded diaper above the perineal opening."
    2. "Place plastic wrap or duct tape around the perineal edges."
    3. "Wipe the cast with a wet cloth and sprinkle it with baby powder."
    4. "Do the best you can because it will get soiled no matter what you do."

429. Three days after the application of a spica cast a child has a temperature of 101.4° F. Suspecting an infection, what clinical finding does the nurse anticipate?
    1. A foul odor from the cast
    2. An irregular respiratory pattern

3. Itching around the top of the cast

4. Complaints of tingling in the toes

430. A nurse is assessing an infant with talipes equinovarus (clubfoot) who had a corrective boot cast applied. Which peripheral vascular assessment cannot be determined while the cast is in place?

1. Pulse

2. Color

3. Warmth

4. Blanching

431. The nurse is teaching the parents of an infant who will have frequent cast changes about cast care. What suggestion should be included in the teaching?

1. Apply lotion to the skin at cast edges

2. Check the skin at the edges of the cast

3. Immerse the cast briefly during the tub bath

4. Cover the damp cast edges with adhesive petals

432. A nurse is preparing to teach a 7-year-old child about crutch-walking. What should be included in the plan?

1. Demonstrating a four-point gait

2. Exploring the child's fear of falling

3. Explaining the reason for rubber tips on crutch ends

4. Discovering how much the child knows about using crutches

433. A 16-year-old adolescent sustains an ankle injury while playing soccer. Crutches with no weight-bearing are ordered by the practitioner. What must the nurse ensure when adjusting the crutches?

1. They reach to 1 inch below the axillae

2. They extend to 6 inches from the side of each foot

3. The elbows are extended when the crutches are held by the crossbars

4. The shoulders are slightly stooped when the crutches are bearing body weight

434. A nurse is teaching an adolescent with a sprained ankle how to use one crutch when walking. What statement indicates that no further teaching is necessary?

1. "Crutches should not be used on stairs."

2. "After a month I can stop using the crutch."

3. "The crutch should be placed in front of my bad ankle."

4. "The crutch will be used on the side of my good ankle."

435. A child hospitalized with juvenile idiopathic arthritis (JIA) complains of pain in the knees. What intervention should help to relieve the discomfort?

1. Immobilizing the affected joints

2. Massaging the swollen areas gently

3. Placing several pillows under the knees

4. Applying warm, moist compresses to the knees

436. A nurse is caring for a child with juvenile idiopathic arthritis (JIA). What is most important for the nurse to attempt to prevent?

1. Infection

2. Hemarthrosis

3. Contracture deformities

4. Delayed intellectual development

437. A nurse is helping a child with juvenile idiopathic arthritis (JIA) perform range-of-motion exercises. What outcome indicates that the exercises have been effective?

1. Knees are more mobile

2. Pedal pulses become stronger

3. Statement that there is less pain

4. Subcutaneous nodules at the joints recede

438. A nurse is teaching a school-age child with juvenile idiopathic arthritis (JIA) activities to prevent the loss of joint function. What should the nurse caution the child to avoid?

1. Bicycle riding

2. Walking to school

3. Isometric exercises

4. Sedentary activities

439. When assessing a child who has just had a short arm cast applied to a fractured right wrist the nurse discovers that the fingers of the right hand are cool. What should the nurse do first?

1. Compare the temperature of each hand

2. Clip the edge of the cast to reduce pressure

3. Elevate the right arm to reduce the swelling

4. Inform the practitioner of the circulatory impairment

440. During the initial assessment of a 7-year-old child with a compound fracture of the wrist the nurse identifies a dark, wet area on the cast. What is the nurse's next action?

1. Notify the practitioner about the stain

2. Remove the stain with soap and water

3. Check if the child was playing with a coloring pen

4. Circle the area with a pen, noting the date and the time

441. A child sustains a fractured femur in a bicycle accident. The admission x-ray films reveal evidence of fractures of other long bones in various stages of healing. What does the nurse suspect is the cause of the fracture?

1. Child abuse

2. Vitamin D deficiency

3. Osteogenesis imperfecta

4. Inadequate calcium intake

442. How should a nurse turn a 10-year-old child in a spica cast?

1. Log-roll the body as one unit

2. Use the crossbar between the legs

3. Ask the child to sit up when changing position

4. Teach the child how to assist by using the overhead trapeze

443. A teenage boy with a diagnosis of osteosarcoma is to have the affected leg amputated. What should the nurse do to promote psychological adjustment and early functioning immediately after surgery?

1. Allow him to change the first dressing

2. Help him adjust to the temporary prosthesis

3. Assign him to a room with another adolescent

4. Have him meet with a member of a cancer survivor organization

444. After an above-the-knee amputation for bone cancer an adolescent male is returned to his room. He is monitored closely because there is a potential for hemorrhage from the residual limb. What should the nurse plan to keep at the bedside?
1. Hemostat
2. Tourniquet
3. Pressure dressing
4. Protamine sulfate

445. A school nurse is screening children for scoliosis. In what age group is it usually identified?
1. Adolescence
2. Preadolescence
3. Early school years
4. Middle school years

446. During a routine physical examination a 10-year-old girl is discovered to have scoliosis. The curve is diagnosed as mild and functional. A daily exercise program is established. The next month, at the follow-up visit, the nurse evaluates that the child is complying with the exercise program. The statement that supports the nurse's conclusion is, "I:
1. like doing my exercises with my brother so he can get stronger."
2. think my exercises will make me a better baseball and soccer player."
3. do my exercises every day while my mother stays with me and watches."
4. count out loud when I do my exercises so my mother can hear that I'm doing them all."

447. The mother of a 10-year-old boy with mild scoliosis asks the nurse, "How long will my son have to continue his exercises before he is better?" How should the nurse respond?
1. "At your son's age the exercise program is done for several months."
2. "Wearing a brace daily probably will lead to a quicker improvement."
3. "Surgery may be necessary, but it will be less involved if the exercises are done."
4. "Even if he continues to exercise, improvement will not be known until he is fully grown."

448. A nurse is teaching a high school student about scoliosis treatment options. What should be the nurse's focus?
1. Effect on body image
2. Least invasive treatment
3. Continuation with schooling
4. Maintenance of contact with peers

449. A spinal fusion is performed on an adolescent with scoliosis. What postoperative nursing intervention is specifically related to surgery for scoliosis?
1. Log-rolling every 2 hours
2. Checking the dressing frequently
3. Supervising deep breathing exercises
4. Maintaining the supine position for 3 days

450. While performing preoperative teaching, a nurse explores a young adolescent's concern about changes in appearance after surgery to correct scoliosis. What is the most appropriate statement by the nurse?
1. "After surgery your back will be much straighter."
2. "You are concerned about how you will look after surgery."
3. "Many teenagers who have this type of surgery do very well."
4. "Your parents think it is important for you to have this surgery."

DRUG-RELATED RESPONSES

451. A nurse is caring for a 3-month-old infant who was admitted to the pediatric unit with severe dehydration caused by diarrhea. After fluid and electrolyte balance is restored, lactobacilli granules (Lactinex) are prescribed. The nurse expects this medication to:
1. Help expel gas
2. Relieve pain caused by hyperacidity
3. Recolonize flora in the intestinal tract
4. Diminish inflammatory mucosal edema

452. Mebendazole (Vermox) is prescribed for a 3-year-old with pinworms. What information should the nurse include when teaching the parents about this medication?
1. It may precipitate transient diarrhea
2. One dose will eliminate the infestation
3. Rectal itching will be relieved the next day
4. Other family members will not need to take it

453. Acetaminophen (Tylenol), 15 mg/kg, is prescribed for a child who weighs 44 pounds. Each 5 mL contains 160 mg. How many mL of acetaminophen should the nurse administer?
Answer: _____ mL

454. A school nurse teaches a 13-year-old child with hay fever that the prescribed phenylephrine (Neo-Synephrine) nasal spray must be used exactly as directed. What complication can occur if the nasal spray is used incorrectly?
1. Tinnitus
2. Nasal polyps
3. Bleeding tendencies
4. Increased nasal congestion

455. A nurse is teaching the parents of an 8-year-old child who is taking a high dose of predniSONE (Meticorten) for asthma. What critical information about predniSONE should be included?
1. It protects against infection
2. It should be stopped gradually
3. An early growth spurt may occur
4. A moon-shaped face will develop

456. A 2-year-old boy with hemophilia A is to start receiving prophylactic intravenous infusions of the recombinant form of factor VIII three times a week. At what time should the nurse instruct the parents to administer the factor on the designated days?
1. At bedtime
2. After lunch

3. Before dinner
4. Upon awakening

457. A 15-year-old adolescent is admitted to the hospital with a diagnosis of status asthmaticus. An intravenous infusion of methylPREDNISolone (Solu-Medrol) is initiated. What adverse effect requires the nurse to intervene immediately?
1. Polyuria
2. Tinnitus
3. Drowsiness
4. Hypotension

458. A nurse is caring for a 15-year-old adolescent who was admitted to the hospital after taking an acetaminophen (Tylenol) overdose. Which diagnostic study is most important for the nurse to monitor at this time?
1. Blood gas levels
2. Liver function tests
3. Complete blood counts
4. Glycosylated hemoglobin findings

459. An infant is to receive an IV antibiotic via piggyback. The prescription is 10 mg/kg of body weight in 24 hours to be administered in equal doses every 12 hours. The infant weighs 22 pounds. How many mg of the antibiotic should the infant receive per dose?
Answer:_____ mg

460. A 3-year-old child with nephrotic syndrome has been receiving predniSONE (Meticorten) for 1 week. The nurse reviews the child's progress record and determines that the medication has been effective. What information supports this conclusion? Select all that apply.
1. _____ Weight loss
2. _____ Lower blood pH
3. _____ Shorter rest periods
4. _____ Increased urinary output
5. _____ Decreased blood pressure

461. A nurse is completing the discharge protocol for a 14-year-old adolescent with osteomyelitis. The nurse teaches the parents how and when to administer the intravenous antibiotic at home. The schedule for administration is four times a day. At what times should the parents administer the antibiotic?
1 8 AM, 12 PM, 4 PM, and 8 PM
2. 8 AM, 4 PM, 12 AM, and 4 AM
3. 10 AM, 2 PM, 10 PM, and 2 AM
4. 6 AM, 12 PM, 6 PM, and 12 AM

462. Digoxin (Lanoxin) is prescribed for a 1-month-old infant. At the next clinic visit the nurse palpates the apical pulse at 88 beats per minute. What is the nurse's responsibility regarding this pulse rate?
1. Notify the practitioner immediately
2. Tell the mother to continue the digoxin
3. Expect the practitioner to lower the dose
4. Ask the mother if this is the infant's usual heart rate

463. A nurse is reviewing medication instructions with the parents of an infant who is receiving digoxin (Lanoxin) and spironolactone (Aldactone). What parental response concerning their infant's care indicates that the instructions are understood?
1. Activity should be restricted
2. Orange juice must be offered daily
3. Vomiting should be reported to the practitioner
4. Anti-inflammatory drugs will not be given with spironolactone

464. A nurse in the pediatric clinic receives a call from the mother of an infant who is receiving digoxin (Lanoxin). The mother states that she forgot whether she had given the morning dose of digoxin. How should the nurse respond?
1. "Give the dose immediately."
2. "Wait 2 hours before giving the medication."
3. "Omit the dose and give it at the next prescribed time."
4. "Take the baby's pulse and give the medication if it is more than 90 beats/minute."

465. An infant with congenital heart disease is to be discharged with prescriptions for digoxin (Lanoxin) and furosemide (Lasix). The nurse discusses the danger signs of digoxin toxicity with the parents. What danger sign requires a call to the practitioner?
1. Difficulty feeding with vomiting
2. Cyanosis during periods of crying
3. Daily naps lasting more than 3 hours
4. Pulse rate greater than 100 beats per minute

466. An infant with a seizure disorder is receiving Phenobarbital (Luminal) at home. The mother calls the pediatric clinic and states that the infant has become lethargic and sleeps for long periods. What should the nurse respond to reduce the mother's anxiety?
1. "There is a drug that will prevent this problem."
2. "This means your baby's medication dose needs to be adjusted."
3. "This is a temporary response to the drug that usually stops after a few weeks."
4. "Many infants experience the same problem but your baby needs the medication."

467. A nurse teaches the parents of a 7-year-old girl on long-term phenytoin (Dilantin) therapy about care pertinent to this medication. Which statement indicates that the teaching was effective?
1. "We give the medication between meals."
2. "Her gums are massaged and teeth flossed frequently"
3. "She is eating high-calorie foods and we encourage fluids."
4. "We will call the clinic if the color of her urine becomes pink."

468. Ferrous fumarate (Feostat) 30 mg is prescribed for an infant. The ferrous fumarate solution contains 45 mg/0.6 mL. How much solution should the nurse administer?
Answer: _____ mL

469. An adolescent who is receiving predniSONE (Meticorten) and vinCRIStine (Oncovin) for leukemia tells the nurse that he is very constipated. What should the nurse explain about the probable cause of the constipation?

1. It is a side effect of the vinCRIStine
2. The spleen is compressing the bowel
3. It is a toxic effect from the predniSONE
4. The leukemic mass is obstructing the bowel

470. A nurse is admitting a 2-year-old toddler to the pediatric unit who has a tentative diagnosis of cystic fibrosis (CF). Pilocarpine (Pilocar) is used as part of the diagnostic process. The nurse anticipates that the pilocarpine will stimulate the:

1. Secretion of mucus
2. Activity of sweat glands
3. Excretion of pancreatic enzymes
4. Release of bile from the gallbladder

471. A nurse in the pediatric clinic evaluates that the pancreatic enzyme replacement being taken by a child with cystic fibrosis is inadequate. What clinical finding supports this conclusion?

1. Anorexia
2. Constipation
3. Sudden weight gain
4. Abdominal cramping

472. A 12-year-old child with cystic fibrosis is to receive four pancrelipase (Pancrease) capsules five times a day. The nurse explains that the medication should be taken with meals and snacks because this will:

1. Enhance oxygenation
2. Limit excretion of fats
3. Facilitate nutrient utilization
4. Prevent iron deficiency anemia

473. A nurse is reviewing discharge instructions with the parent of an infant with cystic fibrosis. What statement indicates that the parent knows how to administer the pancreatic enzyme replacement?

1. "The medication should be given with feedings."
2. "Crushed enteric-coated pills should be given in the formula."
3. "The medication should be given every six hours even during the night."
4. "Granules from the capsule should be eaten in applesauce every morning."

474. A 6-year-old child who had abdominal surgery complains of incisional pain. The nurse administers the prescribed acetaminophen (Tylenol). The mother asks the nurse why her child isn't receiving ibuprofen (Advil). The nurse considers the pharmacokinetics of ibuprofen before responding and replies, "It:

1. may prolong the bleeding time."
2. is contraindicated for young children."
3. can suppress the healing of the incision."
4. becomes ineffective when given for long periods."

475. A nurse is caring for a child who had a craniotomy. The parents ask what effect mannitol (Osmitrol) has. The nurse responds that this medication is given to:

1. Relieve cerebral pressure
2. Increase the bladder's filtration rate

3. Reduce glucose excretion in the urine
4. Decrease the peripheral retention of fluid

476. A 5-year-old child is receiving dactinomycin (Cosmegen) and DOXOrubicin (Adriamycin) therapy following a nephrectomy for Wilms tumor. What should the nursing care include?

1. Administering aspirin for pain
2. Offering citrus juices with meals
3. Ensuring meticulous oral hygiene
4. Eliminating spicy foods from the diet

477. A nurse is caring for a child receiving predniSONE (Meticorten). What outcome does the nurse expect with adrenocorticosteroid therapy?

1. Accelerated wound healing
2. Development of hyperkalemia
3. Increased antibody production
4. Suppressed inflammatory process

478. What is an important nursing intervention for a child who is receiving long-term steroid therapy?

1. Monitoring pulse for irregularities
2. Frequent testing of stools for occult blood
3. Repeated observations of urine for mucous threads
4. Persistent checking of oral mucous membranes for ulcers

479. A nurse is caring for a child with acute poststreptococcal glomerulonephritis (APSGN). What medications does the nurse expect the practitioner to prescribe? Select all that apply.

1. _____ Penicillin
2. _____ Morphine
3. _____ Furosemide
4. _____ Hydralazine
5. _____ Phenobarbital

480. What is a nurse's most important consideration when formulating a plan of care for a child receiving chemotherapy?

1. Preventing infection
2. Increasing caloric intake
3. Limiting nausea and vomiting
4. Monitoring hematoma formation

481. A child newly diagnosed with acute lymphocytic leukemia (ALL) is to receive induction therapy with predniSONE (Meticorten), vinCRIStine (Oncovin), and asparaginase (Elspar). After several days the child becomes constipated. What does the nurse suspect is the cause?

1. Diet, which lacks bulk
2 Inactivity, which results from illness
3. VinCRIStine, which decreases peristalsis
4. PredniSONE, which causes gastric irritability

482. A nurse is assessing the status of a child with leukemia who is receiving vinCRIStine (Oncovin). Which laboratory value indicates that fluid intake needs to be increased?

1. Increased blood uric acid level
2. Urine specific gravity of 1.026
3. Decreased creatinine clearance
4. Blood urea nitrogen of 17 mg/dL

483. A child is receiving chemotherapy. How can the nurse best manage a common side effect of chemotherapy?
   1. Restricting fluid intake
   2. Instituting contact precautions
   3. Keeping the hair closely cropped
   4. Providing meticulous oral hygiene

484. An 8-year-old girl who is receiving methotrexate (Trexall) and cranial radiation is very weak. Her mother asks the nurse if she may give her daughter vitamins. How should the nurse respond?
   1. "That is an excellent idea. I'll try to get an order for her."
   2. "Unfortunately vitamins won't make her feel any better now."
   3. "This won't be possible. Vitamins interfere with the action of methotrexate."
   4. "After we receive the laboratory reports your daughter will be getting vitamins."

485. When considering the side effects of dactinomycin (Cosmegen) and DOXOrubicin (Adriamycin) therapy, the nurse can suggest to the parents of a child receiving these medications that the child:
   1. Wear a baseball cap
   2. Eat three meals daily
   3. Avoid dairy products
   4. Dress in light clothing

486. An adolescent with acute lymphocytic leukemia (ALL) completes parenteral chemotherapy and the practitioner prescribes mercaptopurine (6-MP). The nurse teaches the adolescent about this medication. What statement indicates that the adolescent understands the information?
   1. "This will help prevent a relapse."
   2. "I guess I'll need an IV for this drug."
   3. "I guess this drug is a substitute for brain radiation."
   4. "This will stop the cancer from spreading to my stomach."

487. After receiving levothyroxine (Synthroid) for 3 months for congenital hypothyroidism an infant is brought to the pediatric clinic for a checkup. What does the mother tell the nurse about her baby that indicates that the drug is effective?
   1. Stools are soft
   2. Skin is cool to the touch
   3. Fine tremors have stopped
   4. Activity level has decreased

488. A 1-year-old infant is receiving zidovudine (AZT) for management of HIV infection. The nurse evaluates that the infant is exhibiting signs of life-threatening zidovudine toxicity. What clinical finding supports this conclusion?
   1. Weight loss
   2. Extreme lethargy
   3. Bruises over the body
   4. Increased urine output

489. The mother of a child with type 1 diabetes asks why it was recommended that her child use an insulin pump rather than insulin injections. What should the nurse tell the mother concerning the greatest advantage of the insulin pump?
   1. Independence is fostered
   2. Fear of daily injections is allayed
   3. Dietary restrictions are minimized
   4. Blood glucose monitoring can be eliminated

490. A nurse is teaching a child how to use an insulin pump. What is essential for the child to understand?
   1. The needle must be changed every day
   2. Glucose monitoring is necessary once daily
   3. The pump is an attempt to mimic the way a healthy pancreas works
   4. Subcutaneous pockets near the abdomen are used to implant the pump

491. An adolescent with type 1 diabetes is taking a combination of regular insulin (Novolin R) and an intermediate-acting insulin (Novolin N) before breakfast. The nurse teaches the adolescent about the time of day that is most appropriate for the self-administration of the second dose of intermediate-acting insulin. What time of day does the adolescent identify that indicates the teaching is understood?
   1. Before lunch
   2. Before dinnertime
   3. One hour after lunch
   4. One hour after dinner

492. The mother of a 7-month-old infant who becomes irritable when teething tells the nurse, "My aunt said to wipe my baby's gums with wine to ease the pain." What is the nurse's best response?
   1. "You can try the wine, but be sure it is diluted."
   2. "Your aunt means well, but this is not a good idea."
   3. "The wine will help kill the pain, but don't use it too often."
   4. "An over-the-counter topical gel can be used, but make sure it's for teething."

493. A chelating agent is prescribed for a child with lead poisoning. Because chelating agents may cause hypocalcemia, the nurse encourages the child to eat foods that are high in calcium. Which meals contain the most calcium? Select all that apply.
   1. _____ Beef broth, glazed ham, green beans, and cookies
   2. _____ Chicken noodle soup, liver and onions, and fruit salad
   3. _____ Vegetable soup, roast beef, baked potato, and apple juice
   4. _____ Cream of mushroom soup, macaroni and cheese, broccoli, and milk
   5. _____ Pea soup, roast chicken breast, mashed potatoes, creamed spinach, and orange juice

494. What is the priority nursing intervention for children with lead poisoning who are receiving chelation therapy?
   1. Scrupulous skin care
   2. Provision of a high-protein diet

3. Careful monitoring of intake and output
4. Drawing blood daily for liver function tests

495. Ampicillin (Omnipen) 160 mg IV every 4 hours is ordered. A vial containing 250 mg per 5 mL is available. How many milliliters should the nurse administer?

Answer:_____ mL

496. A nurse determines that the teaching about the side effects of azithromycin (Zithromax) is understood when an adolescent tells the nurse that the most common side effects of this medication is:
1. Tinnitus
2. Diarrhea
3. Dizziness
4. Headache

497. A teenager has a prescription for levofloxacin (Levaquin) to treat a sinus infection. The nurse explains when the medication should be taken. The nurse identifies that the teaching is effective when the teenager says, "I should take the medication:
1. at mealtime."
2. just before a meal."
3. 1 hour before a meal."
4. 30 minutes after a meal."

498. A nurse is planning to screen a child for impaired hearing because the child is receiving an antibiotic that affects hearing. Which medication does the nurse suspect may have caused impaired hearing?
1. Amoxicillin (Amoxil)
2. Ciprofloxacin (Cipro)
3. Clindamycin (Cleocin)
4. Gentamicin (Garamycin)

499. Penicillin G (Bicillin) and probenecid (Benemid) are prescribed for an adolescent who has syphilis. The adolescent asks the nurse why two medicines are needed. What should the nurse explain about the rationale for this combination therapy?
1. "Penicillin treats the syphilis and the probenecid relieves the inflammation in the urethra."
2. "Probenecid delays excretion of penicillin, thereby maintaining blood levels for longer periods."
3. "Probenecid decreases the potential for an allergic reaction developing to the penicillin, which treats the syphilis."
4. "Penicillin attacks the organism during one stage of cell multiplication and the probenecid attacks it at another stage."

500. A 7-year-old boy with the diagnosis of attention deficit hyperactivity disorder (ADHD) is receiving methylphenidate (Concerta). His mother asks about its action and side effects. What is the nurse's initial response?
1. "This medicine increases the appetite."
2. "This medicine must be continued until adulthood."
3. "It is a short-acting medicine that must be given with each meal."
4. "It is a stimulant that has a calming effect on children with your son's disorder."

Additional review questions can be found on the enclosed companion CD.

CHILD HEALTH NURSING
ANSWERS AND RATIONALES

NURSING PRACTICE

1. **2 In most states, the age of majority is 18 years; however, mothers younger than 18 years are considered emancipated minors and can sign consents for themselves and their children.**
   1 Consent is always needed; because the mother is present she can give consent.
   3 The court is not needed because the mother is an emancipated minor, which confers adult status.
   4 The grandmother does not have the legal right to give consent; the mother is present and can give consent.

2. **3 Regardless of age, parenthood confers the rights of an adult to the teenager.**
   1 It is not legal for the grandmother to sign the consent; the father is present and should sign the consent.
   2 The hospital administrator may sign the consent if neither parent is available.
   4 The mother has a legal right to give consent but she is not available.

3. **2 Most injuries to abused children are not life threatening; protection takes priority.**
   1 Treatment of major injuries is the responsibility of the medical staff, not the nurse.
   3 An accurate diagnosis of child abuse may take time and must be fully investigated.
   4 The nurse is often the first person to see the abused child and must establish protection before the practitioner arrives.

4. **1 Children's as well as adults' confidentiality is protected by privacy laws.**
   2 Although health classes may address medication as part of its curriculum, the information should be taught on a general, not personal, level.
   3 Children and their teachers should not be encouraged to divulge private information.
   4 Children and their teachers should not be encouraged to divulge private information.

5. **1 The nurse is responding to the child's feelings. If the child starts to discuss feelings, there may not be a need to inform him that he is too young to refuse treatment.**
   2 Abruptly telling the child that his parents have given their consent disregards the child's feelings.
   3 Although the child is too young to make a decision about treatment, this response is insensitive to the child's feelings.
   4 This response is demeaning and the nurse is misinforming the child by stating he is old enough to refuse treatment.

6. **2 Further assessment is needed. The mother should be supported and options should be explored on how to help address the family's problems.**
   1 The disabled adolescent requires attention. A 13-year-old disabled adolescent should not be given the responsibility of caring for an infant.
   3 This expense is not necessary. Household objects can serve as toys to provide stimulation.
   4 Telling the mother the consequences of emotional neglect is threatening and not constructive; it may cause guilt and anxiety.

7. **3 The child must first be assessed for injuries caused by exposure and treated if necessary.**
   1 Child Protective Services may be called after further assessment and the determination that neglect may be involved.
   2 A warm liquid may be offered after the child's physical status is assessed and it is determined that fluids may be ingested.
   4 Questions about the child's family dynamics may be asked after the status of the child is evaluated.

8. **4 The nurse must validate the presence of physical injury and potential abuse before initiating other interventions.**
   1 Child Protective Services should not be notified until signs of possible abuse are verified.
   2 The school principal should not be notified until signs of possible abuse are verified.
   3 The parents should not be notified until signs of possible abuse are verified.

9. **4 Gloves should be worn when the nurse is exposed to blood and body fluids; this provides a barrier and protects the nurse.**
   1 A mask is not required unless the vomiting is projectile.
   2 A gown is necessary only if there is a risk of contaminating the nurse's clothing.
   3 A face shield or goggles are not required unless the vomiting is projectile.

GROWTH AND DEVELOPMENT

10. **1 A coin can become dislodged and the infant may put it into the mouth, creating a safety issue.**
   2 A tightly placed diaper around the waist will not endanger the infant; cultural beliefs that do not place the infant at risk should not be discouraged.
   3 Binders do not endanger the infant; cultural beliefs that do not place the infant at risk should not be discouraged.
   4 Adhesive tape over the umbilicus will not endanger the infant; cultural beliefs that do not place the infant at risk should not be discouraged.

11. **2**   **The Babinski reflex remains evident throughout the first 12 months of life.**
   1   The Moro or startle reflex disappears by 4 months of age.
   3   The tonic-neck reflex disappears by 4 months of age.
   4   The palmar grasp reflex lessens at 3 months and is replaced by the voluntary pincer grasp by 8 months.

12.   **Answer: 1, 2, 5**
   1   **This is a typical behavior of an 8-month-old. Stranger anxiety (stranger fear) indicates healthy parent-child attachment.**
   2   **This is a typical behavior of an 8-month-old. The infant understands that a person is still there even when out of sight.**
   3   This skill requires coordination that develops around 12 months of age.
   4   This skill requires coordination that develops around 18 months of age.
   5   **This is a typical behavior of an 8-month-old. Walking while holding on to furniture with one hand occurs around 11 to 12 months of age.**

13. **3**   **This is an accurate, nonjudgmental conclusion based on the weight charts of the National Center for Health Statistics. An infant's weight gain at the end of the first year should be 3 times the birth weight.**
   1   This inference is a judgmental reaction; more evidence is needed to come to this conclusion.
   2   This is the expected weight for a 6-month-old infant weighing 7.5 pounds at birth.
   4   There are not enough data to arrive at this conclusion.

14.   **Answer: 2, 3**
   1   This is beyond the ability of a 1-year-old child; a 15-month-old child can jump with both feet but may fall.
   2   **A 1-year-old child has the physical ability to attempt to climb stairs; this skill will not be accomplished until 15 months of age.**
   3   **A 1-year-old child may still have some stranger anxiety but will begin to wander away from a parent and explore the environment.**
   4   A 1-year-old child's vocabulary is limited to one word at a time.
   5   This is beyond the ability of a 1-year-old child; a 15-month-old child can build a tower of several blocks.

15. **4**   **Most 15-month-old toddlers are not ready for toilet training. Voluntary sphincter control develops between 18 and 24 months of age.**
   1   This demonstrates autonomous behavior, typical of a 15-month-old toddler.
   2   This demonstrates separation anxiety, common in 15-month-old toddlers.
   3   This demonstrates autonomous behavior, typical of a 15-month-old toddler.

16. **1**   **Mouthing is a typical activity of young children from 18 to 36 months; thus toddlers are at the highest risk for lead ingestion and other problems related to poisoning.**
   2   There is no evidence of pica practice in the older population.
   3   Children from 3 to 6 years of age may mouth objects, but not as frequently as toddlers.
   4   Some pregnant women engage in pica practice, but it is most often associated with toddlers.

17. **2**   **Children who are spanked tend to use aggressive behavior; as they grow older they learn their own behavior through their parents' behavior.**
   1   Age is not significant in terms of the effectiveness of spanking.
   3   Spanking is a form of child abuse and should be avoided.
   4   Research studies dispute that spanking is an effective disciplinary technique.

18. **1**   **The palmar grasp reflex is expected at 6 weeks of age, begins to fade at 2 months, and disappears by 4 months.**
   2   The pincer grasp is a fine motor voluntary behavior that begins at about 8 months of age.
   3   Grasping is involuntary behavior; it is a reflex response that is not expected in older infants.
   4   The palmar grasp reflex is typical, not atypical, for a 6-week-old infant.

19. **2**   **The comfort measures of close physical contact, the gentle rhythm of rocking, and the reduction of stimuli in a quiet room are conducive to a young infant's rest and sleep.**
   1   Although offering a bottle will satisfy the sucking reflex, if the infant is not hungry, this is a temporary measure that will not ease the discomfort felt by the infant.
   3   Although the diaper should be inspected and changed if needed, emotional comfort should be offered before returning the infant to the crib.
   4   Wrapping the infant snugly in a blanket does not substitute for close physical contact when trying to soothe a crying infant.

20.   **Answer: 3, 4**
   1   A 3-month-old infant is too young for this toy.
   2   A 3-month-old infant is too young for this toy.
   3   **A 3-month-old infant is interested in self-recognition and playing with the baby in the mirror.**
   4   **A colorful mobile will provide visual stimulation for a 3-month-old infant.**
   5   A 3-month-old infant is too young for this toy.

21. **1**   **During the oral stage, infants tend to complete the exploration of an object by putting it into the mouth.**
   2   This is the momentary grasp reflex of neonates before the development of eye-hand-mouth coordination.

3 Infants 9 to 10 months old play this way as they learn that objects continue to exist even though they are not visible.

4 These are the random reflexive movements of 1- to 2-month-old infants whose voluntary control of distal extremities is not developed.

22. 1 **This behavior is within the expected range; a 7-month-old can sit without assistance by extending the legs to the side and leaning forward on the hands. By 8 months an infant should sit steadily unsupported.**

2 Sitting alone is not a predictor of when the infant will walk.

3 Most infants can sit without assistance by 7 to 8 months of age.

4 Most infants can sit without assistance by 7 to 8 months of age.

23. 4 **Eight-month-old infants have the ability to use their fingers and thumbs in opposition (pincer grasp); this enables them to pick up small objects and put them into their mouths and aspirate them.**

1 Although an infant's skin is fragile, this is not the major concern.

2 The danger is not that the items may be hidden but that they may be put into the mouth.

3 The floor is not an infectious health hazard if it is clean.

24. Answer: 1, 3, 5

1 **A textured book promotes tactile stimulation and touch discrimination.**

2 Modeling clay is an unsafe toy for an 8-month-old infant. This age infant continues to explore the environment by placing objects into the mouth.

3 **A stuffed animal promotes manipulative play.**

4 An 8-month-old infant is too young for a play telephone; it is an appropriate toy for a toddler to promote imitative play.

5 **A hanging mobile promotes visual stimulation.**

25. Answer: 1, 2, 4

1 **Nine-month-old infants enjoy the interaction associated with push-pull toys.**

2 **Sitting steadily occurs by 8 months of age.**

3 Self-feeding is accomplished by 2-year-old children, not infants.

4 **Nine-month-old infants respond to simple commands such as "no." Also they try to please their parents.**

5 A 2- to 3-word vocabulary is expected of 12-month-old children.

26. 3 **One way toddlers explore their environment is by putting objects into their mouths.**

1 An expected decline in appetite occurs during this period; it is called physiologic anorexia.

2 The sense of taste is developed at birth.

4 Toddlers assert themselves but are not rebellious of adult authority; adolescents rebel against adult authority.

27. 3 **Brief messages, with only essential words included (telegraphic speech), a vocabulary of 20 words, and frequent use of the word "me" are the expected assessments of a child 18 months to 2 years of age.**

1 A child with a developmental delay has a smaller vocabulary than 20 words and does not use phrases.

2 A child advanced for this age will have a vocabulary of more than 20 words and will use 3- or 4-word sentences rather than telegraphic speech.

4 This speech pattern is age appropriate, not pathological.

28. 4 **Toddlers have not yet developed a concept of time. The child should be warned just before giving the injection, then acceptance is shown when the child cries and is comforted.**

1 Children are sensitive to a dishonest approach; this results in their losing trust in the caregiver.

2 Toddlers' attention span is too short and their cognitive ability is too limited to watch a demonstration and listen to an explanation.

3 Toddlers are too young to participate in therapeutic play; this approach is more appropriate for the preschooler.

29. 4 **Growth slows during the toddler years and these children generally do not eat as much as during infancy; this is called physiologic anorexia, which is typical of this age group.**

1 Toddlers may try to manipulate as they assert their autonomy, but usually not through eating behaviors unless the parents express anxiety and concern over their food intake.

2 Although toddlers have difficulty withstanding frustration and are prone to temper tantrums, these eating behaviors are within the norm for toddlers.

3 Eating disorders usually do not occur in children this young; these behaviors are typical of healthy toddlers.

30. 1 **As the child gets older, growth slows. Toddlers develop physiologic anorexia because their appetite decreases along with their growth rate.**

2 Although the toddler may be too busy to eat, this is not why the growth rate slows.

3 This growth pattern can be interpreted now.

4 Although this may occur, it is not common among toddlers.

31. 2 **Preschool children use imitation of adult situations to help learn social skills; they enjoy make-believe play.**

1 Abstract thinking does not develop until adolescence.

3 Same-gender play is common among preschoolers.

4 Magical thinking is expected in toddlers, preschoolers, and early school-age children.

32. 4 **Giving the child a gift will minimize feelings of being ignored. The child can role-play with the new doll, which is an age-appropriate activity.**

1 Ignoring the child's comments will reinforce insecurity and may promote acting-out behavior.
2 The child is too young to be left alone with an infant.
3 This may increase the child's feelings of jealousy if told that the mother must stay with the baby rather than with her.

33. 1 **Thumb sucking reaches its peak from 18 to 20 months and then subsides to times when comfort is most needed, such as at bedtime and when ill. Most children give it up by age 4. The nurse should reassure the mother by explaining that it is not unusual to thumb suck at age 3.**
2 It is best not to draw attention to the habit by trying to force the child to stop.
3 It is doubtful that other 3-year-olds will notice the thumb sucking.
4 Thumb sucking at age 3 in a healthy, emotionally stable child does not require psychotherapy.

34. 4 **This response may reduce the toddler's level of stress without loss of self-esteem. A light allows the toddler to see familiar objects in the room and reduces fears associated with a dark environment. Toddlers see their parents as capable of all things and will be accepting of this house rule.**
1 Telling the child that monsters do not exist denies the toddler's concerns and is beyond the concrete thinking of a toddler.
2 Sleeping with the parents may interfere with their ability to get a restful night's sleep. With additional emotional support the child should be encouraged to remain in his or her own bed.
3 A toddler thinks in concrete terms and this may not relieve the fear of monsters; it also denies the toddler's concerns.

35. 2 **Four-year-old children can put on a shirt and can close it if the buttons are large.**
1 Four-year-old children will be able to comb, but not part, their hair.
3 Four-year-old children can handle a fork and spoon but cannot hold the meat with the fork while cutting it with the knife; children usually are 7 years old before this task is managed.
4 Four-year-old children old can put on shoes, but usually are unable to tie them until age 5.

36. Answer: 2, 5
1 The use of appropriate grammar does not develop until about 9 to 12 years of age.
2 **Because of developing cognitive abilities, 4-year-old children can form 6- to 8-word sentences.**
3 By 5 to 6 years of age, children ask the definitions of new words; 4-year-old children have not yet achieved this level of development.
4 By 4 to 5 years of age children's speech is intelligible although sounds such as CH, TH, SH, Z, R, and L frequently are imperfect.

5 **Because of expanded experiences and developing cognitive ability, the 4-year-old child should have a vocabulary of approximately 150 to 200 words.**

37. 3 **Imaginary friends are typical of children of this age; children who have few social contacts with peers are more likely to be involved with imaginary friends.**
1 There is no evidence that the parents are having difficulty with childrearing.
2 Disciplining the child is inappropriate. The child was protecting an imaginary friend, and having imaginary friends is typical of a 4-year-old child.
4 Referral to a specialist is unnecessary; this is typical behavior for a 4-year-old child.

38. 3 **Stuttering occurs because the child's advancing mental ability and level of comprehension exceed the vocabulary acquisitions in the preschool years.**
1 Stuttering is common in the preschool years; it is not a problem at this age.
2 Stuttering is common in the preschool years; it is not a problem at this age.
4 Stuttering is common in the preschool years; it is not a problem at this age.

39. 3 **Current practice encourages parents to stay with the child as long as possible; this helps reduce stress related to a frightening experience.**
1 Toys, especially a favorite one, should accompany the child until sedation is induced.
2 The child is too young to climb onto a gurney. Some hospitals allow the child to walk to the operating suite, usually accompanied by the parents.
4 Current theory is consistent with parents remaining with their child during the administration of a sedative, which usually takes place at or near the operating room. Not all institutions allow parents to stay with the child during the induction of anesthesia. Based on parents' positive feedback the practice is becoming more common.

40. 2 **Preschoolers are developing a sense of their body integrity and their sexuality resulting in fears of mutilation and loss of body parts.**
1 Fear of separation from significant others is most prominent in late infancy and during the toddler years.
3 Fear of strangers is most prominent in late infancy and during the toddler years.
4 Preschoolers have not yet reached the age when they become concerned with their dependency needs or their need for independence.

41. 4 **Cooperative play is typical of 5-year-olds as they learn to share and take turns without becoming frustrated.**
1 Team play is typical of older, school-age children who play games with other children and learn to abide by the rules.

2 Parallel play is typical of the toddler age group; they have not yet learned to interact with other toddlers in a social situation.

3 Initiative play does not typify any age group; it is not a recognized term of social play.

42. **Answer: 1, 3**

1 **Imitating adults by playing adult roles in society is at its peak in children 5 years of age; activities strongly identify with same-sex parent.**

2 Older children in the middle childhood years need conformity and rituals whether they play games or amass collections. Rules to games are fixed, unvarying, and rigid. Knowing the rules means belonging.

3 **A 5-year-old is able to negotiate and use make-believe to play. These children are able to follow some rules but may cheat to win.**

4 The use of a pacifier for oral satisfaction is typical of infants.

5 Parallel play occurs in children ages 2 to 3 years.

43. 3 **This action provides adult supervision for all the children.**

1 This is unsafe; 7-year-olds should not be without supervision.

2 This puts too much responsibility on children who are too young and who may get lost or hurt.

4 This puts too much responsibility on children who are too young and who may get lost or hurt.

44. 4 **Schoolwork provides the child with a familiar routine; it encompasses the age-appropriate developmental tasks of industry vs inferiority.**

1 Drawing pictures is an appropriate activity for the preschooler.

2 Although social interaction and mental stimulation are important at this age, continuing with schooling is the priority.

3 Television watching is satisfactory but should not replace active participation.

45. 3 **Several meetings with an adolescent provide an opportunity to develop trust and establish a relationship.**

1 Relating on a peer level is unrealistic because the nurse is not an adolescent's peer.

2 Using teenage language is not necessary and may even impede the establishment of a relationship.

4 It is not necessary to use concrete terms because the adolescent is capable of abstract thought.

46. 4 **During infancy is the preferred age, before the development of body image and fear of castration.**

1 The phallus is not developed enough for surgery to be done shortly after birth.

2 Children 4 to 5 years of age are in the stage of development that is accompanied by fear of mutilation.

3 Having corrective surgery just beyond the onset of puberty is too late. Corrective surgery should be done before the child has to use bathrooms with other boys. The lack of a normal stream of urine

can cause psychological and self-esteem issues for a child this age.

47. 3 **The infant has not yet recognized boundaries between self and mother and is not particular about who meets and resolves needs.**

1 A social smile does not indicate recognition of a specific person but only a human face.

2 The infant does not yet differentiate familiar faces from those of strangers.

4 Because the concept of self-boundaries has not yet developed, the infant does not understand or fear separation from the mother.

48. 3 **A 7-month-old infant is used to having the perineal area exposed and cared for and is not in a developmental stage in which fears related to sexuality are present.**

1 A clean-catch specimen at this age may be contaminated. The order is for a catheterized specimen.

2 Although the mother does have the right to refuse, her concern is not realistic for an infant at this age. The mother needs to be educated.

4 The priority is to assure the mother that a catheterization will not result in an emotional problem for her infant.

49. 2 **The average infant doubles birth weight at 6 months.**

1 Twelve pounds is too low; it may confirm a diagnosis of failure to thrive.

3 Eighteen pounds is too high.

4 Twenty-two pounds is too high; the average infant triples birth weight at 1 year of age.

50. 3 **Typically, infants respond to social play by 10 months of age.**

1 A six word vocabulary is typical of a 15-month-old.

2 Standing without support is typical of a 15-month-old.

4 Building a 2 cube tower is typical of a 15-month-old.

51. 2 **The eustachian tube in young children is shorter and wider, allowing a reflux of nasopharyngeal secretions.**

1 Immunological differences are not a factor in the development of otitis media.

3 There is no difference in the functioning of the eustachian tube among age groups.

4 The size of the middle ear does not play a role in the occurrence of otitis media in young children.

52. 4 **The canal curves upward in children younger than 3 years of age; pulling the pinna down straightens the canal so that medication will reach the eardrum.**

1 The ear canal is not cleansed before instilling ear drops; this can exacerbate the infection.

2 Applying ear wicks is contraindicated because it increases pressure within the ear.

3 This is unnecessary; pressing on the tragus several times will help disburse the drops.

53. 3 **Attributing lifelike qualities to inanimate objects (animism) is associated with preconceptual thought.**
    1 Concrete operational thought is achieved in school-age children.
    2 Concept of reversibility is a phase of concrete operations achieved by school-age children.
    4 Sensorimotor development is related to infants.

54. 3 **Changes in the daily routines in the home and grief expressed by family members lead to anxiety in toddlers.**
    1 The toddler does not have a reality-based concept of death.
    2 Although this may be a bid for more attention, the primary motivation for the behavior is a response to the family's grief.
    4 This is not typical developmental behavior; it is a response to the familial environment.

55. 1 **Hospitalization is traumatic to the preschooler because of separation from significant family members. When parents are unable to visit the nurse should make arrangements with the parents for daily contact.**
    2 Preschoolers are not interested in food; children with nephrotic syndrome often have decreased appetites.
    3 Preschoolers are not concerned about attitudes of peers; it is too early in their social development to have this concern.
    4 Massive edema results in easy fatigability and a lack of interest in play.

56. 1 **Although the local anesthetic will help minimize the discomfort, the needle insertion may still hurt. This is an honest, simple answer that is appropriate for a 3-year-old child.**
    2 This is a judgmental response that is inappropriate for a 3-year-old child; children sometimes need to cry to express their feelings.
    3 Although the child should hold still, there is no guarantee that it will hurt less. This is false reassurance.
    4 There is no guarantee of success despite the nurse's self-proclaimed expertise. This is a form of false reassurance.

57. 3 **Preschoolers can tolerate brief periods of separation from their parents; however, emotions associated with separation and perhaps anger at being left are difficult to hide when the parents arrive or leave.**
    1 Preschoolers usually are quite docile and cooperative because they are afraid of being totally abandoned.
    2 The child will demonstrate despair long before the week is over.
    4 The presence of other children's parents in the playroom does not discourage them from playing with their peers.

58. 3 **The child with abdominal pain may assume the side-lying position with the knees flexed to the abdomen and/or may self-splint when moving.**
    1 A 4-year-old may be unable to identify the exact location of the pain; in addition, the pain may be generalized rather than localized.
    2 Auscultation may be included in the physical assessment, but it is not specific to the assessment of pain.
    4 Questioning the parents may be included when taking the health history, but it is not specific to the current assessment of pain.

59. 3 **Preschool children fear procedures that intrude on their body integrity.**
    1 Separation anxiety is more common in toddlers.
    2 Preschool children are too young to understand the concept of altered family roles; this is a fear that adults experience.
    4 Enforced dependency is a fear that school-age and adolescent children experience.

60. 4 **Preschool children engage in imitative, imaginative, and dramatic play, often using play to simulate household activities.**
    1 Although some preschoolers try to read, most of them are not ready until they are 6 years old.
    2 Preschoolers engage in associative play with other children; they are not ready to learn the rules of a game.
    3 Although family visits should be encouraged, the family's presence is not needed to meet preschoolers' developmental needs because they are now able to tolerate separation better than when they were toddlers.

61. 3 **Playing with age-appropriate puzzles is intellectually stimulating and can be done with the arm that is not immobilized.**
    1 Watching television is a passive activity and not especially stimulating.
    2 The child needs both hands for cutting paper.
    4 Looking at comic books is a passive activity and not especially stimulating.

62. 1 **Finger painting is appropriate for this age child; it provides the child an opportunity for free expression and its free-form nature can give the child a sense of mobility.**
    2 Coloring within lines of pictures in a coloring book requires more skill than most 4-year-olds possess; also this does not allow freedom of expression or movement.
    3 Checkers is a game with too many rules for a 4-year-old to comprehend.
    4 Playing dominos requires the ability to count and conserve numbers, which most 4-year-olds do not possess.

63. 4 **A coloring book with crayons is appropriate for the child's age and suited to the child's limited mobility.**

1   The child is too young for a game of checkers; children of 7 years or older are able to play checkers.
2   Building blocks require a large area and are difficult to play with while on bed rest.
3   The child will not have enough mobility to engage in a game of jacks and is too young for this activity.

64.   **Answer: 2, 5**
1   Playing with a hula hoop requires energy that a child in the acute phase of nephritic syndrome does not have.
2   **Age-appropriate video games do not require excessive energy to play and will help a 6-year-old child avoid boredom.**
3   Large puzzles are more appropriate for toddlers who are developing fine motor skills.
4   A stuffed animal is more appropriate for an infant or toddler. It is a passive toy that will not be stimulating for a 6-year-old child.
5   **Children's books are appropriate for 6-year-old children because at this age they are beginning to read. Also the parents can read to the child. This activity does not require energy.**

65.   1   **Allowing the child to talk about what is frightening provides an opportunity to ventilate feelings and fears.**
2   It is not therapeutic to belittle the child's fears.
3   It is not therapeutic to belittle the child's fears.
4   It is not therapeutic to belittle the child's fears.

66.   1   **School-age children have reached the cognitive level of concrete operations that enables them to understand relationships between things and ideas. They can conceptualize what head lice look like, and if they see them they will recognize them by the description.**
2   Teaching them how to prevent getting head lice should be presented after the students understand the basic information about head lice.
3   Telling them how easily head lice spreads from person to person should be presented after the students understand the basic information about head lice.
4   Telling them how easily head lice spreads from person to person should be presented after the students understand the basic information about head lice.

67.   4   **According to Piaget, an 8-year-old child's level of development is in the stage of concrete operations; the child will benefit from simple concrete examples.**
1   The preschooler and younger child, not the school-age child, require repetition.
2   Therapeutic needle play is more appropriate if and when the child is to receive an injection.
3   The child who is in the period of concrete operations cannot think in the abstract; the ability to do this occurs during adolescence.

68.   1   **Bicyclists are required to follow the rules of the road; they must ride with traffic, obey traffic signs and lights, and signal when turning.**

2   Walking the bicycle at intersections helps prevent accidents.
3   Riding close to the curb helps prevent accidents.
4   Staying in single file helps prevent accidents.

69.   3   **Adolescents are very aware of their changing bodies and become especially concerned with any alteration.**
1   Discussing complications may cause unnecessary concern about the daughter's physical condition.
2   Discussing hypochondriasis may reinforce the mother's concern.
4   This is not a transference situation. The adolescent's behavior is typical; there is no reason to cause guilt in the mother.

70.   2   **Striving to attain identity and independence are tasks of the adolescent and rebellion against established norms may be exhibited.**
1   Nonadherence to a regimen is not a bid for attention; rather it is an attempt to establish an identity, which is a developmental task of adolescence.
3   Although the adolescent may be using denial, denial is not developmentally related to adolescence.
4   Noncompliance is not a sign of regression; it is an attempt to attain identity by rebellion against established norms.

71.   4   **The 15-year-old is preoccupied with appearance. The side effects of the antineoplastics and prednisone may result in the adolescent feeling different, which affects body image.**
1   Although missing school may be a concern, it is not the primary concern.
2   Although limiting social activities is a concern, it is not the primary concern. Socialization can be facilitated.
3   A 15-year-old enjoys and strives for independence and does not enjoy the sick role.

72.   3   **The adolescent is concerned with body image and fears change or mutilation of body parts. The occlusions in the microvasculature associated with sickle cell anemia can cause bone deformities.**
1   Restriction of movement is not a major problem because when the pain is relieved and the crisis is over activity is resumed.
2   Teenagers can tolerate extended periods of separation from the family.
4   Although learning interruptions may be a concern for a teenager, altered body image is a more feared threat.

EMOTIONAL NEEDS RELATED TO HEALTH PROBLEMS

73.   4   **This action provides a familiar, consistent caregiver with whom the child can relate.**
1   Although this may provide some comfort, the child needs to receive love and attention from an adult.

2 This may increase the parents' guilt and anxiety; data given indicate that the parents have been unable, not unwilling, to visit the child.

3 Although this may provide some comfort, the child needs to receive love and attention from an adult.

74. 4 **The 9-year-old child needs an opportunity to express emotions in private; talking about feelings is therapeutic.**

1 This is not of great concern to the child at this moment.

2 This action gives the child the impression that crying is wrong.

3 This does not meet the child's need for expressing emotions.

75. 2 **Toddlers who are separated from their parents for a prolonged period develop separation anxiety; there are three phases: protest, despair, and detachment. This child is exhibiting an early stage of detachment.**

1 Although the child appears to have adjusted to the environment and forms superficial relationships with the new caregivers, in reality the child is trying to avoid the emotional pain caused by the parents' absence.

3 Separation anxiety is not a sign of maturity.

4 Separation anxiety is not a sign of a short memory.

76. 2 **Accepting the parents' need to distance themselves indicates empathy for this adaptive response to grief.**

1 Asking the parents why they don't visit more often is confrontational and may precipitate or increase feelings of guilt.

3 Teaching the parents how to relate with their child may precipitate or increase feelings of guilt.

4 Telling the parents how to relate with their child may precipitate or increase feelings of guilt.

77. 3 **The parents need assistance in exploring their feelings and their family relationships with a professional.**

1 Bringing gifts is an attempt to relieve guilt feelings; the father may still feel responsible for the child's illness.

2 The promise of a special trip may help the parents relieve their guilt feelings.

4 The mother's assumption of the martyr role may help relieve the anxiety caused by feelings of guilt.

78. 2 **The parents need to express and work through their feelings before they can move forward with other coping strategies.**

1 Explanations of the diagnosis do not focus on the needs of the parents at this time.

3 Participation in a support group eventually may be suggested; however, this is not the priority at this time.

4 This is false reassurance; there is no assurance that the surgery will be successful.

79. 3 **This response is accepting of the individual and encourages communication.**

1 There are no data to indicate that the injuries were caused by abuse.

2 It is the nurse's responsibility and should not be transferred immediately to the client's family.

4 This response interprets the client's statement as guilt, which may or may not be the true interpretation.

80. 4 **Suggesting to enlist a surrogate accepts the mother's concern and offers an option.**

1 This direct question may be confrontational and may precipitate a defensive response.

2 Although the mother's presence with the baby is important, the other child and the mother's concerns are ignored by this response.

3 Having the mother divide her time between her two children is an unrealistic option and may increase guilt feelings regarding her care of both children.

81. Answer: 1, 2, 4

1 **The child cringes when approached because past experiences with adults have inflicted pain rather than comfort.**

2 **Evidence of past injuries may exist but the parents do not discuss them because this would be an admission of child abuse.**

3 Abusive parents are unable to provide any emotional support.

4 **Abused children are always on the alert for potential future abuse. Lying motionless prevents bringing attention to them; also, in the past resisting abuse often precipitated more abuse.**

5 Because abusing parents try to hide the fact of abuse, explanations about injuries usually are fabricated, inconsistent, and vague.

82. 1 **The child has not stated why the teasing occurred; asking for clarification in a nonthreatening manner is the first step of the assessment process.**

2 This may be the next question after the situation is clarified.

3 This question is not relevant to the teasing incident at this time.

4 This response minimizes the child's experience. Assuring the child that being teased is not unique may be helpful later.

83. 4 **This response points out reality and does not promote false hope. The nurse should emphasize that everything possible is being done because the outcome cannot be predicted.**

1 The outcome is still in doubt; encouraging the mother's positive interpretation of the child's reflexive behavior raises false hope.

2 The outcome is still in doubt; encouraging the mother's positive interpretation of the child's reflexive behavior raises false hope.

3   The outcome is still in doubt; encouraging the mother's positive interpretation of the child's reflexive behavior raises false hope. The mother's statement did not ask for the nurse's religious viewpoint.

84. 2   **Abused children distrust anyone who touches them because it may be a precursor to abuse.**
1   Abused children are fearful of others and do not smile when approached.
3   Abused children usually do not cry because they have learned not to expect comforting from others.
4   Abused children are acutely aware of anyone at the bedside; they are alert to the possibility of an attack.

85. 2   **People living in poverty feel powerless because they do not have the buying power or social status to influence change.**
1   Their anger is covert and not direct; in addition, the anger rarely resolves their situation, resulting in feelings of powerlessness and hopelessness.
3   They are less likely to postpone gratification because they focus on the present, not the future.
4   Health recommendations may be misunderstood, confusing, or perceived as of little value, and are frequently ignored.

86. 4   **Transferring her anger to an inanimate object indicates the potential for increased impulse control; this is important for the prevention of further abuse.**
1   This is unrealistic because all parents become angry with their children at some time or another.
2   Placing the blame on the child rather than on the mother's behavior indicates lack of progress toward controlling anger.
3   Placing the blame on the spouse rather than the self indicates lack of progress toward controlling anger.

87. 3   **These withdrawn behaviors are associated with separation anxiety; parental contact should be encouraged.**
1   Separation anxiety can be minimized by increasing contact with parents, not by distraction with toys.
2   Toddlers are too young for peer interaction.
4   Assigning a variety of caregivers increases feelings of anxiety; one nurse should care for the child as much as possible to promote consistency, continuity, and the development of trust.

88. 4   **The parents are the most significant people in the young child's life; their involvement in comforting the child is the most supportive intervention for the toddler.**
1   Distraction does not provide an outlet for the toddler's feelings.
2   An explanation of treatment is required and expected, but the priority is for the parents to comfort their child.
3   This type of choice is not a viable option. The medication should be administered as prescribed.

89. 4   **Adherence to dietary restrictions can prevent future complications and celiac crisis.**
1   Celiac crisis usually develops as a result of nonadherence to the diet, so adherence to the diet is a primary objective.
2   Respiratory involvement is not a primary problem with celiac disease.
3   Regardless of adherence to the diet, there may be an interference with the expected growth rate.

90. 1   **This is an honest statement that tells the toddler what to expect and the nurse's expectation that the toddler should stay still during the procedure.**
2   Emphasizing the child's fears will exacerbate the child's fears.
3   Having two nurses present is too threatening for the child.
4   Asking the child to be brave puts unrealistic expectations on the child.

91. 1   **The child is too young to learn colostomy care. It is important that the parents learn this and give feedback demonstrations before the child is discharged.**
2   Increased fluid intake is needed to compensate for fecal fluid loss.
3   The diet should not be restricted at the time of discharge. Both parents and child will learn which foods are poorly tolerated and they will adjust the diet accordingly.
4   Contact games may be restricted, but other physical activities should be encouraged.

92. 4   **Stating that the recovery is progressing is a realistic and optimistic appraisal of the child's status.**
1   Concluding that the illness has resolved is premature.
2   Concluding that the child is no longer critically ill is premature.
3   Concluding that the child has escaped complications is premature.

93. 1   **This is a direct question that should elicit the desired information.**
2   This question can be answered with a yes or no and does not elicit what the child knows or feels about the situation.
3   This question can be answered with a yes or no and does not elicit what the child knows or feels about the situation.
4   This question can be answered with a yes or no and does not elicit what the child knows or feels about the situation.

94. 2   **Wearing a hat until her hair regrows meets the child's present need while assuring her that her hair loss is temporary.**
1   Removing the doll's hair demeans the child's feelings.
3   This response denies the child's feelings.
4   This response demeans the child's feelings; it implies that the hair loss is unsightly.

95. 2 **The child learned to think and solve problems in a different culture and language and may feel helpless in the new classroom.**
    1 There are no data to substantiate that social immaturity is the precipitating factor for the child's behavior.
    3 There are no data to substantiate that discrimination is the precipitating factor for the child's behavior.
    4 There are no data to substantiate that disinterest in school activities is the precipitating factor for the child's behavior.

96. 2 **This response identifies the concern and presents an appropriate protective intervention. Checking for and prompt removal of ticks decreases the chances of the spread of Lyme disease to humans.**
    1 This is an inappropriate response because it focuses on the wrong fear.
    3 This response centers on camping, not on the fear of ticks. Also, it belittles the child's fears.
    4 This response belittles the child's feelings.

97. 4 **This allows the child to volunteer information first and thus feel in control; the nurse can ask validating questions later.**
    1 This is a flippant, insensitive statement.
    2 This focuses the assessment on vomiting, thus predisposing the child to think of vomiting during this treatment.
    3 This is an unfeeling question because it reminds the child and mother that there are more sessions in the future.

98. 1 **The child is old enough to respond when asked a direct question.**
    2 The parents may be too emotionally involved to effectively help their child communicate feelings.
    3 Younger children benefit from this projective technique.
    4 Younger children benefit from this projective technique.

99. 1 **Negotiation of goals is essential to successful learning; mutual goal-setting provides a focus for learning.**
    2 A rapport should have developed before teaching the adolescent about diabetes.
    3 This is premature. If the client does not identify a specific need or set a goal, motivation may be minimal.
    4 This is premature. If the client does not identify a specific need or set a goal, motivation may be minimal.

100. 2 **This is a truthful answer that offers some hope without false reassurance.**
    1 The adolescent is not concerned about escaping death; this statement will cut off communication.
    3 Telling the adolescent that it is too early to anticipate scarring is misinformation.
    4 Ignoring the adolescent's concerns is not therapeutic and cuts off communication.

BLOOD AND IMMUNITY

101. 4 **The passive antibodies to DTaP received from the mother are diminished by 8 weeks of age and no longer interfere with the development of active immunity after this age.**
    1 Vaccines contain attenuated viruses; they may cause irritability and fever, but they do not cause the related disease.
    2 Infants are exposed to infectious diseases; passive immunity from the mother offers some protection.
    3 The spleen does not produce antibodies.

102. 4 **A temperature of 105° F or higher after a DTaP immunization is a contraindication for further DTaP immunizations.**
    1 An allergy to eggs is not a contraindication for the administration of DTaP because eggs are not used in the production of DTaP.
    2 Lactose intolerance is not a contraindication for the administration of DTaP.
    3 Infectious dermatitis is not a contraindication for the administration of DTaP.

103. 1 **Mild reactions are redness and induration at the injection site, slight fever, and irritability.**
    2 Serious reactions are not common.
    3 Induration at the injection site may occur, but not ulceration.
    4 Permanent brain damage is not a likely occurrence after an immunization.

104. 1 **A warm compress will promote circulation, reduce swelling, and relax muscles, thus lessening the inflammation.**
    2 Witch hazel will not lessen inflammation or promote muscle relaxation.
    3 Fever is not an expected response; therefore, the cooling effect of a sponge bath is not necessary.
    4 Cool applications will not provide relief because they reduce circulation to the area.

105. 4 **Between 12 and 15 months is the optimum age because maternal antibodies to measles are no longer present to block the formation of the child's own antibodies.**
    1 The measles vaccine is not given between 2 and 5 months because of the questionable efficacy of the vaccination due to the presence of maternal antibodies.
    2 The measles vaccine is not given between 6 and 8 months because of the questionable efficacy of the vaccination due to the presence of maternal antibodies.
    3 The measles vaccine is not given between 9 and 11 months because of the questionable efficacy of the vaccination due to the presence of maternal antibodies.

106. 3 **The MMR vaccine contains live attenuated viruses and should not be administered when receiving chemotherapy because of the child's compromised immune system.**

1 There are no contraindications for administering Hib vaccine to children who are immunosuppressed.

2 There are no contraindications for administering HepB vaccine to children who are immunosuppressed.

4 There are no contraindications for administering DTaP vaccine to children who are immunosuppressed.

107. 2 **Because chemotherapy can cause nausea, vomiting, and anorexia, the child should be offered any food that is requested. Even if the nutritional quality is minimal, the child will be receiving needed calories.**

1 Fried foods can be eaten because generally they do not cause nausea and vomiting.

3 Fried foods can be eaten because generally they do not irritate the mouth.

4 Food, if prepared adequately, should not be contaminated and cause a problem for a child receiving chemotherapy.

108. 3 **A high white blood cell count causes spinal fluid to appear cloudy and possibly milky white; it is a sign of infection.**

1 Healthy spinal fluid is clear.

2 Elevated glucose levels do not affect the color of the spinal fluid.

4 Red blood cells make the spinal fluid appear sanguineous, not cloudy.

109. 1 **Potatoes and whole milk are not adequate sources of iron; at 8 months of age fetal iron stores are depleted and exogenous iron sources are needed.**

2 Milk contains vitamins A, C, and D.

3 Potatoes are a rich source of potassium.

4 There are amino acids in milk because it is an animal protein.

110. Answer: 1, 2, 3

1 **Conservation of energy is important because anemic children usually are fatigued. There is an inadequate amount of RBCs and hemoglobin to carry oxygen to body cells.**

2 **Anemic children are prone to infection.**

3 **Parents should know which foods are high in iron. Iron promotes the formation of RBCs.**

4 The time and amount of feedings are not as important as the quality of foods that are offered.

5 Usually anemia results from drinking unfortified milk and little else; there should be an increase in the variety and quality of the foods offered.

111. 4 **Gingerbread cookies made with molasses are an excellent source of iron. They can be eaten as a finger food, which toddlers prefer.**

1 Pumpkin pie provides some protein and iron but has a spicy taste that generally is not a favorite of toddlers.

2 Although grapes contain iron, a cup is an excessive amount for an 18-month-old child to ingest.

3 Apples, although nutritious, are low in protein and iron.

112. 2 **Children with leukemia are immunosuppressed; the chickenpox virus can cause death in the individual with a suppressed immune system. The child cannot go home while the sibling has chickenpox.**

1 The vaccine against chickenpox is a live virus and should not be given to an immunosuppressed child.

3 PredniSONE (Meticorten) does not confer immunity to the chickenpox virus.

4 It is unsafe for the child to go home. Chickenpox can be spread by airborne droplets in the prodromal stage and by fomites that have come into contact with oozing vesicles.

113. 2 **Tonsillectomy may result in hemorrhage because of the vascularity of the oropharynx; adequate clotting function must be present.**

1 The potassium level is not significant for this type of surgery if the child is otherwise healthy.

3 The RBC count is not significant for this type of surgery if the child is otherwise healthy.

4 The erythrocyte sedimentation rate (ESR) is not significant for this type of surgery if the child is otherwise healthy.

114. 2 **Increased swallowing occurs with bleeding in the oropharynx.**

1 Signs of respiratory distress, not increased swallowing, are associated with pharyngeal edema.

3 Tenacious secretions may cause gagging, not increased swallowing.

4 There is decreased, not increased, saliva production after a tonsillectomy.

115. Answer: 3, 5

1 Edema is not expected with ALL.

2 Alopecia is not related to the disease process; it occurs as a result of chemotherapy.

3 **Anorexia occurs as a result of catabolism.**

4 The red blood cells are decreased because of bone marrow depression; the child will be lethargic and sleep excessively.

5 **The platelets are decreased because of bone marrow depression resulting in bleeding tendencies; petechiae and ecchymoses result.**

116. Answer: 1, 3, 5

1 **Anorexia is a presenting symptom of ALL and may be the result of enlarged lymph nodes, areas of inflammation in the intestinal tract, and catabolism.**

2 Sores in the mouth are not a presenting sign of ALL but often result from chemotherapy.

3 Pallor is a presenting sign of ALL; the number of red blood cells are decreased (anemia) because of bone marrow depression.

4 Because of bone marrow depression there is a reduced number of red blood cells and therefore less oxygen being carried to body cells. The child will be lethargic and sleep excessively.

5 Decreased platelet production results in bleeding tendencies; petechiae often are a presenting sign of ALL.

117. 2 Anesthesia is used for procedures such as bone marrow aspiration in children.

1 This is a painful procedure. The child will not have pain during the procedure because anesthesia will be used. The site may be sore afterward.

3 The child should be placed prone with a towel roll under the hips for aspiration of marrow from the posterior iliac crest.

4 The child can handle some of the equipment as part of the explanation of the procedure; however, the child will be sedated during the procedure.

118. 3 A vaso-occlusive crisis (painful episode) often precipitates a pooling of blood in the liver and in the spleen, resulting in enlargement of the spleen (splenomegaly).

1 Splenomegaly is not common during infancy.

2 An enlarged spleen is easily palpable in a child.

4 Splenomegaly is not common during late childhood; the spleen of a child with sickle cell anemia usually autoinfarcts by late childhood.

119. Answer: 2, 3, 4, 1

The child is experiencing an allergic reaction. First, the antibiotic should be stopped to prevent anaphylactic shock. Maintaining respiratory functioning is a priority; therefore, it should be assessed immediately and monitored routinely. The continuation of hydration is important to dilute the effect of the allergen and to keep the vein open if emergency medication is required. After the immediate needs of the child are met, the practitioner should be notified.

120. 2 Thalassemia is a hemolytic anemia that is not communicable. Roommates with infectious diseases should be avoided because a child with sickle cell anemia is susceptible to infections. These childrens' spleens become infarcted and gradually are replaced by fibrous tissue by 5 years of age. The spleen filters bacteria thereby triggering phagocytosis; without this trigger these children are prone to infection.

1 The child with sickle cell anemia is susceptible to infection; pneumonia is an infection of the lung.

3 The child with sickle cell anemia is susceptible to infection; pharyngitis is an upper respiratory infection.

4 The child with sickle cell anemia is susceptible to infection; chronic osteomyelitis is an infection of the bone.

121. 4 The red blood cells in sickle cell anemia are fragile. When hypoxia or dehydration occurs the cells become crescent shaped; they then clump together and occlude blood vessels.

1 The platelet count is not severely depressed in vaso-occlusive crisis.

2 This is called an aplastic crisis resulting in severe anemia.

3 This is known as a splenic sequestration crisis.

122. 3 The nurse should teach the parents what the maintenance fluid requirements are for their child. The goal is one and one-half to two times maintenance to ensure adequate hydration. Adequate hydration promotes hemodilution, which helps prevent sickling and thrombus formation.

1 Sunshine may cause dehydration and hemoconcentration, resulting in increased sickling.

2 Muscle contraction increases oxygen demands, which decreases oxygen tension, resulting in increased sickling.

4 Ice causes vasoconstriction and enhances sickling.

123. 1 Seizures and swallowing difficulties are characteristics of a rabies infection, which affects the nervous system; it usually is fatal if untreated.

2 Rabies is not a bacterial infection.

3 Rabies is not a bacterial infection.

4 Although rabies is a viral infection it is not characterized by immunosuppression and opportunistic infections. Immunosuppression and opportunistic infections are associated with AIDS.

124. 2 The current polio vaccine is the inactivated polio vaccine (IPV) (Salk vaccine) that is injectable.

1 This is the *Haemophilus influenzae* type b (Hib) vaccine.

3 This is the oral polio vaccine (OPV) (Sabin vaccine); it is no longer administered because it is related to vaccine-associated polio paralysis (VAPP). However, it is used in the world-wide effort to eliminate the virus in countries where it is endemic.

4 This is the diphtheria, tetanus, and acellular pertussis (DTaP) vaccine.

125. 2 Joints are the most commonly involved areas because of weight bearing and their constant movement.

1 The brain is not the most common site.

3 The intestines are not the most common site.

4 The pericardium is not the most common site.

126. 1 The platelet count is reduced as a result of the bone marrow depression associated with leukemia and chemotherapy. Bleeding will result from the decreased clotting ability of the blood.

2 Neutrophils are white blood cells; they do not influence bleeding.

3 The red blood cell count is an indirect indicator of hematocrit and hemoglobin levels, neither of which provides the reason for or cause of the bleeding.

4 Lymphoblasts may be found in the blood of children with leukemia but they do not influence bleeding.

127. 4 **An electric toothbrush vigorously massages the gums; this may be irritating and cause the gums to hemorrhage.**

1 Cotton swabs can be used because they will not injure the mucous membranes.

2 A mild toothpaste can be used because it will not injure the mucous membranes.

3 A saline mouthwash is isotonic and will not injure the mucous membranes.

128. 2 **Overwhelming infection is the leading cause of death because of the depressed immune system resulting from chemotherapy.**

1 Although promoting growth and development is important, it is not the priority.

3 Although improving nutritional statue is important, it is not the priority.

4 Although providing emotional support is important, it is not the priority.

129. 4 **Meticulous toilet hygiene is essential to prevent infection and promote comfort.**

1 Changing positions is preferable.

2 Underpants keep the area moist and promote bacterial growth; it is preferable to leave the area exposed to air even if under bed linens.

3 Ointments tend to occlude and trap organisms, thus promoting infection.

130. 4 **The child with a low white blood cell count does not show the usual signs of infection, including fever, inflammation, and drainage. Any low-grade temperature or other subtle sign or symptom must be reported immediately so that an antibiotic can be prescribed.**

1 An electric toothbrush may damage the oral mucous membranes. A soft toothbrush or mouth swabs should be used to cleanse the mouth.

2 These children receive therapy for extended periods, and prolonged isolation from their peers may lead to destructive social isolation. The exposure to peers depends on the child's white blood cell levels and an absence of signs and symptoms of infection in the peer.

3 Nausea commonly occurs with this therapy. Antiemetic measures usually are instituted, but the chemotherapeutic medication is continued. Withholding medication should be discussed with the practitioner.

131. 1 **Adequate nutrition is extremely important to the child's overall health; best results are attained when a child receiving chemotherapy is allowed to eat as desired.**

2 Although activities are important to the child's health, these should be planned according to the child's interest and they need not be structured.

3 Mouthwashes can irritate the fragile mucosa; isotonic saline solution should be used.

4 The child should be isolated only from children with known or possible infections.

132. 4 **Effective handwashing helps prevent infection. This is the most important intervention when caring for a child with a suppressed immune system.**

1 Although purchasing a wig may be important for the child's self-image, it is not the priority.

2 Although providing rest is important, it is not the priority.

3 Although offering sufficient fluids is important, it is not the priority.

133. 4 **The production of antibodies is directly related to the number of pathogens to which an individual is exposed. Because adults have lived longer than children they have been exposed to more antigens and therefore produced more antibodies.**

1 The immune systems of children are as capable of producing antibodies as are those of adults.

2 Exposure to pathogens in the environment does not differ significantly between children and adults.

3 The pathophysiological mechanism of AIDS is the same in children and adults.

134. 4 **The Centers for Disease Control and Prevention recommend standard precautions when caring for those who have HIV infection and/or AIDS without opportunistic infections.**

1 Droplet precautions are not necessary because HIV is not transmitted by large-particle respiratory droplets.

2 Contact precautions are not necessary unless the HIV or AIDS is complicated by the presence of disease or infection, necessitating the addition of these precautions to standard precautions.

3 Airborne precautions are unnecessary because HIV is not spread by airborne droplet nuclei; these precautions are used in addition to standard precautions if an opportunistic infection such as *Mycobacterium tuberculosis* is present.

135. 1 **Children with a chronic illness should not be exposed to the additional stress of an infection.**

2 Subsequent to frequent transfusions, the child may have iron overload. An iron-rich diet is contraindicated.

3 Fluid intake can be according to the child's wishes. Because the child is chronically anemic, the child should regulate fluid intake.

4 The child should be encouraged to lead an active life during periods of well-being.

136. 2 **Tetanus immunoglobulin (TIG) contains antibodies, not the live or attenuated virus; it confers short-term passive immunity.**

1 The passive immunity is temporary.

3 Passive, not active, protection is provided.

4 Tetanus toxoid stimulates the production of antibodies, not tetanus immunoglobulin.

137. **4** **Low oxygen tension may precipitate sickling; therefore, adequate oxygenation is desirable.**
    1 The intake of oral iron may contribute to iron overload. Some children with sickle cell anemia receive frequent transfusions to suppress the production of the red cells containing the sickle hemoglobin.
    2 Hemoconcentration results in increased viscosity, which promotes thrombus formation and sickling.
    3 Quiet play is desirable during a painful episode, but it is not used routinely to prevent a crisis.

138. **4** **Motorboating is a relatively passive activity that will not increase the child's oxygen demands, which can precipitate sickling resulting in a painful episode.**
    1 Mountain lakes are usually cold; temperature extremes can contribute to sickling that may precipitate a painful episode.
    2 Playing soccer may lead to increased cellular metabolism and increased tissue hypoxia, which can precipitate sickling that may progress to a painful episode.
    3 High altitudes should be avoided because the lower oxygen concentration of the air might trigger a painful episode.

139. **1** **Dehydration precipitates sickling of red blood cells and therefore is a major causative factor for painful episodes associated with sickle cell anemia.**
    2 An inadequate number of platelets (thrombocytes) is unrelated to painful episodes associated with sickle cell anemia.
    3 Iron intake is unrelated to the sickling phenomenon.
    4 An inadequate number of white blood cells is unrelated to painful episodes associated with sickle cell anemia.

140. **1** **Activity usually is not restricted after the child recovers from the conscious sedation.**
    2 The practitioner probably will use conscious sedation as well as a local anesthetic. The child should not feel discomfort, pain, or pressure while the bone marrow is withdrawn. There may be some discomfort after the procedure when the sedation/anesthetic wears off.
    3 A tight dressing prevents bleeding from the puncture site.
    4 The anterior or posterior iliac crest is the site most often used for bone marrow aspiration in children.

141. **2** **Eosinophils increase to inhibit the inflammatory response to histamine, which is released in allergic reactions.**
    1 Platelets are unrelated to an allergic reaction.
    3 Lymphocytes are unrelated to an allergic reaction.
    4 Immunoglobulins increase, not decrease, in response to an allergic reaction.

142. **3** **The tetanus immunoglobulin (TIG) provides immediate protection, whereas the tetanus toxoid initiates an active immune response.**
    1 Both are effective alone; the combination is preferred.
    2 They do not confer lifelong immunity. After the initial routine immunizations and boosters, it is recommended that the tetanus toxoid be administered every 10 years.
    4 The tetanus immunoglobulin does not have major side effects because it is derived from human serum.

143. **4** **It is recommended that infants be given the measles, mumps, and rubella (MMR) combination vaccine at 12 to 15 months of age.**
    1 The first dose of hepatitis B (HepB) vaccine is given at birth, the second 4 weeks later, and the third 24 weeks after the second dose.
    2 Inactivated poliovirus vaccine (IPV) is given at 2 months, 4 months, and 6 to 18 months of age; the next booster (fourth) will be at 4 to 6 years of age.
    3 Tetanus toxoid is given at 2 months, 4 months, and 6 to 18 months of age; the next booster (fourth) will be at 4 to 6 years of age.

CARDIOVASCULAR

144. **3** **Because infants with heart failure become extremely fatigued while sucking, small frequent feedings with adequate rest periods can improve their total intake.**
    1 Infants with heart failure usually have fluids restricted to reduce the cardiac workload.
    2 Lying flat restricts lung expansion and should be avoided; positioning with the upper body elevated facilitates respirations.
    4 Infants with heart failure are not prone to developing hydrocephalus and do not need to have their head circumference measured again if the initial newborn assessment is within expected limits.

145. **2** **A calibrated syringe or dropper provides the most accurate measurement of the medication.**
    1 Using a nipple is not an accurate way to measure medication.
    3 Using a spoon is not an accurate way to measure medication.
    4 If the dose of medication is diluted and the infant does not drink the entire ounce, the resulting dose will be insufficient.

146. **4** **By using this method the infant remains with the head elevated and the nurse obtains an accurate weight while adhering to the practitioner's orders. This position prevents cardiopulmonary complications.**
    1 Placing the infant in the supine position, even for a short time, may compromise the infant's cardiopulmonary status, and it contradicts the practitioner's order.

2 This is a secondary source of information that is not current. This infant should be weighed on admission to obtain a baseline weight.

3 This is not the most accurate method of weighing the infant. Movements by the parent or infant may influence the result.

147. 4 **Because the mechanism of heart failure is the same in children and adults, the same medications such as cardiac glycosides, angiotensin-converting enzyme (ACE) inhibitors, and diuretics are used, although the dosage will be adjusted for the infant and for the child.**

1 Open heart surgery may or may not be necessary; there are other treatments that may be successful.

2 Multiple operations may or may not be necessary; there are other treatments that may be successful.

3 The treatment of heart failure is basically the same whether the client is an infant, child, or an adult.

148. 1 **The nurse should know how much information the parent has before responding. Pulmonic stenosis is a narrowing of the pulmonic valve at the entrance to the pulmonary artery and may vary in severity. Treatment may vary from balloon angioplasty to valvotomy.**

2 The mother must know by this time that her infant has a problem with the heart. This response is too vague and blunt.

3 The parent is concerned or the question would not have been asked.

4 Referring the mother back to the practitioner abdicates the nurse's role.

149. 4 **Because the infant tires so easily, it is difficult to consume sufficient calories for adequate weight gain. Increased caloric intake is needed to meet the infant's nutritional needs.**

1 Although there is cyanosis, it may not lead to cerebral changes. Cyanosis is not directly related to inadequate weight gain.

2 Although decreased Po_2 does lead to polycythemia, it does not affect the ability to gain adequate weight.

3 Although there is pulmonary hypertension, it is not directly related to inadequate weight gain.

150. 2 **The mixing of oxygenated and deoxygenated blood results in tissue hypoxia; clubbing occurs as a result of additional capillary development and tissue hypertrophy of the fingertips.**

1 The respirations are rapid, not slow.

3 The child's problems are related to decreased oxygenation, not to a clotting defect.

4 The body attempts to compensate for the hypoxemia associated with tetralogy of Fallot by increased erythropoiesis.

151. 1 **Flexing the hips and knees decreases venous return to the heart from the legs. When venous return to the heart is decreased, the cardiac workload is decreased.**

2 Although the orthopneic position reduces pressure of the abdominal organs on the diaphragm, it does not put enough pressure on the femoral veins and vena cava to sufficiently reduce venous return to the heart.

3 The lateral Sims position does not reduce venous return to the heart. It does not put enough pressure on the femoral veins and vena cava to sufficiently reduce venous return to the heart.

4 Although the semi-Fowler position reduces pressure of the abdominal organs on the diaphragm, it does not put enough pressure on the femoral veins and vena cava to sufficiently reduce venous return to the heart.

152. 1 **Tachycardia results from sympathetic stimulation when heart failure occurs; it is the body's attempt to increase cardiac output and increase oxygen to body cells.**

2 Distended neck veins occur only in adults when heart failure has progressed to systemic congestion.

3 The respirations will increase, not decrease, when heart failure occurs.

4 Urinary output is decreased as a result of sodium and water retention.

153. 2 **The body responds to the chronic hypoxia caused by the heart defect by increasing the production of red blood cells in an attempt to increase the oxygen-carrying capacity of the blood.**

1 The red blood cell count will be elevated because the body increases erythrocyte production in an attempt to make more cells available to carry oxygen.

3 Agranulocytosis does not result from hypoxia; it occurs when the white blood cells decrease to very low levels and neutropenia becomes pronounced.

4 Thrombocytopenia (low platelet count) does not result from hypoxia; it occurs in disease processes in which platelet production is suppressed, platelet survival is decreased, or platelet destruction is increased.

154. 4 **During a bowel movement the Valsalva maneuver can occasionally initiate a hypercyanotic spell (tet spell, blue spell). The Valsalva maneuver causes increased intrathoracic pressure, decreased return of blood to the heart, increased venous pressure, and decreased heart rate.**

1 Burping does not influence cardiovascular functioning.

2 Although feeding can cause fatigue and increase the heart rate it will not precipitate such an immediate response as described in the situation.

3 A position change will not precipitate such an immediate response as described in this situation.

155. 4 **This murmur is the most characteristic finding in infants and children with a ventricular septal defect (VSD). A left-to-right shunt is caused by the flow of blood from the higher-pressure left ventricle to the lower-pressure right ventricle.**

1. Children with a VSD generally have tachycardia.
2. Children with a VSD usually are acyanotic.
3. A bounding peripheral pulse is not a usual finding in children with a VSD.

156. 3 **When the child squats, blood pools in the lower extremities because of flexion of the hips and knees; less blood returns to the heart, decreasing the cardiac workload.**
    1. Squatting does not relieve muscle aches.
    2. Squatting is not related to the pull of gravity.
    4. Squatting decreases blood return to the heart.

157. 1 **A cardiac catheterization visualizes the exact location of the ventricular septal defect; also it measures pulmonary pressures.**
    2. Murmurs can be heard with a stethoscope placed at the left lower sternal border.
    3. Cardiomegaly is demonstrated by electrocardiographic and echocardiographic examinations.
    4. Ventricular hypertrophy is demonstrated by electrocardiographic and echocardiographic examinations.

158. 2 **Postprocedure hemorrhage at the catheter insertion site is a life-threatening complication that may occur after a cardiac catheterization because arterial blood is under pressure and the catheter has entered an artery.**
    1. Rest should be encouraged. Flexion of the insertion site should be avoided for several hours to prevent disturbance of the clot. Also the child may have a cardiac problem that causes an oxygen deficit.
    3. It is unnecessary to compare blood pressures in the extremities; the distal pulses are monitored.
    4. The blood pressure should not be unstable unless a problem has developed; fluids should be offered as prescribed.

159. 2 **Range-of-motion exercises to the limb with the catheterization site might cause the dislodging of a clot and hemorrhage.**
    1. Intake should start with fluids and progress as tolerated.
    3. The apical pulse is monitored because a common complication after cardiac catheterization involves disturbances of cardiac rate and rhythm.
    4. The peripheral pulses are assessed because formation of thrombi is a complication of cardiac catheterization.

160. 2 **The catheter insertion site should not be submerged in water; sponge baths limit trauma and infection at the insertion site.**
    1. Fluids should be encouraged to enhance excretion of the contrast medium used during the procedure.
    3. The child is sent home without a pressure dressing.
    4. Ice compresses are contraindicated because they will cause vasoconstriction and may compromise circulation.

161. 3 **The increased blood volume and pressure in the lungs resulting from impaired myocardial**

function results in pulmonary edema causing dyspnea; it is a sign of heart failure.
    1. Polycythemia, not anemia, is more common because there is increased RBC production to counteract hypoxia.
    2. Hypervolemia, not hypovolemia, is related to heart failure and pulmonary edema.
    4. Respiratory, not metabolic, acidosis can develop because of pulmonary insufficiency resulting in retention of carbon dioxide.

162. 1 **Fluid retention is reflected by an excessive weight gain in a short period. Inadequate cardiac output decreases blood flow to the kidneys, thus leading to increased intracellular fluid and hypervolemia.**
    2. Although this assessment may add information to the data regarding kidney function, other assessments such as hourly urine output, blood urea nitrogen (BUN) value, and creatinine level more significantly reflect kidney functioning.
    3. Weight gain resulting from nutritional intake is gradual and will not vary greatly on a day-to-day basis.
    4. Although weight is used to determine medication dosages, the dosage does not need to be recalculated according to changes in daily weights.

163. 3 **A positive antistreptolysin titer is expected with rheumatic fever because of a previous streptococcal infection.**
    1. A positive, not a negative, C-reactive protein is expected with rheumatic heart disease. A positive C-reactive protein is indicative of an inflammatory process.
    2. An increased reticulocyte count is unexpected. An elevated reticulocyte count usually is related to anemia, which stimulates the bone marrow to produce so many red blood cells that more immature blood cells (reticulocytes) enter the circulation.
    4. The erythrocyte sedimentation rate (ESR) is increased, not decreased, with rheumatic heart disease, indicating the presence of an inflammatory process.

164. 1 **The vital signs are taken first to determine the child's postoperative status and to compare results with the previously recorded vital signs.**
    2. Testing for level of consciousness can be done later during the assessment process and after the nurse obtains information about the anesthesia used and if any postoperative sedation was administered.
    3. Measuring the drainage can be done later during the assessment process.
    4. Care related to the nasogastric tube can be done later during the assessment process.

165. 4 **Prophylaxis before an invasive procedure can prevent subacute bacterial endocarditis, which may occur in children and adults with heart abnormalities. The endocardium is the lining**

membrane of the cavities of the heart and the connective tissue bed on which it lies.

1 Gingivitis, an inflammation of the gums, frequently is related to the accumulation of food particles in the crevices between the gums and teeth. Antibiotics are not given to prevent this condition, although they may be prescribed in the presence of an infection of the gums.

2 The endocardium is more susceptible to infection than the pericardium. The pericardium is the fibroserous sac enclosing the heart. The myocardium is the middle layer of the heart wall, composed of cardiac muscle.

3 This is an infection of the myocardium, which is an unlikely sequela of dental procedures.

ENDOCRINE

166. 3 **Pizza contains complex carbohydrates and protein; children can include a slice in their diets on special occasions.**

1 Although candy bars can be low in fat and calories, they may still have a high simple sugar content, which is contraindicated.

2 Diet, not regular, soft drinks are preferred for an individual with type 2 diabetes; regular soft drinks are high in simple sugars.

4 A euglycemic fasting blood glucose should be 70 to 105 mg/dL.

167. 2 **Adequate inspection of the feet should become a habit; it is the quickest and easiest measure to identify pressure sites and prevent infection.**

1 Hot water should never be used because it can cause injury by burning the skin.

3 The feet should be patted dry, not rubbed; rubbing can cause abrasions and injure the skin.

4 Strong antiseptics are too harsh and should not be used because they can cause injury to the skin.

168. 3 **The adolescent is exhibiting signs of hypoglycemia; the blood glucose level should be determined to document the client's status so that appropriate treatment can be instituted.**

1 It may be necessary to offer food rather than withhold it if the client is having a hypoglycemic reaction.

2 A glass of milk may be offered if the blood glucose level indicates that the client is hypoglycemic.

4 Covering the client with a blanket is unnecessary.

169. **Answer: 3, 5**

1 Although the child with diabetes is at risk for developing an infection, surgical aseptic technique should prevent an infection from occurring.

2 Ketoacidosis is associated with type 1, not type 2, diabetes.

3 **The stress of surgery causes the release of epinephrine and glucocorticoids, which increase blood glucose levels.**

4 Urine test results are affected by many variables and therefore they are not reliable indicators of blood glucose levels.

5 **Most individuals with type 2 diabetes who control their diabetes through diet and exercise require insulin during the recovery period based on blood glucose levels. The stress of surgery stimulates the release of epinephrine and glucocorticoids, which increase blood glucose levels.**

170. 4 **A fast-food exchange list allows the diabetic teenager to participate in postgame activities without feeling different from peers; this is important to the adolescent.**

1 The nutritional benefits of fast-foods are not the issue.

2 The adolescent needs to learn how to select appropriate foods when away from the home environment; this promotes social interaction with peers.

3 Eating a food other than pizza when all the friends are eating it will make the adolescent feel different from peers; the temptation not to adhere to the diet may be too great to resist.

171. 4 **The nurse must plan teaching based on the child's present and future cognitive abilities. Piaget describes age-related cognitive abilities that progress through sensorimotor, preoperational, concrete operational, and formal operational stages. Each stage builds on the accomplishments of the previous stage.**

1 Adolescents, not preschool children, are concerned about being different from their peers.

2 Five-year-olds are not emotionally ready to use the defense mechanism of denial.

3 This skill is beyond the ability of a 5-year-old child. Preschoolers think in terms of one idea but cannot understand that a single idea is part of a whole concept. It is not until they enter the school-age years that they have the cognitive and psychomotor abilities to self-test blood glucose.

172. 4 **The glycosylated hemoglobin (GHb) test provides an accurate long-term index of the child's average blood glucose level for the 10- to 12-day period before the test; the more glucose the RBCs were exposed to, the greater the GHb percent.**

1 A high blood pH may indicate developing ketoacidosis, but it reflects short-term variations.

2 Serum protein levels do not reflect the effectiveness of glucose management.

3 Serum glucose levels reflect short-term (hours) variations.

173. 1 **The stress of an infection increases the body's metabolism; the presence of glucocorticoids results in hyperglycemia.**

2 Exercise causes a decrease in insulin needs resulting in hypoglycemia, not hyperglycemia and ketoacidosis.

3 Rapid weight loss causes a decrease in insulin needs resulting in hypoglycemia, not hyperglycemia and ketoacidosis.

4 Excessive insulin results in hypoglycemia, not hyperglycemia and ketoacidosis.

174. 2 **Deep, rapid breathing (hyperpnea) is an attempt by the respiratory system to eliminate excess carbon dioxide; it is a compensatory mechanism associated with metabolic acidosis.**

1 Sweating is a physiological response to hypoglycemia.

3 Tachycardia, not bradycardia, results from the hypovolemia caused by the polyuria associated with ketoacidosis.

4 Hypotension, not hypertension, may result from the decreased vascular volume caused by the polyuria associated with ketoacidosis.

175. **Answer: 1, 4, 5**

1 **At 7 years of age, children are curious and ready to learn when a simple explanation is offered.**

2 The child is too young to be given reading materials to take home; readiness for this is determined at future meetings as the child gets older and reading skills improve.

3 The presence of friends is too distracting.

4 **Seven-year-old children are able to manipulate objects and learn from doing.**

5 **Children learn best when learning is interactive; a return demonstration provides an opportunity for the nurse to evaluate what is learned.**

176. 3 **A check of the blood glucose level will confirm whether the child is hypoglycemic.**

1 A blood pH is not a reliable measure of blood glucose.

2 Although orange juice is appropriate to counter hypoglycemia, it should not be offered until the blood glucose level is determined.

4 Asking the child when food was last ingested does not determine if the child has hypoglycemia.

177. 4 **The child's problem is caused by perceptual difficulties; the preset syringe removes the need to differentiate between 24 and 42 units.**

1 Having the child write the numbers down does not solve the transposition of numbers problem.

2 Having the child use a tuberculin syringe does not solve the transposition of numbers problem.

3 The problem is not caused by the inability to see the numbers but by the child's perception of them.

178. **Answer: 1, 3, 5**

1 **Because clients with type 1 diabetes have little or no endogenous insulin, they must take insulin; dietary control and exercise reduce the amount of exogenous insulin needed.**

2 Although infection increases insulin requirements, prophylactic antibiotics are not needed.

3 **Blood glucose monitoring is an important aspect of therapy because it helps evaluate the effectiveness of diabetic control.**

4 Oral hypoglycemics are ineffective in stimulating insulin secretion in clients with type 1 diabetes.

5 **Although adhering to the diabetic regimen is difficult, especially for adolescents who need to identify with their peers, its importance in promoting euglycemia should be discussed.**

179. 3 **Glucagon promotes liver glycogenolysis, resulting in the release of glucose into the blood.**

1 ACTH is not directly related to glycogenolysis; it is released from the anterior pituitary.

2 Insulin production is not directly related to glycogenolysis; in healthy individuals the level of insulin will increase as the glucose level increases.

4 Epinephrine is not directly related to glycogenolysis; it is released from the adrenal medulla and sympathetic nerve endings.

180. 2 **Negotiation of goals precedes and is essential to successful learning; mutual goal-setting provides a focus for learning.**

1 If the child does not identify this need or set a goal, there may be little motivation to learn the task.

3 If the child does not identify this need or set a goal, there may be little motivation to learn the task.

4 A trusting relationship should have been established during the assessment phase, before beginning the teaching-learning process.

181. **Answer: 4, 5**

1 Irritability is an autonomic nervous system response to hypoglycemia, not hyperglycemia.

2 Headache is a symptom associated with hypoglycemia, not hyperglycemia; it is caused by impaired cerebral function.

3 Sweating with pale, cool skin is an autonomic nervous system response associated with hypoglycemia, not hyperglycemia.

4 **Hyperglycemia acts as an osmotic diuretic resulting in increased urine output (polyuria) and dehydration. Thirst is a compensatory mechanism that causes a person to drink increased amounts of fluid (polydipsia).**

5 **Deep, rapid breathing (Kussmaul breathing) is the body's effort to blow off carbon dioxide in an attempt to correct the metabolic acidosis associated with hyperglycemia and ketoacidosis.**

182. 2 **Rapid breathing is an attempt by the respiratory system to eliminate excess carbon dioxide; it is a characteristic compensatory mechanism to correct metabolic acidosis.**

1 An increased temperature will occur if an infection is present; it is not a response to hyperglycemia.

3 Tachycardia, not bradycardia, results from the hypovolemia of dehydration.

4 Hypotension, not hypertension, may result from the decreased vascular volume associated with hyperglycemia.

183. 1 **Thorough handwashing is the best infection prevention technique and should always precede preparation of an injection.**
2 Shaking insulin causes air bubbles, which can interfere with preparing the dosage accurately; the bottle should be rotated gently.
3 Although sites should be rotated, the abdomen, not the extremities, is the preferred site for self-administration of insulin.
4 The injection site should not be rubbed because this affects absorption of the insulin and causes a reaction at the site.

184. 4 **Practice using a syringe builds confidence. The child's confidence, readiness, and skill for giving self-injections are essential for long-term management of diabetes.**
1 The sites must be rotated at all times.
2 Learning responsibility for injections should be a gradual process with continual support and guidance.
3 Insulin glargine should not be mixed with other insulins; it should be prepared and administered separately.

185. 1 **Insulin glargine is released continuously throughout the 24-hour period; a bedtime snack will prevent hypoglycemia during the night.**
2 This is unsafe because it intensifies hyperglycemia; if hyperglycemia is present, the child needs insulin.
3 Because insulin glargine is a long-acting insulin, bedtime snacks are recommended to prevent a hypoglycemic episode during the night.
4 When hypoglycemia develops, the child will be asleep; the snack should be eaten before going to bed.

FLUIDS AND ELECTROLYTES

186. 3 **Metabolic acidosis occurs with loss of alkaline fluid through diarrhea and is manifested by lethargy and Kussmaul breathing; all of the assessments indicate severe dehydration.**
1 The infant has not urinated because excessive amounts of fluid have been lost via the loose stools; this indicates that the kidneys are functioning by compensating for the fluid loss.
2 All data indicate that there is a severe, not mild, fluid volume deficiency.
4 Respiratory alkalosis is caused by an excessive loss of carbon dioxide, not diarrhea.

187. Answer 1, 3
1 **A baseline assessment of vital signs is essential when planning care.**
2 Assessment of skin turgor is too inaccurate a parameter to be used to plan care.
3 **The amount of weight lost correlates directly with the degree of dehydration.**
4 Although it is helpful to know the infant's urinary output, it is difficult to measure accurately unless the infant has an indwelling catheter.

5 The neurological status is not expected to be pathologic with dehydration.

188. 2 **It is most important for the mother to learn that immediate treatment is necessary for an infant with vomiting and/or diarrhea. Because infants have a greater proportion of body fluid to tissue, they cannot maintain fluid balance when there is a large loss of fluid via vomiting and/or diarrhea.**
1 An infant's diet consists almost totally of milk; teaching about a well-balanced diet is irrelevant at this time.
3 Although cleanliness is important, diarrhea can be contracted despite cleanliness.
4 Antibiotics are not administered for viral gastroenteritis.

189. 4 **Signs of rehydration are an increased urine output and a dilution of the urine, thus lowering its specific gravity. A classic sign of dehydration is oliguria and a concomitant increase in the urine specific gravity as the body attempts to compensate for the fluid loss by releasing antidiuretic hormone.**
1 With rehydration the heart rate should decrease and return to the expected range.
2 With rehydration the blood pressure should increase and return to the expected range.
3 With rehydration the capillary refill time should decrease and return to the expected range.

190. **Answer: 88.5 mL**
2.2 lb = 1 kg; 13 lb = 5.9 kg; 15mL × 5.9 kg = 88.5 mL

191. 3 **Assessment is the first step in the nursing process. Before diagnosing the problem and planning and implementing nursing care, data must be collected to determine the cause of the problem.**
1 This intervention is unsafe without a practitioner's order.
2 Assessment may indicate that an independent nursing intervention is required or it may provide significant information that should be communicated to the practitioner.
4 Oral intake is not related to intravenous intake. Also there may be an order for nothing by mouth.

192. 1 **It is critical to infuse the prescribed fluid over the prescribed time to gradually restore fluid and electrolyte balance.**
2 Cuddling should be offered, preferably by the significant caregiver because after the infant's physical needs have been met, the emotional needs become the priority.
3 Documenting should be done after the infusion is instituted and the infant's response is assessed.
4 Although explaining the purpose of the infusion is important, it is secondary to the physiological safety of the infant.

193. 4 **Loss of weight is the most accurate measurement for evaluation of the magnitude of fluid loss; 1 liter of fluid weighs 2.2 pounds.**
1 Determining dehydration by assessing tissue turgor is subjective and not as accurate as a comparison with the pre-illness weight.

2 Although an increased hematocrit indicates dehydration, it is not an effective monitoring method for assessing the amount of fluid loss.

3 Although dry mucous membranes indicate dehydration, it is not an effective monitoring method for assessing the amount of fluid loss.

194. **2 Daily weights provide an objective measurement because a weight loss indicates a loss of fluid; approximately 1 kg (2.2 pounds) is equal to 1 liter of fluid.**

1 Although a wet diaper count is an objective measure, it is necessary to weigh the diapers before and after the infant voids to estimate the amount of fluid loss.

3 Intake can be measured accurately; however, output, especially with diarrhea, is difficult to measure.

4 Assessing tissue turgor is subjective and has a variety of interpretations. Also the site that should be assessed is over the sternum, not the abdomen.

195. **4 Tissue turgor, although subjective, is one indicator of fluid balance. Tenting of the skin indicates severe dehydration. Increased depth of respirations and scanty urine, in conjunction with prolonged vomiting, reflect dehydration and metabolic alkalosis. Metabolic alkalosis results from hydrochloric acid and potassium depletion.**

1 Although assessments of the vomitus are important, they are not the priority.

2 Although assessment of the abdominal mass is important and the result should be documented, it is not the priority.

3 Although assessments related to feedings are important and they should be documented, they are not the priority.

196. **3 The risks of surgery are greatly increased unless dehydration and metabolic alkalosis from prolonged vomiting are corrected.**

1 Although adequate hydration must be attained, electrolyte balance must be restored as well.

2 Although chloride levels are low, the fluid imbalance must be corrected as well.

4 Malnutrition will be corrected after surgery when the infant retains feedings. Respiratory problems are not associated with pyloric stenosis.

197. **1 In nephrotic syndrome a large proportion of the child's body weight is composed of retained fluid; the loss of fluid is reflected by a loss of weight.**

2 It is difficult to obtain an accurate recording of output in a child who is not toilet trained.

3 It is difficult to evaluate a return to fluid balance by measuring the abdominal circumference because the edema is generalized, not concentrated, in the abdomen.

4 Although increased appetite is a sign of improvement, it is not an indicator of fluid balance.

198. **2 The shift of fluid from the intravascular to the interstitial compartment predisposes**

to hypovolemia; a weak, thready pulse and hypotension are signs of impending shock.

1 Heart failure usually is not a complication of nephrotic syndrome; however, it is a major complication of glomerulonephritis.

3 The development of a pulmonary embolus is not a complication of nephrotic syndrome. Chest pain and dyspnea are signs of a pulmonary embolus.

4 Hypokalemia, not hyperkalemia, occurs. Tubular reabsorption of sodium is increased to replenish the vascular volume; therefore, potassium is excreted.

199. **1 At 15 pounds the infant weighs about 7 kg; 4 mL × 7 kg is 28 mL.**

2 This amount is too much.

3 This amount is too much.

4 This amount is too much.

200. **3 An infant weighing 15½ pounds (7 kg) should have a minimum urine output of 1 mL/kg/hr, or 7 mL/hr. This infant's output is only 2 mL/hr. A decreased urinary output will result in retention of potassium, causing hyperkalemia.**

1 Intractable crying is the expected response of an ill 6-month-old infant.

2 Inadequate tissue turgor is an indication of dehydration, which is the reason for the IV infusion.

4 There is no reason to question the prescription because the IV infusion is supplementing the oral rehydration therapy (ORT).

201. **3 Rapid absorption of acetylsalicylic acid (aspirin) causes the stomach contents to become more acidic, leading to metabolic acidosis.**

1 Hyperventilation is the body's attempt to blow off excess hydrogen ions; carbon dioxide is converted to hydrogen ions via the carbonic anhydrase reaction.

2 The pH of the stomach contents decreases with aspirin toxicity, becoming more acidic, leading to metabolic acidosis.

4 Although an increased renal excretion of bicarbonate can contribute to metabolic acidosis, this is not the mechanism associated with aspirin toxicity. With metabolic acidosis associated with aspirin toxicity the kidneys attempt to decrease the renal excretion of bicarbonate.

202. **3 Hyperpyrexia (elevated temperature) is a manifestation of acute aspirin poisoning; this leads to increased oxygen consumption and heat loss.**

1 Blood pressure is not directly affected by aspirin ingestion.

2 Ascites does not occur as a result of aspirin ingestion; it may occur if the child develops liver failure.

4 Aspirin ingestion does not affect the serum glucose level.

203. **1 Dry mucous membranes and weight loss are classic signs of dehydration. The nurse should calculate the infant's fluid requirements, then obtain an order from the practitioner to increase either free water or the amount of the feedings, as needed.**

2 The findings are not expected; documenting them without notifying the practitioner is an unsafe action.

3 The nurse cannot change the composition of the feeding without a practitioner's order.

4 The nurse cannot change the composition of the feeding without a practitioner's order.

204. 3 **Depressed fontanels related to decreased cerebral spinal fluid are a classic sign of fluid volume deficiency in infants.**

1 A 5% weight loss indicates mild dehydration; a severely dehydrated infant will have a 15% weight deficit.

2 Dehydration is unrelated to allergic reactions.

4 This specific gravity is within the expected limits of 1.005 to 1.020.

205. 2 **Sodium lactate is converted to sodium bicarbonate; it helps correct the sodium deficiency and the metabolic acidosis.**

1 Normal saline results in the chloride combining with the hydrogen ion, intensifying the acidosis.

3 Albumin is a colloid found in blood plasma; it is not used in the treatment of metabolic acidosis.

4 Potassium is not administered until urinary function is restored.

206. 1 **The extremities must be restrained because the infant will use them in an attempt to dislodge the intravenous catheter.**

2 Scalp veins used for intravenous infusions are not located in this area.

3 Pupillary responses are unrelated to dehydration and fluid replacement.

4 The parents can be taught how to hold their infant while there is an IV infusing via a scalp vein.

207. 2 **The present caloric intake for a 24-hour period is 8 ounces, five times each day. This is 40 ounces. Infant formula contains 20 calories per ounce. The infant is consuming 800 calories per day. The infant is 5.6 kg. The recommended daily intake is 108 calories for each kg weight or 605 calories for this infant. Thus, the infant is receiving 195 calories per day over the recommended caloric intake for body weight.**

1 The present caloric intake exceeds the daily recommended requirements by 195 calories.

3 The present caloric intake exceeds the daily recommended requirements by 195 calories.

4 There are enough data to calculate the infant's daily caloric intake (oz × calories × number of feedings).

208. 2 **Fluid retention is reflected by an excessive weight gain in a short period of time; inadequate cardiac output decreases blood flow to the kidneys, thus leading to increased intracellular fluid and hypervolemia.**

1 Daily weights are appropriate if renal disease or hypovolemia is present; however, other assessments such as hourly urinary output, blood urea nitrogen,

and creatinine values provide a more accurate assessment of kidney function.

3 Weight is helpful in determining medication dosages, but daily weights are not used to diagnose digitalis toxicity.

4 Weight gain or loss resulting from nutritional intake is gradual and will not vary on a day-to-day basis.

209. 3 **A child who weighs 15 kg should receive 100 mL daily for the first 10 kg (1000 mL) and 25 mL daily for the additional 5 kg (125 mL). The total daily intake should be approximately 1125 mL. There are 30 mL per ounce and the child will ingest 4 ounces (30×4) which is 120 mL per serving. The child will be receiving 10 servings (1200mL), therefore the child will be receiving an adequate amount of fluid.**

1 Two quarts measure approximately 2000 mL; this is an excessive amount of fluid.

2 A small glass of fluid measures from 4 to 6 ounces depending upon the parents' perception of glass size; the nurse cannot evaluate their understanding from this vague response.

4 Six ounces is equal to 180 mL. Four times 180 mL is equal to 720 mL. This is an insufficient amount of fluid.

210. 4 **Both hypertonic glucose and mannitol (Osmitrol) cause diuresis; the child should be monitored for excessive fluid loss.**

1 Hypertonic glucose and mannitol will cause a fluid loss, not gain.

2 Seizure activity is not anticipated as a result of this infusion.

3 An increased fluid volume can lead to heart failure; however, hypertonic glucose and mannitol cause a fluid loss, not gain.

211. 1 **The IV infusion should be maintained at the slowest rate possible to keep the circulatory access patent until the practitioner can be reached to order the desired rate.**

2 After surgery all previous orders are canceled and new orders must be written.

3 The practitioner, not the nurse in the operating room, must be contacted to obtain a current order.

4 Changing the flow rate of intravenous fluids requires a practitioner's order.

212. 4 **It is imperative that the nurse monitor the IV site and tubing for patency. Signs of obstruction or infiltration must be detected and if needed a new circulatory access must be obtained quickly.**

1 Oral fluids are not administered after abdominal surgery until peristalsis returns.

2 There is no reason to limit handling the infant as long as the IV site is not disturbed. Parent-infant contact should be encouraged.

3 Although an accurate output record, which includes the number of voidings, is important, maintenance of the IV infusion is the priority.

213. **Answer: 2, 4**

1 Lipids are not restricted; usually fats are a prime source of calories.

2 **Sodium is restricted in that salt is not added to foods and processed meat and salty snacks are avoided.**

3 Glucose is not restricted; it is a prime source of calories.

4 **Potassium is always restricted in the presence of oliguria to prevent cardiac dysrhythmias associated with hyperkalemia. Potassium is found in fruit such as bananas, oranges, and apples and in white potatoes.**

214. 1 **One cup equals 8 ounces; therefore, ½ cup equals 4 ounces. The child drank 2, 4, 4, 3, 8, 3, 4, and 2 ounces, which equals 30 ounces.**

2 This volume is too low; it is an incorrect calculation.

3 This volume is too high; it is an incorrect calculation.

4 This volume is too low; it is an incorrect calculation.

215. 4 **Offering fluids in a full 1-ounce medicine cup allows the child to drink without a long time between drinks; a full container, even if it is small, creates the illusion of receiving more.**

1 Although fluids can be limited during sleeping hours, 12 hours is too long for a young child to tolerate without fluids.

2 When fluid is limited, a smaller amount should be apportioned to sleeping hours.

3 If the child is allowed to drink as much as desired until the limit is reached, 15 to 20 hours might elapse before any fluid is permitted again.

216. 4 **Metabolic acidosis results from an excess concentration of hydrogen cations. The kidneys cannot convert ammonium to ammonia and there is inadequate base bicarbonate to maintain an appropriate acid-base balance.**

1 With Kussmaul respirations there is an excess of hydrogen ions, the opposite of an excess of base bicarbonate.

2 Carbonic acid blown off as carbon dioxide is a compensatory mechanism to counter the present metabolic acidosis.

3 There is an excess of hydrogen ions from a metabolic problem rather than an excess of carbonic acid resulting from retained carbon dioxide.

217. 3 **NPO is maintained during the early emergent/ resuscitative phase because of the probability of developing paralytic ileus.**

1 It is unsafe to offer ice chips because the fluid that is ingested interferes with monitoring and controlling the child's fluid and electrolyte status.

2 It is unsafe to offer oral fluids, not only because of the danger of paralytic ileus, but because they interfere with monitoring and controlling the child's fluid and electrolyte status.

4 It is unsafe to offer oral fluids, not only because of the danger of paralytic ileus, but because they interfere with monitoring and controlling the child's fluid and electrolyte status.

218. 4 **Because of the location and degree of burns, an IV line for fluid restoration and access for pain medications is the priority.**

1 Oxygen is not needed because the airway is not involved and oxygen deprivation has not been identified.

2 The insertion of a urinary catheter is a secondary action after fluid administration begins.

3 Although giving pain medication is important, an IV infusion for fluid restoration to prevent hypovolemic shock is the priority. Pain medication for both children and adults with burns usually is administered through an intravenous catheter.

219. 2 **1010 mL is the correct amount of intake. 125 mL× 8 hours = 1000 mL; one dose of the reconstituted antibiotic is administered at 1 PM = 10 mL; 1000 mL + 10 mL = 1010 mL.**

1 1000 mL is an incorrect calculation of the client's intake.

3 1020 mL is an incorrect calculation of the client's intake.

4 1030 mL is an incorrect calculation of the client's intake.

220. 3 **The child has metabolic acidosis; the lungs compensate by blowing off excess carbonic acid in the form of carbon dioxide.**

1 Diaphoresis is a compensatory mechanism to reduce fever by evaporation, not to compensate for metabolic acidosis.

2 Fever is not a compensatory mechanism to counter metabolic acidosis; fever with dehydration results from inadequate fluid for perspiring and cooling.

4 The kidneys excrete hydrogen and ammonium ions to compensate for metabolic acidosis.

221. 3 **Oral rehydration therapy (ORT) is important because the percentage of fluid to body mass is higher in young children than adults, and fluid and electrolyte imbalance with shock can occur quickly.**

1 The BRAT diet (bananas, rice, applesauce, and tea/toast) is no longer recommended. ORT and a regular diet should be encouraged.

2 There are no antiviral agents for treating viral-related diarrhea.

4 Antidiarrheal agents, such as Kaopectate or Imodium, may be harmful because they slow the course of the disease by retaining the virus-containing stool in the intestine.

222. 1 **The child should receive 60 mL from 3 PM to 11 PM. 40 mL + 140 mL = 180 mL per day. There are three eight hour segments in a day; 180 divided by 3 equals 60 mL for the 8 hour segment from 3 PM to 11 PM.**

2 This is more than the amount of fluid the child can receive.

2   This is more than the amount of fluid the child can receive.

4   This is more than the amount of fluid the child can receive.

223.   **Answer: 2, 4, 3, 1**
Respiratory compensation to acidosis involves hyperventilation with increased CO2 elimination. As carbon dioxide is blown off there is a decrease in the hydrogen ions in the blood, leading to an increase in pH to expected limits.

GASTROINTESTINAL

224.   2   **Because of the cleft (opening) in the lip, the infant tends to suck in excessive air; burping helps prevent regurgitation of formula.**
1   Thickened formula is given to infants with reflux problems, such as vomiting after each feeding.
3   The semi-Fowler position may be used for infants with reflux problems; this infant should be held during feedings.
4   The infant should be held during feedings; the bottle should never be propped because aspiration may occur.

225.   2   **Because of the anomalous structure of the upper lip, the infant may have difficulty sucking on a nipple. Adaptive shields are available for breastfeeding. Haberman feeders and other modified devices are used for formula feeding.**
1   Avoiding crying is not an immediate concern; after surgery it is necessary to prevent tension on the suture line.
3   Cleft palate, not cleft lip, may predispose the infant to infection.
4   The infant should be cuddled and held.

226.   3   **Feeding with a syringe provides nutrition without placing stress on the suture line.**
1   Sucking stresses the suture line.
2   A spoon may injure the suture line.
4   Nasogastric feedings are unnecessary because fluid can be ingested orally.

227.   2   **Meticulous care of the suture line is necessary because inflammation and sloughing of tissue disrupt healing.**
1   Burping should be done throughout the feeding.
3   Placing on the abdomen is contraindicated not only because the infant may rub the face on the sheet and irritate the suture line, but because of its relationship to SIDS.
4   The infant can be held at any time.

228.   2   **It is important to minimize crying because crying puts tension on the suture line.**
1   The infant should be out of restraints periodically when a caregiver is present.
3   The infant should not have respiratory difficulty and does not need oxygen.

4   The infant should be cuddled; parents are encouraged to hold their baby as much as possible.

229.   2   **Galactosemia results from an absence of the hepatic enzyme that converts galactose to glucose, a step in carbohydrate metabolism.**
1   Intolerance to grains is found in children with celiac disease.
3   An inability to metabolize an essential amino acid (phenylalanine) describes phenylketonuria.
4   When parasympathetic ganglion cells are absent from the colon, megacolon (congenital aganglionic megacolon) develops.

230.   **Answer: 1, 3**
1   **Milk and dairy products have high lactose content and should be eliminated from the diet.**
2   Both meat and eggs are permitted because neither contains lactose.
3   **Soybean-based formulas are permissible because they do not contain lactose.**
4   Cereals containing wheat products are eliminated from the diet of children with celiac disease.
5   Pancreatic enzymes are prescribed for children with cystic fibrosis, not galactosemia.

231.   2   **If the infant is dehydrated and rehydration therapy is successful, followed by surgery, the result is full recovery.**
1   Medical treatment is not widely used because the success rate with surgery is excellent.
3   After surgery these infants usually tolerate small feedings in 4 to 6 hours; if these are tolerated they can resume regular feedings in 24 hours.
4   Hypertrophic pyloric stenosis is not caused by a metabolic deficiency.

232.   1   **Bicycling increases abdominal relaxation, enabling the examiner to palpate the abdomen easily.**
2   Muscular anomalies of the abdomen are detected by palpation, but first the abdomen must be relaxed.
3   Abdominal contour is assessed by inspection, not palpation; bicycling does not improve its visualization.
4   Abdominal rebound is assessed by palpation, but first the abdomen must be relaxed.

233.   4   **Hypertrophic pyloric stenosis (HPS) occurs when the circumferential muscle of the pyloric sphincter of the stomach becomes thickened. This thickening may be palpated as an olive-like mass in the upper right quadrant to the right of the umbilicus.**
1   This area is over the cardiac sphincter where the esophagus and stomach are connected, which is unrelated to HPS.
2   This area is over the spleen, which is unrelated to HPS.
3   The olive-like mass of HPS is on the right, not left, side of the umbilicus.

234. 1 **Surgery is the treatment of choice for hypertrophic pyloric stenosis HPS. After surgery the infant usually has a rapid recovery with an excellent prognosis.**
    2 HPS is not caused by a chromosomal mutation, it is a structural defect. Hypertrophy of the circular muscle of the pylorus causes obstruction at the pyloric sphincter.
    3 The infant will be tolerating regular feedings within 24 hours after surgery.
    4 A special diet is not required once fluids are tolerated.

235. 1 **Postoperatively, initial feedings consist of an electrolyte solution, such as Pedialyte, until tolerance for progressive feedings is determined.**
    2 An increase in feeding osmolarity is attempted after the tolerance for clear liquids is assessed.
    3 An increase in feeding osmolarity is attempted after the tolerance for clear liquids is assessed.
    4 Thickened cereal is used when an infant experiences gastroesophageal reflux.

236. 2 **The semi-Fowler position allows gravity to aid in emptying the stomach's contents, thereby limiting vomiting.**
    1 Rocking increases the chance of vomiting.
    3 Keeping the infant awake increases the chance of vomiting.
    4 Positioning horizontally increases the chance of vomiting.

237. 2 **The nurse must assess if the infant is eating solid foods and receiving vitamin and mineral supplements. Although orange juice has vitamin C, it is too high in simple sugars and contains insufficient amounts of iron, calcium, and other essential vitamins and minerals.**
    1 It is inappropriate to comment on the infant's weight.
    3 It is insufficient to comment on just one aspect of the infant's diet history.
    4 This is a judgmental and accusatory question. It is insufficient to comment on just one aspect of the infant's diet history.

238. 2 **A 15-month-old child's liver should be palpable 1 to 2 cm below the right costal margin.**
    1 The anterior fontanel closes completely at about 18 months of age.
    3 Abdominal or diaphragmatic breathing is expected in children younger than 7 years of age.
    4 This pulse rate is within the expected range (100 to 110 beats per minute) for a 15-month-old child.

239. 3 **The aspirate should be returned to ensure that the gastric enzymes and acid-base balance are maintained. The amount of the aspirate returned should be subtracted from the volume to be administered in the next feeding.**
    1 Withholding the feeding will compromise the infant's fluid and electrolyte balance.
    2 Discarding the aspirate from the full feeding will compromise the infant's fluid and electrolyte balance.
    4 Both actions will compromise the infant's fluid and electrolyte balance.

240. **Answer: 3, 4, 1, 2**
    Before performing any care, the hands must be washed to prevent contamination, then the package may be opened. The distance that the tube has to be passed is determined before insertion. After tube insertion, stomach contents should be aspirated to determine placement of the tube within the stomach.

241. 1 **Sucking and swallowing (the infant's response to a pacifier) reduce gagging and facilitate the insertion of the nasogastric tube.**
    2 A small amount of gastric fluid is always present and will appear in the tube.
    3 The tube is passed the distance from the ear to the tip of the nose to the distal end of the sternum.
    4 Coughing, gagging, and cyanosis indicate that the tube has passed into the larynx, not the stomach.

242. 2 **The semi-Fowler position limits the potential for aspiration; the child will be partially upright and fluid will remain in the stomach by gravity.**
    1 The supine position allows gastric reflux and may lead to aspiration.
    3 The Trendelenburg position allows gastric reflux and may lead to aspiration.
    4 The side-lying position allows gastric reflux and may lead to aspiration.

243. 2 **For some infants the thickened formula decreases the number of vomiting episodes. Breast milk can be placed in a bottle and cereal can be added to thicken it.**
    1 A 6-week-old infant cannot take food from a spoon and swallow it.
    3 For infants with gastroesophageal reflux this method of positioning has been replaced by the prone position with the head of the mattress elevated. This position may prevent aspiration. These infants should not be left alone after feeding.
    4 This is appropriate; surgery will be done only if complications, such as respiratory distress, esophagitis, or esophageal stricture, occur.

244. 3 **Reflux of gastric contents to the pharynx predisposes the infant to aspiration and the development of respiratory problems.**
    1 There is no risk for a bowel obstruction; the problem is an incompetent esophageal sphincter.
    2 An increased hematocrit is not expected unless there is severe dehydration.
    4 Abdominal distention does not occur because gastric contents are forcefully vomited.

245. 4 **Although the palate can be repaired during the neonatal period, performing the repair so early is controversial. However, the surgical repair should**

be done before the child talks so that the child can learn to speak coherently.

1   Although both cleft lip and palate may occur with other birth defects, it is not always so; most birth defects are diagnosed at the time of birth.

2   Focusing on the disfigurement may raise anxiety and increase guilt.

3   There is a specific reason why the two surgeries are done separately, not merely to minimize complications.

246. 3   **The suture lines in the mouth must be protected. Because the toddler uses the mouth to explore the environment, elbow restraints are needed to prevent placing fingers or objects in the mouth.**

1   The child should have time to play with toys, but with supervision to prevent mouthing activities that may disrupt the suture line.

2   The supine position is acceptable; the toddler should be able to move freely when asleep.

4   A nasogastric tube is not used.

247. 1   **Feeding with a small cup is best because liquids can be given slowly without stress on the suture line; also, using a cup is age appropriate for a toddler.**

2   Sucking on a nipple may cause pressure on the suture line; also, a cup is more age appropriate.

3   Feeding with a syringe increases the chances of damage to the suture line and may result in aspiration.

4   Feeding with a spoon increases the risks of damage to the suture line.

248. 4   **The organisms causing gastroenteritis are eliminated in the feces. The gloves should be removed and the hands washed after giving direct care. New gloves should be donned if the parents are to remain with the child.**

1   A mask is required for airborne precautions.

2   Weighing the diapers is not a requirement of contact precautions; this technique may be used to measure intake and output.

3   This is not necessary. The baby's room door should be closed if airborne precautions are necessary.

249.   Answer 1, 3, 5

1   **Poached eggs are nutritious and are easily digested.**

2   Creamed foods contain milk, which may irritate the GI tract in some children.

3   **Carrots help replace the sodium lost in diarrhea.**

4   Puddings contain milk, which may irritate the GI tract in some children.

5   **Animal crackers are not irritating to the GI tract.**

250. 2   **The infant's daily intake should be approximately 27 ounces. The infant weighs 11 pounds (5 kg). An infant's daily caloric need is 108 calories per kg of body weight. 108 calories × 5 kg = 540 calories per day; since there are 20 calories per oz, 540 ÷ 20 = 27 ounces.**

1   21 ounces is inadequate.

3   33 ounces is excessive.

4   39 ounces is excessive.

251. 3   **Whole grains, legumes, and meat are excellent sources of thiamine, an essential coenzyme factor in carbohydrate metabolism.**

1   Eggs are a fair source of thiamine.

2   Fruits do not contain thiamine.

4   Vegetables are a fair source of thiamine.

252.   Answer: 1, 2, 5

1   **Assessment and documentation of fluid balance are critical aspects of all postoperative care.**

2   **Laparoscopic surgery involves insufflating the abdominal cavity with air, which is painful until it is absorbed. The amount of pain should be measured and documented. Pain can be measured using numbers 1 to 10 for the older child and Wong's FACES for the younger child.**

3   A special diet is not indicated after this surgery.

4   After a laparoscopic appendectomy there is little drainage and no dressings.

5   **Auscultating for bowel sounds and documenting their presence or absence evaluate the child's adaptation to the intestinal trauma caused by the surgery.**

253. 3   **Dishwashing powder is a caustic chemical that requires a specific antidote and the personnel at the poison control center are best qualified to advise the mother.**

1   Syrup of ipecac induces vomiting. It is contraindicated for children.

2   Washing the child's lips may provide comfort, but it will not prevent injury.

4   Neither burnt toast nor milk is recommended as an antidote for poisoning caused by dishwasher powder.

254. 3   **Gagging and vomiting may indicate an esophageal stricture, requiring dilations.**

1   Seizures are not expected after the ingestion of a corrosive substance.

2   Jaundice is not expected after the ingestion of a corrosive substance.

4   Abdominal pain and diarrhea are not expected after the ingestion of a corrosive substance.

255. 3   **Meat is the best source of the complete protein that is needed to maintain nitrogen balance.**

1   Oranges are high in vitamin C, which is needed for healing but not for nitrogen balance.

2   Although there is protein in a bacon sandwich, it is not a significant amount.

4   Although there is protein in chicken soup, it is not a significant amount.

256.   Answer: 3, 4

1   Dairy products carry many microorganisms, but not specifically *Salmonella*.

2   *Salmonella* infection usually is not associated with vegetables.

3 *Salmonella* is present in animal sources such as meat and poultry, but is destroyed when cooked adequately.

4 *Salmonella* is present in animal sources such as eggs, but is destroyed when cooked adequately.

5 *Salmonella* is not associated with processed products such as cheese, nor with grains such as bread.

257. 3 **Bismuth subsalicylate (Kaopectate) has adsorbent and demulcent effects; stool will stay in the intestine longer, which will allow the organism to infect the intestinal mucosa.**

1 Diarrheal stools should be tested for occult blood to determine if the upper GI tract is affected.

2 Oral rehydration therapy (ORT) is an appropriate intervention because it will replace fluid and electrolyte losses.

4 Acetaminophen (Tylenol) should be administered to promote comfort if the child has a fever.

258. **Answer: 3, 4**

1 The prone position will increase pressure on the abdominal area; also it is contraindicated because of its relationship to SIDS.

2 The Trendelenburg position will exert pressure on the colostomy area and may impede respiratory excursion.

3 **Placing the infant onto the back prevents pressure on the abdominal area.**

4 **Placing the infant onto the side prevents pressure on the abdominal area.**

259. 4 **Necrotizing enterocolitis (NEC) is an inflammatory disorder of the gastrointestinal mucosa related to several factors including prematurity, hypoxemia, and high-solute feedings.**

1 Meconium ileus is an intestinal obstruction present at birth usually related to cystic fibrosis.

2 Imperforate anus is the failure of fetal tissue to develop appropriately early in gestation and is present at birth.

3 Duodenal atresia is a genetic defect that occurs early in gestation and is present at birth.

260. 4 **Intussusception creates an intestinal obstruction because the intestine telescopes and becomes trapped within its lumen; stools are red and currant jelly–like from the mixing of stool with blood and mucus.**

1 Bowel sounds may not be significantly affected.

2 High-pitched crying is a result of cerebral irritation; this is not expected with intussusception.

3 Accurate fluid intake and output records are important, but they are not essential to confirming this diagnosis.

261. 1 **Children with celiac disease are unable to digest the gliadin component of gluten, resulting in fatty, foul-smelling diarrheal stools.**

2 Phenylketonuria (PKU) is caused by the absence of phenylalanine; it is not related to celiac disease.

3 Excessive salt in the sweat glands is related to cystic fibrosis.

4 Increased mucous gland secretion viscosity is related to cystic fibrosis.

262. 1 **Steatorrhea (fatty, foul-smelling, frothy, bulky stools) occurs with celiac disease because of an intolerance to gluten; as a result toxic substances, which can damage the intestinal mucosal cells, accumulate and cause diarrhea.**

2 Drinking large amounts of fluid is a response to dehydration. With celiac disease some thirst may occur but it is not continuous.

3 Although these infants are irritable, this sign is too vague to evaluate accurately. Irritability is symptomatic of a variety of problems ranging from cutting teeth to leukemia.

4 Concentrated urine is associated with a urinary tract infection or dehydration; this sign is too vague to evaluate accurately.

263. 2 **The biopsy of the small intestine of a child with celiac disease reveals mucosal irritation, crypt hyperplasia, and villous atrophy.**

1 Fatty plaques do not occur in celiac disease.

3 Superficial ulcerations do not occur in celiac disease.

4 The pancreatic acini degenerate in cystic fibrosis, not celiac disease.

264. **Answer: 4, 5**

1 Lack of gluten in the diet is not the cause of the anemia.

2 The anemia is caused by inadequate absorption rather than the quantity consumed.

3 Lack of the intrinsic factor causes pernicious anemia, not the anemia associated with celiac disease.

4 **Because mucosal lesions limit nutrient absorption, there is inadequate iron for hemoglobin synthesis, causing anemia.**

5 **Because mucosal lesions limit nutrient absorption, there is inadequate folic acid for hemoglobin synthesis, causing anemia.**

265. **Answer: 2, 3, 4**

1 Primary sources of gluten are wheat, rye, barley, and oats; oatmeal is made from oats.

2 **Ice cream, if it does not contain wheat fillers, is acceptable on the celiac diet.**

3 **Rice is a gluten-free grain and is tolerated by the child with celiac disease.**

4 **Corn is a grain that is gluten free and can be tolerated by the child with celiac disease.**

5 Primary sources of gluten are wheat, rye, barley, and oats; whole-wheat bread contains wheat flour and wheat byproducts.

266. 1 **The disappearance of steatorrhea accompanied by formed bowel movements occurs with adherence to the diet.**

2 The ability or inability to cope with stressful situations is not a cause of celiac disease; it is caused by a toxic reaction to gluten.

3 Even when the child understands the disease process, adherence to the diet may be relaxed; as a result of this relaxation, signs and symptoms may recur.

4 Although it is important to assess what the child knows about the diet, it does not guarantee the child will select the foods on the diet.

267. **2** **The labels of foods such as gravy, sauces, and other prepared foods must be checked for hidden gluten.**

1 Rice and corn are virtually gluten free.

3 Although the diet should be high in calories, it compensates for the lack of carbohydrates (e.g., wheat, rye, barley, and oats), not protein.

4 The diet will be continued at least through adolescence, if not for one's entire life.

268. **4** **A low-residue diet should have minimum roughage; eggs prepared any way but fried are permitted; refined bread and toast also are permitted.**

1 Although meat is permitted, spicy, fried, or tough meats are not. Most frankfurters have fillers that interfere with the goal of low residue.

2 Raw fruits are not permitted because they contain roughage.

3 Nuts and jams are not permitted because they contain roughage.

269. **1** **Keeping the bag clean limits odor and promotes cleanliness. The part of the drainage appliance that is attached to the skin is not removed routinely, only when the integrity of its adherence to the skin is compromised.**

2 Milk and milk products do not have to be limited.

3 Only 50 to 100 mL of saline solution should be used for irrigation to prevent fluid reabsorption and retention.

4 Slight bleeding is expected in the immediate postoperative period; it should be reported on the next routine visit.

270. **1** **With enterobiasis the adult worm lays her eggs around the anal opening, producing an irritation and thus an itch.**

2 Scaly skin patches are commonly seen with eczema or dermatitis.

3 A maculopapular rash may be seen with hookworm (*Necator americanus*), not pinworm (*Enterobius vermicularis*), infestation.

4 A bald spot is produced by ringworm of the scalp (tinea capitis), a fungal infection of the skin.

271. **Answer: 2, 3, 4**

1 Pinworms (*Enterobius vermicularis*), not the eggs, are visible to the naked eye.

2 **Reinfestation is common because pinworms easily spread to family members who are in close contact with the child.**

3 **All family members must take the medication to help prevent reinfestation.**

4 **Toddlers touch dirt and then put their hands in their mouths; handwashing for all family members before eating can help prevent reinfestation.**

5 There is no reason for obtaining a stool specimen from the child because the diagnosis is confirmed. The diagnosis is made with a tape test, not a stool specimen.

272. **Answer: 3, 5**

1 Cats do not transmit pinworms.

2 Disinfecting surfaces does not help prevent transmission.

3 **Washing clothing and bed linens daily will help limit transmission.**

4 Toilets are not the usual mode of transmission; the rectal-oral cycle must be completed for an infestation to occur.

5 **Medications, such as mebendazole (Vermox), pyrantel pamoate (Antiminth), and pyrvinium (Povan) are effective, but must be repeated in 2 weeks to prevent reinfestation.**

273. **4** **It is not necessary to wash the bedding daily because roundworm is not transmitted via fomites.**

1 Because the organism is not transmitted from person to person, the family does not have to be medicated.

2 It is advisable to keep small children from playing in areas where there is dirt because young children explore their environment by putting their hands and objects into their mouths.

3 Cooking vegetables should destroy the organism if present and therefore is advisable.

274. **4** **Scheduling toileting before meals does not take advantage of the gastrocolic reflex; after meals probably will be more successful.**

1 Increasing fluid intake may help to relieve or allay constipation; no additional teaching is needed.

2 High-fiber foods help prevent constipation; no additional teaching is needed.

3 One bowel movement per day makes scheduling easier; no additional intervention is needed.

275. **Answer: 1, 2, 3, 4**

First a physical cause of the encopresis should be investigated. This includes the toilet-training process and changes in bowel habits or routines. If there are no changes in bowel patterns, a nutrition history may reveal any changes in the child's eating habits that caused the encopresis. Then the nurse should explore psychosocial factors that may have influenced the development of the encopresis. Finally a physical examination should be performed.

276. **3** **The American Dietetic Association has indicated that the food in fast-food restaurants is calorie dense and higher in fat, sugar, and sodium than the food served at home or in other restaurants.**

1 Although fast-food restaurants encourage patrons to eat quickly, this is not the major reason why eating their food is discouraged.

2 Portions in fast-food restaurants are not large; they are smaller than those in diners and many other restaurants.

4 Fast-food restaurants encourage safe food handling to meet the standards of the local health department.

INTEGUMENTARY

277. **4** **The skin integrity of these children is compromised because of their constant scratching; they are prone to streptococcal and staphylococcal infections.**

1 Although ensuring growth is important, it is not the priority.

2 An exact cause may never be identified.

3 Although providing adequate hydration is important, it is not the priority.

278. **1** **The baby's nails should be cut very short to minimize injury from scratching.**

2 Woolens and synthetic fabrics tend to further irritate the eczematous rash.

3 Non-human milk can exacerbate eczema.

4 Cotton clothing seems to be tolerated the best by infants with eczema.

279. **Answer: 2, 3**

1 Appetite does not play a role in the occurrence of eczema.

2 **Wearing cotton clothing indicates that the parents understand and are trying to minimize their child's allergic reaction.**

3 **Eczema is a common manifestation of allergies in the young child and is often related to foods and clothing. Tolerating new foods is a positive sign that the child is outgrowing some food allergies.**

4 Eczema is an allergic manifestation; it is not contagious.

5 Eczema is an allergic manifestation; it is not contagious.

280. **3** **Scratching can break the integrity of the skin, leaving it vulnerable to infection.**

1 Dermatitis is a response to an allergen; it is not contagious.

2 Scratching will not cause the dermatitis to spread.

4 There are no data to indicate that scratching or dermatitis is a precursor to skin cancer.

281. **1** **The microorganism causing the patches should be determined; commonly they are caused by candidiasis (thrush), a fungal infection.**

2 The patches should not be removed forcibly because it may further injure the delicate oral mucosa.

3 A further assessment of the oral cavity should be conducted immediately.

4 Although teaching the mother to rinse the mouth after a feeding is advisable, the microorganism causing the problem should be identified first.

282. **2** **Air-drying promotes healing; moisture macerates the skin and provides a medium for the growth of microorganisms.**

1 There are no data to indicate that the infant has a fever.

3 Preventing the diaper from adhering to the skin is not the reason for exposing the area.

4 Although the nurse can monitor the infant's passage of stool, this is not the reason the area is left exposed.

283. **2** **Low Fowler or the supine position prevents the incision from coming into contact with the mattress and is the preferred position for infants.**

1 Lying prone causes frictional contact with the mattress and can cause stress on the suture line. It is not recommended for any infant because of its relationship to sudden infant death syndrome (SIDS).

3 Both left and right side-lying positions may cause stress on the suture line.

4 Although holding the infant is recommended, positioning on the caregiver's shoulder may cause friction on the suture line if the baby's head should drop forward.

284. **1** **Touching and cuddling provide a sense of well-being and relieve strain on the suture line that results from restlessness and crying.**

2 It is inappropriate to sedate an infant for its calming effect or to decrease activity.

3 Careful handling will not damage the suture line.

4 Arm movement can be controlled by applying elbow restraints to prevent the infant's hands from touching the suture line.

285. **2** **White spots (Koplik's spots) and the rash with a mucus discharge from the nose (coryza) are clinical indicators of rubeola (measles).**

1 Rubella (German measles) does not cause Koplik's spots.

3 Pertussis (whooping cough) does not cause Koplik's spots.

4 Varicella (chickenpox) does not cause Koplik's spots.

286. **1** **Rubeola (measles) starts with a discrete maculopapular rash on the face and spreads downward, eventually becoming confluent.**

2 Scaly skin occurs with eczema or dermatitis.

3 Bald patches occur with tinea capitis (ringworm).

4 Vesicular skin lesions occur with varicella (chickenpox).

287. **4** **Drying the lesions relieves the itching (pruritus). Patting the lesions will not disturb them, and calamine lotion is an effective drying agent.**

1 Mittens may minimize injury caused by scratching but will not relieve pruritus.

2 An antibiotic ointment prevents secondary infection but does not relieve the itching because it does not have a drying effect. An antibiotic requires a practitioner's order.

3 Dressings may disrupt the vesicles and lead to scar formation.

288. 1 **When all the vesicles have dried, varicella (chickenpox) is no longer transmissible; dried vesicles do not harbor the varicella virus.**

2 Dry scabs do not transmit the virus.

3 Varicella is not associated with a fever unless a bacterial complication such as pneumonia is present.

4 Vesicles that are surrounded by an areola occur in successive crops; they contain the varicella virus.

289. 1 **The estimation of the TBSA that is burned is 5.25% for each anterior portion of the arm and hand (10.5% total) and 6.5% for the upper half of the chest; 17% is the TBSA burned.**

2 12% percent is too low for the TBSA of the burns.

3 20% percent is too high for the TBSA of the burns.

4 15% percent is too low for the TBSA of the burns.

290. 4 **If there is no subsequent infection of the burned areas, wound healing should be uneventful.**

1 Although partial-thickness burns are painful, they usually heal with little or no scarring.

2 Regeneration will occur unless there is further insult to the burn injury such as infection; grafting should not be necessary.

3 Occlusive dressings may be applied to minimize the discomfort of frequent dressing changes; hydrotherapy is not required for partial-thickness burns.

291. 3 **Implementing a pain management plan is the priority action of the medical and nursing staff. There is less physiological stress when the child's pain is managed, which allows healing to occur.**

1 Although monitoring I&O is important and will be done, it is not the priority.

2 Although this is important and it will be done, pain management is the priority.

4 Although maintaining nutrition is important and will be done, it is not the priority.

292. **Answer: 1, 4, 5**

1 **The cheese increases protein intake, that is needed for tissue repair, and the crackers contain carbohydrates that provide calories for the increased metabolism.**

2 Although bread and honey increase caloric intake, they furnish little protein needed for tissue repair.

3 Although orange juice and cookies increase vitamin and fluid intake, they do not supply protein, which is needed for tissue repair.

4 **The milk in the pudding contains protein and whipped cream contains fat. The banana is high in potassium. All of these nutrients are essential for tissue repair.**

5 **Frozen yogurt contains both protein and calories.**

293. 2 **The radial pulses are a reflection of how the child is adapting to the eschar formation. Eschar is rigid and may restrict circulation, leading to loss of perfusion to the limbs.**

1 Blisters are a protective adaptation and should not be disturbed.

3 There are no data to indicate that the child has a respiratory infection.

4 Although range-of-motion exercises are important, adequate arterial perfusion is the priority.

294. 2 **These grafts use tissue from the individual's own body; there is minimal chance of rejection.**

1 This is not part of the therapy for skin grafts.

3 These grafts use tissue from genetically different members of the same species, usually a cadaver; they are used as a temporary graft.

4 This is not part of the therapy for skin grafts.

295. **Answer: 1, 3, 4**

1 **Once a sterile paper field becomes wet it allows microorganisms on the surface of the table to contaminate the field.**

2 Sterile objects below the waist are considered contaminated.

3 **A 1-inch border around the outer edge of a sterile field is considered contaminated because the edges touch the table.**

4 **Once a sterile object comes into contact with any object that is not sterile, it is no longer considered sterile.**

296. **Answer: 2, 3, 5**

1 A skin sensor is accurate as long as the instructions provided by the product are followed.

2 **Rectal temperatures are considered invasive by the preschool-age child; however, it is not the only reason to avoid taking this child's rectal temperature.**

3 **Oral temperatures are accurate, provided the child can hold the thermometer in the mouth correctly.**

4 Tympanic temperatures are accurate.

5 **Chemotherapy causes alterations in mucous membranes; a rectal thermometer may damage delicate rectal tissue.**

297. 2 **A child receiving radiation therapy usually has dry, sensitive skin; the nurse should use plain water to remove perspiration and cellular debris on the skin.**

1 Oil-based products are contraindicated because they can cause the radiation beam to scatter, resulting in tissue damage and inadequate radiation to the tumor site.

3 Soap may remove the marks on the skin that provide accurate directions for the radiation therapist; also soap is drying and should be avoided.

4 Soap may remove the marks on the skin that provide accurate directions for the radiation therapist; also soap is drying and should be avoided.

298. 4 **Soft bristles are less irritating to the oral mucosa and less likely to cause trauma than irritating substances.**

1 Baking soda can be caustic and may irritate the mucosa.

2 Mouthwash can be caustic and may irritate the mucosa.

3 Hydrogen peroxide is a caustic substance that may irritate the mucosa.

299. 4 **Pediculosis capitis (head lice) are common among enclosed groups of children in nursery and primary schools. The eggs (nits) adhere to the hair shafts about an inch from the scalp. They commonly are found behind the ears and at the nape of the neck.**

1 Brownish lines are typical of scabies, which is a mite infestation.

2 Scaly patches in areas with no hair are associated with childhood atopic dermatitis (eczema).

3 Blisters are typical of tinea capitis (ringworm), which is caused by a fungal infection.

300. 2 **Impetigo may develop as a secondary bacterial infection because of breaks in the skin from scratching.**

1 Eczema is an allergic response, not an infection.

3 Cellulitis is an extended inflammation that is not commonly found in children with pediculosis.

4 Folliculitis is a pimple or an infection of the hair follicle; it does not occur secondary to pediculosis.

301. 2 **Permethrin 5% cream (Elimite) is rubbed on all skin surfaces and left in place from 8 to 14 hours before it is washed off.**

1 Permethrin is applied once and should remain on for at least 8 hours.

3 Washing the medication off in less than 8 hours does not provide an adequate dose.

4 A week of treatment is not necessary; one liberal application usually is sufficient to be curative.

302. Answer: 3, 4, 5

1 It is not necessary to know when the child is expected back in school; this information is unrelated to the situation.

2 The child's problem is unrelated to sports activities.

3 **It is important to know if the signs and symptoms are related to a history of allergies, a communicable infection contracted during the trip, or some other factor.**

4 **The nurse must gather information regarding the duration of signs and symptoms because they can be related to a variety of factors that may or may not be related to the camping trip.**

5 **It is important to determine if the child was exposed to a known allergen so that appropriate treatment can be initiated.**

303. 3 **Telling the child that a tick bite caused the disease and it is curable is a straightforward, truthful answer at a level that a 12-year-old child will comprehend.**

1 Just identifying a feeling disregards the fact that the child has asked a question that requires an answer.

2 The child might not understand scientific terminology.

4 Telling the child not to worry is demeaning and avoids answering the question.

304. 2 **The tick must be carefully removed with tweezers or forceps so that the body and head are both removed; this technique prevents further inoculation of the individual.**

1 Using a lighted cigarette is unsafe because the child may be burned; the tick may further inoculate the individual, and the method may hurt the child.

3 Using ammonia is unsafe; the tick may further inoculate the child, and the method may hurt the child.

4 Spraying with insect repellent is unsafe; the tick may further inoculate the child, and the method may hurt the child.

305. 2 **To make effective decisions, baseline information on the child's condition, extent of the injury, and significant past health history are required.**

1 Hyperimmune antirabies serum is not a preferred treatment; it is not necessary to obtain this information.

3 Inoculation for establishment of short-term, passive immunity to rabies follows initial care of injuries; the priority is assessment and treatment of the injury.

4 Authorities should be notified after the injured child has received care.

NEUROMUSCULAR

306. 1 **Organisms that cause meningitis are often harbored in the spinal fluid. The lumbar puncture helps determine if meningitis is present and if the causative agent is bacterial or viral.**

2 Although some blood may be found in the spinal fluid, its presence is not a finding that confirms the diagnosis of meningitis.

3 More conservative measures, such as medications or positioning, are used to reduce intracranial pressure.

4 Although testing for spinal fluid glucose level may be done, it will not determine the causative agent.

307. 4 **The side-lying position with the head and hips flexed separates the vertebrae so that needle insertion is easier; also it provides for better restraint by the nurse.**

1 The sitting position is used at times for adults; it is not recommended for infants or children because of the difficulty with keeping them still.

2 The prone position prevents the head from being flexed and the spine curved outward for the insertion of the needle.

3 The lateral recumbent position is unacceptable; it does not curve the spine.

308. 1 **A positive Kernig sign is indicative of meningitis; it is demonstrated by a spasm of the hamstring muscles when the legs are extended.**

2   A positive Babinski reflex is a dorsiflexion and fanning of the toes resulting from stroking the sole of the foot; adults with neuromuscular impairment and healthy infants exhibit this sign.

3   Chvostek sign is elicited by tapping on the facial nerve in the region of the parotid gland; spasm indicates tetany.

4   In a male, the cremasteric reflex is elicited by stroking on the inner thigh causing the testes to retract into the scrotal sac.

309. 4   **The meningococcal organism is rendered inactive after 24 to 72 hours of antibiotic therapy; isolation is not required after this time.**

1   Meningitis is not evident during the incubation period.

2   The presence of a fever is not the influencing factor indicating the need for isolation.

3   After the diagnosis of meningitis is confirmed, isolation is required for 24 to 72 hours after the institution of antibiotic therapy.

310. 1   **Droplet precautions reduce the transmission of infection from the child to other individuals (cross-infection). The microorganisms are transmitted to others via respiratory droplets.**

2   Droplet precautions do not interrupt the infectious process; they protect those in contact with the child from contracting the infection.

3   Droplet precautions do not protect the child from developing secondary infections; they protect others from being exposed to the child's pathogens.

4   Thorough handwashing and aseptic techniques, not droplet precautions, limit hospital-acquired infections.

311. 2   **Physical contact provides security for a distressed infant.**

1   Feeding to provide comfort is not always an option because the infant may have been fed recently, be anorexic, or be NPO.

3   Music may not always have a calming influence because infants frequently are not aware of the environment.

4   A quiet environment may not always have a calming influence because infants frequently are not aware of the environment.

312. 4   **Down syndrome (trisomy 21) results from extra chromosomal material on chromosome 21.**

1   Down syndrome does not result from a maternal infection.

2   Down syndrome is not related to an X-linked or Y-linked gene.

3   An autosomal recessive gene is not the cause of Down syndrome, although translocation of chromosomes 15 and 21 or 22 is a genetic aberration found in some children with Down syndrome.

313. 3   **Many children with Down syndrome have cardiac anomalies, most often ventricular septal defects, that can be life threatening.**

1   Renal disease is not a characteristic finding in children with Down syndrome.

2   Hepatic defects are not a characteristic finding in children with Down syndrome.

4   Endocrine gland malfunction is not a characteristic finding in children with Down syndrome.

314. 3   **Failure of neural tube closure during the first 3 to 5 weeks of fetal development results in neural tube defects. Myelomeningocele is the most severe form; these children usually have lower extremity and bladder dysfunction.**

1   Hydrocephalus can occur after the repair of either a meningocele or a myelomeningocele.

2   A saclike cyst containing meninges and spinal fluid may be present in either defect.

4   Infection is possible with either defect because of the exposure of the meninges.

315. 4   **Hydrocephalus is a major complication of myelomeningocele, typically after surgical correction. Measuring the head circumference daily provides an accurate basis for a day-to-day comparison.**

1   Although important, daily weights are not specific to monitoring for developing hydrocephalus.

2   An infant's output is unrelated to hydrocephalus.

3   Vital signs should be taken every 2 to 4 hours after surgery.

316. 1   **A tense or bulging fontanel is indicative of increased intracranial pressure, which is caused by the fluid accumulation associated with hydrocephalus.**

2   Conjugate gaze does not occur until 3 to 4 months of age when eye muscles are mature.

3   The head is the largest part of the body at this age; the head circumference should be about 1 inch larger than the chest.

4   An infant cannot support the head before 1 to 1½ months of age.

317. 1   **Because the infant cannot be held, tactile stimulation helps meet the infant's needs and fosters bonding with the parents.**

2   An infant with an unrepaired myelomeningocele cannot be held in the arms.

3   Referrals will be more appropriate at a later time.

4   Although special feeding techniques are important in the postoperative period, they may not improve the parent-infant relationship.

318. 4   **The parents must be taught to identify signs of increased intracranial pressure because this can develop if shunt malfunction occurs; immediate intervention is essential.**

1   The prone position places too much pressure on the shunt; the infant should be flat and turned onto the unaffected side.

2   Dry, sterile dressings are applied postoperatively to prevent infection.

3   Cerebrospinal fluid is not expected to drain from the incision.

319. 4 **The side-lying position on the unoperated side and use of supports avoid pressure on the shunt; the horizontal position prevents too rapid drainage of cerebrospinal fluid.**
    1 This is unsafe. Placing the infant in any position is inappropriate in the immediate postoperative period.
    2 Neck supports should not be used for infants because they flex the neck, which may cause airway occlusion.
    3 The prone position is contraindicated; the head turned to the side puts pressure on the shunt.

320. 1 **Marked irritability may be a sign of malfunction of the shunt or infection and should be reported immediately.**
    2 Complaints of pain are expected after surgery.
    3 A low-grade fever is expected after the stress of surgery.
    4 A pulse rate of 100 beats per minute is within the expected range (70 to 110) for children between the ages of 2 and 10 years.

321. 4 **After the initial safety measures and notification of the practitioner, documentation is a priority; continued monitoring is essential.**
    1 Covering the infant will increase the temperature because heat loss will be reduced; excess clothing should be removed.
    2 Alcohol should never be used for infants or children; it causes severe chilling, which can lead to increased metabolic activity and a higher temperature.
    3 This high fever requires more frequent readings; usually at least every hour or less.

322. 3 **Children with cerebral palsy are especially prone to muscle tone disorders, including spasticity, which can lead to joint contractures.**
    1 The therapy program must be balanced to promote progress in all areas of growth and development.
    2 Splinting limbs is contraindicated because immobility promotes the development of joint contractures.
    4 Although these infants tend to gag and choke during feedings, a special formula is not necessary unless there is an allergy to dairy products.

323. 4 **The athetoid type of cerebral palsy (CP) consists of slow, wormlike, writhing movements.**
    1 The ataxic type of CP is characterized by rapid, repetitive movements.
    2 The spastic type of CP is characterized by hypertonicity of muscles.
    3 The dystonic type of CP is a combination of the spastic and athetoid types.

324. 3 **The infant is too young for specific long-term plans; different problems may manifest as the child grows older.**
    1 Children with cerebral palsy may or may not have cognitive impairments.

2 Cerebral palsy does not get progressively worse; placement outside the home depends on the child's needs and the parents' abilities and desires.
    4 There is no relationship between cerebral palsy and a lowered immune response.

325. 3 **Safety is the priority during the seizure. The child should not be touched except to maintain safety; removing objects that may harm the child is the priority.**
    1 It is unsafe to leave the child having the seizure.
    2 Attempting to open clenched jaws during a seizure may result in injury to the child's teeth and jaw.
    4 The supine position may prevent the drainage of secretions and a pillow may cause airway occlusion by flexing the neck.

326. 3 **The clonic phase of a tonic-clonic seizure is associated with the rapid rhythmic extension and relaxation of muscle groups throughout the body.**
    1 Rigidity occurs during the tonic phase of a seizure.
    2 Loss of consciousness is not specific to the clonic phase; it occurs at the beginning of the tonic phase and continues into the clonic phase.
    4 The movements during the clonic episode are more marked than the movements of a tremor and occur throughout the body, not just the extremities.

327. Answer: 1, 3, 4
    1 **Therapeutic management is based on an accurate description of the seizure.**
    2 It is impossible to take vital signs during a seizure.
    3 **Placing the child onto the side allows for drainage of secretions that cannot be swallowed during the seizure.**
    4 **The first safety precaution is to prevent injury by raising the padded side rails.**
    5 Administering oxygen is useless because the child does not breathe during a seizure.

328. 3 **An inward moving eye (tropia) is one form of strabismus.**
    1 A drooping eyelid is called ptosis; it may be congenital or caused by trauma.
    2 Cloudy eyes are associated with congenital cataracts.
    4 Blinking eyes may be a tic.

329. 1 **Cosmetic improvement is a major goal for children because with crossed eyes they may be teased by their peers.**
    2 The child may still need glasses because surgery does not always correct the defect and there may be other visual problems.
    3 Strabismus does not affect vision to the extent of blindness.
    4 Peripheral vision is intact with strabismus.

330. 2 **Behavioral disturbances such as clumsiness are important clues to early identification of lead poisoning.**
    1 Nosebleeds (epistaxis) are not a clinical sign of lead poisoning.

3   Excessive salivation is not a clinical sign of lead poisoning.

4   Bradycardia is not a clinical sign of lead poisoning.

331. 2   **Adequate hydration is needed because the lead complexes, released during chelation therapy, are excreted by the kidneys.**

1   There is no basis for restricting salt in the diet of children with lead poisoning.

3   There is no basis for restricting refined sugar and flour except for improving the nutrition of all children.

4   There is no reason to increase caloric intake unless the child is underweight; it is unnecessary to restrict protein.

332. 3   **Percodan is a combination drug that contains aspirin as well as oxycodone. Aspirin should not be given after surgery because it affects platelets, prolonging bleeding. In addition, it should not be given to children because it is associated with the occurrence of Reye syndrome. Also it is available only in tablet form, which is difficult to administer to a toddler.**

1   Acetaminophen (Tylenol) is not contraindicated for a child who had oral surgery.

2   Codeine is not contraindicated for a child who had oral surgery.

4   Morphine is not contraindicated for a child who had oral surgery.

333. 3   **There is a strong relationship between Reye syndrome and an antecedent viral infection, especially if treated with aspirin.**

1   A rash is not specifically related to Reye syndrome.

2   Tonsillitis is not specifically related to Reye syndrome.

4   High fevers are not specifically related to Reye syndrome.

334. 4   **It is known that Reye syndrome is related to a febrile viral illness and the ingestion of aspirin as an antipyretic. There is no specific therapy and care is based on treating signs and symptoms.**

1   Reye syndrome is not a genetic disorder.

2   Reye syndrome is not caused by a bacterium.

3   Although the etiology is obscure, its relationship between a febrile viral illness and the ingestion of aspirin as an antipyretic has been documented.

335. 2   **Black lines on the teeth at the gumline are a common finding in lead poisoning (plumbism) attributable to the deposition of lead.**

1   Perthes disease is characterized by pain and hip dysfunction.

3   Salicylate toxicity affects the eighth cranial nerve, causing tinnitus.

4   Neonatal tetracycline administration may cause yellow-brown discoloration of the teeth.

336. 4   **Deaf infants commonly babble until they are 6 months old; if they cannot hear, their vocalizations are not reinforced and they often stop at this time.**

1   Learning to say one word starts at about 11 to 12 months of age.

2   Infants with no hearing impairment do not respond to their name all the time.

3   The Moro reflex is not expected at 7 months; it usually disappears when the infant is 3 to 4 months old.

337. 1   **It is important to determine the infant's feeding patterns because drinking formula from a bottle while in a recumbent position may lead to pooling of fluid in the pharyngeal cavity, which hinders eustachian tube drainage.**

2   Although knowing the frequency of the infection is important, the factor that precipitated the otitis media is more significant.

3   Although it is important to ascertain what medication is taken for otitis media, it is more important to determine its cause.

4   Asking about the other family members is irrelevant because otitis media is an inflammatory response, not an hereditary-related disease.

338. 2   **The incision allows for drainage, which produces relief of pressure and results in immediate relief of pain.**

1   This incision does not leave a scar because healing by primary intention occurs within 24 hours.

3   A myringotomy is performed to prevent the trauma of perforation.

4   The incision is small and heals spontaneously within 24 hours.

339. 2   **Positioning with the affected ear down facilitates drainage by gravity.**

1   Frequent swallowing after a tonsillectomy, not a myringotomy, may be a sign of bleeding.

3   Bleeding is rare and should not occur from this type of incision.

4   Pain is not expected and should be reported if it occurs.

340.   Answer: 1, 2

1   **Lack of drainage may indicate the need for a repeat myringotomy because promoting drainage is the reason for the surgery.**

2   **Pain occurs if drainage is not flowing through the incision; a repeat myringotomy may be needed.**

3   Bleeding is not expected in otitis media or after a myringotomy.

4   Hearing loss is characteristic of otitis media and does not indicate a complication.

5   Fever is not an expected complication of a myringotomy.

341.   Answer 2, 3, 4

1   Swallowing should not be affected because this ability is not related to the operative area.

2   **Adenoids can obstruct nasal breathing, interfering with the sense of taste. After surgery the sense of taste should improve.**

3 Adenoids can obstruct nasal breathing, interfering with the sense of smell. After surgery the sense of smell should improve.

4 Adenoids can obstruct nasal breathing, causing speech to have the typical adenoid sound After surgery the quality of speech should improve.

342. 4 **Range-of-motion exercises are essential to help achieve the primary objectives of maintaining optimum muscle function for as long as possible and preventing the development of contractures.**

1 A high-calorie diet can result in obesity, which may accelerate the time when a wheelchair will be necessary.

2 Seizures are not associated with Duchenne muscular dystrophy.

3 Restricting the use of large muscles can result in disuse atrophy and contractures.

343. 4 **Muscular degeneration is advanced in the adolescent. The disease process involves the diaphragm, auxiliary muscles of respiration, and the heart, resulting in life-threatening respiratory infections and heart failure.**

1 Central nervous system functioning is not affected by Duchenne muscular dystrophy.

2 The integumentary system is not affected.

3 Nutritional problems related to the gastrointestinal system are less significant than cardiopulmonary problems.

344. 3 **A headache is a sign of increased intracranial pressure; lying supine increases the blood flow to the brain, adding to the brain and tumor mass.**

1 There is no evidence that the child is fasting; however, if this were so she would complain of hunger and perhaps a headache, at times other than when she was in the supine position.

2 Although children at this age still suffer from a milder form of separation anxiety, the child's behavior does not indicate this type of anxiety.

4 Although children of this age fear mutilation, the child's behavior does not indicate this fear.

345. **Answer: 2, 3**

1 This is unsafe. The child should not be fed until the practitioner reassesses the child.

2 **When there are signs of increasing intracranial pressure the practitioner must be notified.**

3 **When there are signs of increasing intracranial pressure the child should be reassessed by the practitioner.**

4 If the cause of the vomiting is increased intracranial pressure, antiemetics are not effective.

5 There is no indication that an IV is in place and increasing an IV flow rate is a dependent function of the nurse. Also additional fluids may further increase intracranial pressure.

346. 2 **Motor function is part of a neurological assessment and provides information about cerebral functioning.**

1 Blood pressure is not a direct measure of neurological status.

3 Temperature is not a direct measure of neurological status.

4 Head circumference provides information as to skeletal development and brain growth, not neurological data. A change in head circumference as a result of increased intracranial pressure is not expected in a 4-year-old whose cranial bones are fused.

347. 2 **Raising the foot of the bed increases blood flow to the brain, thereby increasing intracranial pressure.**

1 Temperature elevations may occur after a craniotomy because of stimulation of the hypothalamus. A hypothermic blanket should be ready if the temperature becomes precipitously elevated.

3 Monitoring vital signs is a critical component of postoperative care.

4 IV infusions must be regulated precisely to minimize the possibility of cerebral edema.

348. 3 **Pressure on the hypothalamus, the temperature-regulating mechanism of the brain, causes temperature imbalances.**

1 Infection after surgery is not expected, even if the child has diabetes; infection occurs when there is a break in aseptic technique.

2 After an operation, a temperature caused by an inflammatory response rarely exceeds 101° F; a high fever is not expected after surgical procedures.

4 Viscid secretions do not cause an elevated temperature unless an infection is present.

349. 2 **Immobilization of the spine is most important to minimize additional injury while the child is being assessed.**

1 Placing a pillow under the head is contraindicated because the vertebral column and spinal cord might move, resulting in additional damage to the spinal cord.

3 Log-rolling is unsafe without first immobilizing the spine.

4 Moving the child without first immobilizing the spine is unsafe.

350. **Answer: 2, 4**

1 Because there is no change warranting care by health professionals, hospitalization is unnecessary.

2 **A decreasing level of consciousness is a sign of neurological impairment, and medical attention is required.**

3 Telling the mother not to worry is false reassurance; a change in the child's condition is possible.

4 **Telling the mother why she should awaken her son during the night reassures her that there is no danger in allowing the child to sleep as long as responsiveness is periodically evaluated.**

351. 3 **A declining level of consciousness (LOC) reflects increased intracranial pressure precipitated by injury to the brain.**
  1 Ocular signs are less definitive for increased intracranial pressure than a lowered LOC.
  2 Muscular strength is less definitive for increased intracranial pressure than a lowered LOC.
  4 Injuries on the scalp do not cause increased intracranial pressure because the injuries are outside the cranium.

352. 3 **Motor responses are tested by strength of hand grasps, movement, and strength of upper and lower extremities.**
  1 Drawing is used for assessing hand-eye coordination.
  2 Balancing on one foot is part of the Romberg test; it helps evaluate cerebellar integrity.
  3 Gait and posture are indicators of cerebellar integrity.

353. 1 **Evidence of a subdural hemorrhage may take hours or days to develop; a decreasing level of consciousness is an early indication of neurological damage.**
  2 Although promoting rest is important, early recognition of neurological damage is the priority.
  3 Taking a history at this time is not appropriate nor is it a priority.
  4 Administering an opioid is contraindicated because it may mask the signs and symptoms of increasing neurological injury.

354. 3 **Children who are mentally challenged can learn concrete concepts faster than they can learn abstract concepts.**
  1 Love vs. hate is an abstract concept that children begin to learn between the ages of 7 and 11 years.
  2 Life vs. death is an abstract concept that children begin to learn between the ages of 7 and 11 years.
  4 Right vs. wrong is an abstract concept that children begin to learn between the ages of 7 and 11 years.

355. 1 **During the preschool years speech dysfluency is a typical characteristic of language development; it will resolve if the child is spoken to clearly and is not corrected.**
  2 Avoiding eye contact is demeaning; it may decrease self-esteem and increase stuttering.
  3 Supplying the correct word is demeaning; it may decrease self-esteem and increase stuttering.
  4 Drawing attention to the stuttering is demeaning; it may decrease self-esteem and increase the stuttering.

RESPIRATORY

356. 2 **Continuous assessments are vital to determine the infant's oxygenation and hydration status and responses to the disease process.**
  1 The infant needs the parents' presence to enhance the developmental goal of infancy, the establishment of trust.

  3 Respiratory syncytial virus (RSV) is the most common etiology of bronchiolitis in an infant. Contact precautions are recommended for an infant with bronchiolitis; airborne precautions are not necessary.
  4 The infant is too ill to be involved in stimulating activities; energy should be conserved and oxygen demands kept at a minimum.

357. 2 **Administering oxygen via nasal cannula limits the energy required for breathing; this allows the child to conserve energy that can be used for fluid and nutrient intake.**
  1 Congealed mucus will obstruct air passageways and increase respiratory distress.
  3 Oxygen administration does not trigger the cough reflex.
  4 Oxygen administration through a nasal cannula will have a drying effect.

358. 3 **Cool mist provides humidification.**
  1 Postural drainage probably will increase the child's anxiety.
  2 There is no relationship between eating and the onset of spasmodic croup.
  4 It is useless to attempt to give instruction while the child is fighting to inhale air.

359. 1 **Swelling and edema in airways with small diameters lead to the signs and symptoms of croup.**
  2 It is the small airways that become edematous that cause the problem, not mouth breathing.
  3 An immature immune system is too general a statement; it depends on the specific resistance of the individual child.
  4 This causative factor does not explain why only small children get croup.

360. 1 **The medulla oblongata contains the respiratory center, and the neurons that supply the respiratory muscles originate here; they produce the rhythmic pattern of inspiration and expiration.**
  2 The cerebellum helps control skeletal muscles.
  3 The hypothalamus links the nervous system to the endocrine system and functions as a relay station between the cerebral cortex and lower autonomic centers.
  4 The cerebral cortex is unrelated to respirations. The cerebral cortex is the thin layer of gray matter on the surface of the cerebrum that integrates higher mental functions.

361. 4 **A catheter that is larger than half the diameter of the child's trachea can block the airway.**
  1 Although the child should be hyperoxygenated before suctioning, this procedure does not affect the trachea.
  2 The practice of instilling sterile saline into the tracheostomy tube before suctioning is outdated and potentially harmful.

3 Using negative pressure when inserting the suction catheter may traumatize the trachea.

362. 3 **Because the cause of the child's diagnosis has not been determined, airborne precautions should be instituted.**

1 Droplet precautions are inadequate because they do not include airborne precautions.

2 The child's adaptations do not warrant the need for contact precautions.

4 Neutropenic precautions protect an immunosuppressed child from exposure to microorganisms from others.

363. 2 **The presence of abdominal viscera in the thoracic cavity impinges on the lungs and affects their ability to expand, thus limiting the amount of air that can enter the lungs and alveoli. In addition, these newborns tend to have underdeveloped lungs.**

1 An incarcerated hernia, although a medical emergency, does not impair gas exchange on a long-term basis.

3 The basal metabolic rate is not increased with a diaphragmatic hernia.

4 Excessive secretions do not occur with a diaphragmatic hernia.

364. 4 **The supine position keeps pressure off the operative site. Elevating the head of the bed allows the abdominal organs to move downward away from the diaphragm, promoting respiratory excursion.**

1 Using a contour seat will not promote maximal aeration of the lungs because hip flexion adds tension to the abdominal muscles.

2 Placing the infant onto the unoperated side limits gas exchange in the lung on the unoperated side.

3 The prone position increases the effort of breathing because respiratory excursion is impeded by the weight of the body.

365. 4 **Bilateral breath sounds indicate that the lungs are expanded and functioning.**

1 Lack of crying is not a reliable indicator that the respiratory status is improving; it may indicate that the infant is hypoxic and too fatigued to cry.

2 An expected pH is 7.35 to 7.45; a decreasing pH indicates respiratory acidosis, which can be attributed to decreased gas exchange.

3 Retention of formula is unrelated to gas exchange.

366. 2 **When the chest was opened during surgery for the sternal repair, air entered the thorax; the air must be removed to allow the lungs to reexpand.**

1 Chest tubes may be uncomfortable; also this response discounts the importance of the chest tube to the infant's respiratory status.

3 The tube was inserted for a specific reason; the infant should not be subjected to this discomfort without a specific purpose for the tube's insertion.

4 Placement of the chest tube is unrelated to the infant's ability to retain feedings.

367. 3 **The airway must be cleared of secretions for effective air exchange.**

1 Taking vital signs is unsafe because valuable time is lost while the infant's brain is deprived of oxygen.

2 Oxygenation is ineffective if secretions are not first cleared from the airway.

4 The side-lying position assists in promoting drainage of secretions only after the airway is cleared.

368. 3 **The course of action is to empty the fluid from the tubing and reconnect it because accumulated fluid may flood the trachea.**

1 Removing condensation from the tubing does not require help from a physician's assistant; the nurse or respiratory therapist, depending on hospital protocol, is responsible for this remedial action.

2 Humidity is necessary to preserve moistness of the respiratory tract.

4 The amount of condensation is irrelevant in terms of recording intake and output.

369. **Answer 1, 3, 5**

1 **Bronchiolitis in most infants is caused by the respiratory syncytial virus (RSV). Wheezing occurs as the air passages narrow resulting in the typical whistling sound.**

2 As a result of increased respiratory effort and decreased oxygen exchange, tachycardia, not bradycardia, develops.

3 **As breathing becomes more difficult, the infant must expend more energy and use accessory muscles of respiration to breathe.**

4 Breath sounds are diminished because of edema of the bronchiolar mucosa and filling of the lumina with mucus and exudate.

5 **The infectious and inflammatory changes narrow the bronchial passage, making it difficult for air to leave the lungs.**

370. 2 **Heat and inhaled smoke-related irritants may cause fluid to shift from the intravascular compartment into the interstitial compartment, resulting in edema, which obstructs the airway.**

1 Although monitoring for infection is important, a patent airway is the priority.

3 Although monitoring for posttraumatic stress disorder is important, this might occur later and maintaining a patent airway is the priority.

4 Although monitoring for physical and emotional responses to stress is important, maintaining a patent airway is the priority.

371. 3 **The child may have inhalation burns; respiratory tract injury may result in edema, causing an airway obstruction.**

1 An increase in temperature indicates the presence of an infection. It is too early for an infection to occur.

2 Increased activity is promising because it indicates that the burns were not severe.

4 Edema distal to burns of the extremities is expected.

372. 4 Research has identified that the presence of the common household cockroach is an allergen that can trigger an asthmatic attack in susceptible children.

1 The spider is not identified as an allergen for children who are prone to asthmatic attacks.

2 The centipede is not identified as an allergen for children who are prone to asthmatic attacks.

3 The carpenter ant is not identified as an allergen for children who are prone to asthmatic attacks.

373. 2 Audible wheezing that is heard without a stethoscope is an indication that the airways are significantly compromised; this requires immediate medical intervention.

1 Barrel chest is a sign of chronic asthma. Repeated attacks result in a fixed hyperaerated thoracic cavity; this clinical finding does not require intervention.

3 A heart rate of 105 beats per minute is expected in an 8-year-old child.

4 A respiratory rate of 30 breaths per minute is expected in an 8-year-old child.

374. 1 The goal for teaching a child with asthma breathing exercises is to lengthen expiratory time and expiratory pressure. This activity focuses on inhalation, not exhalation.

2 Singing songs with long phrases forces the child to exhale until each phrase is completed.

3 Activities such as puffing through a straw encourage exhalation.

4 Activities such as blowing through a pipe encourage exhalation.

375. 4 Hardwood floors can be cleansed more easily than rugs. They are more hypoallergenic than outdoor carpeting.

1 Stuffed toys are frequent sources of dust and mold.

2 Out-of-season clothing harbors dust and should not be stored in the allergic child's room.

3 Using a plastic slipcover reduces the child's exposure to dust generated by the mattress.

376. 1 Albuterol (Proventil) relaxes smooth muscles in the respiratory tract, resulting in bronchodilation. The priority is to facilitate respirations. This intervention follows the ABCs of emergency care—Airway, Breathing, Circulation.

2 Obtaining a blood specimen is not the priority. The results will not influence the priority intervention.

3 Notifying the respiratory therapist is not the priority. Chest physical therapy is performed after the respiratory airways are opened. In many facilities chest physical therapy is the responsibility of the nurse, not a respiratory therapist.

4 The use of an incentive spirometer can be taught after the acute episode of respiratory distress. It will take time to receive the device and teach the child regarding its use. It should be used after the respiratory airways are opened.

377. 4 To obtain the peak expiratory flow rate (PEFR), a peak expiratory flow meter (PEFM) is used. This is an objective tool that measures the maximum flow of air that can be forcefully exhaled in 1 second. The PEFM individualizes data for the child because after a personal best value is established, this baseline can be compared with current values to determine progress or lack of progress regarding the child's respiratory status.

1 Although auscultating breath sounds may be done, it is not as objective as a PEFR result.

2 Although monitoring the child's respiratory pattern may be done, it is not as objective as a PEFR result.

3 Although assessing the color of the lips may be done, it is not as objective as a PEFR result.

378. 3 Dysfunction of the exocrine glands leads to mucus that is thicker and more tenacious than expected. The characteristics of the mucus contribute to pooling in the lungs and difficult expectoration. In addition to airway obstruction, these children are more likely to have respiratory infections.

1 Airway irritability is associated with hyperactive airway disease.

2 Inflamed lung parenchyma is associated with pneumonia; this a secondary complication related to stasis of secretions.

4 The endocrine glands are not directly affected in cystic fibrosis.

379. 3 Chest physiotherapy is done midway between feedings to lessen the risk of vomiting and to increase drainage, which is then suctioned.

1 Doing chest physiotherapy before feedings will tire the infant and can lead to inadequate nutritional intake.

2 Chest physiotherapy during a feeding is contraindicated because the infant may vomit and aspirate.

4 Doing chest physiotherapy after feedings may cause the infant to vomit and aspirate.

380. 2 There is more than one gene that can cause cystic fibrosis (CF); genetic analysis is done to test for known alleles.

1 The results of a chest x-ray will not determine whether the individual is a carrier of CF; this may be one of the tests that are conducted when an individual is suspected of having CF.

3 A sweat chloride test is done to diagnose CF, not to determine whether the adolescent is a carrier

4 CF does not result from a chromosomal anomaly.

381. 2 Repeated infections in children with cystic fibrosis, over time, contribute to the development of insulin resistance and the development of type 1 diabetes.

1 Increased irritability is not related to chronic infections.

3 Changes in academic ability are not related to chronic infections.

4 Bone marrow depression is not related to chronic infections.

382. 3 **The oxygen concentration must be closely monitored to minimize side effects.**
    1 Oxygen does not ignite and is not flammable, but it supports fire.
    2 Oxygen is not warmed before administration; it is cool when routinely administered.
    4 Oxygen is considered a medication and therefore must be prescribed when administered routinely.

383. 3 **A child will more likely enjoy using an incentive spirometer as a game rather than using deep breathing techniques as a chore. Children learn best by doing.**
    1 Showing the child a pamphlet is not as effective as practicing the technique.
    2 Blowing focuses on exhalation rather than inhalation; inhalation is more desirable because it expands the lungs, which helps prevent atelectasis.
    4 Showing the child a videotape is not as effective as practicing the technique.

384. 4 **The side-lying position will allow emesis or other obstructive fluid to drain from the mouth and prevent aspiration.**
    1 Tongue blade insertion will not prevent aspiration.
    2 Nasotracheal suction used routinely will traumatize the posterior pharynx and trachea; suctioning should be used only if needed.
    3 The supine position predisposes the child to aspiration of blood, mucus, or vomitus.

385. 1 **Capillary beds are closest to the surface in a finger or earlobe; this proximity allows for accurate measurement of the arterial oxygen saturation.**
    2 The pulse oximeter is designed for use on a finger, earlobe, or toe, not on the abdomen or upper thigh.
    3 Rotating sites is unnecessary.
    4 An instant accurate readout is obtained with a pulse oximeter.

386. 1 **The degree of hypoxia the child experienced will determine the extent of neurological, liver, and renal damage.**
    2 The child was hypothermic, not hyperthermic.
    3 Although emotional trauma can be overwhelming, it usually does not influence the ultimate physical prognosis as does the extent of the hypoxia.
    4 Although aspiration pneumonia may be severe initially, it does not result in long-term sequelae as does the extent of the hypoxia.

387. 3 **An upright position helps prevent aspiration; gravity facilitates movement of food down the esophagus and into the stomach. Metal tableware is safer than plastic tableware because it is unbreakable. Encouraging participation, with socialization, and treating the child with dignity should be part of the meal.**
    1 Although the child might assume an upright position, using a syringe is a form of forced feeding; in addition, the child should be encouraged to eat solid foods.

    2 Feeding in the supine position puts the child at risk for aspiration and choking.
    4 Solid, not chopped, food should be encouraged. A mentally challenged child can easily bite down on plastic tableware and cause it to break. An upright position helps prevent aspiration.

388. 2 **The gag reflex is elicited by pressing on the posterior pharynx, resulting in glossopharyngeal stimulation; inserting the tongue blade on the side of the mouth limits this stimulation.**
    1 Although preventing damage to the rear teeth is important, it is not the reason for inserting the tongue blade on the side of the tongue.
    3 The probability of obstructing the airway is minimal, especially in a conscious child.
    4 This is not the purpose of placing the tongue blade to the side of the child's tongue. By avoiding the gag reflex with this technique, the throat will be visualized.

389. 1 **Infants younger than 1 year of age who develop an airway obstruction should be held with the head down and given five back blows. If the obstruction is not removed, the infant is turned and given five chest thrusts. This is done alternately until the obstruction is dislodged or the infant becomes unconscious.**
    2 Infants and children should not have blind finger-sweeps because the finger may push the obstruction farther down the pharynx or trachea.
    3 The abdominal thrust (Heimlich maneuver) is the first action for children older than 1 year and adults.
    4 If the infant becomes unconscious a modified head-tilt–chin-lift is done before initiating resuscitation.

REPRODUCTIVE AND GENITOURINARY

390. 2 **Dark, frothy urine is characteristic of a child with nephrotic syndrome; large amounts of protein in the urine cause it to have a dark, frothy appearance.**
    1 The child may be somewhat, not severely, lethargic.
    3 Blood pressure is normal or decreased; hypertension is associated with glomerulonephritis.
    4 Children with nephrotic syndrome usually have a pale complexion and are not flushed and ruddy in appearance.

391. 3 **The low-Fowler position decreases pressure on the diaphragm from the abdominal organs and the ascites, thereby increasing respiratory excursion.**
    1 Frequent feedings may lead to fatigue and increased respirations, which will further distress the child.
    2 Placing the child in a well-ventilated room will not alleviate the cause of the respiratory problem, which is pressure on the diaphragm from the ascites.
    4 Oxygen therapy is not necessary; the dyspnea results from pressure on the diaphragm, not lack of oxygen.

392. **3 Severe edema is usually present and changes of position are necessary to prevent skin breakdown.**
    1 A high-protein diet should be offered, although there is no evidence that it alters the outcome of the disorder. A low-protein diet is used for children with azotemia resulting from renal failure.
    2 Fluids are not encouraged and may even be curtailed during periods of edema.
    4 Active play periods are permitted during remission but not during the acute phase; these children tend to self-limit energy expenditure.

393. **3 A child with nephrotic syndrome is at risk for infection. The child with thalassemia is noninfectious and therefore is an appropriate roommate. In addition, the closeness of age will provide for preschool socialization.**
    1 Impetigo is caused by a pathogen; the child with nephrotic syndrome will be exposed to infection, which should be avoided.
    2 Pneumonia is caused by a pathogen; the child with nephrotic syndrome will be exposed to infection, which should be avoided.
    4 Conjunctivitis is caused by a pathogen; the child with nephrotic syndrome will be exposed to infection, which should be avoided.

394. **1 The massive edema, typical of nephrotic syndrome, predisposes the child to skin breakdown.**
    2 The child requires more fluid than 4 ounces each shift to maintain hydration.
    3 Carbohydrates and proteins are not restricted.
    4 Children with nephrotic syndrome usually do not receive blood transfusions.

395. **1 Weight gain is not expected when a child with nephrotic syndrome is discharged. Weight gain must be monitored carefully and reported to the practitioner because it can be indicative of an accumulation of fluid and an exacerbation of the nephrosis.**
    2 Steroids are given with food or milk to prevent gastric irritation.
    3 Testing the urine for protein helps determine whether kidney function is impaired.
    4 The child should be monitored for periorbital edema.

396. **1 The anemia associated with renal failure accounts for the pallor and decreased energy; the decreased appetite and decreased energy are related to the accumulation of toxic wastes.**
    2 Excessive activity should not cause the signs and symptoms identified by the mother if the child is in remission.
    3 An elevated temperature probably will be present with an infection; an infection does not cause a muddy pallor.
    4 Discontinuing the corticosteroids and diuretics, if prescribed, might result in a recurrence of edema in the steroid-dependent child; it is not a sign of renal failure.

397. **3 Lengthening the time between each voiding is a short-term goal that can be measured in increments of 1 or more hours between each voiding.**
    1 There are no data to indicate that the child has a groin rash.
    2 Remaining continent is a long-term goal.
    4 Enhanced self-esteem is a long-term goal and can be measured only indirectly by evaluating behavior.

398. **4 Sterile nonadherent dressings help prevent infection and ulceration of the surrounding skin as well as keep the covering from adhering to the mucosa.**
    1 Seepage of urine will prevent ointment from remaining on the exposed mucosa; also, ointment may irritate the mucosa and result in bleeding.
    2 A urine collector will not adhere because of the moist environment; also, the adhesive backing will be irritating to the skin.
    3 Warm moist compresses are contraindicated because they increase the moisture and temperature in the area, which will enhance the growth of microorganisms and the potential for infection.

399. **Answer: 3, 4, 1, 2**
    Kinking or twisting of the tubing can result in an obstruction of urine flow; the parents can solve this problem by unkinking the tube. If the tubing is not kinked, the bladder should be checked for distention. Slight pressure on the abdominal wall just above the bladder may increase intra-abdominal pressure promoting urine flow. Fluids should be offered because the child should be kept hydrated to produce urine. If no urine is produced within 1 hour, the practitioner should be called because the parents have been unable to solve the problem.

400. **1 The critical period of organogenesis occurs during the first trimester when fetal development is most likely to be adversely affected.**
    2 The fetus is less vulnerable after the first trimester because organ development is complete.
    3 The fetus is less vulnerable to major anomalies during the second 16 weeks because all major organ systems already are formed.
    4 At the time of implantation cellular differentiation has not occurred; the genital bud appears in the seventh week.

401. **4 The parents need to know why a circumcision should not be done. The foreskin may be needed for repair and reconstruction of the penis.**
    1 A cystotomy tube is not inserted because there is no interference with voiding.
    2 Hypospadias is not a genetic disorder, although there appears to be some evidence that it may be familial.
    3 The penis generally is wrapped in petrolatum gauze after, not before, a surgical correction for hypospadias.

402. 2 **Although analgesia is important to minimize pain, it relaxes the infant who may be immobilized to maintain the position of the urethral stent and to ensure optimum healing of the newly formed urethra.**

1 Infants are accustomed to a lack of privacy because of the need to expose the perineum and touch the genitalia when cleaning the area.

3 Fluid intake should be encouraged, not restricted.

4 The indwelling catheter is not clamped because backup pressure may disturb the suture line.

403. 4 **The presence of an uncorrected chordee can affect a child's future sexual capabilities because of the inability to penetrate the vagina.**

1 Kidney function is not affected.

2 The incidence of testicular cancer is not increased.

3 The risk of testicular torsion is not increased.

404. 4 **The smoky urine and the stated symptoms lead the nurse to suspect glomerulonephritis, which usually occurs after a recent streptococcal infection.**

1 A rash on the hands and feet is associated with scarlet fever, not glomerulonephritis.

2 Shoulder and knee pain is associated with rheumatic fever, not glomerulonephritis.

3 Weight loss generally occurs with children who have type 1 diabetes, not glomerulonephritis.

405. 3 **An elevated antistreptolysin O (ASO) titer indicates the presence of a previous streptococcal infection; levels are highest with acute glomerulonephritis, bacterial endocarditis, and scarlet fever.**

1 The sedimentation rate is elevated with glomerulonephritis; it signifies an inflammatory process.

2 Reduced serum complement (C3) activity occurs early in the disease process of glomerulonephritis; it increases as the child improves.

4 The blood urea nitrogen level is increased, not decreased, with glomerulonephritis because of impaired glomerular functioning, resulting in azotemia.

406. Answer: 1, 4, 5

1 **Anorexia occurs as a result of malaise caused by the disease process.**

2 Glycosuria is not associated with acute poststreptococcal glomerulonephritis (APSGN).

3 Hypertension, not hypotension, occurs because of impaired kidney function.

4 **An early sign of APSGN is an edematous face, especially around the eyes, caused by the retention of sodium and fluid.**

5 **Elevated creatinine and blood urea nitrogen levels reflect the presence of nitrogenous bodies especially urea in the blood (azotemia) caused by impaired glomerular filtration.**

407. 3 **The beta-hemolytic streptococcus immune complex becomes trapped in the glomerular capillary loop, causing acute poststreptococcal**

glomerulonephritis. It usually is precipitated by a localized pharyngitis.

1 Clots do not form in the small renal tubules with APSGN.

2 Prevention depends on treating an individual with a group A beta-hemolytic streptococcus infection with antibiotics to eliminate the organism before there is an immune response.

4 APSGN is an acquired, not inherited, disorder.

408. 3 **Corn, chicken, rice, apples, and milk are permitted on a low-sodium, low-potassium diet that the child should be following.**

1 Bananas and potatoes are high in potassium and pretzels are high in sodium.

2 Only the peaches are low in sodium and all but the butter are fairly high in potassium.

4 Processed foods are high in sodium and fairly high in potassium.

409. 1 **Headache, drowsiness, and vomiting can occur if the blood pressure remains elevated, leading to cerebral edema.**

2 Drowsiness, not restlessness, will occur; generalized edema and anorexia are not specific to cerebral edema.

3 Although a fever and confusion can occur, anuria is not specific to cerebral edema.

4 Although the pulse may be altered and vomiting can occur, cardiac decompensation is not related to cerebral involvement.

410. 1 **Foods high in sodium and salty treats usually are limited to control or prevent edema and/or hypertension until the child is asymptomatic.**

2 The child should not be kept active for long periods because rest is needed; the child usually does not need a long convalescence.

3 Glomerulonephritis usually does not cause such severe kidney damage that a kidney transplant is necessary.

4 The mother should contact the practitioner, not the nurse on the unit, for follow-up care.

411. Answer: 3, 4, 5

1 Lethargy occurs in children with nephrotic syndrome (NS) because the gross edema increases oxygen demands. Children with acute glomerulonephritis (AGN) become irritable and lethargic because of malaise, hypertension, and headaches.

2 Gross hematuria occurs in children with AGN because capillary lumens of the affected glomeruli become occluded, altering the permeability of the capillary membrane, which allows large molecules to pass through.

3 **The child with NS is grossly edematous because the glomerular membrane becomes permeable, leading to decreased filtration of plasma and resulting in the accumulation of fluid and sodium. Although the child with AGN has edema the**

nephritic edema is most noticeable in the face, especially around the eyes.

4 Massive proteinuria occurs mainly in children with NS because the permeable capillary membrane allows protein to be excreted by the kidneys.

5 The blood pressure of a child with NS is unchanged or may be decreased. Hypertension is typical of children with AGN most likely because of renal arteriole vasospasm.

412. 1 **Surgery before age 2 reduces concerns about body image that occurs at an older age.**

2 Maturation of testes starts about age 5; surgery should be done before maturation to prevent sterility.

3 Malignancy may develop with or without surgical correction.

4 The puboscrotal ring is not associated with the outcome of this surgical procedure.

413. 1 **Discomfort when urinating (dysuria) is a symptom of a urinary tract infection (UTI) that is common with vesicoureteral reflux. When voiding, urine is swept up the ureters and then flows back to the bladder, resulting in a residual that provides a medium for a UTI.**

2 Oliguria usually does not occur with vesicoureteral reflux.

3 Glycosuria usually does not occur with vesicoureteral reflux.

4 Proteinuria usually does not occur with vesicoureteral reflux.

414. 3 **Wilms tumor is a nephroblastoma that is first observed as an intra-abdominal mass that is firm and painless and located on one side of the abdomen.**

1 Periorbital edema is a sign of glomerulonephritis, not Wilms tumor.

2 Projectile vomiting is indicative of central nervous system problems or a gastrointestinal obstruction, not Wilms tumor.

4 A low-grade fever is a nonspecific sign of many illnesses, not necessarily Wilms tumor.

415. 4 **Because the child has one kidney, efforts to identify signs and symptoms of a urinary tract infection (UTI) must be ongoing. A UTI can compromise kidney function; therefore, it should be identified in the early stage and treated immediately.**

1 A kidney transplant is not necessary because the child has a functioning kidney.

2 Sodium usually is not restricted.

3 Fluids are not restricted; adequate fluid intake is encouraged to prevent a UTI.

416. 4 **High potassium levels can cause cardiac dysrhythmias; the expected range for serum potassium in a child is 3.4 to 4.7 mEq/L.**

1 The expected range for serum sodium is 136 to 146 mEq/L. Hyponatremia is expected with acute renal failure.

2 In a child the expected range for both total and direct bilirubin is 0.2 to 0.8.mg/dL; indirect bilirubin is 0.1 to 1.0 mg/dL. Bilirubin levels are not related to renal failure.

3 The expected range for serum creatinine is 0.3 to 0.7 mg/dL. An increase is expected with acute renal failure.

417. 4 **Taking the blood pressure on the arm with the arteriovenous fistula is contraindicated because the pressure of the inflated cuff can disrupt the integrity of the fistula.**

1 Ingesting more fluids is desirable because an inadequate fluid intake can result in dehydration and an acid-base imbalance.

2 Calling the clinic is desirable because vomiting or diarrhea can lead to dehydration and an acid-base imbalance.

3 Not only should the pulse be monitored to assess vascular functioning distal to the arteriovenous fistula, but it should be done on both extremities and the results compared.

418. 3 **The return of the dialysate solution should be clear; cloudy return dialysate solution is indicative of infection.**

1 Petechiae do not occur during dialysis treatments.

2 There is no danger of an abdominal bruit developing during dialysis.

4 Dialysis does not affect blood glucose levels.

419. 3 **This provides quiet activity that will not jeopardize placement of the peritoneal catheter; also, it is appropriate for the child's cognitive level and allows for social interaction with a peer.**

1 Chess requires cognitive abilities beyond the scope of a 7-year-old child.

2 Although constructing a model airplane is a quiet activity, it probably is too difficult for a 7-year-old to do without help from an adult.

4 Playing catch may result in displacement of the peritoneal catheter.

420. 4 **If the gonococcus organism is present in the genitourinary tract of males, a culture of the urethral exudate provides a definitive diagnosis.**

1 Fever is not a specific diagnostic tool because it occurs with other infections.

2 Although urine may contain gonococcus organisms, the urine dilutes the concentration; the organisms are more concentrated in the urethral discharge.

3 The gonococcus organism is in the genitourinary tract, not the blood; a complete blood count will not provide information to diagnose gonorrhea.

421. 2 **A chancre is the earliest sign of syphilis; a dark-field examination of the scraping will reveal the treponema organism.**

1 A rash occurs in the secondary stage of syphilis.

3 A genital discharge is associated with gonorrhea.

4 Multiple lesions are late manifestations of syphilis.

422. 2 **The condom should be positioned after the penis is erect to maintain the desired fit.**
   1 Vaseline may break down the material used for the condom; a water-based lubricant can be used.
   3 A space should be left at the tip of the penis to provide room for the ejaculate and prevent breakage of the condom.
   4 The penis should be withdrawn immediately after ejaculation while the penis is still erect; if the penis is allowed to become flaccid, semen may leak from the loose-fitting condom.

SKELETAL

423. 3 **For an optimum outcome the harness should be worn continuously; some practitioners permit its removal for bathing.**
   1 The harness should be worn continuously.
   2 Application of the harness will probably waken the infant. The harness should be worn continuously.
   4 The harness should be worn continuously; naps should not be limited.

424. 2 **Difficulty with abduction may indicate developmental dysplasia of the hip.**
   1 Flexion of extremities is a young infant's typical position when sleeping.
   3 Flat feet are an expected finding in a young infant.
   4 Failure to straighten the legs is an expected finding in a young infant.

425. 1 **The affected leg appears to be shorter because the femoral head is displaced upward.**
   2 There is a limited ability to abduct, not adduct, the affected leg.
   3 An anal stricture is not expected with developmental dysplasia of the hip.
   4 When the femoral head slips out of the acetabulum, it is easily palpable.

426. 1 **When standing and bearing weight on the affected hip, the pelvis tilts downward instead of upward, indicating a positive Trendelenburg sign.**
   2 The supine position does not accomplish the desired effect because weight bearing is needed to tilt the pelvis.
   3 The side-lying position does not accomplish the desired effect because weight bearing is needed to tilt the pelvis.
   4 The sitting position does not accomplish the desired effect because weight bearing is needed to tilt the pelvis.

427. 4 **The cartilaginous hip joints are the basis for the use of abduction devices (e.g., Pavlik harness) and spica casts when the infant is very young.**
   1 Congenital hip dysplasia does not limit ambulation for the young child, although the gait will be affected.
   2 Traction is not used to correct developmental dysplasia of the hip.

   3 Although casted infants are easier to manage than toddlers, this is not the reason for early treatment.

428. 2 **Suggesting the use of a protective nonabsorbent material is supportive, constructive, practical, and factual.**
   1 Placing a diaper above the perineal area will not protect the area beneath the perineum.
   3 Although water may or may not cause dissolution of cast material, the infant may inhale powder dust, which can cause respiratory difficulties.
   4 This negative response gives neither a suggestion nor support to the mother.

429. 1 **A foul smell from the cast usually is indicative of an infection under the cast that may be the cause of a fever.**
   2 Respirations may increase but do not become irregular with a fever.
   3 Itching around the top of the cast should not cause a fever; it may indicate neurovascular impairment.
   4 Tingling toes are not a sign of infection; this may indicate a neurovascular complication.

430. 1 **The pedal pulse cannot be palpated under a boot cast.**
   2 Assessing color of the toes is an appropriate neurovascular check and it is measurable.
   3 Assessing warmth of the toes is an appropriate neurovascular check and it is measurable.
   4 Assessing blanching of the toes is an appropriate neurovascular check and it is measurable.

431. 2 **Rough cast edges can cause skin irritation and breakdown.**
   1 Lotions applied to the skin at the edges of a cast can promote skin breakdown.
   3 The skin under the cast may become macerated from inadequate drying after water immersion.
   4 Adhesive petals will not adhere to a damp cast even if the cast is composed of fiberglass; it takes about a half-hour for it to dry.

432. 2 **Fear of falling is a common, realistic fear of a child at this age; the child should be encouraged to verbalize concerns.**
   1 The gait depends on the needs and abilities of the child; the gait used will be the one with the widest base of support.
   3 A 7-year-old child who is about to learn how to walk with crutches is not interested in how the crutch is constructed. Later, when crutch-walking is mastered, the natural curiosity of the school-age child may lead to learning the purpose of rubber tips on crutch ends.
   4 Before determining how much the child knows about crutch-walking, fears about falling must be resolved.

433. 2 **Having the crutches extend to 6 inches from the sides of the feet ensures the maximum base of support when the adolescent ambulates.**

1 Having the crutches reach to 1 inch below the axillae may cause trauma to the brachial plexus; the crutches should be 2 inches below the axillae.

3 The elbows should be flexed, not extended, when holding the crossbars.

4 Causing the shoulders to hunch indicates that the crutches are too short, resulting in trauma to the brachial plexus.

434. 4 **The crutch is positioned on the unaffected side and advanced with the affected leg; the crutch supports the body's weight while the client is walking on the affected leg.**

1 The crutch should be used on the stairs to provide a wide base and extra support when going up or down the stairs.

2 A sprained ankle should heal in less than 1 week and the crutch should no longer be needed.

3 Positioning the crutch in front of the affected foot will place that foot in a weight-bearing position without support, defeating the purpose of the crutch.

435. 4 **Moist heat increases circulation to the involved areas, thereby reducing the swelling and relieving joint pain and stiffness.**

1 Immobilization until pain is gone contributes to contracture deformity.

2 Massaging the swollen areas will aggravate the inflammation and cause more pain.

3 Supporting the knees on pillows is contraindicated because it will promote flexion contractures.

436. 3 **Severe joint pain and swelling cause the child to immobilize the affected parts for prolonged periods, resulting in joint deformities.**

1 The disease process is inflammatory but usually noninfectious.

2 Bleeding into the joints (hemarthrosis) is not part of the disease process.

4 Juvenile idiopathic arthritis is not related to the mental development of the child, but it may contribute to a physical developmental delay.

437. 1 **The exercises are done to preserve function by mobilizing restricted joint motion.**

2 Circulation is not affected by the arthritic process.

3 Exercises are done to restore joint function; they do not necessarily relieve pain.

4 Exercising does not affect the subcutaneous nodules in the joints.

438. 4 **Prolonged sitting in one position can lead to stiffness and flexion contractures and should be avoided.**

1 Riding a bicycle helps maintain joint mobility, which is advantageous.

2 Walking promotes functional movement and is beneficial.

3 Isometric exercises are beneficial because they help maintain muscle tone.

439. 1 **Cool fingers are a sign of circulatory impairment caused by the pressure of the cast; however, if both hands feel cool, it indicates some factor other than circulatory impairment is responsible.**

2 Adjusting the cast should not be done without an order.

3 Further assessment to determine the cause of temperature change is indicated before taking remedial action.

4 Further assessment is needed before informing the practitioner.

440. 4 **The dark stain indicates that there is bleeding. By circling the area, the nurse can determine that more bleeding has occurred if the stained area spreads. It is too soon to report the stain; a compound fracture may bleed initially and the site should continue to be monitored frequently.**

1 This is premature. A compound fracture may bleed initially and the site should continue to be monitored. If the stain extends beyond the initial stain, then the practitioner should be notified.

2 This is inappropriate. The blood is from inside the cast and is impossible to remove. The stain is circled with a pen to provide a baseline for future assessments.

3 The professional nurse should understand that the stain is blood, not coloring ink.

441. 1 **Injuries in various stages of healing are the classic sign of child abuse.**

2 Vitamin D deficiency can be investigated after child abuse is ruled out.

3 Osteogenesis imperfecta can be investigated after child abuse is ruled out.

4. Inadequate calcium intake can be investigated after child abuse is ruled out.

442. 1 **The child should be rolled as one unit with shoulders and hips turned at the same time to prevent injury.**

2 The crossbar is not used to turn because it may dislodge and weaken the cast.

3 The child will not be able to sit up because the cast immobilizes the hips.

4 The overhead trapeze is used for lifting, not turning.

443. 2 **A temporary prosthesis attached to a cast with a metal extension can be applied immediately after surgery this allows the adolescent to walk within several hours and helps start the adjustment process.**

1 The first dressing change usually is done by a member of the surgical team; also, this is too early to expect the adolescent to be ready to observe the surgical site.

3 Assigning the adolescent to a particular room usually is done out of necessity rather than to promote psychological adjustment.

4 It is too early to have another cancer survivor visit; this can be done later in the recovery process.

444. 3 **A pressure dressing will control hemorrhage until surgical intervention can be instituted.**
    1 A hemostat is not practical because bleeding can be internal.
    2 Although a tourniquet can be applied quickly, it may damage the residual limb.
    4 Protamine sulfate is the antidote for an excessive amount of heparin; the client is not receiving heparin.

445. 2 **Preadolescence is the time when scoliosis is most likely to become evident because of the growth spurt that occurs at this time.**
    1 Although scoliosis may occur at any age, idiopathic scoliosis, the most common type, tends to become evident during the preadolescent growth spurt.
    3 Although scoliosis may occur at any age, idiopathic scoliosis, the most common type, tends to become evident during the preadolescent growth spurt.
    4 Although scoliosis may occur at any age, idiopathic scoliosis, the most common type, tends to become evident during the preadolescent growth spurt.

446. 2 **The child is anticipating improvement; this reflects positive internal motivation, which helps maintain the child's interest and willingness to continue with the program.**
    1 Motivation may diminish if the focus is on the brother rather than the child's need to do them.
    3 The exercises are done to please the mother; this is external motivation, which is not as desirable as internal motivation.
    4 The exercises are done to please the mother; this is external motivation, which is not as desirable as internal motivation.

447. 4 **As the child grows the curvature may progress despite the exercise program. The child should be checked often because a brace or surgery may become necessary.**
    1 The younger the child is, the longer the need to exercise; the program should be continued until growth is complete.
    2 A brace may or may not be necessary; specific daily exercises may be all that are necessary to correct functional scoliosis.
    3 Surgery may not be necessary if the exercises are done regularly and the curvature is not severe. Maintaining the exercise program does not guarantee that if surgery becomes necessary it will be less involved.

448. 1 **Establishing an identity is the major developmental task of the adolescent and is related to the affirmation of self-image. To achieve this task there is a need to conform to group norms, one of which is appearance.**
    2 The type of treatment is not an issue.
    3 Although it is important to continue schooling, the effect on body image is more important.
    4 Although it is important to maintain contact with peers, the effect on body image is more important.

449. 1 **Log-rolling is necessary to prevent movement of the newly aligned and instrumented vertebrae and should be done frequently to prevent skin breakdown.**
    2 Checking the dressing is done for all postoperative clients; this action is nonspecific.
    3 Coughing and deep breathing are done by most postoperative clients; this action is nonspecific.
    4 The client who had a spinal fusion can be turned and still be protected from injury by log-rolling. Remaining in one position for 3 days can lead to skin breakdown from unrelieved pressure.

450. 2 **The nurse is using the technique of paraphrasing to encourage the adolescent to expand on personal concerns, which may relieve anxiety.**
    1 Adolescents tend to be present, not future oriented; the nurse should focus on the adolescent's present concerns.
    3 Focusing on others is not client-centered care; the nurse should focus on the adolescent.
    4 Focusing on others is not client-centered care; the nurse should focus on the adolescent.

DRUG-RELATED RESPONSES

451. 3 **The purpose of administering lactobacillus (Lactinex) is to recolonize the bacilli expelled with the diarrheal stools.**
    1 Lactobacillus does not help expel gas.
    2 Lactobacillus does not relieve pain.
    4 Lactobacillus does not have an anti-inflammatory action.

452. 1 **Diarrhea is expected; parents should be informed so that they do not become alarmed.**
    2 Reinfestation is common; the medication should be taken again in 2 weeks.
    3 The medication will not affect rectal itching; it will eliminate the pinworms, and this takes time to accomplish.
    4 All family members should take the medication because cross-contamination frequently occurs.

453. **Answer: 9.4 mL.** Use ratio and proportion to solve the problem.
    One kilogram = 2.2 pounds; 44 pounds divided by 2.2 pounds = 20 kilograms; 15 mg x 20 = 300 mg.

$$5 \text{ mL} : 160 \text{ mg} :: x : 300 \text{ mg}$$
$$160 x = 1500$$
$$x = 1500 \div 160$$
$$x = 9.375 \text{ or } 9.4 \text{ mL}$$

454. 4 **Frequent and continued use of phenylephrine (Neo-Synephrine) can cause rebound congestion of mucous membranes.**
    1 Tinnitus is not a side effect of phenylephrine nasal spray; however, hypotension, tachycardia, and tingling of the extremities may occur.

2 Nasal polyps may be associated with allergies but are unrelated to phenylephrine nasal spray.

3 Bleeding tendencies are unrelated to the use of phenylephrine nasal spray.

455. **2 Gradual weaning from predniSONE (Meticorten) is necessary to prevent adrenal insufficiency or adrenal crisis.**

1 PredniSONE depresses the immune system, thus increasing susceptibility to infection.

3 PredniSONE usually causes a suppression of growth.

4 A moon face may occur, but it is not a critical, life-threatening side effect.

456. **4 Factor VIII is administered once in the morning on designated days. The half-life of factor VIII is short. If administered later in the day, protection will not be adequate during the day when the child is most active and more vulnerable to bleeding.**

1 Administering it at bedtime will not protect the child from injury during the child's activities throughout the day.

2 Administering it after lunch will not protect the child from injury during the child's activities throughout the day.

3 Administering it before dinner will not protect the child from injury during the child's activities throughout the day.

457. **1 Intravenous administration of a steroid can cause a rapid rise in blood glucose levels. An early sign of hyperglycemia is increased urine output. Blood glucose should be monitored frequently and insulin administered as needed.**

2 Tinnitus is associated with some antibiotics and with aspirin (ASA), not steroids.

3 Drowsiness is associated with sedatives, not steroids.

4 Hypertension, not hypotension, is associated with steroid administration.

458. **2 Acetaminophen (Tylenol) is metabolized by the liver and an excess may result in an elevated aspartate aminotransferase (AST) and bilirubin levels and prothrombin time. Hepatic involvement may last up to 7 days and liver damage may be permanent.**

1 Blood gas results are not the priority at this time. They will become important if the adolescent develops hepatic failure or respiratory distress.

3 The hematological components measured in a complete blood count are not profoundly affected by an acetaminophen overdose.

4 Glycosylated hemoglobin is a measure of diabetic control, not a measure of response to an acetaminophen overdose.

459. **Answer: 50 mg.** The infant weighs 22 pounds; divide 22 by 2.2 kg to determine that the child weighs 10 kg; 10 mg/day are ordered for each kg of body weight. Solve by using ratio and proportion.

$$10 \, mg : 1 \, kg :: x \, mg : 10 \, kg$$
$$x = 10 \times 10$$
$$x = 100 \, mg/day; \text{ when divided into two doses,}$$
the infant should receive 50 mg/dose.

460. **Answer: 1, 3, 4**

1 **Children with nephrotic syndrome are grossly edematous. Those who have the steroid-sensitive form of nephrotic syndrome respond to corticosteroids by diuresing within 7 to 21 days after therapy is started and the edematous weight is lost.**

2 Steroid therapy does not affect the blood pH.

3 **Once the child feels better, lethargy decreases and the activity level increases.**

4 **Children who have the steroid-sensitive form of nephrotic syndrome respond to corticosteroids by diuresing within 7 to 21 days after therapy is started.**

5 There is no increase in the blood pressure of children with nephrotic syndrome; therefore, there is no change in blood pressure when the child improves.

461. **4 Intravenous antibiotics should be administered with doses equally spaced over 24 hours so that a constant blood level of the drug is maintained.**

1 The 12 hours between the 8 PM and 8 AM doses is too long; the blood level of the antibiotic will drop and the therapy will not be as effective.

2 The doses are not equally spaced over 24 hours, and the blood level of the antibiotic will not remain constant.

3 The doses are not equally spaced over 24 hours, and the blood level of the antibiotic will not remain constant.

462. **1 Bradycardia (pulse rate less than 90 to 110 beats per minute in infants) is an early sign of toxicity.**

2 Additional doses of digoxin will increase the toxicity.

3 The medication should be stopped; when bradycardia is no longer present, the practitioner may modify the dose.

4 The mother is not a reliable source; the nurse should rely on pulse readings before the digoxin was prescribed.

463. **3 Vomiting is a classic sign of digoxin (Lanoxin) toxicity, and the practitioner must be notified.**

1 Infants regulate their own activity based on their energy level.

2 Orange juice is rarely needed because spironolactone (Aldactone) spares potassium.

4 There is no restriction on giving anti-inflammatories with spironolactone.

464. **3 An additional dose may cause overdosage, leading to toxicity; it is better to omit the dose.**

1 Giving the dose without waiting may cause overdosage, leading to toxicity.

2 Even waiting 2 hours may cause overdosage, leading to toxicity.

4 This is not a reliable method for determining a missed dose; 90 to 110 beats per minute is within the expected range for this age.

465. 1 **Vomiting and feeding issues are early signs of digoxin (Lanoxin) toxicity.**
    2 Cyanosis is expected in a crying infant with heart disease because the energy expenditure exceeds the body's ability to meet the oxygen demand.
    3 Long naps are expected; infants routinely require several naps, and an infant with heart disease requires long rest periods.
    4 The pulse rate of an infant receiving digoxin should remain greater than 100 beats per minute.

466. 3 **Drowsiness frequently is a side effect of barbiturate therapy because it depresses the central nervous system; the infant will adapt to this over time.**
    1 Stimulants are not routinely administered because they counteract the desired effect of seizure reduction.
    2 The dosage does not need adjustment; this response demonstrates little understanding of barbiturate therapy.
    4 The mother's concern is with her own baby; the medication's side effects should be explained.

467. 2 **A common side effect of phenytoin (Dilantin) is gingival hyperplasia. Meticulous oral hygiene may reduce the risk of this occurring.**
    1 Phenytoin is strongly alkaline and should be administered with meals to avoid gastric irritation.
    3 Avoidance of overeating and overhydration may result in better seizure control.
    4 Pink urine may be observed during drug excretion; it is expected and does not require treatment.

468. **Answer: 0.4 mL.** Use ratio and proportion to solve the problem.

$$45 \, mg : 0.6 \, mL :: 30 \, mg : x \, mL$$
$$45 \, x = 18.0$$
$$x = 0.4 \, mL$$

469. 1 **Constipation is a side effect of vinCRIStine (Oncovin) because it slows gastrointestinal motility.**
    2 An enlarged spleen will put pressure on the stomach and diaphragm, not on the large bowel.
    3 Constipation is not a toxic effect of predniSONE (Meticorten).
    4 It is unlikely that leukemia is causing an obstruction.

470. 2 **Pilocarpine (Pilocar) is a cholinergic that is applied to the skin to stimulate sweat production; the sweat is then tested to confirm the diagnosis of CF.**
    1 Pilocarpine does not stimulate the secretion of mucus.
    3 Pilocarpine does not stimulate the excretion of pancreatic enzymes.
    4 Pilocarpine does not stimulate the release of bile from the gallbladder.

471. 4 **Abdominal cramping and distention are associated with inadequate pancreatic enzyme replacement because foods are inadequately digested.**
    1 The opposite of anorexia occurs; the appetite is voracious.
    2 Diarrhea, not constipation, results.
    3 Weight loss, not gain, occurs because of decreased digestion and absorption of nutrients.

472. 3 **Pancreatic enzyme replacement is needed because children with cystic fibrosis cannot release pancreatic enzymes that promote the digestion of food. This results in large amounts of fat in the stool, which can cause bloating and abdominal cramping.**
    1 Increased oxygenation is not the effect of pancrelipase (Pancrease); pancrelipase contains enzymes to break down fats, proteins, and carbohydrates.
    2 Pancrelipase promotes the body's ability to metabolize and absorb fat rather than limit its excretion.
    4 The purpose of pancrelipase is not related to the prevention of anemia.

473. 1 **Pancreatic enzyme replacements are given just before or with every meal to aid digestion.**
    2 Breaking up and dissolving the medication will hasten its degradation by gastric secretions and interfere with its efficiency.
    3 The medication must be given just before or with every meal to aid digestion.
    4 The medication must be given just before or with every meal to aid digestion.

474. 1 **Ibuprofen (Advil), a nonsteroidal anti-inflammatory drug (NSAID), prolongs the bleeding time. In the postoperative period medications that interfere with clotting and prolong bleeding are contraindicated.**
    2 Ibuprofen is safe for young children when administered in appropriate doses.
    3 Ibuprofen has an anti-inflammatory action. This does not interfere with the healing process.
    4 Tolerance for ibuprofen does not develop.

475. 1 **Mannitol (Osmitrol) is an osmotic diuretic used to relieve cerebral edema.**
    2 The bladder is a storage basin and is not involved with filtration; mannitol acts in the kidneys.
    3 Mannitol is an osmotic diuretic that does not affect the body's excretion of glucose.
    4 Mannitol is an osmotic diuretic that does not reduce peripheral edema.

476. 3 **Oral hygiene is essential, especially during the administration of medications that have a negative effect on the oral mucosa.**
    1 Although pain may be present, aspirin is avoided because DOXOrubicin (Adriamycin) also is being used, and a side effect of this medication is thrombocytopenia. In addition, aspirin is contraindicated for children because it is associated with Reye syndrome.

2 Citrus juice will aggravate the stomatitis, which is a common side effect of dactinomycin (Cosmegen).

4 Spicy foods may aggravate the stomatitis that occurs with chemotherapy. However, usually any food that the child requests is permitted.

477. **4 Because of the suppression of the inflammatory process, the nurse must be alert to the subtle symptoms of infection, such as changes in appetite, sleep patterns, and behavior.**

1 Adrenocorticosteroid therapy delays, not accelerates, wound healing.

2 Adrenocorticosteroid therapy may cause hypokalemia, not hyperkalemia, because of the retention of sodium and fluid.

3 Adrenocorticosteroid therapy decreases, not increases, the production of antibodies.

478. **2 Because steroids are irritating to the gastric mucosa, GI bleeding may occur; stools should be checked for frank and occult blood.**

1 Steroids do not cause pulse irregularities.

3 Steroids do not cause mucus in the urine.

4 Steroids do not cause ulcerated mucous membranes.

479. **Answer: 3, 4**

1 Penicillin is administered if there is evidence of a streptococcal infection; however, the strep infection is usually not active when the acute poststreptococcal glomerulonephritis (APSGN) develops.

2 Children with APSGN do not have pain and therefore morphine is not needed.

3 **The child with APSGN is oliguric; diuretics are used to increase urinary output.**

4 **The child with APSGN is hypertensive. Antihypertensives are used to reduce the blood pressure.**

5 If the hypertension is controlled, seizures are not expected and phenobarbital is not necessary.

480. **1 Chemotherapy suppresses the immune system; the child is in danger of contracting an overwhelming infection.**

2 Although increasing caloric intake is important, it is not the priority.

3 Although nausea and vomiting are side effects of chemotherapy; they can be minimized with appropriate pharmacological therapy.

4 Although it is important to check for hematomas, it is not as important as preventing infection; gentle handling helps to prevent hematomas.

481. **3 Constipation, which can progress to paralytic ileus, is a side effect of vinCRIStine (Oncovin).**

1 Lack of bulk can contribute to constipation, but it is not the prime cause of this child's constipation.

2 Inactivity can contribute to, but is not the prime cause of this child's constipation.

4 PredniSONE (Meticorten) may cause nausea and vomiting, but it does not cause constipation.

482. **1 Elevated uric acid levels from destroyed cells may lead to renal problems; increased fluid intake helps dilute urine.**

2 Although the specific gravity should be monitored, it is not of primary importance at this time. The specific gravity is within the acceptable range for a child (1.005 to 1.030).

3 Although the creatinine clearance should be monitored, it is not of primary importance at this time.

4 Although the blood urea nitrogen (BUN) should be monitored, it is not of primary importance at this time. The BUN is within the acceptable range for a child (5 to 20 mg/dL).

483. **4 Children receiving chemotherapy are prone to mucosal cell damage that can produce ulcers throughout the GI tract; oral ulcers are a common side effect causing extreme discomfort.**

1 Increased fluid intake is encouraged to enhance the excretion of uric acid crystals.

2 Chemotherapy acts as an immunosuppressant; contact precautions protect the care provider; it is the child who needs to be protected.

3 Keeping the hair short will not prevent it from falling out while the child is receiving chemotherapy.

484. **3 Many vitamin supplements contain folic acid which negates the action of methotrexate (Trexall), a folic acid antagonist.**

1 Vitamin therapy is contraindicated.

2 Although vitamins do not contribute to well-being, this response does not answer the question.

4 Vitamin therapy is contraindicated.

485. **1 Antineoplastic drugs exert their effect on rapidly dividing tissues such as hair follicles, resulting in alopecia.**

2 Eating regular meals is not related to the side effects of the antineoplastics that are being used.

3 Dairy products are not related to the side effects of the antineoplastics that are being used.

4 Types of clothing are not related to the side effects of the antineoplastics that are being used.

486. **1 The objective for giving mercaptopurine (6-MP) is maintenance therapy to prevent relapses.**

2 Mercaptopurine is an oral medication.

3 Oral chemotherapy is an adjunct to other therapies in childhood leukemia, not an alternative for other therapies.

4 The prime site of metastasis of ALL is to the central nervous system.

487. **1 Because levothyroxine (Synthroid) increases the basal metabolic rate, an absence of constipation is a therapeutic response to the medication.**

2 Cool skin is a clinical sign of hypothyroidism that is related to a slow basal metabolic rate.

3 Fine hand tremors are related to hyperthyroidism and are not present in an infant with hypothyroidism, even one who is stabilized with levothyroxine.

4 Decreased activity is a sign that the levothyroxine was not effective.

488. 3 **Zidovudine (AZT) can cause life-threatening blood dyscrasias including thrombocytopenia.**

1 Weight loss is a response to the disease rather than the therapy.

2 With zidovudine toxicity the infant will demonstrate agitation, restlessness, and insomnia, not lethargy.

4 Urinary output is unrelated to zidovudine toxicity.

489. 1 **Continuous insulin therapy allows the child to become independent of parental control and anxiety regarding insulin injections. The pump can be programmed to give a bolus of insulin, which corresponds to food eaten, rather than needing an injection because of a sudden rise in blood glucose.**

2 The pump requires a subcutaneous needle insertion site that needs periodic changing (e.g., every third day or as necessary).

3 The child must still adhere to the recommended diet; dietary control minimizes the amount of exogenous insulin needed.

4 Blood glucose monitoring is required regardless of the method of insulin administration.

490. 3 **The basal infusion rate mimics the low rate of insulin secretion during fasting and the bolus before meals mimics the high output after meals.**

1 The subcutaneous needle and tubing may be left in place for as long as 3 days.

2 Blood glucose monitoring is performed a minimum of four or more times a day.

4 Most insulin pumps are battery-driven syringes external to the body.

491. 2 **The second dose of the intermediate-acting insulin (Novolin N) should be given at dinnertime. Novolin N insulin peaks in 4 to 12 hours. A second dose is often prescribed approximately 10 to 12 hours after the first dose. A blood glucose reading at bedtime will determine the evening dose of regular insulin (Novolin R).**

1 Before lunch is too early because it may precipitate a hypoglycemic reaction.

3 One hour after lunch is too early because it may precipitate a hypoglycemic reaction.

4 One hour after dinner is too late.

492. 4 **Providing information is a nonjudgmental way to address unsafe child care practices. There are safe over-the-counter (OTC) analgesic products specifically formulated to ease the discomfort of teething.**

1 This advice is unsafe. Alcohol ingestion is contraindicated and illegal for all children.

2 Being judgmental about the aunt's approach may close communication; the nurse should offer acceptable alternatives.

3 This advice is unsafe. Alcohol ingestion is contraindicated and illegal for all children.

493. **Answer: 4, 5**

1 None of the foods in this meal are high in calcium.

2 None of the foods in this meal are high in calcium.

3 None of the foods in this meal are high in calcium.

4 **This meal is high in calcium. The creamed soup, cheese on the macaroni, broccoli, and milk are high in calcium.**

5 **This meal is high in calcium; the white meat chicken, creamed spinach, and orange juice are high in calcium; mashed potatoes are made with milk, which is high in calcium.**

494. 3 **Kidney function must be adequate to excrete the lead; if kidney function is not adequate, nephrotoxicity or kidney damage may result.**

1 Skin breakdown is not associated with chelation therapy.

2 A high-protein diet is not necessary.

4 Liver damage does not occur with chelation therapy.

495. **Answer: 3.2 mL.** Use ratio and proportion to solve this problem.

$$160\,\text{mg} : x :: 250\,\text{mg} : 5\,\text{mL}$$
$$250\,x = 800$$
$$x = 800 \div 250$$
$$x = 3.2\,\text{mL}$$

496. 2 **Diarrhea is initially related to GI irritation, then later, to loss of intestinal flora, which may lead to overgrowth of drug-resistant microbes resulting in superinfection. This also causes diarrhea.**

1 Tinnitus may occur, but it is not the most common side effect.

3 Dizziness (vertigo) may occur, but it is not the most common side effect.

4 Headache may occur, but it is not the most common side effect.

497. 3 **Absorption of levofloxacin (Levaquin) is enhanced when the stomach is empty.**

1 Food in the stomach will interfere with absorption.

2 If the medication is taken just before a meal, food in the stomach shortly afterward will interfere with absorption.

4 If the medication is taken 30 minutes after a meal, food remaining in the stomach will interfere with absorption.

498. 4 **Gentamicin (Garamycin) can be ototoxic because of its effects on the eighth cranial nerve.**

1 Amoxicillin (Amoxil) reactions usually are allergic responses.

2 Impaired hearing does not occur with ciprofloxacin (Cipro).

3 Impaired hearing does not occur with clindamycin (Cleocin).

499. 2 Probenecid (Benemid)results in better utilization of the penicillin G (Bicillin) by delaying its excretion by the kidneys.

1 Probenecid is not prescribed to treat urethritis.

3 Probenecid does not prevent allergic reactions.

4 Penicillin destroys treponema during all stages of its development; the probenecid does not attack the organism during a stage of multiplication.

500. 4 Although the exact mechanism is unknown, clinical improvements have been reported with sympathomimetic amines such as methylphenidate (Concerta). After the purpose and action of the drug are explained, the nurse should review side effects with the parent.

1 The child's appetite usually diminishes.

2 The child should be medicated for as short a period as possible. Each child is evaluated individually.

3 The duration of methylphenidate is 3 to 6 hours and 8 hours with the extended release form. It should be taken 30 to 45 minutes before meals.

CHILD HEALTH NURSING
QUIZ

1. A 2-month-old infant is admitted to the pediatric unit for observation after an automobile collision. Family members are unable to stay. How can the nurse best provide psychological comfort for the infant?
   1. Assign the same nurse to the infant
   2. Follow a routine to which the infant is accustomed
   3. Have the infant listen to the parents' voices over the phone
   4. Ensure that a staff member stays with the infant at all times

2. A 13-month-old child is admitted with a tentative diagnosis of bacterial meningitis and the practitioner schedules a lumbar puncture. What is the most important action the nurse should take in preparation for the lumbar puncture?
   1. Ask the parents what they were told about the test
   2. Use a doll to demonstrate the procedure to the child
   3. Tell the parents they may stay with their child during the test
   4. Obtain a pacifier for the child to suck on during the procedure

3. A nurse initiates preparation of a 9-year-old child for an infratentorial craniotomy. What should the nurse include in the plan?
   1. Encourage doll play with simulated surgical equipment
   2. Have the child draw a picture of a brain and briefly clarify misconceptions
   3. Schedule role-playing with other children who also have had brain surgery
   4. Offer an explanation of the brain's anatomy and how the surgery is performed

4. An infant with bronchiolitis caused by the respiratory syncytial virus (RSV) is admitted to the pediatric unit. What does the nurse expect the prescribed treatment to include?
   1. Humidified air and adequate hydration
   2. Postural drainage and oxygen by hood
   3. Bronchodilators and cough suppressants
   4. Corticosteroids and broad-spectrum antibiotics

5. An 8-year-old child is being discharged after recovery from a sickle cell vaso-occlusive (painful crisis) episode. The nurse teaches the parents the "do's and don'ts" concerning the child's care. The nurse is satisfied that the parents understand the principles of care when they state that they are planning to:
   1. Have the child schooled by a private tutor
   2. Restrict the child's fluid intake during the night
   3. Permit the child to play with just one peer at a time
   4. Encourage the child to engage in low-intensity activities

6. A nurse teaches the parents of an infant with a cardiac defect about how to decrease the workload on their baby's heart. What should the teaching plan include?

1. How to organize care to support uninterrupted sleep
2. Reasons that the infant should not be held when cuddled
3. Reasons that a regular feeding schedule should be maintained
4. How to stimulate the infant periodically to promote respiratory excursion

7. The mother of a 4-week-old boy states, "He cries all the time and always acts hungry, but he throws up everything. He looks like a skinny old man." Based on this information, what is the focus of the nurse's assessment?
   1. Observe the anus to confirm rectal prolapse
   2. Obtain the elimination history to confirm celiac disease
   3. Note the color of vomitus to confirm a bile duct obstruction
   4. Palpate the abdomen to confirm hypertrophic pyloric stenosis

8. A 6-year-old child is admitted to the pediatric unit with a tentative diagnosis of leukemia. What information is essential for the nurse to obtain during the assessment?
   1. Parents' knowledge concerning the diagnosis
   2. Parents' ability to cope with stressful situations
   3. Child's experience with illness and hospitalization
   4. Child's growth percentile and developmental abilities

9. A nurse is caring for an 11-year-old child with type 1 diabetes. Two hours after breakfast the child becomes pale, diaphoretic, and shaky. What action should the nurse take?
   1. Notify the practitioner
   2. Administer supplemental insulin
   3. Obtain a current blood glucose level
   4. Give orange juice with a slice of bread

10. A nurse is obtaining a health history of a 5-year-old child admitted to the child health unit with acute glomerulonephritis (AGN). The nurse expects the child's mother to report that the:
    1. Child had a sore throat a few weeks ago
    2. Child has just recovered from the measles
    3. Child's father has a family history of urinary tract infections
    4. Child's immunizations were administered at the start of school

11. A nurse is helping an adolescent with type 1 diabetes establish a consistent meal pattern. What feedback information indicates that further teaching is needed?
    1. Weighs portion sizes for several months
    2. Reads nutrition labels on prepared foods
    3. Avoids complex carbohydrate substitutes
    4. Limits sugar alternatives containing sorbitol

12. An adolescent is admitted to the unit with a tentative diagnosis of a bone tumor of the left femur. During the admission procedure the adolescent casually asks, "Do they ever have to cut off a leg if someone has bone cancer?" How should the nurse respond?

1. "Sometimes it is necessary. What do you think about such a treatment?"
2. "Most times the leg can be saved although sometimes it may be necessary."
3. "I don't understand why you're asking. Why, do you think this will happen to you?"
4. "The decision can't be made now because the kind of bone cancer must be determined first."

13. A father calls the clinic because he wants information about how to care for his child's severe diaper rash. The nurse asks the father what he has been doing so far. The nurse identifies that the father needs further teaching when he says, "I:
    1. expose the buttocks to the air."
    2. direct a heat lamp to the buttocks."
    3. do not use soap to clean the diaper area."
    4. apply a medicated ointment to the diaper area."

14. While in the hospital's playroom, a male toddler suddenly has a nosebleed that spreads blood on the play table. What is the nurse's first response in this situation?
    1. Take him back to his room for care
    2. Provide nursing care to stop his nosebleed
    3. Call the housekeeping department to clean the room
    4. Secure an order for the blood to be tested for pathogens

15. The parents of a 14-month-old boy with bilateral cryptorchidism ask the nurse in the pediatric clinic why it is important for him to have surgery before he is 2 years old. Before responding, the nurse takes into consideration that uncorrected cryptorchidism can result in:
    1. Infertility
    2. Hydrocele
    3. Varicocele
    4. Epididymitis

16. A nurse is teaching a mother how to care for her toddler who is in a spica cast. In what position should the nurse suggest the mother place the toddler during a feeding?
    1. Upright while on the mother's lap
    2. Recumbent with a pillow under the head
    3. Semi-Fowler on a padded, adjustable tilt board
    4. Side-lying in the football hold facing the mother

17. After surgery a 2-month-old infant returns to the pediatric unit with an intravenous infusion and a nasogastric tube in place. What is the initial nursing action?
    1. Assessing the infant's status
    2. Giving the infant a mild sedative
    3. Connecting the nasogastric tube to wall suction
    4. Placing the intravenous tubing through an infusion pump

18. A 4-year-old child is admitted to the pediatric unit with a diagnosis of Wilms tumor. Considering the unique needs of a child with this diagnosis, the nurse should place a sign on the child's bed that states:
    1. Keep NPO
    2. No IV medications
    3. Record intake and output
    4. Do not palpate the abdomen

19. A nurse in the pediatric unit is admitting an 8-year-old child with asthma after an exacerbation at home. The child is short of breath. In what position should the child be placed to facilitate breathing and to promote respiratory drainage?
    1. Supine
    2. Left lateral
    3. High Fowler
    4. Trendelenburg

20. A toddler is placed in a bilateral hip spica cast for developmental dysplasia of the hip (DDH). The nurse should teach the parents to monitor their child and report to the practitioner the occurrence of:
    1. Warm toes
    2. Leg numbness
    3. Skin desquamation
    4. Generalized discomfort

21. What clinical signs should lead a nurse to suspect that a 1-year-old child has rubella (German measles)?
    1. Bulging fontanel and nuchal rigidity
    2. Conjunctivitis and sensitivity to light
    3. Koplik's spots on soft palate and buccal mucosa
    4. Enlarged posterior-cervical and postauricular nodes

22. A 4-year-old child is diagnosed with acute lymphocytic leukemia (ALL) and induction therapy includes vinCRIStine (Oncovin). What side effect that is unique to this medication is important for the nurse to monitor?
    1. Alopecia
    2. Anorexia
    3. Paresthesia
    4. Constipation

23. A 4-year-old abused child, after being hospitalized for severe injuries, is placed in temporary foster care. The foster family comes to the hospital to meet the child. What action should the nurse take to facilitate their first meeting?
    1. Decorate the child's room with welcome signs
    2. Provide the child and foster family with a private room
    3. Encourage the child to draw a picture of the foster family
    4. Answer the child's questions and add details before the meeting

24. A nurse is caring for an infant with hydrocephalus after the insertion of a shunt. How should the nurse evaluate the effectiveness of the shunt?
    1. Palpate the anterior fontanel
    2. Assess for periorbital edema
    3. Determine the frequency of voiding
    4. Observe for symmetry of the Moro reflex

25. The mother of a 17-year-old adolescent who is going to be a foreign exchange student asks the nurse why her child must have a tetanus toxoid immunization instead of the tetanus immunoglobulin. The nurse responds that the tetanus toxoid immunization provides:
    1. Lifelong passive immunity
    2. Longer-lasting active immunity

3. Temporary active natural immunity
4. Temporary passive natural immunity

26. A nurse confers with the nutritionist about the diet of a child with spina bifida who spends many hours in a wheelchair. What should the nurse encourage the mother to increase in her child's diet? Select all that apply.
    1. _____ Fat
    2. _____ Fiber
    3. _____ Protein
    4. _____ Calories
    5. _____ Carbohydrates

27. Abdominal surgery is planned for a 2-month-old infant. What should the nurse provide for the infant on the day of surgery?
    1. Rattle to shake
    2. Pacifier to suck
    3. Mobile for watching
    4. Music box for listening

28. A 3-week-old infant has surgery for esophageal atresia. What is the immediate postoperative nursing care priority for this infant?
    1. Giving the oral feedings slowly
    2. Reporting vomiting to the practitioner
    3. Checking the patency of the nasogastric tube
    4. Observing for signs of infection at the incision site

29. A 4-year-old child is admitted with burns over the entire right arm and the anterior and posterior aspects of both legs. Using the percentage of total body surface area (TBSA) that was burned, the nurse estimates that the TBSA affected is approximately:
    1. 36%
    2. 41%
    3. 47%
    4. 52%

30. The alkylating chemotherapeutic agent cyclophosphamide (Cytoxan) is prescribed for a child with cancer. What is the most important nursing assessment while the child is receiving this medication?
    1. Extent of alopecia
    2. Changes in appetite
    3. Hyperplasia of gums
    4. Daily intake and output

31. A child with a diagnosis of tuberculosis is admitted to the pediatric unit. Which location should the nurse select as the best placement for the child?
    1. Private room
    2. Isolation room
    3. Four-bed room
    4. Semiprivate room

32. A 5-year-old child has a cardiac catheterization. The child is in the postcardiac catheterization unit for 2 hours when the incoming nurse receives the report from the outgoing nurse. Which part of the child's report should the incoming nurse question?
    1. Vital signs every 30 minutes
    2. Voided 100 mL since admission

3. Pressure dressing over entry site
4. Bed rest with bathroom privileges

33. After corrective surgery for hypertrophic pyloric stenosis, the mother is asked to offer her baby boy his first feeding. He sucks it eagerly and vomits immediately. What is the nurse's explanation to the mother?
    1. "This often occurs after the first feeding."
    2. "He is ridding himself of postoperative mucus."
    3. "Your feeding technique may need to be changed."
    4. "Feedings will have to be stopped until peristalsis improves."

34. A 2-year-old toddler has a hearing loss caused by recurrent otitis media. What treatment does the nurse anticipate the practitioner will recommend?
    1. Ear drops
    2. Myringotomy
    3. Mastoidectomy
    4. Steroid therapy

35. A practitioner prescribes inhaled corticosteroids for a child with asthma. The nurse identifies that the mother understands the teaching about the side effects of this medication when the mother says, "I will monitor my child for:
    1. frequent urination."
    2. white patches in the mouth."
    3. increased blood glucose levels."
    4. short episodes of not breathing."

36. Which reactions does a nurse expect of a 4-year-old child in response to illness and hospitalization?
    1. Anger, resentment over depersonalization, and loss of peer support
    2. Boredom, depression over separation from family, and fear of death
    3. Out-of-control behavior, regression to over-dependency, and fear of bodily mutilation
    4. Intense panic, loss of security over separation from parents, and low frustration tolerance

37. What feeding instruction should a nurse give the mother of a 2-month-old infant with the diagnosis of heart failure?
    1. Use double-strength formula
    2. Avoid using a preemie nipple
    3. Refrain from feeding until crying from hunger begins
    4. Feed slowly while allowing for adequate periods of rest

38. A nurse is caring for an infant with a cleft lip and palate. What should the nurse include when giving the parents information about this diagnosis?
    1. Anticipation that these children will have psychological problems
    2. Emphasis that the two defects follow the laws of Mendelian genetics
    3. Assurance that the defect is rare and probably will not happen twice in the same family
    4. Expectation that these children will have no other defect and otherwise will be healthy

39. A nurse is caring for a child in the postanesthesia care unit (PACU) after a craniotomy for the removal of an

astrocytoma. Suddenly the child develops right pupillary dilation. The nurse concludes that this is a sign of:

1. Fear
2. Severe pain
3. Neurosurgical emergency
4. Reduced intracranial pressure

40. A nurse on the pediatric unit is planning to teach the parents of a child requiring complex care. Both parents are employed full-time. How should the nurse arrange the instructional program?

1. Provide information in short sessions
2. Schedule a whole evening for teaching
3. Offer explanations when the parents visit
4. Require that both parents attend the sessions

41. A nurse is caring for an infant after a cleft lip repair. What should the nurse use to feed the infant for several days after the surgery?

1. Preemie nipple
2. Nasogastric tube
3. Gravity-flow nipple
4. Rubber-tipped syringe

42. A nurse is planning the discharge of a child who had a tonsillectomy. The nurse informs the parents that their child may have a mouth odor, slight ear pain, and a low-grade fever for a few days. In addition to the prescribed analgesic, what should the nurse recommend to limit their child's pain?

1. Warm saline gargles
2. Heating pad to the neck
3. Lemon flavored ice pops
4. Peppermint candy for sucking

43. A 16-month-old toddler is having large, frothy, foul-smelling stools since the introduction of table foods, and is irritable and apathetic. The child is diagnosed with celiac disease and a gluten-free diet is prescribed. What response does the nurse anticipate in the child after 2 days on the diet?

1. Return of appetite
2. Increase in weight
3. Improved behavior
4. Cessation of diarrhea

44. Chelation therapy with succimer (Chemet) is instituted for a child with lead poisoning. What change does the nurse expect when the therapy is effective?

1. Fecal elimination of lead
2. Elevated blood-lead levels
3. Increased urinary excretion of lead
4. Decreased deposition of lead in the bones

45. A nurse anticipates that dialysis will be necessary for a child with chronic kidney disease when the child develops:

1. Hypotension
2. Hypokalemia
3. Hypervolemia
4. Hypercalcemia

46. A nurse must administer an intramuscular injection to a 15-month-old child. What is the reason that the nurse does not administer the injection into the gluteal muscle?

1. Muscle mass in this area is undeveloped
2. Intrusive procedures in this area are feared
3. Toddlers associate this area with punishment
4. Toddlers wiggle away when positioned to access the area

47. What is the best method for a nurse to assess an infant's response to oral rehydration therapy?

1. Observe the color of the stools
2. Monitor the skin turgor frequently
3. Obtain the weight at the same time every day
4. Measure the abdominal girth over the umbilicus

48. A nurse in the daycare center is teaching a group of assistants why toddlers are prone to develop lead poisoning. What factor primarily contributes to their risk for lead poisoning?

1. Lead is easily available to children
2. Their vascular system is very fragile
3. Motor vehicle pollution has increased
4. They have a high level of oral activity

49. A 4-year-old boy with acute lymphocytic leukemia (ALL) is to have a bone marrow aspiration. While involving the child in therapeutic play prior to the procedure the nurse should help him understand that:

1. He needs to have a positive attitude
2. His parents are concerned about him
3. He did nothing to cause his present illness
4. His problem was caused by an environmental factor

50. A practitioner prescribes an initial loading dose of 75 mcg of oral digoxin (Lanoxin). The medication is supplied as an elixir, 50 mcg/mL. How much solution should the nurse administer?

Answer: _____mL

CHILD HEALTH NURSING
QUIZ ANSWERS AND RATIONALES

1. **2 Very young infants gain security from having their needs met consistently.**
   1 Assigning one nurse to care for the infant is ideal although unrealistic. It is not critical at this age because the infant does not yet seek security from a significant caregiver.
   3 Although the infant may recognize the parents' voices, it will not ensure psychological comfort.
   4 Having a staff member stay with the infant is ideal although unrealistic; consistent observation is adequate.
   Client Needs: Psychosocial Integrity; **Cognitive Level:** Application; **Integrated Process:** Caring; **NP:** Planning

2. **1 An informed consent is required. The procedure should be explained to the parents by the practitioner and the nurse should confirm the patient's comprehension and have them sign the consent form.**
   2 The child is too young to comprehend a demonstration of the procedure.
   3 Although staying with the child may be important to the parents, it is not the priority.
   4 Although a pacifier may keep the child calm, this is not the priority.
   Client Needs: Management of Care; **Cognitive Level:** Application; **Integrated Process:** Communication and Documentation; **NP:** Planning

3. **2 Having the child draw a picture indicates the child's level of understanding; an explanation can then proceed.**
   1 Therapeutic play is more appropriate for younger children; it is inappropriate for a 9-year-old child.
   3 Role-playing is inappropriate and nontherapeutic at this time.
   4 Although the school-age child appreciates some detail, extensive detail is inappropriate.
   Client Needs: Health Promotion and Maintenance; **Cognitive Level:** Application; **Integrated Process:** Teaching/Learning; **NP:** Planning

4. **1 Humidified air and hydration are essential to facilitate improvement in the child's physical status.**
   2 Postural drainage is not effective with this disorder; oxygen is used only if the infant has severe dyspnea and hypoxia.
   3 Bronchodilators are not used because the bronchial tree is not in spasm; cough suppressants are ineffective.
   4 Corticosteroids are ineffective; antibiotics are ineffective because the etiological agent is viral.
   Client Needs: Physiological Adaptation; **Cognitive Level:** Application; **NP:** Planning

5. **4 Low-intensity activities should be encouraged because strenuous exercise leads to increased cellular metabolism, causing tissue hypoxia, which can precipitate sickling.**
   1 Hiring a tutor is detrimental to the child's developmental needs and may result in social isolation.
   2 Some parents restrict fluids at night to discourage bedwetting. However, fluids should not be restricted because keeping the child well hydrated helps prevent sickling.
   3 Restricting the child's play activities is unnecessary unless other children have an infectious disease; a variety of peer relationships should be encouraged.
   Client Needs: Physiological Adaptation; **Cognitive Level:** Application; **Integrated Process:** Teaching/Learning; **NP:** Evaluation

6. **1 Long periods of rest must be promoted; activities should be organized to minimize interruptions.**
   2 Parents should be encouraged to cuddle their infant, both for emotional development and to induce sleep.
   3 The feeding plan should be flexible to accommodate the infant's sleep and wake needs and patterns.
   4 Stimulation should be minimized to decrease the workload of the heart.
   Client Needs: Reduction of Risk Potential; **Cognitive Level:** Application; **Integrated Process:** Teaching/Learning; **NP:** Planning

7. **4 With a history that strongly suggests hypertrophic pyloric stenosis (HPS), the nurse should assess the abdomen for an olive-shaped mass and visible peristalsis.**
   1 The data presented are not consistent with rectal prolapse.
   2 The data are not consistent with celiac disease, which includes diarrhea resulting from a reaction to gluten; the infant is too young to have ingested grains.
   3 Although the color of vomitus is important for a diagnosis of HPS, bile duct obstruction is not indicated by the history.
   Client Needs: Physiological Adaptation; **Cognitive Level:** Application; **NP:** Assessment

8. **3 Positive and negative experiences connected with previous illness or hospitalization will influence the child's response and adaptation to this and subsequent hospitalizations.**
   1 Although the parents' knowledge of leukemia is important, the priority care at this time should be directed toward the child's needs.
   2 Although knowing the parents' abilities to cope is important, the child's needs are the focus of care.
   4 Although knowing the child's growth and developmental abilities are important, the priority care at this time should be directed toward the child's immediate needs.
   Client Needs: Psychosocial Integrity; **Cognitive Level:** Application; **Integrated Process:** Caring; **NP:** Assessment

NP, Nursing process.

9. **3 Although the child is demonstrating signs and symptoms of hypoglycemia, a blood glucose level must be determined to guide therapy.**
   1 The practitioner should be notified after the blood glucose level is known and after emergency intervention is implemented, if required.
   2 Administering insulin will exacerbate the hypoglycemia and endanger the child.
   4 If there is hypoglycemia, low-fat milk is preferred as a simple carbohydrate and a slice of bread with peanut butter provides complex carbohydrates.
   Client Needs: Reduction of Risk Potential; **Cognitive Level:** Application; **NP:** Implementation

10. **1 Acute poststreptococcal glomerulonephritis (APSGN) is associated with a history of streptococcal infection of the throat.**
    2 A streptococcal infection, not the measles virus, is associated with the development of APSGN.
    3 APSGN is not an inherited disease.
    4 There are no immunizations that can cause glomerulonephritis.
    Client Needs: Physiological Adaptation; **Cognitive Level:** Application; **Integrated Process:** Communication and Documentation; **NP:** Assessment

11. **3 Complex carbohydrates can be substituted based on caloric content and amount eaten per serving. Flexibility is needed to promote adherence to any dietary regimen.**
    1 Using consistent portion sizes is a key to maintaining diabetic control. By weighing and measuring portion sizes for several months the adolescent learns to recognize the acceptable amount to be eaten at a glance.
    2 The adolescent should read nutrition labels carefully, especially for their carbohydrate and caloric content.
    4 Most dietetic foods contain sorbitol. Sorbitol metabolizes to fructose and then glucose, so its use should be restricted when possible.
    Client Needs: Basic Care and Comfort; **Cognitive Level:** Application; **Integrated Process:** Teaching/Learning; **NP:** Evaluation

12. **1 Acknowledging that amputation may be necessary and asking an open-ended question encourages further discussion of feelings.**
    2 This response is evasive, gives false reassurance that the leg may be saved, and does not address feelings.
    3 This response is demeaning. A direct response not only does not address feelings but also attacks the basis of the adolescent's feelings.
    4 Telling the adolescent that the tumor is cancerous before a diagnosis is made is misinformation that is unsafe nursing practice.
    Client Needs: Psychosocial Integrity; **Cognitive Level:** Application; **Integrated Process:** Caring; **NP:** Implementation

13. **2 Heat lamps are not used because of the potential for burns.**

1 Exposing the diaper area will promote drying and healing.
3 Soap can irritate skin that is excoriated.
4 Ointment protects the buttocks from the irritating contents of stool.
Client Needs: Safety and Infection Control; **Cognitive Level:** Application; **Integrated Process:** Teaching/Learning; **NP:** Evaluation

14. **2 The nurse's priority is to care for the child. Once the child's problem is resolved, the nurse can address the problem of the blood on the play table.**
    1 The child's needs must be met immediately, even if the intervention must be performed in the playroom.
    3 Cleaning up the blood in the playroom is done after the child's immediate needs are met. The hospital's protocol for the removal of the blood should be followed.
    4 Having the blood tested for pathogens is unnecessary unless the nurse or another individual has direct contact with the blood. The hospital's protocol should be followed.
    Client Needs: Physiological Adaptation; **Cognitive Level:** Application; **NP:** Implementation

15. **1 Undescended testes (cryptorchidism) is the failure of the testes to move down the inguinal canal into the scrotum; this migration begins around the 25th to 30th week of gestation. Undescended testes are exposed to body heat that can destroy the sperm-producing ability of the testes, resulting in sterility.**
    2 A hydrocele is an enlargement of the scrotum with fluid; it is not related to cryptorchidism.
    3 A varicocele is a dilation and tortuosity of the scrotal veins; it is not caused by undescended testicles.
    4 Inflammation of the epididymis may occur whether or not cryptorchidism is corrected.
    Client Needs: Physiological Adaptation; **Cognitive Level:** Comprehension; **Integrated Process:** Communication and Documentation; **NP:** Analysis

16. **3 Because of the child's age, lying on a tilt board is the best position; it permits upright feeding while fostering growth and development.**
    1 Positioning on the mother's lap is difficult and unsafe for both mother and child because the combination of the child and the cast is too cumbersome and can cause a fall.
    2 The recumbent position makes feeding and digestion difficult; also it may increase the risk of aspiration.
    4 The football hold is appropriate for an infant, not a toddler.
    Client Needs: Reduction of Risk Potential; **Cognitive Level:** Application; **Integrated Process:** Teaching/Learning; **NP:** Implementation

17. **1 Assessment is the first step of the nursing process and is the priority because it influences all future interventions.**
    2 Administering a sedative may or may not be done and requires a prescription.

3 Although it is important to attach the nasogastric tube to a suction device, this can be done after the infant's status is assessed.

4 Although it is important to connect the IV to a pump, this can be done after the infant's status is assessed.

Client Needs: Reduction of Risk Potential; **Cognitive Level:** Application; **NP:** Implementation

18. **4 Palpation increases the risk of rupturing the tumor mass and is contraindicated.**

1 There are no data to indicate that surgery is scheduled; therefore, there is no reason to maintain NPO.

2 There is no contraindication for IV medication.

3 Recording of intake and output may or may not be ordered; it is not specific only for children with Wilms tumor.

Client Needs: Reduction of Risk Potential; **Cognitive Level:** Application; **Integrated Process:** Communication and Documentation; **NP:** Implementation

19. **3 The high Fowler position allows the lungs more room to expand, thus promoting respirations and affording more comfort.**

1 The supine position will increase dyspnea; it does not allow for chest expansion.

2 The left lateral position will increase dyspnea; it does not allow for chest expansion.

4 The Trendelenburg position will increase dyspnea; it does not allow for chest expansion.

Client Needs: Physiological Adaptation; **Cognitive Level:** Application; **NP:** Implementation

20. **2 Numbness is a neurological symptom that should be reported immediately because it indicates pressure on the nerves and blood vessels.**

1 Warm toes indicate intact circulation to the lower extremities.

3 Peeling skin is the result of inadequate skin care but can be managed easily with lotion or oil.

4 Some degree of discomfort is expected after cast application.

Client Needs: Reduction of Risk Potential; **Cognitive Level:** Application; **Integrated Process:** Teaching/Learning; **NP:** Implementation

21. **4 Lymphadenopathy and the development of a rash after a day of fever, sneezing, and coughing characterize rubella (German measles).**

1 A bulging fontanel and nuchal rigidity are associated with meningitis and encephalitis, not rubella.

2 Conjunctivitis and light sensitivity are associated with rubeola (measles), not rubella.

3 Koplik's spots are present with rubeola, not rubella.

Client Needs: Physiological Adaptation; **Cognitive Level:** Analysis; **NP:** Assessment

22. **4 It is important to monitor for constipation because it may be a forerunner of paralytic ileus and requires treatment.**

1 Alopecia is a common side effect of many classes of chemotherapeutic agents; it is not unique to vinCRIStine (Oncovin).

2 Anorexia is a common side effect of many classes of chemotherapeutic agents; it is not unique to vinCRIStine.

3 Paresthesia is a common side effect of many classes of chemotherapeutic agents; it is not unique to vinCRIStine.

Client Needs: Pharmacological and Parenteral Therapies; **Cognitive Level:** Application; **NP:** Evaluation

23. **2 A private room provides a secure environment for the child and the family to get to know one another.**

1 Printing welcome signs is not therapeutic because it may make the child feel guilty about leaving the biological family.

3 Encouraging the child to draw a picture of the foster family is not therapeutic because it may make the child feel guilty about leaving the biological family.

4 Although some information may be given, too much information about the family may promote preconceived ideas that may be inaccurate.

Client Needs: Psychosocial Integrity; **Cognitive Level:** Application; **Integrated Process:** Caring; **NP:** Implementation

24. **1 A bulging fontanel is the most significant sign of increased intracranial pressure in an infant.**

2 Periorbital edema is not an indicator of increased intracranial pressure.

3 The frequency of voiding is not an indicator of increased intracranial pressure.

4 Symmetry of the Moro reflex is not an indicator of increased intracranial pressure.

Client Needs: Reduction of Risk Potential; **Cognitive Level:** Application; **NP:** Evaluation

25. **2 Toxoids are modified toxins that stimulate the body to form antibodies that can last up to 10 years against the specific disease. Because the adolescent will be in a foreign country, the tetanus toxoid is given prophylactically.**

1 The tetanus toxoid provides active, not passive immunity; all passive immunity is short acting.

3 Only by having the disease can natural immunity occur.

4 Only by having the disease can natural immunity occur. Toxoids confer active, not temporary passive, immunity.

Client Needs: Health Promotion and Maintenance; **Cognitive Level:** Application; **Integrated Process:** Communication and Documentation; **NP:** Implementation

26. **Answer: 2, 3**

1 Of this child's dietary intake, 25% should consist of fat; this is the lowest recommended daily intake for fat. It should not be increased because more fat calories may lead to obesity in an immobilized child.

2 **Extra fiber is needed to prevent constipation resulting from immobility.**

3 **Extra protein is needed for maintaining muscle mass and to help prevent pressure ulcers.**

4 Calories should be limited because energy needs are less for immobile children than children who are active.

5 Carbohydrates, especially simple sugars, should be limited to prevent obesity.

Client Needs: Basic Care and Comfort; **Cognitive Level:** Analysis; **Integrated Process:** Teaching/Learning; **NP:** Implementation

27. 2 **The infant is NPO, and satisfying the sucking need is the priority at this age.**

1 Although a rattle is age appropriate, the sucking need is the priority.

3 Although a mobile is age appropriate, the sucking need is the priority.

4 Although listening to music is age appropriate, the sucking need is the priority.

Client Needs: Health Promotion and Maintenance; **Cognitive Level:** Application; **Integrated Process:** Caring; **NP:** Planning

28. 3 **A nasogastric tube is used postoperatively to decompress the stomach and limit tension on the suture line.**

1 To limit pressure on the suture line, oral feedings should not be implemented in the immediate postoperative period when the nasogastric tube is in place.

2 Vomiting indicates obstruction of the nasogastric tube; that is why the initial action should be to check the patency of the tube.

4 It is too soon for signs of infection to occur.

Client Needs: Reduction of Risk Potential; **Cognitive Level:** Application; **NP:** Evaluation

29. 2 **Using the total body surface area (TBSA) percentage for a child between 1 and 5 years of age, the total arm is 8.5% and each total leg is 16.25%; thus, 32.5% for both legs and 8.5% for the arm equals a total of 41% of TBSA burned.**

1 This percentage is too small.

3 This percentage is too large.

4 This percentage is too large.

Client Needs: Reduction of Risk Potential; **Cognitive Level:** Analysis; **NP:** Assessment

30. 4 **Hemorrhagic cystitis is a potentially serious adverse reaction to cyclophosphamide (Cytoxan) that can sometimes be prevented by an increased fluid intake because the fluid flushes the bladder. Assessment of the extent of hydration can be measured by monitoring and documenting hourly intake and output.**

1 Alopecia is expected; however, it is a benign side effect and hair will regrow when therapy is completed.

2 A change in appetite is expected, but is not a serious side effect of cyclophosphamide administration.

3 Hyperplasia of the gums is unrelated to cyclophosphamide administration; it occurs with phenytoin (Dilantin) therapy.

Client Needs: Pharmacological and Parenteral Therapies; **Cognitive Level:** Application; **NP:** Evaluation

31. 2 **An isolation room is a private room that has special air handling and ventilation to prevent the transmission of airborne droplet nuclei ≤5 μm. It has monitored negative pressure to prevent air from moving from the room into the corridor of the facility. Room air is exchanged 6 to 12 times an hour to the outdoors or through a monitored high-efficiency filtration system.** *Mycobacterium tuberculosis* **remains suspended in the air for prolonged periods and is transmitted via air currents.**

1 A private room does not have the technical equipment to manage airborne droplet nuclei ≤5 μm. Other children and people on the unit will be exposed to the infected individual's pathogens that travel through air currents.

3 A four-bed room will expose the children and other people on the unit to the infected individual's pathogens.

4 A semiprivate room will expose the children and other people on the unit to the infected individual's pathogens.

Client Needs: Safety and Infection Control; **Cognitive Level:** Analysis; **NP:** Planning

32. 4 **Children are kept on complete bed rest for 4 to 6 hours after a cardiac catheterization to reduce the risk of bleeding or trauma to the insertion site; the report about bathroom privileges should be questioned.**

1 Frequent monitoring of vital signs is part of routine postcatheterization care.

2 This urinary output is within acceptable limits for a child of this age; oral fluids are encouraged to promote hydration and urination.

3 A pressure dressing is placed over the insertion site to prevent bleeding. This is routine postcatheterization care.

Client Needs: Management of Care; **Cognitive Level:** Application; **Integrated Process:** Communication and Documentation; **NP:** Evaluation

33. 1 **Explaining that the first postoperative feeding usually induces vomiting provides correct information while supporting the anxious parent.**

2 Vomiting is not caused by mucus accumulation.

3 Questioning the mother's feeding technique may cause guilt; although the feeding techniques may need to be changed, discussing this at this time is inappropriate.

4 When the vomiting subsides, the feeding is continued.

Client Needs: Reduction of Risk Potential; **Cognitive Level:** Application; **Integrated Process:** Communication and Documentation; **NP:** Implementation

34. 2 **Myringotomy is a surgical opening into the eardrum to allow for drainage of accumulated fluid associated with otitis media.**

1 Ear drops are not used because they will obscure the view of the tympanic membrane.

3 Removal of the mastoid will not relieve pressure within inflamed ears.

4 Antibiotics, not steroids, are used for an infectious process.

Client Needs: Physiological Adaptation; **Cognitive Level:** Application; **NP:** Planning

35. **2 Oral candidiasis is a potential side effect of inhaled steroids because of steroids' anti-inflammatory effect; the child should be taught to rinse the mouth after each inhalation.**

1 Frequent urination is not a side effect of steroid therapy.

3 Hyperglycemia is not a side effect of inhaled steroid therapy; it can occur when steroids are administered for a systemic effect.

4 Apneic episodes are not a side effect of steroid therapy.

Client Needs: Pharmacological and Parenteral Therapies; **Cognitive Level:** Analysis; **Integrated Process:** Teaching/Learning; **NP:** Evaluation

36. **3 Piaget's preoperational stage focuses on egocentricity and concrete thoughts, and Freud's phallic stage supports this response.**

1 These feelings are typical of the adolescent.

2 These feelings are typical of the school-age child.

4 These feelings are typical of the toddler.

Client Needs: Health Promotion and Maintenance; **Cognitive Level:** Application; **NP:** Assessment

37. **4 Because of a limited exercise tolerance and fatigue, infants with heart failure become too tired to feed; allowing for rest and feeding slowly limit the fatigue associated with feeding.**

1 Although the infant may receive a formula with a higher caloric value (30 calories per ounce rather than 20 calories per ounce), double-strength formula is too high an osmotic load for the infant.

2 A soft nipple used for preterm infants or a regular nipple with an enlarged opening is preferred to conserve the energy required for sucking.

3 Crying consumes energy and is exhausting. The infant should be fed when exhibiting signs of hunger, such as sucking on a fist.

Client Needs: Physiological Adaptation; **Cognitive Level:** Application; **Integrated Process:** Teaching/Learning; **NP:** Implementation

38. **4 Children with a cleft lip and palate are otherwise healthy, and once a successful feeding technique is established, they feed, gain weight, and thrive as expected, even without corrective surgery.**

1 The way the young child responds to these defects depends on parental responses.

2 Mendelian laws of inheritance do not apply to these defects.

3 These defects are familial; however, an exact pathogenesis has not been identified.

Client Needs: Physiological Adaptation; **Cognitive Level:** Application; **Integrated Process:** Communication and Documentation; **NP:** Planning

39. **3 When one pupil rapidly dilates it is an emergency situation; sudden pressure is exerted on the third cranial nerve on the affected side caused by displacement of the tentorium or uncus.**

1 An autonomic response to fear does not result in pupillary dilation.

2 A response to severe pain will affect both pupils equally.

4 Reduced pressure does not cause one pupil to dilate; more likely, increasing pressure causes this response.

Client Needs: Reduction of Risk Potential; **Cognitive Level:** Application; **NP:** Evaluation

40. **1 The parents probably will be anxious and benefit most from short teaching sessions and written material to review at their leisure.**

2 A whole evening of teaching is overwhelming; the parents may not be able to retain everything presented.

3 The most effective teaching and learning sessions occur in an area with minimal distractions. Being in the room with their child at this time will present a major distraction to the parents.

4 The nurse may recommend, but not insist, that both parents attend the teaching sessions.

Client Needs: Health Promotion and Maintenance; **Cognitive Level:** Application; **Integrated Process:** Teaching/Learning; **NP:** Planning

41. **4 A rubber-tipped syringe minimizes sucking and is not irritating to the suture line.**

1 Using a preemie nipple is one method of feeding before surgery.

2 A nasogastric tube is unnecessary; the infant is hungry enough to feed even if deprived of sucking.

3 Using a gravity-flow nipple is one method of feeding before surgery.

Client Needs: Basic Care and Comfort; **Cognitive Level:** Application; **NP:** Planning

42. **3 Ice pops or ice chips provide a cool liquid that may be soothing to the oropharynx. Red, orange, or brown liquids are contraindicated because they mask the occurrence of bleeding.**

1 Gargling is contraindicated because it may traumatize the operative site, resulting in bleeding. Also warm fluids promote capillary dilation, which may promote bleeding.

2 A heating pad produces vasodilation, which may increase pain and promote bleeding.

4 Hard candies can traumatize the operative site and cause bleeding.

Client Needs: Basic Care and Comfort; **Cognitive Level:** Application; **Integrated Process:** Teaching/Learning; **NP:** Implementation

43. **3 A favorable change in behavior occurs in 2 to 3 days and attests to the effectiveness of the diet; other improvements take longer.**

1 A return of appetite takes more than several days of therapy; anorexia redevelops during episodes of diarrhea.

2 An increase in weight takes more than several days of therapy.

4 Cessation of diarrhea takes more than several days of therapy.

Client Needs: Basic Care and Comfort; **Cognitive Level:** Application; **NP:** Evaluation

44. **3 Succimer (Chemet), a chelating agent, binds with ions of lead to form a water-soluble complex that is excreted by the kidneys.**

1 The elimination of lead via the GI tract is less than via the urinary tract and is an unsatisfactory measure of the success of the chelation therapy.

2 Elevated blood-lead levels are expected when lead initially equilibrates to the blood. Until the lead is excreted in the urine the treatment is not considered a success.

4 A decreased amount of lead in the bones is a desirable effect, but it does not determine the success of therapy; also the amount is difficult to determine.

Client Needs: Pharmacological and Parenteral Therapies; **Cognitive Level:** Comprehension; **NP:** Evaluation

45. **3 Hypervolemia results when kidneys have failed and are no longer able to maintain homeostasis, the blood pressure is high, and cardiac overload is imminent.**

1 Hypertension, not hypotension, is present when kidney failure occurs.

2 Hyperkalemia, not hypokalemia, occurs with kidney failure.

4 Hypocalcemia, not hypercalcemia, is present when kidney failure occurs.

Client Needs: Physiological Adaptation; **Cognitive Level:** Analysis; **NP:** Analysis

46. **1 Infants and small children have small buttocks with a proximal sciatic nerve. In a 15-month-old child, the vastus lateralis is a larger muscle, can tolerate larger quantities of fluid, and is easily accessible if the child is supine, side-lying, or sitting.**

2 Children of this age fear the procedure no matter which site is chosen.

3 Preschoolers, not toddlers, tend to associate many treatments, and illness itself, with punishment.

4 Children who are adequately restrained can be held still when accessing any muscle.

Client Needs: Health Promotion and Maintenance; **Cognitive Level:** Application; **NP:** Planning

47. **3 Weighing daily is the most objective and accurate way to assess fluid loss or gain; weights measured at the same time each day provide daily comparisons.**

1 The color of stools is unrelated to fluid balance; noting consistency is more important although subjective.

2 Although checking the skin turgor is done, it is a subjective finding.

4 Measuring the abdominal circumference is appropriate for assessing the progression of ascites, not for assessing rehydration.

Client Needs: Basic Care and Comfort; **Cognitive Level:** Application; **NP:** Evaluation

48. **4 Toddlers have an increased propensity for putting things into their mouths; these children use this activity as a means of exploring the environment.**

1 Although lead may be found in older homes or in some inner-city dwellings, it is not the primary reason that toddlers are at risk for developing lead poisoning.

2 Toddlers do not have a fragile vascular system; children with a fragile vascular system are severely compromised.

3 Although gas fumes in areas of heavy traffic have increased pollution, most gasoline used does not contain lead.

Client Needs: Health Promotion and Maintenance; **Cognitive Level:** Application; **NP:** Assessment

49. **3 Preschoolers (age 3 to 5 years) are in the preoperational stage of cognitive development; it consists of the preconceptual phase that involves egocentric thought and the phase of intuitive thought, which transitions to the more logical thought of school-age children. 4-year-old children often believe that they cause their illnesses. Emphasizing that they did not cause the illness will help to elicit any fantasy they may have; it helps them understand that treatment is not a punishment.**

1 Telling a 4-year-old to have a positive attitude is inappropriate and does not elicit feelings.

2 Although parental concern is important, it does not address the developmental concerns of a 4-year-old child.

4 Environmental factors are not currently supported as a cause of ALL; it is an inappropriate discussion for a 4-year-old child.

Client Needs: Health Promotion and Maintenance; **Cognitive Level:** Application; **Integrated Process:** Caring; **NP:** Implementation

50. **Answer: 1.5 mL.** Use ratio and proportion to solve the problem.

$$75 : x :: 50 : 1$$
$$50 x = 75$$
$$x = 75 \div 50$$
$$x = 1.5 \text{ mL}$$

Client Needs: Pharmacological and Parenteral Therapies; **Cognitive Level:** Application; **NP:** Implementation

CHAPTER

6

Comprehensive Examination

PART A QUESTIONS

1. The hypertonicity of the muscles in an infant with cerebral palsy causes scissoring of the legs. The nurse teaches the mother that the preferred way to carry the infant is in a sitting position:
   1. Astride one of her hips
   2. Strapped in an infant seat
   3. Wrapped tightly in a blanket
   4. Under the arm using a football hold

2. The nurse administers 2 units of salt-poor albumin to a client with portal hypertension and ascites. The nurse explains to the client that this is administered to:
   1. Provide nutrients
   2. Increase protein stores
   3. Elevate the circulating blood volume
   4. Divert blood flow away from the liver temporarily

3. A 31-year-old client is seeking contraceptive information. Before responding to the client's questions about contraceptives, the nurse obtains a health history. What factor in the client's history indicates to the nurse that oral contraceptives are contraindicated?
   1. More than 30 years of age
   2. Had two multiple pregnancies
   3. Smokes 1 pack of cigarettes a day
   4. Has a history of borderline hypertension

4. While observing a mother visiting her preterm son in the neonatal intensive care nursery (NICU), the nurse identifies that the mother has not yet begun the bonding process. Which statement by the mother supports the nurse's conclusion?
   1. "It looks like such a tiny baby."
   2. "Do you think he will make it?"
   3. "Why does he need to be in an incubator?"
   4. "My baby looks so much like my husband."

5. After a mastectomy, a client returns from surgery with a closed suction drainage system in place and a dry sterile dressing covering the incision. What should the nurse do when observing this client for signs of bleeding?
   1. Empty the output in the portable suction unit hourly
   2. Inspect the bedclothes under the client's axillary area for signs of drainage
   3. Turn the client onto the affected side to inspect for blood that may flow backward
   4. Reinforce the operative site with a pressure dressing if drainage appears on the dressing

6. A nurse is caring for a client who has a portable wound suction device after abdominal surgery. What is the reason why the nurse empties the device when it is half full?
   1. Emptying the unit is safer when it is half full
   2. Accurate measurement of drainage is facilitated
   3. Negative pressure in the unit lessens as fluid accumulates, interfering with further drainage
   4. Fluid collecting in the unit exerts positive pressure, forcing drainage back up the tubing and into the wound

7. Before discharge after a myocardial infarction, a male client asks the nurse how long he should wait before having sexual relations with his wife. What is the best response by the nurse?
   1. "Two weeks is the usual waiting time."
   2. "How long do you think you should wait?"
   3. "Have you discussed this with your physician?"
   4. "You should wait until your heart feels stronger."

8. The laboratory report of a client receiving long-term treatment with lithium carbonate indicates a level of 1.5 mEq/L. The nurse should:
   1. Observe for signs of lithium toxicity
   2. Expect an increase in manic behavior
   3. Administer the next dose of lithium as prescribed
   4. Question whether the client has been taking the medication

9. A client who weighs 176 pounds is being immunosuppressed by daily maintenance doses of cyclosporine (Sandimmune) to prevent organ transplant rejection. The dose prescribed is 8 mg/kg each day. How many milligrams should the nurse administer each day?
   Answer: _____ mg

10. A male cocaine addict remanded for rehabilitation by the court is angry at being hospitalized. When his wife comes to visit he is furious and curses at her. He refuses to visit with her and tells her to go home. The wife leaves in tears. What should the nurse say to the client?
    1. "You are very angry right now."
    2. "Let's talk about what just happened."
    3. "Let's go to your next scheduled activity."
    4. "You should go to the gym to use the punching bag."

11. A nurse administers albuterol to a child with asthma. For what common side effect should the nurse monitor the child?
    1. Flushing
    2. Dyspnea

3. Tachycardia

4. Hypotension

12. An infant with diarrhea requires contact precautions. What is the most effective nursing action to control the spread of this infant's pathogens?

1. Wearing a gown, mask, and gloves during care

2. Allowing only registered nurses to give direct care

3. Restricting visitors to the infant's immediate family

4. Washing hands before and after contact with the infant

13. Which factor identified by the nurse while obtaining the client's health history predisposes a client to type 2 diabetes?

1. Having diabetes insipidus

2. Eating low-cholesterol foods

3. Being twenty pounds overweight

4. Drinking a daily alcoholic beverage

14. A client is admitted to the hospital with a tentative diagnosis of Guillain-Barré syndrome and a nurse is obtaining the client's health history. Which nurse's question will best elicit information that supports this diagnosis?

1. "Have you experienced an infection recently?"

2. "Is there a history of this disorder in your family?"

3. "Did you receive a head injury during the past year?"

4. "What medications have you taken in the last several months?"

15. A couple arrives at the newborn nursery requesting to take their newborn grandson to his mother's room. What is the nurse's best response?

1. "I'll get your grandchild. You must be very excited."

2. "Please go on to see your daughter. I'll bring the baby to her room."

3. "Show me your identification. I need to see it before I can give you the baby."

4. "Only the mother can ask for the baby. Tell her to call us to bring the baby to her."

16. The parents of a child who is receiving chemotherapy for acute lymphocytic leukemia (ALL) ask the nurse about the prognosis of children with this diagnosis. The nurse bases the response on the information that the expected outcome for children with this type of leukemia is:

1. Guarded, but the therapy keeps them pain-free

2. Limited to a few months in most of the children affected

3. Positive, with a probable cure in 95% of the children affected

4. Extended to at least 5 years in more than 75% of the children treated

17. A nurse arrives at the scene of an accident in which a 5-month-old infant is found unconscious. After performing the initial steps of cardiopulmonary resuscitation, the nurse plans to locate the infant's pulse. Which pulse site in the accompanying figure should be palpated?

1. a

2. b

3. c

4. d

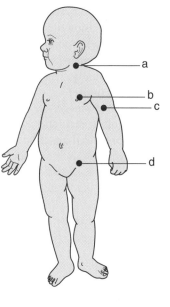

18. A client with malabsorption syndrome is admitted to the hospital for medical intervention. A subclavian catheter is inserted and the client is started on total parenteral nutrition (TPN). What should the nurse teach the client to prevent the most common complication of TPN?

1. Avoid disturbing the dressing

2. Keep the head as still as possible whenever moving

3. Regulate the flow rate on the infusion pump as necessary

4. Monitor daily weights at the same time while wearing the same clothing

19. A 16-year-old male with a diagnosis of adolescent adjustment disorder and his family are beginning family therapy. What is the best initial nursing approach?

1. Set long-term goals for the family

2. Let the client ventilate his feelings first

3. Have the parents explain their rationale for setting firm limits

4. Encourage each family member to share how the problem is perceived

20. A client is admitted to the hospital with the diagnosis of Parkinson's disease. What medication should the nurse expect the practitioner to order to relieve the client's physiological responses to this disease?

1. Levodopa (L-Dopa)

2. Isocarboxazid (Marplan)

3. DOPamine (Intropin)

4. Pyridoxine (vitamin B_6)

21. After a transurethral prostatectomy, a client returns to the postanesthesia care unit with a three-way indwelling catheter with continuous bladder irrigation. What nursing action is the priority?

1. Monitoring for signs of confusion

2. Observing the suprapubic dressing for drainage

3. Maintaining the client in the semi-Fowler position

4. Encouraging fluids by mouth as soon as the gag reflex returns

22. Five days after a client has abdominal surgery a nurse assesses the client's incision site for signs of dehiscence. Which clinical finding supports the nurse's conclusion that the client is experiencing wound dehiscence?
    1. Increased bowel sounds
    2. Loosening of the sutures
    3. Serosanguineous drainage
    4. Purplish color of the incision

23. The mother of a preschool-age child tells the nurse that her husband is dying of cancer and she is worried about how her child will cope. As part of their discussion the school nurse includes that preschool-age children view death as:
    1. Universal
    2. Irreversible
    3. A form of sleep
    4. A frightening ghost

24. A 40-year-old client scheduled for a hemicolectomy because of ulcerative colitis asks if having a hemicolectomy means wearing a pouch and having bowel movements in an abnormal way. Which is the best response by the nurse?
    1. "Yes, hemicolectomy is the same as a colostomy."
    2. "Yes, but it will be temporary until the colitis is cured."
    3. "No, that is necessary when a tumor is blocking the rectum."
    4. "No, only part of the colon is removed and the rest reattached."

25. A client is admitted to the hospital for the implantation of radon seeds in the oral cavity. Which intervention is most important, when the nurse is caring for this client after the procedure?
    1. Providing a regular diet within 2 days
    2. Administering nursing care in a short period
    3. Giving frequent mouth care at least 4 times daily
    4. Having a member of the family stay with the client continually

26. A client with a diagnosis of bipolar I disorder, depressive episode, is receiving lamotrigine (Lamictal). The nurse evaluates that the medication is effective when the client becomes:
    1. More high-spirited
    2. Able to laugh off criticism
    3. Involved in performing activities of daily living
    4. Able to spend the morning entertaining several quiet clients

27. A child is admitted to the pediatric intensive care unit (PICU) with acute bacterial meningitis. What is the nurse's priority intervention?
    1. Offering clear fluids whenever awake
    2. Checking level of consciousness hourly
    3. Assessing the blood pressure every four hours
    4. Administering the prescribed oral antibiotic medication

28. A neonate develops hyperbilirubinemia and phototherapy is begun. What should the plan of care include for an infant receiving phototherapy?
    1. Taking vital signs every hour
    2. Keeping the eye shields on continuously
    3. Giving additional fluids every two hours
    4. Covering the neonate with a lightweight blanket

29. A nurse is caring for an 8-year-old child who is admitted to the pediatric unit with a tentative diagnosis of acute poststreptococcal glomerulonephritis (APSGN). Diagnostic tests are ordered. Which tests will help confirm the diagnosis? Select all that apply.
    1. _____ ASO titer
    2. _____ Urinalysis
    3. _____ Blood chemistry
    4. _____ Intravenous pyelogram
    5. _____ Chest x-ray examination

30. A shy withdrawn male adolescent newly admitted to the psychiatric unit asks one of the female psychiatric nurses for a date. What is the best initial response by the nurse?
    1. Question the client about his sexual identity
    2. Restate the purpose of the nurse-client relationship
    3. Suggest that other staff members care for this client
    4. Review her interactions with the client for flirtatious comments

31. A child diagnosed with Wilms tumor is receiving a chemotherapy protocol including vinCRIStine (Oncovin) and DOXOrubicin hydrochloride (Adriamycin). Which common side effect unique to DOXOrubicin should the nurse expect to observe in the child?
    1. Hair loss
    2. Vomiting
    3. Red urine
    4. Stomatitis

32. The practitioner prescribes a low-fat, 2-gram sodium diet for a client with hypertension. The nurse should explain to the client in language that can be understood that a low-sodium diet will:
    1. Chemically stimulate the loop of Henle
    2. Diminish the thirst response of the client
    3. Prevent reabsorption of water in the distal tubules
    4. Cause fluid to move toward the interstitial compartment

33. A client who had an open reduction and insertion of a prosthesis for a fracture of the femoral neck is stable after surgery and is returned to the orthopedic unit. What is most important for the nurse to do when positioning this client?
    1. Maintain both legs in abduction
    2. Keep both legs in functional body alignment
    3. Avoid placing the client in the supine or prone position
    4. Prevent adduction and external rotation of the affected extremity

34. A client with mild preeclampsia is instructed to rest at home. She asks the nurse, "What do you mean by rest?" What is the most appropriate response?

1. "What do you consider to be rest?"
2. "Take three or four naps each day."
3. "Stay off your feet as much as possible."
4. "Would you like to know what I think it means?"

35. A pregnant woman is admitted in active labor. What should the nurse instruct her coach to do when the client complains of back pain?
    1. Position her with her legs elevated
    2. Apply pressure to the sacrum during contractions
    3. Encourage performance of a panting-breathing pattern
    4. Encourage her to do Kegel exercises between contractions

36. After an infant who was born with talipes equinovarus (clubfoot) has the cast removed, the nurse teaches the mother how and when to exercise the baby's foot. The nurse identifies that the mother understands the instructions when she says that she will exercise the foot:
    1. With each diaper change
    2. Once a day in the morning
    3. Twice a day after each nap
    4. Every four hours during the day

37. A nurse is reviewing the health history and laboratory report of a child with lead poisoning. What complications does the nurse expect in relation to lead toxicity? Select all that apply.
    1. _____ Anemia
    2. _____ Proteinuria
    3. _____ Heart failure
    4. _____ Encephalopathy
    5. _____ Gastrointestinal bleeding

38. Six hours after major abdominal surgery a male client complains of severe abdominal pain; is pale and perspiring; has a thready, rapid pulse; and states he feels faint. The nurse checks the client's medication administration record and determines that the client can receive another injection of pain medication in an hour. What is the most appropriate action by the nurse?
    1. Explain to the client that it is too early to have an injection for pain
    2. Call the practitioner, report the client's symptoms, and obtain further orders
    3. Reposition the client for greater comfort and turn on the television as a distraction
    4. Prepare the injection and administer it to the client early because of the severe pain

39. A client returns from surgery after a total laryngectomy with a laryngectomy tube in the permanent stoma. In which position should the nurse place this client to facilitate respirations and promote comfort?
    1. Side-lying position
    2. Orthopneic position
    3. High-Fowler's position
    4. Semi-Fowler's position

40. A 20-year-old homeless client at 38 weeks' gestation visits the prenatal clinic for the first time. She is accompanied by her 21-year-old boyfriend who is the father.

While they are in the waiting room the nurse becomes concerned because they are sneezing and yawning and have teary eyes. With what substance are these withdrawal signs associated?
    1. Heroin
    2. Cocaine
    3. Morphine
    4. Phenobarbital

41. An infant born with a cleft lip is to have a surgical repair of the lip. What should the nurse teach the parents in preparation for the postoperative period?
    1. Have the infant drink from a cup
    2. Keep the infant's arms in restraints for as long as possible
    3. Tell the parents to burp the infant as little as possible after a feeding
    4. Instruct the parents about different strategies that protect the infant's suture line

42. A couple interested in delaying the start of a family discuss the various methods of family planning. Together they decide to use the basal body temperature method. The nurse explains that the length of the fertility period surrounding ovulation lasts from:
    1. 12 hours before to 24 hours after ovulation
    2. 72 hours before to 24 hours after ovulation
    3. 72 to 80 hours before to 72 hours after ovulation
    4. 24 to 48 hours before to 48 hours after ovulation

43. A 65-year-old client is receiving amitriptyline (Elavil). What is the most important nursing recommendation to make to this client concerning this medication?
    1. Obtain a complete cholesterol and lipid profile
    2. Have an eye examination to assess for glaucoma
    3. Monitor daily temperature for nighttime elevations
    4. Assess for excessive sweating and possible weight loss

44. A nurse is caring for a client who is experiencing the second (acute) phase of burn recovery. The common client response the nurse expects to identify during this phase of burn recovery is an increase in:
    1. Serum sodium
    2. Urinary output
    3. Hematocrit level
    4. Serum potassium

45. A nurse is caring for a client with a history of chronic obstructive pulmonary disease who develops a pneumothorax and a chest tube is inserted. What is the primary purpose of the chest tube?
    1. Lessens the client's chest discomfort
    2. Restores negative pressure in the pleural space
    3. Drains accumulated fluid from the pleural cavity
    4. Prevents subcutaneous emphysema in the chest wall

46. A nurse is caring for a client with the diagnosis of right ventricular failure. Which condition unrelated to cardiac disease is the major cause of right ventricular failure?
    1. Renal disease
    2. Hypovolemic shock
    3. Severe systemic infection
    4. Chronic obstructive pulmonary disease

47. After gastrointestinal surgery, a client's condition improves and a regular diet is ordered. Which food, included on a regular diet, generally is best tolerated with little discomfort?
    1. Fresh fruit
    2. Baked fish
    3. Bran cereal
    4. Whole milk

48. A pregnant client's last menstrual period was on February 11. By July 18, a physical assessment of the client should indicate that the top of the fundus is:
    1. Even with the umbilicus
    2. Just above the symphysis pubis
    3. Two finger-breadths above the umbilicus
    4. Halfway between the symphysis and umbilicus

49. A postpartum nurse is reviewing principles related to automobile infant restraint systems with parents of a newborn who is to be discharged in the morning. What information should be included in the teaching session? Select all that apply.
    1. _____ Use a forward-facing infant car seat
    2. _____ Secure the infant seat so that it is facing the rear
    3. _____ Position the seat between the driver and passenger seats in the front seat
    4. _____ Follow the manufacturer's directions to secure the infant seat in the back seat

50. When talking with a client in crisis, the crisis intervention nurse should first:
    1. Assist the client in deciding what will be done and how it will be done
    2. Identify problems for the client, putting them in the proper perspective
    3. Explain that the center has helped many clients with the same problem
    4. Explore religious and cultural beliefs so the interventions support the client's values

51. A client at 39 weeks' gestation arrives in the birthing suite stating she is having regular contractions. A vaginal examination determines that the presentation is a double-footling breech. The practitioner decides to proceed to a cesarean birth under regional anesthesia. What is an important intervention to prevent maternal postoperative complications?
    1. Providing scrupulous skin care
    2. Maintaining adequate hydration
    3. Monitoring the vital signs frequently
    4. Teaching how to use an incentive spirometer

52. An obese adult develops an abscess after abdominal surgery. The wound is healing by secondary intention and requires repacking and redressing every 4 hours. Which diet should the nurse expect the practitioner to order to best meet this client's immediate nutritional needs?
    1. Low in fat and vitamin D
    2. High in calories and fiber
    3. Low in residue and bland
    4. High in protein and vitamin C

53. A client has a colon resection with an anastomosis. What assessments by the nurse support a suspicion of impending shock? Select all that apply.
    1. _____ Oliguria
    2. _____ Lethargy
    3. _____ Irritability
    4. _____ Hypotension
    5. _____ Slurred speech

54. A client with newly diagnosed hyperthyroidism is treated with propylthiouracil (PTU), an antithyroid drug, along with potassium iodide. The nurse teaches the client about these medications with the understanding that:
    1. Iodide solutions must be diluted in water and taken on an empty stomach
    2. Monitoring for signs of infection or bleeding is necessary while on this drug regimen
    3. Postoperative hemorrhage is a common complication if these drugs are used before a thyroidectomy
    4. These drugs will be discontinued as soon as the temperature and pulse rate return to the expected range

55. During a well-baby clinic visit the nurse assesses an 18-month-old's growth and development. What observation indicates that the toddler is within the expected range?
    1. Pedals a tricycle easily
    2. Climbs up several stairs
    3. Says 150 different words
    4. Builds a tower of 8 blocks

56. A young adolescent is diagnosed as having anorexia nervosa. The nurse identifies that the anorexia nervosa was probably precipitated by:
    1. The acting out of aggressive impulses, which results in feelings of hopelessness
    2. An unconscious wish to punish a parent who tries to dominate the adolescent's life
    3. The inability to deal with being the center of attention in the family and a desire for independence
    4. An inaccurate perception of hunger stimuli and a struggle between dependence and independence

57. Shortly after an amniotomy a nurse determines that the fetal heart rate has decreased from 140 to 80 beats per minute. What is the priority nursing action?
    1. Inspect the vagina
    2. Administer oxygen
    3. Notify the practitioner
    4. Place in the knee-chest position

58. When planning interventions to help a client with bipolar I disorder, manic episode, meet needs for rest and sleep the nurse should consider that the manic client:
    1. Experiences few sleep pattern disturbances
    2. Requires less sleep than the average person
    3. Is easily stimulated, which interferes with sleep
    4. Needs to expend energy to be tired enough to sleep

59. A nurse is caring for a child with developmental dysplasia of the hip. What is the primary intervention for this child?

1. Flexion of the hip
2. Extension of the hip
3. Adduction of the hip
4. Abduction of the hip

60. A nurse in the pediatric clinic is teaching the parents of a toddler how to prevent accidental poisoning. What should the nurse emphasize?
    1. Importance of setting limits
    2. Child's need for exploration
    3. Child's need for parental approval
    4. Importance of labeling medications

61. A nurse is counseling the family of a child with AIDS. What is the most important concern the nurse should discuss with the parents?
    1. Risk for injury
    2. Susceptibility to infection
    3. Inadequate nutritional intake
    4. Altered growth and development

62. A client in preterm labor is to receive a tocolytic medication and bed rest is prescribed. Which position should the nurse suggest that the client maintain while on bed rest?
    1. Lateral
    2. Supine
    3. Fowler's
    4. Semi-Fowler's

63. A neighbor who is a nurse is called on to assist with an emergency home birth. What should the nurse do to help expel the placenta?
    1. Put pressure on the fundus
    2. Ask the mother to bear down
    3. Have the mother breastfeed the newborn
    4. Place gentle continuous tension on the cord

64. A 22-year-old woman is admitted to the emergency department with nausea and vomiting, colicky abdominal pain, and some vaginal spotting. What question is most significant when assessing for a tubal pregnancy?
    1. "Are you sexually active?"
    2. "Does the pain come and go?"
    3. "Did you miss your last period?"
    4. "When did the nausea and vomiting start?"

65. A nurse is caring for a client with dysuria. A urinary tract infection is the presumed medical diagnosis and a urine specimen in sent to the laboratory for a culture and sensitivity examination. Which component found in the client's urine indicates the presence of a urinary tract infection?
    1. Nitrate
    2. Protein
    3. Bilirubin
    4. Erythrocytes

66. A practitioner prescribed divalproex (Depakote) for a client with the diagnosis of bipolar I disorder, manic episode. During a follow-up visit, what side effects from this medication might the client report?
    1. Dizziness, nausea, and vomiting
    2. Photosensitivity, agitation, and restlessness
    3. Abdominal cramps, tremors, and muscular weakness
    4. Weight gain, drowsiness, and decreased concentration

67. A nurse is caring for a child with a diagnosis of cystic fibrosis. Which schedule is best when planning for chest physical therapy?
    1. Three times a day before meals
    2. Three times a day halfway between meals
    3. Two times a day, on awakening and at bedtime
    4. Two times a day, after breakfast and after dinner

68. A nurse is teaching the parents of a 3-year-old child who has a diagnosis of cystic fibrosis about their child's special needs. What statement indicates that the parents need further teaching about the issues related to cystic fibrosis?
    1. "We will air-condition our entire house."
    2. "We will have to move to a very warm climate."
    3. "Our child will be taking pancreatic enzymes with meals."
    4. "Our child will need skin care after each bowel movement."

69. A client who is to begin continuous ambulatory peritoneal dialysis asks the nurse what this entails. What information should the nurse include when answering the client's question?
    1. Hemodialysis and peritoneal dialysis will be done together
    2. Peritoneal dialysis is performed in an ambulatory care clinic
    3. About a quarter of a liter of dialysate is maintained in the peritoneal cavity
    4. Constant contact is maintained between the dialysate and the peritoneal membrane

70. A nurse is assessing a malnourished client with a history of cirrhosis. The client is experiencing nausea, ascites, and gastrointestinal bleeding. The primary cause of the client's ascites is a decrease in:
    1. Vitamins to maintain cell coenzyme functions
    2. Iron to maintain adequate hemoglobin synthesis
    3. Sodium to maintain its concentration in tissue fluid
    4. Plasma protein to maintain adequate capillary-tissue circulation

71. A client at 38 weeks' gestation is experiencing painless vaginal bleeding and is diagnosed with placenta previa. The client is concerned that she may have done something to cause the bleeding. How should the nurse respond?
    1. "It's not your fault; these things happen."
    2. "Don't worry, it's just a sign of beginning labor."
    3. "Your uterus may be weak, causing the vaginal bleeding."
    4. "You have a low-lying placenta that separates when the cervix dilates."

72. A nurse is planning activities for a withdrawn client who is hallucinating. What is the most therapeutic activity for this client?
    1. Going for a walk with the nurse
    2. Watching a movie with other clients
    3. Playing a board game with a group of clients
    4. Playing a game of cards alone in the dayroom

73. A nurse is caring for a client with type 1 diabetes who developed ketoacidosis. Which laboratory value supports the presence of diabetic ketoacidosis?
    1. Increased serum lipids
    2. Decreased hematocrit level
    3. Increased serum calcium levels
    4. Decreased blood urea nitrogen level

74. A client returns from surgery after a right below-the-knee amputation with the residual limb elevated on a pillow to prevent edema. In which position should the nurse place the client after the first postoperative day?
    1. With the residual limb immobilized
    2. For short periods in the prone position
    3. For short periods in the right side-lying position
    4. With the residual limb elevated for a total of three days

75. A client is admitted to the hospital for medical management of acute pancreatitis. Which nursing action is most likely to reduce the pancreatic and gastric secretions of a client with pancreatitis?
    1. Encouraging clear liquids
    2. Obtaining a prescription for morphine
    3. Assisting the client into a semi-Fowler's position
    4. Administering prescribed anticholinergic medication

PART B QUESTIONS

76. A 66-year-old woman who has a history of a 30-pound weight loss in 3 months as well as periods of constipation and diarrhea, is diagnosed with cancer of the colon. The nurse should incorporate into the client's teaching plan that malignant tumors of the colon and rectum are:
    1. Easily detected
    2. Usually localized
    3. Found more frequently in women than in men
    4. Among the third most common cause of cancer in women

77. A 37-year-old client who has type 1 diabetes and has been maintaining glycemic control is pregnant for the third time. Her first child is 4 years old and her second pregnancy resulted in a stillbirth. She is seen in the antepartum testing unit for a nonstress test (NST) at 33 weeks' gestation. What is the primary risk factor in the client's history that indicates a need for the NST?
    1. Her age is more than 35 years
    2. She is at risk for placenta previa
    3. She is at risk for placental insufficiency
    4. Her last pregnancy resulted in a stillbirth

78. A client is worried about what to expect after having a pancreatoduodenectomy (Whipple procedure) for cancer of the pancreas. What is most important for the nurse to know when helping this client plan for the future?
    1. Any history of alcohol or tobacco use
    2. The stage and grade of the client's cancer
    3. Any previous exposure to known carcinogens
    4. The survival rate for individuals with pancreatic cancer

79. After a modified radical mastectomy, the nurse identifies that a 36-year-old female client understands the schedule for self-examination of her remaining breast when she states she will examine her breast:
    1. Seven days after each menstrual period
    2. Several days before an expected menstrual period
    3. Halfway between menstrual periods, preferably after showering
    4. On the same date every month, regardless of when menstruation occurs

80. A nurse is assessing a child with leukemia who is receiving chemotherapy. Which side effect should the nurse anticipate?
    1. Epistaxis
    2. Tachycardia
    3. Flushed skin
    4. Elevated temperature

81. During the administration of total parenteral nutrition (TPN), an assessment of the client reveals a bounding pulse, distended jugular veins, dyspnea, and cough. What is the best intervention by the nurse?
    1. Restart the client's infusion at another site
    2. Slow the rate of the client's infusion of the TPN
    3. Interrupt the client's infusion and notify the practitioner
    4. Obtain the vital signs and continue monitoring the client's status

82. A nurse is caring for a client with pulmonary tuberculosis who is to receive more than one antitubercular medication. Which of the first-line antitubercular medications is associated with a history of damage to the eighth cranial nerve?
    1. Isoniazid (INH)
    2. Rifampin (Rifadin)
    3. Streptomycin (Streptomycin)
    4. Ethambutol (Myambutol)

83. An adolescent girl with a seizure disorder refuses to wear a medical alert bracelet. What should the nurse tell the girl that may help her adhere to wearing the bracelet?
    1. Hide the bracelet under long-sleeved clothes
    2. Wear the bracelet when engaging in contact sports
    3. Ask her friends to wear bracelets that look like hers
    4. Select a bracelet that is similar to those worn by her peers

84. After an automobile collision, a client who sustained multiple injuries is oriented to person and place but is confused as to time. The client complains of a headache and drowsiness, but assessment reveals that the pupils are equal and reactive. Which nursing action takes priority?
    1. Moving the client as little as possible
    2. Preparing the client for mannitol administration
    3. Stimulating the client to maintain responsiveness
    4. Monitoring the client for increasing intracranial pressure

85. A school nurse is teaching a 12-year-old child recently diagnosed with type 1 diabetes about the action of

insulin injections. What statement indicates that the child understands how insulin works in the body?

1. "Glucose is released as fats break down."
2. "It prevents glucose from being stored in the liver."
3. "Glucose is carried into cells where it is burned for energy."
4. "It prevents wasting blood glucose by converting it to glycogen."

86. After an uneventful pregnancy, a client gives birth to an infant with a meningocele. The neonate has 1 minute and 5 minute Apgar scores of 9/10. What is the priority nursing care for this newborn?

1. Protecting the sac with sterile, moist gauze
2. Removing buccal mucus and administering oxygen
3. Placing name bracelets on both the mother and infant
4. Transferring the newborn to the neonatal intensive care unit

87. A nurse in the mental health clinic is counseling a client with the diagnosis of depression. During the counseling session the client states, "Things always seem the same. They never change." The nurse suspects that the client is feeling hopeless. For what indication of hopelessness should the nurse assess the client?

1. Outbursts of anger
2. Focused concentration
3. Preoccupation with delusions
4. Intense interpersonal relationships

88. A fetal scalp pH sample is ordered because of persistent abnormal fetal heart rate patterns. Which fetal pH value indicates to the nurse that the fetus may be compromised?

1. 7.18
2. 7.26
3. 7.31
4. 7.35

89. A client who is scheduled for a muscle biopsy tells the nurse, "They better give me a general anesthetic. I don't want to feel anything." What is the most therapeutic response by the nurse?

1. "You seem to be worried about the test."
2. "This test is done under local anesthesia."
3. "Tell them when you have pain so they can take care of it."
4. "You probably will not have pain so try not to think about it."

90. While in the playroom of a pediatric unit the nurse observes several toddlers seated at a table trying to copy the same picture from a book. They are not talking to each other or sharing their crayons. What does the nurse conclude about this behavioral interaction?

1. It is a typical expression of toddlers' social development
2. This is an example of antisocial behavior found in some children
3. It is a lack of parental role models to demonstrate acceptable behavior

4. This is an illustration of separation anxiety typical of hospitalized toddlers

91. The condition of a child dying from leukemia deteriorates and the child becomes comatose. The parents state that a relative said they should not allow the child to be resuscitated, but they are unsure about this. Which response by the nurse best demonstrates recognition of the ethical issues involved?

1. "Let me tell you about the implications of a DNR order, then you decide."
2. "Perhaps you should talk with your practitioner first; I'll be happy to make the call."
3. "You should discuss this thoroughly with your practitioner and with your religious adviser."
4. "The final decision must be made by you and your practitioner, but it is important to talk about it."

92. Before a postpartum client is discharged, the nurse advises her about problems that should be reported. Which problem identified by the client indicates that the teaching is effective?

1. Breast engorgement with feelings of fullness
2. Urgency, frequency, and burning on urination
3. Increased amount of lochia after physical activity
4. Dryness and tenderness when intercourse is first resumed

93. A client with a diagnosis of polyarteritis nodosa asks the nurse for information about this disorder. What information should the nurse include in the response?

1. Clients with this disease have an excellent prognosis
2. The disorder affects males and females in equal numbers
3. The disorder is considered one of hypersensitivity and the exact cause is unknown
4. Clients with this disease have problems with only the kidneys and the retina of the eyes

94. A slightly overweight client is to be discharged from the hospital after a cholecystectomy. What is most important for the nurse to include in teaching the client about nutrition?

1. Listing those fatty foods that may be included in the diet
2. Explaining that fatty foods may not be tolerated for several weeks
3. Teaching the importance of a low-calorie diet to promote weight reduction
4. Encouraging the client to join a weight reduction program in the local community

95. A client is admitted to the hospital for acute gastritis and ascites secondary to alcoholism and cirrhosis. It is most important for the nurse to assess this client for:

1. Blood in the stool
2. Food intolerances
3. Complaints of nausea
4. Hourly urinary output

96. A client is at high risk for developing ascites because of cirrhosis of the liver. How should the nurse assess for the presence of ascites?

1. Observe the client for signs of respiratory distress
2. Percuss the client's abdomen and listen for dull sounds
3. Palpate the lower extremities over the tibia and observe for edema
4. Listen for decreased or absent bowel sounds while auscultating the abdomen

97. The mental health nurse is facilitating a therapy group. How can the nurse further develop trust among members in the group?
    1. Discuss the importance of everyone trusting each other
    2. Reveal some personal data as a role model for trusting behavior
    3. Have group members reveal some personal information about themselves
    4. Remind group members about the need for confidentiality within the group

98. A client is admitted to the hospital with a tentative diagnosis of infectious pulmonary tuberculosis. What intervention is unique to the isolation precautions related to a client with this diagnosis?
    1. Don an N95 respirator mask and then enter the room
    2. Put on a nonpermeable gown before entering the room
    3. Wear nonsterile gloves when touching the client's body
    4. Maintain separation of 3 feet between the client and other individuals

99. A nurse is admitting a 4-year-old child to the pediatric unit. When helping this child adjust to the unit, the nurse expects that a 4-year-old child's greatest fear related to hospitalization is a fear of:
    1. Bodily harm
    2. Lack of control
    3. Loss of independence
    4. Separation from mother

100. Nursing care for a child admitted with acute glomerulonephritis should be directed toward:
    1. Enforcing bed rest
    2. Promoting diuresis
    3. Encouraging fluids
    4. Removing dietary salt

101. A 5-month-old infant is brought to the pediatric clinic because of exposure to an adolescent sibling with measles. The infant's mother asks the nurse whether her baby can be vaccinated against measles at this age. What should the nurse consider before replying?
    1. The infant's immunizations
    2. The infant's previous viral illnesses
    3. Maternal diseases and immunizations
    4. Maternal exposure to tuberculosis and herpes genitalis

102. A client has an open reduction and internal fixation of the hip. The client is to be transferred to a chair for a half hour on the second postoperative day. What should the nurse do before transferring the client?

1. Assess the strength of the affected leg
2. Explain the transfer procedure step by step
3. Instruct the client to bear weight evenly on both legs
4. Encourage the client to keep the affected leg elevated

103. A nurse assesses a 3-month-old infant who was just hospitalized for dehydration caused by vomiting. What clinical finding does the nurse anticipate?
    1. Weight loss
    2. Dilute urine
    3. Flushed skin
    4. Bulging fontanels

104. A nurse is caring for a client who is receiving IV magnesium sulfate for preeclampsia. At 37 weeks' gestation she gives birth to an infant weighing 4 pounds. What clinical finding in the newborn may indicate magnesium sulfate toxicity?
    1. Pallor
    2. Tremors
    3. Hypotonia
    4. Tachycardia

105. A client sustained a large open wound during an occupational accident. The practitioner prescribes a daily sterile dressing change. What should the nurse do to maintain sterility when changing the dressing?
    1. Put the unopened sterile glove package carefully on the sterile field
    2. Remove the sterile drape from its package by lifting it by the corners
    3 Don sterile gloves before opening the package containing the field drape
    4. Pour irrigation liquid from a height of at least three inches above the sterile container

106. A client who has always been active is diagnosed with atherosclerosis and hypertension. The client is interested in measures that will help promote and maintain health. What recommendation by the nurse will help the client maintain blood vessel patency?
    1. Practice relaxation techniques
    2. Lead a more sedentary lifestyle
    3. Decrease the amount of exercise
    4. Increase saturated fats in the diet

107. A nurse is teaching a client with hypertension about a sodium-restricted diet. What information should the nurse emphasize?
    1. Using salt-free natural seasonings can taste the same as salt
    2. Desiring the taste for salt is inherent but can be overcome with practice
    3. Liking the taste of table salt is learned but it is not a biological necessity
    4. Substituting table salt with potassium chloride-based can be done freely

108. A nurse in the birthing room is assessing a newborn. Which newborn characteristic should be assigned an Apgar value of 2?
    1. A strong cry
    2. Legs and arms slightly flexed

3. Body pink and extremities blue

4. A heart rate of ninety beats per minute

109. Two nurses are planning to help a client with one-sided weakness to move up in bed. What should the nurses do to conform to a basic principle of body mechanics?

   1. Instruct the client to position one arm on each shoulder of the nurses

   2. Direct the client to extend the legs and remain still during the procedure

   3. Have both nurses shift their weight from the front leg to the back leg as they move the client up in bed

   4. Position the nurses on either side of the bed with their feet apart, gather the pull sheet close to the client, turn toward the head of the bed, and then move the client

110. A child recently diagnosed with idiopathic scoliosis has a mild structural curve. The child's mother asks whether the problem can be corrected with exercise. What should the nurse tell the mother concerning an exercise program?

   1. This is used in conjunction with a brace

   2. It can be used if the child appears highly motivated

   3. It might exaggerate the curvature if the curve is severe

   4. This is needed to correct the curvature without requiring a brace

111. A nurse is counseling a client who is experiencing substance abuse delirium. What communication strategies should be used by the nurse when working with this client?

   1. Encourage the client to practice self-control

   2. Use humor when communicating with the client

   3. Offer a self-introduction to the client at each meeting

   4. Approach the client from the side rather than the front

112. A nurse is caring for a client with chronic obstructive pulmonary disease (COPD). Which clinical finding supports the nurse's suspicion that the client is developing cor pulmonale?

   1. Peripheral edema

   2. Productive coughing

   3. Twitching of the extremities

   4. Lethargy progressing to coma

113. A nurse is caring for a client who has chest tubes inserted to treat a hemopneumothorax that resulted from a crushing chest injury. A commonality of the various stationary chest tube drainage systems is that the first chamber is designed to:

   1. Collect drainage

   2. Ensure adequate suction

   3. Maintain negative pressure

   4. Sustain a continuance of the water seal

114. Two 14-year-old girls are best friends and always eat lunch together at school. One of the girls eats rapidly and then immediately leaves to go to the girls' restroom. After a week or so the other girl suspects her friend may be using self-induced vomiting to keep her weight

down. Because the friend is not sure what to do, she speaks with a relative who is a nurse, who encourages her to:

   1. Confront her friend with her suspicions

   2. Talk to the school nurse about her concerns

   3. Inform the girl's mother about her daughter's behavior

   4. Watch a while longer before doing anything that may spoil the friendship

115. A client with the diagnosis of obsessive-compulsive disorder who has a need to wash the hands about 50 to 60 times a day tearfully tells the nurse, "I know my hands are not dirty, but I just can't stop washing them." What is the nurse's best response?

   1. "Let's talk about why you feel you must wash your hands."

   2. "I think you're getting better; you're beginning to understand your problem."

   3. "Don't worry about it; these actions are part of your illness, and these feelings will pass."

   4. "I understand that and maybe we can work together to limit the number of times you wash them."

116. An 18-month-old toddler who has received the appropriate immunizations on time, is visiting the pediatric clinic for the next scheduled immunization. What vaccine should the nurse administer?

   1. Second hepatitis B (Hep B) vaccine

   2. Fifth inactivated polio vaccine (IPV)

   3. First pneumococcal vaccine (PCV) and influenza vaccine (Hib)

   4. Fourth diphtheria toxoid, tetanus toxoid and acellular pertussis (DTaP) vaccine

117. A nurse is assessing a client and suspects diabetic ketoacidosis (DKA). What clinical findings support this conclusion?

   1. Nervousness and tachycardia

   2. Erythema toxicum rash and pruritus

   3. Diaphoresis and altered mental state

   4. Deep respirations and fruity odor to the breath

118. A mental health nurse is participating in a therapy group. The nurse concludes that the group has reached the working stage when the members:

   1. Appear happy in their group interactions

   2. Focus on a variety of needs and concerns

   3. Say what is expected and wanted by the others

   4. Show concern for the feelings of the group leaders

119. A client who is pregnant for the first time questions the nurse about the changes in her body. While describing the changes in each body system, the nurse includes that the system that undergoes the most profound change of all during pregnancy is the:

   1. Urinary system

   2. Endocrine system

   3. Cardiovascular system

   4. Gastrointestinal system

120. Without knocking, a nurse enters the room of a young male client with the diagnosis of panic disorder and

observes him masturbating. What should the nurse do next?

1. Say, "Excuse me," and leave the room
2. Tactfully assess why he needs to masturbate
3. Pretend nothing was seen and carry out whatever task needs to be done
4. Explain in a calm, quiet manner that his behavior is inappropriate in the hospital

121. After a modified radical mastectomy a client tells the nurse, "This diagnosis is as good as a death sentence, and I would rather go now than to suffer." What is the most important nursing intervention at this time?
1. Recommend that the client admit herself to the psychiatric unit of the hospital
2. Determine whether the client has experienced self-destructive suicidal thoughts
3. Encourage the client to focus on the good things in her life to promote positive thinking
4. Explore the possibility of a vacation after hospitalization to reduce the client's stress level

122. A nurse is assessing a client with Crohn disease who is to have an upper gastrointestinal series. Which condition necessitates the cancellation of the upper gastrointestinal series?
1. Hemorrhoids
2. Hyperkalemia
3. Inflamed colon
4. Colon perforation

123. A nurse is obtaining a health history from a client newly diagnosed with cervical cancer. What aspect of the client's life is it most important for the nurse to explore at this time?
1. Sexual history
2. Support system
3. Obstetric history
4. Elimination patterns

124. A nurse is caring for a high-risk pregnant client who had a positive contraction stress test (CST). The nurse determines that a positive test:
1. Indicates the need to perform a nonstress test
2. Indicates the need for an immediate cesarean birth
3. Shows late decelerations of the fetal heart rate with each contraction
4. Shows a fetal heart rate that ranges within the expected limits for the average fetus

125. A male client with the diagnosis of schizophrenia, paranoid type, often displays overt sexual behavior toward female clients and nurses. What is the nurse's best response when the client displays a sexually explicit behavior?
1. Refusing to speak with the client until he stops the behavior
2. Sending the client to his room when the behavior is observed
3. Ignoring this behavior until the client is more in control of his responses
4. Telling the client in a matter-of-fact manner that his behavior is unacceptable

126. A client is admitted to the hospital for medical treatment of bronchopneumonia. What test result should the nurse examine to help determine the effectiveness of the client's therapy?
1. Bronchoscopy
2. Pulse oximetry
3. Pulmonary function studies
4. Culture and sensitivity tests of sputum

127. A nurse is administering an enema to a client who is scheduled for gastrointestinal surgery. What should the nurse do when the client complains of abdominal cramps during the enema?
1. Reduce the rate of flow of the infusion
2. Discontinue the enema and try again later
3. Lower the container below the level of the rectum
4. Close the lumen of the tubing and wait until the discomfort subsides

128. A mother whose infant was diagnosed with cerebral palsy at 6 months of age asks why she was not told that her baby had cerebral palsy when the infant was born. How should the nurse respond?
1. "The neurological lesions changed as your baby matured."
2. "Joint deformities do not appear until after six months of age."
3. "The staff members did not want to alarm you until it was necessary."
4. "Until there is control of voluntary movements a diagnosis cannot be confirmed."

129. A 2-year-old child is admitted with gastroenteritis and dehydration. Peripheral intravenous fluids are prescribed. What is the most appropriate site for the first intravenous insertion?
1. Scalp vein near the fontanel
2. Venous arch on top of the foot
3. Dorsal metacarpals of the hand
4. Basilic vein at the antecubital fossa

130. A grand multipara at 34 weeks' gestation is brought to the emergency department because of vaginal bleeding. The nurse suspects that the client has a placenta previa. What characteristic typical of placenta previa supports the nurse's conclusion?
1. Painful vaginal bleeding in the first trimester
2. Painful vaginal bleeding in the third trimester
3. Painless vaginal bleeding in the first trimester
4. Painless vaginal bleeding in the third trimester

131. A female client who has been hallucinating suddenly rises and shouts, "Stop saying that. Who do you think you are?" What is the most therapeutic response by the nurse?
1. Instruct the client that if she ignores the voices they will disappear
2. Take the client to her room so she can have a quiet place to think away from other clients
3. Tell her the voices she hears are not heard by others, then offer to listen to music with her
4. Point out to her the inappropriateness of her behavior in a nonthreatening, nonjudgmental manner

132. A female client has terminal cancer. Her family members are concerned because she appears to be accepting less and less responsibility for her own care. What should the nurse do to help family members plan for the client's care?
    1. Encourage them to accept her regression until she can cope more effectively
    2. Explain that her anger is normal and identify ways to deal with the behavior
    3. Point out that denial is an expected response and generally is only temporary
    4. Assist them to identify coping strategies to give her more control over the situation

133. A client has a paracentesis, and the practitioner removes 1500 mL of fluid. What clinical finding is most important for the nurse to assess after this procedure?
    1. Dry mouth
    2. Tachycardia
    3. Hypertensive crisis
    4. Increased abdominal distention

134. A client is scheduled for an amniocentesis. What should the nurse do before the procedure?
    1. Give the client the prescribed sedative
    2. Remind the client to empty her bladder
    3. Prepare the client for an intravenous infusion
    4. Encourage the client to drink three glasses of water

135. An episiotomy is performed during a vaginal birth. Sitz baths are ordered three times a day after the first 24 hours. The nurse should include in the teaching plan that sitz baths enhance healing by:
    1. Promoting vasodilation
    2. Cleansing perineal tissue
    3. Softening the incision site
    4. Tightening the rectal sphincter

136. A client with osteoporosis is encouraged to drink milk. The client refuses the milk, explaining that it causes gasiness and bloating. Which food should the nurse suggest that is rich in calcium and digested easily by clients who do not tolerate milk?
    1. Eggs
    2. Yogurt
    3. Potatoes
    4. Applesauce

137. A client receiving steroid therapy states, "I have difficulty controlling my temper, which is so unlike me, and I don't know why this is happening." What is the nurse's best response?
    1. Tell the client it is nothing to worry about
    2. Encourage the client to talk further about this problem
    3. Instruct the client to attempt to avoid situations that cause irritation
    4. Interview the client to determine whether other mood swings are being experienced

138. A nurse is caring for a client who had a femoral-popliteal bypass graft. Four hours after surgery the client's blood pressure is 200/110. What potential complication should motivate the nurse to notify the practitioner?
    1. Rupture of the graft
    2. Anaphylactic reaction
    3. Hypovolemic episode
    4. Occlusion of the graft

139. A nurse has been working for the past 3 months with a 10-year-old child who has a diagnosis of conduct disorder. What is the best long-term goal for this child?
    1. Avoid verbally aggressive behavior for 3 months
    2. Verbalize 10 alternative methods to address anger
    3. Be sent to the principal's office less than 3 times in 5 weeks
    4. Have no physically aggressive episodes during the next 3 months

140. A client who has a history of several myocardial infarctions is admitted to the hospital for an unrelated medical condition. Because of the client's history, the nurse is concerned about the possibility of the client experiencing right ventricular failure. For what early common indication of right ventricular failure should the nurse monitor the client?
    1. Chest pain
    2. Bradypnea
    3. Bradycardia
    4. Peripheral edema

141. An older female client with diarrhea is admitted to the hospital from a nursing home. A stool specimen confirms a diagnosis of a methicillin-resistant *Staphylococcus aureus* (MRSA) infection. The daughter of the client asks why her mother has been placed in a room with another client who is on isolation. How should the nurse respond?
    1. "The other person's infection is not contagious."
    2. "This is the usual practice when antibiotic therapy is started."
    3. "It is safe to place people with the same infection in one room."
    4. "As soon as a private room becomes available we will move her."

142. A 9-year-old child is admitted to the pediatric unit with a tentative diagnosis of an infratentorial brain tumor. What presenting sign does the nurse anticipate when assessing the child?
    1. Ataxia
    2. Papilledema
    3. Cranial enlargement
    4. Generalized seizures

143. One morning a male client whose thought processes are marked by ideas of reference and persecutory ideation appears very upset. The client tells the nurse that the reporter on television told everyone that the client is "a queer." What is the most therapeutic response by the nurse?
    1. "It sounds to me like you're having some frightening feelings."
    2. "I will call the station to ask why the reporter said that about you."

3. "You seem upset by this. Why do you think the reporter said that about you?"

4. "Sometimes we are unsure of ourselves. Could you be projecting feelings onto others?"

144. A nurse is preparing a teaching plan for the parents of a child with celiac disease. The nurse includes that the basic problem in celiac disease is the:
1. Presence of green stools
2. Inability to digest gliadin
3. Absence of intestinal villi
4. Susceptibility to severe dehydration

145. A nurse is caring for an observant Jewish client 1 day after surgery. The diet is increased from full liquid to regular diet as tolerated. What should the nurse consider about Jewish dietary laws when caring for this client?
1. Eating beef and veal is prohibited
2. Consumption of fish with scales is forbidden
3. Meat and milk at the same meal are forbidden
4. Consuming alcohol, coffee, and tea are prohibited

146. A nurse is caring for a mother and a neonate who was just born. What is the priority nursing action to prevent heat loss in the neonate immediately after birth?
1. Place the naked newborn under a radiant warmer
2. Dress the newborn in a shirt and gown immediately
3. Bathe the newborn in warm water as soon as possible
4. Put the naked newborn on the mother's skin and cover with a blanket

147. A client at 20 weeks' gestation visits the prenatal clinic for the first time. Assessment reveals T, 98.8° F; P, 80; BP, 128/80; weight, 142 pounds (prepregnancy weight was 132 pounds); FHR, 140 beats per minute; urine negative for protein; and fasting blood glucose, 92 mg/dL. What should the nurse do after making these assessments?
1. Report the findings because the client needs immediate intervention
2. Document the results because they are expected at twenty weeks' gestation
3. Prepare the client for an emergency admission because these findings may jeopardize the mother and fetus
4. Record the findings in the medical record because they are not within the norm but are not critical

148. A male client with a history of schizophrenia comes to the emergency department accompanied by his wife. What should be the emergency department nurse's priority intervention?
1. Observe and evaluate his behavior
2. Write a plan of care for the mental health team
3. Obtain a copy of the client's past medical records
4. Meet separately with his wife and explore why he came to the hospital

149. A nurse assesses a new mother who is breastfeeding. The client asks how to care for her nipples. What should the nurse recommend?
1. Put lanolin cream on the nipples after breastfeeding
2. Apply a vitamin E gel to the nipples before breastfeeding
3. Use soap and water to clean the breasts and nipples at least once a day

4. Spread breast milk on the nipples after the feeding and allow them to air dry

150. A nurse who is caring for a 32-week appropriate-for-gestational-age (AGA) neonate develops a plan of potential interventions for the neonate. What is the priority intervention?
1. Promoting bonding
2. Preventing infection
3. Supporting temperature
4. Maintaining respirations

151. After several days on bed rest, a preschool-age boy with the diagnosis of a liver laceration becomes demanding and will not listen to the nurses. The child was found in the playroom twice on the previous shift. How can the nurse best meet the needs of this child?
1. Tell the child why remaining on bed rest will enhance recovery
2. Have a television set moved into the child's room as soon as possible
3. Place soft restraints on the child when family members cannot be present
4. Move the child into a room with another preschooler with whom he can play

152. A client is admitted to the hospital with the diagnosis of cancer of the thyroid and a thyroidectomy is scheduled. What is important for the nurse to consider when caring for this client during the postoperative period?
1. Hypercalcemia may result from parathyroid damage
2. Hypotension and bradycardia may result from thyroid storm
3. Tetany may result from underdosage of thyroid hormone replacement
4. Hoarseness and airway obstruction may result from laryngeal nerve damage

153. A client who had extensive pelvic surgery 24 hours ago becomes cyanotic, is gasping for breath, and complains of right-sided chest pain. What should the nurse do first?
1. Obtain the vital signs
2. Initiate a cardiac arrest code
3. Administer oxygen using a face mask
4. Encourage the use of an incentive spirometer

154. A client with cancer of the stomach is admitted to the hospital and scheduled for a subtotal gastrectomy. The nurse is providing preoperative teaching. What should the nurse teach the client to do postoperatively to minimize the complication of dumping syndrome?
1. Ambulate after every meal
2. Remain on a diet low in fat
3. Eat in a semirecumbent position
4. Increase fluid intake when eating food

155. A nurse is teaching a group of nursing assistants how to help disabled clients stand and transfer from the bed to a chair. To protect the caregivers from injury, the nurse teaches them to lift the client by first placing their arms under the client's axillae and next:
1. Bending and then straightening their knees
2. Bending at the waist and then straightening the back

3. Placing one foot in front of the other and then leaning back

4. Placing pressure against the client's axillae and then raising their arms

156. An 11-year-old preadolescent has just been diagnosed with type 1 diabetes. The child, who likes sweets, asks about sugar and sugar substitutes in the diet. What information should the nurse and the dietitian give the child?
1. Honey can be used as a natural sugar substitute
2. The simple sugars such as sucrose or fructose should be avoided
3. The sweet taste habit can be broken by eliminating sweets entirely
4. Sugar substitutes such as saccharin, aspartame, or sucralose can be used

157. The wife of a client enters the hospital to visit her husband who just had surgery. She slips and falls on a recently washed floor in the hallway leading to her husband's room. What action is required to meet the criteria of ethical practice?
1. Initiating an agency incident report
2. Reporting the fall to the state health department
3. Writing a brief description of the incident to be kept by the nurse manager
4. Ignoring the need to document the event because the visitor is not a client in the hospital

158. A 2½-year-old boy who had surgery to revise a ventriculoperitoneal shunt is to be discharged. The nurse advises the parents to call the clinic if the child:
1. Appears drowsy after a nap and becomes irritable
2. Talks incessantly regardless of the presence of others
3. Becomes angry when frustrated and has a temper tantrum
4. Starts arguments with playmates claiming that their toys are his

159. The nurse manager of the unit comes to work obviously intoxicated. The staff nurse's ethical obligation is to:
1. Call the security guard
2. Tell the nurse manager to go home
3. Have the supervisor validate the observation
4. Offer the nurse manager a large cup of coffee

160. A nurse is concerned about a client's mother-infant bonding when on the first postpartum day she is reluctant to:
1. Undress the newborn
2. Breastfeed her newborn
3. Look at her newborn's face
4. Attend classes for newborn care

161. A nurse is caring for a client who had head and neck surgery. Postoperatively, the nurse positions the client's head in functional alignment to prevent the complication of:
1. Cervical trauma
2. Laryngeal spasm
3. Laryngeal edema
4. Wound dehiscence

162. When checking the cervical dilation of a client in labor, a nurse observes that the umbilical cord has prolapsed. What is the priority nursing action?

1. Take the fetal heart rate
2. Turn the client onto her side
3. Cover the cord with a sterile saline cloth
4. Put the client in the Trendelenburg position

163. After abdominal surgery a goal is to have the client achieve alveolar expansion. The nurse determines that this goal is most effectively achieved by:
1. Postural drainage
2. Pursed-lip breathing
3. Incentive spirometry
4. Sustained exhalation

164. A practitioner prescribes a standard walker (pick-up walker with rubber tips on all four legs). What clinical findings does the nurse identify that indicate the client is capable of using a standard walker?
1. Weak upper arm strength and impaired stamina
2. Weight bearing as tolerated and unilateral paralysis
3. Partial weight bearing on the affected extremity and kyphosis
4. Strong upper arm strength and non–weight bearing on the affected extremity

165. A client with advanced cancer of the bladder is scheduled for a cystectomy and ileal conduit. What intervention does the nurse anticipate the practitioner will prescribe to prepare the client for surgery?
1. Intravesicular chemotherapy
2. Instillation of a urinary antiseptic
3. Administration of neomycin sulfate
4. Placement of an indwelling catheter

166. When caring for a client with bulimia nervosa, the nurse expects that bulimia nervosa follows a cyclic pattern. List the following statements in order of progression through this cycle.
1. Hunger results from food deprivation and stress
2. Dieting is an attempt to maintain control of one's life
3. Binge eating numbs physical and emotional discomforts
4. Purging is another attempt to regain control and alleviate guilt
Answer: _____

167. A 9-year-old child sustains a fractured femur in a motor vehicle collision. Two days after surgery for repair of the fracture the nurse identifies a slight decrease in the child's hemoglobin level. What should the nurse do first concerning this clinical finding?
1. Notify the practitioner immediately
2. Schedule blood typing and crossmatching
3. Order additional meat on the child's menu
4. Assess the child's abdomen for internal bleeding

168. At 37 weeks' gestation a client's membranes spontaneously rupture but she does not have contractions. What is most important to include in the nursing plan of care for this client?
1. Monitor for the presence of fever
2. Observe for signs of preeclampsia
3. Assess for heavy vaginal bleeding
4. Prepare for fetal scalp pH sampling

169. A practitioner prescribes cholestyramine (Questran), an anion exchange resin, to treat a client's persistent diarrhea. What vitamin does the nurse anticipate may become deficient because cholestyramine reduces the absorption of fat?
    1. Thiamine
    2. Vitamin A
    3. Riboflavin
    4. Vitamin B_6

170. A primary nurse receives orders for a newly admitted client and has difficulty reading the practitioner's writing. Who should the nurse ask for clarification of this order?
    1. Nurse practitioner
    2. House doctor on call
    3. Practitioner who wrote the order
    4. Nurse manager familiar with the practitioner's writing

171. When assessing a client during the fourth stage of labor, a nurse observes that the perineal pad is soaked end to end with approximately 75 mL of lochia rubra. What is the priority nursing action?
    1. Palpate the uterine fundus
    2. Document the amount and type of lochia
    3. Accompany the client to the bathroom to empty her bladder
    4. Call the laboratory to test for hemoglobin and hematocrit levels

172. A terminally ill client is furious with one of the staff nurses. The client refuses the nurse's care and insists on doing self-care. The next day a different nurse is assigned to care for the client. What should be the newly assigned nurse's initial step in revising the client's plan of care?
    1. Get a full report from the first nurse and adjust the plan accordingly
    2. Ask the practitioner for a report on the client's condition and plan appropriately
    3. Tell the client about the change in staff responsibilities and assess the client's reaction
    4. Assess the client's present status and include the client in a discussion of revisions to the plan of care

173. A nurse is caring for a client who was admitted with the diagnosis of severe preeclampsia and is now receiving an intravenous infusion of magnesium sulfate. What is the classification of this medication?
    1. Diuretic
    2. Oxytocic
    3. Antihypertensive agent
    4. Central nervous system depressant

174. A nurse is caring for a client who is admitted to the birthing unit with a diagnosis of abruptio placentae. For what complication associated with this problem should the nurse monitor this client?
    1. Brain attack
    2. Pulmonary edema
    3. Impending seizures
    4. Hypovolemic shock

175. When developing a plan of care for an older client with a diagnosis of dementia, a nurse should:
    1. Explain to the client the details of the regimen
    2. Demonstrate interest in the client's various likes and dislikes
    3. Be firm when dealing with the client's attitudes and behaviors
    4. Provide consistency in carrying out nursing activities for the client

176. While supervising a smallpox vaccination program, a nurse manager observes a nurse cleansing the arm of a client with an alcohol swab before giving the vaccination. The nurse manager's first reaction should be to:
    1. Continue observing the vaccination
    2. Stop the nurse from giving the vaccination
    3. Give the nurse a povidone-iodine swab to use instead
    4. Notify the members of the team about the need to use antiseptic swabs

177. An older adult client is demonstrating mild confusion after surgical repair of a hernia. What should the nurse do to provide for this client's safety?
    1. Use a nightlight in the client's room
    2. Secure an order for a soft vest restraint
    3. Activate the position-sensitive bed alarm
    4. Raise the four side rails on the client's bed

178. A 6-week-old infant has surgery for hypertrophic pyloric stenosis (HPS). When encouraged to participate in caring for her infant the mother readily assists with all aspects of care but is reluctant to resume feeding her baby. The probable reason that the mother does not feed her infant is because she is:
    1. Afraid that her baby's vomiting will resume
    2. Unaware that she is allowed to feed her baby
    3. Not sure how to feed her baby with a special nipple
    4. Uncertain if her baby will tolerate the thickened formula

179. A client with a fractured tibia and fibula is to be discharged from the emergency department with a right leg cast and crutches. What should the nurse teach the client to do in addition to the technical aspects of crutch walking?
    1. Double the intake of vitamin C
    2. Remove loose rugs from the environment
    3. Avoid taking showers until the cast is removed
    4. Increase weight bearing on the injured leg gradually

180. X-ray films reveal that a client has closed fractures of the right femur and tibia. Also multiple soft-tissue contusions are present. What is the most important nursing intervention?
    1. Perform a neurovascular assessment of the extremity
    2. Reassure the client that these injuries are not that serious
    3. Gather equipment needed for the application of skeletal traction
    4. Prepare the client for a surgical reduction of the injured extremity

181. A client with bilateral varicose veins of the lower extremities questions the nurse about the brownish

discoloration of the lower legs. The best response by the nurse is, "This is probably the result of:
1. inadequate arterial blood supply."
2. delayed healing of tissues after an injury."
3. increased production of melanin in the area."
4. leakage of red blood cells through the vascular wall."

182. The nurse teaches the mother of an infant who is to have a cleft lip repair about postoperative care. What postoperative action by the mother indicates that she understands her infant's postoperative needs?
1. Allows crying for short periods
2. Cleanses the suture line after each feeding
3. Offers a pacifier when the infant becomes restless
4. Gives the feeding with the infant propped on the side

183. A pregnant client has class II cardiac disease. To best plan the client's care, the nurse should consider that the client:
1. Can participate in as much activity as she desires
2. Should be hospitalized if there is evidence of cardiac decompensation
3. Will have to maintain bed rest for most of the day throughout her pregnancy
4. May have to consider a therapeutic abortion if there is evidence of cardiac decompensation

184. A client comes into the emergency department with neurologic deficits after falling off a ladder. What client assessment is included in the Glasgow Coma Scale?
1. Breathing patterns
2. Deep tendon reflexes
3. Eye accommodation to light
4. Motor response to verbal commands

185. A client comes to the medical clinic complaining of headaches. The nurse measures the blood pressure at 172/114. What should the nurse do first?
1. Page the on-call practitioner and monitor the blood pressure
2. Administer ibuprofen and have the client rest quietly for twenty minutes
3. Elevate the head of the bed, provide reassurance, and reassess the blood pressure
4. Place the client in the supine position, administer oxygen, and notify the practitioner

186. The results of a biopsy indicate that a client has a malignant sarcoma of the liver and chemotherapy via regional perfusion is the treatment of choice. The nurse teaches the client that this method of drug administration probably was selected because:
1. Drug therapy can be continued at home with little difficulty
2. Larger doses of drugs can be delivered to the actual site of the tumor
3. Toxic effects of the chemotherapeutic drugs are confined to the area of the tumor
4. Combinations of drugs are used to attack neoplastic cells at various stages of the cell cycle

187. A nurse is caring for a toddler in acute respiratory distress precipitated by laryngotracheobronchitis. The child has a temperature of 103° F. What is the priority nursing intervention?
1. Delivering humidified oxygen
2. Initiating measures to reduce fever
3. Monitoring respiratory status continuously
4. Providing support to diminish apprehension

188. A client is admitted to the hospital with a head injury sustained while playing soccer. For which early sign of increased intracranial pressure should the nurse monitor this client?
1. Nausea
2. Lethargy
3. Sunset eyes
4. Hyperthermia

189. A nurse is caring for an older adult who had an open reduction and internal fixation of a fractured hip. What clinical finding requires the nurse to notify the practitioner?
1. Lack of a productive cough 2 days postoperatively
2. Rectal temperature of 100.2° F 3 days postoperatively
3. Complaints of right-sided chest pain 6 days postoperatively
4. Fatigue in the leg on the unaffected side 5 days postoperatively

190. A client scheduled for surgery has a history of methicillin-resistant *Staphylococcus aureus* (MRSA) since developing an infection in a surgical site 9 months ago. The site is healed and the client reports having received antibiotics for the infection. What should the nurse do to determine if the infecting organism is still present?
1. Notify the infection control officer
2. Inform the operating room of the MRSA
3. Obtain an order to culture the client's blood
4. Call the surgeon for an infectious disease consultation

191. A 13-year-old child with sickle cell anemia is experiencing a painful episode (vaso-occlusive crisis). The nurse assesses the child, obtains the child's vital signs, and reviews the child's laboratory test results. What is the priority nursing intervention?
1. Providing oxygen therapy
2. Administering an analgesic

CLIENT CHART
Laboratory Tests
Hematocrit: 23.2%
Hemoglobin: 8.1 g/dL
Vital Signs
Temperature: 99.6° F, oral
Pulse: 94, regular rhythm
Respirations: 22 breaths per minute, unlabored
Blood pressure: 132/80
Physical Assessment
Fatigue
Anorexia
Irritability
Pulse oximetry of 92% on room air
Pain in the knees, 9 on a scale of 1 to 10
Painful swollen feet, 4 on a scale of 1 to 10

3. Initiating a blood transfusion
4. Monitoring intravenous fluids

192. A nurse is concerned when an 11-month-old infant is brought to the pediatric clinic weighing 9 pounds, 3 ounces. The nurse suspects that the infant is suffering from physical and emotional neglect. What observations lead the nurse to suspect that the child may be maltreated? Select all that apply.
    1. _____ Stranger anxiety
    2. _____ Inappropriate clothing
    3. _____ Social unresponsiveness
    4. _____ Frequent rocking motions
    5. _____ Adequate personal hygiene

193. When auscultating the lungs of a client admitted with severe preeclampsia, the nurse identifies the presence of crackles. What inference does the nurse make when considering the presence of crackles in the lungs?
    1. Seizure activity is imminent
    2. Pulmonary edema has developed
    3. Bronchial constriction was precipitated by the stress of pregnancy
    4. Impaired diaphragmatic functioning was caused by the enlarged uterus

194. After surgery for repair of a myelomeningocele, the nurse places the infant in a side-lying position with the head slightly elevated. The unique reason why the nurse places the infant in this position is because it:
    1. Prevents aspiration
    2. Promotes respiration
    3. Reduces intracranial pressure
    4. Maintains cleanliness of the suture site

195. A highway accident involving 25 vehicles occurs during a foggy, snowy winter day. At the scene of the accident a triage nurse is identifying and labeling victims according to triage acuity principles. What color tag should the nurse label a person who has a simple fracture of the right humerus and several lacerations of the face?
    1. Red
    2. Green
    3. Yellow
    4. Orange

196. A client develops subcutaneous emphysema after the surgical creation of a tracheostomy. What assessment by the nurse most readily detects this complication?
    1. Palpating the neck or face
    2. Evaluating the blood gases
    3. Auscultating the lung fields
    4. Reviewing the chest x-ray film

197. A client who complains of memory loss, nervousness, insomnia, and fear of going out of the house is admitted to the hospital after several days of increasing incapacitation. What nursing action is the priority considering this client's history?
    1. Evaluating the client's adjustment to the unit
    2. Providing the client with a sense of security and safety
    3. Exploring the client's memory loss and fear of going out

4. Assessing the client's perception of reasons for the hospitalization

198. After gastric surgery a client has a nasogastric tube in place. What should the nurse do when caring for this client?
    1. Monitor for signs of electrolyte imbalance
    2. Change the tube at least once every 48 hours
    3. Connect the nasogastric tube to high continuous suction
    4. Assess placement by injecting 10 mL of water into the tube

199. A 10-year-old child recently diagnosed with type 2 diabetes attends the Center for Diabetic Teaching with the parents. The nurse interviews the child before the class begins. What is the usual major concern these children have?
    1. How much school might be missed
    2. Whether the diabetes can be controlled
    3. How the parents will react to the diagnosis
    4. Whether having diabetes means future sterility

200. A client comes to the clinic complaining of a productive cough with copious yellow sputum, fever, and chills for the past 2 days. The first thing the nurse should do when caring for this client is to:
    1. Encourage fluids
    2. Administer oxygen
    3. Take the temperature
    4. Collect a sputum specimen

201. A nurse admits a client with a diagnosis of cholelithiasis for surgery. The client asks many questions about the postoperative course after laparoscopic surgery. What is most important for the nurse to include in the teaching plan?
    1. Need for long-term dietary restrictions
    2. Type of surgical incisions and wound care
    3. Explanation of abdominal and scapular pain
    4. Encouragement to perform abdominal exercises

202. A client is admitted to the burn unit with partial-thickness burns over 30% of the body surface area. Twenty-four hours later the client, who has an IV of 5% dextrose in saline running, has tremors, twitching, and signs of disorientation. During the past hour the urinary output was 110 mL. What should the nurse do next?
    1. Slow the IV rate and notify the practitioner
    2. Slow the IV rate and check the last chest x-ray film
    3. Increase the IV rate and assess the arterial blood gases
    4. Increase the IV rate and request a prescription for calcium gluconate

203. When planning for a client's care during the detoxification phase of acute alcohol withdrawal, the nurse anticipates the need to:
    1. Monitor the client frequently
    2. Keep the client's room lights dim
    3. Address the client in a loud, clear voice
    4. Restrain the client during periods of agitation

204. A client with Hodgkin's disease is to receive the cyclic antineoplastic vinCRIStine (Oncovin) as part of a therapy protocol. The client asks how this medication

works. The nurse responds in language that the client will understand that vinCRIStine helps destroy the malignant cells by:

1. Arresting mitosis in metaphase
2. Inhibiting the synthesis of thymidine
3. Alkylating nucleic acids needed for mitosis
4. Inactivating DNA while inhibiting RNA synthesis

205. A nurse is counseling a client with the diagnosis of bulimia nervosa. The client states that at times she feels helpless in relation to her eating disorder. The nurse is assisting the client to set goals. The most appropriate short-term goal for this client is, "The client will:
1. practice effective socialization skills."
2. perceive her body shape as acceptable."
3. decrease preoccupation with delusional thoughts."
4. verbalize the desire to increase control over stressful situations."

206. A postpartum client is scheduled to have a tubal ligation. She has requested that her husband not be told about the procedure because she has told him she is having exploratory surgery. The client's husband asks the nurse why his wife needs to have exploratory surgery. How should the nurse respond?
1. "What has the physician told you?"
2. "I don't know the answer to that question."
3. "I'm not allowed to give you that information."
4. "Have you talked to your wife about your concerns?"

207. A client with recurrent episodes of depression comes to the mental health clinic for a routine follow-up visit. The nurse suspects that the client may be at an increased risk for suicide. What is a contributing factor to the client's potential risk for suicide?
1. Psychomotor retardation
2. Decreased physical activity
3. Deliberate thoughtful behavior
4. Overwhelming feelings of guilt

208. A 16-year-old girl with sickle cell anemia is experiencing a painful episode (vaso-occlusive crisis) and has a patient-controlled analgesia (PCA) pump. She complains of pain (5 on a scale of 1 to 10) in her right elbow. The nurse observes that the pump is "locked out" for another 10 minutes. What action should the nurse implement?
1. Turn on the television for diversion
2. Call the practitioner for another analgesic order
3. Place the ordered prn warm wet compress on the elbow
4. Inform her gently that she must wait until the pump reactivates

209. When lithium therapy is instituted, the nurse should teach the client to maintain an adequate daily intake of:
1. Iron
2. Sodium
3. Potassium
4. Magnesium

210. A client is admitted to the hospital after having a tonic-clonic seizure and is diagnosed with a seizure disorder.

What is most important for the nurse to include in a teaching program?
1. Outline ways that prevent physical trauma from occurring during a seizure
2. Teach that anticonvulsant medications should be taken on an empty stomach
3. Teach the client that the symptoms and treatment of seizure disorders are similar, regardless of the cause
4. Explain to the client that it is not necessary to tell others of the illness because medication will control seizures

211. After surgery for a myelomeningocele, an infant is being fed by gavage. When checking placement of the feeding tube, the nurse is unable to hear the air injected because of noisy breath sounds. What should the nurse do next?
1. Notify the practitioner
2. Advance the tube 1 cm
3. Insert 1 mL of formula slowly
4. Try aspirating stomach contents

212. A practitioner orders 10 mL of a 10% solution of calcium gluconate for a client with a severely depressed serum calcium level. The client also is receiving digoxin (Lanoxin) 0.25 mg daily and an IV solution of D_5W. The nurse's next action is based on the fact that calcium gluconate:
1. Can be added to any IV solution
2. Must be administered via an IVPB
3. Is nonirritating to surrounding tissues
4. Potentiates the action of the digoxin preparation

213. A nurse in the postanesthesia care unit identifies a progressive decrease in blood pressure in a client who had major abdominal surgery. What clinical finding supports the conclusion that the client is experiencing internal bleeding?
1. Oliguria
2. Bradypnea
3. Pulse deficit
4. High potassium levels

214. A 7-pound newborn is admitted to the nursery with an order for phytonadione (vitamin K) (AquaMEPHYTON) 1 mg IM. The nurse explains to the parents that this vitamin is administered to:
1. Facilitate bilirubin excretion
2. Promote clotting of the blood
3. Increase liver glycogen stores
4. Stimulate growth of bowel flora

215. After surgery to create an ileal conduit, a client awakens and asks for a sip of water. The nurse informs the client that water by mouth cannot be given until the:
1. Ileal loop begins to drain
2. Intestinal anastomosis heals
3. Nasogastric suction is discontinued
4. Client leaves the postanesthesia care unit

216. A 20-year-old male college student tells the nurse at the college health clinic that he has become increasingly anxious, cannot sleep, and has lost his appetite. He also

states that he cannot concentrate and his grades have dropped. What question should the nurse ask?

1. "With whom have you shared your feelings of anxiety?"
2. "What have you identified as the cause of your anxiety?"
3. "It must be difficult for you. How long has this been going on?"
4. "Sounds like you're having problems adjusting. Shall we talk about it?"

217. A postoperative male client complains that the client in the next room sings all night and keeps him awake. The singing client has dementia and is awaiting transfer to a nursing home. How can the nurse best handle this situation?
    1. Tell the client to stop singing
    2. Close the doors to both clients' rooms at night
    3. Give the complaining client the prescribed prn sedative
    4. Move the singing client to a room at the end of the hall

218. A client with active genital herpes has a cesarean birth. The nurse teaches the mother how to limit transmission of the virus to her newborn. The nurse evaluates that the instructions are understood when the mother states, "I:
    1. should avoid kissing my baby on the lips."
    2. must wear gloves when I'm holding my baby."
    3. should wash my clothes and my baby's clothes separately."
    4. must wash my hands with soap and water before handling my baby."

219. The son of a terminally ill woman is concerned about his mother's condition. He asks the nurse, "Will she get better?" What is the nurse's most appropriate response?
    1. "Her vital signs are stable. Right now she is holding her own."
    2. "Of course she will. You can't give up. You must hope for the best."
    3. "Her condition is very serious. It might help you if we discuss your concerns."
    4. "I don't know. You'll have to ask the practitioner. I'll leave a note that you are here."

220. A nurse is caring for a terminally ill client who is angry with everything and everyone. The nurse has been encouraging the client to make decisions about daily activities. The nurse identifies that some of the anger may have resolved when the client states:
    1. "Leave me alone! I want to do it by myself."
    2. "You've got a busy morning ahead of you! I'm really a mess."
    3. "I can do my face, hands, arms, and chest today, but I think you'd better do the rest."
    4. "It's so hard to let someone do so much for me. I don't like it when others do things for me."

221. A nurse is hired to work in a facility where the nurse assumes responsibility for a number of clients' needs. This nursing care delivery system is called:
    1. Team nursing
    2. Modular nursing
    3. Functional nursing
    4. Primary care nursing

222. An IV of 800 mL/24 hours is ordered for a 2½-year-old child. At how many milliliters per hour should the nurse set the volume control device?
    1. 38 mL
    2. 33 mL
    3. 28 mL
    4. 23 mL

223. A client is admitted to the emergency department with head and chest injuries sustained in an automobile collision. What clinical findings indicate that the client is responding to medical intervention and is ready to be transferred from the emergency department to a critical care unit?
    1. Stable vital signs and pain
    2. Pale and alert but restless
    3. Increasing temperature and apprehension
    4. Fluctuating vital signs and drowsy but easily roused

224. A nurse is caring for a 26-year-old client recently diagnosed with HIV. The client needs an update on immunizations and asks which ones are needed. Which vaccines are required to comply with the recommended immunization schedule for a client with HIV?
    1. Influenza, MMR, varicella, and hepatitis A vaccines
    2. Pneumococcal, MMR, influenza, and varicella vaccines
    3. Diphtheria, tetanus, hepatitis A, and hepatitis C vaccines
    4. Tetanus, hepatitis B, influenza, and pneumococcal vaccines

225. A client had a suction curettage for the removal of a hydatidiform mole. What should the nurse emphasize when planning for the client's discharge?
    1. Necessity for follow-up care for at least six weeks
    2. Risk factors for developing another hydatidiform mole
    3. Reasons for postponing another pregnancy for an entire year
    4. Basis for chemotherapy if the chorionic gonadotropin hormone level falls slowly

226. A 63-year-old woman with the diagnosis of estrogen-receptor positive cancer of the breast had a lumpectomy and radiation therapy. Tamoxifen (Nolvadex) is prescribed. The client asks the nurse how long she has to take this medication. The nurse responds, "It will be given for:
    1. the rest of your life."
    2. 10 days, like an antibiotic."
    3. 5 years, after which it will be discontinued."
    4. several months until the bone pain subsides."

227. A client had a surgical fusion of the fourth and fifth lumbar vertebrae. When the nurse and nursing assistant enter the room to provide evening care on the day of surgery, the client becomes anxious about being moved. What should the nurse do?
    1. Reassure the client that they will be careful
    2. Explain that this surgery is not life threatening

3. Describe the need for numerous personnel during turning
4. Suggest that the client can turn on the television for diversion

228. A male client with a history of ulcerative colitis is admitted to the hospital because of severe rectal bleeding. He is engaging in angry outbursts and places excessive demands on the staff. One day the nursing assistant tells the nurse, "I've had it with that man and his behavior. I'm not going in there again." What is the best response by the nurse?
    1. "You need to try to be patient with him. He's going through a lot right now."
    2. "I'll talk with him. Maybe I can figure out the best way for us to handle this."
    3. "Just ignore him and get on with your work. I'll assign someone else to take a turn."
    4. "He's frightened and taking it out on the staff. Let's think of ways we can approach him."

229. A 28-year-old male client is undergoing tests to confirm the diagnosis of Hodgkin's lymphoma. The client and his wife are worried that he may have cancer. The wife states, "Don't you think it is unlikely for someone like my husband to have cancer?" The nurse's response is based on the information that Hodgkin's lymphoma is:
    1. More likely to affect women than men
    2. Diagnosed during adolescence and young adulthood
    3. Typically a disease of older rather than younger adults
    4. Usually occurs frequently among populations of Asian heritage

230. A primigravida asks the nurse, "What caused the blotchy skin on my face, my dark nipples, and the dark line down the middle of my stomach?" The nurse explains that the gland that causes these expected changes during pregnancy is the:
    1. Adrenal gland
    2. Thyroid gland
    3. Anterior pituitary gland
    4. Posterior pituitary gland

231. A client who is formula feeding her infant complains of discomfort in her engorged breasts. What should the nurse recommend that the client do?
    1. Express milk from each breast manually
    2. Apply cold packs and a binder to the breasts
    3. Restrict oral fluid intake to less than a quart a day
    4. Use towels that are warm and moist as compresses

232. A client with schizophrenia who has been taking clozapine (Clozaril) is to be started on 10 mg of olanzapine (Zyprexa) instead. The nurse explains to the client, in terms that can be understood, that olanzapine is being substituted for clozapine because it does not produce the side effect of:
    1. Hypotension
    2. Gastric upset
    3. Agranulocytosis
    4. Metabolic syndrome

233. A client who is suspected of having had a silent myocardial infarction has an electrocardiogram (ECG) ordered by the practitioner. While the nurse prepares the client for this procedure, the client asks, "Why was this test ordered?" The best reply by the nurse is, "This test will:
    1. detect your heart sounds."
    2. reflect any heart damage."
    3. help us change your heart's rhythm."
    4. tell us how much stress your heart can tolerate."

234. Twelve hours after sustaining full-thickness burns to the chest and thighs a client who is NPO is complaining of severe thirst. The client's urinary output has been 60 mL/hr for the past 10 hours. No bowel sounds are heard. What should the nurse do?
    1. Give the client orange juice by mouth
    2. Offer the client 4 oz of water by mouth
    3. Increase the client's intravenous flow rate
    4. Moisten the client's lips with a wet 4 × 4 gauze

235. A client is admitted to the hospital with partial- and full-thickness burns of the chest sustained in a house fire. What is the nurse's priority concern?
    1. Limited physical mobility caused by bed rest
    2. Inadequate gas exchange due to smoke inhalation
    3. Susceptibility to infection as a result of tissue trauma
    4. Decreased fluid volume because of inadequate oral intake

236. A nurse is considering the family's role in discharge planning for an adult client who has been in a psychiatric facility. What is the most appropriate nursing action after the nurse obtains the client's consent?
    1. Inform the family when discharge will occur
    2. Include the family when making specific discharge plans
    3. Answer family members' questions about the client's illness
    4. Have family members help assess the client's readiness for discharge

237. A practitioner prescribes an antidepressant for a hospitalized client who has been severely depressed. Eight days later the nurse observes that the client is neatly dressed and well groomed. The client smiles at the nurse and states, "Things sure look better today." What nursing response is appropriate based on the client's statement?
    1. Compliment the client's appearance
    2. Begin preparing the client for discharge
    3. Arrange for constant supervision of the client
    4. Add privileges to the client's plan of care as a reward

238. On the morning of a scheduled visit the parents of a client hospitalized for incapacitating obsessive behavior call to say that they cannot come because of problems with the accountant for their small business. The client appears upset and goes into elaborate detail about the parents' business and the monthly visit of the accountant. What is the nurse's best response?
    1. "It's disappointing to have plans change at the last minute."

2. "Would you like to talk about what you had planned to do today?"

3. "Would you like to make new plans now that they are not coming?"

4. "It's good that you can recognize that your parents are sometimes busy."

239. A young female client comes to the trauma center stating that she was raped. She is disheveled, pale, and staring blankly. Considering what has occurred, the nurse asks the client to describe what happened. What is the nurse's rationale for asking the client to describe what happened?

1. It will help the nursing staff in giving legal advice and providing counseling

2. Talking about the assault will help her see how her behavior may have led to the event

3. The victim can put the event in better perspective and it helps begin the resolution process

4. Discussing details will prevent the victim from concealing the intimate happenings during the assault

240. A client's respiratory status may be affected after abdominal surgery. The nurse documents the behavioral objective for this client. What statement is a behavioral objective?

1. Demonstrates the technique of coughing and deep breathing

2. Respirations will improve with coughing and deep breathing

3. Coughing and deep breathing will facilitate output of secretions

4. Will cough and deep breathe five or six times every hour while awake

241. An older, confused client is being cared for at home by an adult child who works full-time. The client has lost weight and is wearing soiled and inappropriate clothing. The home care nurse suspects elder neglect. What should the nurse do?

1. Discuss the situation with the adult child

2. Ask the client if the adult child is neglectful

3. Avoid reporting the situation to prevent alienation of the adult child

4. Report suspected neglect by the adult child to adult protective services

242. During the assessment of a client who was admitted to the hospital because of a productive cough, fever, and chills, the nurse percusses an area of dullness over the right posterior lower lobe of the lung. The nurse determines that the client's signs and symptoms may be indicative of:

1. Pleurisy

2. Bronchitis

3. Pneumonia

4. Emphysema

243. A male client with aortic stenosis is scheduled for a valve replacement in 2 days. He tells the nurse, "I told my wife all she needs to know if I don't make it." What response is most therapeutic?

1. "Men your age do very well."

2. "You are worried about dying."

3. "I know you are concerned, but your surgeon is excellent."

4. "I'll get you a sleeping pill tonight because I know you will need it."

244. What should a nurse do to decrease or control the sensory and cognitive disturbances that can occur after a client has open heart surgery?

1. Restrict family visits

2. Withhold analgesic medications

3. Plan for maximum periods of rest

4. Keep the room light on most of the time

245. A client complains of pain 4 hours after a liver biopsy. The nurse identifies that there is a leakage of a large amount of bile on the dressing over the biopsy site. What should the nurse do first?

1. Tell the client to remain flat on the back

2. Medicate the client for pain as prescribed

3. Notify the client's practitioner immediately

4. Monitor the client's vital signs every ten minutes

246. A 13-year-old girl tells the school nurse that she took a pregnancy test and it was positive. She adds that her grandfather has been molesting her for the past 3 years. When the nurse asks if anyone else knows about this, she replies, "Yes, but my mother doesn't believe me." Legally, who must the nurse notify?

1. Police concerning a possible sex crime

2. Child Protective Services for immediate intervention

3. The clinic for an examination to confirm the pregnancy

4. The girl's mother about the pregnancy test's positive result

247. A client is admitted for induction of labor. An IV infusion of oxytocin (Pitocin) is started. When the client's contractions begin they are 1½ to 2 minutes in duration. While the nurse is in the room, one contraction lasts 3 minutes. What should the nurse do first?

1. Give oxygen by nasal cannula

2. Turn off the oxytocin infusion

3. Reposition the monitoring belts

4. Place a call light next to the client

248. A client with heart failure is digitalized and placed on a maintenance dose of digoxin (Lanoxin) 0.25 mg by mouth daily. What responses does the nurse expect the client to exhibit when a therapeutic effect of digoxin is achieved?

1. Diuresis and decreased pulse rate

2. Increased blood pressure and weight loss

3. Regular pulse rhythm and stable fluid balance

4. Corrected heart murmur and decreased pulse pressure

249. An 80-year-old client with a history of coronary artery disease is admitted to the hospital for observation after a fall. During the night the client has an episode of paroxysmal nocturnal dyspnea. In what position should the nurse place the client to best decrease preload?

1. Contour

2. Orthopneic

3. Recumbent

4. Trendelenburg

250. A nurse on the community's terrorism response team is reviewing triage protocols. In contrast to triage policies in local emergency situations, triage in mass casualty events does not give care to clients who have:

1. Multiple fractures

2. Closed head injuries

3. Internal abdominal trauma

4. Radiation/chemical exposures

251. A client has a permanent colostomy. During the first 24 hours there is no drainage from the colostomy. The nurse concludes that this is a result of the:

1. Edema after the surgery

2. Absence of intestinal peristalsis

3. Decrease in fluid intake before surgery

4. Effective functioning of the nasogastric tube

252. A client is admitted to the hospital for surgery for rectosigmoid colon cancer, and the nurse is obtaining a health history as part of the admission process. What clinical findings associated with rectosigmoid colon cancer does the nurse expect the client to report? Select all that apply.

1. _____ Rectal bleeding

2. _____ Inability to digest fat

3. _____ Change in the shape of stools

4. _____ Feeling of abdominal bloating

253. An infant who had been receiving humidified oxygen because of dyspnea caused by acute spasmodic laryngitis is being discharged. The parents ask the nurse about caring for their baby at home. How should the nurse respond?

1. "There are no restrictions after your baby goes home."

2. "Do not allow visitors in your home for several days."

3. "Give two ounces of water after each formula feeding."

4. "Allergen producers such as animals should be avoided."

254. A nurse applies prescribed elbow restraints to prevent a confused client from pulling out a nasogastric tube and indwelling urinary retention catheter. What is most important for the nurse to do?

1. Have the order renewed every 48 hours

2. Assess the client's condition every hour

3. Provide range of motion to the client's elbows every shift

4. Document output from the tube and catheter every 2 hours

255. An emergency tracheotomy is performed on a toddler in acute respiratory distress from laryngotracheobronchitis (viral croup). What early signs of respiratory distress indicate that it is necessary for the nurse to suction the tracheotomy? Select all that apply.

1. _____ Stridor

2. _____ Cyanosis

3. _____ Restlessness

4. _____ Increased pulse rate

5. _____ Substernal retractions

256. A primary nurse is leaving the unit for lunch and gives a verbal report to another nurse on the unit. The primary nurse states that a client has a prescription for morphine 2 mg IV every 3 hours for abdominal pain because the client had major abdominal surgery that morning. While the primary nurse is still at lunch, the client complains of pain on a level 8 on a pain scale of 1 to 10. What should the covering nurse do first?

1. Determine when the pain medication was last given

2. Verify the pain medication prescription in the clinical record

3. Employ nonpharmacological measures initially to relieve the pain

4. Explain that the primary nurse will be back from lunch in a few minutes

257. A client is diagnosed with psoriasis and the nurse is providing health teaching concerning skin care at home. What recommendation does the nurse include in the teaching?

1. Shower twice a day

2. Soak the affected areas in hot water

3. Apply moisturizing lotion several times a day

4. Cover affected areas when in contact with others

258. The black parents of a newborn ask the nurse about several areas of deep blue coloring on their baby's lower back and buttocks. The nurse's response is based on the information that:

1. These areas usually are found on dark-skinned newborns

2. Color changes represent transient mottling that occurs when the baby is cold

3. These are characteristic of the harlequin color change that occurs when the newborn lies on the side

4. Discolorations are probably bruises requiring observation of the infant for the development of jaundice

259. A client who had a brain attack (CVA) frequently cries when family members visit and they are obviously upset by the crying. The nurse explains to the family members that the client is:

1. Having difficulty controlling emotions

2. Demonstrating a premorbid personality

3. Mourning the loss of functional abilities

4. Conveying unhappiness about the situation

260. A nurse is caring for two clients. One has Parkinson's disease and the other has myasthenia gravis. For what common complication associated with both disorders should the nurse assess these clients?

1. Cogwheel gait

2. Impaired cognition

3. Difficulty swallowing

4. Non-intention tremors

261. After a basal cell carcinoma is removed by fulguration, a client is given a topical steroid to apply to the surgical site. The nurse evaluates that the teaching regarding steroids and skin lesions is effective when the

client states that the primary purpose of the medication is to:
1. Prevent infection of the wound
2. Increase fluid loss from the skin
3. Reduce inflammation at the surgical site
4. Limit itching around the area of the lesion

262. A nurse is reviewing a list of current medications with an 80-year-old client who has developed gastrointestinal bleeding. Which medication prescription should the nurse discuss with the practitioner because it is contraindicated for a person who is experiencing gastrointestinal bleeding?
1. Ibuprofen (Advil)
2. Digoxin (Lanoxin)
3. Furosemide (Lasix)
4. Spironolactone (Aldactone)

263. A client is admitted to the hospital with the diagnosis of a right-sided brain attack (CVA). The client is right-handed. Which task will be most difficult for this client?
1. Eating meals
2. Writing letters
3. Combing the hair
4. Dressing every morning

264. A client with type 1 diabetes is diagnosed with diabetic ketoacidosis and initially treated with intravenous fluids followed by an IV bolus of regular insulin. The nurse anticipates that the practitioner will prescribe a continuous infusion of:
1. Novolin L insulin
2. Novolin R insulin
3. Novolin N insulin
4. Novolin U insulin

265. A nurse is caring for a client with a diagnosis of catatonic schizophrenia. What clinical finding does the nurse expect the client to exhibit?
1. Crying
2. Self-mutilation
3. Immobile posturing
4. Repetitious activities

Additional review questions can be found on the enclosed companion CD.

COMPREHENSIVE EXAMINATION

PART A ANSWERS AND RATIONALES

1. **1 Straddling the hip prevents scissoring by keeping the infant's legs abducted.**
   2 An infant seat will not prevent scissoring.
   3 Tight wrapping maintains the infant's legs in a scissored position.
   4 When the football hold is used, the infant is carried in a supine position with the legs adducted, which promotes scissoring.
   Clinical Area: Child Health Nursing; **Client Needs:** Safety and Infection Control; **Cognitive Level:** Application; **Integrated Process:** Teaching/Learning; **NP:** Implementation

2. **3 Increasing oncotic pressure increases the client's circulating blood volume; salt-poor albumin pulls interstitial fluid into the blood vessels, restoring blood volume and limiting ascites.**
   1 Nutrients are provided by total parenteral nutrition, not salt-poor albumin.
   2 Salt-poor albumin is not given to increase protein stores.
   4 Salt-poor albumin has no effect on diverting blood flow away from the liver.
   Clinical Area: Medical-Surgical Nursing; **Client Needs:** Pharmacological and Parenteral Therapies; **Cognitive Level:** Analysis; **Integrated Process:** Communication and Documentation; **NP:** Implementation

3. **4 Oral contraceptives may cause or exacerbate hypertension; this places the client at risk for a brain attack.**
   1 Oral contraceptives are not contraindicated for women older than 30 years of age if there are no known risk factors.
   2 There is no relationship between oral contraceptives and multiple births.
   3 Clients should be strongly cautioned about smoking even 15 cigarettes a day; if this client were older than 35 years of age and smoking cigarettes, oral contraceptives would be contraindicated.
   Clinical Area: Childbearing and Women's Health Nursing; **Client Needs:** Health Promotion and Maintenance; **Integrated Process:** Communication and Documentation; **Cognitive Level:** Application; **NP:** Analysis

4. **1 By failing to acknowledge the infant as a person, the client indicates that she has not released her fantasy baby and accepted the real baby.**
   2 The mother has acknowledged the infant by using "he," and her question denotes a relationship.
   3 The mother has acknowledged the infant by using the word "he."
   4 This response indicates that the mother has incorporated the infant into the family.

Clinical Area: Childbearing and Women's Health Nursing; **Client Needs:** Psychosocial Integrity; **Cognitive Level:** Application; **NP:** Analysis

5. **2 Drainage from the incision may occur even with a wound suction drainage system in place; therefore, the area dependent to the surgical site should be checked for bleeding because drainage will flow by gravity.**
   1 The drainage is emptied either once per shift or when the collection device is half full.
   3 Turning the client onto the affected side is painful and should be avoided; the client may turn to the unaffected side.
   4 If drainage on the dressing is excessive, the surgical staff should be notified.
   Clinical Area: Childbearing and Women's Health Nursing; **Client Needs:** Reduction of Risk Potential; **Cognitive Level:** Application; **NP:** Evaluation

6. **3 As drainage collects and occupies space, the original level of negative pressure decreases; the less the negative pressure, the less effective the drainage.**
   1 A portable wound suction device is easy and safe to empty regardless of the amount of drainage in the unit.
   2 Drainage can be measured accurately by the calibrations on the unit or in a calibrated container after emptying.
   4 A one-way valve between the tubing and the collection chamber prevents drainage from entering the tubing and causing trauma to the wound.
   Clinical Area: Medical-Surgical Nursing; **Client Needs:** Reduction of Risk Potential; **Cognitive Level:** Application; **NP:** Planning

7. **3 The practitioner should be consulted because the decision depends on the amount of damage to the heart muscle and extent of healing.**
   1 It is false reassurance to determine an exact time and date; 2 weeks may be too early.
   2 Although the client's feelings should be considered, this is a medical decision that depends on the amount of damage to the heart muscle.
   4 This response is too vague and does not involve information from the practitioner.
   Clinical Area: Medical-Surgical Nursing; **Client Needs:** Management of Care; **Cognitive Level:** Application; **Integrated Process:** Communication and Documentation; **NP:** Implementation

8. **1 A lithium plasma level of 0.8 to 1.2 mEq/L is appropriate for mood stabilization; the client's level is above the recommended level.**
   2 An increase in manic behavior is unexpected. The client should be monitored for signs and symptoms

of lithium toxicity such as nausea, vomiting, diarrhea, increased tremor, vertigo, and blurred vision.

3 Administering another dose will further increase the plasma level of lithium, which is already elevated beyond the therapeutic range.

4. The client has been taking the medication because the lithium level is too high.

Clinical Area: Mental Health Nursing; **Client Needs:** Pharmacological and Parenteral Therapies; **Cognitive Level:** Application; **NP:** Evaluation

9. **Answer: 640 mg per day.** First compute the client's weight in kilograms and then compute the dosage. Solve the problem using ratio and proportion.

$$\text{Desired Have } \frac{176 \text{ pounds}}{2.2 \text{ pounds}} \times \frac{x \text{ kg}}{1 \text{ kg}}$$

$$2.2\,x = 176$$

$$x = 176 \div 2.2$$

$$x = 80 \text{ kg}$$

$$\text{Desired Have } \frac{80 \text{ kg}}{1 \text{ kg}} \times \frac{x \text{ mg}}{8 \text{ mg}}$$

$$1\,x = 80 \times 8$$

$$1\,x = 640 \text{ mg}$$

Clinical Area: Medical-Surgical Nursing; **Client Needs:** Pharmacological and Parenteral Therapies; **Cognitive Level:** Application; **NP:** Implementation

10. **2 This does not allow the client to escape responsibility for his behavior, a common characteristic of the addicted person.**

1 The client's behavior, not feelings, is the issue that must be addressed in this situation.

3 Ignoring the client's behavior may be interpreted as approval of the behavior.

4 Although this may provide an outlet for the anger, it supports acting-out rather than control of feelings.

Clinical Area: Mental Health Nursing; **Client Needs:** Psychosocial Integrity; **Cognitive Level:** Application; **Integrated Process:** Communication and Documentation; **NP:** Implementation

11. **3 Albuterol produces sympathetic nervous system side effects such as tachycardia and hypertension.**

1 Pallor, not flushing, is a common side effect.

2 Dyspnea is not a common side effect; this medication is given to decrease respiratory difficulty.

4 Hypertension, not hypotension, is a common side effect.

Clinical Area: Child Health Nursing; **Client Needs:** Pharmacological and Parenteral Therapies; **Cognitive Level:** Application; **NP:** Evaluation

12. **4 The most effective method of preventing the spread of infection is handwashing not only before and after care but also before and after using gloves.**

1 A mask is not required for contact precautions.

2 The level of education of the caregiver does not guarantee the correct technique for preventing the spread of infection.

3 The risk for spread of infection is not in the number of visitors but the aseptic technique practiced by these visitors.

Clinical Area: Child Health Nursing; **Client Needs:** Safety and Infection Control; **Cognitive Level:** Application; **NP:** Planning

13. **3 Excessive body weight is a known predisposing factor to type 2 diabetes; the exact relationship is unknown.**

1 Diabetes insipidus is caused by too little ADH and has no relationship to type 2 diabetes.

2 High-cholesterol diets and atherosclerotic heart disease are associated with type 2 diabetes.

4 Alcohol intake is not known to predispose a person to type 2 diabetes.

Clinical Area: Medical-Surgical Nursing; **Client Needs:** Health Promotion and Maintenance; **Cognitive Level:** Application; **NP:** Assessment

14. **1 Symptoms usually appear 1 to 3 weeks after an acute infection; this syndrome is linked to diseases such as viral hepatitis, the Epstein-Barr virus, and infectious mononucleosis.**

2 There is no known familial tendency that exists in the development of Guillain-Barré syndrome.

3 This syndrome is unrelated to head trauma.

4 Drug therapy is not implicated as a contributing factor in Guillain-Barré syndrome.

Clinical Area: Medical-Surgical Nursing; **Client Needs:** Physiological Adaptation; **Cognitive Level:** Application; **Integrated Process:** Communication and Documentation; **NP:** Assessment

15. **2 This response maintains the nurse's legal responsibility of providing for the infant's safety and it promotes a positive interaction with the client's family.**

1 Giving the infant to another person without the mother's knowledge or consent is illegal.

3 Legally, the nurse cannot give the infant to the grandparents.

4 Although insisting that only the mother can ask for the infant may follow legal policy, it is an abrupt nontherapeutic response to the grandparents.

Clinical Area: Childbearing and Women's Health Nursing; **Client Needs:** Management of Care; **Cognitive Level:** Application; **Integrated Process:** Communication and Documentation; **NP:** Implementation

16. **4 Five-year disease-free survival rates for children with acute lymphocytic leukemia are currently 75% to 85%.**

1 This projected prognosis is too fatalistic.

2 This projected prognosis is too fatalistic.

3 This long-term prognosis of a 95% cure rate is too favorable, although this percentage of children achieves the first remission.

Clinical Area: Child Health Nursing; **Client Needs:** Physiological Adaptation; **Cognitive Level:** Application; **NP:** Planning

17. **3 The brachial pulse is recommended for infants and can be palpated on the inner aspect of the arm midway between the elbow and the shoulder; this site is most readily accessible for this age group.**

   1 The carotid artery is difficult to palpate in infants because of their short, fat necks. The carotid artery is the most accessible and central site for individuals more than 1 year of age.

   2 Obtaining a pulse at this site during CPR is not recommended for any age group.

   4 Obtaining a pulse at this site during CPR is not recommended for any age group.

   Clinical Area: Child Health Nursing; **Client Needs:** Physiological Adaptation; **Cognitive Level:** Application; **NP:** Evaluation

18. **1 Disturbing the dressing may expose the area to pathogens. Infection is the most common complication; sterile technique at the catheter insertion site must be maintained.**

   2 Keeping the head still is not necessary; the catheter is sutured in place, and reasonable movement is permitted.

   3 The client should be taught to leave the infusion pump set at the rate prescribed by the practitioner and to call the nurse if the alarm rings.

   4 Excessive weight gain or loss is not a complication of total parenteral nutrition.

   Clinical Area: Medical-Surgical Nursing; **Client Needs:** Pharmacological and Parenteral Therapies; **Cognitive Level:** Application; **Integrated Process:** Teaching/Learning; **NP:** Implementation

19. **4 Family therapy must include the whole family. Each member must be considered individually from his or her perspective as well as a member of the whole. Identification of the problem by the people involved is the priority.**

   1 The family, not the nurse, sets goals. The nurse assists the family to set goals by acting as a facilitator.

   2 Feelings should be shared eventually, but this is not the initial focus.

   3 Setting limits may or may not be a problem within the family.

   Clinical Area: Mental Health Nursing; **Client Needs:** Health Promotion and Maintenance; **Cognitive Level:** Application; **Integrated Process:** Communication and Documentation; **NP:** Implementation

20. **1 Levodopa (L-Dopa) crosses the blood-brain barrier and converts to dopamine, a substance depleted in Parkinson's disease.**

   2 Isocarboxazid (Marplan) is an MAO inhibitor used for the treatment of severe depression, not symptoms of Parkinson's disease.

   3 DOPamine (Intropin) is not given because it does not cross the blood-brain barrier.

4 Pyridoxine (vitamin B_6) can reverse the effects of some antiparkinsonian medications and is contraindicated.

   Clinical Area: Medical-Surgical Nursing; **Client Needs:** Pharmacological and Parenteral Therapies; **Cognitive Level:** Analysis; **NP:** Planning

21. **1 Confusion is a response to cerebral edema. Cerebral edema is a complication of continuous bladder irrigation because of an excessive absorption of irrigating solution by the venous sinusoids during surgery.**

   2 The surgery is performed through the urinary meatus and urethra; there is no suprapubic incision.

   3 It is unnecessary to keep the client in the semi-Fowler's position.

   4 The client is initially NPO and then advanced to a regular diet as tolerated. Continuous irrigation supplies enough fluid to flush the bladder.

   Clinical Area: Medical-Surgical Nursing; **Client Needs:** Reduction of Risk Potential; **Cognitive Level:** Application; **NP:** Planning

22. **3 Serosanguineous drainage from the wound or on the dressing forewarns separation of the wound edges (dehiscence); dehiscence may progress to movement of abdominal organs outside of the abdominal cavity (evisceration).**

   1 Bowel sounds have no relationship to wound status; bowel sounds are expected around the third or fourth postoperative day as intestinal peristalsis returns.

   2 Loosening of sutures may occur after the initial wound edema subsides but is not a sign of failure of the suture line.

   4 A purplish incision is the expected coloration of a healing wound.

   Clinical Area: Medical-Surgical Nursing; **Client Needs:** Physiological Adaptation; **Cognitive Level:** Application; **NP:** Evaluation

23. **3 Between the ages of 3 and 5 years death is viewed as a departure or sleep, which is reversible.**

   1 This is the concept of death held by children starting at 8 to 9 years of age.

   2 This is the concept of death held by children starting at 8 to 9 years of age.

   4 The early school-age child of 6 or 7 years personifies death and sees it as horrible and frightening; this is consistent with the concrete thinking present at this age.

   Clinical Area: Child Health Nursing; **Client Needs:** Health Promotion and Maintenance; **Cognitive Level:** Comprehension; **NP:** Analysis

24. **4 Hemicolectomy is removal of part of the colon with an anastomosis between the ileum and transverse colon; a colostomy is not necessary.**

   1 With a colostomy the intestine opens on the abdomen, whereas in a hemicolectomy a portion of the intestine is resected and the ends reconnected.

2 This is the description of a temporary colostomy; a cure occurs only when the entire colon is removed.

3 A colostomy is done for a variety of reasons other than a tumor; a colectomy with a colostomy is only one intervention that may be used to treat a tumor.
Clinical Area: Medical-Surgical Nursing; **Client Needs:** Reduction of Risk Potential; **Cognitive Level:** Application; **Integrated Process:** Communication and Documentation; **NP:** Implementation

25. **2 Nursing care should be organized and administered efficiently so that the nurse's exposure to radiation is kept to a minimum.**

1 A regular diet is contraindicated until the radon seeds are removed because chewing can dislodge the seeds.

3 Frequent mouth care is contraindicated because it can dislodge the seeds; drying of the mucous membranes cannot be prevented.

4 A family member should not be in attendance continually because this will expose the family member to excessive radiation.
Clinical Area: Medical-Surgical Nursing; **Client Needs:** Safety and Infection Control; **Cognitive Level:** Application; **NP:** Implementation

26. **3 The client will be able to attend to the activities of daily living because lamotrigine (Lamictal), an anticonvulsant, stabilizes neuronal membranes by inhibiting sodium transport and psychomotor hyperactivity.**

1 A high-spirited attitude does not reflect an effective response to lamotrigine.

2 The ability to laugh off criticism does not reflect an effective response to lamotrigine.

4 Entertaining other clients does not reflect an effective response to lamotrigine.
Clinical Area: Mental Health Nursing; **Client Needs:** Pharmacological and Parenteral Therapies; **Cognitive Level:** Application; **NP:** Evaluation

27. **2 Checking the level of consciousness is part of a total neurological check. It assesses for increasing intracranial pressure, which may occur secondary to cerebral inflammation.**

1 The child is too ill to ingest anything by mouth; also vomiting is likely to occur. Hydration is maintained intravenously.

3 Taking the blood pressure and other vital signs every 4 hours is insufficient monitoring; many changes can occur in this time span.

4 The child is too ill to ingest anything by mouth. In addition, intravenous antibiotics have a rapid systemic effect, which is preferable to the oral route.
Clinical Area: Child Health Nursing; **Client Needs:** Reduction of Risk Potential; **Cognitive Level:** Application; **NP:** Planning

28. **3 Insensible and intestinal fluid losses are increased during phototherapy; extra fluid prevents dehydration.**

1 Taking the vital signs every hour is unnecessary unless a change from the baseline occurs.

2 The eye shields should be removed for feeding and when holding the infant.

4 The total body needs to be exposed to the light.
Clinical Area: Childbearing and Women's Health Nursing; **Client Needs:** Physiological Adaptation; **Cognitive Level:** Application; **NP:** Planning

29. **Answer: 1, 2, 3**

1 **The ASO titer (antistreptolysis O) identifies a previous streptococcal infection.**

2 **A urinalysis identifies hematuria and proteinuria caused by impaired glomerular filtration.**

3 **A blood chemistry identifies azotemia, elevated blood urea nitrogen (BUN), and creatinine levels caused by impaired glomerular filtration.**

4 An intravenous pyelogram does not help confirm a diagnosis of APSGN.

5 A chest x-ray does not help confirm a diagnosis of APSGN.
Clinical Area: Child Health Nursing; **Client Needs:** Reduction of Risk Potential; **Cognitive Level:** Analysis **NP:** Assessment

30. **2 Clients who are inexperienced in psychiatric care may have confusion about the nurse-client relationship. The nurse should differentiate this professional relationship from a social relationship.**

1 Although this behavior may be a sign of a sexual identity problem because these clients may mask their concerns with overt masculine actions, this response by the nurse is premature because there are not enough data to come to this conclusion.

3 This response may be interpreted by the client as rejection.

4 Although nurses should always examine their relationships with their clients, it is unlikely that an experienced nurse would communicate inappropriately. This is more likely to be a problem of the client's misinterpretation of his interactions with the nurses.
Clinical Area: Mental Health Nursing; **Client Needs:** Management of Care; **Cognitive Level:** Application; **Integrated Process:** Communication and Documentation; **NP:** Implementation

31. **3 Red urine is a common response to DOXOrubicin (Adriamycin). The red drug is not metabolized and is excreted in the urine. The genitourinary responses to vinCRIStine (Oncovin) are nocturia, oliguria, urinary retention, and gonadal suppression.**

1 Hair loss occurs with both medications.

2 Vomiting occurs with both medications.

4 Stomatitis occurs with both medications.
Clinical Area: Child Health Nursing; **Client Needs:** Pharmacological and Parenteral Therapies; **Cognitive Level:** Application; **NP:** Assessment

32. 3 **Sodium absorbs water in the kidneys' renal tubules. When dietary intake of sodium is decreased, water is not reabsorbed and edema is reduced.**
    1 A decrease in sodium will prevent the reabsorption of water. Furosemide stimulates the loop of Henle to inhibit the reabsorption of sodium and chloride at the proximal and distal tubules.
    2 Adequate hydration is the major factor that diminishes the thirst response.
    4 A low-sodium diet will help move fluid from the interstitial compartment to the intravascular compartment.
    Clinical Area: Medical-Surgical Nursing; **Client Needs:** Basic Care and Comfort; **Cognitive Level:** Application; **NP:** Analysis

33. 4 **Adduction may cause dislocation of the new prosthesis and external rotation increases tension on the suture line.**
    1 Only the operated leg needs to be kept abducted.
    2 Keeping both legs in functional body alignment positions the affected leg too close to the midline and increases the danger of hip dislocation.
    3 The supine position is permitted as long as the affected leg is abducted and external rotation avoided, which help keep the prosthesis firmly in the acetabulum. The prone position is not advised because it puts excessive stress on the operative site.
    Clinical Area: Medical-Surgical Nursing; **Client Needs:** Physiological Adaptation **Cognitive Level:** Application; **NP:** Implementation

34. 1 **This reflects the client's statement and permits clarification, which provides information that can be used in planning.**
    2 This response is too specific an interpretation of a rest requirement; there is more to maintaining rest than naps.
    3 This response is a vague interpretation of a rest requirement; there is more to maintaining rest than staying off the feet.
    4 What the nurse thinks it means does not give a clear picture of what the client interprets as rest.
    Clinical Area: Childbearing and Women's Health Nursing; **Client Needs:** Physiological Adaptation; **Cognitive Level:** Application; **Integrated Process:** Teaching/Learning; **NP:** Implementation

35. 2 **Counterpressure helps alleviate some discomfort.**
    1 Elevating the legs will increase tension on the back and increase discomfort.
    3 Panting may lead to hyperventilation, which may cause maternal respiratory alkalosis and fetal acidosis.
    4 Kegel exercises do not help relieve back pain, they tone the pelvic musculature.
    Clinical Area: Childbearing and Women's Health Nursing; **Client Needs:** Health Promotion and Maintenance; **Cognitive Level:** Application; **Integrated Process:** Teaching/Learning; **NP:** Implementation

36. 1 **Exercising should be done often; association with a specific activity makes it easier to incorporate it into the lifestyle.**
    2 Once a day is not frequent enough.
    3 Twice a day is not frequent enough.
    4 Although every 4 hours is frequent enough, such a rigid schedule is difficult to follow with an infant and compliance may falter.
    Clinical Area: Child Health Nursing; **Client Needs:** Reduction of Risk Potential; **Cognitive Level:** Application; **Integrated Process:** Teaching/Learning; **NP:** Evaluation

37. Answer 1, 2, 4
    1 **Exposure to high levels of lead predisposes the child to anemia. The lead interferes with synthesis of heme.**
    2 **Exposure to high levels of lead predisposes the child to proteinuria and glycosuria because the lead damages the cells of the proximal renal tubules.**
    3 There is no direct relationship between lead toxicity and heart failure.
    4 **Exposure to high levels of lead predisposes the child to encephalopathy caused by increased membrane permeability leading to tissue ischemia and atrophy.**
    5 Gastrointestinal bleeding does not occur with lead toxicity.
    Clinical Area: Child Health Nursing; **Client Needs:** Physiological Adaptation; **Cognitive Level:** Analysis; **NP:** Assessment

38. 2 **The client's signs and symptoms suggest the possibility of shock; the practitioner must be alerted to this possible life-threatening condition.**
    1 The client has unmet needs that must be addressed first.
    3 Distraction is effective with mild, not severe, pain.
    4 This is outside the scope of nursing practice. Practitioner prescriptions must be followed as prescribed or the practitioner should be notified.
    Clinical Area: Medical-Surgical Nursing; **Client Needs:** Management of Care; **Cognitive Level:** Analysis; **Integrated Process:** Communication and Documentation; **NP:** Implementation

39. 4 **The semi-Fowler position helps maintain the head in functional body alignment and facilitates respiration; gravity moves the abdominal organs down and away from the diaphragm, facilitating respiratory excursion.**
    1 The side-lying position, unless the head is elevated, inhibits respiratory excursion.
    2 The orthopneic position may cause flexion of the neck, which will inhibit respirations and place pressure on the suture line; also rest is difficult to maintain in this position.
    3 The high-Fowler's position may cause flexion of the neck, which will inhibit respirations and place pressure on the suture line; also rest is difficult to maintain in this position.

Clinical Area: Medical-Surgical Nursing; **Client Needs:** Physiological Adaptation; **Cognitive Level:** Application; **NP:** Implementation

40. 1 **Research indicates that these are the first physical signs that accompany withdrawal from heroin.**
    2 Depression and irritability accompany withdrawal from cocaine.
    3 Restlessness, shakiness, hallucinations, and possibly coma accompany withdrawal from morphine.
    4 Insomnia, seizures, weakness, sweating, and anxiety accompany withdrawal from phenobarbital.
    Clinical Area: Mental Health Nursing; **Client Needs:** Psychosocial Integrity; **Cognitive Level:** Analysis; **NP:** Analysis

41. 4 **The mother must learn comfort strategies to prevent crying and how to care for the suture line.**
    1 The infant is too young to drink from a cup and will miss oral gratification with this method.
    2 Restraint of the arms can be injurious if left on continuously. The restraints can be removed periodically while being held by the parents or nurse to ensure that the infant does not touch the mouth.
    3 All infants should be burped thoroughly to prevent regurgitation. After cleft lip repair regurgitated milk products can contaminate the suture line.
    Clinical Area: Child Health Nursing; **Client Needs:** Reduction of Risk Potential; **Cognitive Level:** Application; **Integrated Process:** Teaching/Learning; **NP:** Implementation

42. 2 **The ovum is fertilizable for 12 to 24 hours and sperm remain motile for about 72 hours. Therefore, the period of fertility is a total of 96 hours (72 hours before ovulation plus 24 hours after ovulation).**
    1 The fertility period before ovulation is longer than 12 hours.
    3 This time period is too long before and after ovulation.
    4 The period of fertility is longer than 48 hours before ovulation and shorter than 48 hours after ovulation.
    Clinical Area: Childbearing and Women's Health Nursing; **Client Needs:** Health Promotion and Maintenance; **Cognitive Level:** Analysis; **Integrated Process:** Teaching/Learning; **NP:** Implementation

43. 2 **In addition to baseline laboratory tests, an older adult should have an eye examination with glaucoma testing performed when taking amitriptyline (Elavil). Amitriptyline causes dilation of the pupil (mydriasis), which interferes with drainage of aqueous humor through the canal of Schlemm. Interfering with the outflow of aqueous humor will increase intraocular pressure and may cause a progressive loss of vision in clients with glaucoma.**
    1. Amitriptyline is not a drug that affects cholesterol production in the body.
    3. Amitriptyline does not affect temperature regulation.

4. Amitriptyline does not cause excessive perspiration or weight loss; it can increase appetite, especially for sweets, and cause a weight gain.
Clinical Area: Mental Health Nursing; **Client Needs:** Pharmacological and Parenteral Therapies; **Cognitive Level:** Application; **Integrated Process:** Teaching/Learning; **NP:** Implementation

44. 2 **As fluid returns to the vascular system, increased renal flow and diuresis occur.**
    1 An increase in the serum sodium level (hypernatremia) is not a common response identified during the second (acute) phase of burn recovery.
    3 An increase in the hematocrit level indicates hemoconcentration and hypovolemia; in the second phase of burn recovery, hemodilution and hypervolemia occur.
    4 During the second phase of burn recovery, potassium moves back into the cells, decreasing serum potassium.
    Clinical Area: Medical-Surgical Nursing; **Client Needs:** Physiological Adaptation; **Cognitive Level:** Application; **NP:** Assessment

45. 2 **Negative pressure is exerted by gravity drainage or by suction through the closed system.**
    1 Though the discomfort may be lessened as a result of the insertion of the chest tube, this is not the primary purpose.
    3 There is an accumulation of air, not fluid, when a pneumothorax occurs in a client with COPD.
    4 Subcutaneous emphysema in the chest wall is most commonly associated with clients receiving air under pressure, such as that received from a ventilator.
    Clinical Area: Medical-Surgical Nursing; **Client Needs:** Reduction of Risk Potential; **Cognitive Level:** Application; **NP:** Planning

46. 4 **COPD causes destruction of capillary beds around the alveoli, interfering with blood flow to the lungs from the right side of the heart. As the heart continues to strain against this resistance, heart failure eventually results.**
    1 Renal disease causes stress on the left side of the heart.
    2 Hypovolemic shock will not cause stress on the right side of the heart.
    3 Severe systemic infection probably will produce greater stress on the left side of the heart.
    Clinical Area: Medical-Surgical Nursing; **Client Needs:** Physiological Adaptation; **Cognitive Level:** Analysis; **NP:** Analysis

47. 2 **Baked fish is a low-residue, low-fat, high-protein, and non–gas-producing food that usually is well tolerated.**
    1 Fresh fruit has fiber that irritates the gastrointestinal tract.
    3 Bran cereal has fiber that irritates the gastrointestinal tract.
    4 Whole milk irritates the gastrointestinal tract and stimulates mucus production.

Clinical Area: Medical-Surgical Nursing; **Client Needs:** Basic Care and Comfort; **Cognitive Level:** Analysis; **NP:** Evaluation

48. 1 **At about the 22nd week of gestation, the top of the fundus is at the level of the umbilicus.**
   2 Just above the symphysis pubis is too low for a pregnancy between the fifth and sixth months of gestation.
   3 Two finger-breadths above the umbilicus is too high for 20 to 22 weeks' gestation.
   4 Halfway between the symphysis pubis and umbilicus is too low for a pregnancy between the fifth and sixth months of gestation.
   Clinical Area: Childbearing and Women's Health Nursing; **Client Needs:** Health Promotion and Maintenance; **Cognitive Level:** Application; **NP:** Assessment

49. Answer: 2, 4
   1 An infant seat should face the rear, not the front, of the automobile because the head and neck are better protected from a whiplash injury in the event of an accident.
   2 **An infant seat that faces the rear, not the front, of the automobile better protects an infant from head and whiplash injuries in the event of an accident.**
   3 An infant seat should be secured in the rear, not the front, seat. Research demonstrates that passengers in the front seat sustain more serious injuries than individuals in the rear seat in most accidents.
   4 **The manufacturer's instructions state that an infant seat should face the rear, not the front, of the automobile because the infant's head and neck are better protected from a whiplash injury in the event of an accident.**
   Clinical Area: Childbearing and Women's Health Nursing; **Client Needs:** Safety and Infection Control; **Cognitive Level:** Analysis; **Integrated Process:** Teaching/Learning; **NP:** Planning

50. 1 **Although problem-solving potential is increased when clients are involved in exploring alternatives that will affect the direction of their own lives, clients in crisis may be overwhelmed and initially need assistance in making decisions.**
   2 The client, not the crisis intervention practitioner, should identify the problem; the practitioner facilitates the process.
   3 This is useless information because the client is unable to empathize with others at this time.
   4 Identifying the client's religious and cultural beliefs is not the priority at this time.
   Clinical Area: Mental Health Nursing; **Client Needs:** Management of Care; **Cognitive Level:** Application; **Integrated Process:** Communication and Documentation; **NP:** Implementation

51. 2 **Because of the administration of regional anesthesia and the potential for blood loss associated with a cesarean birth, the client should be well hydrated before surgery to maintain adequate blood volume.**

1 Scrupulous skin care is not relevant; just before surgery the skin will be cleansed.
3 Only routine monitoring of vital signs is necessary.
4 The use of an incentive spirometer is important after general, not regional, anesthesia.
Clinical Area: Childbearing and Women's Health Nursing; **Client Needs:** Reduction of Risk Potential; **Cognitive Level:** Application; **NP:** Planning

52. 4 **Protein and vitamin C promote wound healing; this is a postoperative priority.**
   1 Although a low-fat diet is preferred for an obese client, vitamin D, as well as other vitamins, should not be limited.
   2 A high-calorie diet can increase obesity, and there is no indication that this client is at risk for constipation requiring a high-fiber diet.
   3 A low-residue bland diet can cause constipation; the priority is for nutrients to promote healing.
   Clinical Area: Medical-Surgical Nursing; **Client Needs:** Basic Care and Comfort; **Cognitive Level:** Application; **NP:** Planning

53. Answer: 1, 3, 4
   1 **Decreased blood flow to the kidneys leads to oliguria or anuria.**
   2 Restlessness, not lethargy, usually occurs because of decreased cerebral blood flow.
   3 **Irritability, along with restlessness and anxiety, occurs because of a decrease in oxygen to the brain.**
   4 **Hypotension and a narrowing of the pulse pressure occur because of declining blood volume.**
   5 There are various changes in sensorium, but slurred speech is not a manifestation of shock.
   Clinical Area: Medical-Surgical Nursing; **Client Needs:** Reduction of Risk Potential; **Cognitive Level:** Analysis; **NP:** Evaluation

54. 2 **Propylthiouracil (PTU) can cause depression of leukocytes and platelets.**
   1 Propylthiouracil and potassium iodide should be given with milk, juice, or food to prevent gastric irritation.
   3 Drug therapy decreases the risk of postoperative hemorrhage because this drug regimen decreases the size and vascularity of the thyroid gland.
   4 Drug therapy is continued for at least 6 to 8 weeks, even if the client's temperature and pulse return to the expected range.
   Clinical Area: Medical-Surgical Nursing; **Client Needs:** Pharmacological and Parenteral Therapies; **Cognitive Level:** Application; **Integrated Process:** Teaching/Learning; **NP:** Implementation

55. 2 **Climbing stairs is expected developmental behavior for 18-month-old toddlers; however, they may have difficulty coming down the stairs.**
   1 Pedaling a tricycle is above the ability level of an 18-month-old child.

3 A 150-word vocabulary is above the ability level of an 18-month-old child.

4 Building a tower of eight blocks is above the ability level of an 18-month-old child.

Clinical Area: Child Health Nursing; **Client Needs:** Health Promotion and Maintenance; **Cognitive Level:** Application; **NP:** Assessment

56. 4 **These are theoretical explanations for the development of anorexia nervosa.**

1 This does not play a role in the development of anorexia nervosa.

2 This does not play a role in the development of anorexia nervosa.

3 The basis is the struggle between dependence and independence, not a desire for independence alone. The inability to be the center of attention in the family has not been correlated with anorexia nervosa.

Clinical Area: Mental Health Nursing; **Client Needs:** Psychosocial Integrity; **Cognitive Level:** Application; **NP:** Analysis

57. 1 **Inspection seeks to identify the cause for the decreased fetal heart rate; the cord may have prolapsed.**

2 Administering oxygen may be done later, but it is not the priority.

3 The practitioner should be notified after further assessment reveals more information.

4 Placing the client in the knee-chest position is an intervention that can be implemented once it is determined that the umbilical cord is prolapsed. It relieves pressure on the cord, which increases the flow of oxygen and nutrients to the fetus.

Clinical Area: Childbearing and Women's Health Nursing; **Client Needs:** Reduction of Risk Potential; **Cognitive Level:** Application; **NP:** Evaluation

58. 3 **These individuals readily respond to environmental cues. Increased stimulation increases activity; decreased stimulation decreases activity.**

1 Sleep pattern disturbances characteristically occur because of psychomotor activity.

2 All individuals require adequate rest and sleep; hyperactive clients may become exhausted because of their high activity level.

4 Expending energy only increases the tendency to remain awake.

Clinical Area: Mental Health Nursing; **Client Needs:** Psychosocial Integrity; **Cognitive Level:** Application; **NP:** Assessment

59. 4 **Abduction will enable the head of the femur to fit into the acetabulum, thereby correcting the dysplasia.**

1 Flexion causes the head of the femur to move away from the acetabulum.

2 Extension causes the head of the femur to move away from the acetabulum.

3 Adduction causes the head of the femur to move away from the acetabulum.

Clinical Area: Child Health Nursing; **Client Needs:** Basic Care and Comfort; **Cognitive Level:** Comprehension; **NP:** Planning

60. 2 **The toddler's increased physical abilities and curiosity contribute to the high incidence of accidents in this age group; all poisonous substances should be kept out of reach and behind locked doors.**

1 Toddlers are too immature to understand or follow the limits needed to prevent accidents.

3 Although toddlers seek parental approval, their need for autonomy takes precedence.

4 The presence of medication labels is unimportant because most toddlers cannot read.

Clinical Area: Child Health Nursing; **Client Needs:** Safety and Infection Control; **Cognitive Level:** Application; **Integrated Process:** Teaching/Learning; **NP:** Planning

61. 2 **Children with AIDS have a dysfunction of the immune system (depressed or ineffective T cells, B cells, and immunoglobulins) and are susceptible to opportunistic infections.**

1 All children are subject to injury because of their curiosity, inexperience, and lack of judgment.

3 Although inadequate nutrition can be a problem for children with AIDS, the prevention of infection is the priority.

4 Although children with AIDS are usually small for their ages, altered growth and development is not as life threatening as an infection.

Clinical Area: Child Health Nursing; **Client Needs:** Safety and Infection Control; **Cognitive Level:** Application; **Integrated Process:** Teaching/Learning; **NP:** Planning

62. 1 **The lateral position relieves pressure on the vena cava, thus promoting venous return and increasing placental perfusion.**

2 The supine position promotes hypotension because the pressure of the gravid uterus on the vena cava interferes with the return of blood from the lower extremities.

3 The Fowler's position promotes hypotension because the pressure of the gravid uterus on the vena cava interferes with the return of blood from the lower extremities.

4 The semi-Fowler's position promotes hypotension because the pressure of the gravid uterus on the vena cava interferes with the return of blood from the lower extremities.

Clinical Area: Childbearing and Women's Health Nursing; **Client Needs:** Pharmacological and Parenteral Therapies; **Cognitive Level:** Application; **Integrated Process:** Teaching/Learning; **NP:** Implementation

63. 3 **Suckling will induce neural stimulation of the posterior pituitary gland, which in turn will release oxytocin and cause uterine contractions.**

1 Fundal pressure should not be used; this can cause a uterine prolapse.

2 Having the mother bear down can cause a uterine prolapse.

4 If the placenta is still attached to the uterine wall, this may disconnect the cord from the placenta or cause uterine prolapse.

Clinical Area: Childbearing and Women's Health Nursing; **Client Needs:** Health Promotion and Maintenance; **Cognitive Level:** Application; **NP:** Implementation

64. 3 **The nurse must first determine if the client is pregnant. If the client states that she missed her last menses, a pregnancy test should be performed. If positive, the vaginal spotting and the colicky abdominal pain are indicative of a tubal pregnancy that might not have yet ruptured. Further assessments should be made for a definitive diagnosis.**

1 Asking the client if she is sexually active is an intrusive question and the response will not offer relevant information.

2 The pain associated with a tubal pregnancy is constant, not intermittent. The pain may be unilateral, bilateral, or diffuse over the abdomen.

4 Asking when the gastrointestinal upset started will yield information that is too vague to help in determining the problem.

Clinical Area: Childbearing and Women's Health Nursing; **Client Needs:** Physiological Adaptation; **Cognitive Level:** Application; **Integrated Process:** Communication and Documentation; **NP:** Assessment

65. 1 **The presence of nitrate in the urine is characteristic of a urinary tract infection. Nitrates are a byproduct of the breakdown of some pathogens associated with a urinary tract infection.**

2 Protein in the urine may occur for a variety of reasons; it is not specific to a urinary tract infection.

3 Bilirubin in the urine is abnormal, but it is not related to a urinary tract infection.

4 This may occur with various problems, including infection; however, it is not exclusive to infection.

Clinical Area: Medical-Surgical Nursing; **Client Needs:** Reduction of Risk Potential; **Cognitive Level:** Analysis; **NP:** Analysis

66. 1 **Divalproex (Depakote), an anticonvulsive, causes gastric irritation and should be taken with food; it is available in an enteric-coated form. It may cause nausea, vomiting, indigestion, hypersalivation, diarrhea or constipation, anorexia or increased appetite, dizziness, headache, and confusion.**

2 These are common side effects of the phenothiazines.

3 These are signs and symptoms of lithium toxicity.

4 These are common side effects of tricyclic antidepressants.

Clinical Area: Mental Health Nursing; **Client Needs:** Pharmacological and Parenteral Therapies; **Cognitive Level:** Application; **NP:** Evaluation

67. 2 **Chest physiotherapy (CPT) is done several hours after meals to avoid regurgitation and several hours before meals so that unpleasant odors and tastes do not affect the appetite.**

1 CPT should not be done before meals because the unpleasant odors and tastes may interfere with the appetite and eating.

3 CPT should be done more frequently than two times a day. CPT should not be performed before breakfast because the unpleasant odors and tastes may interfere with the appetite and eating.

4 CPT should be done more frequently than two times a day. CPT performed after a meal may result in vomiting.

Clinical Area: Child Health Nursing; **Client Needs:** Management of Care; **Cognitive Level:** Comprehension; **NP:** Planning

68. 2 **Hot climates are contraindicated for children with cystic fibrosis because sweating precipitates an excessive loss of sodium chloride.**

1 Air conditioning is advisable because it will keep the child from sweating.

3 Pancreatic enzymes are essential to help in the digestion of nutrients so that they can be absorbed by the intestinal mucosa.

4 After passage of the feces associated with this disorder, the perianal area may become inflamed if not adequately cleaned.

Clinical Area: Child Health Nursing; **Client Needs:** Physiological Adaptation; **Cognitive Level:** Application; **Integrated Process:** Teaching/Learning; **NP:** Evaluation

69. 4 **Dialysate is introduced into the peritoneal cavity where fluids, electrolytes, and wastes are exchanged through the peritoneal membrane.**

1 Hemodialysis is not necessary with continuous ambulatory peritoneal dialysis.

2 The client can dialyze alone in any location without the need for continuous technical supervision.

3 About 2 liters, not a quarter of a liter, of dialysate are maintained intraperitoneally and can be instilled and drained by the client.

Clinical Area: Medical-Surgical Nursing; **Client Needs:** Physiological Adaptation; **Cognitive Level:** Application; **Integrated Process:** Communication and Documentation; **NP:** Implementation

70. 4 **Malnutrition and liver damage lead to a reduced serum albumin level and failure of the capillary fluid shift mechanism, resulting in ascites.**

1 Vitamins are unrelated to ascites.

2 Iron promotes hemoglobin synthesis, which is unrelated to cirrhosis.

3 The sodium level usually is excessive with cirrhosis.

Clinical Area: Medical-Surgical Nursing; **Client Needs:** Physiological Adaptation; **Cognitive Level:** Application; **NP:** Analysis

71. **4 This response presents facts that help reduce feelings of guilt.**
    1 This response is an inadequate explanation that does not offer any information.
    2 Labor may not be beginning at this time.
    3 Placenta previa can occur in a woman with a healthy uterus.
    Clinical Area: Childbearing and Women's Health Nursing; **Client Needs:** Physiological Adaptation; **Cognitive Level:** Application; **Integrated Process:** Communication and Documentation; **NP:** Implementation

72. **1 Walking with the nurse facilitates a one-to-one interaction and the development of a trusting relationship.**
    2 Watching a movie will allow the client to withdraw further.
    3 Playing a game with others is beyond the client's ability at this time.
    4 Playing cards alone will allow the client to withdraw further.
    Clinical Area: Mental Health Nursing; **Client Needs:** Psychosocial Integrity; **Cognitive Level:** Application; **Integrated Process:** Communication and Documentation; **NP:** Planning

73. **1 With diabetic ketoacidosis serum lipid levels are high because of the increased breakdown of fat. Serum lipid levels can go so high that the serum appears opalescent and creamy.**
    2 With diabetic ketoacidosis the hematocrit level generally is increased because of dehydration.
    3 The calcium level is unrelated to diabetic ketoacidosis.
    4 With diabetic ketoacidosis the blood urea nitrogen level generally is increased because of dehydration.
    Clinical Area: Medical-Surgical Nursing; **Client Needs:** Reduction of Risk Potential; **Cognitive Level:** Application; **NP:** Assessment

74. **2 Positioning the client in the prone position for short periods helps prevent hip flexion contractures.**
    1 The client's residual limb should not be immobilized. Exercises to prevent contractures are begun as soon as possible.
    3 Positioning the client in the right side-lying position can cause trauma to the incision site and should be avoided.
    4 The client's residual limb should not be elevated for more than 48 hours because hip flexion contractures can result.
    Clinical Area: Medical-Surgical Nursing; **Client Needs:** Physiological Adaptation; **Cognitive Level:** Application; **NP:** Implementation

75. **4 Anticholinergic drugs block the neural impulses that stimulate pancreatic and gastric secretions; they inhibit the action of acetylcholine at postganglionic cholinergic nerve fibers.**
    1 Oral fluids stimulate pancreatic secretion and are contraindicated.

2 Morphine sulfate is an analgesic and therefore does not decrease gastric secretions; in the past morphine sulfate was contraindicated for pain control with pancreatitis because it can precipitate spasms of the smooth musculature of the pancreatic ducts and the sphincter of Oddi; however, recent research indicates that it is the drug of choice over meperidine hydrochloride (Demerol) because the metabolites of Demerol can cause CNS irritation and seizures.
3 The semi-Fowler position decreases pressure against the diaphragm; it will not decrease pancreatic secretions.
Clinical Area: Medical-Surgical Nursing; **Client Needs:** Pharmacological and Parenteral Therapies; **Cognitive Level:** Application; **NP:** Implementation

PART B ANSWERS AND RATIONALES

76. **4 Colorectal cancer in women is common in the United States; approximately 68,000 women are diagnosed each year.**
    1 In the early stages, symptoms of cancer of the colon are vague or absent.
    2 Malignancy means a tendency to progress in virulence; a localized tumor usually is benign.
    3 Colorectal cancer is more common in men than women.
    Clinical Area: Medical-Surgical Nursing; **Client Needs:** Health Promotion and Maintenance; **Cognitive Level:** Knowledge; **Integrated Process:** Teaching/Learning; **NP:** Analysis

77. **3 Pregnant women with diabetes are prone to placental insufficiency, which can threaten fetal well-being.**
    1 Advanced maternal age alone is not an indicator for an NST.
    2 Although advanced maternal age increases the risk of placenta previa, this is not the primary reason for having an NST.
    4 There are not enough data to determine the cause of the client's stillbirth, so a conclusion cannot be reached concerning the need for the NST.
    Clinical Area: Childbearing and Women's Health Nursing; **Client Needs:** Reduction of Risk Potential; **Cognitive Level:** Analysis; **NP:** Analysis

78. **2 This individualized information is the best basis for predicting the outcome of therapy.**
    1 This information is not helpful in understanding the likelihood of additional problems associated with the current cancer.
    3 This information is not helpful in understanding the likelihood of additional problems associated with the current cancer.
    4 This information is useful, but it is not specific for this client.
    Clinical Area: Medical-Surgical Nursing; **Client Needs:** Management of Care; **Cognitive Level:** Application; **NP:** Planning

79. 1 **Seven days after each menstrual period breast engorgement is minimal; also this provides a regular examination cycle.**
    2 Premenstrual breast engorgement may cause the breast to feel lumpy.
    3 Ovulation is occurring and hormones may influence breast consistency.
    4 Breast consistency is altered by the menstrual cycle; the same date each month will occur in a different stage of the menstrual cycle. Performing breast self-examination on the same day each month is recommended for women who are postmenopausal.
    Clinical Area: Childbearing and Women's Health Nursing; **Client Needs:** Health Promotion and Maintenance; **Cognitive Level:** Comprehension; **Integrated Process:** Teaching/Learning; **NP:** Evaluation

80. 1 **Nosebleeds (epistaxis) are expected in a child with leukemia who is receiving chemotherapy because the bone marrow is depressed and the number of platelets decreases substantially.**
    2 Tachycardia is not expected unless there is severe anemia.
    3 Usually children with leukemia have pale skin.
    4 An elevated temperature occurs only if there is an infection secondary to the leukemia.
    Clinical Area: Child Health Nursing; **Client Needs:** Pharmacological and Parenteral Therapies; **Cognitive Level:** Application; **NP:** Evaluation

81. 3 **The client is experiencing pulmonary edema because of a fluid volume excess. The high concentration of TPN precipitates a fluid shift from the interstitial compartment into the intravascular compartment.**
    1 Fluid will continue to be infused, which will continue to increase the intravascular volume.
    2 Fluid will continue to be infused, which will continue to increase the intravascular volume.
    4 Fluid will continue to be infused, which will continue to increase the intravascular volume.
    Clinical Area: Medical-Surgical Nursing; **Client Needs:** Pharmacological and Parenteral Therapies; **Cognitive Level:** Application; **NP:** Implementation

82. 3 **Streptomycin is ototoxic and can cause damage to the eighth cranial nerve, resulting in deafness. Assessment for ringing or roaring in the ears, vertigo, and hearing acuity should be made before, during, and after treatment.**
    1 Isoniazid (INH) does not affect the ear; however, blurred vision and optic neuritis, as well as peripheral neuropathy, may occur.
    2 Rifampin (Rifadin) does not affect hearing; however, visual disturbances may occur.
    4 Ethambutol (Myambutol) does not affect hearing; however, visual disturbances may occur.
    Clinical Area: Medical-Surgical Nursing; **Client Needs:** Pharmacological and Parenteral Therapies; **Cognitive Level:** Analysis; **NP:** Evaluation

83. 4 **Because adolescents have a developmental need to conform to their peers, the teenager should be able to select a bracelet with a similar configuration to those worn by her peers.**
    1 Hiding the bracelet under long-sleeved clothes might be acceptable in cool weather but not when it is warm and friends are wearing T-shirts.
    2 The bracelet should be worn at all times when not with responsible family members.
    3 Asking friends to wear a similar bracelet may be difficult, especially if the girl does not wish to tell her friends why she needs the bracelet.
    Clinical Area: Child Health Nursing; **Client Needs:** Safety and Infection Control; **Cognitive Level:** Application; **Integrated Process:** Teaching/Learning; **NP:** Implementation

84. 4 **Limiting increasing intracranial pressure and resulting brain damage depends on frequent, systematic assessments to identify this complication early.**
    1 There is no indication that movement should be restricted.
    2 Mannitol is administered to reduce cerebral edema; there is no indication at this time that this is needed.
    3 Stimulating the client to maintain responsiveness is unrealistic; the state of consciousness should be monitored but otherwise rest is not contraindicated.
    Clinical Area: Medical-Surgical Nursing; **Client Needs:** Management of Care; **Cognitive Level:** Application; **NP:** Assessment

85. 3 **Specialized insulin receptors on insulin-sensitive cells transport glucose through cell membranes, making it available for use.**
    1 Insulin does not break down fats, thereby releasing glucose.
    2 Insulin does not prevent glucose from being stored in the liver.
    4 Insulin does not convert glucose into glycogen.
    Clinical Area: Child Health Nursing; **Client Needs:** Pharmacological and Parenteral Therapies; **Cognitive Level:** Knowledge; **Integrated Process:** Communication and Documentation; **NP:** Evaluation

86. 1 **Preventing infection and trauma is the priority; rupture of the sac may lead to meningitis.**
    2 The Apgar scores are 9/10; oxygen is not needed.
    3 Placing name bracelets on both mother and infant can be done before the infant leaves the birthing room; the priority is care of the infant's sac.
    4 The infant's sac must be protected before the infant is transferred to the neonatal intensive care unit. With Apgar scores of 9/10 the neonate is stable.
    Clinical Area: Childbearing and Women's Health Nursing; **Client Needs:** Management of Care; **Cognitive Level:** Application; **NP:** Planning

87. 1 **Clients who are depressed and feeling hopeless also tend to manifest inappropriate expressions of anger.**
2 Depressed clients frequently have a diminished ability to think or concentrate.
3 Preoccupation with delusions usually is associated with clients who have schizophrenia rather than with clients experiencing depression and hopelessness.
4 Clients who are depressed and feeling hopeless tend to be socially withdrawn and do not have the physical or emotional energy for intense interpersonal relationships.
Clinical Area: Mental Health Nursing; **Client Needs:** Psychosocial Integrity; **Cognitive Level:** Application; **Integrated Process:** Communication and Documentation; **NP:** Assessment

88. 1 **A pH of 7.18 indicates fetal hypoxia; any reading less than 7.2 is dangerous and an emergency birth is indicated.**
2 Any reading greater than 7.2 is not considered life threatening.
3 Any reading greater than 7.2 is not considered life threatening.
4 Any reading greater than 7.2 is not considered life threatening.
Clinical Area: Childbearing and Women's Health Nursing; **Client Needs:** Reduction of Risk Potential; **Cognitive Level:** Application; **NP:** Analysis

89. 1 **This acknowledges the client's apprehension and encourages further communication.**
2 This does not address the client's feelings and may cause more anxiety.
3 This is perhaps true, but it does not foster communication; the client may focus on the word "pain."
4 This negates the client's feelings and promotes false reassurance.
Clinical Area: Medical-Surgical Nursing; **Client Needs:** Psychosocial Integrity; **Cognitive Level:** Application; **Integrated Process:** Communication and Documentation; **NP:** Implementation

90. 1 **As part of the socialization process, toddlers enjoy playing beside other children (parallel play); they are not developmentally ready for interactive (cooperative) play that begins in the preschool years.**
2 This is not antisocial behavior; it is a misinterpretation of parallel play that is typical of toddlers' behavior.
3 This is not an example of an ineffective parental role model; it is a misinterpretation of parallel play that is typical of toddlers' behavior.
4 There are no data to indicate that the children are experiencing separation anxiety.
Clinical Area: Child Health Nursing; **Client Needs:** Health Promotion and Maintenance; **Cognitive Level:** Application; **NP:** Analysis

91. 4 **This ethically sound response clearly defines who is involved in the decision making and allows for parental expression of ideas and thoughts.**
1 Discussion of the implication of a DNR order should not take place until after the family has spoken with the practitioner.
2 Although the answer promotes the practitioner-client relationship, it stops the nurse-client interaction.
3 This response abdicates nursing responsibility. A religious advisor may or may not become involved in the decision making.
Clinical Area: Child Health Nursing; **Client Needs:** Management of Care; **Cognitive Level:** Application; **Integrated Process:** Communication and Documentation; **NP:** Implementation

92. 2 **These clinical findings are indicative of a urinary tract infection and should be reported immediately.**
1 Engorgement is expected and should subside in a few days.
3 An increase in lochial flow or reappearance of lochia after it has ceased is an indication that activity may be too demanding. The client should be advised that this can occur and rest is indicated; it need not be reported to the practitioner.
4 Dryness and tenderness when intercourse is first resumed are expected; the client may find it helpful to use a water-soluble lubricant initially.
Clinical Area: Childbearing and Women's Health Nursing; **Client Needs:** Health Promotion and Maintenance; **Cognitive Level:** Application; **Integrated Process:** Teaching/Learning; **NP:** Evaluation

93. 3 **An autoimmune response plays a role in the development of polyarteritis, although drugs and infections may precipitate it.**
1 The disorder often is fatal, usually as a result of heart or renal failure.
2 Men are affected three times more often than women.
4 Arteriolar pathology can affect any organ or system.
Clinical Area: Medical-Surgical Nursing; **Client Needs:** Physiological Adaptation; **Cognitive Level:** Application; **Integrated Process:** Communication and Documentation; **NP:** Implementation

94. 2 **Bile, which aids in fat digestion, is not as concentrated as before surgery. Once the body adapts to the absence of the gallbladder the client should be able to tolerate a regular diet that contains fat.**
1 Initially the client should avoid fatty foods unless otherwise indicated.
3 Although teaching the client about a low-calorie diet to promote weight reduction is important, it is not as important as temporary avoidance of fatty foods with the gradual resumption of a regular diet.
4 Encouraging participation in a weight reduction program is inappropriate at this time; a temporary

avoidance of fatty foods with the gradual resumption of a regular diet is the priority.
Clinical Area: Medical-Surgical Nursing; **Client Needs:** Basic Care and Comfort; **Cognitive Level:** Application; **Integrated Process:** Teaching/Learning; **NP:** Implementation

95. **1 Erosion of blood vessels may lead to hemorrhage, a life-threatening situation further complicated by decreased prothrombin production, which occurs with cirrhosis.**
    2 Although food intolerances should be identified, there is no immediate threat to life.
    3 Although increased intra-abdominal pressure because of ascites may precipitate nausea, there is no immediate threat to life.
    4 Hourly urine output measurements are unnecessary.
    Clinical Area: Medical-Surgical Nursing; **Client Needs:** Physiological Adaptation; **Cognitive Level:** Application; **NP:** Assessment

96. **2 Percussing over the client's abdomen will produce a dull, not tympanic, sound if fluid is present.**
    1 Respiratory distress occurs with ascites, but it is not an early sign; the client does not have ascites but is at risk for ascites at this time.
    3 Palpating the lower extremities assesses for dependent edema, not ascites. Ascites is fluid within the peritoneal cavity.
    4 Bowel sounds may be heard with developing ascites; when ascites is extensive, bowel sounds may diminish.
    Clinical Area: Medical-Surgical Nursing; **Client Needs:** Physiological Adaptation; **Cognitive Level:** Application; **NP:** Assessment

97. **4 Members must feel comfortable to discuss things in the group; there must be an understanding that what is discussed in the group will remain in the group.**
    1 Talking about trust does little to foster it.
    2 Revealing personal data about oneself will not establish trust and may increase anxiety because the members may feel their turn for exposure will come whether they want it or not.
    3 Having group members reveal some personal information about themselves will not establish trust and may increase anxiety because the members may feel their turn for exposure will come whether they want it or not.
    Clinical Area: Mental Health Nursing; **Client Needs:** Psychosocial Integrity; **Cognitive Level:** Application; **Integrated Process:** Communication and Documentation; **NP:** Implementation

98. **1 A N95 respirator mask is unique to airborne precautions. It is unique for clients with a diagnosis such as tuberculosis, varicella, or measles.**
    2 Donning a nonpermeable gown is not unique to airborne precautions.
    3 Wearing clean gloves when touching the client's body is not unique to airborne precautions.
    4 Maintaining separation of 3 feet between the client and another is necessary with droplet precautions, not airborne precautions.
    Clinical Area: Medical-Surgical Nursing; **Client Needs:** Safety and Infection Control; **Cognitive Level:** Application; **NP:** Planning

99. **1 The psychosexual development of a preschooler focuses on the fear of invasive procedures.**
    2 Hospitalization threatens the toddler's autonomy more than the preschooler's.
    3 The adolescent may be threatened with the loss of independence when hospitalized.
    4 Separation from the mother is most critical during infancy and toddlerhood.
    Clinical Area: Child Health Nursing; **Client Needs:** Health Promotion and Maintenance; **Cognitive Level:** Application; **NP:** Analysis

100. **2 With the reduction of edema the child's health improves, the appetite increases, and the blood pressure normalizes.**
    1 Ambulation does not have an adverse effect on this disorder; most children voluntarily restrict their activities and remain in bed during the acute phase.
    3 Fluids are not encouraged because the kidneys are inflamed and cannot tolerate large amounts of fluid.
    4 Sodium intake is decreased, not eliminated; sodium restriction is not tolerated well by children and may further decrease their appetite.
    Clinical Area: Child Health Nursing; **Client Needs:** Physiological Adaptation; **Cognitive Level:** Application; **NP:** Planning

101. **3 It is important to determine whether the infant has maternally transmitted antibodies against measles.**
    1 Vaccination against measles is done when the infant reaches 12 to 15 months of age.
    2 The infant's previous viral illnesses have no relationship to the present exposure to measles.
    4 Maternal exposure to tuberculosis and herpes genitalis is not relevant when determining if the infant has passive immunity to measles.
    Clinical Area: Child Health Nursing; **Client Needs:** Health Promotion and Maintenance; **Cognitive Level:** Application; **Integrated Process:** Communication and Documentation; **NP:** Assessment

102. **2 The client should understand the steps in the transfer to assist appropriately and avoid injury.**
    1 Assessing strength in the affected leg is not advisable because it may disrupt the repair of the affected hip; also weight bearing initially is not permitted on the operative leg.
    3 Bearing weight on the affected leg is contraindicated initially. The client may touch the floor with the foot of the affected leg but may not bear weight on the affected leg.

4 Elevating the leg will cause hip flexion, which is contraindicated initially because it may precipitate hip dislocation.
Clinical Area: Medical-Surgical Nursing; **Client Needs:** Reduction of Risk Potential; **Cognitive Level:** Application; **Integrated Process:** Teaching/Learning; **NP:** Implementation

103. 1 **Vomiting leads to weight loss, a sign of dehydration. Weighing daily is an accurate measure to assess fluid loss or gain.**
2 Concentrated, not dilute, urine is associated with dehydration because the kidneys reabsorb fluid from the circulation in an attempt to establish fluid balance; this causes the urine to be concentrated.
3 The skin of a dehydrated infant is pale and gray.
4 Depressed, not bulging, fontanels are associated with dehydration.
Clinical Area: Child Health Nursing; **Client Needs:** Basic Care and Comfort; **Cognitive Level:** Application; **NP:** Assessment

104. 2 **Hypotonia occurs with magnesium sulfate toxicity because of skeletal and smooth muscle relaxation.**
1 Pallor is not a sign of magnesium sulfate toxicity.
3 Tremors are not a sign of magnesium sulfate toxicity.
4 Tachycardia is not a sign of magnesium sulfate toxicity.
Clinical Area: Childbearing and Women's Health Nursing; **Client Needs:** Pharmacological and Parenteral Therapies; **Cognitive Level:** Application; **NP:** Evaluation

105. 2 **The outer 1 inch of the sterile field is considered contaminated and can be touched without wearing sterile gloves.**
1 The outside of an unopened sterile glove package is not sterile. The field will become contaminated if the unopened package is placed on the sterile field.
3 The outer package, which contains a sterile field drape, is not sterile; if it is touched with sterile gloves, the sterile gloves will become contaminated.
4 Liquids should be poured from a height of 4 to 6 inches; this ensures that the solution bottle does not contaminate the sterile container.
Clinical Area: Medical-Surgical Nursing; **Client Needs:** Safety and Infection Control; **Cognitive Level:** Application; **NP:** Implementation

106. 1 **Research has shown that decreasing stress will slow the rate of atherosclerotic development.**
2 Exercise is thought to decrease atherosclerosis and the formation of lipid plaques.
3 Exercise is thought to decrease atherosclerosis and the formation of lipid plaques.
4 Saturated fats in the diet are contraindicated because they increase the risk for atherosclerosis.
Clinical Area: Medical-Surgical Nursing; **Client Needs:** Health Promotion and Maintenance; **Cognitive Level:** Application; **Integrated Process:** Teaching/Learning; **NP:** Implementation

107. 3 **The taste for salt is learned from habitual use and can be unlearned or reduced with health improvement motivation and creative salt-free food preparation.**
1 Substitutes do not taste the same as salt.
2 The taste for salt is learned.
4 Using salt substitutes containing potassium chloride may be unsafe; excessive use can produce abnormally high serum potassium levels.
Clinical Area: Medical-Surgical Nursing; **Client Needs:** Basic Care and Comfort; **Cognitive Level:** Application; **Integrated Process:** Teaching/Learning; **NP:** Implementation

108. 1 **A strong cry indicates effective respiratory function and is assigned a value of 2.**
2 If the flexion of the arms and legs is slight and movement is diminished, the value assigned is 1.
3 A value of 1 is assigned when the body is pink and the extremities are blue.
4 The heart rate should be more than 100 beats per minute and therefore 90 beats per minute is assigned a value of 1.
Clinical Area: Childbearing and Women's Health Nursing; **Client Needs:** Reduction of Risk Potential; **Cognitive Level:** Analysis; **NP:** Analysis

109. 4 **This places both nurses in a stable position in functional alignment thereby minimizing stress on muscles, joints, ligaments, and tendons.**
1 The client should be instructed to fold the arms across the chest. This keeps the client's weight toward the center of the mass being moved and keeps the arms safe during the move up in bed.
2 The nurses should assist the client in flexing the knees and placing the feet flat on the bed. This enables the client to push the body upward using a major muscle group. The client's assistance to the best of one's ability reduces physical stress on the nurses as they move the client up in bed.
3 On the count of three, weight should be shifted from the back to the front leg, not the front to the back leg. This action generates movement in the direction that the client is being moved.
Clinical Area: Medical-Surgical Nursing; **Client Needs:** Safety and Infection Control; **Cognitive Level:** Application; **NP:** Analysis

110. 1 **An exercise program and a brace are the treatments of choice for mild structural scoliosis.**
2 Although compliance will affect the ultimate outcome of treatment, exercises alone are not helpful in this type of scoliosis.
3 Exercises are to be encouraged, regardless of the type or extent of scoliosis.
4 Exercises alone are used only with postural-related, not structural-related, scoliosis.
Clinical Area: Child Health Nursing; **Client Needs:** Management of Care; **Cognitive Level:** Application;

Integrated Process: Communication and Documentation; **NP:** Implementation

111. **3 Clients with delirium have a short-term memory loss; therefore, it is necessary to reinforce information.**

1 Clients experiencing delirium are unable to participate in a discussion about self-control.

2 Humor is inappropriate and may cause the client to feel uncomfortable.

4 Approaching the client from the side rather than the front may initiate a startle response and the client may become fearful.

Clinical Area: Mental Health Nursing; **Client Needs:** Psychosocial Integrity; **Cognitive Level:** Application; **Integrated Process:** Communication and Documentation; **NP:** Planning

112. **1 Cor pulmonale is right ventricular failure caused by pulmonary congestion; edema results from increasing venous pressure.**

2 A productive cough is symptomatic of the original condition, COPD.

3 Although twitching of the extremities may be caused by alterations in oxygen and hydrogen ion levels and their effects on the central nervous system, it is the sign of peripheral edema that directly indicates increasing venous pressure secondary to cor pulmonale.

4 Although lethargy progressing to coma is caused by alterations in oxygen and hydrogen ion levels and their effects on the central nervous system, the sign of peripheral edema directly indicates increasing venous pressure secondary to cor pulmonale.

Clinical Area: Medical-Surgical Nursing; **Client Needs:** Physiological Adaptation; **Cognitive Level:** Application; **NP:** Assessment

113. **1 The chamber closest to the client in a three-chamber system is the first chamber; it collects drainage. Chamber 2 is the water seal that ensures that air does not enter the pleural space. Chamber 3 is the suction control chamber of the system.**

2 The third chamber in a three-chamber system is the suction regulator when it is attached to a source of suction.

3 Chamber 1, the chamber closest to the client in a three-chamber system, does not maintain negative pressure.

4 The second chamber is the water-seal chamber that prevents air from entering the client's pleural space.

Clinical Area: Medical-Surgical Nursing; **Client Needs:** Physiological Adaptation; **Cognitive Level:** Application; **NP:** Planning

114. **2 The adolescent is exhibiting signs of bulimia nervosa. The school nurse is an appropriate resource for the friend. The school nurse has the responsibility to intervene because purging can lead to malnutrition and electrolyte imbalances, which are life threatening.**

1 The friend does not have the expertise to intervene.

3 The friend should seek out a professional with whom to share this information. The friend does not have the expertise to intervene.

4 Waiting any longer may jeopardize the health of her friend.

Clinical Area: Mental Health Nursing; **Client Needs:** Management of Care; **Cognitive Level:** Application; **Integrated Process:** Communication and Documentation; **NP:** Implementation

115. **4 The nurse shows an understanding of the client's needs by not totally restricting the handwashing and by working with the client to set limits on the behavior.**

1 At this time the client is still too anxious and is incapable of coping with the reasons for handwashing.

2 Continued handwashing does not reveal an understanding of the underlying problem nor is it a sign of progress.

3 This response denies the client's feelings and may close off communication.

Clinical Area: Mental Health Nursing; **Client Needs:** Psychosocial Integrity; **Cognitive Level:** Application; **Integrated Process:** Caring; **NP:** Implementation

116. **4 The recommended age for the fourth dose of DTaP is 15 to 18 months.**

1 The recommended age for the second dose of Hep B is 4 weeks after the first dose given immediately after birth.

2 Four, not five, doses of IPV are recommended.

3 The initial dose of PCV and Hib are given at 2 months.

Clinical Area: Child Health Nursing; **Client Needs:** Health Promotion and Maintenance; **Cognitive Level:** Analysis; **NP:** Implementation

117. **4 Deep respirations and a fruity odor to the breath are classic signs of DKA because of the respiratory system's attempt to compensate by blowing off excess carbon dioxide, a component of carbonic acid.**

1 Nervousness and tachycardia are indicative of an insulin reaction (diabetic hypoglycemia). When the blood glucose level decreases, the sympathetic nervous system is stimulated, resulting in an increase in epinephrine and norepinephrine. This causes clinical findings such as nervousness, tachycardia, palpitations, sweating, tremor, and hunger.

2 Erythema toxicum rash and pruritus are unrelated to diabetes; they indicate a hypersensitivity reaction.

3 Although an altered mental state is associated with both hypoglycemia and DKA, diaphoresis is associated only with hypoglycemia. Diaphoresis occurs when the blood glucose level decreases and stimulates an increase in epinephrine and norepinephrine.

Clinical Area: Medical-Surgical Nursing; **Client Needs:** Physiological Adaptation; **Cognitive Level:** Application; **NP:** Assessment

118. 2 **Focusing on a variety of needs and concerns is typical of the working stage of the group; trust has been established, and a willingness to discuss any problems or needs is present.**

    1 Satisfaction with group interactions may occur at any stage; satisfaction occurs in social, as well as therapeutic, relationships.

    3 Saying what is perceived as being expected occurs in the early stages of group therapy before trust is established and when everyone is trying to adapt.

    4 Showing concern for the feelings of group leaders occurs in the early stages of group therapy before trust is established.

    Clinical Area: Mental Health Nursing; **Client Needs:** Psychosocial Integrity; **Cognitive Level:** Analysis; **Integrated Process:** Communication and Documentation; **NP:** Evaluation

119. 3 **Total blood volume increases 50%, which necessitates the heart to pump harder and work more to accommodate this increase.**

    1 Although the renal threshold is lowered, the major changes occur in the cardiovascular system.

    2 Changes in hormone levels occur but they are not as profound as changes in the cardiovascular system.

    4 Pressure from the growing uterus can result in digestive discomfort and altered patterns of elimination, but these changes are not as significant as those in the cardiovascular system.

    Clinical Area: Childbearing and Women's Health Nursing; **Client Needs:** Health Promotion and Maintenance; **Cognitive Level:** Knowledge; **Integrated Process:** Communication and Documentation; **NP:** Implementation

120. 1 **The client has the right to privacy; the behavior is acceptable in the privacy of his room.**

    2 Masturbation is a sexual outlet; assessment is unnecessary unless the act is practiced to excess or in public.

    3 Ignoring the situation can cause needless embarrassment to the client and may close off communication.

    4 The behavior is not inappropriate because the client was in the privacy of his own room.

    Clinical Area: Mental Health Nursing; **Client Needs:** Psychosocial Integrity; **Cognitive Level:** Application; **Integrated Process:** Communication and Documentation; **NP:** Implementation

121. 2 **When clients in obvious crisis appear depressed, anxious, and desperate, the nurse should question them regarding the presence of suicidal thoughts.**

    1 Further assessment and exploration are needed before encouraging the client to admit herself to a psychiatric facility.

    3 When clients are overwhelmed with problems, it is difficult for them to think positively.

    4 Running away from problems does not help solve them, nor will escaping bring lasting relief.

    Clinical Area: Mental Health Nursing; **Client Needs:** Psychosocial Integrity; **Cognitive Level:** Application; **Integrated Process:** Communication and Documentation; **NP:** Assessment

122. 4 **When a client has a perforated viscera, barium can leak out of the intestinal tract and cause inflammation and/or an abscess.**

    1 Although hemorrhoids may be irritating, this does not contraindicate barium studies.

    2 Serum potassium is unaffected; barium is insoluble and will not affect blood content.

    3 Barium studies are not contraindicated when the bowel is inflamed. An upper gastrointestinal series is useful in diagnosing ulcerative colitis and Crohn disease.

    Clinical Area: Medical-Surgical Nursing; **Client Needs:** Safety and Infection Control; **Cognitive Level:** Analysis; **NP:** Analysis

123. 2 **During a health crisis the client will need support from significant others.**

    1 The sexual history was important to know to assist in the diagnosis; it is not the priority at this time.

    3 Although the obstetric history is important to know as part of the medical history, it is not the priority at this time.

    4 Although elimination patterns are important to know, it is not the priority at this time.

    Clinical Area: Childbearing and Women's Health Nursing; **Client Needs:** Psychosocial Integrity; **Cognitive Level:** Application; **NP:** Assessment

124. 3 **This is the definition of a positive CST result.**

    1 A CST is performed after an NST is nonreactive or equivocal, not before.

    2 A positive CST result does not dictate a cesarean birth; an expeditious vaginal birth may be attempted.

    4 These variations in the fetal heart rate are expected in a healthy fetus.

    Clinical Area: Childbearing and Women's Health Nursing; **Client Needs:** Reduction of Risk Potential; **Cognitive Level:** Comprehension; **NP:** Assessment

125. 4 **This response rejects the behavior, not the client; it helps separate the client from the behavior.**

    1 This response does not help the client learn self-control; it rejects both the client and the behavior.

    2 Isolating the client limits learning more acceptable responses.

    3 Part of recovery is learning acceptable behavior; ignoring inappropriate behavior is not therapeutic.

    Clinical Area: Mental Health Nursing; **Client Needs:** Psychosocial Integrity; **Cognitive Level:** Application; **Integrated Process:** Communication and Documentation; **NP:** Implementation

126. 4 **The aim of therapy is to eliminate the causative agent, which is determined from culture and sensitivity tests of sputum.**
   1 Bronchoscopy shows the appearance of the bronchi but does not indicate the presence or absence of microorganisms.
   2 Pulse oximetry is used to assess for hypoxemia; it does not provide data on the condition of the lung tissue itself or the presence or absence of microorganisms.
   3 Pulmonary function studies indicate air volume that may be within the expected range despite the presence of bronchopneumonia.
   Clinical Area: Medical-Surgical Nursing; **Client Needs:** Reduction of Risk Potential; **Cognitive Level:** Application; **NP:** Evaluation

127. 4 **Stopping the flow reduces cramping caused by distention of the intestinal lumen. Distention results from the volume of fluid instilled.**
   1 Reducing the rate of flow of the enema fluid still infuses fluid into the intestine, which will increase the discomfort.
   2 There is no need to discontinue the enema. An effective enema must be administered before gastrointestinal surgery.
   3 Lowering the container several inches below the anus will result in the fluid flowing back out through the rectal tube into the container. This is the principle used when administering a return-flow enema (also known as Harris flush). The purpose of the preoperative enema is to evacuate the bowel of feces, not just flatus.
   Clinical Area: Medical-Surgical Nursing; **Client Needs:** Basic Care and Comfort; **Cognitive Level:** Application; **NP:** Implementation

128. 4 **Cortical control of voluntary muscles occurs between 2 and 4 months of age.**
   1 The neurological lesions are fixed and will neither progress nor regress.
   2 Cerebral palsy is not diagnosed by the presence of joint deformities; these may develop later because of spastic muscle imbalance.
   3 Parents have a right to be informed of their child's diagnosis as soon as possible.
   Clinical Area: Child Health Nursing; **Client Needs:** Management of Care; **Cognitive Level:** Application; **Integrated Process:** Communication and Documentation; **NP:** Implementation

129. 3 **The first insertion site should be distal (low) on the periphery of an extremity and progress proximally (upward) toward the trunk; the upper extremities are the most appropriate sites for intravenous insertions for adults and children older than 1 year.**
   1 Scalp veins are used for infants only if peripheral veins are inaccessible.
   2 Foot veins should not be used once a child is walking.

   4 The antecubital fossa should be avoided because the arm will have to be immobilized to stabilize the intravenous insertion site to prevent an infiltration.
   Clinical Area: Child Health Nursing; **Client Needs:** Pharmacological and Parenteral Therapies; **Cognitive Level:** Comprehension; **NP:** Planning

130. 4 **As the lower uterine segment stretches and thins, tearing and bleeding occur at the low implantation site.**
   1 First-trimester bleeding is associated with spontaneous abortion or inadequate implantation, not placenta previa.
   2 Painful vaginal bleeding in the third trimester usually is associated with abruptio placentae rather than placenta previa.
   3 First-trimester bleeding is associated with spontaneous abortion or inadequate implantation, not placenta previa.
   Clinical Area: Childbearing and Women's Health Nursing; **Client Needs:** Physiological Adaptation; **Cognitive Level:** Comprehension; **NP:** Analysis

131. 3 **This response presents the reality of the situation and helps distract the client during a threatening hallucination.**
   1 This is not therapeutic. It will be difficult for the client to ignore the voices.
   2 This response encourages withdrawal and isolation and will not stop the hallucination.
   4 This response will have little effect on the client's behavior and will not stop the hallucination.
   Clinical Area: Mental Health Nursing; **Client Needs:** Psychosocial Integrity; **Cognitive Level:** Application; **Integrated Process:** Caring; **NP:** Implementation

132. 1 **Regression to a more immature, helpless developmental level is not unusual and should be supported at this time.**
   2 The client's behavior does not indicate anger.
   3 Denial is not the response described.
   4 The client's behavior is inconsistent with the need for more control.
   Clinical Area: Mental Health Nursing; **Client Needs:** Management of Care; **Cognitive Level:** Application; **Integrated Process:** Caring; **NP:** Planning

133. 2 **Fluid may shift from the intravascular space to the abdomen as fluid is removed, leading to hypovolemia and compensatory tachycardia.**
   1 Dry mouth may occur with dehydration, but it is not as vital or immediate as signs of shock. Dry mouth is a subjective symptom that cannot be objectively measured.
   3 The fluid shift can cause hypovolemia with resulting hypotension, not hypertension.
   4 A paracentesis decreases the degree of abdominal distention.
   Clinical Area: Medical-Surgical Nursing; **Client Needs:** Reduction of Risk Potential; **Cognitive Level:** Application; **NP:** Evaluation

134. 2 **An empty bladder reduces the risk of bladder puncture during the procedure.**
    1 Sedation is not necessary.
    3 An IV is not necessary.
    4 Encouraging a client to drink three glasses of water is done before a sonogram, not an amniocentesis.
    Clinical Area: Childbearing and Women's Health Nursing; **Client Needs:** Reduction of Risk Potential; **Cognitive Level:** Application; **Integrated Process:** Teaching/Learning; **NP:** Implementation

135. 1 **Heat causes vasodilation and an increased blood supply to the area, which enhances healing.**
    2 Cleansing is done immediately after voiding and defecating, usually with a squeeze bottle filled with cleansing solution or water.
    3 Softening the incision site is not the purpose of sitz baths.
    4 Relaxation, not tightening, of the rectal sphincter is promoted by sitz baths; relaxation provides for comfort but it does not enhance healing.
    Clinical Area: Childbearing and Women's Health Nursing; **Client Needs:** Health Promotion and Maintenance; **Cognitive Level:** Application; **Integrated Process:** Teaching/Learning; **NP:** Planning

136. 2 **Yogurt, which contains calcium, is more easily digested because it contains the enzyme lactase, which breaks down milk sugar. Yogurt contains approximately 274 to 415 mg of calcium for an 8-oz container depending on how it is prepared.**
    1 Eggs contain approximately 22 mg of calcium.
    3 One potato contains approximately 7 to 20 mg of calcium depending on how it is prepared.
    4 Eight ounces of applesauce contain approximately 3 mg of calcium.
    Clinical Area: Medical-Surgical Nursing; **Client Needs:** Basic Care and Comfort; **Cognitive Level:** Analysis; **Integrated Process:** Teaching/Learning; **NP:** Implementation

137. 4 **Steroids increase the excitability of the central nervous system, which can cause labile emotions manifested as euphoria and excitability and/or depression.**
    1 This response denies the value of the client's statement and offers false reassurance.
    2 The client has already stated the problem and does not know why this is happening.
    3 Instructing the client to attempt to avoid situations that cause irritation is difficult to do because the mood swings may occur without an overt cause.
    Clinical Area: Medical-Surgical Nursing; **Client Needs:** Pharmacological and Parenteral Therapies; **Cognitive Level:** Application; **Integrated Process:** Communication and Documentation; **NP:** Evaluation

138. 1 **Hypertension increases pressure on the suture lines of the graft and is a serious risk factor in causing a rupture of the graft.**

2 A sign of anaphylactic shock includes a decrease, not increase, in BP as a result of peripheral vascular collapse manifested by massive vasodilation, pallor, imperceptible pulse, and circulatory failure, leading to coma and death.
    3 Hypovolemia is indicated by a decrease, not an increase, in blood pressure.
    4 Occlusion of the graft is indicated by absent pedal pulses, not an increase in blood pressure.
    Clinical Area: Medical-Surgical Nursing; **Client Needs:** Management of Care; **Cognitive Level:** Application; **Integrated Process:** Communication and Documentation; **NP:** Implementation

139. 4 **A child with a conduct disorder is physically aggressive; no physical aggression in 3 months demonstrates that treatment is successful; the physical aggression differentiates it from oppositional defiant disorder.**
    1 Controlling verbal aggression alone is not appropriate for this child; this outcome more correctly addresses the problems of a child with oppositional defiant disorder.
    2 This is an appropriate short-term, not long-term, goal for this child.
    3 This demonstrates a negative outcome for this child.
    Clinical Area: Mental Health Nursing; **Client Needs:** Management of Care; **Cognitive Level:** Analysis; **Integrated Process:** Communication and Documentation; **NP:** Planning

140. 4 **Increased venous pressure resulting from backup of blood, as the right ventricle of the heart fails, forces capillary fluid to seep into interstitial spaces, resulting in peripheral edema.**
    1 Chest pain may be present with a myocardial infarction or cardiovascular insufficiency, not heart failure.
    2 Tachypnea and dyspnea, not bradypnea, occur with right ventricular failure.
    3 Bradycardia does not occur; the heartbeats may vary in intensity, a pulse deficit may be present, or a bounding pulse may be felt.
    Clinical Area: Medical-Surgical Nursing; **Client Needs:** Physiological Adaptation; **Cognitive Level:** Application; **NP:** Assessment

141. 3 **There is no need to separate one client with MRSA from another client with the same infection.**
    1 MRSA infections are highly contagious.
    2 MRSA infections are resistant to most antibiotics, especially methicillin.
    4 Clients with the same infection can remain in the same room; contact precautions are necessary to protect visitors and staff members.
    Clinical Area: Medical-Surgical Nursing; **Client Needs:** Safety and Infection Control; **Cognitive Level:** Application; **Integrated Process:** Communication and Documentation; **NP:** Implementation

142. 1 **An early sign of an infratentorial tumor is ataxia. The parents describe it as clumsiness that becomes progressively worse.**
    2 Papilledema is a very late sign of tumor involvement.
    3 At 9 years of age cranial sutures are completely closed and the cranium does not get larger.
    4 Seizures usually occur with cerebral or supratentorial tumors.
    Clinical Area: Child Health Nursing; **Client Needs:** Physiological Adaptation; **Cognitive Level:** Application; **NP:** Assessment

143. 1 **This response encourages exploration of the client's concerns and feelings.**
    2 This response validates ideas of reference and is an inappropriate response.
    3 The anxious client may not be able to handle being confronted with feelings; this may precipitate a panic reaction.
    4 This response attempts to provide insight prematurely and may increase anxiety.
    Clinical Area: Mental Health Nursing; **Client Needs:** Psychosocial Integrity; **Cognitive Level:** Application; **Integrated Process:** Communication and Documentation; **NP:** Implementation

144. 2 **Celiac disease is an immunological small intestine enteropathy characterized by the inability to metabolize the gliadin component of gluten found in grains, such as wheat, barley, rye, and oats; this results in excessive glutamine that is toxic to the mucosal cells.**
    1 The stools are fatty and yellow.
    3 The intestinal villi are present, but will atrophy if subjected to foods containing gluten.
    4 Fluid balance is not the basic problem with celiac disease; however, dehydration can occur in celiac crisis.
    Clinical Area: Child Health Nursing; **Client Needs:** Physiological Adaptation; **Cognitive Level:** Comprehension; **NP:** Analysis

145. 3 **Jewish dietary laws prohibit any combination of milk and meat at the same meal.**
    1 The Hindu, not Jewish, religion prohibits the ingestion of beef and veal; many Hindus believe that the cow is sacred.
    2 Fish that have scales and fins are considered clean, and therefore allowed in the diet.
    4 Seventh Day Adventists, Baptists, Mormons, and Muslims prohibit some or all of these beverages.
    Clinical Area: Medical-Surgical Nursing; **Client Needs:** Psychosocial Integrity; **Cognitive Level:** Application; **NP:** Planning

146. 4 **Skin-to-skin contact between mother and infant is most effective in maintaining the infant's body temperature; heat is transferred by conduction.**
    1 A radiant warmer is effective if the mother or newborn is unable to have immediate skin-to-skin contact.
    2 Dressing the newborn in a shirt and gown immediately is not effective; also a blanket and radiant warmer are necessary if skin-to-skin contact with the mother is not possible.
    3 Bathing the infant should be delayed until the newborn's body temperature is stabilized.
    Clinical Area: Childbearing and Women's Health Nursing; **Client Needs:** Health Promotion and Maintenance; **Cognitive Level:** Application; **NP:** Implementation

147. 2 **All data presented are expected for a client at 20 weeks' gestation and should be documented.**
    1 There is no need for immediate intervention because all data are expected.
    3 There is no evidence to suggest the need for an emergency admission; all findings are expected.
    4 All data presented are expected for a client at 20 weeks' gestation and should be recorded.
    Clinical Area: Childbearing and Women's Health Nursing; **Client Needs:** Health Promotion and Maintenance; **Cognitive Level:** Application; **Integrated Process:** Communication and Documentation; **NP:** Implementation

148. 1 **The client and his needs are the priority, and assessment is the first step of the nursing process.**
    2 Writing a plan of care for the mental health team is done after a thorough assessment is completed.
    3 The nurse must deal with the present, not the past.
    4 Although meeting separately with the wife should be done, it is not the priority.
    Clinical Area: Mental Health Nursing; **Client Needs:** Management of Care; **Cognitive Level:** Application; **NP:** Assessment

149. 4 **Breast milk is a natural lubricant for the nipples and obviously is not toxic for the infant.**
    1 Products containing lanolin are not recommended to be applied to the nipples because they may be ingested by the infant.
    2 Products containing vitamin E are not advised because they may be ingested by the infant.
    3 Soap should not be used on the nipples because it has a drying effect, which may precipitate cracked nipples.
    Clinical Area: Childbearing and Women's Health Nursing; **Client Needs:** Health Promotion and Maintenance; **Cognitive Level:** Application; **Integrated Process:** Teaching/Learning; **NP:** Implementation

150. 4 **If the airway is not patent and gas exchange is inadequate, life cannot be sustained; thus maintaining respirations is the priority.**
    1 Although bonding is important to the parent-child relationship, without oxygen life is not sustained.
    2 Although preventing infection is important, without oxygen life is not sustained.
    3 Although body temperature is important because the preterm neonate is lacking brown fat and other defense mechanisms needed to maintain temperature, without oxygen life is not sustained.

Clinical Area: Childbearing and Women's Health Nursing; **Client Needs:** Management of Care; **Cognitive Level:** Application; **NP:** Planning

151. **4 Preschoolers are active, sociable individuals who enjoy the company of peers and become bored when isolated.**
    1 Preschoolers have a limited ability to understand complex explanations of cause and effect; they use concrete thinking.
    2 Although a TV set will provide some distraction, encouraging peer contact is preferred.
    3 Restraints will increase agitation, and it is punitive.
    Clinical Area: Child Health Nursing; **Client Needs:** Management of Care; **Cognitive Level:** Application; **NP:** Implementation

152. **4 Laryngeal nerve injury can cause laryngeal spasms, resulting in airway obstruction.**
    1 Parathyroid damage results in hypocalcemia, not hypercalcemia.
    2 Thyroid storm (thyroid crisis) is characterized by the release of excessive levels of thyroid hormone, which increases the metabolic rate. An increase in the metabolic rate increases vital signs resulting in hypertension, not hypotension, and tachycardia, not bradycardia.
    3 Tetany is caused by a decrease in parathormone, a parathyroid hormone, not a thyroid hormone.
    Clinical Area: Medical-Surgical Nursing; **Client Needs:** Reduction of Risk Potential; **Cognitive Level:** Analysis; **NP:** Analysis

153. **3 The client is exhibiting the classic signs and symptoms associated with the postoperative complication of pulmonary embolus. Initially oxygen should be administered to increase the amount of oxygen being delivered to the pulmonary capillary bed.**
    1 Obtaining the vital signs should be done after oxygen therapy is instituted.
    2 The client is not experiencing a cardiac arrest and, therefore, a code should not be initiated.
    4 After more definitive medical intervention, deep breathing and coughing or use of an incentive spirometer may be done to prevent or treat atelectasis.
    Clinical Area: Medical-Surgical Nursing; **Client Needs:** Physiological Adaptation; **Cognitive Level:** Application; **NP:** Implementation

154. **3 Eating in a semirecumbent position slows gastric emptying, thereby helping to prevent premature passage of gastric contents into the duodenum.**
    1 Ambulating after meals speeds gastric emptying and should be avoided.
    2 A diet low in fat speeds gastric emptying and should be avoided.
    4 Increasing fluid intake when eating food speeds gastric emptying and should be avoided.

Clinical Area: Medical-Surgical Nursing; **Client Needs:** Reduction of Risk Potential; **Cognitive Level:** Application; **Integrated Process:** Teaching/Learning; **NP:** Implementation

155. **1 The leg bones and muscles are used for weight bearing and are the strongest in the body. Using the knees for leverage while lifting the client shifts the stress of the transfer to the caregiver's legs. By using the strong muscles of the legs the back is protected from injury**.
    2 Bending at the waist and then using the back for leverage is how many caregivers and people who must lift heavy objects sustain back injuries. The anatomical structure of the back is equipped only to bear the weight of the upper body.
    3 By leaning back, the client's weight is on the caregiver's arms, which are not equipped for heavy weight bearing.
    4 The caregiver's arms are not strong enough to lift the client. In the struggle to lift the client, the client and caregiver may be injured.
    Clinical Area: Medical-Surgical Nursing; **Client Needs:** Safety and Infection Control; **Cognitive Level:** Application; **Integrated Process:** Teaching/Learning; **NP:** Implementation

156. **4 Saccharin (Sweet'N Low), aspartame (Equal), and sucralose (Splenda) are non-nutritive sweeteners recommended for individuals with diabetes.**
    1 Honey is not a sugar substitute. Honey, a fructose, provides 1.3 times as many calories as does table sugar and must be calculated into the diet.
    2 Simple sugars may be used in controlled amounts and must be calculated into the diet.
    3 Foods do not have to taste sweet to contain sugar; individuals who enjoy sweetened foods do not break the sweet-taste habit.
    Clinical Area: Child Health Nursing; **Client Needs:** Basic Care and Comfort; **Cognitive Level:** Application; **Integrated Process:** Teaching/Learning; **NP:** Implementation

157. **1 Health care agencies document the occurrence of any event out of the ordinary that results in or has the potential to harm a client, employee, or visitor**.
    2 Falls by visitors are not required to be reported to state health departments. However, incident reports are required to be presented to accrediting agencies for review when an agency is in the process of being accredited.
    3 This action is not a requirement of ethical practice. However, a nurse who is involved in an incident or is a witness to an incident should write an accurate description of the event along with the names of individuals involved. This documentation should be kept by the nurse at home. Lawsuits may take several years before they come to trial and personal notes may help the nurse recall the event. The documentation must accurately contain the same elements included in the formal incident report.

4 No action is irresponsible. All events out of the ordinary that result in or have the potential to harm a visitor should be documented in an agency incident report.
Clinical Area: Medical-Surgical Nursing; **Client Needs:** Safety and Infection Control; **Cognitive Level:** Application; **Integrated Process:** Communication and Documentation; **NP:** Planning

158. 1 **Drowsiness and irritability are characteristic signs of increasing intracranial pressure; other signs and symptoms include nausea, projectile vomiting, headache, and diminished physical activity.**
2 Incessant talking is expected behavior of a 2½-year-old toddler.
3 Temper tantrums are expected of a 2½-year-old toddler.
4 An inability to share is expected behavior of a 2½-year-old toddler
Clinical Area: Child Health Nursing; **Client Needs:** Physiological Adaptation; **Cognitive Level:** Application; **Integrated Process:** Teaching/Learning; **NP:** Implementation

159. 3 **The staff nurse should call the supervisor to confirm and deal with the problem.**
1 The security guard has no authority in this situation.
2 Although this removes the nurse manager from the clinical setting, it does not provide for documentation of the situation; also the nurse manager may be in no condition to go home independently.
4 Drinking coffee does not make a person less intoxicated.
Clinical Area: Medical-Surgical Nursing; **Client Needs:** Management of Care; **Cognitive Level:** Application; **Integrated Process:** Communication and Documentation; **NP:** Implementation

160. 3 **Looking at the face or seeking eye-to-eye contact with the infant is an early sign of beginning bonding with the infant.**
1 Mothers may feel inept or worry about upsetting the nurse by undressing their infant; new mothers need encouragement to undress their infant.
2 Refusing to breastfeed her newborn may indicate that the mother is worried that she does not have enough milk, a common concern.
4 The client may have attended prenatal classes, may be otherwise occupied, may not be feeling well enough to attend the class, or feels that she has enough experience to care for her infant without attending a class for newborn care.
Clinical Area: Childbearing and Women's Health Nursing; **Client Needs:** Health Promotion and Maintenance; **Cognitive Level:** Application; **NP:** Assessment

161. 4 **Maintaining functional alignment of the head prevents flexion and hyperextension of the neck, both of which place tension on the suture line; tension on the suture line can precipitate wound dehiscence.**
1 The cervical vertebrae are designed to flex and hyperextend; there should be no ill effects.

2 Flexion and hyperextension of the neck do not cause laryngeal spasms.
3 Flexion and hyperextension of the neck do not cause laryngeal edema.
Clinical Area: Medical-Surgical Nursing; **Client Needs:** Safety and Infection Control; **Cognitive Level:** Application; **NP:** Planning

162. 4 **Placing the client in the Trendelenburg position may prevent further prolapse and should relieve pressure on the umbilical cord.**
1 Taking the fetal heart rate will be done later; the priority is to relieve pressure on the umbilical cord.
2 Turning the client onto her side will not relieve pressure on the umbilical cord, although it promotes placental perfusion.
3 Covering the cord with a sterile saline cloth will not relieve pressure on the umbilical cord.
Clinical Area: Childbearing and Women's Health Nursing; **Client Needs:** Management of Care; **Cognitive Level:** Application; **NP:** Implementation

163. 3 **Incentive spirometry expands collapsed alveoli and enhances surfactant activity, thereby preventing atelectasis.**
1 Postural drainage helps clear accumulated secretions from the pulmonary tree; it does not directly promote alveolar expansion.
2 Pursed-lip breathing promotes sustained exhalation, not inhalation.
4 Sustained exhalation promotes the collapse, not expansion, of alveoli.
Clinical Area: Medical-Surgical Nursing; **Client Needs:** Management of Care; **Cognitive Level:** Analysis; **NP:** Planning

164. 4 **A walker with four rubber tips on the legs requires more upper body strength than a rolling walker. A client who is non–weight bearing on the affected extremity is able to use a standard walker.**
1 A rolling walker is more appropriate for this client. A client with weak upper arm strength and impaired stamina is less able to lift up and move a walker with four rubber tips.
2 A client with unilateral paralysis is not a candidate for a standard walker. The client must be able to grip and lift the walker with both upper extremities and move the walker forward.
3 A rolling walker is more appropriate for this client. A client with kyphosis is less able to lift up and move a walker with four rubber tips.
Clinical Area: Medical-Surgical Nursing; **Client Needs:** Safety and Infection Control; **Cognitive Level:** Application; **NP:** Analysis

165. 3 **Intestinal antibiotics and a complete cleansing of the bowel with enemas until returns are clear are necessary to reduce the possibility of fecal contamination when the bowel is resected to construct the ileal conduit.**

1   Intravesicular chemotherapy is unnecessary because the urinary bladder is removed with this surgery.

2   Instillation of a urinary antiseptic is not necessary. There is no evidence of a urinary tract infection.

4   The urinary bladder will be removed, so there is no need for an indwelling urinary catheter. No data indicate that the client is experiencing urinary retention before surgery.

Clinical Area: Medical-Surgical Nursing; **Client Needs:** Pharmacological and Parenteral Therapies; **Cognitive Level:** Application; **NP:** Planning

166.   **Answer: 2, 1, 3, 4**

Ineffective coping skills and body image issues lead to dieting in an attempt to maintain control; deprivation of food and psychosocial stressors cause hunger and anger that precipitate binge eating, which numbs discomforts; guilt about eating and panic about weight gain and loss of control precipitate purging.

Clinical Area: Mental Health Nursing; **Client Needs:** Psychosocial Integrity; **Cognitive Level:** Analysis; **NP:** Analysis

167.   4   **Internal bleeding after a traumatic injury may be gradual. The priority is to assess for internal bleeding and then initiate nursing care based on the findings.**

1   The practitioner should be notified if the assessment reveals a slow internal bleed.

2   Preparing for a blood transfusion may be necessary if the assessment reveals a slow internal bleed.

3   Although meat, an iron-rich food, is appropriate for mild anemia, adding iron-rich foods to the child's menu is not the priority at this time.

Clinical Area: Child Health Nursing; **Client Needs:** Management of Care; **Cognitive Level:** Application; **Integrated Process:** Communication and Documentation; **NP:** Implementation

168.   1   **The possibility of an ascending infection increases when membranes have ruptured and birth is not imminent; the client must be monitored for signs of infection.**

2   Preeclampsia is unrelated to spontaneous rupture of the membranes.

3   Heavy vaginal bleeding is a sign of placenta previa, which generally is diagnosed before membranes rupture.

4   Fetal scalp pH sampling is not indicated with spontaneous rupture of membranes; it is indicated if persistent late decelerations are observed on the fetal monitor during labor.

Clinical Area: Childbearing and Women's Health Nursing; **Client Needs:** Management of Care; **Cognitive Level:** Application; **NP:** Planning

169.   2   **Cholestyramine is a fat-binding agent; it binds with and interferes with all the fat-soluble vitamins (A, D, E, and K).**

1   Thiamine is not a fat-soluble vitamin and is unaffected.

3   Riboflavin is not a fat-soluble vitamin and is unaffected.

4   Vitamin B_6 is not a fat-soluble vitamin and is unaffected.

Clinical Area: Medical-Surgical Nursing; **Client Needs:** Pharmacological and Parenteral Therapies; **Cognitive Level:** Application; **NP:** Evaluation

170.   3   **The practitioner who wrote the order should be called for clarification. The nurse is liable and responsible if the order is misinterpreted.**

1   Only the practitioner who wrote an undecipherable order can correctly clarify the order.

2   Only the practitioner who wrote an undecipherable order can correctly clarify the order.

4   Only the practitioner who wrote an undecipherable order can correctly clarify the order.

Clinical Area: Medical-Surgical Nursing; **Client Needs:** Management of Care; **Cognitive Level:** Application; **Integrated Process:** Communication and Documentation; **NP:** Implementation

171.   1   **The fundus should be palpated to determine if it is boggy. A boggy uterus reflects uterine atony; it should be massaged until firm.**

2   Documenting the amount of lochia without correcting the problem will place the client in physical jeopardy because the client may hemorrhage.

3   Although a full bladder decreases uterine contractility and should be emptied, allowing the client to ambulate to the bathroom to void before massaging her fundus may cause increased bleeding.

4   Requesting laboratory tests without first intervening will place the client in physical jeopardy because the client may hemorrhage.

Clinical Area: Childbearing and Women's Health Nursing; **Client Needs:** Health Promotion and Maintenance; **Cognitive Level:** Application; **NP:** Assessment

172.   4   **Because the client is feeling a loss of control, it is most important to include the client in revision of the plan of care.**

1   These responses do not consider changes in the client or obtain the client's input.

2   Planning nursing care is within the nurse's function and judgment, not the practitioner's; also, the client should be included.

3   This is an authoritarian approach and does not include the client is planning future care.

Clinical Area: Medical-Surgical Nursing; **Client Needs:** Management of Care; **Cognitive Level:** Application; **Integrated Process:** Communication and Documentation; **NP:** Planning

173.   4   **Magnesium sulfate is a central nervous system depressant; it decreases cerebral irritability, thus preventing seizures.**

1   Magnesium sulfate is not a diuretic; however, adequate kidney function is necessary to promote its excretion, otherwise toxicity will result.

2 Magnesium sulfate is not an oxytocic; oxytocin is used to promote uterine contractions and can cause an increased blood pressure.

3 Magnesium sulfate is not an antihypertensive; however, it may cause a transient decrease in blood pressure because of its peripheral dilating effect.

Clinical Area: Childbearing and Women's Health Nursing; **Client Needs:** Pharmacological and Parenteral Therapies; **Cognitive Level:** Knowledge; **NP:** Planning

174. **4 With abruptio placentae, uterine bleeding can result in massive internal hemorrhage, causing hypovolemic shock.**

1 A brain attack may occur with a dangerously high blood pressure; there is no information indicating the presence of a dangerously high blood pressure.

2 Pulmonary edema may occur with severe pre-eclampsia or heart disease; there is no information indicating the presence of these conditions.

3 Seizures are associated with severe preeclampsia; there is no information indicating the presence of severe preeclampsia.

Clinical Area: Childbearing and Women's Health Nursing; **Client Needs:** Physiological Adaptation; **Cognitive Level:** Application; **NP:** Planning

175. **4 Familiarity with situations and continuity add to the client's sense of security and foster trust in the relationship.**

1 Detailed explanations will be forgotten; instructions should be simple and to the point and given when needed.

2 Although demonstrating interest in the client's likes and dislikes helps individualize care, continuity is the priority.

3 Some degree of flexibility by the nurse helps individualize care.

Clinical Area: Mental Health Nursing; **Client Needs:** Management of Care; **Cognitive Level:** Application; **Integrated Process:** Communication and Documentation; **NP:** Planning

176. **2 Alcohol deactivates the smallpox vaccine. Cleansing of the arm should not be done before the immunization is given unless the arm is dirty; if dirty, only water should be used to cleanse the site.**

1 Observation is insufficient; the nurse manager must intervene to ensure that the vaccine is given using the correct technique.

3 Povidone-iodine (Betadine) will deactivate the smallpox vaccine.

4 Cleansing of the arm is unnecessary unless it is dirty; if so, only water should be used to cleanse the site. The site should be dry before administering the vaccine.

Clinical Area: Medical-Surgical Nursing; **Client Needs:** Management of Care; **Cognitive Level:** Application; **Integrated Process:** Communication and Documentation; **NP:** Implementation

177. **3 A positional bed alarm is a noninvasive devise to protect a client who attempts to get out of bed unassisted. Staff members must immediately respond to the alarm to ensure that clients are protected from potential injury.**

1 Although a nightlight may help orient a client at night it does not help during the daylight hours.

2 A vest restraint is a measure of last resort when all other less restrictive measures have proven to be ineffective.

4 Confused clients often become more agitated when all the side rails are raised, posing an increased, not a decreased, risk of injury. Confused clients may try to climb over the side rails or try to exit from the end of the bed, placing them at risk for entrapment or a fall.

Clinical Area: Medical-Surgical Nursing; **Client Needs:** Safety and Infection Control; **Cognitive Level:** Application; **NP:** Planning

178. **1 Previous experiences with projectile vomiting are frightening; the nurse should explain that this should not recur and encourage the mother to resume feeding her baby.**

2 The data indicate that the mother knows she is allowed to feed her baby but is reluctant to do so.

3 A special nipple is not required.

4 Thickened formula is not necessary after surgery.

Clinical Area: Child Health Nursing; **Client Needs:** Basic Care and Comfort; **Cognitive Level:** Application; **NP:** Analysis

179. **2 Loose rugs can interfere with crutch walking and cause a fall; they should be removed to prevent further injury.**

1 Calcium rather than vitamin C is encouraged to enhance bone healing; vitamin C minimizes capillary fragility. It is not within the legal role of the nurse to encourage the client to increase the dose of any medication without a practitioner's order.

3 The client may shower if the cast is protected from becoming wet.

4 Decisions regarding weight bearing is a medical, not a nursing, responsibility.

Clinical Area: Medical-Surgical Nursing; **Client Needs:** Safety and Infection Control; **Cognitive Level:** Application; **Integrated Process:** Teaching/Learning; **NP:** Implementation

180. **1 Identifying the status of the damage is the priority. Before a treatment protocol is determined, the presence of nerve and/or vascular damage and compartment syndrome must be identified.**

2 False reassurance is never appropriate.

3 Skeletal traction is rarely used. Closed fractures in the absence of soft tissue damage generally are reduced by manipulation. Closed fractures with soft tissue damage may require an external fixation device to reduce the fracture, immobilize the bone, and allow for treatment of the soft tissue damage.

4 Preparing the client for surgery is premature; more data are necessary before a treatment option is determined.

Clinical Area: Medical-Surgical Nursing; **Client Needs:** Reduction of Risk Potential; **Cognitive Level:** Application; **NP:** Assessment

181. 4 **Increased venous pressure alters the permeability of the veins, allowing extravasation of RBCs; hemolysis of RBCs releases a pigment called hemosiderin, which causes a characteristic brownish discoloration (brawny appearance).**
    1 The arterial circulation is not affected by the pathology of varicose veins.
    2 Although tissue healing may be delayed, the brownish discoloration is the result of the hemolysis of RBCs, not trauma.
    3 There is no increase in melanocyte activity in the skin surrounding varicose veins.

    Clinical Area: Medical-Surgical Nursing; **Client Needs:** Physiological Adaptation; **Cognitive Level:** Application; **Integrated Process:** Communication and Documentation; **NP:** Implementation

182. 2 **Cleansing after feeding keeps the suture line from becoming infected.**
    1 Crying exerts pressure on the suture line and may cause wound separation (dehiscence).
    3 Sucking exerts pressure on the suture line and may cause wound separation (dehiscence).
    4 The infant should be held and cuddled during feedings.

    Clinical Area: Child Health Nursing; **Client Needs:** Safety and Infection Control; **Cognitive Level:** Application; **Integrated Process:** Teaching/Learning; **NP:** Evaluation

183. 2 **Clients with cardiac disease should be taught the signs and symptoms of cardiac decompensation; if they occur, the client should stop the activity that precipitated them and notify the health care provider.**
    1 Participating in as much activity as she desires is acceptable behavior for a client with class I cardiac disease.
    3 Maintaining bed rest is the treatment for a client with class III cardiac disease.
    4 Considering a therapeutic abortion is the recommendation for a client with class IV cardiac disease.

    Clinical Area: Childbearing and Women's Health Nursing; **Client Needs:** Management of Care; **Cognitive Level:** Application; **NP:** Planning

184. 4 **The three areas of assessment to determine the level of consciousness using the Glasgow Coma Scale are motor response to verbal commands, eye-opening in response to speech, and verbal response to speech.**
    1 Assessing breathing patterns is not included in the Glasgow Coma Scale.
    2 Assessing deep tendon reflexes is not included in the Glasgow Coma Scale.

3 Assessing eye accommodation is not included in the Glasgow Coma Scale.

Clinical Area: Medical-Surgical Nursing; **Client Needs:** Reduction of Risk Potential; **Cognitive Level:** Analysis; **NP:** Assessment

185. 3 **Blood pressure increases with pain and stress; reevaluation is critical before determining if the practitioner should be notified.**
    1 Assessment should be completed before notifying the practitioner.
    2 Prescribing medications is a dependent function of the nurse, and medication should not be administered until the cause of the headache is determined.
    4 Oxygen is not indicated. The head of the bed should be elevated. The practitioner should be notified if a second blood pressure reading remains elevated.

    Clinical Area: Medical-Surgical Nursing; **Client Needs:** Reduction of Risk Potential; **Cognitive Level:** Application; **NP:** Assessment

186. 2 **Regional perfusion therapy permits relative isolation of the tumor area and saturation with the drug(s) selected.**
    1 This method of drug administration requires medical and nursing supervision.
    3 Although toxic effects are mainly confined to the treated area, some migration may still occur.
    4 Combinations of chemotherapeutic drugs are administered via intravenous or oral routes, not via regional perfusion.

    Clinical Area: Medical-Surgical Nursing; **Client Needs:** Pharmacology and Parenteral Therapies; **Cognitive Level:** Application; **NP:** Planning

187. 3 **Laryngeal spasms can occur abruptly; patency of the airway is determined by continuous monitoring for signs of respiratory distress.**
    1 Providing oxygen is important, but maintenance of respirations is the priority.
    2 The fever should be treated, but it is not critical at 103° F; maintenance of respirations is the priority.
    4 Offering support is important, but maintenance of respirations is the priority.

    Clinical Area: Child Health Nursing; **Client Needs:** Management of Care; **Cognitive Level:** Application; **NP:** Planning

188. 2 **Lethargy is an early sign of a changing level of consciousness; it is one of the first signs of increased intracranial pressure.**
    1 Nausea is a subjective symptom, not a sign, that may be present with increased intracranial pressure.
    3 Sunset eyes are a late sign of increased intracranial pressure that occurs in children with hydrocephalus.
    4 Hyperthermia is a late sign of increased intracranial pressure that occurs as compression of the brainstem increases.

Clinical Area: Medical-Surgical Nursing; **Client Needs:** Reduction of Risk Potential; **Cognitive Level:** Application; **NP:** Assessment

189. 3 **Chest pain, along with dyspnea, cough, hemoptysis, and apprehension, is a classic sign of a pulmonary embolism. Six days postoperatively is a prime time for symptoms of a pulmonary embolus to occur because decreased mobility promotes the development of deep vein thrombosis.**
    1 The lack of a productive cough does not require nursing intervention; a productive, not nonproductive, cough indicates a respiratory infection requiring intervention.
    2 An increase in temperature can result from the inflammatory process; the temperature-regulating mechanisms in older adults may be compromised slightly, and they may show a slight elevation in body temperature for a longer period of time after surgery than a younger client.
    4 Weight bearing is being done by the unaffected leg at this time, and fatigue is expected.
    Clinical Area: Medical-Surgical Nursing; **Client Needs:** Management of Care; **Cognitive Level:** Application; **NP:** Evaluation

190. 3 **Obtaining cultures is the most reliable method of determining the presence of an infecting microorganism.**
    1 Although notifying the infection control officer should be done, the presence of an infecting microorganism should be identified first.
    2 Informing the operating room personnel of the MRSA is usual when an infecting microorganism is present; however, it is not yet confirmed that the infecting microorganism is present.
    4 Although calling the surgeon for an infectious disease consultation may be done, the presence of an infecting agent should be identified first.
    Clinical Area: Medical-Surgical Nursing; **Client Needs:** Management of Care; **Cognitive Level:** Application; **Integrated Process:** Communication and Documentation; **NP:** Assessment

191. 2 **The pain caused by vascular occlusion is often described as excruciating, and analgesics should be administered immediately after a pain assessment.**
    1 Oxygen is not helpful in reversing the sickling, which is causing the pain.
    3 Although a blood transfusion may be needed to treat the anemia and reduce the viscosity of the sickled blood, it is not the priority.
    4 Although intravenous fluid is important, it is not the priority.
    Clinical Area: Child Health Nursing; **Client Needs:** Physiological Adaptation; **Cognitive Level:** Analysis; **NP:** Planning

192. Answer: 2, 3, 4
    1 Stranger anxiety begins at about 5 to 6 months when infants become responsive to the caregivers who have met both physical and emotional needs. When strangers speak to them or reach out to hold them they seem fearful, cling to their caregiver, and cry. Infants whose needs have not been met adequately have no reason to be fearful of others.
    2 A typical sign of physical neglect is the wearing of dirty clothes or clothing that is not suitable to the environment.
    3 The infant who has not experienced social responsiveness from the caregiver has not learned how to be socially responsive to others.
    4 Infants who experience emotional deprivation resort to self stimulating behaviors in an effort to meet their emotional needs.
    5 Infants who experience physical neglect are more likely to be unclean with signs of unattended skin lesions such as a diaper rash or bruises.
    Clinical Area: Mental Health Nursing; **Client Needs:** Psychosocial Integrity; **Cognitive Level:** Analysis; **NP:** Assessment

193. 2 **Pulmonary edema is associated with severe preeclampsia; as vasospasms worsen capillary endothelial damage results in capillary leakage into the alveoli.**
    1 Crackles are not an indication of an impending seizure; signs of an impending seizure include hyperreflexia, developing or worsening clonus, severe headache, visual disturbances, and epigastric pain.
    3 Pregnancy does not precipitate bronchial constriction although the hormones associated with pregnancy can cause nasal congestion.
    4 Impaired diaphragmatic functioning is a discomfort associated with pregnancy that may result in shortness of breath or dyspnea, not crackles.
    Clinical Area: Childbearing and Women's Health Nursing; **Client Needs:** Physiological Adaptation; **Cognitive Level:** Application; **NP:** Analysis

194. 3 **The side-lying position with the head slightly elevated promotes venous return by gravity, which helps reduce intracranial pressure, a problem after myelomeningocele repair.**
    1 Although preventing aspiration is important, the reason for this position that is unique with this type of surgery is that it minimizes intracranial pressure.
    2 Although promoting respiration is important, the reason for this position that is unique with this type of surgery is that it minimizes intracranial pressure.
    4 Although maintaining cleanliness of the suture site is important, the reason for this position that is unique with this type of surgery is that it minimizes intracranial pressure.
    Clinical Area: Child Health Nursing; **Client Needs:** Physiological Adaptation; **Cognitive Level:** Application; **NP:** Planning

195. 3 **A yellow tag (priority II) indicates injuries that need treatment within 2 hours. Although clients who have sustained simple fractures, lacerations,**

or fever can wait for treatment for 2 hours, they need to be reassessed every 30 minutes to ensure that their condition did not deteriorate. If their condition deteriorates they should be relabeled with a red tag (priority I) indicating the need for immediate treatment.

1 A red tag (priority I) indicates a client with respiratory distress, trauma or bleeding, or neurological deficits that need immediate treatment.

2 A green tag (priority III) indicates a client who needs care that can wait for hours. Although clients with sprains, rashes, and minor pain can wait hours for treatment, they need to be reassessed every 1 to 2 hours to ensure that their condition did not deteriorate. If their condition deteriorates they should be relabeled according to their level of need.

4 An orange tag indicates a nonemergent psychiatric situation.

Clinical Area: Medical-Surgical Nursing; Client Needs: Safety and Infection Control; Cognitive Level: Application; Integrated Process: Communication and Documentation; NP: Implementation

196. 1 **Subcutaneous emphysema refers to the presence of air in the tissue that surrounds an opening in the normally closed respiratory tract; the tissue appears puffy, and a crackling sensation is detected when trapped air is compressed between the nurse's palpating fingertips and the client's tissue.**

2 Gas exchange and thus blood gases are not affected.

3 The lungs are not affected.

4 The lungs are not affected.

Clinical Area: Medical-Surgical Nursing; Client Needs: Reduction of Risk Potential; Cognitive Level: Application; NP: Evaluation

197. 2 **The client is anxious and afraid of leaving home; the priority is provision for safety and security needs.**

1 Unless the client is provided with a sense of security, adjustment probably will be unsatisfactory because the anxiety will most likely escalate.

3 Exploring the client's memory loss and fear of going out cannot be done until anxiety is reduced.

4 The client is experiencing memory loss and may not be able to remember what precipitated admission to the hospital; some memory loss may be a result of high anxiety and thought blocking.

Clinical Area: Mental Health Nursing; Client Needs: Safety and Infection Control; Cognitive Level: Application; Integrated Process: Caring; NP: Planning

198. 1 **Gastric secretions, which are electrolyte rich, are lost through the nasogastric tube; the imbalances that result can be life threatening.**

2 Changing the nasogastric tube every 48 hours is unnecessary and can damage the suture line.

3 High continuous suction can cause trauma to the suture line.

4 Injecting 10 mL of water into the nasogastric tube to test for placement is unsafe; if respiratory intubation has occurred aspiration will result.

Clinical Area: Medical-Surgical Nursing; Client Needs: Reduction of Risk Potential; Cognitive Level: Application; NP: Evaluation

199. 1 **School-age children are most concerned about school, if not for the academics, for the social aspects.**

2 School-age children generally live in the present; there is little concern about the future.

3 The parents' reaction may be of some concern but not as much as school.

4 School-age children generally live in the present; there is little concern about the future.

Clinical Area: Child Health Nursing; Client Needs: Health Promotion and Maintenance; Cognitive Level: Application; Integrated Process: Communication and Documentation; NP: Assessment

200. 3 **Baseline vital signs are extremely important; physical assessment precedes diagnostic measures and intervention.**

1 This is done after the practitioner makes a medical diagnosis; this is not an independent function of the nurse.

2 This might be done after it is determined whether a specimen for blood gases is needed; this is not usually an independent function of the nurse. Oxygen is administered independently by the nurse only in an emergency situation.

4 A sputum specimen should be obtained after vital signs and before administration of antibiotics.

Clinical Area: Medical-Surgical Nursing; Client Needs: Reduction of Risk Potential; Cognitive Level: Application; NP: Assessment

201. 3 **Mild shoulder pain is commonly a response to nerve irritation from insufflating the abdomen with carbon dioxide gas to permit visualization and introduction of instruments. Understanding what to expect supports control and decreases fear.**

1 There are no long-term dietary restrictions related to this surgery.

2 Although it is important for the client to understand that generally there are one or more small puncture wounds made through the abdominal wall and how to care for them after surgery, it is more important for the nurse to explain about the mild shoulder pain, which may frighten the client if it is unexpected.

4 Postoperative abdominal exercises are not necessary.

Clinical Area: Medical-Surgical Nursing; Client Needs: Reduction of Risk Potential; Cognitive Level: Application; Integrated Process: Teaching/Learning; NP: Planning

202. 1 **These are signs of water intoxication, which may proceed to pulmonary edema; the practitioner should be notified.**

2 Chest x-ray findings lag behind clinical manifestations; the last chest x-ray film does not reflect the client's current status.

3 Although the arterial blood gases may be monitored, increasing the IV rate should never be done, particularly if water intoxication is suspected.

4 Increasing the IV rate should never be done, particularly if water intoxication is suspected. Calcium gluconate is a calcium product to treat hypocalcemia. During the resuscitation/emergent phase of burn recovery the client will experience hyperkalemia, hyperchloremia, and hyponatremia.

Clinical Area: Medical-Surgical Nursing; **Client Needs:** Pharmacological and Parenteral Therapy **Cognitive Level:** Analysis; **NP:** Implementation

203. 1 **During detoxification this provides for safety and prevents suicide, which is a real threat.**

2 Bright light is preferable to dim light because it minimizes shadows that can contribute to misinterpretation of environmental stimuli (illusions).

3 The client who is experiencing the detoxification phase of acute alcohol withdrawal usually does not lose the sense of hearing, so there is no need to shout.

4 Restraints may upset the client further; they should be used only if the client is a danger to oneself or others.

Clinical Area: Mental Health Nursing; **Client Needs:** Psychosocial Integrity; **Cognitive Level:** Application; **NP:** Planning

204. 1 **VinCRIStine (Oncovin) is a plant alkaloid that is cell-cycle specific. It affects cell division during metaphase by interfering with spindle formation and causing cell death.**

2 Inhibiting the synthesis of thymidine is the typical action of antimetabolites, not plant alkaloids.

3 Alkylating nucleic acids needed for mitosis is typical of the action of alkylating agents, not plant alkaloids.

4 Inactivating DNA and RNA synthesis is the typical action of antineoplastic antibiotics, not plant alkaloids.

Clinical Area: Medical-Surgical Nursing; **Client Needs:** Pharmacological and Parenteral Therapies; **Cognitive Level:** Comprehension; **NP:** Implementation

205. 4 **The client needs to learn to cope with stressful life situations effectively, rather than resort to binge-purge behaviors. The first step toward achieving control is expressing a desire to do so.**

1 Most clients with bulimia nervosa are socially adept and do not need to focus on improvement in this area.

2 This is a long-term, not short-term, goal for a client with bulimia nervosa.

3 Clients with bulimia nervosa do not tend to experience delusional thoughts.

Clinical Area: Mental Health Nursing; **Client Needs:** Management of Care; **Cognitive Level:** Application;

Integrated Process: Communication and Documentation; **NP:** Planning

206. 4 **This response protects the wife's confidentiality while fostering open communication between the couple.**

1 This response does not foster communication between the client and the client's husband.

2 This abrupt statement is not true and does not support the wife or the husband.

3 This abrupt statement does not support the wife or the husband.

Clinical Area: Childbearing and Women's Health Nursing; **Client Needs:** Management of Care; **Cognitive Level:** Application; **Integrated Process:** Communication and Documentation; **NP:** Implementation

207. 4 **Overwhelming feelings of guilt are factors that contribute to the client's risk for suicide. The client may ruminate over past or present failings and extreme guilt can assume psychotic proportions.**

1 Psychomotor retardation is a clinical finding associated with depression and usually does not lead to suicide because the client does not have the energy for self-harm.

2 Decreased physical activity is a clinical finding associated with depression and usually does not lead to suicide because the client does not have the energy for self-harm.

3 Impulsive behaviors, not deliberate thoughtful behaviors, are factors that contribute to the client's risk for suicide.

Clinical Area: Mental Health Nursing; **Client Needs:** Psychosocial Integrity; **Cognitive Level:** Application; **NP:** Analysis

208. 3 **Vasodilation should help reduce pain from cellular clumping; this will address the pain until the pump can be activated.**

1 Television may be an adequate distractor for mild pain, not moderate or severe pain.

2 Nursing measures should be attempted first to relieve the pain before calling the practitioner.

4 Telling the adolescent to wait provides no comfort for a person in pain.

Clinical Area: Child Health Nursing; **Client Needs:** Basic Care and Comfort; **Cognitive Level:** Application; **Integrated Process:** Caring; **NP:** Implementation

209. 2 **Decreased sodium intake can accelerate lithium retention with subsequent toxicity.**

1 Iron is unrelated to the administration of lithium.

3 Potassium is unrelated to the administration of lithium.

4 Magnesium is unrelated to the administration of lithium.

Clinical Area: Mental Health Nursing; **Client Needs:** Pharmacological and Parenteral Therapies; **Cognitive Level:** Application; **Integrated Process:** Teaching/Learning; **NP:** Implementation

210. 1 **The client may become injured in many ways during a seizure, and trauma prevention is a priority.**
    2 Anticonvulsants can cause GI disturbances, especially early in therapy, and should be taken with food.
    3 Seizures and seizure disorders are not similar; they vary greatly.
    4 Others should understand the condition and be taught how to help in case of a seizure.
    Clinical Area: Medical-Surgical Nursing; **Client Needs:** Safety and Infection Control; **Cognitive Level:** Application; **Integrated Process:** Teaching/Learning; **NP:** Planning

211. 4 **Gastric returns indicate correct placement of the feeding tube.**
    1 Further assessment is necessary before notifying the practitioner.
    2 Advancing the tube even 1 cm may cause undue trauma regardless of where the tube is located.
    3 Inserting even a small amount of formula is unsafe until correct placement is verified; formula may enter the lungs if the tube is not in the stomach.
    Clinical Area: Child Health Nursing; **Client Needs:** Reduction of Risk Potential; **Cognitive Level:** Application; **NP:** Implementation

212. 4 **Toxicity can result because the action of calcium ions is similar to that of digoxin.**
    1 Calcium gluconate cannot be added to a solution containing carbonate or phosphate because a dangerous precipitation will occur.
    2 Calcium gluconate can be added to the IV solution the client is receiving.
    3 If calcium infiltrates, sloughing of tissue will result.
    Clinical Area: Medical-Surgical Nursing; **Client Needs:** Pharmacological and Parenteral Therapies; **Cognitive Level:** Application; **NP:** Implementation

213. 1 **A decreased blood volume leads to a decreased blood pressure and glomerular filtration; compensatory ADH and aldosterone secretion cause sodium and water retention, resulting in decreased urine output.**
    2 The respirations become rapid and shallow to compensate for decreased cellular oxygenation.
    3 The peripheral pulse rate may be rapid and thready, but it is the same rate as the apical rate.
    4 Hypokalemia, not hyperkalemia, occurs because as sodium is retained, potassium is excreted.
    Clinical Area: Medical-Surgical Nursing; **Client Needs:** Reduction of Risk Potential; **Cognitive Level:** Application; **NP:** Evaluation

214. 2 **The newborn's intestinal tract is sterile and therefore does not have intestinal flora to synthesize vitamin K, a precursor to prothrombin that is necessary for clotting.**
    1 Bilirubin excretion is not affected by vitamin K.
    3 Glycogen stores are not affected by vitamin K.
    4 Stimulation of the growth of bowel flora is not affected by vitamin K.

Clinical Area: Childbearing and Women's Health Nursing; **Client Needs:** Pharmacological and Parenteral Therapies; **Cognitive Level:** Comprehension; **NP:** Implementation

215. 3 **Nasogastric suction is maintained to prevent pressure on the intestinal anastomosis; oral fluids are permitted when peristalsis resumes and the nasogastric suction is stopped.**
    1 The ileal loop begins to drain immediately after surgery unless it is a continent conduit; this has no bearing on when oral fluids can be started.
    2 Waiting until the intestinal anastomosis heals is too long to wait to administer fluids; sips of water are permitted when other specific criteria are met.
    4 Leaving the postanesthesia care unit has no bearing on when oral fluids can be started. Sips of water are permitted when other specific criteria are met.
    Clinical Area: Medical-Surgical Nursing; **Client Needs:** Reduction of Risk Potential; **Cognitive Level:** Application; **Integrated Process:** Teaching/Learning; **NP:** Implementation

216. 3 **This response recognizes the client's feelings and attempts to collect data about the duration of the problem.**
    1 This response is irrelevant and will not elicit data about the extent of the anxiety.
    2 The client may not be able to identify the cause of his anxiety. Anxiety is most often a response to a vague, nonspecific threat.
    4 It is too early to identify the cause of the anxiety; crisis intervention with anxious clients requires a more structured approach than "shall we talk."
    Clinical Area: Mental Health Nursing; **Client Needs:** Psychosocial Integrity; **Cognitive Level:** Application; **Integrated Process:** Communication and Documentation; **NP:** Implementation

217. 4 **Moving the client who is singing away from the other clients diminishes the disturbance.**
    1 A client with dementia will not remember instructions.
    2 It is unsafe to close the doors of clients' rooms because they need to be monitored.
    3 The use of a sedative should not be the initial intervention.
    Clinical Area: Medical-Surgical Nursing; **Client Needs:** Management of Care; **Cognitive Level:** Application; **Integrated Process:** Caring; **NP:** Implementation

218. 4 **The virus disintegrates rapidly on contact with soap used with meticulous handwashing.**
    1 The lesion is in the genital area, not on the lips; kissing will not affect the infant.
    2 Wearing gloves when holding the infant is unnecessary.
    3 Washing clothes separately is not necessary.
    Clinical Area: Childbearing and Women's Health Nursing; **Client Needs:** Safety and Infection Control; **Cognitive Level:** Application; **NP:** Evaluation

219. 3 **This response provides the family member with an opportunity to express feelings.**
    1 This statement does not address the family members' concerns.
    2 This response is false reassurance and cuts off communication.
    4 This response shuts off communication and abdicates nursing responsibility toward the client.
    Clinical Area: Mental Health Nursing; **Client Needs:** Psychosocial Integrity; **Cognitive Level:** Application; **Integrated Process:** Communication and Documentation; **NP:** Implementation

220. 3 **This demonstrates the client's diminished anger and is a realistic assessment and acceptance of present capabilities and limitations.**
    1 Anger is still apparent.
    2 This shows dependency; the client either has given up or is being sarcastic.
    4 This shows dependency and suggests the client is still angry.
    Clinical Area: Mental Health Nursing; **Client Needs:** Psychosocial Integrity; **Cognitive Level:** Application; **Integrated Process:** Communication and Documentation; **NP:** Evaluation

221. 4 **This is the definition of primary care nursing.**
    1 In team nursing there is a mix of staff members who provide care along with a team leader who usually is a registered nurse.
    2 In modular nursing clients are assigned according to geographic location and a variety of professionals are involved; this is similar to team nursing, but the teams are smaller.
    3 In functional nursing the nurse manager makes work assignments with specific tasks for each nurse.
    Clinical Area: Medical-Surgical Nursing; **Client Needs:** Management of Care; **Cognitive Level:** Knowledge; **NP:** Analysis

222. 2 **The volume control device should be set at 33 mL/ hr; 800 mL divided by 24 hours equals 33 mL/hr.**
    1 This flow rate is too rapid.
    3 This flow rate is too slow.
    4 This flow rate is too slow.
    Clinical Area: Child Health Nursing; **Client Needs:** Pharmacological and Parenteral Therapies; **Cognitive Level:** Application; **NP:** Implementation

223. 1 **Stable vital signs are the major indicators that transfer will not jeopardize the client's condition. Although complaints of pain are a concern, they do not place the client in physiological jeopardy.**
    2 Restlessness and pallor may be early signs of shock; the client needs further assessment.
    3 An increasing temperature is a signs of increasing intracranial pressure; the client should not be transferred at this time.
    4 The vital signs are not stabilized; therefore, transfer at this time is contraindicated.

Clinical Area: Medical-Surgical Nursing; **Client Needs:** Physiological Adaptation; **Cognitive Level:** Analysis; **NP:** Evaluation

224. 4 **According to recent recommendations, adults with HIV should receive tetanus, influenza, hepatitis B, and pneumococcal vaccines.**
    1 Live pathogen vaccines (MMR, varicella) are contraindicated for individuals who are immunosuppressed.
    2 Live pathogen vaccines (MMR, varicella) are contraindicated for individuals who are immunosuppressed.
    3 Currently there is no immunization for hepatitis C and the diphtheria vaccine is not recommended.
    Clinical Area: Medical-Surgical Nursing; **Client Needs:** Health Promotion and Maintenance; **Cognitive Level:** Analysis; **Integrated Process:** Teaching/Learning; **NP:** Planning

225. 3 **The client is monitored for human chorionic gonadotropin (hCG) levels twice a week until they return to the expected range and remain there for 3 weeks. Monthly measurements are taken for up to 6 months and then are done bimonthly for the remainder of the year. If at any time during the year there is an increasing titer, choriocarcinoma is suspected. If measurements remain within the expected range for a year, another pregnancy may be attempted.**
    1 Follow-up care for only 6 weeks is dangerous; follow-up care should continue for at least 1 year.
    2 Identifying risk factors for developing another hydatidiform mole is not the priority.
    4 Chemotherapy for choriocarcinoma is given if hCG titers increase, not decrease.
    Clinical Area: Childbearing and Women's Health Nursing; **Client Needs:** Reduction of Risk Potential; **Cognitive Level:** Application; **Integrated Process:** Teaching/ Learning; **NP:** Planning

226. 3 **Tamoxifen is an estrogen antagonist antineoplastic medication that has been found to be effective in 50% to 60% of women who have estrogen-receptor–positive cancer of the breast. After 5 years of administration there is an increased risk of complications and it is discontinued.**
    1 Tamoxifen usually is prescribed for 5 years after initiation of therapy, not for the rest of the client's life.
    2 This length of time will not produce positive effects for the client. Tamoxifen usually is prescribed for 5 years after initiation of therapy, not just for 10 days.
    4 Tamoxifen may cause the side effect of bone pain that indicates its effectiveness. If bone pain occurs, medication is given to manage the pain and the drug is continued.
    Clinical Area: Childbearing and Women's Health Nursing; **Client Needs:** Pharmacological and Parenteral Therapies; **Cognitive Level:** Application; **Integrated Process:** Communication and Documentation; **NP:** Implementation

227. 1 **The client's major concern at this time is most likely pain caused by inappropriate handling.**
    2 This statement is false reassurance and should not be given.
    3 The number of personnel will not ensure careful handling; this does not address the client's most likely primary concern.
    4 Diversion is not an appropriate response to the client's primary concern.
    Clinical Area: Medical-Surgical Nursing; **Client Needs:** Basic Care and Comfort; **Cognitive Level:** Application; **Integrated Process:** Communication and Documentation; **NP:** Implementation

228. 4 **This response interprets the client's behavior without belittling the nursing assistant's feelings; it encourages the assistant to get involved with plans for future care.**
    1 Although this response recognizes the client's feelings, it does not address the nursing assistant's feelings nor helps the assistant cope with the client's behavior.
    2 This assumes the nursing assistant has nothing to contribute and only the nurse can deal with the problem.
    3 This response does not help the nursing assistant understand the client's behavior, nor does it demonstrate an understanding of the client's feelings.
    Clinical Area: Medical-Surgical Nursing; **Client Needs:** Management of Care; **Cognitive Level:** Application; **Integrated Process:** Communication and Documentation; **NP:** Implementation

229. 2 **Hodgkin's lymphoma occurs most often during the ages of 15 to 35 years of age and between 50 to 60 years of age.**
    1 Hodgkin's lymphoma affects younger men and women equally and affects more men than women between the ages of 50 and 60 years.
    3 The incidence of Hodgkin's lymphoma is not limited to people in older age groups. The prevalence of Hodgkin's lymphoma is increased in teenagers and young adults (15 to 35 years of age).
    4 Asian populations are less likely to develop Hodgkin's lymphoma than other populations.
    Clinical Area: Medical-Surgical Nursing; **Client Needs:** Physiological Adaptation; **Cognitive Level:** Application; **Integrated Process:** Communication and Documentation; **NP:** Assessment

230. 3 **Hypersecretion of melanocyte-stimulating hormone (MSH) from the anterior pituitary gland causes darkened pigmentations during pregnancy.**
    1 The adrenal glands do not secrete the hormone that causes the excess in pigmentation.
    2 The thyroid gland does not secrete the hormone that causes the excess in pigmentation.
    4 The posterior pituitary gland does not secrete the hormone that causes the excess in pigmentation.

Clinical Area: Childbearing and Women's Health Nursing; **Client Needs:** Health Promotion and Maintenance; **Cognitive Level:** Comprehension; **Integrated Process:** Communication and Documentation; **NP:** Implementation

231. 2 **Application of cold relieves discomfort, and the binder provides support and aids in pressure atrophy of acini cells so that milk production is suppressed.**
    1 Expressing milk manually is suitable for the engorged breastfeeding, not formula feeding, mother because it promotes comfort and stimulates milk production.
    3 Restriction of fluids will not prevent engorgement and may cause dehydration.
    4 Warm, moist compresses are suitable for the engorged breastfeeding mother because it promotes comfort and stimulates milk production.
    Clinical Area: Childbearing and Women's Health Nursing; **Client Needs:** Health Promotion and Maintenance; **Cognitive Level:** Application; **Integrated Process:** Teaching/Learning; **NP:** Implementation

232. 3 **Although neutropenia may occur, agranulocytosis does not occur as a side effect of olanzapine.**
    1 Cardiovascular responses, such as hypotension, are side effects of both medications.
    2 Dyspepsia, nausea, vomiting, anorexia, and other gastrointestinal disturbances occur with both medications.
    4 Metabolic syndrome may occur with olanzapine. Metabolic syndrome is a cluster of conditions including weight gain, increased cholesterol and triglyceride levels, hyperglycemia, and diabetic ketoacidosis.
    Clinical Area: Mental Health Nursing; **Client Needs:** Pharmacological and Parenteral Therapies; **Cognitive Level:** Application; **Integrated Process:** Communication and Documentation; **NP:** Implementation

233. 2 **Changes in an ECG will reflect the area of the heart that is damaged because of hypoxia.**
    1 A stethoscope is used to detect heart sounds.
    3 Medical interventions such as cardioversion or cardiac medications, not an ECG, can alter heart rhythm. An ECG will reflect heart rhythm, not change it.
    4 Identifying how much stress a heart can tolerate is accomplished through a stress test; this uses an ECG in conjunction with physical exercise.
    Clinical Area: Medical-Surgical Nursing; **Client Needs:** Reduction of Risk Potential; **Cognitive Level:** Comprehension; **Integrated Process:** Communication and Documentation; **NP:** Implementation

234. 4 **No bowel sounds are present; therefore, the client must remain NPO. Comfort measures may be helpful until bowel sounds return and the practitioner changes the dietary order.**
    1 Giving the client orange juice is unsafe; the client must be kept NPO until bowel sounds are present.

2 Offering the client 4 ounces of water by mouth is unsafe; the client must be kept NPO until bowel sounds are present.

3 The urinary output is adequate; there is no need to increase IV fluids. Also, the nurse cannot increase the IV flow rate without a practitioner's order.
Clinical Area: Medical-Surgical Nursing; **Client Needs:** Basic Care and Comfort; **Cognitive Level:** Application; **NP:** Implementation

235. 2 **Maintaining a patent airway is the priority; because of the proximity of the chest and nose/mouth, inhalation burns also may have occurred.**

1 Although limited physical mobility caused by bed rest is important, it is not the priority.

3 Although susceptibility to infection as a result of tissue trauma is important, it is not the priority.

4 The client's fluid needs can be met intravenously.
Clinical Area: Medical-Surgical Nursing; **Client Needs:** Management of Care; **Cognitive Level:** Application; **NP:** Planning

236. 2 **Involving the family in the decision-making process usually helps them become more committed to making plans work.**

1 Just providing the discharge date does not ensure appropriate family support.

3 Although increasing the family's understanding of the client's illness is helpful, it does not ensure their support for the client after discharge.

4 The treatment team is responsible for determining the client's readiness for discharge, not the family.
Clinical Area: Mental Health Nursing; **Client Needs:** Management of Care; **Cognitive Level:** Application; **Integrated Process:** Communication and Documentation; **NP:** Planning

237. 3 **A change in behavior that appears positive may indicate that the client has worked out a plan for suicide; the potential for suicide increases when physical energy returns. Increased supervision is needed.**

1 Complimenting the client's appearance may increase the client's feelings of inadequacy because it implies the client did not look good before.

2 It is inappropriate to consider discharge simply because of a change in behavior. Many factors should be involved in the decision for discharge.

4 Adding privileges is not indicated at this time.
Clinical Area: Mental Health Nursing; **Client Needs:** Management of Care; **Cognitive Level:** Analysis; **Integrated Process:** Caring; **NP:** Planning

238. 1 **This intervention recognizes and supports justified feelings and provides an opportunity to ventilate further.**

2 This response ignores the client's feelings and directs communication away from the emotionally charged area.

3 This response ignores the client's feelings and directs communication away from the emotionally charged area.

4 This response ignores the client's feelings and directs communication away from the emotionally charged area.
Clinical Area: Mental Health Nursing; **Client Needs:** Psychosocial Integrity; **Cognitive Level:** Application; **Integrated Process:** Communication and Documentation; **NP:** Implementation

239. 3 **Talking about what actually happened helps the client sort out the truth from confused thoughts and begins to help the client accept what happened as a part of their history.**

1 Legal counselling should come from a legal authority, not the nurse. The victim should be told of the legal services available.

2 Sexual assaults often are planned and are violent acts of the perpetrators who are responsible for their behavior.

4 If the client does not want to discuss intimate details, this should be respected.
Clinical Area: Mental Health Nursing; **Client Needs:** Psychosocial Integrity; **Cognitive Level:** Application; **Integrated Process:** Communication and Documentation; **NP:** Planning

240. 4 **This objective includes observable client behavior, which is specified by amount and time and therefore is measurable.**

1 This objective is not stated in measurable terms.

2 This objective is not stated in measurable terms.

3 This is a statement, not an objective.
Clinical Area: Medical-Surgical Nursing; **Client Needs:** Management of Care; **Cognitive Level:** Application; **Integrated Process:** Communication and Documentation; **NP:** Planning

241. 4 **The nurse has a legal responsibility to report suspicions of neglect to adult protective services, and failure to do so can result in charges being brought against the nurse.**

1 Although the nurse can address concerns with the caregiver, the nurse has a legal responsibility to report suspicions of neglect to the appropriate authorities.

2 The client is confused and may be unable to respond appropriately.

3 Although the nurse may be concerned about preventing alienation of the adult child, the nurse legally must report the situation to the appropriate authorities.
Clinical Area: Mental Health Nursing; **Client Needs:** Management of Care; **Cognitive Level:** Application; **Integrated Process:** Communication and Documentation; **NP:** Implementation

242. 3 **The data presented indicate an infectious process within the lung. The classic clinical findings associated with pneumonia are a productive cough (sputum is purulent, blood-tinged, or rust-colored), fever, chills, pleuritic chest discomfort, and dyspnea. Percussion is dulled over areas of consolidation.**

1 The cardinal clinical findings associated with pleurisy are pain in the lower lobe at the height of inspiration and a pleural friction rub.

2 Although fever and chills can occur later in bronchitis, the cardinal clinical findings associated with bronchitis are irritating cough, chest pain, and shortness of breath.

4 The cardinal clinical findings associated with emphysema are barrel chest, resonance on percussion, and thick, tenacious sputum.

Clinical Area: Medical-Surgical Nursing; **Client Needs:** Physiological Adaptation; **Cognitive Level:** Analysis; **NP:** Analysis

243. 2 **This is a reflective statement that conveys acceptance and encourages further communication.**

1 This response is false reassurance that does not lessen anxiety.

3 This response is false reassurance and cuts off communication; this statement does not encourage the client to discuss feelings.

4 The reliance on a pill to help the client in this instance evades the problem and cuts off further communication.

Clinical Area: Medical-Surgical Nursing; **Client Needs:** Psychosocial Integrity; **Cognitive Level:** Application; **Integrated Process:** Communication and Documentation; **NP:** Implementation

244. 3 **Sleep deprivation alone can cause these disturbances because of the interruption in REM sleep.**

1 Lack of contact with significant others increases anxiety and feelings of isolation, which can lead to disturbances in rest.

2 Pain limits or interrupts periods of sleep and rest. Analgesics should be administered as prescribed.

4 Constant light increases cerebral arousal and limits sleep.

Clinical Area: Medical-Surgical Nursing; **Client Needs:** Basic Care and Comfort; **Cognitive Level:** Application; **NP:** Planning

245. 3 **A small amount of bile-colored spotting is expected, but a large amount is excessive and not expected. The practitioner should be notified.**

1 The client should be on the right side to compress the liver capsule against the chest wall.

2 Medicating the client treats only the pain and disregards the need for medical evaluation of the complication.

4 Although monitoring vital signs is important, the priority is to notify the practitioner.

Clinical Area: Medical-Surgical Nursing; **Client Needs:** Management of Care; **Cognitive Level:** Application; **Integrated Process:** Communication and Documentation; **NP:** Implementation

246. 2 **It is the nurse's legal responsibility to report child abuse to the appropriate agency.**

1 Although the police may be notified, this is not the nurse's responsibility at this time.

3 Arranging for an examination to confirm the pregnancy may be done later; it is not the priority.

4 The nurse has not yet verified the girl's pregnancy; at this time it is most important to protect her from further abuse.

Clinical Area: Mental Health Nursing; **Client Needs:** Management of Care; **Cognitive Level:** Application; **Integrated Process:** Communication and Documentation; **NP:** Implementation

247. 2 **This is a hypertonic contraction. The oxytocin must be stopped before another contraction occurs to prevent uterine rupture and/or fetal hypoxia.**

1 Although giving oxygen is important and eventually may be done, it is not the priority.

3 Although repositioning the monitoring belts may be necessary, it is not the priority.

4 Placing a call light next to the client is unnecessary; the client receiving oxytocin for induction of labor should be continuously attended.

Clinical Area: Childbearing and Women's Health Nursing; **Client Needs:** Pharmacological and Parenteral Therapies; **Cognitive Level:** Analysis; **NP:** Implementation

248. 1 **Digoxin (Lanoxin) slows the heart rate, which is reflected in a slowing of the pulse; it also increases kidney perfusion, which promotes urine formation, resulting in diuresis and decreased edema.**

2 Digoxin will decrease, not increase, the blood pressure; digoxin does promote weight loss through diuresis.

3 Although digoxin produces diuresis as a result of improved cardiac output, which increases fluid output, it does not regulate an irregular pulse.

4 Digoxin will not correct a heart murmur or decrease the pulse pressure.

Clinical Area: Medical-Surgical Nursing; **Client Needs:** Pharmacological and Parenteral Therapies; **Cognitive Level:** Analysis; **NP:** Evaluation

249. 2 The client's paroxysmal dyspnea was probably caused by sleeping in bed with the legs at the level of the heart; this position increases venous return from dependent body areas increasing the intravascular volume. Sitting up and leaning forward while keeping the legs dependent slows venous return as well as increases thoracic capacity.

1 Although the contour position elevates the client's head, it does not place the legs in a dependent enough position to substantially decrease venous return.

3 The recumbent position is contraindicated. Venous return increases when the lower extremities are at the level of the heart. Also the pressure of the abdominal organs against the diaphragm decreases thoracic capacity.

4 The Trendelenburg position is contraindicated. Venous return increases when the lower extremities are higher than the level of the heart. Also

the pressure of the abdominal organs against the diaphragm decreases thoracic capacity.

Clinical Area: Medical-Surgical Nursing; **Client Needs:** Physiological Adaptation; **Cognitive Level:** Application; **NP:** Implementation

250. 2 **Individuals with serious head injuries are not cared for immediately in mass casualty events because the need is to care for the largest number of people who have the least severe injuries.**
    1 People with fractures are cared for in mass casualty events.
    3 People needing uncomplicated abdominal surgeries are cared for in mass casualty events.
    4 People with survivable radiation or chemical exposures are cared for in mass casualty events.

    Clinical Area: Medical-Surgical Nursing; **Client Needs:** Management of Care; **Cognitive Level:** Analysis; **NP:** Planning

251. 2 **Absence of peristalsis is caused by manipulation of abdominal contents and the depressant effects of anesthetics and analgesics.**
    1 Edema will not interfere with peristalsis; edema may cause peristalsis to be less effective, but some output will result.
    3 An absence of fiber has a greater effect on decreasing peristalsis than does decreasing fluids.
    4 A nasogastric tube decompresses the stomach; it does not cause cessation of peristalsis.

    Clinical Area: Medical-Surgical Nursing; **Client Needs:** Physiological Adaptation; **Cognitive Level:** Application; **NP:** Evaluation

252. **Answer: 1, 3, 4**
    1 **Passage of red blood (hematochezia) is one of the cardinal signs of rectosigmoid colon cancer; ulceration of the tumor and straining to pass stool precipitate this clinical finding.**
    2 An inability to digest fat is not specific to rectosigmoid colon cancer.
    3 **A cancerous mass can grow into the lumen of the sigmoid colon, altering the shape of stool; stools may be ribbon-like or pencil thin.**
    4 **Tumors in the rectosigmoid colon cause partial and eventually complete obstruction of the intestinal lumen. Stool in the descending and sigmoid colon is more formed and thus straining to pass stools, gas pains, cramping, and incomplete evacuation commonly occur.**

    Clinical Area: Medical-Surgical Nursing; **Client Needs:** Physiological Adaptation; **Cognitive Level:** Analysis; **Integrated Process:** Communication and Documentation; **NP:** Assessment

253. 1 **Care for an infant after spasmodic croup should be directed toward personal care, optimum nutrition, and stimulation.**
    2 Infants need environmental stimuli; friends and family who do not have a communicable infection should be encouraged to visit.

3 The infant does not require additional fluids if all feedings are consumed.
    4 Croup is not directly related to antigen-antibody responses.

    Clinical Area: Child Health Nursing; **Client Needs:** Health Promotion and Maintenance; **Cognitive Level:** Application; **Integrated Process:** Teaching/Learning; **NP:** Implementation

254. 2 **A restraint impedes the movement of a client; therefore, a client's condition needs to be assessed every hour.**
    1 All restraints are required to be reordered every 24 hours.
    3 Restraints should be removed and activity and skin care provided at least every 2 hours to prevent contractures and skin breakdown.
    4 Output from tubes may be monitored hourly, but generally do not need to be documented as frequently as every 2 hours. Generally output from tubes is emptied, measured, and documented at the end of each shift. A client who is in critical condition or in the immediate postoperative period may have urinary output measured hourly because this reflects cardiovascular status.

    Clinical Area: Medical-Surgical Nursing; **Client Needs:** Safety and Infection Control; **Cognitive Level:** Application; **NP:** Implementation

255. **Answer 3, 4**
    1 Stridor is a late sign of hypoxia; suctioning should be done before stridor occurs.
    2 Cyanosis is a late sign of hypoxia; suctioning should be done before cyanosis occurs.
    3 **Restlessness is an early sign of hypoxia; suctioning is required to keep the airway patent.**
    4 **An increased pulse rate is an early sign of hypoxia; suctioning is required to keep the airway patent.**
    5 Substernal retractions are a late sign of hypoxia; suctioning should be done before substernal retractions occur.

    Clinical Area: Child Health Nursing; **Client Needs:** Physiological Adaptation; **Cognitive Level:** Analysis; **NP:** Analysis

256. 2 **Before administering any medication for the first time the nurse must verify the accuracy of the prescription. The prescription as it appears in the medication administration record is verified against the prescription in the client's medical record. This ensures that the prescription was transcribed accurately.**
    1 Checking when the pain medication was last given is done after the order is verified.
    3 Nonpharmacological measures are used for mild to moderate pain, not pain associated with recent major abdominal surgery.
    4 The client's pain must be immediately addressed. The covering nurse is capable of verifying the pain

medication order and administering it safely at the correct time.

Clinical Area: Medical-Surgical Nursing; **Client Needs:** Safety and Infection Control; **Cognitive Level:** Application; **NP:** Implementation

257. **3** **Moisturizing lotions provide an occlusive film on the skin surface so that usual water loss through the skin is limited allowing the trapped water to hydrate the stratum corneum.**
  1 Excessive exposure to water produces more irritation and scaling.
  2 Excessive exposure to water, particularly hot water, increases irritation and scaling.
  4 Psoriasis is not a communicable disease and affected areas do not need to be covered when in contact with others.

Clinical Area: Medical-Surgical Nursing; **Client Needs:** Basic Care and Comfort; **Cognitive Level:** Application; **Integrated Process:** Teaching/Learning; **NP:** Implementation

258. **1** **Deep blue coloring on the skin often seen on the lower back and buttocks are called Mongolian spots. Mongolian spots are a variation within the norm and disappear in the first year.**
  2 Mottling caused by cold covers the entire body.
  3 The harlequin color change is not purple or blue and involves an entire half of the body.
  4 In this newborn these are expected findings; if the baby were light skinned, the possibility of bruises should be investigated.

Clinical Area: Childbearing and Women's Health Nursing; **Client Needs:** Health Promotion and Maintenance; **Cognitive Level:** Application; **Integrated Process:** Communication and Documentation; **NP:** Analysis

259. **1** **A common complication of a brain attack (cerebrovascular accident) is an inability to control emotional affect; clients may be depressed or apathetic and have a lability of mood.**
  2 There are no data to support the conclusion that the client is demonstrating a premorbid personality.
  3 There are no data to support the conclusion that the client is mourning the loss of functional abilities.
  4 There are no data to support the conclusion that the client is conveying unhappiness about the situation.

Clinical Area: Medical-Surgical Nursing; **Client Needs:** Physiological Adaptation; **Cognitive Level:** Application; **Integrated Process:** Communication and Documentation; **NP:** Implementation

260. **3** **Difficulty swallowing (dysphagia) is a manifestation of both neurological disorders. With Parkinson's disease there is a progressive loss of spontaneity of movement, including swallowing, related to degeneration of the dopamine-producing neurons in the substantia nigra of the midbrain. With myasthenia gravis there is a decreased number of ACh receptor sites at the neuromuscular junction, which interferes with muscle contraction, impairing muscles involved in chewing, swallowing, speaking, and breathing.**
  1 A cogwheel gait is associated with Parkinson's disease, not myasthenia gravis. With Parkinson's disease the decrease in dopamine results in impaired coordinated voluntary movements.
  2 Impaired cognition is associated with Parkinson's disease, not myasthenia gravis. Progressive dementia occurs as a result of a loss of cholinergic cells in the basal nucleus of a Meynert and neuronal loss, senile plaques, and neurofibrillary tangles in the neocortex.
  4 Non-intention tremors are associated with Parkinson's disease, not myasthenia gravis. The non-intention tremors associated with Parkinson's disease result from the loss of the inhibitory influence of dopamine in the basal ganglia, which interferes with the feedback circuit within the cerebral cortex.

Clinical Area: Medical-Surgical Nursing; **Client Needs:** Physiological Adaptation; **Cognitive Level:** Analysis; **NP:** Assessment

261. **3** **Steroids are used for their anti-inflammatory, vasoconstrictive, and antipruritic effects.**
  1 Steroids increase the incidence of infections because they are anti-inflammatory agents and mask symptoms of infection.
  2 Steroids increase fluid retention because they promote the reabsorption of sodium from the tubular fluid into the plasma.
  4 Although steroid ointments have an antipruritic effect, their major purpose after surgery is their systemic anti-inflammatory effect.

Clinical Area: Medical-Surgical Nursing; **Client Needs:** Pharmacological and Parenteral Therapies; **Cognitive Level:** Application; **Integrated Process:** Teaching/Learning; **NP:** Evaluation

262. **1** **Ibuprofen (Advil) is a nonsteroidal anti-inflammatory drug (NSAID) that can cause bleeding in the GI tract; clients with a history of gastrointestinal (GI) bleeding should not take NSAIDs.**
  2 Digoxin (Lanoxin) is an antidysrhythmic used to slow and strengthen the heart rate; it does not contribute to GI bleeding.
  3 Furosemide (Lasix), a commonly used diuretic, is not contraindicated with GI bleeding.
  4 Spironolactone (Aldactone) is a diuretic that often causes potassium retention; it does not cause GI bleeding.

Clinical Area: Medical-Surgical Nursing; **Client Needs:** Management of Care; **Cognitive Level:** Analysis; **Integrated Process:** Communication and Documentation; **NP:** Implementation

263. **4** **If the client is right-handed there will be difficulty with dressing because it requires the use of two hands, and some clothing requires movement of both sides of the body when dressing.**

1 A right-handed client is able to continue to use the right hand because it is the left side that is affected by a lesion on the right side of the brain.

2 A right-handed client is able to continue to use the right hand because it is the left side that is affected by a lesion on the right side of the brain.

3 A right-handed client is able to continue to use the right hand because it is the left side that is affected by a lesion on the right side of the brain.

Clinical Area: Medical-Surgical Nursing; **Client Needs:** Basic Care and Comfort; **Cognitive Level:** Application; **NP:** Assessment

264. 2 **Regular insulin is the only insulin that is administered intravenously.**

1 Novolin L insulin cannot be administered intravenously.

3 Novolin N insulin cannot be administered intravenously.

4 Novolin U insulin cannot be administered intravenously.

Clinical Area: Medical-Surgical Nursing; **Client Needs:** Pharmacological and Parenteral Therapies; **Cognitive Level:** Analysis; **NP:** Planning

265. 3 **Clients with catatonia exhibit rigidity and posturing behaviors.**

1 Most clients with catatonic schizophrenia are unable to express feelings.

2 Self-mutilation is associated with depression.

4 Repetitious activities are associated with obsessive-compulsive disorders.

Clinical Area: Mental Health Nursing; **Client Needs:** Psychosocial Integrity; **Cognitive Level:** Application; **NP:** Assessment